CURRENT THERAPY IN NEONATAL-PERINATAL MEDICINE – 2

Medical Titles in the Current Therapy Series

CURRENT
THERAPY IN
NEONATAL-PERINATAL
MEDICINE – 2

Nicholas M. Nelson, M.D.

Professor of Pediatrics
The Milton S. Hershey Medical Center
Pennsylvania State University
College of Medicine
Hershey, Pennsylvania

1990

B.C. Decker Inc • Toronto • Philadelphia

Publisher   **B.C. Decker Inc**
3228 South Service Road
Burlington, Ontario   L7N 3H8

B.C. Decker Inc
320 Walnut Street
Suite 400
Philadelphia, Pennsylvania   19106

Sales and Distribution

United States and Puerto Rico
The C.V. Mosby Company
11830 Westline Industrial Drive
Saint Louis, Missouri   63146

Canada
McAinsh & Co. Ltd.
2760 Old Leslie Street
Willowdale, Ontario   M2K 2X5

Australia
McGraw-Hill Book Company Australia Pty. Ltd.
4 Barcoo Street
Roseville East 2069
New South Wales, Australia

Brazil
Editora McGraw-Hill do Brasil, Ltda.
rua Tabapua, 1.105, Itaim-Bibi
Sao Paulo, S.P. Brasil

Colombia
Interamericana/McGraw-Hill de Colombia, S.A.
Apartado Aereo 81078
Bogota, D.E. Colombia

Europe
McGraw-Hill Book Company GmbH
Lademannbogen 136
D-2000 Hamburg 63
West Germany

France
MEDSI/McGraw-Hill
6, avenue Daniel Lesueur
75007 Paris, France

Hong Kong and China
McGraw-Hill Book Company
Suite 618, Ocean Centre
5 Canton Road
Tsimshatsui, Kowloon
Hong Kong

India
Tata McGraw-Hill Publishing Company, Ltd.
12/4 Asaf Ali Road, 3rd Floor
New Delhi 110002, India

Indonesia
P.O. Box 122/JAT
Jakarta, 1300 Indonesia

Italy
McGraw-Hill Libri Italia, s.r.l.
Piazza Emilia, 5
I-20129 Milano MI
Italy

Japan
Igaku-Shoin Ltd.
Tokyo International P.O. Box 5063
1-28-36 Hongo, Bunkyo-ku,
Tokyo 113, Japan

Korea
C.P.O. Box 10583
Seoul, Korea

Malaysia
No. 8 Jalan SS 7/6B
Kelana Jaya
47301 Petaling Jaya
Selangor, Malaysia

Mexico
Interamericana/McGraw-Hill de Mexico, S.A. de C.V.
Cedro 512, Colonia Atlampa
(Apartado Postal 26370)
06450 Mexico, D.F., Mexico

New Zealand
McGraw-Hill Book Co. New Zealand Ltd.
5 Joval Place, Wiri
Manukau City, New Zealand

Panama
Editorial McGraw-Hill Latinoamericana, S.A.
Apartado Postal 2036
Zona Libre de Colon
Colon, Republica de Panama

Portugal
Editora McGraw-Hill de Portugal, Ltda.
Rua Rosa Damasceno 11A–B
1900 Lisboa, Portugal

South Africa
Libriger Book Distributors
Warehouse Number 8
"Die Ou Looiery"
Tannery Road
Hamilton, Bloemfontein 9300

Southeast Asia
McGraw-Hill Book Co.
348 Jalan Boon Lay
Jurong, Singapore 2261

Spain
McGraw-Hill/Interamericana de Espana, S.A.
Manuel Ferrero, 13
28020 Madrid, Spain

Taiwan
P.O. Box 87–601
Taipei, Taiwan

Thailand
632/5 Phaholyothin Road
Sapan Kwai
Bangkok 10400
Thailand

United Kingdom, Middle East and Africa
McGraw-Hill Book Company (U.K.) Ltd.
Shoppenhangers Road
Maidenhead, Berkshire
SL6 2QL England

Venezuela
McGraw-Hill/Interamericana, C.A.
2da. calle Bello Monte
(entre avenida Casanova y Sabana Grande)
Apartado Aereo 50785
Caracas 1050, Venezuela

NOTICE

The authors and publisher have made every effort to ensure that the patient care recommended herein, including choice of drugs and drug dosages, is in accord with the accepted standards and practice at the time of publication. However, since research and regulation constantly change clinical standards, the reader is urged to check the product information sheet included in the package of each drug, which includes recommended doses, warnings, and contraindications. This is particularly important with new or infrequently used drugs.

Current Therapy in Neonatal-Perinatal Medicine – 2   ISBN 1–55664–070–6

Library of Congress catalog card number: 89–51065   10   9   8   7   6   5   4   3   2   1

CONTRIBUTORS

DAVID B. ACKER, M.D.

Assistant Professor of Obstetrics and Gynecology, Harvard Medical School; Director of Perinatology, Harvard Community Health Plan, Boston, Massachusetts

Shoulder Dystocia

LINDSAY S. ALGER, M.D., F.A.C.O.G.

Associate Professor of Obstetrics and Gynecology, University of Maryland School of Medicine; Associate Director of Maternal-Fetal Medicine, University of Maryland Medical Systems/Hospital, Baltimore, Maryland

Therapeutic Abortion

PAMELA ARN, M.D.

Assistant Professor of Pediatrics, University of Florida College of Medicine, Gainesville; Attending Physician, Nemours Childrens Clinic, Jacksonville, Florida

Symptomatic Inborn Errors of Metabolism

OM P. ARYA, M.B.B.S., D.T.M.&H., D.P.H., D.I.H., Dip. Ven.

Head, University Department of Genitourinary Medicine, University of Liverpool; Consultant Physician, Royal Liverpool Hospital, Department of Genitourinary Medicine, Liverpool, England

Early Congenital Syphilis

GORDON B. AVERY, M.D., Ph.D.

Professor of Pediatrics, George Washington University School of Medicine and Health Sciences; Chairman, Department of Neonatology, Children's Hospital National Medical Center, Washington, D.C.

Bronchopulmonary Dysplasia

WILLIAM F. BALISTRERI, M.D.

Professor of Pediatrics, University of Cincinnati College of Medicine; Director, Division of Pediatric Gastroenterology and Nutrition, Children's Hospital Medical Center, Cincinnati, Ohio

Chronic Cholestasis

THOMAS V.N. BALLANTINE, M.D., F.A.C.S.

Professor of Surgery and Pediatrics, Pennsylvania State University College of Medicine; Chief, Division of Pediatric Surgery, Pennsylvania State University Hospital, Hershey, Pennsylvania

Circumcision
Hirschsprung's Disease

KJELL R.M. BARLÖV, M.D.

Lecturer, Faculties of Medicine and Theology (Medical Ethics), University of Lund School of Medicine, Malmö; Staff, Department of Obstetrics and Gynecology, Hospital of Ystad, Ystad, Sweden

Breech Presentation

VANESSA A. BARSS, M.D.

Assistant Professor of Obstetrics, Gynecology, and Reproductive Biology, Harvard Medical School; Director of Ambulatory Obstetrics and Director of High Risk Pregnancy Clinic, Brigham and Women's Hospital, Boston, Massachusetts

Intrauterine Transfusion

DENNIS W. BARTHOLOMEW, M.D.

Clinical Assistant Professor of Pediatrics, Uniformed Services Health Science University, Bethesda, Maryland; Staff, USAF Medical Center, Keesler Air Force Base, Mississippi

Hyperammonemia

MARK L. BATSHAW, M.D.

W.T. Grant Professor of Pediatrics, University of Pennsylvania School of Medicine; Physician in Chief, Children's Seashore House and Chief, Division of Child Development, Children's Hospital, Philadelphia, Pennsylvania

Hyperammonemia

GREGORY P. BECKS, M.D., FRCPC

Assistant Professor, Department of Medicine, Division of Endocrinology and Metabolism, St. Joseph's Health Centre/University of Western Ontario, London, Ontario, Canada

Thyrotoxicosis in Pregnancy

HARRY J. BELL, M.D.

Assistant Professor of Pediatrics, The Johns Hopkins University School of Medicine; Director of Pediatric Rehabilitation, Mount Washington Pediatric Hospital, Baltimore, Maryland

Spinal Cord Injury

MARK F. BELLINGER, M.D.

Associate Professor, Department of Surgery, University of Pittsburgh School of Medicine; Chief, Pediatric Urology, Children's Hospital, Pittsburgh, Pennsylvania

Hydronephrosis

D. WOODROW BENSON Jr., M.D., Ph.D.

Professor of Pediatrics, Northwestern University Medical School; Head, Division of Cardiology, Children's Memorial Hospital, Chicago, Illinois

Disturbances of Cardiac Rhythm and Conduction

CHESTON M. BERLIN Jr., M.D.

Professor of Pediatrics and Pharmacology, Pennsylvania State University College of Medicine; Chief of General Pediatrics and Acting Chairman, Department of Pediatrics, The Milton S. Hershey Medical Center, Hershey, Pennsylvania

Phenylketonuria: Experience in Pennsylvania

RAMA BHAT, M.D.

Associate Professor in Pediatrics, Obstetrics, and Gynecology, Abraham-Lincoln School of Medicine; Attending Neonatologist, University of Illinois at the Medical Center, Chicago, Illinois
Tissue pH Monitoring

JOHN M. BISSONNETTE, M.D.

Professor of Obstetrics, Gynecology, Cell Biology, and Anatomy, Oregon Health Sciences University School of Medicine, Portland, Oregon
Chorionic Villus Sampling

KAREN M. BLACKBIRD, R.D.

Manager, Clinical Nutrition and Nutritionist, P.K.U. Program, The Milton S. Hershey Medical Center, Hershey, Pennsylvania
Phenylketonuria: Experience in Pennsylvania

LILLIAN R. BLACKMON, M.D.

Associate Professor of Pediatrics, University of Maryland School of Medicine; Director of Nurseries, University of Maryland Medical Systems/Hospital, Baltimore, Maryland
Chlamydial Infections

DANIELLE K.B. BOAL, M.D.

Associate Professor of Radiology and Pediatrics, Pennsylvania State University College of Medicine and The Milton S. Hershey University Hospital, Hershey, Pennsylvania
Organ Imaging

DESMOND J. BOHN, M.B., B.Ch., F.F.A.R.C.S., M.R.C.P.(UK), FRCPC

Assistant Professor of Anesthesia and Pediatrics, University of Toronto Faculty of Medicine; Assistant Director, Intensive Care Unit, The Hospital for Sick Children, Toronto, Ontario, Canada
Pulse Oximetry

MONICA BOLOGA, M.D.

Division of Clinical Pharmacology, The Hospital for Sick Children, Toronto, Ontario, Canada
Morphine Infusion

JOHN M. BOWMAN, M.D.

Professor, Department of Pediatrics and Child Health and Department of Obstetrics, Gynecology, and Reproductive Sciences, University of Manitoba Faculty of Medicine; Medical Director, Rh Laboratory, Winnipeg, Manitoba, Canada
Rh Prophylaxis

JANE E. BRAZY, M.D.

Associate Professor of Pediatrics and Affiliate Appointment in Obstetrics-Gynecology, University of Wisconsin Medical School; Director, Perinatal Center, Meriter-Madison General Hospital, Madison, Wisconsin
Near Infrared Spectrophotometry

JOHN G. BROOKS, M.D.

Professor of Pediatrics and Director, Division of Pediatric Pulmonology, University of Rochester School of Medicine and Dentistry, Rochester, New York
Apparent Life-Threatening Events

SAUL W. BRUSILOW, M.D.

Professor of Pediatrics, The Johns Hopkins University School of Medicine; Active Staff, Pediatrics, The Johns Hopkins Hospital, Baltimore, Maryland
Symptomatic Inborn Errors of Metabolism

GERARD N. BURROW, M.D.

Professor of Medicine, Vice Chancellor for Health Sciences and Dean, School of Medicine, University of California School of Medicine, San Diego, California
Thyrotoxicosis in Pregnancy

MARY K. BUSER, N.N.P., M.S.

Nursing Director, Emergency Transport Service, Children's Hospital, Denver, Colorado
Infant Transport

L. JOSEPH BUTTERFIELD, M.D.

Clinical Professor of Pediatrics, University of Colorado School of Medicine; Chairman Emeritus, Department of Perinatology, Children's Hospital, Denver, Colorado
Infant Transport

WINSTON A. CAMPBELL, M.D.

Associate Professor, Obstetrics and Gynecology, Associate Director, Maternal-Fetal Medicine, and Director, Maternal-Fetal Medicine Intensive Care Unit, University of Connecticut Health Center, School of Medicine, Farmington, Connecticut
Premature Rupture of the Membranes

WALDEMAR A. CARLO, M.D.

Associate Professor of Pediatrics, Case Western Reserve University School of Medicine; Associate Director, Neonatal Intensive Care Unit, Rainbow Babies and Children's Hospital, Cleveland, Ohio
Weaning From the Respirator

BENJAMIN S. CARSON, M.D.

Assistant Professor of Neurosurgery, Oncology, and Pediatrics, The Johns Hopkins University School of Medicine; Director of Pediatric Neurosurgery, The Johns Hopkins Medical Institutions, Baltimore, Maryland
Hydrocephalus

ALDO R. CASTANEDA, M.D., Ph.D.

William Ladd Professor of Surgery, Harvard Medical School; Surgeon-in-Chief, The Children's Hospital, Boston, Massachusetts
Total Anomalous Pulmonary Venous Connection: Surgical Aspects

VICTOR CHERNICK, M.D., FRCPC

Professor of Pediatrics, University of Manitoba Faculty of Medicine; Head, Section of Pediatric Respirology, Children's Hospital, Winnipeg, Manitoba, Canada
Continuous Distending Pressure

JUDITH L. CHERVENAK, M.D.

Instructor, Department of Obstetrics and Gynecology, New Jersey Medical School, Newark, New Jersey
Multiple Gestation

FRANK A. CHERVENAK, M.D.

Associate Professor, Department of Obstetrics and Gynecology, Cornell Medical Center, New York, New York
Multiple Gestation

RICHARD B. CLARK, M.D.

Professor, Departments of Anesthesiology and Obstetrics/Gynecology and Director, Obstetric Anesthesia, University of Arkansas College of Medicine, Little Rock, Arkansas
Regional Anesthesia

MARVIN CORNBLATH, M.D.

Clinical Professor of Pediatrics, University of Maryland School of Medicine; Lecturer in Pediatrics, The Johns Hopkins School of Medicine, Baltimore, Maryland
Hypoglycemia

ROBERT K. CREASY, M.D.

Emma Sue Hightower Professor and Chairman, Department of Obstetrics, Gynecology, and Reproductive Sciences, University of Texas Medical School; Chief, Obstetrics and Gynecology Service, The Hermann Hospital, Houston, Texas
Advanced Maternal Age
Late Fetal Death
Postdate Pregnancy

FERNAND DAFFOS, M.D.

Department of Medicine and Fetal Biology, Institut de Puericulture, Paris, France
Fetal Blood Sampling

DONALD J. DALESSIO, M.D.

Clinical Professor of Neurology, University of California School of Medicine, San Diego; Chairman, Department of Medicine and Senior Consultant in Neurology, Scripps Clinic and Research Foundation, La Jolla, California
Epilepsy in Pregnancy

JOSEPH DANCIS, M.D.

Professor and Chairman of Pediatrics, New York University Medical Center; Director of Pediatrics, Bellevue and Tisch Hospitals, New York, New York
Maple Syrup Urine Disease

JOHN R. DOIG, B.Sc., M.B., Ch.B., M.R.C.O.G., F.R.N.Z.C.O.G.

Department of Midwifery, University of Glasgow, Glasgow, Scotland
Nuchal Cord

STEVEN DONN, M.D.

Associate Professor of Pediatrics, University of Michigan Medical School; Staff, Section of Neonatology, University of Michigan Medical Center, Ann Arbor, Michigan
Hypoxic-Ischemic Encephalopathy

JOHN H. DOSSETT, M.D.

Associate Professor, Department of Pediatrics, Pennsylvania State University College of Medicine, Hershey, Pennsylvania
AIDS: Perinatal HIV Infection

ROBERT D. EDEN, M.D.

Associate Professor of Obstetrics and Gynecology, Wayne State University School of Medicine, Detroit, Michigan
Uterine Rupture

EDMUND A. EGAN, M.D.

Professor of Pediatrics and Physiology, State University of New York School of Medicine; Attending Physician, Division of Neonatology, Children's Hospital, Buffalo, New York
Wet Lung Syndromes

HENRIK EKBLAD, M.D., Ph.D.

Postgraduate Fellow, Neonatology and Neonatal Intensive Care Unit, Children's Hospital, University of Turku, Turku, Finland
Early Metabolic Acidosis

PATRICIA H. ELLISON, M.D.

Research Professor, Department of Psychology, University of Denver, Denver, Colorado
Transcephalic Impedance

MICHAEL F. EPSTEIN, M.D.

Associate Professor of Pediatrics, Harvard Medical School; Chief, Division of Newborn Medicine, The Children's Hospital, Boston, Massachusetts
Hydrops Fetalis

CAROL I. EWING, M.B., Ch.B., B.Sc., M.R.C.P.(UK), D.C.H., D.R.C.O.G.

Pediatric Senior Registrar, St. Mary's Hospital, Manchester, England
Early Congenital Syphilis

LAWRENCE J. FENTON, M.D.

Professor and Chairman, Department of Pediatrics, University of South Dakota School of Medicine; Attending Neonatologist, Sioux Valley Hospital, Sioux Falls, South Dakota
Nurse Clinicians

ROBERT M. FILLER, M.D.

Professor of Surgery, University of Toronto Faculty of Medicine; Surgeon-in-Chief, The Hospital for Sick Children, Toronto, Ontario, Canada
Meconium Ileus

NEIL N. FINER, M.D., FRCPC

Professor of Pediatrics, University of Alberta Faculty of Medicine; Director, Newborn Medicine and Pediatric Intensive Care Unit, Royal Alexandra Hospital, Edmonton, Alberta, Canada
Computerized Databases on Personal Computers

LORETTA P. FINNEGAN, M.D.

Professor of Pediatrics, Psychiatry, and Human Behavior, Jefferson Medical College of Thomas Jefferson University; Director of Family Center, Thomas Jefferson University Hospital, Philadelphia, Pennsylvania
Neonatal Abstinence Syndrome

RICHARD S. FOX, M.D.

Plastic Surgeon, Private Practice, North Dartmouth, Massachusetts
Cleft Disorders

IVAN D. FRANTZ III, M.D.

Professor of Pediatrics, Tufts University School of Medicine; Chief, Division of Newborn Medicine, New England Medical Center Hospitals, Boston, Massachusetts
High-Frequency Ventilation

JOHN M. FREEMAN, M.D.

Professor, Department of Neurology and Pediatrics, The Johns Hopkins University School of Medicine; Director of Pediatric Neurology Services, The Johns Hopkins Medical Institutions, Baltimore, Maryland
Hydrocephalus

EMANUEL A. FRIEDMAN, M.D., Sc.D.

Professor of Obstetrics, Gynecology, and Reproductive Biology, Harvard Medical School; Obstetrician/Gynecologist-in-Chief, Beth Israel Hospital, Boston, Massachusetts
Shoulder Dystocia

FREDRIC D. FRIGOLETTO Jr., M.D.

William Lambert Richardson Professor of Obstetrics, Harvard Medical School; Chief of Obstetrics, Brigham and Women's Hospital, Boston, Massachusetts
Intrauterine Transfusion

BARBARA L. GEORGE, M.D.

Associate Clinical Professor of Pediatrics/Cardiology and Director, Pediatric Cardiac-Surgical Intensive Care, University of California, UCLA School of Medicine, Los Angeles, California
Congestive Heart Failure

WELTON M. GERSONY, M.D.

Professor of Pediatrics, Columbia University College of Physicians and Surgeons; Director, Division of Pediatric Cardiology, Babies Hospital and Presbyterian Hospital, New York, New York
Total Anomalous Pulmonary Venous Connection
Transposition of the Great Arteries

BOYD W. GOETZMAN, M.D., Ph.D.

Professor, Division of Neonatology, Department of Pediatrics, University of California School of Medicine, Davis, California
Umbilical Artery Catheterization

JOHN W. GOLDKRAND, M.D.

Clinical Professor, Department of Obstetrics and Gynecology, Medical College of Georgia School of Medicine, Augusta; Director of Obstetrical Services, Department of Obstetrics and Gynecology, Memorial Medical Center, Savannah, Georgia
Pregnancy-Induced Hypertension

ROBERT C. GOODLIN, M.D.

Professor of Obstetrics/Gynecology, University of Colorado School of Medicine; Assistant Director, Obstetrics/Gynecology, Denver General Hospital, Denver, Colorado
Premature Labor

WILLIAM P. GRAHAM III, M.D.

Clinical Professor of Surgery, Pennsylvania State University College of Medicine, Hershey; Active Surgical Staff, Harrisburg Hospital, Polyclinic Medical Center, Harrisburg and Carlisle Hospital, Carlisle, Pennsylvania
Cleft Disorders

H. GORDON GREEN, M.D., M.P.H., F.A.A.P.

Clinical Associate Professor of Pediatrics, University of Texas Southwestern Medical Center; Director, Dallas County Health Department, Dallas, Texas
Babies Doe: Problems of Severely Handicapped Newborn Infants

PAUL A. GREENBERGER, M.D.

Professor of Medicine, Section of Allergy-Immunology, Northwestern University Medical School; Attending Physician, Northwestern Memorial Hospital, Chicago, Illinois
Asthma in Pregnancy

MICHAEL F. GREENE, M.D.

Assistant Professor of Obstetrics and Gynecology, Harvard Medical School; Chief, Maternal Fetal Medicine, Brigham and Women's Hospital, Boston, Massachusetts
Intrauterine Transfusion

ARTHUR W. GRIX, M.D.

Assistant Professor of Clinical Pediatrics, Department of
Pediatrics, University of California School of Medicine,
Davis, California
Vater Association

JAY L. GROSFELD, M.D.

Professor and Chairman, Department of Surgery, Indiana
University School of Medicine; Surgeon-in-Chief,
James Whitcomb Riley Hospital for Children,
Indianapolis, Indiana
Inguinal Hernia in the Perinatal Period

JOHN H. GROSSMAN III, M.D., Ph.D., F.A.C.O.G.

Professor of Obstetrics, Gynecology, and Microbiology
and Director, Division of Maternal-Fetal Medicine, George
Washington University School of Medicine and Health
Sciences, Washington, D.C.
Herpes Simplex Infection

ALAN B. GRUSKIN, M.D.

Professor and Chairman, Department of Pediatrics, Wayne
State University School of Medicine; Pediatrician-in-Chief,
Children's Hospital of Michigan, Detroit, Michigan
Acute Renal Failure

HUNTER A. HAMMILL, M.D.

Assistant Professor of Obstetrics and Gynecology, Baylor
College of Medicine; Attending Obstetrician and
Gynecologist, Jefferson Davis Hospital, Houston, Texas
Chlamydial Infections During Pregnancy and Infancy

WILLIAM C. HANIGAN, M.D., Ph.D.

Clinical Associate Professor, Section of Neurosurgery,
Department of Neurosciences, University of Illinois
College of Medicine; Pediatric Neurosurgeon, Private
Practice, Peoria, Illinois
Perinatal Magnetic Resonance Imaging

JEFFREY B. HANSON, M.D.

Assistant Clinical Professor of Pediatrics, University of
Colorado School of Medicine; Medical Director,
Emergency Transport Services, Children's Hospital,
Denver, Colorado
Infant Transport

WILLIAM E. HATHAWAY, M.D.

Professor Emeritus of Pediatrics, University of Colorado
School of Medicine, Denver, Colorado
Disseminated Intravascular Coagulation

ALFRED D. HEGGIE, M.D.

Associate Professor of Pediatrics and Pathology, Case
Western Reserve University School of Medicine; Attending
Pediatrician and Associate Director, Virology Laboratory
and Hospital Epidemiologist, University Hospitals of
Cleveland, Cleveland, Ohio
Chlamydial Infections During Pregnancy and Infancy

THOMAS HEGYI, M.D.

Professor of Pediatrics, University of Medicine and
Dentistry of New Jersey, Robert Wood Johnson Medical
School, Piscataway; Director, Division of Neonatology, St.
Peter's Medical Center, New Brunswick, New Jersey
Intraventricular Hemorrhage

HENRY C. HEINS Jr., M.D., M.P.H.

Professor Emeritus, Department of Obstetrics and
Gynecology, Medical University of South Carolina College
of Medicine, Charleston, South Carolina
Eclampsia

JOHN J. HERBST, M.D.

Professor and Chairman, Department of Pediatrics,
Louisiana State University Medical School,
Shreveport, Louisiana
Gastroesophageal Reflux

SUSAN HOU, M.D.

Assistant Professor of Medicine, University of Chicago,
Pritzker School of Medicine; Attending Physician, Michael
Reese Hospital, Chicago, Illinois
Chronic Renal Disease in Pregnancy

BONNIE BOYER HUDAK, M.D.

Fellow, Neonatology and Pediatric Pulmonology, The
Johns Hopkins University School of Medicine,
Baltimore, Maryland
Meconium Aspiration

CARL E. HUNT, M.D.

Professor and Chairman, Department of Pediatrics,
Medical College of Ohio, Toledo, Ohio
Pneumograms

MICHAEL V. JOHNSTON, M.D.

Professor of Neurology and Pediatrics, The Johns Hopkins
University School of Medicine and The Kennedy Institute,
Baltimore, Maryland
Hypoxic-Ischemic Encephalopathy

RICHARD A. JONAS, M.D.

Assistant Professor, Harvard Medical School; Associate in
Cardiac Surgery, The Children's Hospital,
Boston, Massachusetts
*Total Anomalous Pulmonary Venous Connection: Surgical
Aspects*

M. DOUGLAS JONES Jr., M.D.

Professor of Pediatrics, Associate Professor of
Anesthesiology/Critical Care Medicine, and Assistant
Professor of Gynecology and Obstetrics, The Johns
Hopkins University School of Medicine,
Baltimore, Maryland
Meconium Aspiration

AUGUST L. JUNG, M.D.

Associate Professor of Pediatrics and Director, Division of Neonatology, University of Utah School of Medicine, Salt Lake City, Utah
Phototherapy

PENTTI KERO, M.D., Ph.D.

Assistant Professor of Neonatology, University of Turku; Director, Neonatology and Neonatal Intensive Care Unit, Children's Hospital, University of Turku, Turku, Finland
Early Metabolic Acidosis

JERALD D. KING, M.D.

Assistant Clinical Professor of Pediatrics and Director of Education, Division of Neonatology, University of Utah School of Medicine, Salt Lake City, Utah
Phototherapy

JOACHIM G. KLEBE, M.D.

Associate Professor, Department of Obstetrics and Gynaecology and Head of the Diabetes in Pregnancy Study Unit, Aarhus University School of Medicine, Aarhus, Denmark
Diabetes in Pregnancy

JEROME O. KLEIN, M.D.

Professor of Pediatrics, Boston University School of Medicine; Director, Division of Pediatric Infectious Diseases, Boston City Hospital, Boston, Massachusetts
Nosocomial Infections

LEONARD I. KLEINMAN, M.D.

Professor of Pediatrics, State University of New York School of Medicine; Director of Newborn Services, Childrens Medical Center University Hospital, Stony Brook, New York
Renal Cystic Disease

WINSTON W.K. KOO, M.B.B.S., F.R.A.C.P.

Assistant Professor of Pediatrics, University of Alberta Faculty of Medicine; Staff Neonatologist, University of Alberta Hospitals, Edmonton, Alberta, Canada
Rickets in Infants

GIDEON KOREN, M.D., A.B.M.T.

Assistant Professor of Pediatrics and Pharmacology, University of Toronto Faculty of Medicine; Career Scientist, Ontario Ministry of Health, Toronto, Ontario, Canada
Morphine Infusion

EHUD KRONGRAD, M.D.

Associate Professor of Pediatrics (Pediatric Cardiology), Columbia University College of Physicians and Surgeons; Associate Attending Pediatrician, Babies Hospital, New York, New York
Balloon Atrial Septostomy

P. GONNE KÜHL, M.D.

Chief of the Pediatric Intensive Care Unit and Attending Neonatologist, University Children's Hospital, University of Heidelberg, Heidelberg, Federal Republic of Germany
Hypokalemia

ROGER L. LADDA, M.D.

Professor of Pediatrics, Pennsylvania State University College of Medicine; Chief, Division of Genetics, The Milton S. Hershey Medical Center, Hershey, Pennsylvania
Prenatal Genetic Diagnosis

EDMUND F. LA GAMMA, M.D., F.A.A.P.

Associate Professor of Pediatrics, Neurobiology, and Behavior, State University of New York School of Medicine; Attending Neonatologist, University Hospital, Stony Brook, New York
Necrotizing Enterocolitis

ANDRÉ D. LASCARI, M.D.

Professor of Pediatrics, Albany Medical College; Staff, Albany Medical Center, Albany, New York
Breast-Feeding Jaundice

FRANCESCO LAURENTI, M.D.

Professor of Child Health and Chief Researcher in Neonatal Immunology, Institute of Pediatrics, La Sapienza, University of Rome, Rome, Italy
Granulocyte Transfusion

STEWART LAWRENCE, M.D.

Assistant Professor, Department of Pediatrics, University of Florida Health Science Center, Jacksonville, Florida
Intrauterine Growth Retardation: Pediatric Aspects

RALPH A.W. LEHMAN, M.D., F.A.C.S.

Professor of Surgery, Pennsylvania State University College of Medicine; Chief of Neurosurgery, The Milton S. Hershey Medical Center, Hershey, Pennsylvania
Myelomeningocele

JAMES A. LEMONS, M.D.

Professor of Pediatrics, Indiana University School of Medicine; Director, Neonatal/Perinatal Section, James Whitcomb Riley Hospital for Children, Indianapolis, Indiana
Vitamin E Supplementation

GARY R. LERNER, M.D.

Assistant Professor of Pediatrics, Wayne State University School of Medicine; Attending Nephrologist, Division of Pediatric Nephrology, Childrens Hospital of Michigan, Detroit, Michigan
Acute Renal Failure

GRAHAM C. LIGGINS, M.B., Ph.D., F.R.C.O.G.

Emeritus Professor, Department of Obstetrics and Gynaecology, University of Auckland, Auckland, New Zealand
Antenatal Corticosteroids

PHILIP J. LIPSITZ, M.D.

Professor of Pediatrics, State University of New York School of Medicine, Stony Brook; Chief, Division of Neonatal-Perinatal Medicine, Schneider Children's Hospital of Long Island Jewish Medical Center, New York, New York
Exchange Transfusion

GEORGE A. LITTLE, M.D.

Professor of Clinical Maternal and Child Health, Dartmouth Medical School; Staff, Dartmouth-Hitchcock Medical Center, Hanover, New Hampshire
Apnea

MICHAEL D. LOCKSHIN, M.D., F.A.C.P.

Professor of Medicine, Cornell University Medical College; Attending Physician, Hospital for Special Surgery and The New York Hospital, New York, New York
Systemic Lupus Erythematosus in Pregnancy

SCOTT N. MacGREGOR, D.O.

Assistant Professor, Department of Obstetrics and Gynecology, Northwestern University Medical School, Chicago; Attending Perinatologist, Evanston Hospital, Evanston, Illinois
Intrauterine Growth Retardation: Obstetric Aspects

M. JEFFREY MAISELS, M.B., B.Ch.

Clinical Professor of Pediatrics, University of Michigan Medical School, Ann Arbor and Wayne State University School of Medicine, Detroit; Chairman, Department of Pediatrics, William Beaumont Hospital, Royal Oak, Michigan
Hyperbilirubinemia

KEITH H. MARKS, M.B., B.Ch., F.C.P., Dip. Paed., M.R.C.P., Ph.D.

Associate Professor of Pediatrics, Pennsylvania State University College of Medicine; Chief, Division of Newborn Medicine, Department of Pediatrics, The Milton S. Hershey Medical Center, Hershey, Pennsylvania
Pulmonary Interstitial Emphysema
Thermal and Caloric Balance

RICHARD J. MARTIN, M.B., F.R.A.C.P.

Associate Professor of Pediatrics, Case Western Reserve University School of Medicine; Co-Director, Division of Neonatology, Rainbow Babies and Children's Hospital, Cleveland, Ohio
Weaning From the Respirator

EUGENE D. McGAHREN, M.D.

Chief Resident, Department of Surgery, University of Virginia Health Sciences Center, Charlottesville, Virginia
Tracheoesophageal Fistula

JAMES J. McGILL, M.B.B.S., F.R.A.C.P.

Research Fellow, Department of Pediatrics, University of Melbourne; Clinical Geneticist, Department of Genetics, Royal Children's Hospital, Melbourne, Australia
Transient Diabetes

PAUL MERLOB, M.D.

Assistant Professor of Pediatrics, University of Tel Aviv Sackler School of Medicine, Tel Aviv; Director, Neonatal Unit, Department of Pediatrics and Neonatology, Beilinson Medical Center, Petah Tikva, Israel
Craniosynostosis

BRUCE A. MEYER, M.D.

Fellow in Maternal-Fetal Medicine, Department of Obstetrics, Gynecology, and Reproductive Sciences, University of Texas Medical School; Staff Physician, The Hermann Hospital, Houston Texas
Late Fetal Death

RICHARD A. MEYER, M.D.

Professor of Pediatrics, University of Cincinnati College of Medicine; Director, Cardiac Ultrasound and Attending Cardiologist, Children's Hospital Medical Center, Cincinnati, Ohio
Echocardiographic Evaluation of Congenital Heart Disease in the Fetus and Newborn

WILLIAM H. MICHAELS, M.D., F.A.C.O.G.

Staff Perinatologist, Providence Hospital, Southfield, Michigan
Incompetent Cervix

BARBARA A. MILLER, M.D.

Assistant Professor of Pediatrics, Pennsylvania State University College of Medicine; Staff, Department of Pediatrics, The Milton S. Hershey Medical Center, Hershey, Pennsylvania
Thrombocytopenia

JAY M. MILSTEIN, M.D.

Associate Professor, Division of Neonatology, Department of Pediatrics, University of California School of Medicine, Davis; Medical Director, Special Care Nurseries, Sacramento, California
Vater Association

LOUIS L. MIZELL, M.D.

Chief, Pediatric Gastroenterology, USAF Medical Center, Keesler Air Force Base, Mississippi
Gastroesophageal Reflux

ELI M. MIZRAHI, M.D.

Assistant Professor of Neurology (Section of Neurophysiology) and Pediatrics (Section of Pediatric Neurology), Baylor College of Medicine, The Methodist Hospital and Texas Children's Hospital, Houston, Texas
Electroencephalographic/Polygraphic/Video Monitoring

MARK MONTGOMERY, M.D., FRCPC

Assistant Professor, University of Calgary Faculty of Medicine; Pediatric Pulmonologist, Alberta Children's Provincial General Hospital, Calgary, Alberta, Canada
Continuous Distending Pressure

DAVID M. MUMFORD, M.D.

Professor and Associate Dean, Baylor College of Medicine, Houston, Texas
Teenage Pregnancy

RODRIGO A. MUÑOZ, M.D.

Clinical Professor of Psychiatry, University of California School of Medicine, San Diego; Medical Director, Harborview Medical Center, San Diego, California
Postpartum Psychosis

JOHN L. MYERS, M.D.

Assistant Professor of Surgery and Pediatrics, The Milton S. Hershey Medical Center, Pennsylvania State University College of Medicine, Hershey, Pennsylvania
Arterial Switch Operation: Correction of Simple Transposition of the Great Arteries

DAVID J. NOCHIMSON, M.D.

Professor and Vice Chairman, Department of Obstetrics and Gynecology and Associate Dean, School of Medicine, University of Connecticut Health Center, Farmington, Connecticut
Premature Rupture of the Membranes

WILLIAM I. NORWOOD, M.D., Ph.D.

Professor of Surgery, University of Pennsylvania School of Medicine; Chief, Cardiovascular Surgery, Children's Hospital, Philadelphia, Pennsylvania
Hypoplastic Left Heart Syndrome

OSAMU NOSE, M.D., Ph.D

Assistant Professor of Pediatrics, Osaka University School of Medicine; Chief of Pediatric Endocrinology and Nutrition, Osaka University Hospital, Osaka, Japan
Hypothyroidism

DONALD A. NOVAK, M.D.

Assistant Professor, University of South Florida College of Medicine; Chairman, Division of Gastroenterology, University of South Florida Medical Center and Tampa General Hospital, Tampa, Florida
Chronic Cholestasis

MARY E. O'CONNOR, M.D., M.P.H.

Assistant Clinical Professor of Pediatrics, University of California School of Medicine; Staff, Department of Pediatrics, San Francisco General Hospital, San Francisco, California
Hemorrhagic Disease (Vitamin K Deficiency)

WILLIAM OH, M.D.

Professor of Medical Science in Pediatrics and Obstetrics, Brown University Program in Medicine; Pediatrician-in-Chief, Women and Infants Hospital, Providence, Rhode Island
Immunizations
Infant of a Diabetic Mother

PER OLOFSSON, M.D., Ph.D

Associate Professor of Obstetrics and Gynecology, University of Lund School of Medicine; Staff, Department of Obstetrics and Gynecology, University of Lund General Hospital, Malmö, Sweden
Fetal Surveillance in High-Risk Pregnancy

SUSAN OLSON, Ph.D

Assistant Professor of Medical Genetics, Oregon Health Sciences University School of Medicine, Portland, Oregon
Chorionic Villus Sampling

EARL A. PALMER, M.D.

Associate Professor of Ophthalmology and Pediatrics and Chief, Strabismus and Pediatric Ophthalmology, Oregon Health Sciences University School of Medicine; Director, Elks Children's Eye Clinic and Consultant, University Hospitals, Portland, Oregon
Cryotherapy for Retinopathy of Prematurity
Ophthalmoscopy in the Newborn

ALAN M. PEACEMAN, M.D.

Instructor in Clinical Obstetrics and Gynecology and Fellow in Maternal Fetal Medicine, Department of Obstetrics, Gynecology, and Reproductive Sciences, University of Texas Medical School; Staff Physician, The Hermann Hospital, Houston, Texas
Advanced Maternal Age

DALE L. PHELPS, M.D.

Associate Professor of Pediatrics and Ophthalmology, University of Rochester School of Medicine and Dentistry; Staff, Division of Neonatology, Strong Memorial Hospital, Rochester, New York
Retinopathy of Prematurity

JOHN D. PIGOTT, M.D.

Assistant Professor of Surgery, University of Pennsylvania School of Medicine; Assistant Surgeon, Children's Hospital, Philadelphia, Pennsylvania
Hypoplastic Left Heart Syndrome

RICHARD A. PIRCON, M.D.

Clinical Instructor and Fellow, Maternal-Fetal-Medicine, Memorial Women's Hospital, Long Beach, California
Uterine Rupture

RONALD L. POLAND, M.D.

Professor of Pediatrics, Wayne State University School of Medicine; Director of Neonatal Services, Detroit Medical Center Affiliated Hospitals, Detroit, Michigan
Diagnosis-Related Groups

REIJO PUNNONEN, M.D.

Docent and Chief Physician, Department of Obstetrics and Gynecology, University Central Hospital of Tampere, Tampere, Finland
Vacuum Extraction

LUIS M. PRUDENT, M.D.

Clinical Professor of Pediatrics, University of Buenos Aires, Buenos Aires, Argentina
Sepsis

TERESA J. REID, R.N./M.S.N.

Instructor, Department of Pediatrics, University of South Dakota School of Medicine, Sioux Falls, South Dakota
Nurse Clinicians

SALOMON H. REISNER, M.B., Ch.B.

Professor of Pediatrics, University of Tel Aviv Sackler School of Medicine, Tel Aviv; Staff, Department of Pediatrics and Neonatology, Beilinson Medical Center, Petah Tikva, Israel
Craniosynostosis

ROBERT RESNIK, M.D.

Professor and Chair, Department of Reproductive Medicine, University of California School of Medicine, San Diego; Chief, Obstetrics and Gynecology, University of California San Diego Medical Center, San Diego, California
Cord Prolapse

DON M. ROBERTON, M.D., F.R.A.C.P.

Senior Lecturer, University of Melbourne; Pediatric Physician and Director of Clinical Immunology, Royal Children's Hospital, Melbourne, Australia
Transient Diabetes

ALFRED G. ROBICHAUX III, M.D.

Assistant Clinical Professor of Obstetrics and Gynecology, Louisiana State University Medical Center; Co-Director, Division of Maternal Fetal Medicine, Ochsner Clinic, New Orleans, Louisiana
Herpes Simplex Infection

BRADLEY M. RODGERS, M.D.

Professor of Surgery and Pediatrics and Chief, Division of Pediatric Surgery, University of Virginia Health Sciences Center, Charlottesville, Virginia
Congenital Diaphragmatic Hernia
Tracheoesophageal Fistula

MORTIMER G. ROSEN, M.D.

Willard C. Rappleye Professor, Department of Obstetrics and Gynecology, Columbia-Presbyterian Medical Center; Chairman, Department of Obstetrics and Gynecology, Sloan Hospital for Women, New York, New York
Previous Cesarean Section

CHARLES R. ROSENFELD, M.D.

Professor of Pediatrics and Obstetrics/Gynecology and Director, Division of Neonatal-Perinatal Medicine, University of Texas Southwestern Medical Center; Medical-Director of Nurseries, Parkland Memorial Hospital, Dallas, Texas
Intrauterine Growth Retardation: Pediatric Aspects

MARTIN P. SAMUELS, M.B., M.R.C.P.

Research Fellow in Pediatrics, National Heart and Lung Institute; Pediatric Registrar, Bromptom Hospital, London, England
Cyanotic/Apneic Episodes

BARRY S. SCHIFRIN, M.D.

Director, Department of Maternal-Fetal Medicine, AMI-Tarzana Regional Medical Center, Tarzana, California
Fetal Monitoring During Labor
External Cephalic Version

ROBERT E. SCHUMACHER, M.D.

Assistant Professor of Pediatrics, University of Michigan Medical School; Staff, C.S. Mott Children's Hospital, Ann Arbor, Michigan
Bilirubinometry

HANNSJÖRG W. SEYBERTH, M.D.

Professor of Pediatrics and Pharmacology, University of Heidelberg; Hermann and Lilly Schilling Professor for Medical Research and Attending Physician in Neonatology and Pediatrics, Children's Hospital, Heidelberg, Federal Republic of Germany
Hypokalemia

DONALD L. SHAPIRO, M.D.

Professor of Pediatrics, University of Rochester School of Medicine and Dentistry; Director of Neonatology, The Strong Memorial Hospital, Rochester, New York
Group B Streptococcal Infections
Surfactant Replacement Therapy

NANCY F. SHEARD, Sc.D., R.D.

Assistant Professor, Department of Nutrition, University of Massachusetts, Amherst, Massachusetts
Parenteral Nutrition

ROGER E. SHELDON, M.D.

Professor of Pediatrics, University of Oklahoma College of Medicine; Chief, Neonatology Section, Department of Pediatrics and Chief, Nursery Service, Oklahoma Memorial Hospital, Oklahoma City, Oklahoma
Tetany

JAMES R. SHIELDS, M.D.

Department of Maternal-Fetal Medicine, AMI-Tarzana Regional Medical Center, Tarzana, California
External Cephalic Version

BILLIE LOU SHORT, M.D.

Associate Professor of Pediatrics, George Washington University School of Medicine and Health Sciences, Washington and Assistant Professor, The Johns Hopkins Medical Institutions, Baltimore, Maryland; Associate Neonatologist, Children's Hospital National Medical Center, Washington, D.C.
Neonatal Extracorporeal Membrane Oxygenation

AVINOAM SHUPER, M.D.

Lecturer in Pediatrics, University of Tel Aviv Sackler School of Medicine, Tel Aviv; Staff, Department of Pediatrics and Neonatology, Beilinson Medical Center, Petah Tikva, Israel
Craniosynostosis

RICHARD K. SILVER, M.D.

Assistant Professor, Department of Obstetrics and Gynecology, Northwestern University Medical School, Chicago; Director, Perinatal Education, Division of Maternal-Fetal Medicine, Evanston Hospital, Evanston, Illinois
Placenta Previa

PEGGY B. SMITH, Ph.D.

Professor of Obstetrics and Gynecology, Baylor College of Medicine, Houston, Texas
Teenage Pregnancy

SELMA E. SNYDERMAN, M.D.

Professor of Pediatrics, New York University School of Medicine; Attending Physician, University and Bellevue Hospitals and Director, New York University Pediatric Metabolic Disease Center, New York, New York
Maple Syrup Urine Disease
Phenylketonuria

DAVID P. SOUTHALL, M.D., M.R.C.P.

Senior Lecturer in Pediatrics, National Heart Lung Institute; Consultant Pediatrician, Brompton Hospital, London, England
Cyanotic/Apneic Episodes

JAMES A. STANKIEWICZ, M.D.

Associate Professor and Vice Chairman, Department of Otolaryngology–Head and Neck Surgery, Loyola University Medical Center; Attending Physician, Loyola University Medical Center, Maywood and Courtesy Staff, Childrens Memorial Hospital, Chicago, Illinois
Laryngotracheal Stenosis

CHARLES L. STEWART, M.D.

Instructor of Pediatrics, Children's Medical Center, State University of New York College of Medicine; Attending Pediatric Nephrologist, Children's Medical Center, Stony Brook, New York
Renal Cystic Disease

THOMAS M. STUBBS, M.D.

Assistant Professor, Department of Obstetrics/Gynecology, Medical University of South Carolina College of Medicine, Charleston, South Carolina
Eclampsia

ANN M. SUTTON, M.B.B.S., D.C.H., F.R.C.P.

Consultant Pediatrician and Honorary Lecturer, University Department of Child Health, Royal Hospital for Sick Children, Glasgow, Scotland
Copper Deficiency

JUKKA TAKALA, M.D., Ph.D.

Assistant Professor of Anesthesiology, Kuopio University; Director, Critical Care Research Program, Intensive Care Unit, Kuopio University Central Hospital, Kuopio, Finland
Early Metabolic Acidosis

PAUL M. TAYLOR, M.D.

Professor of Pediatrics, Obstetrics/Gynecology, and Psychiatry, University of Pittsburgh School of Medicine; Active Staff, Pediatrics (Neonatology), Magee-Womens Hospital and Children's Hospital, Pittsburgh, Pennsylvania
Bonding and Attachment

BRADLEY T. THACH, M.D.

Professor of Pediatrics, Washington University School of Medicine; Staff, Department of Pediatrics, Division of Newborn Medicine, Children's Hospital, St. Louis, Missouri
Obstructive Apnea

HOWARD O. THOMPSON, M.D.

Instructor and Fellow, Maternal-Fetal Medicine, Strong Memorial Hospital, Rochester, New York
Incompetent Cervix

JAMES A. THORP, M.D.

Fellow in Maternal-Fetal Medicine, Department of Obstetrics, Gynecology, and Reproductive Sciences, University of Texas Medical School; Staff Physician, The Hermann Hospital, Houston, Texas
Postdate Pregnancy

ATTILA TOTH, M.D.

Associate Professor of Obstetrics and Gynecology, Cornell University Medical College; Director, The MacLeod Laboratory for Infertility, The New York Hospital-Cornell Medical Center, New York, New York
Spontaneous Abortion

WILLIAM E. TRUOG III, M.D.

Professor of Pediatrics, University of Washington School of Medicine; Medical Director, Infant Intensive Care Unit, Children's Hospital Medical Center, Seattle, Washington
Resuscitation

REGINALD C. TSANG, M.B.B.S.

Professor of Pediatrics, Obstetrics, and Gynecology, Director, Division of Neonatology, and Vice Chairman, Pediatric Affairs UH, University of Cincinnati/Children's Hospital Medical Center, Cincinnati, Ohio
Rickets in Infants

HIROSHI USHIJIMA, M.D., Ph.D.

Assistant Professor of Pediatrics, Teikyo University School of Medicine; Chief of Special Pathogens, National Institute of Health, Tokyo, Japan
Clostridium difficile Infection

NESTOR E. VAIN, M.D.

Director, Neonatal Intensive Care Unit, Sanatorio Mitre; Co-Director, Neonatal Intensive Care Unit, Sanatorio Anchorena, Buenos Aires, Argentina
Sepsis

DAVID L. VALLE, M.D.

Professor of Pediatrics, The Johns Hopkins University School of Medicine; Active Staff, Pediatrics, The Johns Hopkins Hospital, Baltimore, Maryland
Symptomatic Inborn Errors of Metabolism

KATHLEEN A. VENESS-MEEHAN, M.D.

Senior Instructor in Pediatrics, University of Rochester School of Medicine; Staff, Division of Neonatology, Department of Pediatrics, University of Rochester Medical Center, Rochester, New York
Group B Streptococcal Infections

PANKAJA S. VENKATARAMAN, M.B.B.S.

Associate Professor of Pediatrics, University of Oklahoma College of Medicine, Oklahoma City, Oklahoma
Tetany

ANTHONY M. VINTZILEOS, M.D.

Associate Professor, Obstetrics and Gynecology and Director, Maternal-Fetal Medicine and Obstetrics, University of Connecticut Health Center School of Medicine, Farmington, Connecticut
Premature Rupture of the Membranes

BETTY R. VOHR, M.D.

Associate Professor of Pediatrics, Brown University Program in Medicine; Director, Neonatal Follow-Up Clinic, Women and Infants Hospital, Providence, Rhode Island
Immunizations

RAYMOND B. WAIT, M.D.

Associate Professor of Obstetrics and Gynecology, Baylor College of Medicine, Houston, Texas
Teenage Pregnancy

W. ALLAN WALKER, M.D.

Professor of Pediatrics, Harvard Medical School; Chief, Combined Program in Pediatric Gastroenterology and Nutrition, Massachusetts General Hospital and The Children's Hospital, Boston, Massachusetts
Parenteral Nutrition

ROBERT M. WARD, M.D.

Associate Professor of Pediatrics, University of Utah School of Medicine; Medical Director, Infant Care Services, Primary Children's Medical Center, Salt Lake City, Utah
Persistent Pulmonary Hypertension

STEVEN J. WASSNER, M.D., F.A.A.P.

Associate Professor of Pediatrics, Pennsylvania State University College of Medicine; Chief, Division of Pediatric Nephrology, The Milton S. Hershey Medical Center, Hershey, Pennsylvania
Fluid Therapy

LAWRENCE R. WELLMAN, M.D.

Associate Professor of Pediatrics, University of South Dakota School of Medicine; Attending Neonatologist, Sioux Valley Hospital, Sioux Falls, South Dakota
Nurse Clinicians

ROBERT M. WRIGHT, M.D.

Chief of Radiology, Saint Francis Medical Center, Peoria, Illinois
Perinatal Magnetic Resonance Imaging

STEVEN M. WRIGHT, Ph.D.

Assistant Professor of Electrical Engineering, Department of Engineering, Zachary Engineering Center, Texas A&M University, College Station, Texas
Perinatal Magnetic Resonance Imaging

JEN-TIEN WUNG, M.D.

Associate Clinical Professor of Anesthesiology and Pediatrics, Columbia University College of Physicians and Surgeons; Associate Attending Anesthesiologist and Associate Director, Neonatal ICU, Columbia-Presbyterian Medical Center, New York, New York
Mechanical Ventilation

EDWARD R. YEOMANS, M.D.

Chief of Obstetrics, Department of Obstetrics/Gynecology, Wilford Hall USAF Medical Center (SGHG), Lackland Air Force Base, San Antonio, Texas
Intrauterine Growth Retardation: Pediatric Aspects

DONALD YOUNKIN, M.D.

Associate Professor of Neurology and Pediatrics, University of Pennsylvania School of Medicine; Staff, Division of Neurology, Children's Hospital, Philadelphia, Pennsylvania
Neonatal Seizures

PREFACE

This Second Edition of *Current Therapy in Neonatal-Perinatal Medicine* aims to continue the plan of the first: a horizontal slice through some newer developments of clinical relevance, as well as statements of established personal practice in areas of continuing importance to those whose major professional involvement is with the newborn and his family.

Topics include the late-breaking (cryotherapy) and the heart-breaking (AIDS). The dominance of technology (ECHO, ECMO, EFM, MRI) and its intermingling with art (fetal blood sampling, video electroencephalography) should not surprise a practitioner entering the '90s. This more mercantile era for medicine (at least in North America) is becoming denoted by "DRGs" and computer controls, the latter now becoming manageable at the personal as well as "main frame" level. Surgical topics burgeon, especially concerning the heart. The non-surgeon, reading of such operations as "filleting" or "gusseting" (in the process of "switching" the great arteries), is reminded of the tonsorial traditions from which such advances arose.

The geography of authorship has now widened to include *all* the hemispheres (Near East and Far East, Australasia and Scandinavia, as well as the Americas). Fortunately for the Editor, most modern medical authors, regardless of mother tongue, write English well. The greater challenge has been to resist the temptation to translate these fine manuscripts into *American*!

Despite the occasional vagaries of old-fashioned ("non-FAX") mail service between Pennsylvania and Ontario, Brian Decker's team, especially Julia Ollinger and Mary Mansor (medical editor and fellow Mozart lover), has been most gently effective in bringing all this to pass.

We continue to enjoy the freedom *not* to cover some important topics, on the thesis that either they were covered in the earlier volume (many are updated here by their previous or different authors), or we will get to them in subsequent versions.

Nicholas M. Nelson
Hershey, Pennsylvania
August 7, 1989

PREFACE TO THE FIRST EDITION

When first approached by Brian Decker to undertake the editing of the present volume, I (as a congenital and fervid "lumper") expressed great doubt that it were possible to conjure up the 100 or so clinical topics in neonatal/perinatal medicine necessary to fulfill the established format of the Decker "Current Therapy" series. But then I recalled Dr. Mary Ellen Avery's observation that early editions of the Harriet Lane (pediatric house officer's) Manual had exhaustively presented hard knowledge of proper management of the premature infant in 1 or 2 pages, whereas presently 10 or more pages barely suffice for only superficial treatment, and gained confidence that the total meal might be adequate; the real question was the size and texture of the bites. We hope our readers will agree that this final menu is *al dente* and intellectually nourishing.

Those among the authorship (and readership) of this volume who know me can attest (as could the preceding paragraph) to my enjoyment in pressing the English language to its outer limits. Those less acquainted with this aberration have occasionally been nonplussed by (but in the end always graciously acceded to) such eccentricities as the inclusion of computers, transportation, and bereavement under the general rubric of "treatment." Briefly put, I have for present purposes chosen to interpret current therapy to mean "what's happening" in the field of neonatal-perinatal medicine, here presented to those involved subspecialists who must get things done by those who make things happen. The inclusion of such demonstrably nonperinatal topics as ectopic pregnancy should also serve notice of my continuing intent to present material presumed to be of general interest to those who serve the needs of the pregnant woman and her products of conception.

The final choice of topics will, no doubt, strike many as odd. Why, for instance, is there no chapter on infantile respiratory distress syndrome (née hyaline membrane disease)?— because I took it as a personal challenge to produce a table of contents that did not include these terms, since I regard this "disease" not as an affection of lung, but as a global phenomenon of developmental deficiency among multiple organs. Those who feel bereft need only to look to the chapters on surfactant replacement, mechanical ventilation, parenteral nutrition, patent ductus arteriosus, and parental bereavement for a surfeit of material on the current therapy of hyaline membrane disease—to such a degree has this lumper become a splitter! Beyond this, the final array of topics presented here is the admixed result of my own highly subjective judgment of the general importance or current curiosity inherent to each, as well as the presence of new information, or at least inflammatory opinion ("action," in the vernacular), all balanced against the availability of authoritative and lucid writers whose other commitments and work habits could permit inclusion. Moreover, the fact that this volume is intended for approximately biennial renewal, combined with the ever-sedate pace of true therapeutic advance in clinical medicine, has allowed us the freedom *not* to cover certain topics of unquestioned importance in this first edition.

A personal trip through the cabbage patch of illness during the production of this volume has denied me the ultimate reward of editorship (the massaging of someone else's words), and I am, accordingly, grateful for the high competence herein displayed by Brian Decker's associates, particularly so because I have thus been able to savor these manuscripts more as reader than editor and to note such happy diversity in writing styles. The most gratifying discovery has been that there is so much with which I can agree.

I have gained some personal pearls: that there is a Munchhausen syndrome in obstetrics, that self-examination of the cervix is a concept supported (even taught) by male obstetricians (as well as by the National Organization of Women), that one-half of LBW infants are SGA, that prospects for future child-bearing by the woman who has suffered an ectopic pregnancy are dim.

Some items qualify as "non-news": that physicians don't handle death well, that the provision of contraceptive (or any other) information to teenagers does not guarantee its accurate application (has driver education diminished young male auto accident rates?); but I have felt illuminated by the authors' efforts to look behind these depressing facts.

I find it satisfying that such "hi tech" maneuvers as monitored "kick counts" of fetal activity and patellar reflex bioassay of $MgSO_4$ blood levels (in toxemia/eclampsia) yet survive and still contribute to patient management in the era of fetoscopy and high-frequency ventilation by machines that beep but don't always call home.

I would estimate that the current volume's "not-yet-ready-for-prime-time-players" include the self-same high-frequency ventilation, as well as surfactant replacement and fetal surgery. On the other hand, the passing parade has now clearly seen indomethacin muscle ligation out of pride-of-place in the management of patent ductus; Waterston has changed places with Blalock; arterial puncture has given way to transcutaneous polarography; and exchange transfusion has been all but done in by RhoGam.

As one who, at a high point during pediatric internship in 1955, observed his first exchange transfusion performed by Dr. Alexander Wiener in Bellevue Hospital (it was a Professor's procedure then)—the effluent blood spurting from the infant's nicked radial artery into a waiting (sterile) shot glass—I now read with mixed emotion the attestations herein recorded from Boston and Munich that it has again become, after a brief fluorit, a Professor's procedure.

Years ago, while picking my young son up from Sunday school, I fell into conversation with our minister, in whose choir I had once sung soprano. Taking prideful note of my entry into pediatrics and that of his own son (and my classmate) into the ministry, he reminisced over his early days (1915-) as a young churchman and how his career had chronologically paralleled the major march of modern medicine. Almost mistily he said, "You know, we hardly *ever* have a baby funeral anymore!"

Just so.

Nicholas M. Nelson
Hershey, Pennsylvania
February 4, 1985

CONTENTS

Special Procedures

Neonatal Medicine

General Considerations

Specific Clinical Entities

SPECIAL PROCEDURES

PERINATAL MEDICINE | GENERAL CONSIDERATIONS

ANTENATAL CORTICOSTEROIDS

GRAHAM C. LIGGINS, M.B., Ph.D., F.R.C.O.G.

The obstetrician can contribute to the well-being of the newborn preterm infant in a number of ways, one of which is antenatal corticosteroid treatment. The desirability of avoidance of unnecessary preterm delivery is evident, but when it is unavoidable, every effort must be made to deliver the infant in the best possible condition and in the best possible environment. This means that the delivery should occur close to an intensive care nursery (possibly after referral), that every measure should be taken to avoid intrapartum asphyxia, and that an experienced team of obstetricians and neonatologists should be present at delivery. The last requirement may lead to either the performance of cesarian section or the administration of epidural anesthesia throughout labor. The use of corticosteroids to avoid referral or to justify less than the best available perinatal care is unwarranted and dangerous.

The benefits to the preterm infant of antenatal corticosteroid treatment have been proved beyond doubt in numerous well-controlled trials in several countries. Despite this, such treatment is by no means universal; those opposing it usually argue that treatment of respiratory distress syndrome (RDS) is now associated with low mortality rate and that corticosteroids may have long-term adverse effects. Such arguments against treatment overlook both the serious morbidity of RDS in survivors, particularly bronchopulmonary dysplasia and intellectual or learning handicaps, and the complete absence of long-term adverse effects of corticosteroids, at least up to the age of 6 years, per a study by MacArthur and colleagues in 1982.

THEORETICAL BACKGROUND

Since the first reports in 1969 of accelerated lung maturation in fetal animals exposed to corticosteroids, the mechanisms underlying the response have been very extensively investigated in both human and animal lungs. An extremely complex series of changes has been elucidated. Indeed, every aspect of normal maturation is affected by corticosteroids. Overall, differentiation of the various tissue components of lung is increased at the expense of growth, which is slowed (catch-up growth occurs later). The synthesis of surfactant is increased in various ways, including breakdown of glycogen stores in lung epithelium, enhanced activity of enzymes promoting the synthesis of phosphatidylcholine and phosphatidylglycerol, and increased synthesis of the protein components of surfactant. In addition, corticosteroid treatment alters the collagen and elastin structure of the alveolar walls to make them more distensible. Finally, corticosteroids induce the formation of beta-adrenergic receptors, thereby enhancing the effects of epinephrine in stimulating secretion of surfactant and in resorbing water from the fluid-filled airways.

INDICATIONS

Most infants born before the end of the 34th week of pregnancy benefit from treatment, the exceptions being those in whom pulmonary maturation is already advanced, as demonstrated by the lecithin-sphingomyclin ratio, or in whom it is likely to have occurred as the result of prolonged fetal stress associated with growth retardation. Since infants with prior stress born by elective cesarean section are particularly prone to RDS, consideration should be given to corticosteroid treatment in such pregnancies up to a later gestational age, about 36 weeks. Similarly when there is a history of RDS in a previous infant born near term, whether or not it was associated with maternal diabetes, treatment in subsequent pregnancies is appropriate. There is no known lower limit to the gestational age at which corticosteroid treatment may be beneficial. However, the response becomes less as gestational age decreases for reasons that are discussed below.

CONTRAINDICATIONS

In itself, antenatal corticosteroid treatment has no absolute contraindications. Most complications arise not directly from the steroids but from ancillary management required to accomplish completion of a course of treatment. In particular, maternal complications may accompany tocolysis with beta-adrenergic agents or magnesium sulfate, and fetal complications may develop during the period in which delivery is delayed. In general, corticosteroid treatment is contraindicated in the presence of disorders that normally call for expedited delivery. Fetal hypoxemia, fetal infection, and placental abruption are examples from a more extensive list. In each patient for whom treatment is considered, a careful analysis of risk versus benefit is made before making a decision to treat, bearing in mind that the earlier the gestational age, the greater the potential for benefit and the greater the risk that can be accepted. When in doubt, a compromise may be chosen between the optimal period of 72 hours from the start of treatment to delivery and a shorter period of delayed delivery.

STANDARD PROTOCOL

Any steroid with glucocorticoid activity and in an appropriate dose is probably effective. Usually the choice lies between betamethasone and dexamethasone, since these are the most thoroughly investigated steroids. Treatment regimens vary, but the aim should be to maintain high blood levels in the mother and fetus for a period of 48 hours. My practice is to administer four doses each of betamethasone, 5 mg intramuscularly, at 12-hour intervals. A total dose of 20 to 25 mg of either betamethasone or dexamethasone in divided doses over 36 hours is the most commonly used regimen in other centers. A controlled trial in which betamethasone was compared with hydrocortisone 200 mg times four has been completed in our hospital but data have not yet been analyzed. No obvious differences between the two treatment groups were apparent. If reservations are held about the long-term safety of corticosteroid analogues, the use of the natural hormone, hydrocortisone, could be an acceptable alternative.

Not infrequently the question arises as to whether repeated courses of treatment are desirable when the first course in not followed by delivery but the patient remains at high risk for preterm delivery because of, for example, placenta previa. It is known that the effect of treatment in preventing RDS is lost by the end of a week in pregnancies in which treatment is given before 30 weeks. On the other hand, studies of long-term safety apply only to a single course of treatment. Whether repeat courses are potentially dangerous or whether effects persist in pregnancies in which treatment is given later than 30 weeks is unknown. My practice is to avoid more than two courses of treatment unless the indications are compelling and not to treat again when the previous course was given later than 29 weeks.

CONTROVERSIES

Even among those who favor the use of corticosteroids, certain areas of controversy have remained. The idea that prolonged rupture of the membranes in itself promoted lung maturation led to the conclusion that corticosteroid treatment was ineffective and unnecessary in these circumstances. In our original study (Liggins and Howie, 1972), no distinction could be made between the responses to corticosteroids of those with and without ruptured membranes. Recent work has usually concluded that ruptured membranes are not associated with a reduced incidence of RDS and that corticosteroid treatment is beneficial. Another question concerns the possibility that corticosteroid treatment may increase the risk of death in fetuses compromised by pregnancy-induced hypertension. This arose from the results of our early trial, but subsequent reanalysis showed that factors other than the corticosteroid were related to the excess of deaths. More recent studies report benefit from corticosteroids in such pregnancies without an increase in fetal mortality.

The National Institute of Health–sponsored multicenter trial in the United States found that corticosteroids prevented RDS only in female infants, which has been interpreted by some as indicating that treatment should be given only to female infants after sex is determined by ultrasonography. The results of the multicenter trial differ from those of six other well-controlled trials in which treatment benefit was shared among male and female infants.

It has been suggested that twin pregnancies should be given twice the standard dose of corticosteroid because of the presence of two babies. In fact, the total volume into which the maternally administered hormone is distributed is only slightly (5 percent) increased by the extra fetus. Although the theoretical basis for a higher dose is dubious, evidence suggests that steroids are less effective in twin pregnancies, perhaps because of the greater immaturity of second twins.

THE FUTURE

Even under optimal conditions when a full course of corticosteroid treatment is completed, RDS is not entirely prevented, particularly in very low birth weight infants. Can the results of corticosteroid treatment be improved? Two current lines of research in experimental animals suggest that this may be possible by combining steroids either with other hormones or with the instillation of surfactant into the infant's lungs soon after birth.

In the third trimester, the maturational effects of corticosteroids are expressed in the presence of rising levels of various other hormones (including triiodothyronine and prolactin) in fetal blood. Before 28 weeks, the levels of these hormones are very low, raising the possibility that the relatively poor response to corticosteroids at very early gestational ages is a consequence of deficiency of other hormones. To test this idea, fetal sheep were treated with corticosteroid combined with mixtures of other hormones at an early gestational age when the lungs were entirely unresponsive to physiologic amounts of steroid alone. A remarkable synergistic effect of cortisol, triiodothyronine, and prolactin was found, and the fetal lungs became almost as distensible and stable as term lungs. Since the secretion of both triiodothyronine and prolactin can be stimulated in the fetus by thyrotropin-releasing hormone, and since thyrotropin-releasing hormone readily crosses the placenta after maternal administration, further experiments tested the combination of cortisol and thyrotropin-releasing hormone. The results were as striking as when the individual hormones were given. Controlled clinical trials of corticosteroid and thyrotropin-releasing hormone in very preterm labors are under way in both New Zealand and the United States. Empirical use of this regimen is unjustified until the results are available.

The combination of antenatal treatment with steroids or steroids plus thyrotropin-releasing hormone with instillation of surfactant into the lungs soon after birth has been investigated in rabbits. Preliminary reports show that beneficial effects of each treatment are additive when they are combined. Clinical trials are needed to determine whether similar responses can be achieved in human infants.

Supported by the Medical Research Council of New Zealand.

SUGGESTED READING

Liggins GC, Howie RN. A controlled trial of antepartum glucocorticoid treatment for prevention of the respiratory distress syndrome in premature infants. Pediatrics 1972; 50:515–525.
Little B, Avery ME, De Mets D, et al. Effect of antenatal dexamethasone administration on the prevention of respiratory distress syndrome. Am J Obstet Gynecol 1982; 141:276–287.
MacArthur BA, Howie RN, Dezoete JA, Elkins J. School progress and cognitive development of 6-year-old children whose mothers were treated antenatally with betamethasone. Pediatrics 1982; 70:99–105.
Papageorgion A, Stern L. Antenatal prevention of the neonatal respiratory distress syndrome: benefits and potential risks for the mother and the infant. J Perinat Med 1986; 14:75–86.

FETAL MONITORING DURING LABOR

BARRY S. SCHIFRIN, M.D.

We consider electronic fetal monitoring (EFM) a routine technique that is potentially beneficial in all pregnancies, both high and low risk. EFM predicts the absence of asphyxia with greater accuracy than any other known technique or combination of techniques. It has a lower false normal rate than fetal blood sampling or auscultation. It provides insights into the mechanism of asphyxia and the likelihood with which such insults can be ameliorated by conservative measures. EFM improves perinatal outcome by reducing the risk of intrapartum stillbirth and low Apgar score. Furthermore, perinatal outcome appears enhanced in both high- and low-risk patients. The development of fetal distress in labor is not limited to patients previously designated as high risk. Recently, EFM patterns have been shown to correlate with neonatal and subsequent neurological disability.

The monitor cannot be used as a fancy stethoscope. If the same criteria for distress as used in auscultation are applied to EFM tracings, then the monitor is being misused, and the cesarean section rate will probably rise precipitously. There is little question that bad monitoring is worse than none at all.

Some maintain that the monitor restricts patient movement, diverts attention from the patient, and interferes with the progress and conduct of labor. Unfortunately, the image prevails that EFM requires the patient, once admitted, to have her membranes ruptured, if feasible, to have an electrode applied, a uterine catheter and an intravenous line inserted, and then for her to be anchored, on her back, to the monitor. At our institution we monitor the fetus with external devices at the time the patient is admitted to the hospi-

tal. Once assured that the fetus is in good condition, we allow the patient to walk around with telemetry or even without the monitor until the membranes rupture. She may use the bedpan or the bathroom, unless she detects unusual uterine activity or returns to bed. If the initial EFM pattern is suspect, procedures necessary for definitive diagnosis are undertaken. External surveillance may be maintained as long as the tracing is satisfactory and reassuring.

EFM has a number of limitations. It does not predict (nor does pH) neonatal distress resulting from trauma, sepsis, drugs, or congenital anomaly—factors that account for more than 50 percent of depressed newborns. Nor does it predict fetal distress very well, as a number of apparently normal fetuses demonstrate abnormal fetal heart rate patterns. A new lexicon is required and technical problems await the unwary. If obstetric personnel have not received appropriate training, the pitfalls of relying on EFM and FBS increase drastically. Nevertheless, the insight provided by fetal heart rate and fetal blood sampling into fetal state and condition cannot be matched by auscultation no matter how assiduously it is practiced.

Periodic fetal heart rate decelerations include early, variable, and late decelerations. Early decelerations begin simultaneously with the contraction, reach a nadir near the peak of the contraction, and return to the baseline at the end of the contraction. The amplitude and duration of the deceleration are proportional to the amplitude and duration of the uterine contraction. Early decelerations usually drop 10 to 15 beats per minute (bpm) below baseline at nadir; they rarely exceed 30 bpm or fall to a level below 100 beats per minute. They are most frequently observed in advanced labor after the vertex begins to descend and are believed to be related to head compression.

Variable decelerations, the most common patterns observed, frequently develop without warning late in the first stage of labor and even more frequently during the second stage. During the first stage of labor, they are believed to be related to cord compression. During the second stage of labor, they are more likely due to head compression. Factors that increase the likelihood of variable decelerations include ruptured membranes, oligohydramnios, vasa previa, nuchal cord and short or prolapsed cord, and occiput posterior position. Brief accelerations (so-called "shoulders") may precede or follow the decelerations. The initial fall in rate may be very abrupt, producing a change of 30 bpm or greater over 1 to 2 seconds. Recovery is usually rapid. Variable decelerations may mimic early or late decelerations but can be generally recognized by the subsequent pattern of decelerations.

Deep or prolonged variable decelerations commonly contain a brief episode of bradycardia at about 60 bpm with absent variability, representing nodal rhythm. Uncommonly, such decelerations may contain a brief episode of cardiac asystole (heart block) lasting 2 to 3 seconds. These episodes seem to represent an exuberant vagal response in usually healthy fetuses. They are invariably associated with average or increased baseline variability after the deceleration, and the outcome has uniformly been good. Like the episode of nodal rhythm, they should be treated as any other severe variable deceleration. Variable decelerations that end with small, smooth accelerations ("overshoot") and are associated with persistently absent baseline variability may anticipate subsequent death, congenital anomaly, or neurologic disability. Variable decelerations with "slow return" to previous baseline rate and variability without reactive tachycardia do not represent fetal compromise.

Late decelerations are symmetric, develop after the onset of the contraction, reach a nadir after the peak of the contraction, and return to baseline beyond the end of the contraction. The amplitude may be as small as 5 to 10 bpm to as great as 60 bpm. As in early decelerations, amplitude and duration of late decelerations are proportional to the intensity and duration of the uterine contraction. Late decelerations are thought to represent fetal hypoxia due to impaired uterine blood flow and are frequently associated with excessive frequency of contractions, maternal hypotension, and fetal growth retardation. Although true late decelerations may be subtle, they are, nevertheless, repetitive and invariably but usually transiently raise the heart rate and diminish variability. Isolated late-appearing decelerations, no matter how typical, should not be considered a sign of hypoxia. Similarly, transient, late-appearing decelerations associated with normal variability and no rise in baseline may represent fetal breathing movements.

Prolonged decelerations last longer than 2 minutes and are caused by various maternal provocations during the second stage of labor, including cord compression, vaginal examination, uterine hypertonus, placental abruption, and sustained expulsive efforts.

We estimate the effect of prolonged or repeated variable or late decelerations on fetal condition by examining baseline heart rate and variability in response to the decelerations. If variability and baseline rate remain normal, babies are usually born in good condition irrespective of the frequency or character of the decelerations. No matter what their amplitude, continuing decelerations, associated with decreasing variability and rising baseline rate, indicate fetal deterioration.

THE DIAGNOSIS AND TREATMENT OF FETAL DISTRESS

Much of the benefit of EFM relates to the simultaneous recording of uterine contractions. Uterine contractions may cause pressure on the fetal presenting part or trap the umbilical cord between the fetal body and extremities or between the fetus and the uterine wall. Their most consistent effect, however, is the impairment of uterine blood flow in direct proportion to its duration and amplitude. This decrease in oxygen availability during uterine contractions is usually well tolerated, and there is little evidence that these effects of contractions are cumulative.

The fetal heart rate responses to hypoxia depend upon the rapidity and intensity of the hypoxic episode as well as the frequency and intensity of uterine contractions. In the absence of uterine contractions, the fetus responds to slowly developing hypoxia with rising heart rate and decreased variability. When compensation is no longer possible, the heart rate becomes unstable, slows, and death ensues. During labor, on the other hand, the earliest signs of distress are recurrent late or variable decelerations followed by the changes in baseline rate and variability. If the asphyxial insult is acute and/or profound, the fetus will respond with a prolonged deceleration (bradycardia) irrespective of contractions.

Thus, fetal distress is usually defined in relationship to uterine contractions. In the absence of uterine contractions, the patterns of distress (baseline tachycardia, decreased variability) are far more insidious and less amenable to early detection.

We have divided the clinical signs of fetal evaluation during labor into four categories consisting of reassuring, suspicious, threatening, and ominous. Each category consists of an evaluation of both baseline and periodic changes.

Each of the baseline changes in the suspicious category may reflect fetal hypoxia, but when such changes are unaccompanied by decelerations, the mechanism is usually other than hypoxia. Maternal fever, secondary to amnionitis, is the most common discoverable etiology of fetal tachycardia. Here the fetal and maternal rates rise in proportion to the fever. But tachycardia may represent fetal sepsis long before it has been manifested as maternal fever. Prompt treatment, including cooling when the fever is excessive, has a rapid effect. Fetal tachyarrhythmias may raise the fetal heart rate in excess of 160 bpm. In the absence of deceleration, we do not limit the duration of tachycardia.

The vast majority of babies with persistent heart rates between 90 and 120 bpm average baseline variability, do not demonstrate objective compromise. Baseline bradycardia in the range of 50 to 80 bpm may signal the presence of complete heart block. Severely asphyxiated babies with bradycardia usually have sinus rhythm. Rarely, an apparent fetal bradycardia may represent the maternal heart rate transmitted through the dead fetus. In external mode, the ultrasound transducer may inadvertently detect pulsation in maternal vessels, irrespective of the viability of the fetus. This problem is readily solved by simultaneous monitoring of the maternal and presumed fetal pulse or by noting the absence of the fetal heart motion with Doppler or real-time B-scan ultrasound.

Reassuring Patterns

Baseline features of reassuring patterns include average variability and stable fetal heart rate. Periodic features include absent decelerations, early decelerations, mild variable decelerations, and uniform accelerations.

Early decelerations not caused by hypoxia require no therapy. Mild variable decelerations (often indistinguishable from early decelerations) appear totally innocuous, especially if associated with mild variable accelerations ("shoulders") before and after the deceleration. Uniform accelerations invariably signify a healthy reactive fetus. Most important, normal variability strongly suggests that there is no fetal indication for intervention.

Suspicious Patterns

Suspicious patterns show abnormal baseline features but absent decelerations. These baseline features include tachycardia (>150 bpm), bradycardia (<110 bpm) and decreased variability. Periodic decelerations are absent.

Severely compromised infants invariably show decreased to absent variability along with decelerations. But decreased variability without decelerations is generally a reflection of drugs administered during labor. Narcotics, tranquilizers, and local and general anesthetic agents all diminish both long- and short-term variability. Decreased variability may also reflect fetal sleep or inactivity. These alternating epochs are easily seen during antepartum fetal heart rate testing and may also be seen during labor. Persistently absent variability without decelerations may occasionally reflect a congenital anomaly or pre-existing neurologic deficit.

We recommend that monitoring begin prior to the administration to the mother of any medication that has the potential for altering fetal heart rate patterns. If an asphyxial insult is superimposed on an infant whose heart rate variability is diminished by medications, decelerations will appear.

Suspicious patterns usually require no therapy. A search for the underlying cause should be made and the baby stimulated by means of abdominal palpation or pelvic examination. When there is a suspicious pattern, potentially compromising drugs or anesthetic techniques should be avoided until hypoxia is excluded by fetal blood sampling if necessary.

Threatening Patterns

Baseline features of threatening patterns include stable rate and average variability. Periodic features of threatening patterns include periodic late decelerations or variable decelerations. We include increased baseline variability in this category.

The clinical significance of increased variability (<15 bpm) is not completely understood. In most instances, increased variability is associated with fetal maturity, the administration of ephedrine, variable decelerations, and a short umbilical cord or mild (compensated) fetal hypoxia. Almost invariably, however, it is associated with a normal outcome and requires no therapy.

Threatening patterns represent unequivocal fetal insult

related to impaired uterine blood flow (late decelerations) or impaired umbilical blood flow (variable decelerations). Late decelerations associated with good variability (so-called "reflex late decelerations") are usually found in previously normal patterns during episodes of maternal supine hypotension or excessive uterine activity. More importantly, these episodes are usually correctable with conservative measures.

The management of late decelerations includes (1) turning the patient on her side to eliminate supine hypotension and improve uterine blood flow, (2) administering oxygen by mask (5 L per minute), (3) correction of hypotension if present, and (4) stopping oxytocin infusion. The patient should be examined.

The response of variable decelerations to corrective measures is less predictable than the response of late decelerations. Often these patterns can be corrected or their severity reduced by altering the mother's position between lateral, supine, and Trendelenburg positions. Failing this, we place the patient in the knee-chest position, which occasionally corrects the pattern. If such maneuvers fail and a rising heart rate and loss of variability become superimposed, intervention is considered. Gentle elevation of the vertex may ameliorate the pattern, but this maneuver should be undertaken only in the delivery room. Blood sampling plays little role here.

We emphasize that the interpretation and therapy of variable decelerations are the same in both first and second stages. Except when delivery is imminent, therapy should be governed by the conservative principles elaborated above.

Prevention is more important than therapy. Avoidance of the supine position and judicious use of oxytocin infusion and heightened surveillance during the second stage are appropriate safeguards in all patients. During the expulsive efforts of the second stage, variable and prolonged decelerations are common. With the end of the contraction and cessation of pushing, the deceleration commonly returns promptly to the previous baseline rate and variability. Failure of the fetal heart rate pattern to recover promptly requires refraining from pushing with subsequent contractions until the pattern has resolved.

Ominous Patterns

Baseline features of ominous patterns include absent baseline variability, unstable rate, and bradycardia or tachycardia. Periodic features of ominous patterns include late decelerations and variable decelerations with rebound accelerations (overshoot).

Ominous patterns combine periodic features of the threatening category with the baseline patterns of the suspicious category. These patterns strongly suggest severe fetal compromise and require immediate attention and delivery. (Rebound accelerations (overshoot) are uniform accelerations following variable decelerations of any amplitude and are accompanied by absent baseline variability.) Baseline tachycardia is common but preceding accelerations are rare. More than any other pattern, the combination of decreased variability and variable decelerations with overshoot strongly suggests autonomic imbalance. It may be seen following administration of atropine or in premature fetuses as well as in those who are severely asphyxiated or neurologically compromised.

An unstable rate with absent short-term variability that is occasionally sinusoidal is an added clue that fetal compensatory mechanisms are exhausted. This heart rate pattern consists of regular oscillations with absent short-term variability. This pattern carries a grave prognosis in the untreated anemic fetus, irrespective of etiology. The pattern may be found, however, in fetuses with central nervous system or cardiac anomalies or in otherwise normal fetuses following administration of narcotics to the mother during labor. When a persistent sinusoidal pattern is encountered during labor, scalp blood sampling and ultrasound examination are indicated.

Before fetal death only the ominous baseline changes may be present, and late or variable decelerations may be absent. Bradycardia is common, but the rate may occasionally lie in the normal range. Heart rate changes in the terminally ill fetus are rarely dramatic. Cardiac arrest may occur, but unlike those seen with variable decelerations, these are predictable, associated with sinus rhythm, and invariably fatal.

Although the same conservative measures advocated for threatening patterns should be applied to the patient with ominous patterns, preparations should be made for expeditious delivery, as recovery is unlikely. Beta-sympathomimetics continue to gain popularity as a temporizing measure in the treatment of fetal distress. Bicarbonate and glucose infusions have no value. During the second stage, refraining from pushing may have a salutary effect on the deceleration pattern.

Ultrasonic transducers tend to exaggerate short-term variability but have little effect on long-term variability. But it is unreasonable to believe that variability cannot be estimated from a satisfactory external tracing. In the analysis of variability with external devices, we consider the area of least variability as the most representative. If oscillations in the rate are seen, variability is probably present. We stress that if decelerations are present or accelerations are absent, direct monitoring should be undertaken. In addition, under certain circumstances the maternal rate may be counted or the true rate (maternal or fetal) may be doubled or halved. In this instance auscultation of the fetal heart rate will reveal the error.

Acid-Base Sampling

We recommend fetal blood sampling under only a few circumstances. We consider normal patterns and ominous patterns relative contraindications to fetal blood sampling.

With reassuring patterns we rarely find low pH values. With ominous patterns, and the failure to improve them with conservative measures, we prefer immediate delivery. Threatening patterns warrant conservative measures that are usually corrective. We see no indication for fetal blood sampling if the baseline rate is stable and adequate variability is confirmed by a direct electrode. With suspicious patterns we reserve fetal blood sampling for decreased variability in the presence of meconium or when there is a suspicion of post-term pregnancy or intrauterine growth retardation.

Prerequisites for fetal blood sampling are ruptured membranes, minimal cervical dilatation of about 2 to 3 cm, and an accessible fetal pole. Fetal blood should not be obtained from the face, genitals, brow, or over a fontanelle. In about 10 to 15 percent of cases, a sample cannot be obtained either because of peripheral vasoconstriction or because of other technical difficulties. A single value is rarely conclusive.

The ideal time to sample is before the contraction, but blood flows better and is easier to obtain during a contraction. If sampling is done during a variable deceleration, the absolute pH can be in the acidotic range. Frequently, however, this represents only a respiratory acidemia from which the fetus will quickly recover.

Although we use scalp sampling infrequently, we often perform acid-base analysis on umbilical artery and vein blood immediately after delivery. We restrict such testing to (1) the depressed newborn, and (2) those infants in whom depression is expected (irrespective of outcome). This strategy provides insight into the cause of neonatal depression and should eliminate the inappropriate designation of perinatal asphyxia as a cause of neonatal depression.

Most records demonstrating fetal distress are self-limited or respond promptly to conservative measures, and intervention is rarely necessary. The indication for intervention on behalf of the fetus is nonremediable fetal distress. This philosophy represents an attempt to use the monitoring pattern to determine whether or not the maternal placental unit is capable of sustaining the fetus. If patterns of distress are not remediable, then intervention should be undertaken as quickly as is consistent with maternal and fetal safety. This way of thinking holds that it is not possible to define a single, critical interval of time between onset of distress and optimal delivery. Nor can we safely state how much hypoxia is tolerable without compromise. Rather, it seems appropriate to minimize such exposure.

FETAL SURVEILLANCE IN HIGH-RISK PREGNANCY

PER OLOFSSON, M.D., Ph.D.

The ultimate aim of all obstetric care in high-risk pregnancy is to decide the optimal time for delivery, or when extrauterine life is safe for a baby at risk. Is it justifiable to allow a pregnancy to continue in the hope of reducing the risks associated with prematurity, even when the first signs of fetal jeopardy appear? This is the challenge facing the obstetrician.

A more liberal attitude toward intervention at a very early gestational age has posed the question of limits. What is the earliest limit for extrauterine life? The survival rates of infants at the University of Lund in the period 1981 to 1984 were 55 percent in the weight range of 500 to 700 g, 52 percent for 701 to 800 g, 66 percent for 801 to 900 g, 75 percent for 901 to 1,000 g, and 90 percent in the 1,001 to 1,500 g range.

Fetal weight estimation is difficult, however, even with ultrasonic fetometry. It is more accurate and relevant to calculate in terms of gestational age. Since fetal maturation is a more important measure than weight, exact dating is important.

Until 24 weeks of gestation, the prospect of extrauterine survival is virtually nonexistent. In the 25th week, the outlook begins to improve. This is the best time for transfer to a hospital with facilities for neonatal intensive care. It allows a few days for re-evaluation of diagnosis and full obstetrical intervention to be considered by a gestational age of 25 completed weeks. Before 32 weeks, it is best to transport the parturient in the undelivered state, since the transportation itself may be fatal for an infant of very low birth weight (<1,500 g).

METHODS OF FETAL SURVEILLANCE

Ultrasonography

Obstetric ultrasonography has simplified many problems. First, the problem of fetal dating, since postmenstrual gestational age is a vague concept when dealing either with extreme prematurity or with prolonged pregnancy. Gestational age is better ascertained by ultrasonic fetometry. Biparietal measurement in the 17th week gives a precise result plus or minus 6.4 days (± 2 standard deviations). All obstetric departments in Sweden now use ultrasonic fetometry for fetal dating.

Gestational age is best described in completed weeks and days. For example, the first day of prolonged pregnancy is given as 42+0 (42 completed weeks but 0 completed days in week 43; equal to the 295th day of pregnancy, or the 15th day after the expected day of birth).

Second, ultrasonography provides an improved possibility of detecting intrauterine growth retardation (IUGR). Longitudinal measurements are then a prerequisite, making a second routine examination necessary. Fewer than 20 percent of all obstetric departments in Sweden carry out a second examination, however. At most clinics, a second sonogram is indicated by a clinical suspicion of growth retardation. It is a mistaken belief that one routine examination instead of two also means one examination less per woman. Screening with one examination leads to 1.9 examinations (mean) per woman, but two examinations lead to only 2.3 (mean).

A second examination in the 32nd to 33rd week would seem optimal. Since both growth acceleration and retardation often occur late in pregnancy, the cutoff levels for further evaluation have to be liberal (see section on IUGR). A disadvantage is then that a third examination will be necessary, in a considerable number of cases, for selection of fetuses with true abnormal growth.

Ultrasonography also makes it possible to detect fetal malformations, placenta previa, and hydramnios. Fetal morphology and placental localization should have already been evaluated at the first routine examination, in the 17th week.

An early diagnosis of low placental localization is important for prevention of fatal bleeding from a placenta previa. A low placenta should be checked on in the 28th to 30th week. By then an anterior uterine wall placenta has often retracted due to elongation of the lower uterine segment, whereas a posterior wall placenta usually remains low.

Estriol Assays

Among the estrogen assays used to assess fetal condition, the estriol fraction is considered to be the most reliable. It is disputed whether it should be done in conjugated or unconjugated form, in urine or in plasma. Short-term and daily fluctuations in estriol excretion and errors in urine sampling make the interpretation even more difficult.

Estriol assays were introduced in Lund in 1964. In a series of 183 diabetic pregnancies monitored with urinary estriol assays, normal values predicted a normal Apgar score in 89 percent and, if lethal malformations were excluded, a survival rate of 99 percent. Among 17 cases (9 percent) with subnormal or decreasing values, three intrauterine deaths occurred.

How could three intrauterine deaths have been allowed to occur when the estriol curves clearly indicated fetal jeopardy? The explanations are, first, that the determinations were performed only once or twice a week and then only on inpatients, and, second, that the results were not available the same day. In high-risk pregnancy, and in diabetic pregnancy in particular, such a delay in obtaining actual information on fetal status may prove fatal, since fetal compromise can occur rapidly. These three intrauterine deaths might have been prevented by making more frequent determinations, with immediate reporting of the results. Owing to such a lack of immediate information, confusing reports in the literature, and, particularly, introduction of routine antenatal electronic fetal heart rate

(FHR) monitoring, estriol determinations were abandoned in Lund in 1981.

Fetal Movement Counting

Maternal recognition of fetal activity is suggested as a simple test of fetal well-being. A decrease in fetal movements can precede intrauterine death by several days. The methodologic problems are considerable, however. The inter-and intraindividual variations are wide, which makes it difficult to agree on an alarm signal. Strong and rapid day-to-day fluctuations in fetal activity should indicate fetal jeopardy. When fetal movement counting is used in low-risk pregnancies, the false-positive test rate is high. Fetal movement counting might be more useful in high-risk pregnancies, but then rather as a trigger for further evaluation of fetal status together with other methods. The alarm signal is neither a sensitive nor a very specific diagnostic test of fetal jeopardy. The value of such counting in inpatients is doubtful, since these cases are carefully monitored with other methods, and there is often not much more to be gained from counting. Fetal activity monitoring may be valuable as a part of a biophysical profile score, however.

Electronic Fetal Heart Rate Monitoring

Electronic fetal heart rate monitoring has required the development of a new attitude toward a more active obstetric management and intervention for the good of the fetus. Antenatal electronic fetal heart rate monitoring, performed as a nonstress test or as an oxytocin challenge test, is a well-documented method for safe fetal surveillance.

The nonstress test is simple, inexpensive, and provides an immediate test result. This makes it superior to other tests for fetal surveillance. A *normal* nonstress test has a high predictive value for various parameters of fetal outcome, and its specificity is good as well. On the other hand, the predictive value and sensitivity of an *abnormal* nonstress test are poor. The test is therefore best used when deciding not to intervene.

The oxytocin challenge test is thought to give a better estimation of the uteroplacental reserve capacity. Generally speaking, the oxytocin challenge test is no better than the nonstress test for routine fetal surveillance, however. In one series of diabetic pregnancies, no significant advantages were found by performing the oxytocin challenge test when both tests were done within 1 week ante partum. The oxytocin challenge test has a lower false-positive rate and might thus be worth performing in some uncertain cases. Precautions should be taken in cases of IUGR, since the stress of undergoing an oxytocin challenge test may further jeopardize the fetus.

Various scoring systems have been applied to evaluate the nonstress test. In the American literature, it is most often classified as either reactive or nonreactive. In the classification used in Lund, baseline fetal heart rate, long-term variability, accelerations, and decelerations are all evaluated in relation to fetal and uterine activity (Table 1). This four-scale classification system is well suited to the

TABLE 1 Classification of the Nonstress Test

Class 1 Normal

At least two accelerations with fetal movements or uterine contractions
Baseline heart rate 120–160 beats per minute
Baseline variability 10–25 beats per minute
No decelerations

Class 2 Suspect pathology

No accelerations
Baseline heart rate 100–120 or 160–180 beats per minute
Baseline variability 5–10 or > 25 beats per minute for > 20 minutes

Class 3 Slight pathology

Baseline heart rate < 100 or > 180 beats per minute
Occasional moderate variable decelerations

Class 4 Severe pathology

Silent pattern/sinusoidal
Late decelerations
Severe variable decelerations

clinical situation. A severely pathologic nonstress test calls for immediate termination of the pregnancy. One must make certain that such a pathologic pattern is not temporary, however. For example, decreased variability is common during fetal inactivity and the registration time must then be extended over 1 to 2 hours. Otherwise, a 20 to 30 minute registration is long enough for routine use.

A scheme for nonstress testing is shown in Figure 1. It is not possible to state how often a test should be repeated to ensure reliable surveillance. A decade ago, it was the general opinion that a normal nonstress test was safe for a week. Today, we know that intrauterine death can occur within a few hours after a normal test. The recommendation for practical use is that a nonstress test should be repeated one to three times a week on outpatients and one to two times per day on inpatients, depending on the com-

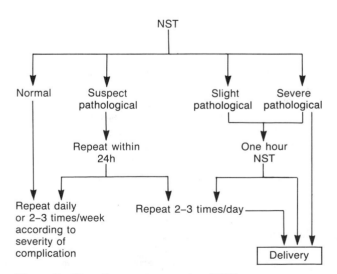

Figure 1 Chart for nonstress testing (NST).

plication. A normal nonstress test might sometimes be misinterpreted as abnormal and lead to intervention. In dubious cases, the nonstress test should therefore be supplemented by other tests, such as the oxytocin challenge test, combined real-time/Doppler ultrasound fetal blood flow measurement, and biophysical profile.

Ultrasonic Fetal Blood Flow Measurements

By using a recently developed technique that combines pulsed Doppler ultrasound and real-time linear array ultrasound, simultaneous measurement of fetal blood flow velocity and vessel imaging is possible. This makes measurement possible not only of flow velocity but also of flow volume in the fetal aorta, carotids, and umbilical vessels. The method has been applied in high-risk pregnancies, for example in pre-eclampsia, IUGR, Rh isoimmunization, diabetes, and fetal cardiac arrhythmia.

The shape of the flow velocity waveform is evaluated and classified. In the umbilical artery, certain waveform characteristics may predict the development of fetal distress. The systolic-diastolic flow ratio is an indicator of the vascular resistance distal to the point of measurement. A high ratio in the umbilical artery—and thus a high placental bed vascular resistance—is correlated to an increased risk of fetal distress.

A very low (or even negative) diastolic blood flow is an ominous sign. According to the diastolic flow, the velocity waveforms have been classified into different blood flow groups. Abnormal blood flow groups often precede the occurrence of pathologic electronic fetal heart rate patterns. The measuring of fetal blood flow might thus be a method for the early detection of fetal jeopardy. Further studies may establish whether the method is better able to predict fetal distress than is electronic fetal heart rate monitoring.

By calculating the volume blood flow (which is possible when both flow velocity and vessel diameter can be measured) in different fetal vessels, the redistribution of blood flow within the fetus can be determined under different conditions. The effects of, for example, fetal hypoxia, medication, and analgesia can then be evaluated. It is hoped that this will improve the safety of some medical or obstetric interventions under consideration. Further studies are needed before the method can be considered suitable for clinical use, however. It will then be imperative to prevent such misinterpretations and needless interventions as occurred with the introduction of electronic fetal heart rate monitoring in the 1970s.

Biophysical Profile

The biophysical profile score can be described as an "intrauterine Apgar score." Its original components include scoring of the nonstress test, amount of amniotic fluid, fetal breathing movements, fetal tone, and fetal movements. In Lund, the test has been modified by replacing the nonstress test with fetal reactivity.

The biophysical profile has the same disadvantages as the Apgar score—it is difficult to standardize and is a subjective estimation of signs and symptoms, each of which is accorded equal importance in the final score sum. Amniotic fluid volume and fetal reactivity are better correlated with fetal outcome than are other parameters. When evaluating the biophysical profile score, oligohydramnios and hypoactivity in particular should be observed. The biophysical profile should seldom be the sole determinant of when to interrupt a pregnancy, although it is most valuable when making a decision in doubtful cases when other tests are not decisive.

SPECIAL CONSIDERATIONS

Pre-eclampsia

The frequency of hypertension during pregnancy (blood pressure $\geq$ 140/90 mm Hg) is 8.8 percent in Lund. Albuminuria in addition (i.e., pre-eclampsia) is a prognostically ominous sign. Edema is a normal condition during pregnancy, but since an excessive or rapid weight gain often precedes the development of hypertension, one should be particularly watchful for such a development.

A diastolic blood pressure of 95 mm Hg or higher often requires antihypertensive therapy. A diastolic blood pressure of 100 mm Hg or higher, or symptoms such as headache, epigastralgia, and blurred vision, warrant immediate referral to a specialist.

Before medication is started, the patient should rest in bed for 2 to 3 days in the hospital in order to stabilize her blood pressure. At term, and in cases of epigastralgia and deep tendon reflex hyperactivity, termination of the pregnancy should be considered. If the cervical status is unfavorable, intracervical application of 0.5 mg of prostaglandin E_2 jelly can be used to accelerate cervical ripening.

Attention to fetal distress and fetal growth retardation is mandatory. If an ominous electronic fetal heart rate pattern appears, or if fetal growth ceases, the best advice is to interrupt pregnancy. But if the decision is to continue pregnancy, cautious maternal and fetal surveillance is imperative. As mentioned earlier, maternal symptoms and complaints are of great significance. A high hematocrit level and absence of edema may be ominous signs of hemoconcentration and impaired peripheral circulation. In such cases, continued diuresis (minimum 50 ml per hour) is important. A low urine output is a bad sign.

A low or decreasing platelet count can be a symptom of microthrombosis and platelet consumption and risk of disseminated intravascular coagulation. It often parallels increasing subjective maternal symptoms. This is a dangerous condition that requires immediate treatment and prompt delivery to eliminate the trigger factor. Prednisolone (10 to 30 mg daily) is often effective for prevention of further platelet consumption and should be considered when the count falls below 100,000 per cubic millimeter. Cortisone therapy is not contraindicated, even in cases of severe pre-eclampsia. Maternal recovery and stabilization of the condition are often seen when prednisolone therapy is initiated.

If the platelet count falls below 50,000 to 60,000 per cubic millimeter, operative delivery is dangerous because of the risk of profuse bleeding. It is not only the quantity but also the quality of platelets that is defective. A platelet transfusion might then be indicated. The risk of a low fetal platelet count should also be considered, since in the case of a traumatic delivery it may result in intracerebral hemorrhage. Determination of the fetal platelet count is possible by sampling fetal scalp blood during labor.

Medication is controversial. Cardioselective beta$_1$-adrenoceptor blockade (atenolol) has been used in Lund for more than a decade. Nonselective beta-blockade should be avoided during pregnancy. Caution in using beta$_1$-blockade is also recommended in certain cases, since it can have a depressive effect on the fetal heart (decreased baseline fetal heart rate, decreased long-term variability, reduced acceleration amplitude) and thus obscure signs of fetal distress. Recent unpublished data suggest that beta$_1$-blockade sometimes increases vascular resistance in the placental circulation. More investigations are therefore needed to determine in which cases this occurs. Until more knowledge has been accumulated, beta$_1$-blockers should be used with caution in cases of placental insufficiency and discontinued if ominous fetal heart rate patterns appear.

When the effect of beta$_1$-blockade is poor, hydralazine and chlorpromazine can be given in addition. In the case of a diastolic blood pressure greater than 110 mm Hg, 2.5 mg dihydralazine is given repeatedly intravenously. Higher doses might cause too rapid a fall in blood pressure, which can be injurious to the fetus.

Preterm Premature Rupture of the Membranes

When preterm (36 completed weeks or less) premature rupture of the membranes occurs before 25 weeks, the prognosis is poor, even in cases in which the pregnancy continues for several weeks. In one series from Lund, the survival rate was only 7 of 31 when the membranes ruptured in weeks 19 through 24 compared with 54 of 56 when rupture occurred in weeks 25 through 33. Interruption of pregnancy is therefore recommended when premature rupture of the membranes occurs before the 20th week.

In weeks 20 through 25, management is individualized, sometimes on an outpatient basis. The patient measures her body temperature twice a day and visits the outpatient clinic once a week.

Hospitalization with bed rest is recommended after 25 weeks. The patient is allowed to leave the bed only for reasons of personal hygiene. Fetal surveillance is initiated, with electronic fetal heart rate monitoring daily and ultrasonic fetometry every second week. It should be observed that a manifest intrauterine infection with maternal fever is often preceded by a few hours of fetal tachycardia. Cervical and urethral cultures are performed weekly (nonspecific aerobes and group B streptococci). Antibiotics are not given for prophylaxis, not even in cases of positive culture without clinical infection. The cultures are used as a guide for therapy in cases of clinical infection, when more extensive culturing is performed.

A clinically manifest intrauterine infection is an absolute indication for prompt delivery, irrespective of gestational age, as otherwise severe infection with septicemia may develop within a few hours. When delivery is decided, antibiotics should be given intravenously (e.g., a combination of cefuroxime and clindamycin).

Tocolytic therapy can be considered in the case of uterine contractions, but only in the absence of ablatio placentae and intrauterine infection. If pregnancy continues without complications and without any spontaneous labor, labor is induced in gestational weeks 32 to 34.

Prolonged Pregnancy

Prolonged pregnancy is defined as a gestational age of more than 14 days after the estimated date of birth (295 days or longer). This is an arbitrary limit, established to suit the weekly cycle. The scientific basis for a 2-week limit is weak. The introduction of ultrasound screening has reduced the rate of prolonged pregnancy from 9 to 3 percent.

The management of prolonged pregnancy can vary. It has been quite common to induce labor at 2 weeks after estimated date of birth in primiparas and at 3 weeks in multiparas. Some have been induced only if there is a favorable cervical status. This of course is illogical, since the possible fetal risks of prolonged pregnancy are in no way connected with the cervical score. If labor is not induced and pregnancy is allowed to continue, spontaneous labor will occur within 3 days in 50 percent of cases and within a week in 90 percent.

How dangerous then is prolonged pregnancy? Statistics from Lund can illustrate the problem. During the period from 1970 to 1986, altogether 53,906 infants were delivered. Only five intrauterine deaths occurred in prolonged pregnancies. The frequency of prolonged pregnancy was approximately 9 percent in the period from 1970 to 1980 and 3 percent in 1981 to 1986 (ultrasonic fetometry for dating was introduced in 1980). The stillbirth rate in prolonged pregnancy was then 0.13 percent. When corrected for fetal malformations, the figure was 0.078 percent. It can thus be debated whether the stillbirth rate in prolonged pregnancy may be even lower than in term pregnancy, provided that complicated pregnancies have received adequate attention.

Uncertainty about the risks of prolonged pregnancy is still considerable, but a reliable policy for management can nevertheless be decided on. Pregnancy should be evaluated 2 weeks after the estimated date of birth. Primiparas and multiparas are managed in the same way. Particular attention should be paid to signs of placental insufficiency, e.g., impaired fetal growth and oligohydramnios. Pregnancy can continue in uncomplicated cases, with outpatient clinic visits and nonstress tests performed every second day. When the pregnancy reaches the 44th week, induction of labor is recommended.

Diabetes

Diabetic pregnancy is charged with several complications. Congenital malformation, pre-eclampsia, preterm delivery, respiratory distress syndrome, macrosomia, and neonatal hypoglycemia are among the most serious. The panorama of perinatal and infant mortality in diabetic pregnancy has changed dramatically over the last two decades. In Lund, the perinatal mortality rate declined from 24.3 percent to 1.1 percent over the period from 1960 to 1980, since which time it has approached the figure for the general obstetric population (0.9 percent). The figure is now so low that other standards would be better measures of fetal outcome. During the same period, the cumulative infant (1 year) mortality declined from 31.3 to 4.6 percent. Even so, it is still two to three times as high as in the general population.

Congenital malformations are responsible for about one-half of the perinatal mortality and are currently recognized as the main problem in diabetic pregnancy. Preventive measures, with meticulous metabolic control at the time of conception and embryogenesis, are mandatory to prevent development of malformations. Young diabetic women should be repeatedly informed about the preventive measures and offered a reflectance meter for home blood glucose level monitoring when planning a pregnancy.

Strict metabolic control also is important for normal fetal growth and neonatal glucose homeostasis. Maternal hyperglycemia causes fetal hyperglycemia, fetal hyperinsulinemia, and possibly macrosomia. Ultrasonic fetometry is therefore repeated monthly during the first two trimesters and every 2 to 3 weeks thereafter. Fetal growth acceleration occurs during the last trimester, and it is therefore worthwhile to institute strict control, even when a diagnosis of gestational diabetes is determined late in pregnancy. In the case of macrosomia, a more strict regulation of glucose level, early induction of labor, or cesarean section may be considered. Serial ultrasonography is also necessary to detect IUGR, which frequently occurs in cases of severe diabetes or in connection with preeclampsia.

Hypertension complicates 10 to 25 percent of diabetic pregnancies. The figure in Lund is 22 percent. These women are among the most seriously ill of all high-risk patients.

Since 1976, cardioselective beta$_1$-adrenoceptor blockade has been the preferred medication for hypertension in Lund and in diabetic pregnant women. In a series of 18 women, no serious adverse effects on the blood glucose homeostasis were found. The effects on the fetal heart, as detected by electronic fetal heart rate monitoring, were similar to those found in other pregnancies. There was no proof that this depressive effect was in any case deleterious, although the frequency of pathologic nonstress tests was high. Even though most fetuses were in some jeopardy as a result of their mothers' condition, fetal outcome was successful in 17 of 18 cases. Beta$_1$-blockade is suggested as a safe alternative for antihypertensive therapy in diabetic pregnant women, with caution for those warnings already discussed (see section on pre-eclampsia).

Management can be on an outpatient basis when pregnancy progresses without complications. Spontaneous labor can be awaited, and induction is not performed until weeks 40 to 41. The risk of unexpected intrauterine death should be considered, however, and very careful surveillance is mandatory. Nonstress tests should be performed twice a week from 34 weeks in outpatients and daily in inpatients. The patient is finally hospitalized in the 38th week. It is still not clear whether prolonged pregnancy is safe in a diabetic woman under rigorous control. Until we know more, it is wise to terminate pregnancy at term.

Should complications arise, hospitalization should be liberally recommended and if ominous signs occur, termination of pregnancy should be considered. Amniocentesis and determination of the lecithin/sphingomyelin ratio for estimation of fetal lung maturity no longer have a place in diabetic pregnancy management. A fetus in jeopardy should be delivered if indicated, irrespective of gestational age. Since 1966, no infant of a diabetic mother has died at Lund hospital as a result of respiratory distress syndrome.

Twin Pregnancy

Twin pregnancy is accompanied by an increased risk of preterm labor, hydramnios, pre-eclampsia, placenta previa, ablatio placentae, cord prolapse, transverse lie, and fetal distress. For a successful outcome, it is paramount to identify and treat these complications early.

During the first two trimesters, ultrasonography should be performed in order to identify abnormal fetal growth and hydramnios. When there is a chance of extrauterine life, i.e., between 25 and 26 weeks of gestation, the examinations should be accelerated to every second or third week. A liberal attitude toward sick leave from work during the last trimester is recommended in order to prevent preterm birth. The cervical status should then be examined during frequent checkups. In cases of uterine contractions and cervical dilatations, hospitalization with bed rest and tocolytic therapy is indicated until 36 completed weeks.

Spontaneous labor is awaited and labor is not induced in cases of uncomplicated pregnancy. Twin pregnancies seldom continue beyond full term, but when this happens, labor induction should be considered. In cases of preterm delivery, cesarean section is generally performed before 33 completed weeks. In weeks 32 to 33, however, vaginal delivery might be considered in a multipara with uncomplicated pregnancy and with the first twin in vertex presentation.

From 34 weeks (fetal weight 1,800 to 2,000 g), vaginal delivery is scheduled. The presentation of the second twin is then not considered, since its position can change during labor. In a case of breech presentation of the first twin, management is similar to that for singleton breech presentation.

In cases of IUGR, the circumstances may become troublesome. IUGR often occurs early in twins and sometimes as a discordant growth. This means that only one twin is growth-retarded, whereas the other has normal or even accelerated growth. Oligohydramnios frequently occurs in the amniotic sac of the smaller fetus and hydramnios in the sac of the larger fetus. Discordant growth can occur in monozygotic twins as a transfusion syndrome but also is found in heterozygotic twins. As pregnancy progresses, the divergence becomes more pronounced. In cases of IUGR of both twins, the pregnancy can be terminated on behalf of both twins, but in a case of discordant growth, the situation is quite different. Is it justified to terminate a pregnancy before term on behalf of the smaller fetus and risk the health of the larger fetus? There is no absolute answer to this. The decision must be made in agreement with the parents. Before 32 weeks, termination should be performed only in highly selected cases because of the risk of complications, even in normal-sized infants.

Intrauterine Growth Retardation

Fetal growth is best assessed by ultrasonic fetometry carried out in serial measurements over time. The relationship between gestational age and fetal weight is roughly linear. In Lund, a second ultrasound examination in the 32nd week is included in the screening program. By using this program, the antenatal detection of IUGR has increased from 55 to 75 percent.

Small-for-gestational age is defined as a birth weight of mean weight of −2 standard deviations, but this is too low a cutoff point when ultrasonography is performed in the 32nd week. Only 50 percent of small-for-gestational-age infants will then be identified as having IUGR. The most effective cutoff level for suspicion of IUGR in the 32nd week is mean weight of −1 standard deviation (corresponding to a weight deviation of −12 percent from the mean), although the false-positive rate then becomes high. It is then necessary to make serial measurements to exclude false-positive cases.

It is important to determine whether the IUGR is proportional or disproportional. The proportionately growth-retarded fetus has a subnormal number of cells and a normal head-to-abdomen ratio. This might be due to genetic factors and not necessarily a result of intrauterine malnutrition.

The disproportionately growth-retarded fetus has an increased head-to-abdomen ratio, i.e., a small abdominal diameter is an early sign of IUGR. This condition is merely a result of lack of fetal nutrients and can be compensated for when a normal nutritional status is restored. Disproportional growth is often coincident with oligohydramnios, which should thus be regarded as an ominous sign.

When disproportional IUGR occurs in a fetus genetically predisposed to grow large, ultrasonic screening in the 32nd week may fail. The symphysis-fundal height growth curve and attention to oligohydramnios are then important signals of impaired growth.

The two main types of growth retardation can be distinguished by ultrasonic fetometry. It is then important to evaluate the individual growth curves of the head, abdomen, and femur. In proportional IUGR, in most cases it is probably not necessary to perform any extraordinary fetal surveillance. In disproportional IUGR, close surveillance is mandatory. In severe cases (weight deviation greater than −28 percent, or when growth ceases), hospitalization is recommended. Daily nonstress tests, a weekly biophysical profile, and ultrasonic fetometry every second week are then performed.

A difficult decision is when to interrupt a pregnancy complicated by IUGR. One reason for prolonging pregnancy might be to observe the effect of therapy , such as cortisone administration for acceleration of fetal lung maturation. This might justify prolongation of the pregnancy for a few days. The use of cortisone therapy is doubtful in such cases, however. Cortisone administration might depress the fetal adrenal function, which is probably elevated in many cases of IUGR, and cause hypoadrenocorticism after withdrawal.

PREMATURE LABOR

ROBERT C. GOODLIN, M.D.

The successful management of women in premature labor demands as much skill as any problem in obstetrics. It is often difficult to diagnose the presence of premature labor and/or chorioamnionitis, abruptio placentae, fetal anomalies, uterine contraction rings, and Munchausen's labor syndrome.

MUNCHAUSEN'S SYNDROME OF PREMATURE LABOR

Women who fake premature labor, returning again and again to the labor suite claiming to have painful uterine contractions, are said to have Munchausen's syndrome. These pregnant women learn to mimic uterine contractions with the external uterine activity monitor, to moan appropriately, and, in some cases when the electronic monitor is removed, to reattach the apparatus themselves. This is not an insignificant problem, occurring in an estimated 5 percent of patients claiming to be in premature labor. There is a tremendous loss of hospital time and expense in an effort to stop this premature labor, and in two of my patients, pulmonary edema was caused by this effort. Although some fake only uterine contractions, others put instruments such as darning needles into their vaginas in order to have a "bloody vaginal show," or they bring in undergarments saturated with blood (with a dry vagina). On discharge from the labor suite, they invariably return within 2 or 3 days with the same complaints of premature labor and bloody show. One of our patients has faked uterine contractions and self-inflicted bloody show during three different pregnancies. She has declined postpartum tubal ligation. We have received little if any help from our psychiatric colleagues in these cases, having referred nine such women. They diagnosed all as hysterical and advised us to refuse to admit them or to allow them to achieve any "gain" from their manipulations. In my experience, this is much easier said than done, since it has been unclear what their gain is.

PREMATURE LABOR

The diagnosis of premature labor is difficult. Our criteria consist of contractions and/or significant changes in the cervix, especially effacement. Since frequent vaginal examinations in some pregnant women initiate uterine contractions, there obviously should be a limit on the frequency of pelvic examinations to ascertain whether changes have occurred in the cervix. Our success rate for stopping premature labor for longer than a week is 40 to 50 percent. Those clinics claiming 90 to 100 percent success must be using less stringent criteria for the diagnosis of premature labor. In our experience, the presence of amniotic fluid in the vagina does not necessarily signify premature rupture of hind membranes. A high leak (rupture of hind waters), as after an abdominal amniocentesis, is not labor. Some women can hold urine in their vaginas with voiding, often confusing the picture when large amounts of fluid are found in the vagina.

ASSOCIATED ABNORMALITIES WITH PREMATURE LABOR

In our experience, approximately 50 percent of women in true premature labor are relatively hypovolemic, 25 percent have chorioamnionitis (often silent except for the occurrence of labor), and another 25 to 30 percent have intrinsic uterine problems such as incompetent cervix, immature (hypoplastic) uterus, or uterine anomalies. Obviously, some women have more than a single cause of premature labor. Those women who are relatively hypovolemic almost invariably have a growth-retarded fetus.

Neonatologists in general fail to recognize the tiny newborn as growth retarded, simply because their standards are based on the infants as delivered, and their norms for fetal weight versus gestational age are derived from infants born prematurely. The better data come from routine ultrasonic scanning; if a fetus is seen to be growth retarded at 26 weeks, it is ten times as likely to be delivered before 32 weeks as is the appropriate for gestational age 26-week fetus.

Since the presence of chorioamnionitis is difficult to diagnose in many of these women in premature labor, we assume that it may be present in all. Our drug of choice has been intravenous ampicillin, since it covers most of the offending organisms such as gonococcus, B-hemolytic *Streptococcus, Listeria,* and *Haemophilus influenzae.* Unfortunately, during the past year, six of the nine cases of infection with *Haemophilus influenzae* were not sensitive to ampicillin but required gentamicin. In the future we may have to use both ampicillin and gentamicin. Our policy is to obtain cervical cultures from all women in prema-

ture labor before starting any antibiotic therapy. We have found a good correlation between the predominant cervical bacteria and that grown out of the amniotic fluid. If amniotic fluid cannot be obtained from the vaginal fornix in these women, we perform an abdominal amniocentesis for Gram's stain of the fluid as well as for bacterial culture and studies for fetal lung maturity before starting tocolysis therapy. If there does appear to be chorioamnionitis, a uterine lavage is done with ampicillin, either through a catheter inserted transcervically in cases of premature rupture of the membranes or injected transabdominally at the time of the abdominal amniocentesis. We have used uterine lavage with antibiotics for more than 25 years with success. After lavage, women with obvious chorioamnionitis, a tender uterus, and high fever have almost always become afebrile, with virtual disappearance of their uterine tenderness. When cesarean section is performed in these women, cultures obtained from the uterine cavity fail to grow any bacteria. We also use systemic antibiotics. The occurrence of chorioamnionitis appears to be related to the presence of severe cervicitis and to coitus, both of which can be manipulated on a prophylactic basis.

PRENATAL DIAGNOSIS AND THERAPY

We treat grossly infected cervices for two reasons: (1) with coitus and the associated uterine activity of orgasm, the infected cervix may be the source of the amniotic infection syndrome and/or chorioamnionitis, and (2) the infecting bacteria can be a source of prostaglandins that cause premature labor or premature rupture of the membranes. Treatment in high-risk patients consists of local vaginal antibiotics and abstinence (including orgasm). We make the patient a partner in these decisions, as abstinence can place additional strains on an unstable marriage.

We teach our patients at high risk of premature labor (almost always those who have had a previous premature delivery or known uterine anomaly) to examine their own cervices during the course of their pregnancy. This seems easily accomplished, particularly for those who have previously used a diaphragm as a means of contraception. The clinic staff also routinely examines the cervix of all registered patients at 28 to 30 weeks. We are then left with a significant number of women who have a silently dilated cervix, perhaps 25 to 35 percent of the multigravidas prior to the 33rd week of pregnancy. The question then arises as to what form of therapy these women should be offered. We generally recommend (1) as much bed rest in a lateral position as possible, (2) avoidance of coitus and/or orgasm, and (3) use of tocolysis (terbutaline) until the 34th week. If frequent bed rest is not possible, we offer a McDonald's cervical suture in those dilated more than 2 cm before 30 weeks of pregnancy. For the primigravidas, we strongly recommend cerclage.

In those women with a previous history of membrane rupture or premature birth before 28 weeks, whether with painful labor or not, the antenatal staff examines the cervix every 2 weeks from 14 through 28 weeks and the patient examines herself daily. A clean-catch urine specimen is obtained at each visit for bacterial screening. Ultrasound examination is done at 4-week intervals to check for "tunneling" of the lower segment.

Although this examination program can cause unnecessary concern over misinterpretation, it has detected early significant cervical changes. One learning experience for the staff is the patient's frequent report of changes of the cervix from high and posterior to low and anterior as the day's activity progresses. Therefore, we suggest that the patient check the cervix in the evening for a means of comparison when the most cervical change is likely. Since we have not randomized any of these forms of diagnosis of premature labor, it is difficult to determine their efficacy, but they do seem to be successful.

Above all, our outpatient program is directed toward education and introduction of tranquility. Increased anxiety can produce relative maternal hypovolemia.

IN-HOSPITAL CARE

Since many of these pregnant women in premature labor are relatively hypovolemic, a significant part of our prophylactic therapy consists of efforts to expand maternal plasma volume. In many cases, this requires nothing more than bed rest; in others, it requires 2 to 3 L of intravenous Ringer's lactate solution, or sometimes intravenous 5 or 25 percent albumin. Our first indication that these women in premature labor are hypovolemic is how frequently their hematocrit values show significant drops of 15 to 30 percent with bed rest and successful tocolysis therapy. Therefore, we carefully follow hematocrits, and if a significant drop occurs, we very cautiously observe for pulmonary edema. On the other hand, successful tocolysis therapy requires that a plasma volume expansion occur, as indicated by a 15 percent of greater drop in hematocrit, increasing the risk of pulmonary edema with any successful therapy. Perhaps the most successful means of expanding plasma volume is to induce maternal tranquility, which is, of course, often difficult to achieve. We prescribe a mild tranquilizer (hydroxyzine or Vistaril), if only to keep the patient calm while at bed rest. Vigorous expansion of plasma volume with intravenous 5 percent albumin or Hespan solution appears to be associated with an increase in amniotic fluid volume and rupture of membranes. Therefore, caution is advised in how quickly the attempt is made to achieve maternal plasma volume expansion. Our goal is to make significant changes in maternal hematocrit values over a 24- to 36-hour period.

Tocolysis Therapy

We use magnesium sulfate, ritodrine, and terbutaline, in that order, in order to inhibit labor. We have found that if terbutaline fails, none of the others succeeds, whereas the converse is not true. Intravenous therapy is continued for up to 10 days and oral therapy up to 34 weeks.

Indomethacin, a potent inhibitor of prostaglandin synthesis, has been associated, after prolonged intrauterine exposure, with oligohydramnios and premature closure of the ductus arteriosus in the fetus and ileal perforation in the preterm newborn. We have therefore limited its use to situations where bacterial infection with prostaglandin production is likely, as in premature rupture of the membranes with immature amniotic fluid, and where only 48 hours of tocolytic therapy appears indicated.

Nifedipine, a calcium channel blocker agent, is recommended when maternal serum digoxin (digoxin-like substance) is elevated >0.2 ng/ml in cases of premature labor. Digoxin-like substance (DLS) is presumed to be a steroid and to arise in the fetal area of the fetal adrenal cortex and to modulate the onset of labor, much as fetal cortisol functions in the sheep. In normal pregnancies, digoxin is usually not detected in maternal serum before the 35th week of pregnancy. Nifedepine is a potent antagonist of digoxin and seems to be a particularly effective tocolytic agent when abnormal maternal serum or urine levels of DLS are present. However, we have restricted its use because, in pregnant sheep and monkeys, in utero exposure to nifedipine is associated with fetal acidosis. To date, no adverse effects have been reported in human pregnancies, even with its prolonged use.

Steroid Therapy

We have been vigorous in our treatment of premature labor, with or without premature rupture of the membranes. Our patients receive steroids in order to help the fetus achieve lung maturity. Originally this was offered to all women with infants under 34 weeks' gestation, but we now offer it only to those below 30 weeks. The neonatology care has improved to the point where there seems to be no significant difference in the neonatal course of infants weighing more than 1,300 g with or without steroids. We are most likely to offer steroids to nonwhite than to white patients, based on the collaborative study. Our attempts to select males by Barr body studies of amniotic fluid have failed.

Antibiotic Therapy

As noted, we cover all these patients with antibiotics for 3 days while awaiting the results of cultures. Unless it is a significant organism (*Listeria, Haemophilus influenzae,* gonococcus, or group B *Streptococcus*), the antibiotic is discontinued. We have had bacterial overgrowth with prolonged antibiotic therapy. On the other hand, our house staff is always apprenhensive on the day when antibiotics are discontinued because so many of these patients appear to go back into premature labor once the antibiotics are stopped. If labor does appear to recur after a discontinuance of antibiotics, we continue the antibiotics for another 3-day course of therapy.

REVIEW OF MEDICAL THERAPY FOR PREMATURE LABOR

Our overall success in this vigorous management with steroids, antibiotics, and tocolytic agents has been somewhat discouraging. Although we have forestalled labor in some pregnant women for 10 to 12 weeks after premature rupture of their membranes, when reviewing our past data, we have also had cases of amniotic band syndrome and newborns with hypoplastic lungs born after weeks of hospitalization of the mother for premature rupture of the membranes. We have also had five cases of silent fetal death in utero despite nonstress fetal heart rate monitoring performed every other day and monitoring with the biophysical profile at least once a week. In three of the five, after the diagnosis of no fetal heart tone, we found the cervix silently dilated, and the breech with the prolapsed cord in the vagina. When we compare our success in carrying cases with ruptured membranes from 22 weeks onward with cases in which no effort was made to inhibit labor, we are discouraged. There was no statistical improvement brought about by prolonged therapy over what one would expect if labor had been terminated after an arbitrary time of therapy such as 2 to 3 days, which would still allow time for the antibiotics to have their beneficial effect. We are therefore re-evaluating our policy of attempting to prolong uterine "rent." Our experience suggests that it is not as beneficial as has been suggested, especially in cases of premature rupture of the membranes.

DELIVERY OF THE TINY NEWBORN

Delivery is achieved by the least traumatic means possible. If the patient's membranes are intact and cervical dilation is occurring at a relatively rapid rate (2 cm per hour or greater), we allow vaginal delivery whether breech or vertex presentation. Our numbers are small, but some of our more outstanding neonatal successes with 600- to 800-g fetuses, in terms of survival without significant brain damage, have been with those born "in caul." For the tiny breech in caul, we suggest a hands-off delivery. If membranes are ruptured and labor is progressing at a slow rate, we favor cesarean section for either the breech or the vertex presentation if the estimated fetal weight is less than 1,200 g.

Our technique for cesarean section requires, above all, massive antibiotic coverage prior to beginning the procedure, for many patients have ruptured membranes and others have silent chorioamnionitis. As already noted, we often use intrauterine lavage, either transabdominally or with the uterine pressure catheter placed through the cervix. With the transcervical amniotic fluid injection, 2 g of ampicillin are placed in 1 liter of Ringer's lactate and the fluid is flushed through as quickly as can be accomplished (usually in 20 to 50 minutes). On occasion we have injected radiopaque media, and in most cases the dye (and antibiotics) is distributed throughout the uterine cavity, and interestingly enough, within a few minutes a maternal intravenous pyelogram appears. Apparently, the injected transcervical fluid is picked up very quickly, almost as fast as intravenously administered fluid. But the point is that the antibiotic reaches the amniotic cavity much more quickly than by the intravenous route. As already noted, we also use intravenous ampicillin so that the uterine cavity is exposed to maximum antibiotic coverage.

The technique of cesarean section is debatable. If there appears to be a lower uterine segment, the vertical incision is begun in the lower segment, and efforts are made to deliver the fetus without extension of the incision into the body of the uterus. We do our best to make sure that the incision is ample because our reason for the cesarean section is an atraumatic delivery. The most difficult breech deliveries in my memory are those that have been delivered abdominally because the incisions were in the undeveloped lower uterine segment or because the skin and fascial incisions were inadequate in fat women. There is absolutely no reason to deliver a premature infant by cesarean section if the delivery will be traumatic for the fetus. Often these vertical incisions end up as classic incisions, as the incision is carried up into the body of the uterus. Sometimes we can use a transverse incision in an apparently developed lower segment, but on at least two occasions this has not been a wise decision because the patient had an unrecognized uterine contraction ring. Under these circumstances, a transverse incision in the lower segment is useless.

When the premature infant is born, an attending neonatologist takes the infant immediately to the newborn resuscitation room, which in our institution is adjacent to the operating room. The newborn is not moved from that room until its condition is stabilized; sometimes this takes as long as 45 minutes.

To close the vertical uterine incision, we generally follow the technique described by Potter: single figure-of-X interrupted 2–0 chromic sutures. Although it makes the next delivery difficult, we do attempt to dissect off the uterine serosal surface so that the incision can be covered, and we cover most of the incision with the advanced bladder flap. During closure of the wound, we again lavage heavily with antibiotics and continue the antibiotic therapy for at least 3 days postoperatively. Given this massive antibiotic therapy, we have not had prolonged maternal morbidity, even when there was grossly infected amniotic fluid and chorioamnionitis. When the lavage is omitted, either prior to the section or afterward, or when massive antibiotics are not used in the first 3 days postoperatively, we have had prolonged maternal morbidity of 3 and 4 weeks, ending with hysterectomy. Objections to this massive antibiotic therapy have been raised on grounds of unnecessary sensitization and risk of development of resistant strains, especially with the lavage technique. But our experience indicates that these complications are worth the risk.

The vertical incision in the immature uterus is a risky procedure for subsequent pregnancies. We know of at least two women who have ruptured their uteruses with disastrous results, having had this type of incision with a previous premature delivery. Despite the fact that we repeatedly inform the patients of the type of incisions they have had, in one of these cases, the patient did not indicate to her obstetrician during a subsequent pregnancy that she had had a vertical classic incision, and her previous records had not been obtained. When the rupture occurred, there had been at least 20 hours of symptoms of abdominal pain, which were being treated as a probable renal stone. In this particular case, the fetus, which was lost, weighed nearly 2,500 g, and an emergency hysterectomy was done under most difficult circumstances. Fortunately, the mother survived, but she did bring suit against both us and her more recent obstetrician. After this experience, we have done our best to explain the hazards of a vertical classic incision to both the patient and her husband. We have her sign a detailed informed consent and do our best to make certain that she knows what type of incision she has had. On the other hand, we have had occasion to repeat cesarean sections after a classic incision, and except for difficulty in dissecting down the bladder flap, the uterus has appeared to be essentially normal. Obviously, it is not possible to predict how the incision will heal, particularly in the presence of chorioamnionitis.

PRENATAL GENETIC DIAGNOSIS

ROGER L. LADDA, M.D.

The objective of prenatal diagnosis is to assess the fetal condition. Such testing is usually reserved for couples at high risk for a well-characterized genetic abnormality sufficiently severe to warrant the risks of the test procedure. The tests performed are related to the special presenting features of the heritable condition and the stage in the pregnancy at which the abnormality can be detected. In most clinical situations, the fetus is found to be normal, and the parents are reassured about fetal development. In only a few instances is the fetus found to have an anomaly, and the couple then has the option of considering interruption of the pregnancy.

The events leading to the evaluation of the fetal condition are often convoluted, mandating last-minute referrals and time constraints. The early recognition of a genetic risk is critical and requires the cooperation of family physicians, pediatricians, and obstetricians to place the various risks in appropriate perspective for a particular couple. Highly specialized diagnosticians must be readily available to evaluate fetal images and tissues. The couple electing to proceed with prenatal diagnosis needs to be counseled about the indications for testing and the limitations of the technology to identify specific fetal abnormalities. Prenatal testing is probably one of the most accurate technologies available in medicine, yet there is always the possibility of a missed diagnosis, and in some cases the severity of the defect and its handicapping potential may be difficult to predict.

TECHNOLOGY

Two major technologies are available for evaluating the fetal condition. Observation of the fetus by standard radiologic and ultrasonographic techniques provides a general view of the fetal position, form, and skeletal structure. The other major methods include invasive procedures such as amniocentesis, fetoscopy, and, more recently, chorionic villus sampling. Each of these techniques is applied according to the specific indication.

RADIOLOGIC EXAMINATION

Simple x-ray films of the pregnant abdomen may identify signs of fetal death, anencephaly, hydrocephaly, defects of the limbs, and various skeletal dysplasias. The interpretation of most skeletal peculiarities requires considerable skill and experience that are not always immediately available in the community hospital, and pregnant women with fetuses with suspected defects should be referred to major centers for definition and counseling. These diagnostic radiologic studies pose no threat to fetal development.

ULTRASONOGRAPHY

The ultrasonographic evaluation of the fetus became common in the mid-1970s. In early 1964, the diagnoses of anencephaly and other neural tube abnormalities were achieved before 20 weeks' gestation. Several forms of ultrasonography are used, but the most common is B-mode (real-time),which allows one to obtain views of the entire fetus, observing fetal movement directly, and to focus on specific contours of fetal structures. Fetal biparietal diameter can be measured with ease, and other structures of the fetus, such as heart valves and central nervous system structures also may be identified. A skilled and experienced operator is able to provide information about most fetal structures.

Ultrasonography is an important tool in the evaluation of any pregnancy. There is no known harmful effect of ultrasound energy on the fetal tissues. It is now used nearly routinely early on in the pregnancy to confirm the existence of a fetus and to identify the number of fetuses. The growth of the uterus and fetus, placental size, and location and volume of amniotic fluid may be followed by ultrasonographic studies every 4 to 6 weeks if indicated. Serial ultrasound scans can provide a great deal of information about the quality of fetal growth and identify early intrauterine growth retardation, which is commonly found in many severe heritable conditions.

The types of anomalies that can be identified readily as early as 14 to 15 weeks' gestation include neural tube defects, encephalocele, and various forms of spina bifida. Serial ultrasound examination may provide information about the quality of brain growth and identify microcephaly and hydrocephaly. Ventricular shape and size can be evaluated. Holoprosencephaly and other brain defects such as hydrancephaly and porencephaly may be detected.

External features of the fetus may be readily screened to search for defects such as gastroschisis, omphalocele, and limb reduction abnormalities. It is possible to count digits with detailed ultrasound scanning in the appropriate circumstance; the detection of polydactyly or oligodactyly opens a variety of diagnostic problems for further testing. The humerus and the femur are routinely measured during a diagnostic scan.

Internal anomalies, such as cleft lip and palate, atresia of the esophagus, diaphragmatic hernia, duodenal atresia, and various other intestinal obstructions may be identified. Cardiac malformations may be readily identified and may alert the cardiovascular surgeon to the possible need for early intervention at the time of birth. Another major category of internal anomalies that can be seen early on includes renal agenesis, polycystic kidneys, and hydronephrosis; the latter is often associated with posterior urethral valves.

Essentially every pregnant women in a large metropolitan area has an ultrasound examination to confirm the gestational age of the fetus against the date of the last menstrual period within the first or second trimester. This type of ultrasound scan (level I) is usually limited to measurement of the fetal biparietal diameter, chest circumference, and femur length. It is not a diagnostic examination in the sense of searching for fetal anomalies, and it may often be misconstrued by the pregnant woman or couple as to the depth of the fetal analysis. This general scan commonly reveals a suspicious finding, and a more detailed scan is then required. Detailed high resolution ultrasound scans (level II) only are applied currently in those pregnancies in which a strong suspicion of a fetal anomaly exists. However, advanced level ultrasound scans at 19 to 21 weeks' gestation are becoming more common as public awareness of the frequency of birth defects increases. It is imperative for couples to understand that the ultrasound scan cannot detect all structural defects.

FETOSCOPY

Fetoscopy involves the introduction of a large-bore fiberoptic scope into the amniotic cavity via an abdominal puncture for direct visualization of certain parts of the fetus. One major application of fetoscopy has been in the direct visualization of the umbilical cord for the purpose of obtaining fetal venous blood samples for diagnostic tests. Samples of fetal skin and other tissue may be obtained by fetoscopy. Lamellar ichthyosis, harlequin ichthyosis, and several epidermolysis bullosa syndromes have been detected by fetal skin biopsy. However, fetoscopy is associated with a 5 to 10 percent risk of loss of the pregnancy. The field of vision is also restricted to small areas.

With the availability of high-resolution ultrasound scanning, most fetal tissues can be obtained using a much smaller biopsy needle system under the guidance of ultrasonography with a much-reduced risk of loss of the pregnancy.

AMNIOCENTESIS

In over 90 percent of referrals, prenatal diagnosis involves obtaining amniotic fluid cells for the purpose of evaluating the fetal chromosomal make-up and searching for trisomy 21 anomaly. Fetal cells are sloughed from the fetal skin and from the respiratory, urogenital, and gastrointestinal tracts and circulate in the amniotic fluid. Extra embryonic cells derived from the amniotic membrane also slough into the amniotic fluid. Amniocentesis allows amniotic fluid to be obtained and placed in a special medium to stimulate the growth of the few viable cells contained in the fluid. Amniocentesis may be performed as early as 14 weeks' gestation, but it usually is not technically possible to do so until about 15 to 16 weeks' gestation. This time period is chosen because the amount of amniotic fluid may just become sufficient to allow for easy access. Prior to 14 weeks, the uterus may not be sufficiently large to be entered easily.

Amniocentesis is an outpatient procedure. The woman's abdomen is surgically prepared after a brief ultrasound scan to mark the placenta, fetus, and main "pocket" of fluid. A 20-gauge needle is then placed into the amniotic sac under the guidance of ultrasonography. In our clinic, 2 to 3 ml of amniotic fluid are initially removed in a 5-ml syringe and placed to the side to clear any maternal cells that may have adhered to the interbore of the needle. Then another syringe is attached to the needle, and 25 to 30 ml of amniotic fluid are removed for culture. The amniotic fluid is sent to the cytogenetics laboratory, where a small sample is used for alpha-fetoprotein determination as a general scan to evaluate fetal well-being or to identify open neural tube defects, and the remainder is used to establish cell cultures for chromosomal analysis or biochemical assays.

The cells are separated from the amniotic fluid by gentle centrifugation, resuspended in culture medium, and layered on coverslips or dispersed into culture flasks for bulk cultures. From 25 to 30 ml of amniotic fluid approximately 12 individual coverslip cultures can be established, in addition to two bulk or flask cultures. The in situ colony or coverslip method allows for initial screening of the amniotic fluid fibroblast cultures at approximately 6 to 8 days following the amniocentesis and complete analysis within 14 to 21 days. The amniotic fluid alpha-fetoprotein assay is completed within 1 week of the amniocentesis. Thus, from the time of amniocentesis, at 16 weeks' gestation, to completion of the analysis may require 3 to 4 weeks, bringing the pregnancy to 19 to 20 weeks' gestation. Biochemical assays may require one or two additional weeks.

The risks of amniocentesis include hemorrhage secondary to the puncture of an anterior placenta or a peripheral vessel emanating from the placenta; intrauterine or extrauterine infection (extremely uncommon in our experience —none in 4,000 successive procedures); possible fetal injury from direct puncture, unlikely to occur with ultrasound guidance; and the possibility of spontaneous loss of the pregnancy. It is estimated that one pregnancy in 200 to 300 is lost from complications of the procedure. Massive loss of amniotic fluid vaginally accompanied by bleeding within the first 2 to 3 days following the procedure indicates a high potential risk of abortion. However, it may be difficult at times to relate the procedure to the loss of a particular pregnancy, because many pregnancies may be lost spontaneously during this period of time. Only one pass of the needle is considered appropriate. If fluid is not obtained with a single pass, a second pass may be considered but only after careful discussion with the couple.

CHORIONIC VILLUS SAMPLING

In couples at high risk for bearing a child with genetic abnormalities, fetal tissue (chorionic villi) may be obtained as early as 8 to 11 weeks' gestation for chromosomal and biochemical analyses. Under the guidance of ultrasonography, a small flexible catheter guided by a stylet is passed through a properly prepared cervix into the chorionic tissue. The transabdominal approach is also used and may reduce the risk of infection. The chorionic villi are aspirated into a culture medium. On average, about 5 to 5 chorionic villi ("Christmas tree structures") may be obtained. The chorionic villi have a high rate of mitotic activity, allowing direct in situ preparation of metaphases for chromosomal analysis. In addition, the cells obtained may be used for the extract of DNA for determination of restriction fragment length polymorphisms. The chorionic villi sampling techniques have about a 2 percent risk of inducing loss of pregnancy.

The advantages of chorionic villus sampling are the early stage of fetal assessment before fetal movement is realized and the rapid availability of results. If an anomaly is detected, then termination of the pregnancy may be carried out by suction curettage with much less risk to the mother and before bonding begins to develop.

INDICATIONS FOR PRENATAL TESTING

Maternal age accounts for over 90 percent of the referrals for prenatal testing in most centers. Advanced maternal age has been generally accepted to be 35 years and older, and the risk is related largely to the increased occurrence of chromosomal aneuploidy, such as trisomy 21, trisomy 18, and trisomy 13. The average incidence of trisomy 21 in the general population is about one in 800 live births, the risk usually offered at a maternal age of 30 years. At age 35 years the risk is about one in 250 to 350 and at 40 years about one in 80, with the risk climbing to about one in 10 at 45 years of age.

Another high-risk category includes the couple who has already had a child with trisomy 21. The recurrence risk, based on empiric observation, is 1 to 2 percent independent of maternal age. This predisposition to recurrence of a sporadic trisomy is not understood.

Any couple in which one member is a carrier of a balanced chromosomal translocation has a high risk of having a child with a major chromosomal imbalance. Such couples are generally recognized through the previous loss of one or more pregnancies or the birth of a child with multiple malformations who is found to have a chromosomal imbalance. Although the theoretical risk of a chromosomal imbalance in the fertilized egg is considerable, the most likely outcome in such a pregnancy based on actual observations is a normal-appearing child. Most imbalances appear to be associated with early first trimester losses.

Prenatal diagnosis is also offered to every couple in a subsequent pregnancy following the birth of a child with a chromosomal abnormality. Following the birth of a child with trisomy 13 or 18, the recurrence risk may approach 1 percent.

Neural tube defects represent a major severe category of malformations readily detected by prenatal testing. About one child in 1,000 is born with a neural tube abnormality. Following the birth of one child with a neural tube defect, the recurrence risk may be as high as 5 percent, depending upon the family history and ethnicity. Recurrence risks increase dramatically with each successive affected child. The combination of maternal serum alpha-fetoprotein screening and level II ultrasound scanning should provide a 90 to 95 percent detection rate. However, amniocentesis for amniotic fluid alpha-fetoprotein testing and amniotic fluid acetylcholinesterase activity (specific to the fetal nervous system), in addition to diagnostic ultrasonography, may be indicated to raise the detection rate to near certainty.

Other couples with indications for prenatal testing include those who have had a child with a well-defined inborn error of metabolism. The metabolic defect must be sufficiently well understood so that prenatal diagnostic testing would be considered highly accurate with little or no margin for error. These conditions are most often autosomal recessive traits with a 25 percent recurrence risk, but X-linked recessive traits and other levels of inheritance may be involved. Many defects have been detected or excluded and many more are theoretically detectable.

Other heritable conditions in which the basic defect is unknown are potentially diagnosable by new techniques utilizing recombinant DNA technology. Well-characterized diseases may be more rapidly detected. Using restriction fragment length polymorphisms, sickle cell anemia and many of the thalassemias can be readily diagnosed by direct study of the mutation in the fetus. The extraordinary power of recombinant DNA technology is demonstrated in the application of this technology to the prenatal diagnosis of cystic fibrosis, Duchenne's muscular dystrophy, and hemophilia A, conditions in which the basic metabolic abnormality is still to be defined. Many other conditions such as phenylketonuria, alpha$_1$-antitrypsin deficiency, and Gaucher's disease may be detected prenatally. In Gaucher's disease, the mutation pattern may predict the risk of neurologic manifestations. In specific high-risk families, the predisposition to certain malignancies, such as retinoblastoma, may be determined. The power of this new technology may be appreciated by considering the hypothesis that with about 250 genetic markers evenly spaced throughout the genome, essentially every disease know to humans could be linked to one of these specific markers and the potential for deriving informative restriction fragment length polymorphisms in a given family.

MATERNAL SERUM ALPHA-FETOPROTEIN SCREENING

Maternal serum alpha-fetoprotein screening has become a part of routine obstetric care. Alpha-fetoprotein is produced by the fetal liver and gastrointestinal tract and is excreted into the amniotic fluid via the fetal urine. It diffuses into the maternal circulation at concentrations of only a fraction found in fetal serum and amniotic fluid. A neural tube defect gives rise to leakage of fetal fluids and is associated with elevated alpha-fetoprotein levels in the amniotic fluid and maternal serum. An elevated maternal serum alpha-fetoprotein level detected at 16 to 17 weeks' gestation by general screening triggers concern for additional testing, such as ultrasound scanning, to search for a fetal neural tube defect. Amniocentesis may also be indicated to determine the amniotic fluid level of alpha-fetoprotein.

Low levels of alpha-fetoprotein in maternal serum may be associated with intrauterine growth retardation, fetal distress, or death. Chromosomal trisomies may be associated with relatively low maternal serum values, but the screening assay has low sensitivity and specificity for chromosomal aneuploidy. Routine screening of women under 35 years of age may lead to the detection of about one-third of pregnancies with a trisomic fetus.

FUTURE OF PRENATAL DIAGNOSIS

Great progress has been made since amniocentesis was first introduced for genetic diagnosis in the early 1960s. Technology is rapidly evolving, and the day can be imagined when virtually all structural defects and most inborn errors of metabolism can be detected. The goals are to simplify the technology while increasing specificity and sensitivity of the tests and to minimize the danger to mother and fetus by limiting the invasiveness of procedures. Although it is currently experimental, the separation of fetal cells from a maternal blood sample for assessment of the fetal condition by various tests, including restriction fragment length polymorphisms, is not beyond early realization.

But what is to be done with these defective fetuses? Birth defects detected by prenatal testing are prevented now only by pregnancy interruption. Certainly some modalities of effective treatment will become available, but gene replacement is difficult to conceptualize at present.

Finally, should all pregnancies be screened routinely in the course of normal obstetric care? And if such screening is not performed, should couples be informed of its availability? In this area, as in others, patient education is fundamental to effective care and understanding.

SUGGESTED READING

Milunsky A, ed. Genetic disorders and the fetus: diagnosis, prevention and treatment. New York: Plenum Press, 1986.

PREVIOUS CESAREAN SECTION

MORTIMER G. ROSEN, M.D.

Once again clinical obstetrics is in transition with respect to the management of the patient with a previous cesarean section. This commentary is based on a personal clinical experience in a large hospital and a relatively complete review of the literature. This chapter relates only to the patient with a single previous cesarean birth performed in the transverse manner in the lower uterine segment. Studies relating to vaginal birth following a classic or low vertical incision, or after several cesarean operations, are insufficient in size to allow authoritative statements with respect to medical care. Management of these patients may be individualized, but frequently the result is repeat cesarean birth. Since 90 percent of all cesarean sections are performed through low transverse uterine incisions, this discussion encompasses most of the cesarean patient population. How does one decide the route for delivery? How does one apply appropriate clinical care or alter that care during the management of labor in the patient with a previous cesarean birth?

PATIENT EVALUATION

Selecting the Route of Delivery

Appropriate records must be available for review, including operative notes or a discussion with the physician who was present at the first procedure. A concise review of labor problems during the previous pregnancy is helpful for planning purposes.

In the presence of a low transverse uterine incision, without evidence of uterine lacerations following delivery of the fetus, the choice for vaginal birth route is an option. In my practice, a prior classic or low vertical incision, an observed extension of the original incision (laceration at time of delivery), or a T-shaped incision is a relative contraindication to vaginal birth. Conversely, diagnoses such as puerperal infection of the endometrium, cystitis, or most infections are not contraindications to the vaginal birth route. However, the rare uterine incision that is visualized during the puerperium and documented as the site of severe infection should be considered carefully during a subsequent gestation.

The Hospital Environment

Early in the antepartum period the clinician should discuss with the patient the labor and delivery environment, including available emergency surgical support in the chosen hospital. In the circumstances of a well-equipped hospital environment, the vaginal birth route is an option. However, the choice is limited when the hospital lacks emergency surgical support necessary for a possible cesarean section. The patient should be aware of an alternate hospital within the geographic region that has a more appropriate labor and delivery environment. There is little need to take additional patient risks when choices are available. It is usually suggested that an emergency cesarean should be able to be performed within 30 minutes of when it is needed.

If alternate hospital birth environments are not available, the options for birth route are more limited. The risks of uterine rupture are extremely small, less than 2 percent in labor. Perinatal death relating to rupture is also extremely uncommon and should be balanced against preterm delivery of the nonlaboring patient following elective repeat cesarean section. Maternal risk of death following repeat cesarean is about twice as high as that following successful vaginal birth (20 per 100,000 versus 10 per 100,000 births). However, it is evident that maternal uterine infection rates are higher following failed labor trials that terminate in repeat cesarean births than when section is performed electively in the nonlaboring patient.

Contraindications to Vaginal Birth: Dystocia and Absolute Pelvic Contracture

Absolute pelvic contracture is seen in patients with a history of rickets, scurvy, or bone fracture (with radiologic evidence of a compromised asymmetric pelvis) and in women of short stature, Nägele's pelvis, or an obstructed pelvis due to kidney or fibroid tumors. Trials for cesarean birth are acceptable in patients whose clinical histories include a diagnosis such as dystocia, cephalopelvic disproportion, and failure to progress. Often those clinical situations are influenced by fetal size and position, uterine forces, or other fetal factors that may not be repeated in the next gestation.

Previous diagnoses such as dystocia, cephalopelvic disproportion, and poor progress in labor warrant a subsequent trial of labor. Many babies are born larger than their siblings born by cesarean. Excessive size (9 lb or 4,000 g), a floating vertex (over the pubic symphysis at labor onset), and a long closed cervix with a floating vertex at labor onset are problems that warrant concern. These clinical situations are not absolute contraindications to labor, but they may foreshadow longer labors and a greater chance that vaginal delivery will be complicated.

The absence of a previous labor with cervical dila-

tion does not contraindicate a trial of labor. Similarly, a patient with a history of previous cesarean section for abruptio placentae or placenta previa is an appropriate candidate for labor trial. Patients with previous uterine metroplasties or myomectomies are not candidates for labor trials, since these procedures represent major incisions into the myometrium.

Some physicians suggest that the very low birth weight baby (1,500 g) would benefit from cesarean section by avoiding the vaginal pressures on the vertex and the potential risks for subsequent intracerebral hemorrhage. I believe that birth weight and fetal maturity affect neonatal outcome to a greater degree than the choice of birth route. In the absence of fetal distress or an abnormal fetal lie, the low birth weight fetus in the mother with a previous cesarean section is managed similarly to the term fetus. Labor is not suggested in the case of oblique or transverse fetal lie.

THE CONDUCT OF LABOR

The Onset

Patients are advised to report to the hospital when they think labor has commenced. True labor can be confirmed in the labor suite by observation and electronic monitoring.

If during labor the patient changes her mind about vaginal delivery because of fears relating to the previous labor and birth, I generally defer to her request and proceed with a cesarean. However, in order to minimize fear of labor risk, antepartum care should include educational programs preparing for labor and delivery.

Clinical Care in the Labor Suite

Patients are advised to contact me or to proceed to the hospital *early* after the onset of labor. Upon the patient's entry into the labor suite, the vital signs of the mother and fetus are obtained. Management should include installation of an intravenous line with an 18- or 19-gauge needle, typing and holding blood, and the performance of routine labor studies on urine and blood.

Electronic monitoring should be instituted. External monitoring is acceptable only if the information is comprehensible, since there is no point in obtaining monitoring tracings of poor or useless quality. Patients may be disconnected from the monitors to walk or change position. During ambulatory time auscultation should be carried out every 15 minutes during the active phase of labor and at least every 30 minutes during the latent phase.

Subsequently, with preparations made and monitors in place, the conduct of labor may proceed normally.

Maternal analgesia or regional anesthesia is acceptable; however, I encourage natural birth and try to minimize the use of medications. In the absence of rare, sudden, severe abdominal pain or the association of maternal and fetal distress, the prospective identification of uterine scar separation (rupture) is extremely difficult. Modest amounts of suprapubic pain are normal. Analgesia and anesthesia may be needed to tolerate labor.

In the absence of fetal distress, labor should proceed. If protractions or arrests of labor occur during the active phase, clinical judgment must be used. I am more inclined to terminate the labor in the presence of a floating vertex with a cervix dilated beyond 6 cm and well into the active phase. But if the patient wishes to continue, I may temporize with medication to determine whether analgesia or regional anesthesia encourages more descent and dilation. The use of analgesics or regional anesthetics does not always result in a rapid response time. Results of sedation may not occur for several hours. If no progress occurs, a cesarean is performed.

In the presence of unexplained uterine bleeding (not cervical) during the labor trial, labor is terminated unless delivery is imminent. The bleeding may represent a uterine rupture that cannot be diagnosed except by laparotomy.

The Use of Oxytocin

Many will argue that the use of oxytocin produces contractions of the uterine smooth muscle that are not different from those experienced during normal labor. Although this may be true, originally we maintained a policy of neither inducing nor augmenting labor with oxytocin in order to avoid misuse in obstructed or prolonged labor. We have changed our policy and today accept the judgment of the physician as one guide to use of oxytocin during labor. It is now used both to induce and to augment labor.

Protractions or Arrests During Active Phase of Labor

In general, sedation, rest, and ambulation should be used with caution. In the presence of abnormal labors the cesarean birth option should be considered as an early stage intervention. In contrast, a more prolonged labor trial may be carried out in the unscarred uterus. Termination of any labor during the latent phase should occur only infrequently.

The Second Stage of Labor

As noted earlier, the second stage of labor is managed as in all noncesarean patients. Spontaneous maternal bearing down is acceptable. Obstetric abdominal pushing is not indicated.

The Third Stage of Labor

Following birth the placenta may be delivered spontaneously or manually. I prefer to remove the placenta immediately after cutting the umbilical cord. At that time the dilated cervix and relaxed uterus allow easier examination of the uterine scar.

The patient should be advised of an anticipated uterine exploration. Generally the procedure can be managed without anesthesia. There is little point in trying to deliver a previous cesarean patient vaginally and then using deep anesthesia to relax the uterus for inspection. Anesthesia is one of the operative risks to be avoided when the delivery is vaginal.

Examination of the scar may be confusing. A thickened fundus or body of the uterus and a thin lower uterine segment can be felt. The boundary between thick and thin segments should not be confused with scar dehiscence. If you can feel no discrete hole, pocket, linear defect, or the inside of the mother's umbilicus, and if there is no evidence of bright red uterine bleeding, stop the examination. Too much exploration may cause separation of the segments.

If I feel relatively certain that a defect is present, my policy is to perform a laparotomy *at that time* and repair the incision if a defect is found. In the next pregnancy these patients should have abdominal deliveries.

In contrast to the postdelivery examination of the uterus, I have not found that "gentle" vaginal intracervical exploration or digital exploration is helpful in defining an intact or dehisced scar while labor is in progress.

The Post-term Patient

This patient requires concern and sensitive management. Since the mother is often under greater than usual anticipatory stress about the forthcoming trial of labor, and since a large number of pregnancies extend post-term, emotional support is needed. The eventuality of a post-term gestation should be discussed with the patient early in the pregnancy. The post-term patient is not always or even often like the postmaturity patient (e.g., with a growth-retarded or dysmature fetus) and should be managed similarly to other patients in this clinical situation. Beyond 41 weeks' gestation, I see patients biweekly, and at each visit monitor the fetus with nonstress tests. At our hospital, management policies are not aggressive. Fetal size should be defined if macrosomia is suspected in one post-term patient.

Rh PROPHYLAXIS

JOHN M. BOWMAN, M.D.

An Rh-negative woman, delivered of an ABO compatible Rh-positive baby, has a 16 percent probability of becoming Rh immunized, in 1.5 to 2 percent of instances by delivery, and in a further 7 percent by 6 months after delivery. The remaining 7 percent will show, by mounting a secondary Rh immune response in the second trimester of the next Rh-positive pregnancy, that they were also Rh immunized ("sensibilized") by the first pregnancy, the antibody having been at too low a level to be demonstrated at that time. If her Rh-positive baby is ABO incompatible, the Rh-negative mother is at a 1.5 to 2 percent risk of becoming detectably Rh immunized by 6 months after delivery. The risk of Rh immunization is 2 percent and 4 percent after a spontaneous and an induced abortion, respectively. It is 2.5 percent after ultrasound-directed mid- or third-trimester amniocentesis. Although there are no reported studies to date, since first-trimester chorionic villus sampling carries a risk of fetomaternal transplacental hemorrhage, chorionic villus sampling is also associated with a risk of Rh immunization. The Rh(D) antigen is present in the red cell membrane as early as the fifth to sixth week of gestation.

The development and licensure in 1968 of Rh immune globulin (RhIG) represented a major milestone in preventive medicine. By its use, Rh immunization and its sequelae, Rh erythroblastosis and hydrops fetalis, were prevented. RhIG is always effective in preventing Rh immunization with two provisos: it must be given before Rh immunization has begun and it must be given in a sufficient dose.

The standard prophylactic dose of Cohn cold ethanol manufactured RhIG for intramuscular use, in the United States is 300 μg. Elsewhere, doses of 100 μg to 120 μg of similar preparations have been found to be almost equally protective. In West Germany, Ireland, and Canada, ion exchange chromatography prepared RhIG, for intravenous use, in doses of 120 μg, has proved highly effective.

The outline of Rh prophylaxis presented here is that carried out in the Rh Laboratory of the University of Manitoba, Faculty of Medicine, and the Health Sciences Centre, Winnipeg. The Rh Laboratory is responsible for Rh prophylaxis in the Province of Manitoba, which has 17,000 deliveries annually, of which 2,300 to 2,400 are in Rh-negative women, 1,400 of whom have Rh-positive babies. There are an additional 600 to 650 abortions (spontaneous and induced) in Rh-negative women each year.

POST-DELIVERY Rh PROPHYLAXIS

Postdelivery prophylaxis consists of the administration of one standard dose of RhIG (300 μg intramuscularly in the United States) within 72 hours after delivery to all Rh-negative, unimmunized women delivering Rh-positive babies, irrespective of the ABO status of the baby.

Since rare but documented instances of Rh immunization have first appeared after delivery, within the first 72 hours, our practice is to administer the RhIG as soon as the baby has been determined to be Rh positive and the mother therefore to be at risk.

If for any reason the Rh status of the baby is not known within 72 hours after delivery, we give the mother RhIG despite the one-third chance that her baby is Rh negative and that she is not at risk. *It is preferable to treat a woman who is not at risk than to fail to treat one who is at risk.* Conversely, if a woman at risk is inadvertently not protected within 72 hours after delivery, we give her RhIG up to 28 days after delivery as soon as we have discovered the oversight. There is experimental evidence that some protection against Rh immunization is conferred by administration of RhIG 13 days after exposure to Rh-positive red cells. However, in this circumstance the patient and her physician must understand that the longer after delivery RhIG administration is delayed, the less likely it is that it will be protective.

Because of the 2 to 4 percent risk of Rh immunization following abortion, we administer RhIG to every unimmunized Rh-negative patient who aborts. If a 50-μg (mini) dose of RhIG is available, it will protect against Rh immunization following first-trimester abortion. Since 50 μg only prevents Rh immunization following exposure of up to 2 ml of Rh-positive fetal red cells, we recommend that a standard dose of RhIG (not the minidose) be given if second-trimester therapeutic abortion is carried out.

Postdelivery Rh prophylaxis has been 85 to 90 percent effective in eradicating Rh immunization. Residual problems in Rh prevention are outlined in Table 1.

FAILURE TO CARRY OUT POSTDELIVERY PROPHYLAXIS

Failure to give RhIG to the Rh-negative mother after delivery of an Rh-positive infant may be due to her failure to seek prenatal care, failure of her physician to send her blood for grouping and antibody screening, or failure of the hospital delivery unit to send maternal and cord blood for testing after delivery.

Personnel giving obstetric care must know the Rh and Rh immunization status of all pregnant women in their

---

TABLE 1 Residual Rh Prophylaxis Problems

Failure to administer RhIG after delivery or abortion.

Failure to give RhIG after amniocentesis.

Failure to prevent Rh immunization after massive fetal transplacental hemorrhage.

Rh immunization during pregnancy—antenatal Rh prophylaxis.

Rh immunization in infancy—the "grandmother theory."

The mother with weak Rh antibodies.

The problem of the D^u mother.

unit. The Rh-negative woman, after blood group determination and antibody screen at her initial prenatal visit, should be rescreened at 20, 28, and 32 to 34 weeks' gestation. At delivery, cord and maternal blood should be tested. If the baby is Rh positive and the mother is Rh negative and unimmunized, RhIG must be given. A weakly positive cord blood red cell direct antiglobulin (Coombs') test, in the presence of ABO incompatibility, is not a reason for withholding RhIG. The baby has ABO erythroblastosis. Since ABO incompatibility does not prevent Rh immunization completely, RhIG should be administered.

The Rh-negative woman who becomes Rh immunized following abortion does so after a relatively small fetal red cell transplacental hemorrhage. She is a good responder and often has a severely affected fetus in her next Rh-positive pregnancy. Therapeutic abortions should not be carried out until the Rh and Rh immunization status of the patient are determined. If the patient is Rh negative and unimmunized, RhIG (a standard dose) must be given at the time of therapeutic abortion.

Compliance after spontaneous abortion may be more difficult. Early spontaneous abortion may occur before the first prenatal visit, and the woman may not be hospitalized. Rh-negative women should know their Rh status and that they are at risk of Rh immunization after a spontaneous abortion. Personnel caring for the woman who aborts must determine her Rh status and give her RhIG if she is Rh negative and unimmunized.

Antepartum hemorrhage in the Rh-negative woman is associated with a substantial risk of fetal transplacental hemorrhage and Rh immunization, although there are no reported data to indicate the degree of such risk. We administer a full dose of RhIG (300 μg) to the Rh-negative woman who has an antepartum hemorrhage. If the pregnancy continues, we administer an additional dose every 12 weeks until delivery. Twelve weeks is the longest time interval for which 300 μg of RhIG is likely to remain protective.

FAILURE TO GIVE RhIG AFTER AMNIOCENTESIS

If the placenta is traversed at amniocentesis, there is a significant risk of fetomaternal hemorrhage. In the era before ultrasonography, 10.6 percent of amniocentesis procedures were associated with fetal transplacental hemorrhages. Amniocentesis under ultrasonography direction reduces the risk to 2.5 percent. We give every Rh-negative, unimmunized women a standard 300-μg dose of RhIG at the time of amniocentesis. Again, this dose is repeated every 12 weeks if the woman is undelivered and in 6 weeks if the amniocentesis is repeated. Despite fears to the contrary, RhIG administration at the time of amniocentesis does not harm the fetus.

FAILURE TO PREVENT Rh IMMUNIZATION AFTER MASSIVE TRANSPLACENTAL HEMORRHAGE

One 300-μg dose of RhIG given intramuscularly prevents Rh immunization after exposure to up to 25 ml of Rh-positive blood (12 to 13 ml of Rh-positive red cells). The same dose gives partial protection after a greater exposure, to the extent that after exposure to one unit (450 ml) of Rh-positive blood, 300 μg of RhIG reduce the incidence of Rh immunization from the expected 65 percent to 35 percent.

In three series of Manitoba Rh-negative women, from 1967 to 1987, in whom Kleihauer's acid elution fetal transplacental hemorrhage studies were carried out at delivery, one woman in 416 (38 of 15,795 women studied) had more than 25 to 30 ml of fetal blood in her circulation, an incidence of 0.24 percent. Thus the incidence of Rh immunization attributable to undiagnosed massive fetal transplacental hemorrhage following administration of 300 μg of RhIG would be 0.084 percent (0.24 $\times$ 0.35), one in 1,200 Rh-negative women delivering Rh-positive babies.

Thus failure to diagnose and treat massive fetomaternal transplacental hemorrhage is a rare cause of persisting Rh immunization. Because the Kleihauer acid elution fetal cell screening test, although it is accurate and reproducible in experienced hands, does not lend itself to routine blood bank laboratory screening (the rosetting test of Sebring and Polesky or the enzyme–linked antiglobulin test of Riley and Ness may be better screening tests for such laboratories), and since massive fetal hemorrhage is a rare cause of Rh immunization, it could be argued that screening for massive transplacental hemorrhage is not cost-effective and should not be carried out. Nevertheless, we do screen for transplacental hemorrhage, and both blood transfusion and obstetrics societies recommend it.

If a transplacental hemorrhage greater than 25 ml of fetal blood is diagnosed after delivery, we give two vials of RhIG (600 μg) for a hemorrhage between 25 ml and 50 ml of blood, three vials (900 μg) for a hemorrhage between 50 ml and 75 ml, and so on. If an ion exchange prepared RhIG is given intravenously, as is our custom, the dose is reduced by 40 percent. We give 1,200 μg of RhIG intramuscularly every 12 hours or 300 μg intravenously every 6 hours until the total calculated dose has been administered.

In the very rare, occasionally life-threatening instance in which a transplacental hemorrhage exceeding 75 to 100 ml is diagnosed in the third trimester, the possibility of fetal compromise (even demise) as well as the hazards of Rh immunization must be considered. Immediate ultrasound assessment of the fetal condition should be undertaken. If the pregnancy is past 32 to 33 weeks' gestation, immediate delivery should be carried out with neonatal facilities available for management of an anemic baby who may be in hypovolemic shock. If the baby is Rh positive, the mother should be given RhIG in the appropriate dosage.

If an Rh-negative woman under the age of 45 is inadvertently (or deliberately) transfused with Rh-positive blood, every effort should be made to prevent Rh immunization. If less than 900 ml of blood (400 ml of red cells) has been given, RhIG in the recommended dose should be given. Rh-negative cross-matched blood should be available to treat the anemia that will develop. If the volume transfused is greater than 900 ml, we elect to carry out a 1.5 blood volume exchange transfusion using ABO compatible Rh-negative cross-matched blood, thereby removing 75 percent of the transfused Rh-positive red cells. We then give RhIG in a dose based on 30 percent of the Rh-positive blood volume originally transfused. Differential agglutinations 72 to 96 hours after the final dose should show no remaining Rh-positive red cells, and antibody testing should reveal the presence of passive Rh antibody.

Rh IMMUNIZATION DURING PREGNANCY— ANTEPARTUM PROPHYLAXIS

It has now been shown quite conclusively in Manitoba and elsewhere that 1.5 to 2 percent of Rh-negative women carrying Rh-positive fetuses, who are not Rh immunized at the commencement of their pregnancies will be Rh immunized by the time they delivery their babies and therefore will not be protected by postdelivery Rh prophylaxis. Rh immunization during pregnancy causes 20 times as much residual Rh immunization as untreated massive fetomaternal transplacental hemorrhage. Women who become Rh immunized during pregnancy are "good responders." Subsequently, they frequently have very severely affected erythroblastotic fetuses. Twenty percent of subsequent Rh-positive fetuses in a Manitoba series required either early delivery (8 percent) or intrauterine transfusions and early delivery (12 percent). In the period from March 1979 to March 1984, of 52 women referred from elsewhere to our institution for intrauterine fetal transfusions, 27 percent had been Rh immunized during a previous pregnancy.

Following a successful antenatal prophylactic clinical trial in Winnipeg, carried out from 1968 to 1976, which reduced the Rh immunization rate during pregnancy from 1.8 to 0.1 percent, we began a service program of antenatal Rh prophylaxis during pregnancy. All Rh-negative unimmunized pregnant women whose husbands are Rh positive (or Rh unknown) are given one standard 300-μg dose of RhIG at 28 weeks' gestation. We now use an ion exchange prepared RhIG given intravenously, but in the past and in the clinical trial we used Cohn cold ethanol intramuscular RhIG. Both are equally protective. Because 12 weeks extends the protective effect of 300 μg of RhIG (half-life 21 days) to its very limit, if the woman is undelivered 12.5 weeks after her antenatal injection, we give her a second antenatal injection of RhIG. Then if delivery occurs within 3 weeks (which it usually does), we do not give a postdelivery injection of RhIG unless there is evidence of a fetal transplacental hemorrhage greater than or equal to 0.1 ml of fetal red cells. Currently the antenatal Rh prophylaxis service program protection rate in Manitoba is 95 percent.

Although arguments have been advanced against administration of antenatal RhIG, based on lack of cost effectiveness and potential risk to the fetus, they are entirely without foundation. Antenatal Rh prophylaxis costs 11 times as much for every instance of Rh immunization prevented than does postdelivery Rh prophylaxis. Nevertheless, antenatal Rh prophylaxis is more cost-effective than many other recommended medical procedures.

With respect to fetal damage due to exposure to foreign IgG, all fetuses are exposed to very much larger amounts of foreign (maternal) IgG throughout gestation, which is not harmful to the fetus and is beneficial for the neonate. Although we have not studied the immunologic status of the 25,000 fetuses whose mothers have been given RhIG at 28 weeks' gestation in Manitoba and do no intend to do so, we have not had any cases of suspected damage reported to us.

In 1989, *the physician who neglects to offer his Rh-negative pregnant patient 28 weeks' gestation Rh prophylaxis neglects to do so at the physician's and the patient's peril*.

Rh IMMUNIZATION IN INFANCY— "THE GRANDMOTHER THEORY"

As early as 1953 it had been proposed that reverse passage of Rh-positive maternal red cells into an Rh-negative fetus at the time of birth might occur and cause Rh immunization, later detected during a first Rh-positive pregnancy. Sixty percent of mothers of Rh-negative babies are Rh positive. Careful studies of capillary blood samples taken at 1 or 2 days of age show a 2 percent incidence of reverse maternal fetal transplacental hemorrhage. With one exception (fetal hydrops produced by massive maternal fetal transfusion), the hemorrhages have been minute (0.005 ml, one-twentieth the amount associated with a 3 percent incidence of maternal Rh immunization). We believe that Rh immunization during infancy, if it occurs at all, is an exceedingly rare event. For that reason, we neither recommend nor administer RhIG to Rh-negative female neonates born of Rh-positive mothers.

SUPPRESSION OF WEAK Rh IMMUNIZATION; FACT OR FANCY

Rh-negative women who have Rh antibodies detected only by Auto-Analyzer techniques and not by manual methods may not be truly Rh immunized. From the standpoint of Rh prophylaxis, they should be managed as if they were not Rh immunized. The Rh-negative woman who has a very weak Rh antibody detectable at the very outer limits of sensitivity of manual enzyme or indirect antiglobulin techniques is an entirely different matter. Attempts in Winnipeg to suppress or reverse Rh immunization once it has been demonstrated, no matter how weakly, have been uniformly unsuccessful. We do not give RhIG to women with Rh antibodies weakly demonstrated by enzyme or antiglobulin techniques, nor do we recommend that it be given. However, if screening tests are questionable and if the specificity of the antibody is in doubt, RhIG should be given, with the understanding that it may not be protective.

THE SO-CALLED "D^u" MOTHER

Most D^u mothers are genetically Rh positive with a weakened expression of D due to the presence of the gene for the antigen C on the opposite chromosome. They are not at risk of Rh immunization and need not be given Rh-

IG. Controversy surrounds the less common genetic D^u woman, who is missing part of the D antigen mosaic. On very rare occasions such women do become Rh immunized and in at least one instance hydrops has resulted. If the uncommon genetic D^u mother can be differentiated from the environmental D^u genetic Rh-positive mother, we do recommend that the former be given RhIG after delivery, although the risk of Rh immunization is very, very small.

SPONTANEOUS ABORTION

ATTILA TOTH, M.D.

Spontaneous abortion refers to a clinical condition describing the loss of the intrauterine product prior to the viability of the fetus, conventionally accepted as 20 weeks of intrauterine life, or 500 g of fetal body weight. The term habitual aborter describes a patient who serially miscarries, with three or more miscarriages being taken arbitrarily as the starting point from which a patient is labeled a habitual aborter. The exact frequency of spontaneous abortion in the general population is unknown. With the availability of sensitive beta-human chorionic gonadotropin serum assays, early pregnancies are detected that formerly were written off as simple abnormal prolongations of the menstrual cycle. Five- to 10-day delays in the onset of the menstrual period, followed by sudden, heavier than usual menstrual bleeding, are very frequently diagnosed through the beta subunit as early spontaneous abortions. It is estimated today that more pregnancies are lost spontaneously than are actually carried to term. Therefore, many practitioners believe that it is unnecessary to initiate a full-scale work-up after the first miscarriage. We would like to emphasize, however, that if an infectious condition precipitates the first spontaneous abortion and is allowed to persist without treatment, the subsequent pregnancies often become high risk and thus jeopardize the outcome of the fetus. The actual chance that a woman will experience a subsequent pregnancy loss once she has had two spontaneous abortions has changed drastically during the last 40 years. In the late 1930s, the figure was a staggering 73 percent. By the mid-1970s, this number was reduced to approximately 30 to 35 percent, and in our laboratory, since the introduction of aggressive antibiotic therapy, it has fallen to less than 5 percent.

ETIOLOGY OF SPONTANEOUS ABORTIONS

Chromosomal Abnormalities

A chromosomal abnormality is still believed to be the most common etiologic factor behind spontaneous abortion. Indeed, *up to 50 percent of the examined first trimester losses show some kind of chromosomal abnormality.*

Thus it has been speculated that spontaneous, random errors in meiosis or mitosis occur in sperm or in the ovum or in both germ cells. Another possible hypothesis is that a noxious agent can induce the meiotic or mitotic errors, and that these noxious agents, if they are not eliminated, could repeat the process. A third possibility relies heavily on a defect in parental genes that is either detected or undetected owing to the limitations of currently available techniques. The dramatic rise in the number of Down syndrome cases associated with advanced parental age suggests that spontaneous chromosomal damage can occur with advancing age. During the last 6 years, in our patients not one pregnancy had to be terminated because of chromosomal damage, a record that coincides with our aggressive use of antibiotics, suggesting that bacteria or bacterial toxins present in the environment in which the early embryogenesis takes place could serve as the noxious agents that may induce the meiotic or mitotic errors.

Medical Illnesses

Systemic lupus erythematosus, congenital cardiac disease, and renal disease are among the medical diseases associated with spontaneous abortions. The severity of the underlying disease condition determines the outcome of pregnancy. It has been suggested that the high rate of fetal wastage among patients with systemic lupus erythematosus is due to circulating immune complexes. In pregnant patients with congenital cardiovascular disease, the spontaneous fetal wastage is in excess of 50 percent. With renal disease, especially with coexistent hypertension, the incidence of fetal loss can be extremely high. Individual, uncontrolled studies suggest that diabetes mellitus, especially when there is poor control of the blood glucose level, can lead to increased fetal wastage. Double-blind controlled studies are still unavailable.

The role of a hypoactive thyroid both in infertility and in pregnancy losses is suspected and partially documented by several investigators. Patients with previous abortions who carried pregnancies to term had thyroid test profiles that lagged behind those of the controls. The test profile also was always low in habitual aborters who did not carry their pregnancies to term.

Immunologic Factors

It is believed that women who have repeated spontaneous abortions lack a key serum blocking antibody that is supposed to protect the fetus from rejection by the mother. The blocking factor belongs to the immunoglobulin G class and acts to protect the fetus from maternal antibodies and subsequent immunologic rejection via the coating of fetal antigens on the placenta. It is further believed that homozygosity in the HLA antigen system can prevent the mother from producing blocking antibodies. Desensitization, with a suspension of the husband's white blood cells, is suggested in several publications

Studies dealing with major blood group incompatibilities are contradictory and await further confirmation.

Isolated reports do not show conclusive evidence that antisperm antibodies are associated with habitual abortions.

Endocrine Factors, Luteal Phase Defect

Luteal phase refers to the second part of the menstrual cycle that is dominated by the corpus luteum and its main hormone, progesterone. Progesterone is necessary to support an early pregnancy up to 8 weeks, when the placenta takes over the progesterone production. Sluggish luteal phase hormone production by the corpus luteum is believed to result in early pregnancy losses.

The incidence of luteal phase deficiency varies, depending on the patient population studied. Among infertile couples, luteal phase deficiency is documented in approximately 3 to 5 percent of the cases; among habitual aborters, however, it can reach up to 35 percent. Several years ago, we became aware that a subclinical oophoritis can lead to luteal phase defect, and thus we have found that correction of the condition by antibiotics can be more rewarding than supporting the luteal phase with progesterone or overdriving the entire menstrual cycle with clomiphene or follicle-stimulating hormone (Pergonal) therapy during the first part of the cycle. We resort to progesterone or clomiphene therapy only if and when antibiotic therapy fails to restore the endometrial lining and the proper progesterone level.

Psychological Factors

It is the overall consensus of the medical literature that there is no firm scientific basis to assume that psychogenic factors lead to habitual abortion, and we share this observation.

Radiation, Drugs, and Environmental Pollutants

Radiation. Adequate studies are missing and obviously will not be available until serious nuclear accidents occur and follow-up studies are completed.

Drugs and Other Substances. These (e.g., cigarette smoking, alcohol abuse, and certain psychotropic drugs) have been associated with but not proved to cause spontaneous abortions.

Environmental Pollution. The cases under study are based on associations and projected causal connections without proper scientific evaluation of the data.

Anatomic Causes of Spontaneous Abortion

Uterine and cervical factors can lead to habitual abortion due to malformation of the Müllerian duct system. A wide variety of cases in which there is abnormal fusion of the two ducts have been described. Cases ranging from simple arcuation of the uterine body to complete duplication of the entire uterus and cervix have been seen. The spontaneous abortion usually takes place during the second trimester, when the intrauterine cavity becomes inadequate to support a growing fetus. There are surgical techniques describing the reconstruction of the anatomy to enlarge the uterine cavity to accommodate a full-size infant. In general, anatomic abnormalities account for less than 1 percent of the total number of habitual abortion cases.

Abnormalities of the cervix due to congenital factors can lead to incompetent cervix and typically to second trimester painless dilation followed by spontaneous delivery of a nonviable infant. Surgical procedures are available to correct the condition (Shirodkar or MacDonald).

A separate group of uterine abnormalities, associated with diethylstilbestrol exposure during intrauterine life, is described and documented through hysterosalpingography. These include a T-shaped uterus with a constricted cavity and cervical and tubal abnormalities. The overall surface area of the uterine lining is reduced when compared with that of a control group. Patients who were exposed to diethylstilbestrol while in utero have an overall increased incidence of pregnancy loss.

Uterine Myomata

Uterine fibroids are either subserosal, intramural, or submucosal. Subserosal or intramural fibroids do not endanger intrauterine pregnancy; however, submucosal fibroids lead to repeated losses because of the poor blood supply of the affected endometrium adjacent to the myoma. We do not routinely recommend myomectomies for habitual aborters unless we can document that the location of the myoma is submucosal.

Intrauterine Adhesions

In our experience, intrauterine adhesions are iatrogenic in a great majority of cases (the result of multiple dilation and curettage). A smaller proportion of such adhesions are caused by ascending infections. Both conditions prevent a newly formed lining from covering the anterior and posterior walls of the uterine cavity, and thus the denuded muscular walls will adhere. The condition more frequently leads to infertility than to habitual abortion.

Infections

Implicating infectious agents as the cause of habitual abortions is unfortunately complicated by the lack of properly controlled prospective studies. *We have become convinced during the last 10 years that the single best agent to interrupt a chain of spontaneous abortions is a course of broad-spectrum antibiotics.* Isolated studies in the literature implicate the following bacteria: *Chlamydia trachomatis, Mycoplasma hominis, Ureaplasma urealyticum, Listeria monocytogenes, Salmonella typhosa, Vibrio comma, Plasmodium,* and *Brucella.* The suspected viruses are herpes, cytomegalovirus, variola, and varicella. *Candida albicans* and *Toxoplasma gondii* also have been implicated. From our experience, we have added selective species of a score of anaerobic bacteria to the above list: *Actinomyces, Propionibacterium, Clostridium, Fusobacterium, Bacteroides, Acidaminococcus, Streptococcus,* and *Peptostreptococcus.*

The antibiotics we use cover for *Chlamydia trachomatis, Mycoplasma hominis, Ureaplasma urealyticum,* and a wide group of anaerobic bacteria. It is our belief that one miscarriage should be handled with the same serious care as three or more miscarriages. This view originates from the observation in our laboratory that if the seminal fluid or the endometrial biopsy specimen was found to be positive for any of the above-named bacteria, the pregnancy following a miscarriage without intervening antibiotic therapy had an extremely high chance of becoming a high-risk pregnancy with an unfavorable course, including both maternal and fetal complications. Antibiotics given after the first miscarriage for isolates we believed could be the cause yielded healthier subsequent pregnancies with much more viable fetuses. In our laboratory, the work-up of the habitual aborter is initiated with a meticulous bacterial screening of the male's seminal fluid and the female's endometrial biopsy specimen. No further test is proposed or administered until the implicated bacteria are eradicated with single or multiple antibiotic courses. Our experience shows that the genital flora is one of the most stubborn to be influenced by oral antibiotics. The regimen recommended by our laboratory is 4 to 6 weeks of broad-spectrum antibiotics, composed of doxycycline (Vibramycin), 100 mg three times a day, followed by erythromycin (E-Mycin), 333 mg four times a day, to cover the *Mycoplasma* and *Chlamydia* groups. If a repeat culture still reveals anaerobic bacteria, a course of metronidazole (Flagyl) is offered, 500 mg four times a day for 2 weeks. It is not uncommon for the therapy course to be extended for as long as 8 to 10 weeks in difficult cases. An initial publication from our laboratory shows that the length of antibiotic therapy is inversely related to the chance for a recurrent miscarriage. Not only were we able to reduce the number of miscarriage recurrences, but the outcome of pregnancies was proved to be superior in quality to the pregnancies that were conceived after one or more spontaneous abortions without antibiotic therapy. Larger infants with higher Apgar scores were born to those patients, and there were fewer perinatal maternal and fetal complications. In certain clinical situations in which oral antibiotics failed and the poor obstetric history justified it, our laboratory introduced ambulatory intravenous antibiotic treatment against anaerobic bacteria. The intravenous therapy is complemented with oral antibiotics. The dosage regimen consists of 1,800 mg of clindamycin, 160 mg of gentamicin given to the patient intravenously during office hours, and 200 mg of doxycycline taken in the evening. This regimen is carried out Monday through Friday for 2 consecutive weeks. We are impressed with the benefits of antibiotics not only in the treatment of first trimester losses, but also in managing second trimester incompetent cervices, and we use them as first-line drugs to stop premature labor. The drop in recurrent miscarriage rate in our series is complemented by an improved fetal outcome and markedly reduced maternal complications during the entire pregnancy.

For those patients whose habitual abortions cannot be solved through an anti-infectious approach, a complete preconceptional evaluation should be offered.

SUGGESTED READING

Rock JA, Zacur HA. The clinical management of repeated early pregnancy wastage. Fertil Steril 1983; 39:123–140.

Toth A, Lesser ML, Brooks-Toth CW, Feiner C. Outcome of subsequent pregnancies following antibiotic therapy after primary or multiple spontaneous abortion. Surg Gynecol Obstet 1986; 163:243–250.

TEENAGE PREGNANCY

PEGGY B. SMITH, Ph.D.
RAYMOND B. WAIT, M.D.
DAVID M. MUMFORD, M.D.

SCOPE OF THE PROBLEM

Data from the late 1970s and early 1980s suggest several contemporary trends concerning adolescent pregnancy and live births to teenagers. The absolute number of pregnant teens declined during this time and several related phenomena contributed to this trend. First, a general decline in the adolescent population contributed to a resulting decline in the number of pregnancies among this age group. The post-World War II baby boom peaked in 1957, and the number of American teenagers from ages 15 to 19 grew to 21.4 million in 1976. Since then, there has been a continuous decline to 18.4 million in 1985, with approximately 9.0 million girls and 9.4 million boys.

Moreover, *the availability of birth control and its more effective use among teens also has prevented conception.* Contraceptive use among unmarried, sexually active, adolescent girls increased steadily during the 1970s and then leveled off in the early 1980s. In 1982, approximately 85 percent of sexually active teenagers ages 15 to 19 reported that they had used a contraceptive method, compared with only approximately 66 percent in 1976 and nearly 73 percent in 1979. Concomitantly, the proportion reporting never using any method declined from more than 35 percent in 1976 to less than 15 percent in 1982. Abortion was also a factor in reducing the number of births although it was underutilized by this group. About 30 percent of all abortions performed in the United States each year involve teenagers. Many teens do not have access to abortion services, even though services have expanded dramatically in this country since 1973. In 1980, six percent of United States residents obtaining abortions did so outside their home towns. Teenagers traveled an average of 45 miles from home to obtain such services. In 1982, approximately 443,300 abortions were obtained by women under 20. An estimated 40 percent of all pregnancies of girls ages 15 to 19 end in abortion; among girls under 15, the number of abortions surpassed the number of births as early as 1974, and there are now 1.4 abortions for every live birth among girls in this age group. A resulting decline in the teen pregnancy rate has occurred from 272 births per 1,000 in 1972 for women aged 15 to 19 to 233 births per 1,000 to teens aged 15 to 19 in 1984.

Among those girls who become pregnant, very few, especially among the unmarried, intended the conception. Data from the major surveys indicate that 82 percent of these adolescent girls ages 15 to 19 did not intend to become pregnant, and 31 percent of this group reported that they were practicing a method of contraception.

PROGRAMMATIC INTERVENTION

A variety of primary, secondary, and tertiary programmatic intervention strategies funded from both the public and private sectors have been developed to intervene in the problem of teenage pregnancy. Although educational and community-based programs play a role in this effort, probably the most significant strategies involve a variation of the medical model, in the form of family planning services that include a range of reproductive health services, including pregnancy testing, prenatal care, testing for sexually transmitted diseases (STDs), and treatment, abortion, and sterilization services. The last two services are usually provided on a referral basis.

As utilization patterns for these reproductive clinics have increased among adolescents in the late 1970s and 1980s, several variations have evolved. Growing interest in primary prevention has generated an approach that recommends that reproductive and primary health services actually be housed directly on the middle and secondary school campuses. As a result, in the last 5 years approximately 50 communities have initiated such a health care model. The goals of such school-based models are directed at the overall physical and mental health of teenagers, but because of the incorporation of reproductive health services, many of these programs are sometimes subject to criticism from the conservative sector of the community.

Although initial evaluations indicate that these clinics are effective in maintaining contraceptive regimens and in reducing live births among teenagers, several aspects continue to make the assessment of such programs problematic. First, the reduction in live births cannot be unequivocally attributed to improved contraception rather than to effective utilization of abortion services. In addition, since most school-based clinics follow the school semester, they do not provide full-scale services during the summer vacation. Finally, limited formularies often do not stock any prescription items, so that adolescents must resort to filling prescriptions for treatment of sexually transmitted diseases (STD) and birth control at unsubsidized neighborhood drugstore prices.

MEDICAL ASPECTS

Since the early 1960s, the assessment of the medical consequences of teenage pregnancy continues to remain contradictory. Some studies suggest that the pregnant adolescent who is 16 years of age and under and her newborn are at risk for medical, social, and emotional complications. Other investigations suggest that the primary variable in the enhancement of perinatal outcome is the provision of early prenatal care independent of maternal age.

Reasons for the lack of adequate prenatal care vary. In some localities, especially in the rural South, prenatal care is simply not available. Some adolescents, operating under a "personal fable" approach, actually deny or ignore the pregnancy until the third trimester or the actual onset of labor. Administrative complexities of large public health institutions may also thwart adolescents from completing the requirements for prenatal care enrollment. For example, the currently enacted Medicaid Expansion Act, while broadening the levels of income eligibility, requires an adolescent to verify and produce data concerning her parents' financial status. Such a requirement is a complex and cumbersome deterrent to entering the maternity system. A pregnant teenager needs to enter the health care system with the least amount of delay, and verification of financial status should be secondary to the initiation of timely prenatal care. Financial arrangements can be completed once she is in the system and fortified by positive reinforcement, follow-up care, and emotional support.

The literature indicates that the major cause of poor birth outcome is preterm birth. Of all the preventable causes of perinatal loss, this has been one of the slowest to respond to intervention. It is currently hypothesized that at-risk adolescents can be effectively taught to identify the early signs of labor, allowing them to arrive at the emergency room in a timely manner so that tocolytic drugs can be administered to prevent the onset of active labor. Full-scale evaluations are currently under way. Preliminary results indicate mixed results of such interventions, especially in high-risk, indigent populations. In addition, like the effects of early prenatal care, such instructions may reinforce positive health practices, such as weight control or cessation of smoking, which have a more powerful effect on perinatal outcome.

SEXUALLY TRANSMITTED DISEASES

Although concern over acquired immunodeficiency syndrome has shifted national attention and funding priorities to human immunodeficiency virus (HIV), one must remember that other sexually transmitted diseases (STD), although not as deadly, are significant health problems for adolescents. The serious health problems caused by these diseases include pelvic inflammatory disease, infertility, ectopic pregnancy, adverse pregnancy outcomes, infant pneumonia, death, immune deficiencies, and cancer. The Centers for Disease Control estimates of the sexually transmitted diseases have increased to almost 13 million cases per year. More important for our focus, 65 percent of all STD cases occur in persons under the age of 25. An estimated 2.5 million teenagers are infected each year. Current estimates of incidence of STDs anticipate 4 million new cases of gonorrhea, 100,000 new cases of syphilis, 1 million new cases of venereal warts, and 500,000 new cases of genital herpes each year.

Historically, adolescents have been slow to come to clinics for STDs for treatment. Family planning clinics are strategically positioned to provide STD screening and treatment. Members of groups at high risk for STD (inner-city poor, minorities, and the young) are the predominant patients at these clinics. Although accessibility, continuity, and confidentiality are important characteristics of a clinic for effectively providing health services to teenagers, STD treatment at the same clinic site where the family planning services are also offered appears to contribute to a high treatment rate.

From a public health perspective, prevalence data on chlamydial infection among adolescents should encourage public health professionals to re-evaluate their position on the treatment of this infection. Chlamydial disease is as prevalent as gonorrhea in the adolescent population and is a significant cause of pelvic inflammatory disease. However, the diagnosis and treatment of this infection, especially in the public health sector, are not as aggressive as the protocols designed for gonorrhea. The consequence is that infected individuals remain in the sexually active pool much longer than those infected with gonorrhea. On average, the lapse time from diagnosis to test of cure for infection with *Chlamydia* is double that for gonorrhea.

The reported incidence of human papillomavirus infection of the external genitalia among teens has increased dramatically; 1983 data from the Centers for Disease Control show a 500 percent increase in the incidence of condyloma acuminatum from 1966 to 1981, based on the number of reported visits to private physicians. The number of consultations for this condition rose from 169,000 to 946,000 for men and women combined. Although dermatologists see the largest percentage of men, gynecologists see the largest percentage of women (54.4 percent), with more than 65 percent of the 946,000 consultations in patients aged 15 to 29 years.

NUTRITION

Many teenagers have poor eating habits that may worsen during pregnancy. Intensive nutritional counseling is mandatory, and special attention should be directed toward the unique dietary habits of different racial or ethnic groups. A caloric intake sufficient to produce a total weight gain of 24 to 28 lb during pregnancy is considered optimal. In general, the pregnant teenager requires intake of 45 kcal per kilogram of body weight per day. Restricted diets to control weight gain should be monitored carefully to ensure an adequate intake of protein and other essential nutrients. A minimum of 75 g of protein daily is needed to satisfy fetal and maternal requirements. Since many teenagers begin pregnancy with reduced iron stores, iron supplementation is re-

quired to provide 40 to 60 mg of ferrous iron daily during the last two trimesters of pregnancy. Most prenatal vitamin-mineral supplements provide sufficient iron, vitamins, and essential trace elements in a single daily dose, except for calcium. The average pregnant teenager needs 1.2 to 1.6 g of calcium daily. Since the usual prenatal capsule contains only 15 to 20 percent of the daily requirement, the additional calcium should be obtained from dairy products.

OBSTETRIC COMPLICATIONS

Obstetric complications are significantly higher in pregnant adolescents compared with patients in the 19- to 24-year-old group. These include problems such as increased weight, anemia, pre-eclampsia, prolonged labor, low birth weight infants, and a higher incidence of cesarean sections. However, careful analysis of most studies reveals that obstetric problems may be influenced more by socioeconomic factors than by age. In general, studies of pregnant adolescents have focused on single, poor, and undernourished girls who receive little or no prenatal care in a busy public health care facility that may not be sensitive to teen needs. On the other hand, control teenage groups and older teens have usually been married and of higher socioeconomic standing, and they have received better prenatal care from a private physician. When factors of race, prenatal care, and economic status are controlled in comparing groups, many authorities believe that the alleged obstetric differences between young teenagers and older patients disappear. As noted earlier, most complications apparently can be reduced to insignificant levels by better quality prenatal supervision. Two obstetric complications, pre-eclampsia and cephalopelvic disproportion, seem to persist in the pregnant adolescent (15 years of age) even with good prenatal care.

Some studies have reported twice as many infants under 2,500 g in the teenager as compared with the general population, whereas other investigations have shown no significant differences. Current thinking suggests that when sociodemographics are adequately controlled, differences in mean birth weight between various age groups become much less pronounced.

Unfortunately, certain groups of at-risk adolescents who most require prenatal care services are often reluctant to enroll. Hispanic teenage mothers are more likely to get prenatal care at a later stage of pregnancy than non-Hispanic mothers. National statistics show that in 1982, 24 percent of Hispanic mothers between the ages of 10 and 14 received no prenatal care until the third trimester of pregnancy or none at all, compared with 20 percent of 10- to 14-year-old black mothers. In the 15- to 19-year-old age group, similar patterns exist, with 17 percent of Hispanics receiving late or no care, compared with 10 percent of whites and 15 percent of blacks.

The literature suggests that people of low socioeconomic status and minority populations frequently have a different concept of illness and culturally different attitudes toward health behavior. Manifestations of these differences can take several forms. The poor, in particular, frequently ignore common symptoms of disease and illness. Symptoms such as chronic fatigue, excessive vaginal bleeding, and fainting spells generally are not considered important enough by low-income Mexican-Americans, for example, for them to seek medical care. This group may tend to consult a physician only when they have exhausted home remedies and the illness has become critical enough to interfere with their daily activities. A number of studies have concluded that self-treatment, or treatment within the family unit, is common among Hispanic women.

Many obstetric complications in teenagers are similar to those found in older patients. These include problems such as fetal malpresentations, third trimester bleeding, and postpartum hemorrhage. Medical disorders such as heart disease, diabetes, and thyroid dysfunction are no more common in the pregnant teenager than in the adult maternity patient.

POSTPARTUM CARE

There is no indication that the puerperium is more likely to be complicated in the adolescent than in the older patient. Endometritis, an infected episiotomy, and urinary tract infections are seen with equal frequency in the teenager and the adult.

One important aspect of postpartum care in the teenager is the opportunity to provide age-appropriate information about medically acceptable methods of contraception. Many teenage patients have never been instructed in correct contraceptive methods. The postpartum examination offers an excellent opportunity to provide such instruction. Once a patient maintains a contraceptive regimen for several months, she is more likely to continue.

In addition to contraception, the postpartum period offers a teenager the opportunity to begin a regimen of diagnostic and prophylactic medical care, including weight control, good nutrition, and effective sex hygiene that she may have never utilized prior to her pregnancy. Most important, the postpartum interval provides an opportunity to orient the young mother to her psychosocial and biomedical needs and those of her new infant.

CONTRACEPTIVE USE

The broad availability of birth control methods has been perceived as the complete answer to eliminating teenage pregnancy. However, patterns of adolescent contraceptive use suggest that significant cognitive and emotional barriers may confound birth control method implementation, even among the most motivated teens. Age seems to play an important role. The older the adolescent girl at the time of initiation of sexual activity, the more likely she is to use contraception and to use it regularly and effectively. In addition, the older the adolescent girl, the more likely she is to use a medical method, primarily the birth control pill. Younger girls more often report that they have never used contraception, in part because they have had less time to develop patterns of use. Younger girls are also more likely to be sporadic and ineffective contraceptive users, and they are more likely to rely on methods of their male partners. Estimates suggest that only 30 percent of sexually active females, ages 15 years and under, used contraception at last intercourse.

Concern that abortion may become a substitute for contraception is not supported by available data. In 1979,

teenagers who had terminated an unintended pregnancy by abortion were less likely to have experienced a second pregnancy within 2 years than those girls who carried their first pregnancy to term. Data from the National Center for Health Statistics suggest that about 12 percent of abortions in 15- to 17-year-olds and 22 percent of abortions in 18- to 19-year-olds are repeat abortions. Furthermore, clinic studies show that, 3 weeks following an abortion, less than 10 percent of girls were not using any method of contraception, whereas more than 80 percent were using the pill or intrauterine device.

MARRIAGE AND TEENAGE PREGNANCY

In spite of a recent leveling off in the absolute numbers of pregnant adolescents, concern about teen pregnancy has increased. An important trend in adolescent pregnancy is the increase in unmarried childbearing in this age group. In the early 1980s more than half of all births to adolescents occurred outside marriage, compared with only about one-third in 1970. In 1984 births to unmarried mothers under age 20 numbered more than 270,000. In addition, these trends are influenced by race. Blacks, as compared with certain ethnic groups, have more out-of-wedlock births. However, since 1970 there has been a sharp increase both in the number of pregnancies among white adolescents, and in the number of live births in this group. Older teenagers remained more likely than younger ones to marry in order to legitimate a birth. Between 1980 and 1984, on average, 26 percent of pregnant 15- to 17-year-olds married, compared with 35 percent of pregnant 18- to 19-year-olds and 43 percent of pregnant 20- to 24-year-olds. Nevertheless, as seen in 1984, the proportion of illegitimate births was more than twice as high among blacks than whites. This may reflect individual, community, and societal apprehensions about the social, medical, and financial costs and also the fact that many pregnant adolescents who remain single are locked in a cycle of poverty.

The single adolescent's choice between marriage or single parenthood is not easy. There is no question that a single female head of a household will earn only about 58 percent as much as the male head of a household and will not be able to provide her child with the additional emotional support and role modeling supplied by two parents and by a constant male figure in the home. On the other hand, many surveys suggest that "shotgun" marriages have significant shortcomings. Estimates suggest that 50 to 80 percent of all adolescent couples divorce or separate within the first 5 years of marriage. Under these circumstances, young wives usually have greater difficulty in re-entering school, completing vocational training, and achieving contraceptive compliance because the responsibilities of a home and a husband may take priority over educational and reproductive needs. Thus, adolescents who marry may actually have more difficulty controlling subsequent fertility than their single peers. Our own experience indicates a lesser motivation for family planning and subsequent clinic returns among the married adolescents compared with single girls. The married young women did not refill their birth control prescriptions as frequently and were more likely to experience a repeat pregnancy during the 12 months following delivery.

In addition, they were slower to finish school or vocational training.

FAMILY ROLE IN ADOLESCENT PREGNANCY

The family, whether by design or default, is the primary social-sexual model for the pregnant teenager to whom it conveys sexual attitudes and factual information. This conditioning includes special religious and moral codes, sexual role models, and social-sexual guidelines, including dating patterns, curfews, and in some cases, sexual practices.

The sexual rules, models, and frequent knowledge gaps of the teenager may contribute indirectly to the occurrence of conception. In our experience the most common site for sex leading to conception is in the girl's home during the afternoon. Medical personnel can suggest ways that the family can address the ineffective sexual guidelines previously transmitted and can encourage emotional and financial family support for the adolescent. Communication between the teenager and the family should be fostered whenever possible. Prior to the actual birth of the child, the family should be encouraged to enroll the adolescent in a prenatal clinic. Practitioners should attempt to involve parents in the prenatal care process early, so that medical care can be provided in the first trimester and continued into the postpartum period, emotional support can be given, and financial arrangements can be made for the young mother's needs.

Once the baby is born, the family often becomes a prime element in day-care provision. Many adolescents are unable to secure adequate child care facilities without the family's help. Support services are crucial in the early months of the infant's life. Immediate family care for the infant may allow adolescents to complete an academic year and to minimize the risk of permanent school drop-out. Such services from family members are not without trade-offs or risks, however. In an effort to help the teenager, families may wittingly or unwittingly usurp her parental prerogatives. Thus, the daily routine and health care needs are determined not by the infant's biological mother but by her parents. Such support systems may trap the younger mother within her family unit, limiting her ultimate independence. In extreme cases, the infant may be given temporarily to other family members in a foster care situation. The family and health professional should be aware of the young mother's need to achieve her own parenting status and independence and to complete her educational or vocational requirements.

SUGGESTED READING

Bachrach CA. Contraceptive practice among American women. Fam Plann Perspect 1984; 16:253–259.

Bureau of the Census. Population estimates and projections. Current population reports, Series P-25, No. 965, 917. Washington DC: US Department of Commerce, 1980.

Dryfoos JG. Prevention strategies: A progress report. Report to the Rockefeller Foundation. New York: Rockefeller Foundation, 1984.

Edwards L, Steinman M, Arnold K, Hakanson E. Adolescent pregnancy prevention services in high school clinics. Fam Plann Perspect 1980; 12:6–14.

Hayes CD, ed. Risking the future adolescent. Sexuality, pregnancy, and childbearing. Washington DC: National Academy Press, 1987.

Koenig MA, Zelnik M. The risk of premarital first pregnancy among metropolitan-area teenagers: 1976 and 1979. Fam Plann Perspect 1982; 14:239–248.

Smith PB. Sociologic aspects of adolescent fertility and childbearing among Hispanics. J Dev Behav Pediatr 1986; 7:346–349.

Smith PB, McGill L, Wait RB. Hispanic adolescent conception and contraception profiles—a comparison. J Adolesc Health Care 1987; 8:352–355.

Smith PB, Nenney SW, McGill L. Health problems and sexual activity of selected inner city, middle school students. J Sch Health 1986; 56:263–266.

Smith PB, Wait RB. Adolescent fertility and childbearing trends among Hispanics in Texas. Tex Med 1986; 82:29–32.

Zelnik M, Shah FK. First intercourse among young Americans. Fam Plann Perspect 1983; 15:64–72.

SPECIFIC CLINICAL ENTITIES

ADVANCED MATERNAL AGE

ALAN M. PEACEMAN, M.D.
ROBERT K. CREASY, M.D.

The vast majority of pregnancies occur in the middle portion of the time between menarche and menopause. Over the past decade, however, increasing attention has been paid in the literature, both lay and medical, to the pregnancies of women toward the end of their reproductive years. Much controversy has been stirred as to the implications, risks, and benefits of conceiving at an older age for the woman herself, her family, and society at large. Although the scope of this issue includes psychological, social, and economic aspects, our discussion is limited to the medical aspects of advanced maternal age.

Many names have been used in the past in reference to these women, including postmature, premenopausal, and elderly gravidas. In an effort to avoid a negative connotation or bias, we prefer the term advanced maternal age. By convention, this designation is usually defined as a maternal age of 35 years or older at the time of delivery, but this is obviously an arbitrary assignment. The National Center for Health Statistics data show that in 1985, approximately 6.5 percent of all births in the United States occurred in women aged 35 or older, but in some populations this percentage approaches 10 percent.

The reason that advanced maternal age during pregnancy has become more of an issue in recent years is that it is becoming more common. In the United States, according to the Census Bureau, there has been an increase in the absolute number of women between ages 35 and 44 from 11,856,569 in 1970 to an estimated 16,136,000 in 1985, as well as an increase in the number of births to women in this age group from 230,196 to 242,670 over this same period. Although women of lower socioeconomic status are turning more toward permanent sterilization at younger ages, women of higher socioeconomic levels are postponing having their families for reasons that include career, financial and education opportunities, and control over fertility, all of which are more available today.

Certain risks arise when a woman postpones her family. First, it must be recognized that a couple's fertility decreases as their ages increase. Furthermore, those with underlying fertility problems are not being recognized at early ages, so that therapies to correct them have time constraints. Second, obstetricians have long recognized the increased rates of complications among older gravidas and their fetuses. Although the fertility aspect is important, this discussion is confined to the assessment and management of advanced maternal age pregnancies.

When examining the effects of advancing maternal age on pregnancy outcome, it is important to try to separate out confounding variables. Such things as underlying disease, gravidity, length of infertility, and previous surgery all are more common in a group of patients at older ages and can influence outcome statistics independently. Therefore, in trying to assess the age factor alone for any particular pregnancy outcome, these underlying issues must be controlled for.

Spontaneous Abortions. Most studies on the subject show increased risk for spontaneous abortion with increasing maternal age. The amount of increased risk is unclear because of the difficulties in study designs. The rate of spontaneous loss of recognized pregnancies probably does not exceed 20 percent for women between 35 and 40 years of age and may be somewhat higher at age 40 or older. This is not much above what many experts quote for all age groups.

Chromosomal Abnormalities. Increased incidences of chromosomal aberrations have been associated with advanced maternal age for many years. This is true in spontaneous abortions and stillbirths as well as in live borns. Data collected by different testing techniques are now available for counseling patients as to their specific age-related risk of carrying a fetus with a cytogenetic abnormality (Table 1). As opposed to other complications in which it is unclear whether advancing age is a cause or a cofactor, chromosomal aberrations are directly related to increased maternal age. This is thought to be due to increased rates of nondisjunction in older eggs during meiosis. Prenatal testing by amniocentesis has been available in the United States for over a decade and is now offered to all patients over age 35 and to those who have had a previous offspring with a chromosomal aberration. Also, the recent finding of an association between a low maternal serum alpha-fetoprotein level and Down syndrome in the offspring has brought the determination of these levels into the calculation of risk of an affected fetus. Nevertheless, the majority of live-born infants with chromosomal abnormalities occur in women under age 35 who have no risk factors. The current prenatal testing scheme aimed at women of advanced maternal age therefore misses up to 70 percent of these infants. A recent study by Benacerraf and colleagues reported that an ultrasound screening test looking for a thickened nuchal skin fold or a relatively shortened femur measurement at 15 to 21 weeks' gestation might be an accurate predictor of trisomy 21 syndrome in a fetus. With the sensitivity set at 75 percent, the specificity is 98 percent. If this is true not only for their population but for all women, even those under age 35, the majority of trisomy 21 fetuses could be detected in the middle trimester if this testing scheme were implemented. Also, normal ultrasound screening in women over age 35 might make the possibility of a trisomy 21 fetus so remote that amniocentesis for cytogenetic studies would not be indicated. At present, however, this screening tool is still investigational, and further studies are needed to confirm its clinical usefulness. In the meantime, genetic counseling and amniocentesis should still be offered to all women aged 35 or over.

Underlying Maternal Disease. Women are much more likely to be diagnosed as having hypertension, diabetes, cardiovascular disease, and renal disease as they approach the middle of the fourth decade of life. All these conditions are associated with a marked increase in the perinatal complication rate. Because outcome is directly related to the severity of the underlying disorder and the ability to control it, it is imperative to identify and treat patients with these conditions when appropriate. Attention must be paid to screening techniques in the older population, who are more likely to have positive test findings. This includes a strict protocol for testing for glucose intolerance at several times during the pregnancy.

Perinatal Mortality Rates. Almost all studies show a two- to fourfold increase in the perinatal mortality rate for women over 35 as compared with women aged 20 to 29, even after correction for lethal anomalies. This is attributable more to an increased rate of stillbirths than to neonatal losses. However, in general, these studies have not corrected for underlying maternal disease, and data from low-risk pregnancies (those without underlying maternal diseases) have generally failed to show an increase in the perinatal mortality rate with increasing age. Although further study is necessary, what may indeed be true is that the elevated rate may come almost entirely from the higher incidence of high-risk patients with advancing age, and older patients without underlying disease may be at no higher risk of perinatal loss.

Maternal Mortality. Data compiled from United States statistics for 1968 to 1975 showed a strong relationship between advanced maternal age and risk of maternal death. As compared with pregnant women aged 25 to 29, pregnant women aged 35 to 39 had a mortality rate four times as high (60.0 per 100,000 live births), and women aged 40 to 44 almost eight times as high (102.2 per 100,000 live births). More recent figures from the National Center for Health Statistics for 1983, however, have demonstrated a significant reduction in the maternal mortality rate as advances in diagnosis, eduction, and treatment have become more available. The maternal mortality rates per 100,000 live births for women aged 35 to 39 and 40 to 44 dropped to 20.0 and 27.0, respectively. Since the risk of mortality will never be completely eliminated from complicated pregnancies, those conditions which predispose maternal medical complications—such as advanced maternal age—will always have a mortality rate higher than that of the general population. Most likely, age is not a direct factor in mortality other than by increasing the chances of underlying disease. Women over 35 who have no medical problems may not be at any increased risk of maternal mortality compared with their younger counterparts.

Pre-eclampsia. Many studies have looked at the relationship between increasing maternal age and risk for pre-eclampsia. Although some conflicting data exist, the majority of reports support a positive association. However, the counterargument stating that this is not a reflec-

TABLE 1 Estimated Rates of Cytogenetic Abnormalities by Maternal Age

Maternal Age (At Time of Procedure/Delivery)	Rate of Detection of Cytogenetic Abnormalities (Excluding Balanced Rearrangements and Mosaics)	
	1st Trimester (Chorionic Villus Sampling)	2nd Trimester (Amniocentesis)
35	1/112	1/140
36	1/85	1/111
37	1/65	1/88
38	1/49	1/70
39	1/37	1/56
40	1/28	1/44
41	1/22	1/35
42	1/16	1/28
43	1/12	1/22
44	1/9	1/18
45	1/7	1/14
46	1/5	1/11

Adapted from handout supplement to Hook EB, Cross PK, Jackson LG, et al. Rates of 47, +21 and other cytogenetic abnormalities diagnosed in first trimester chorionic villus samples: comparison with rates from second trimester amniocentesis. Am J Hum Genet 1987; 41(Suppl):A276.

tion of age but rather an underlying vascular disorder is hard to refute. Nevertheless, it is clear that when pre-eclampsia occurs in older gravidas, the perinatal mortality rate is much higher than in their younger counterparts with pre-eclampsia. Older mothers should therefore be observed more closely in the third trimester for signs of pre-eclampsia, and those with the diagnosis should be managed aggressively.

Premature Labor. Increasing maternal age is usually associated with an increase in rates of premature birth. Once again, some conflicting reports have been published, but most of the literature supports a two- to threefold increase in preterm birth rates among women over age 35 as compared with women in their twenties. What is known is that the nulliparous female aged 35 to 39 is at the highest risk for preterm labor of any 5-year age bracket. On the other hand, the multiparous woman in this age bracket with no other risk factors for preterm labor is at one of the lowest risks for preterm delivery. In women over 35 having their first child, early signs and symptoms of premature labor must be searched for and acted on to try to avoid this frequent complication.

Abnormal Labor. After controlling for parity, most studies do not find a significant change in the course of labor with advancing maternal age. There are reports of slightly lengthened second stages, more dysfunctional labor patterns, and an increased incidence of protraction disorders with advancing age, but these findings are not consistent from study to study. What is universally found, however, is an increasing cesarean section rate with advancing maternal age. Some of this can be attributed to the performance of repeat cesarean sections. Even in the primigravida populations, however, the rate is anywhere from two to 10 times as high for women over age 35 as compared with those in their twenties. This increased operative delivery rate cannot be explained solely on the basis of labor abnormalities in the older age group. Most likely, increased cesarean rates reflect all of the following: increased intervention for underlying maternal disease and the resultant fetal compromise, high rates of repeat cesarean sections, some increased incidence of labor abnormalities with age, and physicians' tendencies to intervene earlier with operative delivery in older patients.

MANAGEMENT OF PREGNANCY IN PATIENTS OVER AGE 35

In most aspects, the management of the patient over age 35 is not much different from that of the younger patient. We make an effort at the first prenatal visit to assign an accurate gestational age, and counseling is given in regard to nutrition, exercise, and avoidance of teratogens and unprescribed drugs. A careful history is taken to try to elicit any history of underlying medical diseases, and the physical examination is as thorough as in any prenatal patient. Screening for glucose intolerance is performed at the first visit, and abnormalities are followed up promptly with a full 3-hour glucose tolerance test.

The patient over age 35 is also given information about genetic amniocentesis at the first visit so that appropriate planning and discussion can take place prior to 16 weeks' gestation. The patient is told of her age-specific risk for detection of chromosomal abnormalities and of her choices in the event that an abnormality is found. She is also counseled as to the risks of second trimester amniocentesis. For those who choose to have the procedure, an amniotic fluid alpha-fetoprotein level is determined as well, and a full ultrasound examination is performed, including biometry and a scan for congenital defects in the cardiac, neural tube, and gastrointestinal systems. We do not routinely recommend chorionic villus sampling for chromosome analysis in patients under 40 years of age, unless the patient has a prior affected offspring or carries a genetic condition that can be detected by this procedure. For the patient who declines chromosome testing of her fetus, a notation is made on the chart that she was offered the procedure. These patients are then encouraged to have maternal serum alpha-fetoprotein determinations at 16 to 18 weeks' gestation. Ultrasound examinations are performed at 16 to 20 weeks' gestation on all women with underlying maternal disease as a baseline for comparison, as these women are at increased risk for fetal growth abnormalities.

As the pregnancy of the advanced maternal age patient progresses, careful and frequent surveillance is maintained in those with underlying disease. Glucose tolerance is rechecked at least twice more, at the end of the second trimester and in the middle third trimester. Because of the increased risk of preterm birth in nulliparous women over age 35, these patients are also instructed to watch for signs and symptoms of preterm labor and to report any abnormal findings promptly.

Many patients ask about the specific risks and dangers of pregnancy after age 35. All patients are told of the increased risk of chromosomal anomalies and that there may be a slightly increased risk of spontaneous first trimester abortion. Also explained are the increased chances of finding gestational diabetes and of preterm labor. Those patients with underlying diseases, such as hypertension or diabetes, are counseled that their risks for perinatal mortality are much lower than they were 20 years ago but that they are still much higher than those of the general population. Those patients without underlying disease who have normal chromosomal studies and glucose tolerance tests are told that good perinatal outcome is as likely as in the general population. As long as signs and symptoms of preterm labor do not arise, these patients are encouraged to continue their normal activities and enjoy their pregnancies. All women of advanced maternal age, however, are cautioned that labor abnormalities may be more frequent and that the chances of a cesarean delivery are increased.

SUGGESTED READING

Benacerraf BR, Gelman R, Frigoletto FD. Sonographic identification of second-trimester fetuses with Down's syndrome. N Engl J Med 1987; 317:1371-1376.

Hansen JP. Older maternal age and pregnancy outcome: a review of the literature. Obstet Gynecol Surv 1986; 41:726.

Kirz DS, Dorchester W, Freeman RK. Advanced maternal age: the mature gravida. Am J Obstet Gynecol 1985; 152:7-12.

Martel M, Wacholder S, Lippman A, et al. Maternal age and primary cesarean section rates: a multivariate analysis. Am J Obstet Gynecol 1987; 156:305-308.

ASTHMA IN PREGNANCY

PAUL A. GREENBERGER, M.D.

Uncontrolled asthma during gestation has been associated with maternal and fetal mortality and other complications, such as intrauterine growth retardation; conversely, when repeated episodes of acute asthma are avoided, maternal and fetal outcomes can approximate those seen in gravidas who do not have asthma. The goals of therapy during management of the gravida with asthma are to avoid repeated episodes of acute bronchospasm, emergency room visits and hospitalizations, nocturnal dyspnea, and daily persistent wheezing from asthma. Pharmacotherapy utilized to achieve these goals should be appropriate for the gravida and not harmful for the fetus. The medical literature does not provide information predicting which gravidas with asthma will have improved, unchanged, or worsened severity of asthma during gestation.

Perhaps the most important physiologic alteration in normal pregnancy that is relevant to management of asthma is that the physiologic hyperventilation of pregnancy results in a maternal arterial Pco_2 of 30 to 32 mm Hg, such that the pH increases to about 7.44. In some gravidas without asthma, the Po_2 increases from 90 mm Hg to 100 mm Hg or more. Minute ventilation, which is the product of tidal volume (the volume of air expired during resting ventilation), and respiratory rate may increase by as much as 50 percent. Airway resistance is not thought to change significantly during gestation in the absence of episodes of asthma. During the initial response to acute bronchospasm, the gravida hyperventilates. In that she already has a higher baseline respiratory status than when she is not gravid, her capacity to hyperventilate further may be limited. It is possible that she may have less pulmonary reserve to compensate for the acute bronchospastic event. Thus, she may be more likely to develop alveolar hypoventilation as she "fatigues" during an attack of asthma. This scenario is hypothetical, although it appears to occur in a number of women who come to the hospital with uncontrolled asthma. In any event, try to reverse the acute attack promptly in order to avoid the potential adverse effects of maternal hypoxemia and hypocarbia (which, if marked, may decrease uterine blood flow) or of hypercarbia (which requires transfer of the gravida to the intensive care unit).

PRIOR PLANNING REGARDING MANAGEMENT OF GRAVIDAS WITH ASTHMA

It is advisable to have established previously where in the hospital the gravida will be treated, depending on the severity of the asthma. For example, when hospitalization is indicated in our hospital, all gravidas (even in the first trimester) are admitted to the obstetrics floor and the medical service responsible for ambulatory asthma management is consulted. The logistics of providing unin-terrupted maternal-fetal assessment are preserved. Conversely, when a gravida presents with asthma of such severity that evidence of alveolar hypoventilation is present (Pco_2 in the high 30s or higher), she is transferred to the medical intensive care unit and the obstetrics service is consulted. All physicians involved in the management of gravidas with life-threatening episodes of asthma should determine at what point, if any, a gravida who experiences a respiratory arrest from asthma should have an emergency cesarean section. Fortunately, intervention of this magnitude is uncommon but should be considered whenever a gravida with asthma requires admission to the medical intensive care unit for respiratory failure.

INITIAL ASSESSMENT OF THE ACUTELY DYSPNEIC GRAVIDA

As in any case of acute asthma, one needs to determine the severity of the current episode quickly. The literature contains many investigations of various parameters for evaluation, but controversy remains. Overall clinical assessment should be the initial task. Is there cyanosis, exhaustion, inability to speak more than a few words, or marked dyspnea?

The physical examination includes attention to the observations noted in Table 1. Systolic and diastolic hypertension may occur during acute severe bronchospasm, but following effective emergency therapy the blood pressure returns to baseline values. Similarly, tachycardia (which when greater than 120 beats per minute has been associated with hypoxemia) usually subsides when the acute episode of asthma has been relieved. These two observations are important, since at times one may be tempted to withhold epinephrine in the presence of hypertension or tachycardia during acute severe asthma. I recommend reversing the acute event with epinephrine subcutaneously, which provides beta-adrenergic–mediated bronchodilation and a decrease in tachycardia, hypertension, and tachypnea. Pulsus paradoxus is a danger sign that reflects that the hyperinflation of lung volumes (air trapping) and severe airways obstruction. Similarly, the presence of severe wheezing with marked dyspnea or decreased breath sounds is evi-

TABLE 1 Physical Findings in Severe Asthma

Physical findings often associated with severe asthma
  Labored respirations over 30 breaths per minute
  Pulse rate over 120 beats per minute
  Hypertension
  Pulsus paradoxus
  Use of accessory muscles of respiration
  Decreased breath sounds
  Inability to speak a complete sentence

Physical findings suggesting immediate hospitalization
  Cyanosis
  Po_2 <70 mm Hg
  Pco_2 >38 mm Hg
  Electrocardiographic abnormalities
  Subcutaneous emphysema
  Dyspnea such that only a few words can be spoken
  Fetal distress

dence for a severe asthma attack that should necessitate hospitalization.

The arterial blood gas measurements provide valuable data regarding the extent of alveolar hypoventilation (elevation of Pco_2) and hypoxemia. A scheme for arterial blood gas staging that I have found useful is presented in Table 2. The pertinent information in the initial assessment of the acutely wheezing gravida might best include overall assessment as above, blood pressure with a check for paradoxical pulse, pulse rate, respiration rate, use of accessory muscles of respiration, and examination of the thorax, chest, and heart. The heart may be difficult to examine well in the presence of wheezes or rhonchi. The history may be limited, as the gravida cannot provide lengthy answers to queries as to why and when the acute deterioration appeared to have started. This information may be obtained after acute therapy has relieved some of the dyspnea.

In questioning the gravida regarding triggers of the acute attack, several observations about asthma should be kept in mind. First, asthma is often chronic and not acute; hence, chronic airways obstruction and lung hyperinflation may well have preceded the acute deterioration. Second, one's perception of dyspnea may be altered by gestation; however, it is known that for many nongravidas with asthma, no symptoms are noted until the forced vital capacity is reduced to below 60 percent of that predicted. Third, any gravida who has received emergency therapy for asthma in the last 7 to 14 days on more than two occasions might best be hospitalized immediately upon recurrence.

Although the aerosol route for administration of beta-adrenergic agonists is preferred by some, it provides no greater bronchodilation than subcutaneous epinephrine (0.3 ml of 1:1,000 solution). Doses of epinephrine can be repeated twice at 20-minute intervals. Advantages of subcutaneous epinephrine include (1) ready availability, (2) apparent safety over years of use in pregnancy, and (3) administration of an endogenous chemical. The fear of potential untoward systemic effects from subcutaneous epinephrine has prompted many physicians to administer drugs by the inhaled route. Potential disadvantages of this approach are a possible delay in administration of beta-adrenergic agonists, the cost of respiratory treatments, and the potential dilemma of utilizing pharmacologic agents that have not been demonstrated to be appropriate (or inappropriate) for administration during gestation. If the gravida has not improved markedly after epinephrine, in-

travenous aminophylline or theophylline can be administered, as can corticosteroids.

Regarding methylxanthine therapy, inquire as to when the last dose of theophylline was ingested. The widespread use of long-acting theophyllines emphasizes the need for caution, in order not to over-load the patient who only 3 hours previously ingested a 12-hour theophylline tablet. First, determine when the last dose of theophylline was ingested and consider when the drug is supposed to deliver its peak quantity. It may be helpful to obtain a serum theophylline concentration; a low concentration implies noncompliance in most cases. As a rule, if any 12-hour theophylline tablets have been consumed in the last 12 hours, do not administer the usual loading dose of 5.6 mg per kilogram of aminophylline over 20 minutes. Considering that in the management of acute asthma, theophylline may not be as valuable as beta-adrenergic agonists, one should administer either no theophylline or only a continuous infusion of 0.5 mg per kilogram per hour (lean body weight) until the effects of previously ingested theophylline have been clarified. Occasionally, just as the acutely dyspneic gravida may overuse her beta-adrenergic agonist inhaler and delay appropriate therapy, she may take additional 12- or 24-hour theophylline tablets that may be absorbed in the hours after reaching the hospital. Some drugs or conditions that alter theophylline elimination are listed in Table 3.

If the gravida has not improved after two injections of epinephrine, it is advisable to consider theophylline as discussed and also to administer oral corticosteriods. Although cortisone acetate has been shown to produce cleft palates in rodents when administered in very high doses during gestation, increasing experience with humans has confirmed that corticosteroids are appropriate and not harmful to the fetus or gravida. Depending on the improvement that has been achieved, either the gravida should be discharged to be examined on an ambulatory basis or she should be hospitalized. If she is discharged after receiving two or more injections of epinephrine, prednisone is administered in a dose of 40 to 60 mg per day until she can be re-evaluated in 3 to 7 days. This dose is sufficient to avoid most repeated visits to the emergency area. The fetus should be evaluated by physicians managing the pregnancy before the gravida is released from emergency care. Should initial therapy with epinephrine and theophylline

TABLE 2 Arterial Blood Gas Abnormalities by Stage

Stage	Po_2	Pco_2	pH	Comment
I	→	↓	↑	
II	↓	↓	↑	Typical findings in the emergency room
III	↓	→	→	Alveolar hypoventilation
IV	↓	↑	↓	Respiratory acidosis

→ = within normal limits; ↓ = decreased; ↑ = increased.

TABLE 3 Some Factors Affecting Theophylline Clearance

Increased clearance
  Smoking
  Phenytoin

Decreased clearance
  Congestive heart failure
  Hepatic diseases
  Severe attacks of asthma
  Acute pneumonia
  Macrolide antibiotics
  Cimetidine
  Viral respiratory infections

prove inadequate to reverse the acute episode, hospitalization is indicated, at which time hydrocortisone can be administered at a dose of 200 mg every 4 to 6 hours. Methylprednisolone may be administered instead of hydrocortisone in a dose of 40 to 50 mg every 4 to 6 hours. Arterial blood gas monitoring should be utilized. Supplemental oxygen is recommended as indicated by the arterial blood gas measurements.

An attempt should be made to determine the initiating factor or factors that resulted in need for emergency therapy for asthma. Some causes include (1) IgE-mediated factors such as animal exposure, (2) upper respiratory infections, (3) ingestion of aspirin or other nonsteroidal anti-inflammatory drug, even chewing gum containing aspirin, (4) exposure to fresh paint, (5) noncompliance with physician advice or appointments on an ambulatory basis, (6) occupational exposures, and (7) the "I will be better tomorrow syndrome" in which the patient continues to self-medicate, despite lack of improvement.

MANAGEMENT OF CHRONIC ASTHMA ON AN AMBULATORY BASIS

Management should be on an individual basis, with step-wise increments in pharmacotherapy. Attempts should be made to elicit IgE-mediated causes of asthma which, once identified, may indicate avoidance measures that can reduce the need for medication. Obviously, as little medication as possible should be administered, but one must appreciate the potential untoward effects of repeated episodes of acute asthma or chronic asthma that are associated with maternal hypoxemia or hypocarbia that may decrease uterine-placental blood oxygen delivery. Some general measures to insist on include (1) no smoking, recreational drug use, or ethanol ingestion, (2) avoidance (removal) of animals at home that are triggers of bronchospasm, and (3) communication between physician and gravida when there is a significant change in respiratory status. A list of medications considered appropriate for use throughout gestation is presented in Table 4. For initial pharmacotherapy of mild chronic asthma, theophylline, at a dose of 300 mg every 12 hours, is administered. Some physicians and patients prefer inhaled beta-adrenergic agonists instead of theophylline. A dilemma exists because these newer agents do not have published data to support their use. A cautious approach would be to use either epinephrine by inhalation or ephedrine 25 mg orally up to four times a day. If theophylline is inadequate therapy and beta-adrenergic agonists are either not tolerated or ineffective when used

TABLE 4 Therapeutic Modalities Considered Appropriate for Use During Gestation

Theophylline
Aminophylline
Cromolyn
Ephedrine
Epinephrine

Prednisone
Prednisolone
Methylprednisolone
Hydrocortisone
Beclomethasone dipropionate

Penicillin derivatives
Erythromycin
Influenza immunization in second or third trimester
Allergen immunotherapy (trees, grasses, weeds, dust, mold)

Some therapeutic modalities without published reports regarding use during gestation.*

Albuterol
Metaproterenol
Terbutaline
Fenoterol

* In the absence of experience during gestation, these drugs are not prescribed.

with theophylline, an inhaled corticosteroid such as beclomethasone dipropionate (2 to 4 inhalations up to four times a day) may be added. Some patients who are not wheezing may be given a trial of cromolyn (two inhalations three to four times a day) instead of beclomethasone dipropionate.

Acute exacerbations of chronic asthma may occur in the presence of upper respiratory infections. When the gravida develops dyspnea with significant wheezing in the presence of a viral infection, she may no longer be adequately managed with the regimen that has proved successful on an ambulatory basis. A short effective course of prednisone, such as 30 to 60 mg daily given as a single morning dose for 4 to 7 days, usually results in resolution of the signs and symptoms of asthma, at which time the gravida may continue her "chronic" medications without systemic corticosteroids. In many cases, this recommendation prevents the need for emergency therapy or hospitalization.

Supported by USPHS Grant AI 11403 and the Ernest S. Bazley Grant.

BREECH PRESENTATION

KJELL R.M. BARLÖV, M.D.

As a member of the staff at Danderyd Hospital, Stockholm (4,000 deliveries per year), at the beginning of the 1970s I had the opportunity to work with Björn Westin, an exceedingly talented and creative obstetrician. At the annual meeting of the Swedish Society of Obstetrics and Gynecology in 1974 at Växjö, Westin presented a program for selecting pregnant women with breech presentations into groups for vaginal delivery or for cesarean section, respectively.

In my post as head of the Obstetrics Department at the Central Hospital, Karlskrona, from 1976 to 1983, I sometimes found myself saying to a pregnant woman whose baby was in the breech presentation, "You can give birth to your baby in breech presentation as easily as in vertex presentation," and, in so saying this instantly felt what I will call an obstetric anxiety. But in a 5-year prospective study (1977 to 1982) on term singleton breech delivery after uncomplicated pregnancy, I found that 45 percent of the mothers were delivered vaginally without any perinatal mortality or persistent morbidity.

This chapter deals with my personal methods for handling pregnancies and deliveries in the breech presentation.

There are a number of different causes of breech presentation. Even Hippocrates described different positions of the fetus in the womb and felt that the fetus always stayed in the breech presentation until the seventh month, after which it turned to vertex presentation—"the fetal somersault of Hippocrates." Today we know that about 3 percent of all fetuses are in breech presentation in the last part of the third trimester. Many reasons for this fact have been proposed. Even today, however, we do not fully understand why most fetuses are in vertex presentation at the time of birth (possibly gravitation or accommodation). A list of causes of breech presentation usually includes preterm delivery, placenta previa, hydrocephalus, contracted pelvis, pelvic tumors, and hereditary factors. Dunn suggested that the mobility of the fetus was impaired by the extension of the fetus' legs that occurs in breech presentation, and that the extended legs may relate to impaired mobility of the lower limbs caused by myelomeningocele or some other neuromuscular disease. It can be said that anything that alters the shape of the uterine cavity or the mobility of the fetus may produce a breech presentation.

The so-called intrinsic characteristics of the breech presentation are, among others, preterm delivery, low birth weight, multiple pregnancy, low placental implantation, and uterine and fetal abnormalities. These factors may contribute to the somewhat higher perinatal mortality and morbidity associated with breech delivery. It should be noted that the frequency of congenital malformations for fetuses in breech lie is three times higher than that for fetuses in vertex lie. Therefore when the fetus is in breech presenta-tion, there should be many reasons for alert bells ringing in your mind.

The pregnancy and delivery must be subjected to a total assessment. I call this process "a whole situation analysis," and it involves *all* parameters: medicobiologic, psychological, and social. The Westin scoring system is the basic instrument I use. Also of importance is the future parents' sense of confidence in their future role as mother and father. Most important of all may be the way in which the physician handles the situation. We have the possibility to guide the decision-making process to the point where we want it, but we must listen intently to the human beings we have in front of us. When we, as professionals, have true confidence in ourselves, the couple will recognize that fact and will be secure in their final decision. As a physician you must have both the future parents and the staff on your side whatever is decided. Otherwise, the complication rate will increase.

As a specialist you know the specific problems associated with breech delivery. You know that the largest part of the fetus, the unmolded head, is delivered last, which may contribute to tentorial tears and intracranial hemorrhage. You know the increased risk of umbilical cord prolapse and that a double footling presentation may promote these two complications (the fetus with double footling presentation should be delivered by cesarean section). You know that the arms of the fetus may be retracted over the head, especially when you are forced to extract the baby for whatever reason. You know that the head of the fetus may be hyperextended. (Ultrasound or radiologic examination must be done at the beginning of the labor and cesarean section must be performed if the fetus is "star-gazing".) You know that delivery trauma and asphyxia are the most important causes of increased mortality and morbidity.

However, if you use the whole situation analysis method I am advocating, you will be able to select that mother with breech presentation to whom you can confidently say, "You can give birth to your baby in breech presentation as easily as in vertex presentation." This is, perhaps, a rash statement, but recent experience supports my contentions.

In about 45 percent of cases it is possible to identify the woman with breech presentation who can give birth vaginally without any more increased infant mortality or persistent morbidity beyond what would be expected at any vaginal delivery. Different screening protocols have been worked out for this purpose. The scoring system I use has been presented by Björn Westin. It takes into consideration maternal pelvic data, the estimated weight of the fetus (determined by ultrasound examination and palpation), the soft parts of the delivery canal (e.g., the fat pads inside the pelvis, keeping an eye on the mother's weight), the ripening of the cervix, the condition of the muscular pelvic floor, the type of breech presentation, and the previous obstetric history. Moreover, I take into serious consideration the general physical and mental condition of the mother, her regard for her own body, pregnancy, and future motherhood, her relation to her husband (can he be of help?) and her relationship with us, the staff in the delivery department. I do not limit myself to figures representing centimeters in the pelvis or weights but try to make a whole situation analysis.

When I meet the mother with her fetus in breech presentation in the 36th week of pregnancy, I talk with her about the delivery. During this discussion we talk about the different ways of delivery, vaginal or cesarean section, and even mention the possibility of external cephalic version. I also try to find out her attitude toward her pregnancy and delivery and emphasize that at this point we cannot yet decide the final mode of delivery in her special case. We have to know more—to gather more facts.

Therefore I order a pelvimetry and, eventually, an ultrasonographic weight estimate of the baby. The mother goes home to think over her situation, and I do the same. In a few days we meet again at the delivery department. I fill in the data on the pelvic score index (Westin, maximum 20 points), assess all available facts, estimate the weight of the baby by means of palpation, and listen to the mother and father. If the Westin screening yields a high enough score (over 13 to 15) and no other contraindications rule out a vaginal delivery, and when I feel a positive motivation from the mother's side, I then propose vaginal delivery by saying, "You can give birth to your baby in breech presentation as easily as in vertex presentation."

As regards external cephalic version, you may calculate an estimated frequency of complications (ablatio placentae and umbilical cord complications) of about 1 percent. Therefore my opinion is generally not to try external version when the fetus is in breech presentation except for when the pelvis is too small or the baby too big for a breech delivery, but both are sufficient for a vertex delivery. The external cephalic version is done under tocolysis and above all gently. The mother is prepared for an immediate cesarean section if necessary. My own success rate in external version is about 50 percent. Elective cesarean section, about 55 percent of cases, is recommended when external version fails or is rejected and in all other cases not suitable for vaginal delivery.

As previously mentioned, the most important factor is the mother's confidence in herself and in those who will assist her at the delivery. Informed consent to the recommended method of delivery is of great importance.

The labor may start spontaneously. The mother can be up on her feet as long as possible. Cardiotocography (CTG) is done on admission to the delivery department (the so-called door test) and then intermittently or continuously if needed. Oxytocin infusion is started when labor is weak or insufficient. Routine perineotomy may be of use, but I use it less and less often.

Breech delivery is an obstetric challenge. *In my opinion, the midwife should be the prime assistant at the breech delivery* (as she always is in Sweden for the vertex delivery). The midwife guides the mother through the whole labor, has the closest contact with her, and is the one next to her when the baby is born. The personal contact between the mother and the midwife is of great importance to the sense of security the mother must have in order to rely on her own power at the moment of giving birth to a new life. At that moment the midwife is the professional person closest to her and the obstetrician is backing up the midwife, prepared to take over if needed. The pediatrician is nearby but not in the room until he or she is eventually needed.

Today the mother usually gives birth in the so-called short bed, litothomy position, but in a breech delivery I allow the mother to give birth in whatever position she considers most convenient. In vertex deliveries 75 percent of the women use alternative delivery positions; such as lying on their sides, knee-chest positions, or kneeling or standing on their feet.

During the last 4 years I have been working at Ystads BB, near Lund, where there are 850 deliveries per year. The size of the department is ideal. It is an integrated department, meaning that the same people assist at the delivery as at the patients "lying-in" stay 2 to 7 days afterward in the hospital. Our aim is "home delivery at the hospital," and our theme is that pregnancy and birth are physiologic processes. We attempt to strengthen the vitality and capability that are significant for the future mother and father, and are at hand if anything goes wrong. Ninety-five percent of the mothers and fathers have attended the psychoprophylaxis course held by the midwife. As a physician I meet the pregnant woman at least twice, and all breech deliveries are planned as described. The results at Ystads BB are as encouraging as those from my study at Karlskrona. Therefore I recommend the whole situation analysis for breech presentation delivery. Under this system of management, about 45 percent of such pregnant women can give birth vaginally without increased perinatal mortality or persistent morbidity.

SUGGESTED READING

Barlöv K, Larsson G. Results of a five-year prospective study using a feto-pelvic scoring system for term singleton breech delivery after uncomplicated pregnancy. Acta Obstet Gynecol Scand 1986; 65:315–319.

Barnum C. The effect of gravitation on the presentation and position of the fetus. JAMA 1915; 64:498–502.

Dunn PM. Congenital postural deformities. Br Med Bull 1976; 32:71–76.

Luterkort M. The natural history of breech pregnancy and its consequences. Doctoral dissertation from the Department of Obstetrics and Gynecology, General Hospital, Malmö, University of Lund, Sweden, 1986.

Westin B. Evaluation of a feto-pelvic scoring system in the management of breech presentations. Acta Obstet Gynecol Scand 1977; 56:505–508.

Westin B. Management of breech presentation. In: Breech delivery. Växjö: Proc Swed Gynecol Society 1974; 39–45.

Zatuchni GI, Andros GJ. Prognostic index for vaginal delivery in breech presentation at term. Am J Obstet Gynecol 1967; 98:854–857.

CHLAMYDIAL INFECTIONS DURING PREGNANCY AND INFANCY

ALFRED D. HEGGIE, M.D.
HUNTER A. HAMMILL, M.D.

Chlamydia trachomatis is the most prevalent sexually transmitted pathogen in the United States and western Europe. Genital infection in pregnant women is common, and transmission to the infant during birth is frequent. Almost all infants who become infected develop neonatal chlamydial conjunctivitis and unless infection is eradicated by appropriate treatment, 10 to 20 percent of these infants can be expected to develop chlamydial pneumonia at 1 to 3 months of age. Genital infection in women can result in cervicitis, endometritis, and salpingitis and is an important cause of involuntary sterility. *Treatment of maternal infection prevents perinatal transmission and maternal complications.* Detection and eradication of this infection should be among the goals of prenatal care.

MATERNAL CHLAMYDIAL INFECTION

Maternal chlamydial infection may elude detection because it is usually asymptomatic. In nonpregnant women, mucopurulent cervicitis, defined as the presence of ten or more leukocytes per high-power field in smears of mucopus, has been found to correlate with the presence of chlamydial infection. During pregnancy, recognition of cervicitis may be difficult because physiologic changes at the squamocolumnar junction result in ectopy (eversion of the cervix) and edematous congestion that may be misinterpreted as signs of cervicitis. Although these changes are not caused by chlamydial infection, they may predispose to it, since ectopy increases the degree of exposure of the columnar mucosa of the cervical canal to microorganisms entering the vagina. *Chlamydia trachomatis* preferentially infects columnar epithelia. Hence, cervical infection during pregnancy is frequent if exposure to chylamdiae occurs. Patients who complain of genital itching and malodorous vaginal discharge are more likely to have vaginitis then cervicitis. Bacterial vaginitis in adults is seldom caused by *Chlamydia* because the glycogen-coated squamous epithelium and acid pH of the postpubertal vagina render it relatively resistant to chlamydial infection. Diagnostic evaluation for vaginitis should include tests for other genital pathogens. However, chlamydial vaginitis may occur in young girls. The epithelium of the prepubertal vagina is relatively atrophic and consists of cuboidal cells. Glycogen coating is absent, and the pH is neutral. These conditions are relatively favorable for chlamydial infection. The occurrence of chlamydial vaginitis in a child is highly suggestive of sexual abuse, but the possibility of persistent neonatal infection should be considered in very young children.

Although one study suggests that primary chlamydial infections during pregnancy may predispose to low birth weight infants and premature rupture of the membranes, most studies show no association between chlamydial infection and adverse outcomes of pregnancy. Transplacental infection has not been documented and probably does not occur. *The confirmed risks of chlamydial infection to both mothers and infants occur at parturition.* Passage through an infected birth canal results in infection in 35 to 75 percent of exposed infants. Ascending maternal infection may result in late postpartum chlamydial endometritis, but this appears to be an infrequent event.

Since chlamydial infections of the lower female genital tract are so often either asymptomatic or associated with nonspecific symptoms or signs, a diagnosis can be made with certainty only by antigen detection or isolation of the organism by culture. Ideally, all pregnant women should be tested for genital chlamydial infection, but if this is not possible, efforts should focus on high-risk groups such as unwed teenagers and women with prior histories of other sexually transmitted diseases. Diagnostic testing should be scheduled so that if infection is detected, treatment can be completed before the onset of labor. Although prompt initiation of treatment after detection of infection is desirable, compliance with therapeutic regimens may be poor during the first trimester because of the vomiting of pregnancy that frequently occurs at this time. In patients who are noncompliant because of first-trimester vomiting, treatment can be deferred until the second trimester, since adverse effects of maternal chlamydial infection on the fetus in utero have not been identified. As with other sexually transmitted diseases, a confirmation of cure should be obtained by retesting for infection approximately 2 weeks after completion of therapy. The patient's sexual partner should also be evaluated and treated concurrently. Since women who are treated early in pregnancy may become reinfected, tests for chlamydial infection should be repeated near term.

TREATMENT OF MOTHER AND SEXUAL PARTNER

Recent treatment guidelines from the Centers for Disease Control recommend that *Chlamydia*-infected pregnant women receive erythromycin base, 500 mg four times a day, or erythromycin ethylsuccinate, 800 mg four times a day, by mouth, for 7 days. Unfortunately, gastrointestinal intolerance to oral erythromycin is frequent in pregnant women and may preclude completion of therapy. In intolerant patients, a 14-day course of erythromycin base at the lower dosage of 250 mg four times a day is recommended. In our experience, approximately 50 percent of pregnant women are unable to complete the recommended course of erythromycin therapy. In a pilot study to evaluate alternative treatments, we have been successful in eradicating infection with a 7-day course of clindamycin, 450 mg, by mouth, four times a day. We have not encountered cases of pseudomembranous enterocolitis with this regimen, but it must be recognized that this in one of the complications associated with clindamycin treatment. The relatively short course of therapy probably minimized this risk. Further studies are required to validate the efficacy of this treatment. In addition to treatment of the index patient, vigourous efforts should be made to institute concurrent treatment of her sexual partner with tetracycline hydrochloride, 500 mg, by mouth, four times a day, for 7 days, or doxycycline hyclate, 100 mg, by mouth, twice a day, for 7 days. This reduces the possibility of reinfection of the pregnant woman and treats or prevents chlamydial urethritis or epididymitis in the male partner. Tetracycline or doxycycline should not be used for treatment of pregnant women because it is deposited in the developing bones and teeth of the fetus.

NEONATAL OCULAR PROPHYLAXIS

In recent years, ocular prophylaxis at birth with erythromycin or tetracycline ointments has been used in an effort to prevent neonatal acquisition of chlamydial infection. Initial reports indicated that this treatment prevented chlamydial conjunctivitis but had no effect on nasopharyngeal colonization, a frequent concomitant of ocular infection. Subsequent studies with larger numbers of infants have shown that even prevention of ocular infection by this method is unreliable. Although it is possible that more effective topical antichlamydial medications may be developed, local treatment of the eye cannot be expected to eradicate nasopharyngeal infection. Persistent infection of the nasopharynx can serve both as a source for reinfection of the conjunctivae and for progression of infection to the lower respiratory tract. Reliable protection of the infant against perinatal infection requires prepartum detection and treatment of maternal infection. If this cannot be done, it could be argued that neonatal conjunctivitis is an advantageous outcome of perinatal infection, since it should serve to alert health care providers to the possibility that the infant and his or her parents may have chlamydial infections.

NEONATAL CHLAMYDIAL CONJUNCTIVITIS

Chlamydia trachomatis infection is among the most frequently identified causes of purulent conjunctivitis during the first month of life. In infants from economically deprived urban families, *Chlamydia* is probably a more frequent cause of this disease than any other microorganism. The signs of neonatal chlamydial conjunctivitis usually appear during the second week of postnatal life. This is in contrast to other forms of neonatal conjunctivitis, such as chemical conjunctivitis from ocular prophylaxis with silver nitrate, which usually clears by 3 days of age, and gonococcal ophthalmia, which typically appears at 3 to 5 days of age. Since there is considerable overlap in the time of onset and the clinical severity of conjunctivitis caused by various microorganisms, definitive etiologic diagnosis depends on culture results. *Chlamydia trachomatis* can also be identified by detection of chlamydial antigen is specimens of conjunctival cells by fluorescent antibody or ELISA (enzyme-linked immunosorbent assay) techniques. Neonatal chlamydial conjunctivitis requires treat-

ment with oral erythromycin syrup, 50 mg per kilogram per 24 hours in four divided doses for 14 days. Although the four doses should be given at as evenly spaced intervals as possible, it is not necessary to alter the family's or infant's sleep pattern to administer medication. This regimen eradicates both conjunctival and nasopharyngeal infections. Concurrent treatment with topical ophthalmic antimicrobial medications is unnecessary. Failure of chlamydial conjunctivitis to resolve or recurrence of conjunctivitis after treatment is usually the result of noncompliance. In these cases a repeat course of erythromycin for 1 to 2 weeks should be prescribed.

Some physicians maintain that it is unnecessary to obtain diagnostic bacteriologic tests for neonatal conjunctivitis, including tests for *Chlamydia*. They prefer to treat empirically and topically with sulfacetamide ophthalmic solution or tetracycline ophthalmic ointment. Etiologic investigation is carried out only if the conjunctivitis fails to resolve. We feel that bacteriologic diagnosis is always important. If appropriate testing is not readily available, at least Gram's stained smears of conjunctival swabs should be examined to rule out the presence of gram-negative diplococci indicative of infection with *Neisseria gonorrhoeae*. Gonococcal conjunctivitis requires prompt systemic treatment with penicillin. In the latter disease, bacteriologic cultures not only assist with the diagnosis but are the only means of detecting penicillin-resistant gonococci. Conjunctivitis caused by other common bacterial pathogens, including *Chlamydia*, usually resolves on topical therapy. The problem with chlamydial conjunctivitis, however, is that topical therapy frequently does not eradicate conjunctival infection and has no effect on nasopharyngeal colonization. Therefore, conjunctivitis may recur or chronic, low-grade conjunctival infection may ensue. Although corneal vascularization and conjunctival scarring resulting from persistent neonatally acquired chlamydial infection have been reported, these sequelae do not appear to be frequent outcomes of neonatal chlamydial infection is this country. However, untreated nasopharyngeal infection can spread to the lower respiratory tract and cause interstitial pneumonia. Another consideration that lends importance to bacteriologic diagnosis in cases of chlamydial conjunctivitis is that if chlamydial cultures or antigen detection studies are not done, the opportunity to identify and treat infection in the infant's parents is lost.

CHLAMYDIAL PNEUMONIA

Chlamydial pneumonia is much less frequent than conjunctivitis and occurs in less than 20 percent of infants born vaginally to infected mothers. Disease presentation occurs at 1 to 3 months of age, considerably later than chlamydial conjunctivitis. This delay is probably related to the time required for the organism to traverse the nasopharynx and multiply in the lower respiratory tract. Typically, onset occurs at about 8 weeks of age and is characterized by gradual development of cough and congestion over a 1 to 2 week period. Poor feeding and retarded weight gain are often observed when there has been a delay in medical evaluation. Affected infants are afebrile and often have a prior history of conjunctivitis. Chest x-ray films show bilateral interstitial infiltrates and hyperexpansion. Laboratory findings of eosinophil counts of 300 per mm³ and serum IgG and IgM concentrations of 500 mg per deciliter and 110 mg per deciliter, respectively, are highly correlated with chlamydial pneumonitis. Although life-threatening complications have not been reported, clinical manifestations can persist for weeks and radiologic abnormalities for months if the infection is not treated. Only one long-term follow-up study has been done. It suggests that chlamydial pneumonia, like other respiratory infections during infancy, may cause or predispose to obstructive pulmonary disease later in childhood. The recommended treatment for chlamydial pneumonia is the same as that used for chlamydial conjunctivitis: oral erythromycin syrup, 50 mg per kilogram per 24 hours in four divided doses for 14 days. Clinical improvement occurs within 3 to 5 days. Oral treatment with sulfisoxazole is probably also effective, but there has been much more experience with erythromycin and therefore it is recommended. The use of sulfisoxazole is also complicated by its competi-

tion with bilirubin for binding sites of albumin. In neonates this may contribute to hyperbilirubinemia. Although chlamydial pneumonia seldom occurs during the neonatal period, manufacturers' package inserts advise against use of sulfisoxazole in infants under the age of 2 months.

SUGGESTED READING

Alexander ER, Harrison HR. Role of *Chlamydia trachomatis* in perinatal infection. Rev Infect Dis 1983; 5:713–719.
Centers for Disease Control. *Chlamydia trachomatis* infections. Policy guidelines for prevention and control. MMWR 1985; 34:53S–74S.
Heggie AD, Jaffe AC, Stuart LA, et al. Topical sulfacetamide vs oral erythromycin for neonatal chlamydial conjunctivitis. Am J Dis Child 1985; 139:564–566.
Thompson SE, Washington EG. Epidemiology of sexually transmitted *Chlamydia trachomatis* infection. Epidemiol Rev 1983; 5:96–123.
Tipple MA, Beem MO, Saxon EM. Clinical characteristics of the afebrile pneumonia associated with *Chlamydia trachomatis* infection in infants less than 6 months of age. Pediatrics 1979; 63:192–197.
Weiss SG, Newcomb RW, Beem MO. Pulmonary assessment of children after chlamydial pneumonia of infancy. J Pediatr 1986; 108:659–664.

CHRONIC RENAL DISEASE IN PREGNANCY

SUSAN HOU, M.D.

Pregnancy in women with renal disease is associated with an increase in several serious maternal and fetal complications, including hypertension, proteinuria, and renal failure in the mother and prematurity and death for the fetus. Women with advanced renal failure have decreased fertility, but some pregnancies do occur even in women treated with chronic dialysis. Kidney transplantation frequently restores fertility to women with end-stage renal disease, but pregnancy in these women raises questions about the effect of immunosuppressive drugs and opportunistic infection on the fetus. This chapter addresses treatment strategies for the common problems that arise in pregnant women with renal disease.

HYPERTENSION

Hypertension is the most common and often the most dangerous complication in pregnant women with renal disease. If the data from two large series of pregnant women with renal disease are pooled, we find that hypertension (blood pressure 140/90 mm Hg or higher) was a problem in 85 of the 244 pregnancies. In one series, almost 20 percent of the women experienced severe hypertension with blood pressures of 170/110 mm Hg or higher. When blood

pressure control becomes more problematic, it is difficult to determine whether the patient has developed superimposed pre-eclampsia. Preexisting renal disease can lead to proteinuria, hyperuricemia, worsening renal function, and hypertension, so that the usual clinical parameters by which the diagnosis of pre-eclampsia is made become confusing. When pregnant women with renal disease undergo biopsy because clinically they appear to have superimposed pre-eclampsia, biopsy confirms the clinical impression in only 50 percent of cases. However, biopsy is rarely required, because the decision to terminate the pregnancy usually depends only upon the success of efforts at blood pressure control.

Patients should be taught to take their own blood pressure daily, as abrupt rises may occur between office visits. Although there is debate about the use of antihypertensive drugs in pregnant women with essential hypertension, in women with renal disease blood pressure should be treated aggressively. If blood pressure is consistently higher than 140/90 mm Hg, antihypertensive medication should be started. Methyldopa has a 25-year history of use in pregnancy, and careful follow-up studies of children exposed to methyldopa in utero have shown no ill effects from the drug. It should be started in doses of 250 mg twice daily; the dose can be increased to a total of 2 to 3 g daily, divided into two to four doses. There are several acceptable medication alternatives that do not have the long track record enjoyed by methyldopa. Early fears about the effect of beta-blockers on fetal growth and ability of the fetus to tolerate hypoxic stress have not been borne out, and their safety and efficacy have been demonstrated in two randomized, controlled studies. Clonidine, labetalol, and prazosin have also been used as first-line drugs in pregnancy. If one drug does not control blood pressure, hydralazine can be added in a total daily dose of 200 mg. Used as a single oral agent, hydralazine is a poor antihypertensive drug. For refractory hypertension, oral nifedipine can be used in doses of 10 to 30 mg, three times daily.

For hypertensive crises with either seizures or blood pressure of 170/110 mm Hg or higher, parenteral hydralazine or oral nifedipine can be used. The initial dose of hydralazine should be 5 mg given intravenously, followed by 5 to 10 mg intravenously every 20 to 30 minutes. Oral nifedipine is used in doses of 10 to 30 mg. Intravenous diazoxide in repeated boluses of 30 mg can be used if blood pressure cannot be controlled by hydralazine or nifedipine. Nitroprusside carries a risk of fetal cyanide toxicity, so it should be used only when other agents fail to control life-threatening hypertension. If blood pressure cannot be controlled on an oral regimen and remains 170/110 mm Hg or higher despite maximal treatment, the pregnancy should be terminated.

PROTEINURIA

The development or worsening of proteinuria is common in women with renal disease. Between 15 and 30 percent of women with proteinuria at the onset of pregnancy develop proteinuria in the nephrotic range during pregnancy. Worsening proteinuria does not necessarily reflect worsening of the renal disease or the development of superimposed pre-eclampsia. Proteinuria by itself is not a major threat to the fetus, although there is one study that shows a correlation between serum albumin level and fetal weight, with lower weights in the infants of severely hypoalbuminemic mothers.

When uncomplicated nephrotic syndrome appears during pregnancy, biopsy can often be delayed until after delivery. If hypertension and renal insufficiency appear, biopsy may be necessary to distinguish between pre-eclampsia and primary renal disease. If massive edema and severe hypoalbuminemia occur, biopsy should be done to look for a steroid-responsive lesion. In pregnant women we favor doing an open biopsy, because increased renal blood flow may increase the bleeding complications of a closed biopsy. If disabling edema occurs in a woman with minimal change disease, a course of prednisone, 120 mg every other day for 2 months, can be started. The response rate to alternate-day steroids is somewhat less than to daily steroids but is good enough that a trial of this less toxic regimen is warranted. If edema and hypoalbuminemia are mild, treatment can be delayed until after delivery, as high-dose steroids may aggravate hypertension and hyperglycemia, particularly in the third trimester. In the absence of pre-eclampsia, diuretics can be used to treat severe edema in women with glomerular diseases that are not steroid-responsive. Diuresis should be limited to 1 to 2 pounds daily and, if postural hypotension develops, diuretics can be adjusted to give an even slower diuresis. Patients with nephrotic syndrome usually require loop diuretics. They should be started initially on 40 mg of furosemide daily and the dose increased until diuresis occurs. Sodium restriction alone is rarely successful in reducing edema once it has formed. However, a low-sodium diet should be used in conjunction with diuretics to prevent reaccumulation of edema. In women with impaired renal function, worsening of anemia is the rule. Patients should be transfused to maintain a hematocrit above 25 ml per deciliter, as they are at higher risk for bleeding complications than are healthy women.

LOSS OF RENAL FUNCTION

When renal function is fairly well preserved (serum creatinine concentration less than or equal to 1.4 mg per deciliter), pregnancy does not appear to alter the natural history of the renal disease. However, when more advanced renal insufficiency is present, there is a risk that the renal disease will progress rapidly. If serum creatinine rises, reversible causes of renal failure should be ruled out. Obstruction should be ruled out if there is a solitary kidney or polyhydramnios, as the risk of obstruction is increased in such a setting. Volume contraction should be corrected. Nephrotoxic drugs, especially nonsteroidal anti-inflammatory agents, should be avoided. Once renal function has declined as a result of the underlying disease, it is usually not reversed by either delivery or termination of the pregnancy. When a patient is seen early in pregnancy, she should be made to understand that although her renal function will be closely monitored, there are no interventions that will reliably restore her to her pre-pregnancy baseline if her renal function deteriorates.

It is no longer justifiable to terminate a pregnancy before fetal viability if renal function deteriorates. In many cases, the renal disease is destined to progress eventually, and pregnancy hastens the need for dialysis and transplant but does not cause end-stage renal disease in someone who otherwise would not have reached it. Even with a decline in renal function, the chance of giving birth to a healthy infant is good. In a series we published describing 23 women with moderate renal insufficiency who conceived, 80 percent of the pregnancies resulted in long-term survival of the infant. However, if the decline in renal function occurs after 32 weeks' gestation when the baby's risk for long-term complications of prematurity is small, early delivery is warranted for both maternal and fetal indications.

DIALYSIS IN PREGNANCY

When renal failure is severe, dialysis should be initiated when the blood urea nitrogen level reaches 80 to 100 mg per deciliter. Because limited experience with dialysis during pregnancy has shown a poor outcome for women treated with hemodialysis, at present we favor chronic ambulatory peritoneal dialysis for women needing dialysis during pregnancy. Since dialysis is continuous in patients treated with chronic ambulatory peritoneal dialysis, rapid volume shifts and electrolyte changes are avoided. Abrupt drops in blood pressure are unusual when such dialysis is used, whereas such drops may be difficult to avoid during hemodialysis. Once dialysis is initiated, the frequency is increased to maintain a blood urea nitrogen level of 50 mg per deciliter or below. Dietary restrictions are eliminated to ensure that the mother can have adequate protein intake for maternal and fetal needs. Dialysis frequency generally needs to be increased during the third trimester to offset fetal urea production, which increases to as much as 540 mg per day.

TRANSPLANTATION

Over 1,500 pregnancies have occurred in renal transplant patients. Return of fertility is common following transplantation, and allograft recipients need contraceptive counseling to avoid unplanned pregnancies. The spontaneous abortion rate in the first trimester is 16 percent, similar to the rate in the general population. We advise patients to wait for 2 years after transplantation to conceive. By this time renal function is generally stable and doses of immunosuppressive drugs have been lowered. Hypertension should be well controlled at the time of conception, and the serum creatinine level should be below 2 mg per deciliter. The dose of prednisone should be 15 mg per day or less and that of azathioprine less than 2 mg per kilogram per day. We advise testing for hepatitis antigen and human immunodeficiency virus prior to conception.

We follow the same guidelines for treatment of hypertension as we use for pregnant women with other types of renal disease. Renal function may decrease after a renal transplant during pregnancy. Biopsy is frequently necessary to determine the cause of deterioration. Often rejection, cyclosporine toxicity, and pre-eclampsia can be distinguished from one another only by biopsy.

Transplant patients are at risk for infectious complications affecting both the mother and fetus. Screening urine cultures should be done monthly and asymptomatic bacteriuria treated with antibiotics. Invasive procedures should be minimized, and surgical procedures should be covered with prophylactic antibiotics. Transplant patients are at risk for viral infections that may affect the fetus. Infants of hepatitis carriers should be treated with hepatitis B immune globulin within 48 hours after birth and with hepatitis B vaccine within 1 week after birth. Hepatitis vaccine should be repeated at 1 and 6 months. Cervical cultures for herpes simplex should be done and a cesarean section performed if culture results are positive at the time of delivery. Patients who are positive for human immunodeficiency virus should be advised of the 50 percent risk of passing the virus on to the infant. In caring for the newborn, there should be a high index of suspicion for congenital cytomegalovirus infection. The diagnosis of active infection in the mother may be difficult, and the risk of infection of the infant is not high enough for most women to consider pregnancy termination.

There are several neonatal risks associated with immunosuppressive drugs. In some series a slight increase in congenital anomalies has been noted in patients treated with azathioprine, but the problem is rare when the maternal dose is less than 2 mg per kilogram per day. Chromosomal breaks in lymphocytes have been observed in the infants. To date, there have been no reports of increased malignancy in the offspring of transplant patients. However, animals exposed to 6-mercaptopurine in utero have a dose-related decrease in fertility and an increased incidence of stillbirth. The children of transplant recipients are still too young to determine if their fertility was affected by their exposure to azathioprine in utero. Adrenal insufficiency secondary to prednisone is rare, but infants should be monitored for this complication.

Thymic hypoplasia, leukopenia, and thrombocytopenia have been described in the infants of transplant patients. Data on cyclosporine are still limited, but intrauterine growth retardation has been described. Transplant patients require an increased dose of steroids during labor or cesarean section; 100 mg of hydrocortisone should be given every 8 hours for 24 to 48 hours during labor and after delivery. Maintenance steroid doses in transplant patients are generally too low to promote lung maturation for the infant when premature delivery is anticipated. Transplantation may result in sensitization to some antigens on the allograft. Rh compatibility is not a prerequisite for transplantation. Thus, Rh-negative women may be sensitized by a kidney from an Rh-positive donor. Rh-negative women should be followed for the appearance of antibodies.

LUPUS NEPHRITIS

The patient with systemic lupus erythematosus and renal disease is among the most difficult to manage. There is an increase in frequency of lupus flares during pregnancy and during the postpartum period. The best prognosis for pregnancy is noted when the patient conceives during a period of remission. Even in these cases, between 7 and 33 percent experience a flare of lupus during gestation. Of those who conceive during an active flare, 50 to 60 percent experience a worsening of renal disease. If therapeutic abortions are excluded, fetal survival is about 90 percent for women in remission at conception, but may be as low as 60 percent for those who conceive with active lupus. If lupus flares during pregnancy, the patient should be treated with 60 mg of prednisone daily. If the patient responds, this dose should be continued for 6 weeks and tapered slowly. If severe steroid side effects result, azathioprine can be added at 2 mg per kilogram per day. If renal insufficiency occurs and does not respond to steroids, a biopsy should be done. If the biopsy shows diffuse proliferative disease, cyclophosphamide is the most effective agent. When given during organogenesis, cyclophosphamide is associated with a 50 percent incidence of congenital anomalies. Whenever possible, therefore, its use should be postponed until the postpartum period, and consideration should be given to terminating the pregnancy if cyclophosphamide is required in the first trimester.

The infants of mothers with lupus may have neonatal lupus syndrome with cutaneous manifestations and heart block. This may occur when signs of maternal lupus are minimal or absent.

In women with lupus nephritis, a course of 60 mg of prednisone daily for 2 weeks after delivery minimizes the chance of a postpartum flare.

FETAL OUTCOME

The infants of women with renal disease are at risk for prematurity, growth retardation, and intrauterine fetal death. In women with renal disease whose renal function is well preserved, the combined stillbirths and neonatal deaths account for 10.7 percent of pregnancies. These numbers are drawn from a study done on patients who were pregnant between 1960 and 1980. All those included reached the second trimester. We would expect both stillbirths and neonatal deaths to be decreased with improved antenatal monitoring and improved care of premature infants. Survival for the infants of mothers with moderate renal insufficiency (serum creatinine higher than or equal to 1.4 mg per deciliter) was 80 to 81 percent in two studies describing 43 pregnancies in 41 women. These studies present a contrast to earlier papers that reported a 50 percent fetal loss rate. Survival for infants of transplant patients is 90 percent, if the pregnancy goes beyond the first trimester. The outlook for successful pregnancy remains poor in dialysis patients, with a success rate of only 20 to 25 percent.

Women with a childhood history of acute glomerulonephritis or acute pyelonephritis need not be considered high risk if renal function, blood pressure, and urinalysis are normal. All women with active renal disease should be considered high-risk patients and should have twiceweekly nonstress tests from 26 weeks' gestation despite the difficulties of interpretation between 26 and 30 weeks. A biophysical profile can be done in patients with nonreactive nonstress tests. In dialysis patients oxytocin challenge tests carry a risk of premature labor. In dialysis patients the risk of fetal loss is high enough that elective delivery at 34 to 36 weeks is justified. In other types of renal disease, outcome is good enough that premature delivery should only be done for specific maternal and fetal indications.

Prematurity and premature labor are common in all women with renal disease. Premature labor is most common in dialysis patients. Sixty-five percent of infants are born prematurely, and 45 percent of the premature births are secondary to premature labor. Approximately one-third of dialysis patients have premature labor that does not result in delivery. Forty-five to sixty percent of transplant patients and 50 percent of women with moderate renal insufficiency deliver prior to 37 weeks' gestation, although changes in blood pressure or renal function, rather than premature labor, account for many of the deliveries. If premature labor occurs, the patient should be assessed for concealed placental abruption and for fetal distress. If there is no indication for delivery, an attempt can be made to control premature labor. Terbutaline in doses of 25 mg given subcutaneously can be used if blood pressure is well controlled. Nifedipine, 10 to 30 mg three to four times daily, can also be used.

There is an increased incidence of intrauterine growth retardation in infants of women with renal disease. Fetal growth should be followed by serial ultrasound studies. Even infants who are neither premature nor growthretarded should be followed in a special care nursery for the first 24 hours. Infants of women with azotemia have elevated blood urea nitrogen and creatine levels at birth and an exaggerated diuresis with a risk of electrolyte abnormalities following birth.

Cesarean section need be done only if there are clearcut obstetric indications. In transplant patients, the cesarean section rate is about 25 percent. An increase in cesarean sections done because of fetal distress can be anticipated.

SUGGESTED READING

Davison JM. Renal transplantation and pregnancy. Am J Kidney Dis 1987; 9:374–380.

Hayslett JP, Lynn RI. Effect of pregnancy in patients with lupus nephritis. Kidney Int 1980; 18:207–220.

Hou SH. Pregnancy in women requiring dialysis for renal failure. Am J Kidney Dis 1987; 9:368–373.

Hou S, Grossman S, Madias NE. Pregnancy in women with renal disease and moderate renal insufficiency. Am J Med 1985; 78:185–194.

Katz AI, Linheimer MD. Effect of pregnancy on the natural course of kidney disease. Semin Nephrol 1984; 4:252–259.

CORD PROLAPSE

ROBERT RESNIK, M.D.

Cord prolapse occurs when a portion of the umbilical cord descends into the lower uterine segment or vagina in advance of the fetal presenting part. The frequency of this complication is approximately 1 in every 200 deliveries. Cord prolapse may occur at any time following rupture of the membranes but is most commonly associated with prematurity, malpresentations such as transverse lie and footling or incomplete breech, hydromnios, delivery of the second twin, and a high fetal presenting part.

OVERT CORD PROLAPSE

The most common clinical presentation is that of the overt cord prolapse. Upon diagnosis by visual or vaginal examination, plans should be made to elevate the fetal presenting part in order to avoid umbilical cord compression and then to effect immediate delivery. The patient may be placed in deep Trendelenburg's position or the knee-chest position, and the examining hand prevents the presenting part from occluding umbilical blood flow. Anesthesia and nursing personnel are summoned and preparations made for delivery. A vaginal delivery may be accomplished if it can be performed without maternal or fetal trauma. In the case of a vertex presentation, this requires full dilation of the cervix and a station low enough in the pelvis for an operative vaginal delivery to be safely performed. If a breech presentation is noted and the cervix is fully dilated, consideration may be given to a total breech extraction if the maternal pelvis is felt to be of adequate size and the fetus weights less than 3,500 g. The use of halothane anesthesia may facilitate delivery. If conditions preclude a safe vaginal delivery, cesarean section should be performed immediately. It should be emphasized that cesarean section is the usual safe mode of delivery and that the individual who first makes the diagnosis should continue to decompress the umbilical cord by elevating the presenting part until after abdominal delivery. This requires that surgical drapes be placed over the examiner. All anesthetic and surgical procedures should be carried out without delay but with appropriate maternal intravenous lines and meticulous attention to safe induction of anesthesia with endotracheal intubation.

Although the initial examiner should be able to determine the umbilical cord pulse, occasionally there is a question of whether or not the fetus is still alive. External Doppler or fetal electrocardiogram by scalp electrode is useful under these circumstances. If the fetus has expired or the gestational age is not viable, vaginal delivery should be anticipated.

OCCULT CORD PROLAPSE

Occult cord prolapse occurs when the umbilical cord is compressed between the lower uterine segment and the fetal presenting part but cannot be visualized or palpated by the examining hand. In fact, it is a presumptive diagnosis made by the clinical observation of severe bradycardia by abdominal auscultation and/or severe variable decelerations diagnosed by fetal electrocardiogram. Management is determined by the response of the abnormal fetal electrocardiogram tracing to maternal positional change, including lateral repositioning and Trendelenburg's position. If the variable fetal heart rate decelerations become progressively severe and vaginal delivery is not imminent, cesarean section is indicated. This type of fetal heart rate abnormality is seen in clinical conditions associated with oligohydramnios, such as premature rupture of the membranes, in post-term gestation, and in the growth-retarded fetus. Some have suggested that replacement of intrauterine fluid volume with large infusions of normal saline may correct the umbilical cord compression by providing a "cushioned," more natural environment. Preliminary studies suggest that such infusions decrease the severity and frequency of variable decelerations, but whether this is a safer and more efficacious procedure for the fetus than immediate abdominal delivery has not yet been determined.

FUNIC PRESENTATION

Less commonly observed is the funic presentation, in which the umbilical cord lies in front of the presenting part and the membranes are still intact. This is almost always diagnosed by pelvic examination, although recent reports demonstrate that the skilled sonographer may make this diagnosis if the fetal presenting part is not too low in the maternal pelvis. If the fetus is mature, appropriate management is cesarean section. In the presence of a premature fetus, as documented by amniotic fluid lung maturation studies, bed rest is warranted until fetal maturity is achieved.

Umbilical cord prolapse is a relatively common and dramatic event. Each labor and delivery unit should have a plan prepared in the event that such an emergency occurs so that appropriate therapy can be initiated and carried out in a rapid but controlled manner.

DIABETES IN PREGNANCY

JOACHIM G. KLEBE, M.D.

Diabetes in pregnancy is a problem created almost entirely by human circumstances. Prior to the discovery of insulin there were only a few diabetic women who became pregnant, and of these very few were able to carry through their pregnancies to term. Many diabetic women died late in the period of pregnancy in a diabetic coma; others died while giving birth because of the extremely large size of their babies, and these infants often died soon after birth due to respiratory problems or congenital malformations. Following the discovery of insulin in 1923 by Best and Banting, however, this situation was completely altered. Pregnant diabetic women survived, but there was still an extremely high rate of perinatal mortality—approximately 50 percent. Around 1940, checks on diabetic pregnancies were centralized with a view to improving medical and obstetric treatment. This resulted in a reduction of the perinatal mortality for diabetic pregnancies, which now approaches the mortality rate for nondiabetic pregnancies. However, the diabetic pregnancy is still not without its problems, and these good results have only been achieved by extremely intensive centralized control and teamwork among obstetricians, internists, pediatricians, and an efficient unit with a staff of specially trained nurses, dietitians, social workers, and many others. Apart from all this, it is also important that daily examinations be carried out by as few people as possible.

PREPREGNANCY CONSULTATION

It is important for all diabetic women wishing to become pregnant to take part in *prepregnancy consultation*. Diabetic pregnancies still result in a congenital malformation rate that is twice that of nondiabetic pregnancies. Since such deformities start in the early stages of pregnancy, and since it is certain that good blood glucose regulation can reduce the frequency of malformations, it is of the utmost importance that optimal blood glucose regulation be carried out even prior to conception. This is why all diabetic women should be trained to test their own blood glucose by the finger prick method. Long-term blood glucose regulation is assessed from hemoglobin A_{1c}. Diet and the need for exercise are assessed and balanced. The aim is to achieve mean blood glucose values of approximately 6 mmol per liter, even though such a low mean blood glucose value might make it more difficult to lead a normal daily life. One debatable point is whether conventional injection techniques or the insulin pump or pen technique should be employed. Since a number of pregnant diabetic women have developed late diabetic complications that might be associated with extremely complicated pregnancies and with the deterioration of eye and kidney functions, which might even become permanent, it is important during the prepregnancy consultation to assess eye and kidney functions as well as blood pressure. As part of the eye examination the fundus should be studied and a decision made as to whether or not laser treatment is indicated for retinopathy. In our department we assess kidney function by serum carbamide, serum creatinine clearance, and protein excretion.

Kidney volume is assessed by measuring the kidneys ultrasonographically. Diabetics, as a result of their diabetes and increased glomerular filtration, normally have an increased kidney volume. But a permanent late diabetic nephropathy results in a reduction in kidney volume once again. Our material concerning pregnant diabetic women reveals a deterioration of kidney function, in particular for those with initially small kidney volumes. Similarly, a vigorous proteinuria and hypertension are relatively serious contraindications to pregnancy. Apart from family and social conditions, these clinical parameters must always be considered in any assessment of diabetic women as a feature of prepregnancy consultation.

Once the patient has completed the prepregnancy consultation, an assessment must be made of whether or not pregnancy is advisable. If not, advice must be given as to an effective means of contraception or even sterilization. If pregnancy is recommended, blood glucose control should be intensified, contraception discontinued, and basal body temperature measurements commenced in order to register the time of ovulation. An appointment for an admission to the hospital for the first checkup must be made as early as 10 days after temperature elevation is measured.

ADMISSION TO THE HOSPITAL FOR THE FIRST CHECKUP

All pregnant diabetic women must be admitted to the hospital as soon as pregnancy has been confirmed, whether the pregnancy has been planned or not. If the pregnant woman has not taken part in a prepregnancy consultation, an assessment must be made of whether the pregnancy is contraindicated, whether therapeutic abortion should be advised, or whether the pregnancy can continue with intensive blood glucose control.

If the pregnant woman wishes to continue the pregnancy, even though there are contraindications to doing so, and if the patient has been informed as to the problems, the prognosis, and the risks involved, then she is offered the chance to take part in the normal control program.

At the initial checkup the blood glucose level should be adjusted as optimally as possible, that is, to approximately 6 mmol per liter. All pregnant women should be trained to test blood glucose levels themselves. The most appropriate method of insulin application is established, i.e., the conventional insulin technique, insulin pump treatment, or the pen-injection technique. The clinical dietitian carries out a dietary analysis and works out an individual diet, including a diet number that in our kitchen means serving a special calorie-fixed diet for each patient when she is subsequently admitted to the hospital for checks.

The pregnant woman's kidney function is again assessed, based on serum carbamide, serum creatinine, and creatinine clearance. Ultrasonic measurements of kidney volume are carried out, and protein excretion is measured daily both quantitatively and by determining urinary microalbumin excretion. Kidney volume in nondiabetics increases during pregnancy by approximately 20 percent. Kidney volume in diabetics, however, increases considerably in most cases, and it is by no means uncommon to see increases of 100 percent. However, if kidneys that are relatively undersized are registered without any particular increase during pregnancy, this is always a serious danger signal. Similarly, protein excretion must be assessed. Most pregnant women in White-class F/R have constant proteinuria. For a group of diabetics who either have microalbumin excretion or normoalbumin excretion in their urine, an increase of protein excretion can be measured during pregnancy. Since in several cases of fetal death we have registered a previous increase in protein excretion (even though it was only as microalbuminuria) as early as several weeks before death, protein excretion must also be included as a prognostic parameter.

Retinoscopy is always carried out. If a proliferative retinopathy is starting, laser treatment is commenced to prevent detachment of the retina.

If the patient has taken part in a prepregnancy consultation, the length of the pregnancy can be assessed, based on the basal body temperature graph and on two ultrasonographic scans. The ultrasound picture might also be compared with the menstrual history, even though this method is somewhat more uncertain. Approximately 30 percent of the diabetic fetuses that are *early growth-retarded* have congenital malformations. This method gives us one more prognostic parameter at an extremely early stage in pregnancy.

Once all examinations have been completed, White's classification is carried out, and the outpatient program is planned.

The pregnant woman is introduced to the entire unit and the social worker is contacted with a view to dealing with the special conditions that apply to pregnant diabetics.

Prior to discharge, the pregnant patient has to complete two tests, partly dealing with dietary matters and partly dealing with ordinary features of diabetes and pregnancy. The answers are checked by the dietitian and one of the nurses on the antenatal ward, and the patient is discharged to the ambulatory program only when her answers to the test questions are satisfactory.

The patient may contact the unit 24 hours a day and can always consult with a specialist if the unit is unable to deal with any problems that may arise.

AMBULATORY TREATMENT

All pregnant diabetics are checked every second week and whenever needed in cases of unstable blood glucose levels or pregnancy complications.

All pregnant diabetics carry out tests on blood glucose level themselves with two 24-hour profiles a week and at least five blood glucose values per day on these 2 days. Urine is tested for glucose if necessary, but *we attach relatively little significance to the secretion of glucose in urine*, since kidney thresholds vary considerably in the course of a pregnancy, and not always in any particular pattern. During ambulatory checks, blood glucose is tested simultaneously by the patient and by the laboratory, which can reveal any errors the patient might have made in her tests. Hb A_{1c} is checked once a month. A reduction in Hb A_{1c} values is almost always noted, not surprisingly as a result of the considerable improvement in glucose regulation during pregnancy. As a result of the 24-hour profiles, any necessary adjustment to insulin doses can be made.

Kidney function is assessed every fourth week by serum creatinine, serum carbamide, and creatinine clearance. Protein excretion is assessed by micro-macro albumin excretion at each check. Urine microscopic examination and urine cultures are carried out at least at every second check, as it is well known that infection of the urinary system is the commonest cause of precoma and coma, entailing a considerable increase in perinatal mortality. Kidney volume is determined each trimester, mainly as a means of observing alterations but also as a means of diagnosing any occurrence of hydronephrosis, since this condition very often brings about pyelonephritis and thereby the development of precoma or coma.

Weighing and the measurement of blood pressure are carried out at each examination. An appreciable increase in weight is often the result of too much insulin or of the accumulation of fluid at the start of pre-eclampsia. An appreciable increase in weight or in blood pressure requires hospital admission to the prenatal unit.

The pregnancy is assessed clinically as well as by the measurement of symphysis-fundus length. It is extremely important that the same person or persons check the pregnant woman, since in this way it is possible immediately to register what is often a minimal alteration in the clinical condition. Only this continuity of care can reduce perinatal mortality to one-third of its present level. Ultrasonographic scanning is carried out every fourth week. By the 16th week crown-rump measurements are taken and thereafter the biparietal diameter is determined, and in the 32nd and 36th weeks fetal weight is calculated. In our unit we determine human placental lactogen levels at each examination, and from the 22nd week serum estriol is measured. Even though estriol has only minor importance as a screening tool during an uncomplicated pregnancy, one nearly always notes a fall in estriol values prior to fetal death, meaning that frequent measurements of estriol in a crisis may be important. Human placental lactogen, the equivalent of the placental mass, is always at the upper end of the normal range, although not in diabetics with late diabetic manifestations. Figures should always be assessed based on individual growth graphs. Kidney function must be taken into consideration, since human placental lactogen is broken down in the kidneys. "Falsely" increased human placental lactogen values are seen at the start of kidney insufficiency even before any serious effect on the fetus can be seen as a result of reduced breakdown of human placental lactogen in the kidneys.

From the 32nd week on the patient is checked each week, and apart from the examinations described above, cardiotocography is carried out as a nonstress test at least once a week.

Retinoscopy is performed each trimester and more frequently if a proliferative retinopathy requiring treatment is present.

FINAL ADMISSION

All pregnant women are admitted to the hospital 24 days prior to their estimated delivery, at the latest. A status examination is carried out for both kidney and fetal function in order to determine if induction should be carried out 21 days before term. Even though several other centers aim for later partus than this, we prefer to deliver at the latest 21 days before term in the majority of cases, since the fetus might well be relatively oversized despite careful regulation, and since there is still the risk of fetal death if delivery is postponed, particularly in the higher White classes.

DELIVERY

Delivery is primarily achieved by rupture of the membranes if the cervix is prepared. If unripe, the cervix is matured by prostaglandin gel. Diabetics in White's class R were previously most often delivered by elective cesarean section, since a worsening of eye complications was feared; the attitude of eye specialists at the moment, however, is that only retinopathy is an indication for cesarean section. Elective cesarean section is often carried out on diabetics with previous cesarean section, unless the patient has actually already started a spontaneous delivery that is well under way.

The fetus in breech presentation is always delivered by elective cesarean section. If there are other complications in addition to diabetes, elective section is also carried out. The frequency of section for insulin-treated diabetics at our unit is between 40 and 50 percent.

On delivery day, insulin amounts are reduced to 50 to 60 percent of the amounts administered in the third trimester. Patients fast and a 5 percent glucose drip is set up, running at 20 drops per minute. Blood glucose is measured at least every second hour, and insulin amounts are calculated accordingly. Blood glucose values are kept at approximately 6 to 7 mmol per liter. Blood glucose values that are too high can entail fetal acidosis. Blood glucose values that are too low result in neonatal hypoglycemia.

Following rupture of the membranes, a decision must be taken as to whether the patient should still fast 100 percent or whether a light breakfast may be given. Unless spontaneous labor begins quickly, a prostaglandin drip is used to stimulate labor. Cross-matched blood should always be available. A labor curve ("Partogram") is kept, since one neither wants a birth that is too quick or one that is too protracted. As a result of the reduced intervillous flow and consequently the increased risk of intrauterine asphyxia, all such fetuses are monitored by cardiotocography, either by external registration or by scalp electrode, as soon as this is possible. The least cardiotocographic abnormality means that a decision must be taken as to the scalp pH. Cesarean section is carried out liberally, since infants of diabetic mothers are considerably more vulnerable than those of nondiabetic mothers. If the labor extends for more than 24 hours, and if there is no sign that delivery will soon take place, it is normally terminated by cesarean section under epidural anesthesia, since after fluid correction this has the least effect on placental circulation. Furthermore, patients are more awake and can eat soon after delivery, which is important for their blood glucose regulation.

As soon as the birth has been completed, umbilical cord pH is determined, and the infants are moved to the premature unit for observation, although not until after an infant-mother relationship has been established.

INFANTS OF DIABETIC MOTHERS

Infants of diabetic mothers in White's class A, B, and C are most often larger than those of nondiabetic mothers.

Even though blood glucose regulation has been optimal, with low mean values, too much glucose is still transported via the placenta. For this reason, most fetuses have some degree of hyperinsulinism. This causes increased fetal growth, which means that these children still weigh more than expected. On the other hand, we often see relatively growth-retarded fetuses in diabetics with late diabetic vascular changes (White's class D and F/R). If there has been hyperinsulinism, the infant most often develops a hypoglycemia neonatally, which is best treated by the mother's milk. Treatment with glucose often causes a reactive hypoglycemia. We nearly always recommend early feeding with breast milk. Glucose infusion can nearly always be avoided. Since we still deliver approximately 21 days before term, the infants are premature despite their often relatively high fetal weight.

As a result of increased diffusion path, making placental oxygen diffusion more difficult, the fetuses adapt in utero by an increase in blood volume. At the time of birth infants of diabetic mothers receive a relatively oversized placental transfusion, which can total 50 percent of the child's blood volume. This in turn causes a relatively oversized neonatal blood volume after birth. In the course of a few hours, circulating volume is normalized by an extracellular displacement of plasma volume. This causes large diureses, a tendency to peripheral edema, and the development of a relative lung edema (transient tachypnea) in the course of a few hours after birth, but normally it passes soon after. A few cases may, however, need treatment with continuous positive airway pressure or a respirator. As a result of the reduction in intravascular plasma volume, hematocrit values increase. This causes increased blood viscosity with circulation and diffusion problems. As a result, we recommend that the umbilical cord be cut early on, approximately 10 to 20 seconds following childbirth. In this way, the child avoids receiving part of the large placental transfusion.

As a result of all these complications, all newborns of diabetic mothers need extremely careful observation by trained staff in a special care unit. Most infants of diabetic mothers need temporary oxygen treatment, guided by transcutaneous Po_2 measurements.

The increased erythrocytic mass is broken down in the course of the following days, causing the development of hyperbilirubinemia. Most infants of diabetic mothers thus need neonatal phototherapy.

As a result of the high frequency of deformities, half of the neonatal deaths in children of diabetic mothers are caused by fatal malformations, most often in the cardiovascular system.

PUERPERITY

Shortly after birth, maternal insulin needs fall to approximately half of the insulin amounts needed toward the end of pregnancy. This is a result of alterations in insulin sensitivity. If the amount of insulin is not reduced correspondingly, patients become hypoglycemic, often to such an extent that this can cause serious cerebral symptoms, which do not, however, last long.

It is always important to ensure that the patient in confinement eats as normally as possible in order to normalize her blood glucose. If cesarean section has been carried out, the glucose drip is always held open until the patient is able to eat normally. For this reason, we prefer epidural anesthesia, the advantage of which is that the patient is able to eat immediately after delivery. Early consumption of food also appears to minimize postoperative paralysis of the intestines.

Patients should always be encouraged to breast-feed, since the baby receives important nutrition in this way. In addition, it appears that breast-feeding protects the child to some extent from the development of diabetes in later life. Breast-feeding, however, is not completely without its problems, since the infant is always under observation in a premature unit in the first days of its life, the time at which normal mother-child contact should be established. In such cases milk should be taken from the mother at first. A further complication is that blood glucose status in puerperity is unstable. These factors mean that extra efforts must be made if normal breast-feeding is to be achieved.

Moreover, it seems that the regulation of diabetes is not reasonably stable again until approximately 3 months after birth. This unstable period is caused by an increased need for calories resulting from the increased milk secretion and the altered and less stable way of life a family with a newborn experiences.

After discharge, we check our patients and their infants after approximately 1 month, after 3 months, and after 1 year. The final consultation is with a view to holding a new prepregnancy consultation, since it is advisable to wait a year before a new pregnancy. On the other hand, a diabetic patient should not be too old before she has finished having her children. We advise diabetics to have only two children, partly because of the strain of a pregnancy and partly because of the diabetic's own prognosis.

ECLAMPSIA

THOMAS M. STUBBS, M.D.
HENRY C. HEINS Jr., M.D., M.P.H.

Eclampsia is the presence of seizure activity (1) in a pregnant patient otherwise fulfilling the criteria for pre-eclampsia, and (2) without other known cause, such as epilepsy. In the modern era, better prenatal care and effective magnesium sulfate prophylaxis have made eclampsia a relatively unusual occurrence in most hospitals. Occasional cases of eclampsia still occur, and so the obstetrician must know how to treat this classic obstetric emergency.

GENERAL GOALS

Although its mechanism of action is debated, magnesium sulfate alone almost always controls the convulsions. General goals are shown in Tables 1 and 2. Stabilization requires a complete history and physical examination (with the history from any available sources), appropriate laboratory evaluation, and careful monitoring of the mother and fetus. Pre-eclampsia-eclampsia may involve the central nervous system, heart, lungs, liver, kidneys, and uteroplacental unit (e.g., abruption, infarction), and so complete evaluation of the patient is necessary to avoid overlooking these aspects of the disease process. Once a patient is fully evaluated and stabilized, delivery is indicated.

GIVE MAGNESIUM SULFATE

Magnesium sulfate ($MgSO_4 \cdot 7H_2O$ USP) is the drug of choice to stop the seizures; give 4 g intravenous push at a rate of 1 g per minute. Four grams of magnesium sulfate is 8 ml of a 50 percent solution, which can be diluted with sterile saline to make it easier to control the rate of intravenous injection. When preparing magnesium sulfate for administration, it is helpful to remember that a 1 percent solution of a drug contains 10 mg per milliliter of that drug. It is well known that too much magnesium sulfate or too rapid a rate of administration causes respiratory compromise. A large-bore intravenous catheter is useful in the management of eclampsia. Regular checks of the emergency cart will ensure that the necessary medications are available when needed.

TREAT SEIZURE RECURRENCE

Occasionally seizures recur after the initial 4-g dose treatment and in spite of the usual maintenance therapy.

TABLE 1 Goals of Management

Stop the convulsions
Minimize maternal and fetal hypoxia
Prevent aspiration
Prevent self-inflicted trauma
Prevent intracranial hemorrhage by controlling severe hypertension
Avoid respiratory compromise from injudicious use of magnesium sulfate
Stabilize and evaluate the patient
Lead and coordinate the team of personnel caring for the eclamptic patient
Choose an appropriate time and route for delivery

Table 3 describes the preferred magnesium sulfate management of seizure recurrence. Sodium amobarbital and diazepam both have extended half-lives, and both readily cross the placenta. One must be alert for maternal or neonatal respiratory depression, which may be provoked or augmented by either sodium amobarbital or diazepam.

Table 4 shows two choices for administration of maintenance magnesium therapy.

MONITOR MAGNESIUM THERAPY

Magnesium sulfate therapy is monitored by evaluation of (1) the reflexes, (2) respirations, (3) urine output, and (4) at some institutions, serum magnesium levels (Table 5).

1. The patellar reflex is a valuable bioassay that is immediate, reliable, and free. When giving magnesium sulfate to a patient who initially had reflexes present, loss of the patellar reflex usually indicates levels of

TABLE 2 Immediate Management of the Seizure

Magnesium sulfate: 4 g IV at a rate of 1 g/minute
Tongue blade
Oxygen
Gentle restraint

TABLE 3 Management of Seizure Recurrence

Give another 4 g of magnesium sulfate IV push at a rate of 1 g/minute; reduce this dose to 2 g if the patient is small.
If the above fails, use one of these:
   Sodium amobarbital (Amytal) up to 250 mg IV push
     over 3 minutes, or
   Diazepam (Valium) 5–10 mg IV push at a rate no faster
     than 5 mg/minute
Watch carefully for respiratory compromise.

TABLE 4 Magnesium Sulfate Maintenance Therapy

Choose either of these regimens:
  After a 4-g IV loading dose, give 2 g/hour by continuous
    infusion.
    Pro: Avoids discomfort of IM injection
    Con: Risk of inadvertent IV administration of dangerous
      amounts of magnesium; do not leave the main
      magnesium bottle open to the patient's IV line! Rarely,
      more per hour may be needed.

  Alternatively, use this IM regimen of proven efficacy
    (J.A. Pritchard); this is especially useful when staffing
    is rationed or maternal transport is necessary:
    Start immediately after a 4-g IV loading dose.
    Give 20 ml of 50% magnesium sulfate solution, one-
      half (5 g) injected deeply into the upper outer quadrant
      of both buttocks through a 3-inch long, 20-gauge
      needle, in turn followed by:
    Every 4 hours 10 ml of 50% magnesium sulfate solution
      (5 g) injected deeply into the upper outer quadrant
      in alternate buttocks if reflexes, respirations, and urine
      output are satisfactory.

    For relief of local discomfort, add 1 ml of 2% lidocaine
      to each IM magnesium dose before injecting.

TABLE 5 Monitoring Magnesium Therapy

Be sure:
  Reflexes: present
  Respirations: >12/minute, normal depth
  Urine output: >25 ml/hour
If a serum magnesium level is obtained, seek the
  therapeutic range: 4–6 mEq/L (or 4–7 mg/dl)

magnesium of at least 8 to 10 mg per deciliter, which is above the therapeutic range. The presence of a detectable reflex helps guard against magnesium overdose (see Table 5).

2. Magnesium levels higher than 8 to 10 mg per deciliter (approximately 8 to 10 mEq per liter) are associated with respiratory compromise or arrest. A respiratory rate of less than 12 breaths per minute is likely to represent respiratory depression from dangerous hypermagnesemia. Respirations should return to normal when maintenance magnesium is given.

3. Urine output is an extremely valuable indicator of the patient's general condition and of the appropriate rate for magnesium sulfate administration. Urinary loss of magnesium is normally rapid. If urine output is less than 25 ml per hour, reduce or stop dosage to prevent hypermagnesemia. An increase in the rate of magnesium administration may be necessary to maintain therapeutic levels in the face of improving renal function and urinary output post partum. Insertion of a Foley catheter is almost mandatory. In addition to indicating that the rate of magnesium sulfate administration may need to be decreased, oliguria may be associated with a change in the color of the urine from yellow to a dark brownish hue, representing bilirubinuria secondary to hepatic involvement in the eclampsia or hemoglobinuria resulting from intravascular hemolysis.

4. The serum magnesium level can be a useful complementary test for the evaluation of magnesium therapy, but this level is never a substitute for the evaluation of reflexes, respirations, and urine output. The serum magnesium level can be useful for ensuring the adequacy of magnesium therapy in patients who are hyperreflexive in spite of the usual 2 g per hour intravenous rate of magnesium sulfate administration. A level of 4 to 6 mEq per liter (or 4 to 7 mg per deciliter) indicates a therapeutic level, and there is no need for an increased rate of magnesium sulfate administration in such a patient. Serum magnesium levels also may be useful in monitoring patients who are hyporeflexive before therapy is even started. If a clinician uses serum magnesium levels, it is valuable to know the past clinical correlation between the patient's condition and local laboratory values, whether given in milliequivalents per liter or milligrams per deciliter.

TREAT MAGNESIUM OVERDOSE

The patient who has respiratory depression from magnesium sulfate is given calcium gluconate, 1 g by intravenous push over 3 minutes (Table 6). Calcium

TABLE 6 Management of Magnesium Overdose

Calcium gluconate, 1 g IV over 3 minutes
Oxygen
Airway and ventilatory support as needed

gluconate is frequently packaged by the manufacturer in 1-g vials containing 10 ml of a 10 percent solution. Respiratory support must be given as needed during the episode of respiratory compromise.

STAFF AWARENESS

Other guidelines involve staff awareness as well as the relationship of magnesium sulfate to hypertension, labor, and fetal heart rate variability. Avoidance of the oversimplified abbreviation "MS" prevents confusion of magnesium sulfate orders with morphine sulfate orders. The clinician should beware of changing the concentration of magnesium sulfate in the bottle without alerting the entire staff of that change. The antihypertensive effect of magnesium sulfate is mild and transient; patients with marked hypertension should be treated with hydralazine (Apresoline), as will be described. Although magnesium sulfate can be used as a tocolytic, it has little effect on established labor in the active phase. The effect of magnesium sulfate on fetal heart variability is controversial, but decreased fetal heart rate variability after the first minutes of administration should make the clinician very suspicious of some other cause of decreased variability.

TREAT HYPERTENSION: HYDRALAZINE (APRESOLINE)

Widespread experience has demonstrated that intravenous hydralazine is the drug of choice for preventing intracranial hemorrhage from severe hypertension in eclampsia. Diastolic hypertension higher than 110 mm Hg should be treated as part of the stabilization of eclamptic or pre-eclamptic patients. In most instances, 5 mg of hydralazine can be given intravenously, followed by checks of the blood pressure every 5 minutes. A higher initial dose of 10 mg would risk hypotension in patients who are very sensitive to hydralazine. The goal is a diastolic pressure of 90 to 100 mm Hg, still high enough to prevent significant uterine hypoperfusion and resulting fetal compromise. After 20 minutes, a further 5 to 10 mg can be given intravenously if necessary, depending on the degree of hypertension remaining and the response to the initial 5-mg dose. To achieve initial blood pressure control, a cumulative total of 5 to 20 mg of hydralazine is commonly given intravenously in severely hypertensive eclamptic or pre-eclamptic patients. Eventual return of the diastolic pressure to levels over 110 mm Hg would require repeat therapy.

Continuous intravenous infusion with an electronic pump can be used as an alternative to the intravenous bolus therapy. Table 7 shows dose per minute and dose per hour at various infusion rates of a mixture of 40 mg of hydralazine and 500 ml of 0.45 normal saline. Avoid mixing hydralazine with other medications.

Hydralazine works mainly by a direct effect on the arteriolar smooth muscle. There is little effect on venous capacitance. Knowledge of the peak effect of intravenous hydralazine at 15 to 20 minutes prevents the clinician from giving too much hydralazine before the initial dose has reached its maximum effect.

Studies using invasive monitoring have shown that in the pre-eclamptic patient, the systemic vascular resistance is increased, as are cardiac output, heart rate, and stroke volume. Hydralazine causes a reflex increase in sympathetic nervous system activity resulting in increased heart rate, stroke volume, cardiac output, and myocardial oxygen requirements. Pre-eclamptic and/or eclamptic patients receiving hydralazine therapy should be observed for angina or signs of cardiac failure, such as hypotension, weak pulse, tachycardia, tachypnea, cyanosis, or rales. Side effects of hydralazine therapy include headache, tachycardia, angina pectoris, anorexia, nausea, vomiting, and diarrhea.

In the unusual instance in which hydralazine does not satisfactorily control the hypertension, two other pharmacologic options are diazoxide and nitroprusside. In a patient who has already received hydralazine, diazoxide should be avoided because the two drugs may act synergistically to cause profound maternal hypotension. For sodium nitroprusside, the disadvantage is that significant fetal and maternal levels of cyanide can develop, resulting from combination of the drug with red blood cells or tissue. Because of the limited experience with sodium nitroprusside in pregnancy, the risk of cyanide to the fetus, and the usual severity of the hypertension in a patient for whom hydralazine therapy alone was inadequate, such patients should be delivered promptly. At least in theory, prompt delivery will minimize the danger of cyanide to the fetus and still allow for nitroprusside control of very severe maternal hypertension that is unresponsive to hydralazine.

When using antihypertensive therapy in pre-eclamptic patients, it is vital that a properly functioning intravenous line be maintained. If hypotension does occur, intravascular volume can be promptly increased as a step toward correcting the hypotension.

ANESTHESIA AND ANALGESIA

For analgesia, 25 mg of meperidine (Demerol) may be given intravenously every 1 to 2 hours to the mother of a term fetus. If possible, avoid narcotics in the eclamptic mother of the premature fetus. Time the meperidine dose so that it is given at the beginning of a contraction in order to minimize placental transfer. Avoid narcotics just before delivery when possible. Avoid oversedation of the postictal eclamptic patient.

For delivery, pudendal block or local infiltration offers the least opportunity for alteration in maternal organ perfusion. When more than local infiltration or pudendal block is needed, general anesthesia is a good choice. Epidural anesthesia can be useful if expertly administered, but spinal anesthesia is to be avoided because of the risk of hypotension. "Topping off" the total magnesium dose

TABLE 7 Hydralazine Drip

40 mg of hydralazine in 500 ml 0.45 normal saline
10 ml/hour = .0133 mg/min = 0.8 mg/hour
20 ml/hour = .0266 mg/min = 1.6 mg/hour
30 ml/hour = .0399 mg/min = 2.4 mg/hour
40 ml/hour = .0532 mg/min = 3.2 mg/hour
50 ml/hour = .0665 mg/min = 4.0 mg/hour
60 ml/hour = .0798 mg/min = 4.8 mg/hour

just before delivery may cause hypermagnesemia in the newborn and should be avoided. The pediatrician appreciates being advised of magnesium therapy in the mother so that the newborn can be observed for symptomatic hypermagnesemia. The anesthesiologist usually decreases the amount of succinylcholine given to these patients because of potentiation of the effect of that drug by maternal magnesium levels. The patient should be watched for seizure activity when recovering from general anesthesia. After general anesthesia, magnesium therapy is promptly reinstituted.

TIMING AND MODE OF DELIVERY

If the eclamptic patient undergoes delivery immediately, the mother and the fetus may both be endangered by unresolved hypoxia and acidosis remaining from the eclamptic episode. It is better to delay delivery until the patient's condition has improved and stabilized. Maternal death has been known to result from a cesarean performed on an unstable eclamptic patient, and better maternal oxygenation usually relieves fetal stress. Acidosis usually corrects spontaneously. Emotional support and a dark quiet room facilitate interim management of the patient. Cesarean section may be indicated for problems other than the eclampsia. Labor can usually be successfully induced, even long before term.

POSTPARTUM ECLAMPSIA

Approximately 25 percent of eclampsia occurs post partum. Magnesium sulfate should be continued in the eclamptic patient 24 hours after delivery and even longer if the patient complains of persistent headache and/or scotomata. Monitoring of blood pressure should be continued after magnesium sulfate is stopped.

Rarely, conventional magnesium sulfate treatment does not prevent late-onset postpartum eclampsia (later than 48 hours). If a postpartum patient is admitted with a history of convulsions more than 48 hours after delivery and is hypertensive with proteinuria and/or edema, late postpartum eclampsia should be the primary diagnosis while ruling out other possible causes. Magnesium sulfate or diazepam may be used for seizure control in these patients. Other disorders that should be considered include cerebral edema, thrombosis, intracranial hemorrhage, hypertensive encephalopathy, pheochromocytoma, intracranial tumor, epilepsy, and metabolic disorders such as hypoglycemia.

EPILEPSY IN PREGNANCY

DONALD J. DALESSIO, M.D.

When treating the pregnant epileptic patient, attempt to maintain her in a seizure-free state. When possible, minimize the adverse effects of the seizure disorder in the course of the pregnancy and the possible teratogenic effects of anticonvulsants on the fetus.

There are many different forms of epilepsy, some quite rare. This review focuses on primary generalized seizures (grand mal or tonic-clonic), including partial complex seizures (temporal lobe), which may become generalized. Absence seizures (petit mal) are discussed briefly.

A few simple rules should be followed:

1. If possible, attempt to withdraw anticonvulsant medication from women who wish to become pregnant and who have been seizure-free for at least 2 years. This should be done slowly, tapering the drug or drugs over a period of 60 to 90 days, *before* pregnancy occurs. Do not attempt to withdraw anticonvulsants from an epileptic woman with a long history of seizures who clearly requires medications.
2. When possible, attempt to obtain seizure control using a single drug (monotherapy).
3. Monitor plasma levels of anticonvulsants frequently during pregnancy.
4. Try to ensure medication compliance and good health habits during pregnancy.
5. Informed consent of the pregnant epileptic is mandatory. The patient must understand the relative risks of epilepsy and its treatment for the developing fetus.

SEIZURE FREQUENCY IN PREGNANCY

Pregnant epileptic patients can be divided into two categories: women who have been identified as epileptic prior to conception and in whom a level of seizure control has been established, and women who experience a seizure disorder that is not related to toxemia for the first time during pregnancy. Fewer than one-quarter of women in the latter group have seizures *only* during pregnancy, and the term "gestational epilepsy" has been applied to this situation. The occurrence of gestational seizures in one pregnancy does not imply that they will recur in subsequent pregnancies.

Most studies suggest that approximately 50 percent of pregnant epileptics experience *no change* in their seizure frequency during pregnancy, 40 percent of pregnant epileptics experience *more seizures* than before, and 10 percent of pregnant epileptics have *fewer seizures* while gravid.

SEIZURES AND COMPLICATIONS OF PREGNANCY

There are no differences between epileptic women and controls in the incidence of hyperemesis gravidarum, abruptio placentae, or toxemia. Bleeding at delivery may be increased in the pregnant epileptic, an occurrence related to vitamin K deficiency produced particularly by phenytoin, phenobarbital, primidone, and related compounds (see later on). Induction of labor and intervention during delivery are reported more frequently in epileptics. There is no relationship between eclampsia and epilepsy.

SEIZURES AND THE OUTCOME OF PREGNANCY

The best statistics on seizures and the outcome of pregnancy come from the Collaborative Perinatal Project (NCPP) of the National Institute of Neurological and Communicative Disorders and Stroke. In this study, conducted between 1959 and 1966, 54,000 women were followed in 12 cooperating university hospitals from the first prenatal visit until the children born of these pregnancies reached 7 years. Stillbirth, microcephaly, mental retardation, and nonfebrile seizure disorders occurred with increased frequency in the offspring of women with seizure disorders. Overall, the risk of any unfavorable outcome was *doubled* in the women with seizures. Low birth weight, neonatal seizures, and first year deaths were not increased in the offspring of pregnant epileptics. About 80 percent of women with seizure disorders in this study had infants with none of the unfavorable outcomes studied. The NCPP study, although invaluable, was done at a time when serum anticonvulsant levels of patients were not available. Nor were physicians aware then of the possible need for increased doses of anticonvulsants during pregnancy. Thus, this study is less than satisfactory in providing data regarding the effects of anticonvulsants on either the pregnancy or the fetal outcome.

PREGNANCY AND METABOLISM OF ANTICONVULSANTS

In general, there is a *decline* in plasma levels of anticonvulsants during pregnancy, when the maintenance dose remains constant.

The available data suggest that phenytoin, carbamazepine, and phenobarbital are cleared more rapidly from the plasma during pregnancy. For carbamazepine, primidone,

and chlorazepate, accelerated metabolism of the drugs may be responsible in part; for phenytoin, the data are less clear. Levels of valproic acid decrease by 30 to 40 percent during pregnancy.

Anticonvulsants are transferred across the placenta, and placental transfer and fetal elimination rates are known for phenytoin, phenobarbital, primidone, and carbamazepine. Phenytoin concentrations are identical in cord and maternal serum at term. The half-life of phenytoin in the plasma of the newborn ranges from 55 to 69 hours. Elimination of the drug by the fetus is generally completed by the fifth day.

Phenobarbital concentrations in human umbilical cord plasma are virtually identical to those of the mother's plasma. Phenobarbital is eliminated from newborns within 2 to 7 days; infants born of epileptic mothers may be dependent on phenobarbital and may experience withdrawal symptoms, characterized by hyperexcitability, tremor, restlessness, and difficulty in sleeping.

The half-life of carbamazepine in the newborn, ranging from 8 to 28 hours, is not significantly different from the half-life of the drug in adults.

Despite these facts, breast-feeding should not be discouraged, unless the infant exhibits poor sucking and somnolence, in which case early weaning can be considered.

TERATOGENICITY OF ANTICONVULSANTS

The incidence of congenital malformations in normal infants varies from 1 to 6 percent, depending on the studies surveyed. Hence, an increased malformation rate can be detected in any study group only if the population is large or the rate of malformation is considerable. It has been suggested that the risk of congenital malformations among infants exposed to anticonvulsants in utero is greater than that in the general population. The anomalies appearing most frequently include cleft palate, cleft lip, and cardiac defects. Among the risk factors for teratogenicity that must be considered are the inherent teratogenicity of the anticonvulsants, the occurrence of frequent convulsions during pregnancy, the incidence of complications during pregnancy, and the socioeconomic class of the pregnant epileptic patient. The incidence of congenital malformations is lowest in mothers who are seizure-free during pregnancy and increases sequentially for epileptic mothers who have multiple seizures, whose disorder is difficult to control, and who require several medications.

During the last decade a fetal hydantoin syndrome was reported, suggesting an association between the drug phenytoin and certain patterns of malformation. The syndrome was characterized by craniofacial anomalies, deficient growth, mental retardation, and limb defects. Subsequent studies have not confirmed this relationship. Similar groups of anomalies have been reported in pregnant epileptics who are not treated or who have been treated with anticonvulsants other than phenytoin. Thus, this issue remains in doubt. It seems most likely that the fetal hydantoin syndrome represents an aggregation of unfavorable findings for which all treated pregnant epileptics are at risk rather than a result of specific exposure to phenytoin.

Some drugs do cause specific syndromes and should be avoided. It is clear that a trimethadione syndrome exists. Affected infants have developmental delay, low-set ears, palatal anomalies, irregular teeth, V-shaped eyebrows, and speech disturbances. Some infants have intrauterine growth retardation, short stature, cardiac anomalies, ocular defects, simian creases, hypospadias, and microcephaly.

Another drug that should be avoided in the pregnant epileptic if possible is valproic acid. In animals, valproic acid is teratogenic, causing dose-related morphologic abnormalities, including cleft palate and renal defects. Recent reports have suggested an association between neural tube defects and valproic acid employed during pregnancy. Given the disability produced by neural tube defects, which are often not amenable to surgical correction, it seems prudent to avoid this drug for seizure control during pregnancy, unless absolutely necessary. If it must be used, amniocentesis before the 20th week of gestation is advised, to detect increases on alpha-fetoprotein levels, which are associated with neural tube defects. If defects are found, therapeutic abortion can be considered.

Finally, according to the American Academy of Pediatrics Select Committee on Anticonvulsants in Pregnancy, no woman should receive anticonvulsant medication unnecessarily. This Committee recommends that medication should be withdrawn from a woman who has been seizure-free for "many years" prior to pregnancy. When a woman who has recurrent epilepsy and requires medication asks about pregnancy, she should be advised that she has a 90 percent chance of having a normal child but that the risk of congenital malformations and mental retardation is two times greater than usual because of her disease and its treatment. There is no reason to switch from phenytoin to phenobarbital or to other anticonvulsants, about which even less is known with respect congenital anomalies. If the patient is actively epileptic, discontinuation of therapy is not advised because of the danger of prolonged seizures.

DRUG REGIMENS AND SEIZURE THERAPY IN PREGNANCY

When possible, it is preferable to treat patients adequately with one anticonvulsant, making sure that the *plasma level is in the therapeutic range*. This is particularly the case in the pregnant epileptic, given the decline in plasma antiepileptic drug levels that occurs routinely during pregnancy if the oral dose ingested is constant (Table 1).

TABLE 1 Anticonvulsants Used for Epilepsy in Pregnancy

Drug	Dosage	Side Effects	Toxicity	Tonic-Clonic	Absence	Complex Partial
Phenytoin (Dilantin)	Average 400 mg/day Range 300–1,200 mg/day Therapeutic level 10–20 μg/ml	Ataxia, drowsiness, gum hyperplasia, hypertrichosis, nystagmus	Rash, serum sickness, pseudolymphoma, Stevens-Johnson syndrome, lupus erythematosus, macrocytic anemia, rare hepatic or marrow toxicity, cerebellar degeneration, peripheral neuropathy	+	–	+
Phenobarbital	Average 120 mg/day Range 30–210 mg/day Therapeutic level 10–35 μg/ml	Drowsiness, ataxia, nystagmus	Rare: rash	+	–	+
Primidone (Mysoline)	Average 1,000 mg/day Range 500–2,000 mg/day Therapeutic level 4–12 μg/ml	Drowsiness, nausea, ataxia, nystagmus (tachyphylaxis usual)	Rash, adenopathy lupus erythematosus, macrocytic anemia, arthritis, edema	+	–	+
Carbamazepine (Tegretol)	Average 600 mg/day Range 200–1,200 mg/day Therapeutic level 6–12 μg/ml	Drowsiness, dizziness, blurred vision, ataxia, GI disturbance	Blood dyscrasia (rare)	+	–	+
Ethosuximide (Zarotin)	Average 1,000 mg/day Range 500–2,000 mg/day Therapeutic level 40–100 μg/ml	Nausea, abdominal pain, drowsiness, personality change, headache	Rash, nephropathy, marrow depression	–	+	–
Clonazepam (Clonopin)	Average 3 mg/day Range 1.5–20 mg/day Therapeutic level 0.01–0.07 μg/ml	Drowsiness, dizziness, ataxia	Coma	+	–	+

From Dalessio DJ. Seizure disorders and pregnancy. N Engl J Med 1985; 312:559–563.

For sustained treatment of intermittent generalized seizures, either phenytoin or carbamazepine should be employed. The choice depends on the clinician's familiarity with the drug to be used and his or her own assessment of the relative risks associated with treatment of the pregnant epileptic. The effective dosage of phenytoin is between 300 and 400 mg daily; it may be taken in divided doses in the morning and at bedtime. After approximately 2 weeks, blood level determinations should be obtained. The therapeutic range is between 10 and 20 μg per milliliter of serum, and the dose of the medication should be raised or lowered to maintain adequate blood levels while achieving seizure control. As much as 1,200 mg per day of phenytoin may be required to maintain adequate serum concentrations during pregnancy.

Many physicians prefer to use carbamazepine initially for primarily generalized seizures or for focal seizures, of complex partial type, if that diagnosis can be established with surety. The dosage ranges from 200 to 1,200 mg per day, the average being 600 mg per day. Occasionally, abnormalities of blood cells, such as aplastic anemia, agranulocytosis, thrombocytopenia, and leukopenia, have been reported following treatment with carbamazepine. Thus, this drug should be discontinued if evidence of significant bone marrow depression occurs, although mild leukopenia can be tolerated. Patients with a history of adverse hematologic reactions to any other drug may be particularly at risk for treatment with carbamazepine.

In initiating anticonvulsant therapy for the previously untreated pregnant epileptic, one-half of the usual maintenance dose can be given, increasing weekly until the full maintenance dose is reached. It is assumed that plasma clearance is slow in those who have not used anticonvulsants before, but autoinduction of liver enzymes increases quickly thereafter. Phenytoin is an exception to this general concept, and a single loading dose of 900 mg can be employed on the first day of treatment.

Absence seizures, such as the petit mal type, are rare in adults but may be seen occasionally during pregnancy. Ethosuximide (Zarontin) is the drug of choice, given in amounts of 250 to 500 mg three or four times daily. Clonazepam (Clonopin), 1 mg three times daily, may also be helpful in this situation.

If seizures occur repeatedly during monotherapy with anticonvulsants, careful assessment of the patient's compliance with the drug regimen is in order. A written regimen of anticonvulsant administration specifying time and dose can be provided. The problem of possible sleep deprivation should be addressed and corrective action suggested. Only thereafter should drug doses by increased to the maximum or a second drug employed. When anticonvulsant levels of the second drug reach the therapeutic range, the first drug can be gradually discontinued over the next 7 days. If seizures again persist, a third drug can be added in a similar fashion. If seizures continue, two drugs can be given, attempting to reach the therapeutic range for both medications.

Treatment of grand mal status epilepticus requires immediate hospitalization. The treatment regimen of Delgado-Escueta and Bajorek, as modified, is recommended (Table 2).

MONITORING ANTICONVULSANT LEVELS

Attempt to establish a treatment regimen that provides optimal seizure control using a single-dose anticonvulsant. When possible, this should be done before the inception of pregnancy. The patient should be educated regarding the importance of medication compliance and good health habits through pregnancy. She should be seen at least monthly so the plasma levels of the anticonvulsant can be obtained and the dose adjusted to the required therapeutic range. Again, it may be necessary to increase

TABLE 2   Management of Generalized (Tonic-Clonic) Status Epilepticus in Pregnancy (Modified from Delgado-Escueta and Bajorek)

1. Insert an indwelling intravenous catheter. Draw venous blood for anticonvulsant levels and toxic screen, glucose, blood urea nitrogen, electrolyte, and complete blood count stat determinations. Draw arterial blood for stat pH, Po_2, Pco_2, HCO_3. Monitor respiration, blood pressure, and heart activity (electrocardiogram). If possible, monitor the patient's electroencephalogram. Monitor the fetus.
2. Start intravenous infusion through an indwelling venous catheter with normal saline containing vitamin B complex. Give a bolus injection of 50 ml 50 percent glucose. Give 100 mg thiamine intramuscularly.
3. Infuse diazepam intravenously no faster than 2 mg per minute until seizures stop or to a total of 20 mg.* Also start infusion of phenytoin no faster than 50 mg per minute to a total of 18 mg/kg. If hypotension develops, slow the infusion rate. (Phenytoin, 50 mg/ml in propylene glycol, may be placed in a 100-ml volume control set and diluted with normal saline. The rate of infusion should then be watched carefully. Alternatively, phenytoin may be injected slowly by intravenous push.
4. If seizures persist, two options are now available: intravenous phenobarbital *or* diazepam in an intravenous drip. The two drugs should *not* be given in the same patient. An endotracheal tube should now be inserted. Continue to monitor fetal signs.
5. Intravenous phenobarbital option: Start infusion of phenobarbital no faster than 100 mg per minute until seizures stop or to a loading dose of 20 mg/kg.
6. Diazepam intravenous drip option: 50–100 mg of diazepam are diluted in 500 ml D5W and run in at 40 ml per hour. This ensures diazepam serum levels of 0.2 to 0.8 μg/ml.*
7. If seizures continue, general anesthesia with halothane and neuromuscular junction blockade is instituted. If an anesthesiologist is not immediately available, 50 to 100 mg of lidocaine may be given by intravenous push. If lidocaine is effective, 50 to 100 mg diluted in 250 ml of D5W should be dripped intravenously at a rate of 1 to 2 mg per minute.
8. If lidocaine has not terminated seizures within 20 minutes from the start of infusion, general anesthesia with halothane and neuromuscular junction blockade must be given. Continue to monitor fetal signs.

* Intravenous lorazepam can be considered as a substitute for diazepam. The lack of active metabolites and the longer duration of action in status epilepticus make it a useful alternative. (From Dalessio DJ. Seizure disorders and pregnancy. N Engl J Med 1985; 312:554–563.)

medications during pregnancy; the doses needed for maintenance may reach levels that would be toxic in the nongravid state. These doses may be required for variable periods after delivery, with reductions in dose depending on plasma levels obtained subsequently in the postpartum period. Usually, weekly serum level determination of anticonvulsants are necessary in the postpartum period.

If possible, the trough plasma level, the lowest plasma anticonvulsant level for a 24-hour period, should be obtained. This is usually achieved by testing a sample of fasting blood before the initial anticonvulsant dose of the day.

HEMORRHAGIC DISEASE OF THE NEWBORN AND ANTICONVULSANTS

In newborns exposed to phenytoin or barbiturates in utero, bleeding tendencies may develop during the first day of life after delivery; these are related to decreased levels of vitamin K–dependent clotting factors despite normal levels in the mother. This form of drug-induced vitamin K deficiency should be distinguished from the physiologic deficiency occurring in normal infants between the second and fifth days. The drug-induced bleeding disorder occurs earlier and may be life-threatening; it can be prevented with injections of vitamin K (phytonadione) in the mother prior to delivery, and in the newborn. One milligram should be given routinely to all newborns after delivery. In infants known to be exposed in utero to antiepileptic drugs, clotting studies should be obtained 2 hours after the vitamin K is administered. If the clotting factors continue to be abnormal, consultation with a pediatric hematologist is strongly suggested.

SUGGESTED READING

Dalessio DJ. Seizure disorders and pregnancy. N Engl J Med 1985; 312:559–563.

Delgado-Escueta AV, Bajorek JG. Status epilepticus: mechanisms of brain damage and rational management. Epilepsia 1982; 23 (Suppl. 1):29–41.

Levy RH, Yerby MS. Effects of pregnancy on antiepileptic drug utilization. Epilepsia 1985; 26(Suppl. 1):552–557.

Nelson KB, Ellenberg JH. Maternal seizure disorder, outcome of pregnancy, and neurological abnormalities in the children. Neurology 1982; 32:1247–1254.

Stumpf D. Anticonvulsant use during pregnancy. Clin Ther 1985; 7:258–265.

HERPES SIMPLEX INFECTION

ALFRED G. ROBICHAUX III, M.D.
JOHN H. GROSSMAN III, M.D., Ph.D., F.A.C.O.G.

Herpes simplex virus (HSV) is a double-stranded DNA virus that produces clinical infection in less than 1 percent of all pregnant patients. Most women with HSV infections have a self-limited localized mucous membrane lesion lasting several days to weeks. When *recurrent* HSV complicates parturition, the likelihood of neonatal infection is relatively low (less than 8 percent). Serious perinatal morbidity is substantially more likely (40 percent) when women acquire *primary* genital HSV during pregnancy. Nearly 60 percent of all newborn HSV infections are either disseminated or localized in the central nervous system. Despite antiviral chemotherapy, the mortality 6 months after diagnosis of disseminated neonatal herpes exceeds 50 percent. Of these survivors, only 35 percent will develop normally. Hence, precautions are necessary to prevent these devastating outcomes.

CONGENITAL INFECTIONS

A limited number of congenital HSV infections have been reported. These cases are associated with severe consequences for the fetus, including skin lesions and sores at birth, chorioretinitis, microcephaly, hydrocephalus, and microphthalmia. These cases have been associated with primary, recurrent, and (presumably) asymptomatic maternal infections at varying times during gestation. The risk of in utero transmission of HSV appears to be extremely low. We suspect that this virus is highly destructive to susceptible tissue and that early intrauterine infection most likely results in early pregnancy loss. Such a hypothesis is consistent with the observation that systemic maternal HSV infection during the first trimester is associated with a threefold increased frequency of miscarriage. If the mother does not abort, the obstetrician feels pressured into determining whether intrauterine infection has occurred. Limited experience with HSV culture of amniotic fluid has not consistently correlated with intrauterine infection; therefore, we do not recommend amniocentesis. Experience with prenatal diagnosis of other congenital infections by serologic testing of cordocentesis samples obtained after 21 to 22 gestational weeks has been reported. This approach might be applicable to patients at risk for congenital HSV, provided that they are identified prospectively. Further investigation in this area is needed. Detailed sonographic examination after organogenesis is complete may also be of value.

ANTEPARTUM MANAGEMENT

The most important aspect of antepartum management is the identification of individuals who are truly at high risk. Historical data are of particular importance. A pregnant patient with a history of HSV infection should be questioned regarding (1) the presence of prodromal symptoms, (2) the areas of the body affected, and (3) criteria for previous diagnoses. The reliability of previous diagnoses is an important issue because we are able to document genital herpes by tissue culture in only one-third of all patients who claim to have ongoing problems with HSV by history. If there is clinical suspicion that a herpetic infection may be present, attempts should be made to isolate the virus in tissue culture as soon as possible. Diagnosis dependent on exfoliative cytology lacks sufficient sensitivity and specificity for obstetric management, compared with viral isolation in tissue culture. Papanicolaou smears alone are therefore not acceptable for the diagnosis of genital herpes during pregnancy. Rapid and reliable tests for detection of HSV are being developed. These should be useful in antepartum and intrapartum surveillance for infection. There is insufficient experience at present, however, to assess their value in clinical management.

Successful culture of herpes from a presumed lesion requires careful attention to technique. The patient should point out specific symptomatic target areas. If vesicles or crusted lesions are found, they should first be "unroofed" and then swabbed with a cotton swab until the fibers become discolored by absorbed secretions. This will be uncomfortable for the patient, but it is the only method that ensures reliable recovery of the virus. The endocervical canal should also be gently swabbed to detect silent cervical carriage. Swabbing of the vaginal wall is rarely useful, since heavy bacterial contamination decreases the yield of positive results—although an exception to this is a specific painful vaginal lesion. The purpose of culturing the lesions is to confirm the absence of infection. A complete and properly obtained negative culture in a symptomatic patient is good evidence *against* HSV infection.

The culture swab should be placed immediately in the appropriate transport medium and sent to the laboratory. The medium is a balanced salt solution supplemented with calf serum and antibiotics. It is available in most laboratories and, frozen at $-20°C$, can be stored in the office until use. After a culture is taken, it should be transported promptly to the laboratory; if this is not possible, it may be kept in the refrigerator at $4°C$ (*not* frozen) until transportation can be arranged. Refreezing a newly obtained culture decreases its infectivity almost tenfold and may lead to a false-negative test result. Fifty percent of positive HSV cultures are completed within 24 hours, and 90 percent are positive within 72 hours of sampling.

OTHER GENITAL INFECTIONS

Not every mucocutaneous lesion that brings a woman into the office is caused by herpes infection. Major differential conditions that occur commonly in pregnancy include (1) excoriated lesions from physical trauma, (2) scratching due to allergic reactions, and (3) moniliasis. Several symptomatic office visits lead to one of two outcomes: (1) HSV is present, as indicated by the association of specific signs and symptoms with a positive culture (especially valuable information when the pregnancy is close to term), or (2) HSV cannot be documented. This should reassure both physician and patient that the risk of HSV for the fetus is minimal, as well as prompt investigations of other causes of symptoms.

DELIVERY

If a genital HSV infection is suspected at any time during the pregnancy, culture should be obtained promptly for documentation. Most patients have an average of two to three episodes, with a range of one to nine. Even if a patient has a documented episode of HSV infection during pregnancy, she should be allowed to deliver vaginally, as long as there is no *clinical* evidence of recurrent infection during the interval before delivery.

Data acquired during the last 5 years indicate that weekly cultures near term do not affect the incidence of neonatal herpes and are very expensive, and should therefore be abandoned. If there is no clinical evidence of HSV infection at the onset of labor, vaginal delivery should be permitted. There is reason to believe that maternal antibodies may modify the duration and quantity of virus exposure and may afford partial neonatal protection. Should clinical symptoms develop, attempts must be made promptly to document HSV by culture. At the time of delivery, clinical suspicion of reinfection must take precedence over a negative culture.

In the patient near term with a satisfactory estimate of gestational age and a positive HSV infection by culture, we continue surveillance by culture. As soon as we can verify absence of infection, we discuss with the patient induction of labor as a means of avoiding cesarean delivery. Naturally, before induction is employed, clinical conditions should be favorable for a successful vaginal delivery and fetal maturity should be assured. Conversely, if the patient is at term and has an active genital infection, cesarean delivery is appropriate, provided that both doctor and patient agree to the risks and benefits of this approach and there is a reasonable likelihood that the fetus is mature.

All patients in labor who have active genital HSV infections should have an abdominal delivery. There is no "magic cut-off point" at which patients with prolonged rupture of membranes and active infection should not have an abdominal delivery. In fact, abdominal delivery is recommended regardless of the duration of amniorrhexis, since it cannot be assumed that every infant has acquired the virus by ascending infection.

EXTRAGENITAL HERPES SIMPLEX VIRUS

Extragenital herpetic lesions occasionally prompt management questions. HSV appears to be tightly cell-bound, so that only direct contact with the lesion or infected secretions can lead to transmission. Therefore, simply covering lesions distant from the vulva (e.g., on the buttocks or thighs) with a dressing will secure the area for safe vaginal delivery without risk of infection. Patients with distant lesions that are adequately covered are also suitable candidates for internal monitoring by scalp electrode and intrauterine pressure catheter, if these procedures are indicated for obstetric reasons. Patients are allowed epidural anesthesia, provided that there are no active presacral or lumbar lesions.

POSTPARTUM CARE

We use strict isolation of potentially infected newborns to prevent horizontal spread within the nursery. Rooming-in is allowed and recommended. Breast-feeding is without risk to the newborn, provided that lesions are covered and good hand-washing techniques are followed. Babies should be followed closely for 7 to 10 days by pediatricians alerted to the possibility of HSV infection.

INCOMPETENT CERVIX

WILLIAM H. MICHAELS, M.D., F.A.C.O.G.
HOWARD O. THOMPSON, M.D.

Cervical failure (CF), or more commonly cervical incompetency (CI), is the inability of the internal os of the cervix to contain the products of conception between the 13th and approximately the 25th weeks of gestation. The diagnosis of CI can be difficult and elusive. Since the etiology is multifactorial, successful management requires the skillful use of multiple diagnostic systems to avoid overdiagnosis or misdiagnosis. The condition has been recognized for well over a century, and it is estimated that in the United States 20,000 to 30,000 pregnancies are affected annually. It accounts for up to 15 percent of all second-trimester losses and a significant number of premature births. Every obstetric patient must be considered at potential risk.

Unlike the situation in many other obstetric catastrophes, a highly successful form of intervention has been available for over 30 years: an encircling suture or cerclage can be placed to reinforce the internal os. A major deterrent to a successful operation is failure to make a timely diagnosis. Once advanced membrane protrusion (hourglassing) has developed, the chance of surgical success is greatly diminished.

The timing of cerclage placement after the 12th gestational week avoids the risk of first-trimester abortion, and intervention before the 18th week reduces the possibility of cervical failure when the weight of the conceptus can no longer be supported by the internal os. The contemporary practice of documenting an intact pregnancy with ultrasonography in the early second trimester makes prophylactic placement of a suture possible before 16 weeks when the diagnosis is established by history, diagnostic signs and symptoms in the current pregnancy, or a previously placed cerclage.

Since the age for fetal viability is now 25 to 26 weeks, patients first diagnosed as having CF in the early third trimester are of special concern. Until recently, surgical intervention was rarely recommended after 20 weeks. Sutures placed after this date are traditionally considered to be less successful and associated with a higher incidence of premature rupture of the membranes, infection, and premature labor. Nonetheless, since the availability of second-generation tocolytics, many obstetricians now place sutures up to the 24th week of gestation. Although cerclage placement is possible after 24 weeks, surgical intervention after that time is highly controversial. In selected cases, we have been able to perform cerclage procedures successfully up through the 25th week of gestation when cervical changes are documented without evidence of labor. This is a gray area, for the clinician must determine whether the primary failure of the cervical mechanism or premature labor is the cause of cervical dilatation and/or effacement.

Many authors advocate cerclage placement before definite cervical changes in all patients who are at risk, and maintain that early surgery is less complicated and can avoid the problems of late diagnosis. Higher, although spurious, success rates have been demonstrated for such patients. A positive diagnosis made after traditional cervical changes avoids many unnecessary cerclage procedures. The cerclage operation is not without risk and may increase the incidence of preterm labor and premature rupture of the membranes, which makes the aggressive posture unacceptable to many clinicians, including ourselves. We usually consider previous placement of a cerclage to be an absolute indication for a repeat cerclage when cervical changes and history are well documented. However, selected patients do not exhibit evidence of cervical failure in a subsequent pregnancy because of cervical scarring. A rigorous cervical surveillance protocol (Table 1) is followed when a suspicious but less certain history is noted, or when the patient is at risk because of special circumstances, such as a twin pregnancy, proved diethylstilbestrol (DES) exposure, or cervical abnormalities. Many of these patients will not need surgery. Primigravid patients are a diagnostic dilemma, and special attention must be paid to development of symptoms, changes noted on pelvic examinations, and ultrasound surveillance.

HISTORICAL RISKS

The primigravida has no obstetric history, but a carefully taken gynecologic history may reveal important information. Table 2 shows the histories of a group of 107 at-risk patients. All had at least one historical risk marker. These histories confirm the impression of other authors that cervical incompetency is often acquired through obstetric or gynecologic manipulations of the cervix (Table 3). Although it is not often mentioned, cervical trauma caused by extension of a cesarean incision into the cervix, myomectomy, or metroplasty may place a gestation at increased risk for CI.

Congenital defects involving the lower uterine segment–cervical complex or uterus may also cause CI

TABLE 1 Incompetent Cervix Surveillance Protocol

I. Identification of patients at risk
    A. History
    B. Symptoms
    C. Pelvic findings (initial examination)
    D. Initial ultrasound examination*
    E. Follow-up pelvic examination if A–D positive

II. Alert patients to possible symptoms
    A. Advise immediate physician notification if
        1) increased vaginal or rectal pressure
        2) heaviness in pelvis
        3) increased discharge (watery, serosanguineous)
        4) frank bleeding
        5) sudden change in bowel or bladder habits
        6) sensation of "something falling out" of the vagina
        7) increased uterine irritability
    B. When symptoms develop
        1) treat as an obstetric emergency
        2) arrange for immediate examination

III. If suspicious symptoms, pelvic examination, or history
    A. Weekly pelvic examinations beginning at 14–16 weeks
    B. Initial ultrasound examinations at 14–16 weeks
        1) if normal
            a. weekly pelvic examinations until 26 completed weeks
            b. ultrasound examinations every other week to 26th completed week
        2) if abnormal and
            a. suspicious—repeat in 24 hours
            b. positive—careful pelvic examination and immediate admission for cerclage
            c. if nonconfirmatory ultrasound changes—repeat in 1 week

IV. If cervical incompetency suspected by ultrasound or pelvic examinations or symptoms
    A. Avoid intercourse
    B. Avoid travel
    C. Modify activities as required
    D. Take increased rest, elevate legs
    E. Follow for possible
        1) premature rupture of membranes
        2) preterm labor
        3) incompetent cervix
    F. Admit to ultrasound surveillance protocol

* All ultrasound examinations must include a detailed survey of the lower uterine segment–cervical complex.

TABLE 2 Distribution of Historical Risks for Developing Incompetent Cervix (107 Patients Reporting 192 Risk Factors)*

Rank	Risk Factors	% Risks	% of Patients††	N†
1	Spontaneous second trimester loss	11.5	20.6	22
2	Preterm labor	10.4	18.7	20
3	Induced abortion (any trimester)	9.4	16.9	18
4	Suspicious or poor history	9.4	16.9	18
5	Premature rupture of membranes	8.9	15.9	17
6	Twins	7.8	14.0	15
7	Previous cervical dilatation	6.8	12.1	13
8	Miscellaneous	5.7	10.3	11
9	DES exposure	5.2	9.3	10
10	Previous cerclage	3.6	6.5	7
11	Classic history without cerclage	3.6	6.5	7
12	Habitual pregnancy loss	3.1	5.6	6
13	Short cervix	3.1	5.6	6
14	History of cervical trauma	3.1	5.6	6
15	Cold conization	3.1	5.6	6
16	Labor abnormalities	2.6	4.7	5
17	Myoma	2.6	4.7	5
	Total	100.0	179.5	192

* Modified from Michaels WH, Montgomery C, Karo J, et al. Ultrasound differentiation of the competent from the incompetent cervix: prevention of preterm delivery. Am J Obstet Gynecol 1986; 154:537.
† N = number of patients reporting each risk factor
†† Some patients had more than one risk factor

TABLE 3   Mechanism of Acquired Cervical Incompetency

Obstetric
   Multiple induced abortions
   Second-trimester abortion without *Laminaria*
   Forceps trauma
   Dilatation of immature cervix
   Spontaneous cervical laceration
   Cervical tear at cesarean section

Gynecologic
   Repair of septate uterus
   Deep conization of cervix
   Laser conization
   Cervical myomectomy
   Cervical pregnancy
   Partial vaginectomy

to develop. Until the late 1960s, a congenital disturbance in the ratio of collagen to muscle tissue was thought to be responsible. Our studies demonstrate that one in five patients exposed to DES antenatally develop CI. When an exposed patient had also undergone a partial vaginectomy, the risk rose to one in four.

The diagnosis of a multiple gestation may also increase the risk for premature, passive cervical shortening and CI. Universal placement of a prophylactic cerclage in all multifetal pregnancies has not proved effective in randomized studies. It is well established, however, that a "relative" cervical incompetency can occur. In our experience, CF develops in one in 10 twin pregnancies. It is our opinion that when symptoms and clinical changes are noted and confirmed by ultrasonography, selective cerclage placement before 26 weeks is warranted for some patients.

Induced abortion was the third leading risk factor noted for our patients (see Table 2). We maintain a close vigilance on these patients, especially when the abortion has been performed before a previous term pregnancy or at a very young maternal age. The year in which the abortion occurred may also be important, because studies reviewing abortions performed soon after legalization suggested an increased incidence of CI related to those procedures. Current reviews do not suggest such a risk.

Among our patients, a previous second-trimester loss and preterm labor ranked as the most common historical risks (see Table 2). Premature rupture of the membranes before 36 completed weeks of gestation was also associated with CF. We monitor all patients with similar histories, even if CF has not been previously suspected. Less than one in 10 of our patients studied were at risk because of a previous cerclage procedure. Documentation of all important historical risk factors is the cornerstone to making an early and precise diagnosis of CI.

OBSERVING FOR CLINICAL SYMPTOMS

For the successful management of a patient at risk, the recognition of possible symptoms of CI is extremely important (Table 4). It is worrisome that approximately two-thirds of patients at risk reported no symptoms and that over one-third of the diagnosed patients did not recognize the significance of their symptoms. Over one-half of the positive diagnoses in our clinical experience would have been missed if symptoms alone were used to initiate a pelvic examination. Experience has shown that many patients who experience these symptoms do not have an incompetent cervix, but a delay in performing an examination may lead to an irremediable situation. We have seen more than one patient in consultation for whom this basic examination was omitted or postponed until the next morning, only to find that they had advanced to an untreatable stage or had sustained rupture of the membranes. We teach all at-risk patients to recognize and report symptoms as they occur so that they can be examined immediately.

A bloody discharge was reported by 6.5 percent of our at-risk patients and by almost all of our patients who developed advanced cervical shortening and dilatation. It accounted for about 15 percent of all symptoms and was the most significant symptom since changes were noted on 70 percent of the vaginal examinations. Increased pressure and vaginal discharge were the most frequently reported symptoms among all patients at risk.

TABLE 4   Distribution of Characteristic Symptoms of Incompetent Cervix*

Rank	Symptom	N	% of Symptoms Reported	% of Symptoms Among Population at Risk
1	Increased pressure	24	52.2	22.4
2	Increased discharge	10	21.7	9.3
3	Bloody discharge	7	15.2	6.5
4	Dysuria	2	4.8	1.9
5	Bleeding	2	4.8	1.9
6	Cramps	1	2.3	0.9
	Total	46	100.0	42.9

Seventy-four of 107 at-risk patients (69.2%) had no symptoms; some patients had more than one symptom.

* Modified from Michaels WH, Montgomery C, Karo J, et al. Ultrasound differentiation of the competent from the incompetent cervix: prevention of preterm delivery. Am J Obstet Gynecol 1986; 154:537.
N = number of patients reporting the symptom

TABLE 5   Pelvic Examination

I. Evaluation with large speculum
   A. ? Lacerations
   B. ? Symmetry, shape, position
   C. Longer than 2.5 cm (normal)
   D. Less than 2.5 cm (? short)
   E. Can membranes be seen?
   F. Note DES changes
   G. ? Cervix patulous (redundant)
   H. Evidence of congenital malformation
   I. Nitrazine, fern test
   J. Suspicious lesions
II. Culture cervix
   A. *Chlamydia* culture
   B. Gram stain
   C. Vaginal flora
   D. Gonococcus (GC) culture
   E. Pap smear if not recently done and cervix closed
III. Gentle palpation
   A. Only after speculum examination
   B. ? Fornices well formed
   C. ? Sensation of bulging in the lower uterus
   D. ? External os dilated
   E. ? Effacement
   F. Internal os open?; closed?*

* We do not invade the internal os because dilatation can be demonstrated on ultrasonogram.

PELVIC EXAMINATIONS

Patients at risk should undergo weekly pelvic examination beginning at the 14th or 16th week of gestation (Table 5). Serial examinations are not necessary before 12 weeks since the pressure from the products of conception does not test the competency of the internal os before this time. Ideally, the patient should be examined by the same physician and the degree of dilatation and effacement should be noted. Even when the anatomy is normal, the imprecision and subjectivity of the pelvic examination often leaves the clinician with a feeling of uncertainty.

For patients with abnormal anatomy, a patulous-multiparous cervix, a juvenile cervix, multiple unrepaired lacerations, or an apparently short cervix, the pelvic examination is even more difficult. Slightly over one-third of at-risk patients in the authors' series had short cervices, while almost one-fifth were described as patulous. As noted in Table 6, not all of our patients had significant pelvic findings. Nearly one-third of our diagnosed patients showed positive changes on ultrasonograms when CI was first diagnosed, but had inconclusive histories, symptoms, or pelvic examinations.

ULTRASOUND EXAMINATIONS

Frustrated after examining many patients on a twice-weekly basis only to find visible membranes, advanced shortening, and cervical dilatation at the next examination, we sought a reliable method of earlier diagnosis that could also avoid overtreatment of patients with questionable cervical shortening. The anatomic position of the cervix is ideal for ultrasound examination (Fig. 1). The amniotic fluid allows precise definition of the internal os. When the bladder is moderately distended, the lower uterine segment–cervical complex is displayed between the fluid interfaces. Only the vaginal side of the cervix lacks a natural fluid-filled compartment to improve resolution. This can be overcome by placing a 30-ml, fluid-filled Foley balloon against the cervix, or by introducing approximately 20 ml of sterile saline into the vagina when the patient is in a reclining position, hips up. The syringe is gently held in the vagina by an assistant and acts as an obturator. The cervix is now surrounded on three sides by a fluid medium and is easily displayed using the 3.5-mHz sector transducer. Alternatively, vaginal probes allow visualization of the same anatomy without requiring a distended bladder or vaginal lavage. We have used both techniques and find them to be interchangeable.

The regional anatomy of the lower uterine segment and cervix is dynamic when viewed by real-time ultrasonography. Our initial attempts to diagnose cervical incompetency with ultrasound were unsuccessful when only measurements of cervical length were used (Table 7). A short, stable cervix may be competent, while a longer cervix that is dilated more than 10 mm with some degree of membrane protrusion tends to be incompetent. Depending on the degree of bladder distention, the length and

TABLE 6   Results of Pelvic Examination (107 Patients at Risk)*

Rank	Findings	N	% of Findings	% of Patients at Risk
1	Short cervix	36	51.4	33.6
2	Patulous cervix	20	28.6	18.7
3	Changes of DES exposure	5	7.1	4.7
4	Deformed cervix	5	7.1	4.7
5	Cervical dilatation	2	2.9	1.9
6	Distended lower uterine segment	2	2.9	1.9
	Total	70	100.0	65.5

* Modified from Michaels WH, Montgomery C, Karo J, et al. Ultrasound differentiation of the competent from the incompetent cervix: prevention of preterm delivery. Am J Obstet Gynecol 1986; 154:537.
N = number of patients in whom the finding occurred

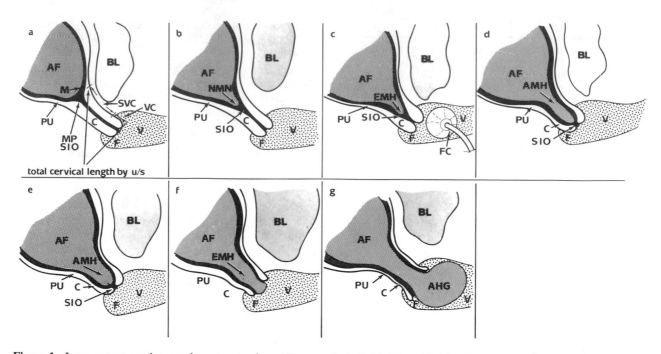

Figure 1 Incompetent cervix: membrane protrusion. AF = amniotic fluid; BL = bladder; C = cervix; F = fornix vagina; PU = posterior uterine wall; SIO = sonographic internal os; V = vagina. *a*, Normal cervix. M = amniotic membranes; MP = mucus plug; SVC = supravaginal portion of cervix; VC = vaginal cervix. *b*, Normal cervix with nipple. NMN = normal membrane nippling. *c*, Early membrane herniation (EMH). FC = Foley catheter bulb against cervix. *d*, Advanced membrane herniation (AMH). *e*, Advanced membrane herniation with further cervical dilatation. *f*, Membranes prolapsed into vagina. EMH = early membrane hourglassing. *g*, Hourglassing of membranes. AHG = advanced hourglassing of membranes.

thickness of the cervix can vary by 20 percent during each examination. If the bladder is overdistended, the anterior and posterior walls of the lower uterine segment are approximated, creating the impression of a long cervix with false membrane protrusion through a pseudointernal os. Movement of the fetus or amniotic fluid into and out of the lower uterine segment can create a similar situation and lead to a false diagnosis of cervical incompetency.

Looking for Membrane Displacement or Herniation

The sonographer must appreciate the dynamics of membrane protrusion through the internal os. Normally, the fetal membranes form a wide, smooth "U" shape as they course over the internal os (Fig. 1*a*). The "U" configuration narrows with excessive bladder filling, decrease in forewaters, or movement of the fetus out of the lower uterus. Increased external pressure from the transducer can cause a similar alteration in shape of the membrane formation. A highly contractile lower uterine segment may also narrow the "U." Under some circumstances, perhaps when the mucus plug is not well formed or snug against the internal os, a nipple-like formation can be seen that by definition measures less than 6 mm (Fig. 1*b*).

Physiologic Principles

When support is lost, the chorioamniotic membrane begins to protrude through the internal os and herniate into the cervix (Fig. 1*c*). The cervix continues to dilate and efface under the influence of gravity, abnormally directed uterine forces, and increasing membrane herniation (Fig. 1*d*). Ultimately, either the tensile strength of the membrane is exceeded and rupture occurs, or it continues to protrude through the cervical canal, causing the mucus plug to be expelled (Fig. 1*e*). Both situations result in increased vaginal discharge, which is commonly serosanguineous. For some patients the membrane does not rupture: it slides through the internal os into the vagina and forms a secondary fluid-filled sac with an hourglass shape (Fig. 1*f*). If large enough, the hourglassed membrane distends the vagina, causing low back, bladder, or rectal pressure (Fig. 1*g*). As these events occur, the patient often has the sensation that the pregnancy is "falling out." Such changes can be readily documented by serial ultrasound examinations.

DIAGNOSIS

The earliest changes of CI do not necessarily occur on the vaginal side of the cervix. Anatomically, 40 to 50 percent of the cervix, the pars supravaginalis, is located above the vaginal vault and is not visualized or palpated on vaginal examination. Sonographic examination of the lower uterine segment–cervical complex visualizes the entire cervix and establishes the diagnosis of CI earlier and more reliably (Fig. 2).

From study of serial sonographic examinations of over 200 patients at risk, we believe dilatation of the internal

TABLE 7 Useful Ultrasound Measurements*

Average Measurements

	Normal	*Postdiagnosis*
Cervical length	44.3 ± 9.2 mm	30.3 ± 11.1 mm
Membrane protrusion	2.7 ± 4.5 mm	20.3 ± 15.9 mm
Cervical dilatation	2.6 ± 5.8 mm	17.1 ± 10.1 mm

Diagnostic Criteria

Cervical length	Approximately 30% decrease in length without labor
	> 25 mm and stable, normal
	< 25 mm, short, at risk
	< 20 mm, suspicious
	< 15 mm, incompetent until proved otherwise
Membrane protrusion	≤ 6 mm, normal
	> 6 mm, abnormal
	> 6 mm with progressive changes, diagnostic of cervical incompetency
Cervical dilatation	< 10 mm, may be normal
	> 10 mm and stable, suspicious
	> 15 mm with herniation of membranes, diagnostic of cervical incompetency

These measurements are a guide only. Serial changes are the most important factor in making the diagnosis of cervical incompetency.

* Modified from Michaels WH, Montgomery C, Karo J, et al. Ultrasound differentiation of the competent from the incompetent cervix: prevention of preterm delivery. Am J Obstet Gynecol 1986; 154:537.

os and membrane protrusion can occur in the days, and sometimes hours, preceding the development of physical symptoms or vaginal changes. Measurements of membrane protrusion, cervical length, and cervical dilatation can serve as guides (see Table 7). Each patient should undergo weekly ultrasound examinations to establish the diagnosis while serving as her own control. Once suspicious changes are observed, ultrasound examinations are repeated in 24 hours. Progressive herniation, dilatation, and decreasing cervical length constitute the ultrasound diagnosis of CI (Table 8).

The natural behavior of the cervix in pregnancy should be understood before one attempts to use ultrasound to assist in making the diagnosis of CI. The cervix is rarely dilated or effaced before the 20th week of gestation. Several studies have demonstrated that the external os dilates 2 to 3 cm after 28 weeks of gestation in about one-third of patients. About 90 percent of these patients have a closed internal os, and most deliver at term. Therefore, any patient in the second and perhaps early third trimester, whose vaginal examination is suspicious should be examined by ultrasound.

ANCILLARY TECHNIQUES

Other than our ultrasound technique and the traditional method of performing serial pelvic examinations, we are not aware of another useful method for diagnosing CI during pregnancy. When the diagnosis is considered before conception, a hysterogram can demonstrate congenital uterine abnormalities or funneling of the uterine cavity at the level of the cervix. Passage of an 8- to 10-mm He-

gar dilator without resistance prior to menses is suggestive of cervical incompetency. These test results are not usually available to the obstetrician when he suspects CI in pregnancy.

SURGICAL TECHNIQUE AND POSTDIAGNOSIS MANAGEMENT PROTOCOL

When the diagnosis of CI is made, the patients are admitted to the hospital, placed in Trendelenburg's position, and prepared for a cerclage. If not already on tocolytics, patients are started preoperatively on subcutaneous terbutaline. Tocolytic therapy is continued for at least 1 week after surgery. It is usually changed to oral therapy (2.5 mg every 4 to 6 hours) 24 hours after the cerclage is placed. Patients are routinely surveyed for anemia and bladder or vaginal infection, and complete cultures are taken, including a *Chlamydia* screen. Antibiotic coverage is used only when cultures are positive.

Our surgical technique is a modification of the procedure taught by Sherman, a pioneer in the management of CI. It combines features of both the McDonald and the Shirodkar cerclages. A precerclage, intraoperative ultrasound is performed. The bladder is distended with normal saline or genitourinary irrigant through a three-way Foley catheter. The cervix is measured, the position of the membranes is noted, and the fetus is evaluated. The bladder is emptied and surgically advanced after the anterior vaginal mucous membrane is incised just in front of the bladder reflexion. A 4-mm Mersilene suture on a 3/4-inch tapered needle is placed intrastromally as close to the internal os as possible. Usually four to six passes into and out of the cervical stroma are required before the suture can be tied. We secure the knot tightly in a purse-string fashion; this closes the cervical canal, and avoids leaving a loop of suture exposed (Fig. 3). The knot is tied anteriorly for ease of removal. Bleeding from the bladder dissection usually stops at this time, because the suture acts as a tourniquet. Any bleeding vessels are clamped and ligated, but this is rarely required. After the suture is tied, the bladder is redistended and the location of the cerclage is noted by ultrasound. If the suture is intrastromal and located no lower than one-half the distance between the external and internal os, the bladder is emptied and

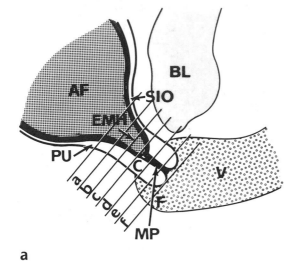

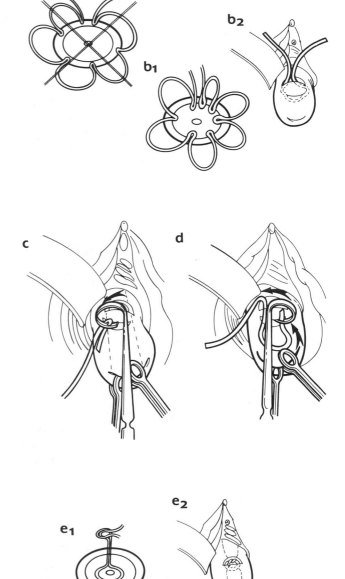

Figure 2 Details of membrane herniation as seen sonographically. *a–f* = level of transverse sections; AF = amniotic fluid; BL = bladder; C = cervix; EMH = early membrane herniation; F = fornix; MP = mucus plug; SIO = sonographic internal os; V = vagina (small circles represent sterile saline). *a*, Lower uterus (LU). M = amniotic membranes; P = posterior placenta. *b*, Lower uterine segment (LUS). MH = membrane herniation. *c*, Upper cervix, dilated internal os (DIO), and canal. *d*, Dilated midcervix. *e*, Residual mucus plug. *f*, External os (EO) and residual plug.

Figure 3 Details of high cerclage placement. *a*, Submucosal suture. b_1, Intrastromal placement of suture. b_2, Intrastromal placement of suture. *c*, Anterior cervical incision; counterclockwise suture placement. *d*, 360-degree circumference of cervix completed. e_1, Knot tied securely, anteriorly. e_2, Anterior cervicovaginal incision closed.

TABLE 8   Ultrasound Protocol

I.   Complete ultrasound examination
   A. BPD, femur length
   B. Abdominal, head circumferences after 24 weeks
   C. Assessment for anomalies
   D. Placental position
   E. Evaluation of adnexae
   F. Evaluation of developing lower uterine segment after 20 weeks
II. Evaluation of lower uterine segment–cervical complex
   A. Differential bladder filling
     1) PO fluid to moderate bladder distention
     2) observe cervix, lower uterine segment
   B. If overdistended, allow partial voiding
   C. If inadequate filling
     1) further PO fluids *or*
     2) retrograde distention with Foley catheter
   D. Measure cervical length: draw a line through the center of the cervical canal, which is often represented sonographically by an anechoic space in the center of the cervix, from the vaginal side of the decidual plate or the base of the membranes in front of the sonographic internal os to the base of the sonographic external os. If the decidual plate is present, the length of the cervix is measured only to the vaginal side of the decidual tissue that separates the membranes from the internal os (Fig. 1).
   E. Measure cervical dilatation
   F. Note position of membranes relative to sonographic internal os
III. Observe for membrane protrusion through internal os
   A. Nipple: protrusion < 6 mm
   B. Herniation: protrusion > 6 mm
   C. If less than 6-mm protrusion, repeat in 24 hours
   D. Progressive protrusion of membranes constitutes ultrasound diagnosis of cervical incompetency and is always associated with cervical dilatation
IV. Measurement of cervix
   A. Includes
     1) vaginal cervix
     2) supravaginal cervix
V.   If significant changes, admit for cerclage procedure

* Placement of a 30-ml Foley balloon against the cervix or instillation of sterile saline or water (20 ml) into vagina with hips elevated in dorsal lithotomy position helps define distal end of cervix and fornices. Syringe held in vagina by assistant acts as an obturator.

the vaginal mucosa closed with a running 2–0 chromic suture. The cerclage can easily be seen to be placed extravesically and intrastromally on transverse and longitudinal scan views. After surgery the three-way catheter is replaced with a No. 16 Fr., 5-ml catheter, which is usually left in situ until the following morning.

Postoperatively, the patient is maintained in Trendelenburg's position until a program of gradual ambulation is started. A Kleihauer-Betke stain is performed on maternal serum to determine if RhoGAM is needed for Rh-negative patients. The patient is usually discharged after 72 to 96 hours. Maternal-fetal surveillance is continued on an outpatient basis. A follow-up ultrasound examination is obtained within 1 week of discharge. Urinalysis and culture screen are repeated at this time. Patients are seen weekly until delivery. Pelvic examinations are not repeated until 36 weeks unless indicated.

The cerclage is removed after 37 completed weeks of pregnancy. If oral tocolytics have been continued, they are stopped. Approximately 20 percent of patients go into labor within 24 hours of cerclage removal. Induction is indicated if the cervix opens more than 3 cm or a history of precipitous labor is noted. In only 5 percent of our patients was labor induced. Cesarean section is carried out for obstetric indications only. For a planned cesarean section, the cerclage is removed after delivery. When pre-term labor unresponsive to tocolytics occurs, or premature rupture of the membranes is noted, the cerclage is removed immediately. Over 90 percent of our patients deliver spontaneously after the onset of labor, usually within 1 week of cerclage removal.

Over 100 cerclages have been placed using the procedure described, which combines ultrasound surveillance with high intrastromal cerclage placement. Most procedures are performed under spinal anesthesia. Cervical necrosis or devascularization have not occurred. We have not experienced intraoperative membrane rupture, cerclage slippage, or the need for a second suture. Only two cases of documented cervical dystocia have occurred. We have achieved a 95 percent success rate defined by intact membranes and delivery after 36 weeks.

SUMMARY OF PROTOCOL

Table 9 outlines our protocol for diagnosing and treating the incompetent cervix. On the initial visit, we emphasize key historical points and establish abnormalities of pelvic anatomy. We recommend initial ultrasound surveillance and pelvic examination for at-risk patients at 14 to 16 weeks. For patients not undergoing ultrasound examinations at this time, we recommend another pelvic examination at approximately 18 to 24 weeks. If the cervix is

TABLE 9 Cerclage Protocol

I.   Diagnosis of incompetency confirmed
   A.   History
   B.   Serial pelvic changes
   C.   Serial ultrasound changes
   D.   Development of significant symptoms
II. Consider emergent procedure
   A.   If membranes are not visualized through speculum, place cerclage within 24 hours
     1) admit to hospital
     2) place in Trendelenburg's position
     3) confirm nonrupture of membranes
     4) culture vagina
     5) CBC, differential, urinalysis
     6) start subcutaneous terbutaline (0.25 mg) 1 hour before surgery
   B.   If membrane herniation exceeds 30 mm or cervix is well effaced, or if membranes can be seen, consider as an obstetric emergency
     1) repeat A (1–5)
     2) start terbutaline immediately
     3) arrange for stat OR
   C.   Avoid hourglassing of membranes
III. Obtain informed consent
IV. Avoid digital manipulation of exposed membranes; limit pelvic examination to speculum surveillance only until cerclage
V.   Administer spinal anesthesia (avoid hypotension)
VI. Arrange for intraoperative ultrasound surveillance
   A.   Place three-way Foley catheter
   B.   Distend bladder
   C.   Measure cervical length, dilatation, membrane protrusion
   D.   Use 30-ml Foley balloon vaginally to help identify distal end of cervix
   E.   Empty bladder
   F.   Observe fetus, fetal heart rate, movement, breathing during cerclage
VII. Placement of cerclage (assistant required)
   A.   Identify mucosal reflexion over bladder
   B.   1¾-inch incision into vaginal mucosa
   C.   Ligate arterial bleeders
   D.   Elevate bladder using either digital pressure or sponge stick; proper plane must be established
   E.   Insert 4-mm Mersilene suture counterclockwise
     1) use long Allis clamps or ring forceps for traction
     2) place patient in steep Trendelenburg's position
     3) tie suture anteriorly
       a. five knots
       b. secure knot with silk ligature (2–0)
   F.   Four to six bites into and out of cervix will be required
     1) ensure intrastromal placement of cerclage
     2) always place cerclage as close to internal os as possible (high suture)
     3) leave no segment of cerclage exposed, except anteriorly
     4) be sure cerclage is placed as high as possible in posterior cervix, as well
     5) If membranes are exposed, insert 30-ml pediatric Foley catheter, distended with 10–20 ml saline into lower cervix to protect membranes
     6) Tie knot as tightly as possible
       a. reduces bleeding
       b. closes canal completely
       c. pull cerclage up as a "pursestring"; be sure all loops are pulled into cervix before tying
     7) take patient out of steep Trendelenburg's position as soon as possible
   G.   Close vaginal incision with running 2–0 chromic suture; inform patient that small strings may be seen in 8–10 days as suture dissolves
   H.   Secure hemostasis

I.   Repeat ultrasound measurements
     1) ensure cerclage is at least 50% of distance toward internal os
     2) ensure cerclage is entirely intrastromal
     3) ensure cerclage is located extravesically
VIII. Postcerclage management, first 24 hours
   A.   Replace three-way Foley catheter with 16 Fr., 5-ml device; leave Foley in place 12–24 hours
   B.   Watch I/O
   C.   Observe for uterine irritability
     1) subcutaneous terbutaline (0.25 mg) every 4–6 hours
     2) if after 20 weeks' gestation, monitor for contractions and fetal heart rate
   D.   Order one-time 50-mg Demerol, if necessary
     1) if further pain medication required, consider possible implications
       a. ? labor
       b. ligated ureter
       c. hematoma
   E.   Pad count 24 hours
   F.   Obtain urinalysis before Foley removed
   G.   Complete bed rest, modified Trendelenburg's position, first 18–24 hours
IX. Second 24 hours postsurgery
   A.   Change to PO terbutaline (2.5 mg) every 4–6 hours
     1) discontinue if no symptoms
     2) if uterine irritability, continue PO terbutaline
   B.   Gradual ambulation
   C.   Observe for fever, bleeding, evidence of bladder infection
X.   At 72 hours, consider for discharge
XI. Ultrasound examination 1 week after cerclage, with pelvic examination
   A.   Ensure nonslippage
   B.   Ensure membranes are intact
   C.   Ensure continued fetal viability
XII. Continue weekly visits
   A.   Observe for
     1) premature rupture of membranes
     2) increased uterine irritability
     3) premature labor
     4) infection
   B.   Culture cervix at 36 weeks
   C.   Repeat urinalysis
   D.   Pelvic examination if symptoms, abnormal discharge
   E.   Ultrasound examination every 4–6 weeks to assess fetal growth and cervical status
XIII. Removal of suture
   A.   Establish fetal maturity by dates
   B.   Amniocentesis if indicated
   C.   Remove cerclage at maturity, or if labor or premature rupture of membranes
   D.   If cesarean section planned, remove cerclage after delivery of fetus
   E.   Observe for 4 hours postcerclage removal
     1) if > 3-cm dilatation and 80% effacement, consider induction, *or*
     2) discharge, await spontaneous labor
XIV. Delivery
   A.   Anticipate spontaneous labor for most patients
   B.   Cesarean section for obstetric indications
XV. Manage concurrent medical or obstetric complications
XVI. Consider all patients at risk or diagnosed to have cervical incompetency as a *high-risk pregnancy*

short or the position of the fetus unusually low, an ultrasound examination should be performed and repeated weekly until the 28th week of pregnancy. If CI has not been established, patients are followed for possible premature labor. If uterine irritability is established by the observation of more than three contractions per hour, patients are placed on oral tocolytics, regardless of the cervical status.

We extend our appreciation to our medical staff; our research associates, Joel Ager, Ph.D. and Faye Schreiber, B.A.; and to John Temple, M.D., and James Karo, M.D., who performed the intraoperative ultrasound studies.

SUGGESTED READING

Michaels WH, Montgomery C, Karo J, et al. Ultrasound differentiation of the competent from the incompetent cervix: prevention of preterm delivery. Am J Obstet Gynecol 1986; 154:537.
Sherman AI. Hormonal therapy for control of the incompetent os of pregnancy. Obstet Gynecol 1966; 28:198.

INTRAUTERINE GROWTH RETARDATION: OBSTETRIC ASPECTS

SCOTT N. MacGREGOR, D.O.

Low infant birth weight may result from two distinct pathologic entities: preterm delivery and failure of normal fetal growth. The recognition of the heterogeneity of this group of infants has enabled the special risks of each subgroup to be appreciated. The small for gestational age (SGA) fetus is at greatly increased risk of perinatal morbidity and mortality compared with fetuses whose birth weights are appropriate for gestational age (AGA). In addition, neurodevelopmental abnormalities are more frequent in SGA as compared with AGA infants. Detection of fetal growth retardation is essential so that intensive fetal surveillance may be instituted and pregnancy intervention accomplished prior to fetal compromise.

Although fetal growth retardation is an accepted clinical entity, it has no universally accepted definition. Any classification of growth-retarded fetuses should reflect differences in sex of the fetus, racial status, maternal parity, and geographic location. Growth retardation is traditionally defined as birth weight less than the tenth percentile for gestational age. However, this definition includes those fetuses with pathologically reduced growth potential (e.g., congenital infections), those with abnormal growth due to inadequate uteroplacental supply of nutrients, and constitutionally small fetuses. The constitutionally small group is normally nourished and probably incurs no increased perinatal risk. Conversely, fetal malnutrition and associated perinatal morbidity may occur in normal birth weight infants. Finally, because the diagnosis of growth retardation relies on infant birth weight, definitive diagnosis must await delivery. Therefore, recognizing the limitations of the definition of in utero growth retardation, the goal of obstetric care should be early identification of diminished fetal growth and institution of appropriate antepartum and intrapartum management.

CLASSIFICATION OF GROWTH RETARDATION

Growth-retarded fetuses are commonly divided into two subgroups: symmetric and asymmetric. These subgroups are related to the time of onset and the duration of the events that caused diminished fetal growth. Symmetric growth retardation results from fetal insult early in gestation, which may cause cell death or retard cell division, leading to symmetric reduction in organ size. These infants are symmetrically small (head circumference, abdominal circumference, length) relative to AGA infants. Therefore, weight-to-length ratios are usually normal. Factors associated with symmetric growth retardation are listed in Table 1.

Asymmetric growth retardation results from a fetal insult or abnormal processes later in gestation. In later gestation, cell number is complete; therefore, these processes affect only cell size. These infants usually have normal head size and length. However, subcutaneous tissue and abdominal circumference (liver size) are reduced and, as a result, weight-to-length ratios are also reduced. Common factors associated with asymmetric growth retardation are listed in Table 1. Although the causes of asymmetric growth retardation are varied, all result in altered uteroplacental blood flow and transfer of oxygen and nutrients to the fetus. Fetal compensation for these alterations, redirecting blood flow to the brain and heart and away from the visceral organs, results in the asymmetric growth pattern. The reductions in subcutaneous fat and liver size are due to increased utilization and decreased storage of fat and hepatic glycogen, respectively. With the exception of fetal chromosomal abnormalities, congenital malformations and infections, symmetric growth retardation may reflect more severe uteroplacental abnormalities than those observed in asymmetric growth retardation.

Finally, an additional subgroup at risk for fetal death and neonatal morbidity may be identified. This group demonstrates a flattening of the fetal growth curve and loss of subcutaneous fat. Birth weights are within the normal ranges; however, these infants are thin and length-to-weight

TABLE 1 Factors Associated with Fetal Growth Retardation

Genetic abnormalities*
Congenital malformations*
Congenital infection*
Teratogen exposure*
Immunologic factors (lupus anticoagulant, anticardiolipin antibody)*
Severe malnutrition
Tobacco smoking
Ethanol abuse
Drug abuse (cocaine, opiates)
Cyanotic heart disease
Chronic hypertension
Pre-eclampsia/eclampsia
Diabetes mellitus (class D-R)
Chronic renal disease
Severe anemia
Placental abnormalities
Multiple gestation
Previous stillbirth or SGA infant

* Primarily associated with symmetric growth retardation.

ratios may be abnormal. These fetuses are classified as manifesting late-onset fetal malnutrition.

SCREENING FOR FETAL GROWTH RETARDATION

Precise estimation of gestational age is essential for identification of the fetus with suspected growth retardation. Lack of accurate gestational age assessment leads to difficulty in determining whether a fetus is growth-retarded or appropriately grown but with inaccurate gestational age assessment. Estimated date of delivery has been shown to be inaccurate in 20 to 40 percent of women with regular menstrual histories. Therefore, early and meticulous establishment of gestational age should be attempted. Some authors have advocated routine ultrasound examination at 16 to 20 weeks of pregnancy to achieve this goal. This recommendation is reasonable in those patients with inaccurate menstrual histories and those who have risk factors associated with fetal growth retardation. *The inability to estimate gestational age reliably in the third trimester by either clinical or ultrasound parameters continues to be a major cause of undiagnosed fetal growth retardation.* Recent data suggest that transverse cerebellum diameter may serve as a reliable indicator of gestational age even in these fetuses with abnormal growth. This implies that the cerebellum is the last region of the fetal brain to be affected by a decrease in blood flow. This measurement may prove to be useful in fetal growth retardation due to uteroplacental aberrations. However, it is unlikely to be reliable in the fetus who is undergrown as a result of either chromosomal abnormalities or congenital infection.

Previous delivery of a growth-retarded infant imparts the highest risk for subsequent fetal growth retardation (see Table 1). However, one-third of the growth-retarded infants have no identifiable antenatal risk factors. Clinically, fetal growth is evaluated by measuring uterine fundal height, which coincides with gestational age between 18 and 34 weeks. Inappropriate growth is suspected if the measurement lags more than 2 cm below the expected height. Although numerous studies have confirmed the usefulness of this measurement as a screening technique, there are several problems associated with relying on fundal height. These include low positive predictive value, inability to differentiate symmetrically and asymmetrically growth-retarded fetuses, and limited usefulness beyond 34 weeks' gestation. As a result, ultrasound techniques have become the cornerstone in screening, diagnosis, and management of abnormal fetal growth. Screening for fetal growth retardation by ultrasound examination should be performed in any pregnancy with risk factors or size-date discrepancies as assessed by fundal height.

ULTRASOUND DIAGNOSIS OF FETAL GROWTH RETARDATION

Advances in ultrasound technology have enabled obstetricians to identify fetal growth retardation more accurately. The majority of ultrasound techniques rely on precise estimation of gestational age. Fetal biometric parameters, ratios of these measurements, amniotic fluid volume, placental grade, estimated fetal weight, and Doppler velocity waveform measurements can all be utilized in the evaluation of fetal growth.

Biparietal diameter (BPD), head circumference (HC), abdominal circumference (AC), and femur length (FL) measurements are routinely obtained during ultrasound examination and compared with normal values. In pregnancies with accurate gestational age assignment, growth retardation may be suspected on the basis of these measurements and classified as symmetric or asymmetric. Abdominal circumference is the most reliable of these measurements in identifying the undergrown fetus, since it is diminished in both types of growth retardation. Furthermore, these measurements may be obtained serially (as frequently as every 14 days) to evaluate continued growth. The ratio of these values may provide additional information. The head circumference to abdominal circumference (HC/AC) ratio can be used to distinguish between symmetric and asymmetric growth retardation. Femur length to abdominal circumference (FL/AC) ratio has been utilized as a fetal "ponderal index." In the neonate, the ponderal index (birth weight $\times$ 100/crown-heel length) is used to identify infants who are undergrown relative to their length. The use of the FL/AC ratio is based on the fact that femur length is related to length and abdominal circumference is related to birth weight. Unlike HC/AC, the FL/AC ratio is constant over a wide range of gestational ages. Similarly, recent studies have calculated fetal midarm circumference to abdominal circumference, a ratio commonly used in the neonate to identify malnutrition. However, these ratios may only identify the asymmetrically growth-retarded fetus.

Estimated fetal weight (EFW) may also be calculated using biparietal diameter, head circumference, abdominal circumference, and femur length measurements. EFW is the value most frequently relied on to diagnose suspected fetal growth retardation, since it relates directly to birth weight, which is used to diagnose growth retardation definitively. Fetal growth retardation is suspected in those pregnancies with EFW less than the tenth percentile for gestational age relative to birth weight tables derived from a similar population. The following formulas are those we commonly use to calculate EFW:

1. $\text{Log EFW} = 1.326 - 0.0034 \, (AC \times FL) + 0.0107 \, (HC) + 0.0438 \, (AC) + 0.158 \, (FL)$.
2. $\text{Log EFW} = -1.7492 + 0.166 \, (BPD) + 0.046 \, (AC) - 0.002646 \, (AC \times BPD)$.
3. $EFW = 1.304 + 0.05281 \, (AC) + 0.1938 \, (FL) - 0.004 \, (AC \times FL)$.

Formulas 2 and 3 are utilized if femur length or biparietal diameter measurements, respectively, are difficult to obtain. The accuracy of these formulas is usually plus or minus 10 percent of EFW.

Additional ultrasound evaluations used to aid in the diagnosis of fetal growth retardation include amniotic fluid volume assessment, placental grading, and distal femoral epiphyseal ossification center identification. Oligohydramnios in the absence of ruptured membranes is associated with a high incidence of fetal growth retardation. However, amniotic fluid volume is normal in more than 80 percent of pregnancies resulting in SGA infants (i.e., low sensitivity). Similarly, grade III placentas (Grannum's classification) in preterm gestations are associated with an increased frequency of fetal growth retardation. Yet, this finding is common in term and post-term pregnancies, and the majority of pregnancies with undergrown fetuses have lesser-grade placentas. Distal femoral epiphyseal ossification center identification by ultrasound examination has been advocated as a method to differentiate between growth-retarded and normal or constitutionally small fetuses. This method requires further confirmation prior to clinical use.

Doppler ultrasound is one of the newest and most promising methods of evaluating pregnancies for fetal growth retardation. Doppler velocity waveform measurements of the umbilical and uterine arteries roughly correlate with blood flow and have been used to evaluate uteroplacental function. In most instances, large reductions in velocity are accompanied by reductions in blood flow. Doppler velocity waveform measurements are based on the relationship between systole and diastole, most commonly expressed as the systolic-diastolic ratio (S/D or A/B). The placental vessels are characterized by continuous diastolic blood flow and progressive fall in resistance as gestation advances. Maternal uterine artery and fetal umbilical artery waveforms reflect placental resistance. Therefore, a progressive fall in the S/D ratio in the uterine and umbilical arteries is observed as pregnancy progresses. After 30 weeks' gestation, the S/D ratio of the umbilical artery should be less than 3.0. Fetal growth retardation due to uteroplacental perfusion abnormalities is associated with increased placental resistance, decreased umbilical blood flow, and elevated S/D ratios. It is logical and has been suggested by some authors that Doppler velocity waveform measurements are abnormal prior to diminution of fetal growth parameters assessed by ultrasound. Fetal prognosis deteriorates as diastolic flow decreases, and absent or reversed flow is associated with the greatest likelihood of fetal demise.

MANAGEMENT OF FETAL GROWTH RETARDATION

Accurate gestational age estimation and history must be obtained at the initial prenatal evaluation. Patients with questionable dates and those who have risk factors associated with fetal growth abnormalities (see Table 1) should have early ultrasound examination to establish expected date of delivery. In addition, those with risk factors or size-date discrepancies by fundal height examination should have serial real-time and Doppler ultrasound evaluations of the fetus. In these pregnancies, ultrasound examination is repeated at least every 3 to 4 weeks. If risk factors are identified that may be treated or eliminated, therapy should be instituted as soon as possible. After identification of an SGA fetus, an intensive effort should be made to (1) classify the growth retardation as symmetric or asymmetric, (2) diagnose the etiology, and (3) ensure delivery of a viable infant when possible.

Classification is accomplished using real-time and Doppler ultrasound methods previously described. Fetal anomalies, abnormal karyotype, and congenital infections should be considered as etiologic factors in symmetrically undergrown fetuses. Extensive sonographic evaluation is performed to exclude fetal structural abnormalities. Fetal cells may be obtained for chromosomal analysis by either amniocentesis or percutaneous umbilical blood sampling. Percutaneous umbilical blood sampling offers the advantage of rapid results (48 hours versus 2 to 3 weeks with amniocentesis). In addition, fetal blood may be examined for total and specific IgM (to evaluate the presence of congenital infection) and blood gas indices (to evaluate fetal acid-base status). If percutaneous umbilical blood sampling is not performed, maternal antibody titers to rubella

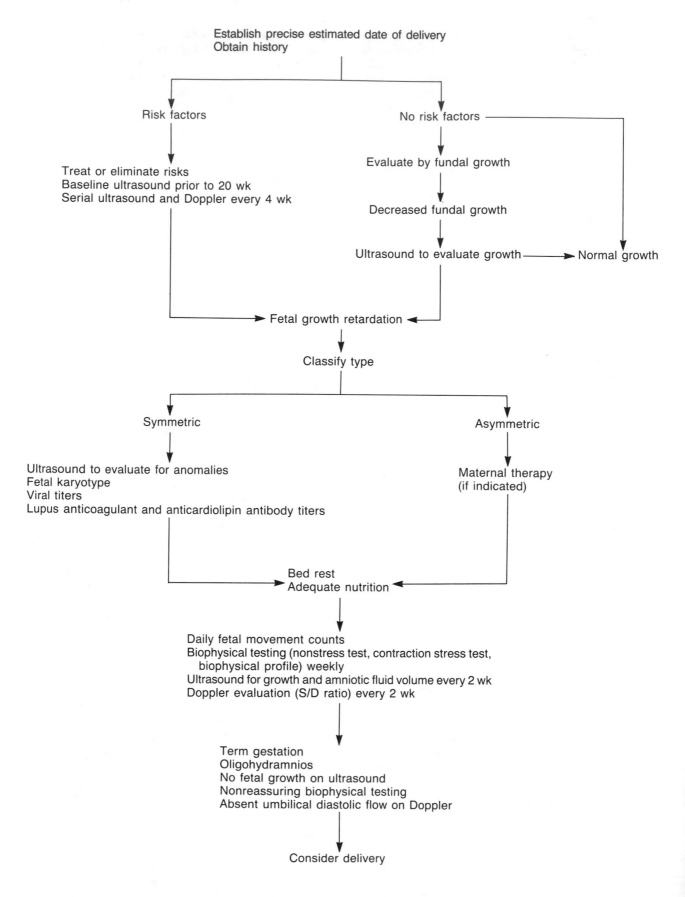

Figure 1 Diagnosis and management of fetal growth retardation.

and cytomegalovirus should be obtained. In both symmetric and asymmetric groups, lupus anticoagulant and anticardiolipin antibody titers should be obtained. Positive test results would be most useful in subsequent pregnancies.

Patients are placed on bed rest (either in the hospital or at home) in order to provide maximal placental perfusion and delivery of oxygen and nutrients to the fetus. In a recent study, humidified oxygen (55 percent) was administered continuously to patients whose pregnancies were complicated by severe growth retardation and fetal hypoxia. This therapy resulted in improved fetal acid-base status (assessed by percutaneous umbilical blood sampling) and decreased placental resistance (assessed by Doppler ultrasonography). Maternal hyperoxygenation may be considered in pregnancies complicated by severe fetal growth retardation at an early gestational age when neonatal survival is low. At a minimum, fetal surveillance includes the following: daily fetal movement counts, ultrasound evaluation of fetal growth and amniotic fluid volume every 2 weeks, and Doppler velocity waveform measurements of the umbilical artery every 2 weeks. In addition, fetal biophysical testing (nonstress test, biophysical profile, or contraction stress test) should be initiated when growth retardation is suspected, and should be repeated at least weekly. These fetal surveillance techniques may be repeated as frequently as every day if severe fetal growth retardation is present.

Delivery should be considered in pregnancies with suspected fetal growth retardation under the following circumstances: diagnosis at term; oligohydramnios; absence of interval fetal growth on serial ultrasound examination (10 to 14 days); nonreassuring fetal biophysical testing; and absent umbilical artery diastolic flow on Doppler evaluation. The decision to proceed to delivery is a matter of ascertaining the risks from continued fetal stay in utero compared with the risks of prematurity. Among growth-retarded infants, those delivered between 37 and 40 weeks' gestation have a better prognosis than those delivered before 37 weeks' gestation. Since uteroplacental insufficiency is commonly associated with fetal growth retardation, these fetuses are more likely to become intolerant of labor. Fetal heart rate should be monitored throughout labor, and preparation for immediate cesarean section should be made if needed. Finally, it is essential that the initial care of the newborn be provided by a skilled pediatrician. A summary of the diagnosis and management of the growth-retarded fetus is outlined in Figure 1.

LATE FETAL DEATH

BRUCE A. MEYER, M.D.
ROBERT K. CREASY, M.D.

Intrauterine fetal demise is one of the most difficult challenges facing the obstetrician. Currently, the World Health Organization defines late fetal death as that occurring after 28 completed weeks of gestation; however, many states define it as death that occurs after gestation of 20 weeks or more, which complicates statistical analysis. Fetal mortality has ranged from 10 to 15 per 1,000 in the United States over the past 5 years. The diagnosis of fetal demise has been significantly simplified by the widespread use of real-time ultrasonography. More sophisticated techniques of fetal and maternal evaluation have led to improved understanding of the myriad causes of this event. However, the cause of a significant proportion of late fetal deaths still remains unexplained. All the skills of the practitioner are demanded in dealing with methods of delivery and in assisting with the process of grieving. Attempts to determine the etiology of the demise are especially important in terms of the counseling of families regarding future pregnancies.

ETIOLOGY

Consideration of the causes of fetal death can be divided into five broad categories: chromosomal abnormalities, congenital malformations, infections, immunologic causes, and obstetric complications, the last of these dealing primarily with maternal disease and placental implantations and functions.

Chromosomal Abnormalities

A large number of chromosomal abnormalities have been extensively studied and catalogued, and the great majority lead to fetal wastage in the first trimester. The largest group of these abnormalities involve either changes in the numbers of a single chromosome or in sets of chromosomes. The most common proven forms associated with late fetal demise are the trisomies, the most well known being trisomy 13, 18, and 21. The remaining autosomal trisomies are thought to be generally incompatible with survival through the first trimester. The monosomy most commonly associated with late demise is monosomy X (or Turner's syndrome), although the overwhelming majority of conceptions with this abnormality terminate spontaneously in the first trimester. Structural chromosomal abnormalities resulting from breakage or rearrangement of chromosomal segments have also been identified, unbalanced translocations being those most commonly involved in late fetal death.

Congenital Malformations

Fetal malformations account for approximately 25 percent of late fetal deaths, one-half of these having a genetic etiology. Death is believed to be related to sudden decompensation of a biochemical or structural nature. Abnormalities of the heart, urinary tract, gastrointestinal system, and neural tube are the most common, although it remains a mystery why some fetuses with the same specific malformation die in utero while others succumb in the neonatal period. Neural tube defects such as spina bifida, anencephaly, and holoprosencephaly are associated with the highest incidence of stillbirth, although disorders of the urinary tract such as obstructive uropathy, cystic or dysplastic kidney, and complete renal agenesis also carry a high rate of in utero demise. Anomalies of the gastrointestinal tract such as omphalocele, gastroschisis, and intestinal atresia have also been noted in stillborn fetuses. Additionally, nonchromosomal skeletal dysplasias, amniotic band syndromes, and some forms of congenital dwarfism (most commonly osteogenesis imperfecta type II and achondrogenesis) have presented as stillbirths. Autopsy is especially important in these cases, as establishment of the specific diagnosis can be of critical value in determining the risk of recurrence.

Infections

Infection is involved in a decreasing proportion of in utero fetal deaths, primarily owing to our increasing ability to treat and thus prevent fetal loss; the most dramatic example is syphilis. Currently, bacterial infections such as group B streptococcal and listerial infections have been clearly linked with fetal demise: the former frequently via ascension from the vagina, and the latter via transplacental infection, with maternal septicemia leading to placental abscess formation. Both of these organisms are exquisitely sensitive to ampicillin (which crosses the placenta in high concentrations) and are thus amenable to early intervention. Although recent data clearly indicate that infection of the amniotic sac with organisms from the vagina or endocervix is possible, the organisms that have been cultured (i.e., *Ureaplasma*, *Mycoplasma*, and *Chlamydia*) have not been clearly shown to cause fetal demise by direct infection. These organisms have been linked to neonatal death via activation of prostaglandin production, premature labor, and subsequent neonatal death due to prematurity. Organisms represented by the TORCH complex of diseases (toxoplasmosis, rubella, cytomegalovirus infection, herpes simplex, and syphilis) have long been established as causes of fetal death in utero. Coxsackie B viruses have been linked to late fetal demise by causing hydrops and subsequent death from myocarditis. Other infectious diseases either have been eradicated (e.g., smallpox) or have not been shown to cause death (e.g., hepatitis, poliomyelitis, varicella).

Immunologic Causes

Autoimmune damage to fetal or placental tissue by maternal antibodies directed against maternofetal antigens has been implicated in late fetal loss. Hemolytic autoimmune losses are primarily due to erythroblastosis fetalis, while nonhemolytic causes of late fetal demise appear to be a consequence of uteroplacental vascular damage, although the direct evidence for an immunologic cause is sparse. It has been documented recently that certain autoantibodies are associated with an increased rate of pregnancy loss, even though clinically evident collagen vascular disease may not be present. Examples of this include antiphospholipid antibodies such as lupus anticoagulant and anticardiolipin. Additionally, antibodies against ribonucleoprotein (anti-SSA) have been associated with congenital heart block and subsequent late fetal loss.

Obstetric Complications and Maternal Disease

A number of other conditions causing late fetal deaths can be linked to maternal diseases or abnormalities of the placenta: specifically, abruptio placentae, placenta previa, twin-twin transfusion, postmaturity, intrauterine growth retardation, and cord accidents such as torsion, thrombosis, knotting, and amniotic band strangulation can cause late fetal losses. Maternal conditions associated with fetal demise in utero include hypertensive disorders (both chronic disease and superimposed pre-eclampsia) and diabetes mellitus. Diabetes has shown a marked decline as an etiology, thanks to insulin usage and aggressive screening of patients for the gestational form of the disease, as well as counseling regarding preconceptual diabetic metabolic control and the subsequent reduction in anomalies.

DIAGNOSIS

The diagnosis of late fetal demise is currently made primarily through the use of ultrasound to demonstrate the absence of cardiac motion with real-time imaging. Doppler evaluation, as well as scalp monitoring, may be misleading owing to confusion with maternal cardiac activity and pulsatile maternal aortic blood flow being transmitted and reflected in the fetus. Radiographic signs of demise include the "halo sign" (representing fluid accumulation between the cranium and scalp). Overlapping of cranial sutures and abnormal angulation of the fetal spine have been described; however, these are presumptive, rather than diagnostic, findings. The accessibility, ease of application, sensitivity, and specificity of ultrasound, along with the absence of radiation, have made it the most important tool in the diagnosis of intrauterine fetal death.

MANAGEMENT

Delivery Timing and Methods

Once the diagnosis of intrauterine fetal demise has been made, management of the delivery can still pose many problems for the practitioner. Although a number of patients have spontaneous onset of labor, some do not, and the emotional pressures to proceed with delivery can be extreme. The potential medical consequences of postponement of delivery after the diagnosis has been made are primarily related to maternal coagulation defects.

The best method for managing late fetal death depends on the gestation of the fetus, the experience of the physician, and maternal medical conditions that may complicate the induction of labor. *The availability of prostaglandin preparations has made expectant management of patients with fetal demise a significantly less common technique.* Prostaglandin E_2 (PGE_2) vaginal suppositories for the treatment of fetal demise up to 28 weeks has been well documented as both efficacious and safe. With dosage intervals of 2 to 6 hours, 20-mg vaginal suppositories have resulted in delivery in more than 90 percent of cases. Primary side effects include nausea and vomiting, diarrhea, pyrexia, uterine hypertonia, and tachycardia, although the frequency of occurrence is related to dosage interval. Premedication is recommended for these symptoms with an antiemetic, an antidiarrheal, and an antipyretic, which have reduced side effects from application. Significant complications of this technique are rare; however, uterine rupture and cervical lacerations have been reported, although the concomitant usage of oxytocin has been implicated in most cases.

In patients with fetal demise occurring after 28 weeks, a number of techniques for delivery have been described, including 10-mg PGE_2 intravaginal suppositories at intervals based on clinical response; 3 mg of PGE_2 in viscous gel as a cervical ripening agent, and subsequent oxytocin infusion; oxytocin infusion alone; intra-amniotic instillation of 40 mg of PGF_2; and intramuscular 15-methyl prostaglandin in doses of 250 mg every 2 hours. The following protocol is currently in use at our institution: If the condition of the cervix is unfavorable, an effort at ripening is made with 3 mg of PGE_2 in viscous gel placed intravaginally. Approximately one-half of these patients go into spontaneous labor and deliver. An interval of at least 6 hours is allowed and if labor is not evident, intravenous oxytocin infusion is begun. Few side effects have been noted and uterine hypertonia has not been encountered. If the condition of the cervix is favorable, oxytocin induction is attempted. If this is unsuccessful, low-dose PGE_2 may be used as long as a sufficient interval between the two techniques has elapsed, since concomitant oxytocin and prostaglandin usage appears to carry a higher risk of uterine rupture and cervical laceration. Absolute contraindications to PGE_2 use include maternal cardiac failure and severe hypertension (PGF_2 is contraindicated with maternal asthma); relative contraindications include renal or hepatic disease, diabetes, a previous vertical uterine scar, or other circumstances that may preclude vaginal delivery. In patients with multiple gestations, no significant body of data is available; however, if both fetuses have died, the above techniques have been used subject to the size of the uterus. When confronted with the demise of a single fetus of a twin gestation, efforts at determining the cause of death are important, as the surviving twin may be exposed to the same risks. Additionally, monozygous twins are at risk of fetofetal exchange of thromboplastic material. This event has been postulated to cause such phenomena as renocortical necrosis and multicystic encephalomalacia. The incidence of these syndromes is unknown.

Coagulopathy

The mother with a dead fetus in utero is at risk of developing disseminated intravascular coagulopathy (DIC), whether the fetus is a singleton or whether one fetus in a set of multiple gestations has died. *The probability that coagulopathy will develop appears to be directly related to the length of time a dead fetus is retained in utero.* Declining plasma fibrinogen levels have been demonstrated, beginning approximately 4 weeks after demise, although instances of clinical DIC have been reported before that time in late fetal deaths. Current methods of diagnosis and induction of labor have significantly reduced the incidence of hypofibrinogenemia and coagulopathy. In the absence of hemorrhage, the coagulation defect can be corrected with heparin therapy. The great majority of coagulopathies resolve within 48 hours of delivery. If the pregnancy is allowed to continue after a diagnosis of in utero demise, monitoring for development of hypofibrinogenemia is indicated.

Postdelivery Evaluation and Treatment

When a stillborn baby has been delivered, evaluation of the infant for the purpose of diagnosis and counseling is critical. Although decisions regarding autopsy can be difficult for patients, it may be the only method of establishing a diagnosis, thereby aiding in the planning and management of future pregnancies. A number of factors need to be taken into account by the physician, including the financial (and emotional) cost to the parents, the ease with which data can be obtained, the sensitivity and specificity of individual tests, medicolegal issues, and the treatability of the determined condition. After appropriate history has been obtained from the parents, a careful physical examination of the baby and placenta should be undertaken, including photographs, which are useful not only for the permanent record but also for the family. When no congenital malformation or hydrops is present, studies such as a Kleihauer-Betke smear to evaluate for evidence of fetomaternal hemorrhage, VDRL test to evaluate for syphilis, and fibroblast culture to evaluate chromosomes and for metabolic storage diseases are specifically indicated. Histologic examination of the tissue for evidence of an infectious etiology should be undertaken. Maternal blood samples for TORCH titers and a partial thromboplastin time test to screen for lupus anticoagulant should be performed.

If there are congenital malformations, it is initially most important to note whether a single malformation or multiple anomalies are present, as recurrence rates may be very different (e.g., bilateral renal agenesis versus adult or infantile polycystic kidney in the presence of Potter's syndrome). Chromosomal analysis is especially important in cases in which malformations are found because in a significant proportion of these stillbirths there are abnormal karyotypes. Additionally, radiographic examination may be indicated in infants with short limbs or bony abnormalities to assist the evaluation of potential skeletal dysplasias. When autopsy has been refused, ultrasonographic evaluation of the urologic system in cases of Potter's syndrome may be of value. Karyotype can be obtained from the chorionic plate of the placenta (if autopsy has been refused), thus emphasizing the importance of placental examination.

A thorough evaluation of stillbirths can be accomplished through this protocol. Although costly and time consuming, examinations such as autopsy, chromosomal analysis, and bacterial and viral culture tests are of significant value in diagnosis. If an etiology can be determined, the findings can be shared with the family and they can be counseled about the risk of recurrence. If no diagnosis can be established, then the risk of a recurrent stillbirth is empirically doubled.

Grief Process

Society underestimates the impact of a fetal loss on families. Intense grieving associated with the loss has been recognized as the most consistent reaction by parents. The process of gradually detaching ties to a loved one has been described in stages that follow a consistent form, but it is not a step-by-step progression. Grieving families often go through an initial phase of shock followed by grief, anger, and subsequent gradual return to normal functioning. The exact circumstances surrounding the loss play an important role, and significant impact on the process can be made if a specific diagnosis can be established. Multiple investigations have shown that *resolution of the grieving process can be aided by allowing and encouraging families to view, hold, and examine the stillborn*. Parents tend to focus on the normality of features rather than the maceration or malformation, which has been used as an argument in the past to discourage families from viewing the fetus (although preparation for the sight of abnormalities is helpful). Pictures or footprints may be useful as tangible reminders of life and can help to resolve grief. The presentation of options regarding autopsy is appropriate before delivery (when possible), but immediate discussion of findings as well as subsequent visits to reaffirm the parents' understanding of diagnoses is important, both for counseling regarding future attempts at pregnancy, and in terms of patient satisfaction with medical care. *Families often require multiple follow-up visits to discuss and reorganize their knowledge of the issues surrounding their loss*. The physician can be especially valuable in allowing a ventilation of emotions, as well as in offering compassion, providing information, and aiding in the resolution of misconceptions and guilt feelings. Many families feel a sense of failure of reproductive ability and are frightened of future attempts at conception, even after counseling. Subsequent pregnancies can be marked by strong ambivalence and anxiety, and testing for subsequent abnormalities can be extremely stressful. Pathologic grief reactions occur most commonly in mothers of a stillborn infant who have poor support systems and a lack of outlets for processing their grief. Many communities have support groups of women and men who have suffered late fetal demise and who can be extremely helpful in dealing with such a loss.

SUGGESTED READING

Berezin N. After a loss in pregnancy. New York: Simon and Schuster, 1982.
Diagnosis and Management of Missed Abortion and Antepartum Fetal Death. ACOG Technical Bulletin, No. 55, 1979.
Kochenow NK. Management of fetal demise. Clin Obstet Gynecol 1987; 30:322–330.

MULTIPLE GESTATION

FRANK A. CHERVENAK, M.D.
JUDITH L. CHERVENAK, M.D.

The management of multiple gestation has long challenged the obstetric profession. In this chapter, we discuss the antepartum and intrapartum management of multiple gestation. It is critical to remember, however, that optimal obstetric management can only be based on the accurate antenatal diagnosis of the multiple gestation. The widespread use of obstetric ultrasonography has greatly facilitated the task. Only 10 years ago it was widely appreciated that only 50 percent of multiple gestations were diagnosed before delivery, whereas current estimates are higher than 90 percent.

ANTEPARTUM MANAGEMENT

Considerations in the antepartum management of multiple gestations include prevention of prematurity, evaluation of fetal growth, fetal assessment, detection of fetal anomalies, and management of fetal death.

Prevention of Prematurity

Probably the greatest cause of perinatal morbidity and mortality associated with multiple gestation is premature birth. Prophylactic bed rest, although widely prescribed, is of uncertain therapeutic benefit. We do not advocate hospitalized bed rest unless warranted for other indications. We believe, however, that modified bed rest at home and/or at work may be of value. Prophylactic cerclage placement and prophylactic use of tocolysis have not been found to be clinically efficacious in the prevention of premature birth for multiple gestations. These interventions should be utilized, of course, when there is clinical evidence of an incompetent cervix or premature labor.

Selective fetal reduction, in order to reduce the risk of premature birth, is a newly described option. This procedure should be considered experimental at present, but probably is of greatest value when an excessive number of embryos (four or more) result from the use of various infertility therapies.

Evaluation of Fetal Growth

Multiple gestations are at substantially increased risk for intrauterine growth retardation. The higher the number of the fetuses, the greater the risk, because of an excessive demand on the uteroplacental circulation. It is rare for intrauterine growth retardation to occur prior to 26 weeks of gestation. Although twin-to-twin transfusion due to placental vascular anastomoses may result in growth retardation of one twin, this phenomenon is responsible for a small minority of cases of growth retardation among multiple gestations. It is impossible to assess individual fetal growth in multiple gestation clinically with fundal height measurements or other manual determinations. It is, therefore, the present standard of care that every mul-

tiple gestation be followed by monthly ultrasound examinations, beginning at about 26 weeks.

Ultrasound examination can then suggest intrauterine growth retardation, based on a decrease in estimated fetal weight or by using other ultrasound parameters. It is important to remember, however, that constitutional differences among fetuses may occur that are not pathologic in nature.

Fetal Assessment

Because fetuses of multiple gestations are at increased risk for uteroplacental insufficiency, fetal assessment at about 28 weeks of gestation is indicated. Although there is no consensus concerning the optimal method of fetal assessment, the nonstress test, a biophysical profile, and Doppler assessment are currently the most widely used methods in this clinical setting.

Certain obstetric conditions, such as fetal hemorrhage due to vasa praevia, cord accident, abnormal placentation, and pre-eclampsia are more common in multiple gestations. The practicing obstetrician should therefore be aware of these associations.

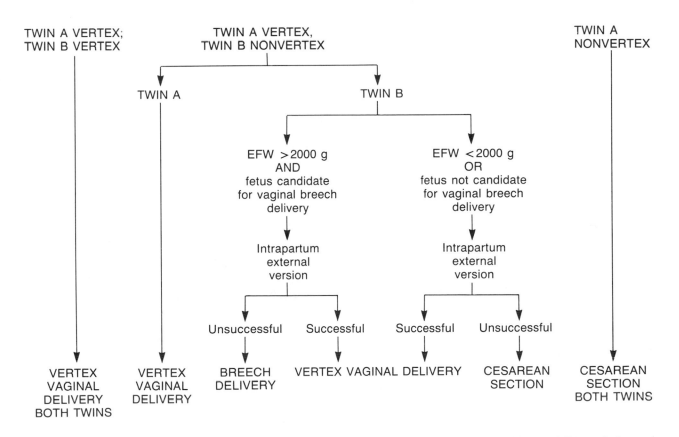

Figure 1 Protocol for the intrapartum management of gestation. (Reprinted with permission from Chervenak FA, et al. Intrapartum management of twin gestation. Obstet Gynecol 1985; 65:119.)

Fetal Anomalies

Among monozygotic twins, there is an increased frequency of fetal anomalies. Two anomalies that are specific to multiple gestations are conjoined twins and the acardiac twin. In the former case, delayed separation of a single zygote is responsible, whereas in the latter, arterial-to-arterial anastomoses permit sustained growth.

In those cases in which fetal anomalies are diagnosed prior to 24 weeks of gestation, termination of the pregnancy may be elected by the parents. Management during the third trimester and during labor is dependent upon the specific anomaly.

Management of Fetal Death

It is not uncommon for one embryo of a multiple gestation to die spontaneously during the first trimester. This phenomenon, termed "vanishing twin," is probably a common occurrence that may be responsible for vaginal bleeding in what then may evolve as a singleton pregnancy or a multiple gestation of a lower order.

Occasionally, death of a single fetus in a multiple gestation may occur during the second or third trimester. In such cases maternal coagulopathy due to the retained dead fetus may result. Weekly surveillance of the maternal clotting status is therefore indicated in any case of second or third trimester fetal demise.

INTRAPARTUM MANAGEMENT

When considering the intrapartum management of multiple gestation, the goal is to avoid traumatic delivery without the need for unnecessary cesarean section. Most authorities believe that when three or more fetuses are present, cesarean section is the management of choice.

When considering twin gestations, a clinically useful classification is (1) twin A vertex with twin B vertex (42.5 percent of the total twin population); (2) twin A vertex with twin B nonvertex (38.4 percent of the total twin population); and (3) twin A nonvertex (19.1 percent of the total twin population). We present a management protocol for these three groups of twin gestations in Figure 1.

Twin A Vertex with Twin B Vertex

Attempted vaginal delivery is appropriate for vertex-vertex twins. Recently, 5-minute Apgar scores have been shown not to correlate with the time interval between twin deliveries. After delivery of twin A there is no urgency to deliver twin B if electronic fetal heart rate monitoring or sonographic visualization of the fetal heart shows no abnormality.

If labor has not resumed within 10 minutes after delivery of the first twin, oxytocin augmentation with careful surveillance of the fetal heart may be valuable. Once the vertex is in the pelvic inlet, amniotomy is recommended.

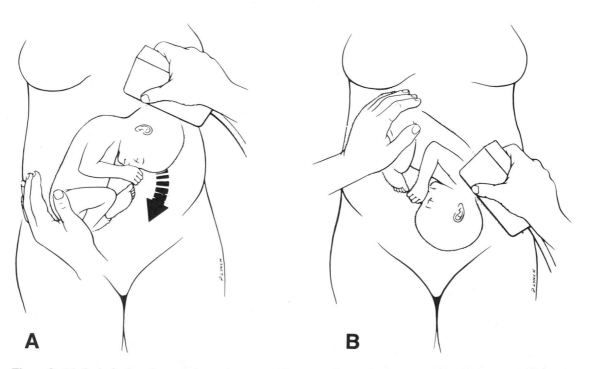

A **B**

Figure 2 Method of using ultrasound transducer to guide vertex of second twin into pelvis. (Reprinted with permission from Chervenak FA, et al. Intrapartum external version of the second twin. Obstet Gynecol 1983; 62:160.)

Cesarean section should be considered the management of choice if deterioration of the fetal heart rate tracing of twin B occurs before atraumatic vaginal delivery is possible.

Twin A Vertex with Twin B Nonvertex

Several authorities have advocated cesarean section as the proper management when the second twin is in a breech presentation or transverse lie. This approach has been justified by reports of an association of increased perinatal mortality and depressed Apgar scores with breech delivery of the second twin.

We believe, however, that routine cesarean section is not necessary for all twins with vertex-nonvertex presentations and the management options of intrapartum external version and breech delivery of the second twin are also important.

The following guidelines for performance of intrapartum external version of the second twin are recommended:

1. Sonographic assessment of the size of both fetuses should be performed. If twin B is larger than twin A and a great size disparity exists, version with an attempt at vaginal delivery is best avoided.
2. Epidural anesthesia is advisable before delivery to provide for abdominal wall relaxation.
3. The procedure should be performed only if immediate back-up cesarean section is possible.
4. A real-time ultrasound machine should be present in the delivery room to determine fetal presentation accurately after delivery of the first twin. Fetal heart rate should be monitored throughout delivery. Also, gentle pressure with the transducer can guide the infant in vertex presentation into the birth canal (Fig. 2).
5. If this is not successful, version can be attempted either as a forward or backward roll. The shortest arc between the vertex and the pelvic inlet should be attempted first. Undue force should always be avoided.
6. If version to the vertex presentation is successful, membranes should be ruptured and oxytocin augmentation may be used.
7. If version is unsuccessful, if the fetal heart tones of twin B show evidence of fetal distress, or if twin B fails to descend after successful version, cesarean section or breech extraction is necessary. We have found that there is not an excessive risk of asphyxia for the vaginally delivered breech second twin.

The documented ill-effects of vaginal delivery for low birth weight (< 1,500 g) singleton breech presentation infants should be considered, however, in a plan of intrapartum management for vertex-nonvertex twin gestations. As no data currently exist that have demonstrated any protection against the hazards of breech delivery for the low-birth-weight nonvertex second twin, we believe that vaginal breech delivery is currently not warranted when a birth weight is less than 1,500 g. Fortunately, fetal weight can be estimated with fair reliability by antenatal sonography, so that 95 percent of the time estimations are accurate within plus or minus 20 percent. Therefore, use of a cutoff of 2,000 g for estimated fetal weight is very unlikely to result in an infant with a birth weight of less than 1,500 g.

Intrapartum management of vertex-nonvertex twins is summarized in Figure 1. During the intrapartum period, sonographic estimation of fetal weight is determined, and assessment is made of the standard criteria for vaginal breech delivery. If the sonographic estimation of fetal weight is higher than 2,000 g and the criteria for vaginal breech delivery are satisfied, external cephalic version is attempted; if this is unsuccessful, a breech delivery is performed.

If the sonographic estimation of fetal weight is less than 2,000 g or the criteria for vaginal breech delivery are not satisfied, external cephalic version is attempted. If this is unsuccessful, a cesarean section is performed. Even in those hospitals where breech delivery is not acceptable under any circumstance, routine cesarean section may not be necessary for vertex-nonvertex twin gestations, as intrapartum external cephalic version of the second twin may be successful.

It should be emphasized that cesarean section is not a panacea and does not preclude the possibility of birth injury. When cesarean section is performed, an adequate uterine incision is mandatory if birth injury is to be avoided.

Twin A Nonvertex

At present, cesarean section seems to be the delivery method of choice when the first twin is nonvertex, as there are no studies to document the safety of vaginal delivery for this group. External cephalic version of a nonvertex first twin would be difficult, if not impossible. Interlocking of fetal heads is a potentially disastrous complication of vaginal breech delivery of the first twin. It is not inconceivable that the second twin might also interfere with breech vaginal delivery of the first twin in more subtle ways, such as deflection of the descending vertex. We recognize, however, that fears of nonvertex vaginal delivery of the first twin may not be warranted and that vaginal delivery may prove to be safe in well-defined cases.

SUGGESTED READING

Acker D, Leiberman M, Holbrook H, et al. Delivery of the second twin. Obstet Gynecol 1982; 59:710.

Berkowitz RL. Multiple gestations. In: Gabbe S, Niebyl JR, Simpson JL, eds. Obstetrics: normal and problem pregnancies. New York: Churchill Livingstone, 1986:739.

Cetrulo CL, Ingardia CJ, Sbarra AJ. Management of multiple gestation. Clin Obstet Gynecol 1980; 23:533.

Chervenak FA, Johnson RE, Youcha S, et al. Intrapartum management of twin gestation. Obstet Gynecol 1985; 65:119.

Chervenak FA, Johnson RE, Berkowitz RL, Hobbins JC. Intrapartum external version of the second twin. Obstet Gynecol 1983; 62:160.

Ganesh V, Apuzzio J, Iffy L. Clinical aspects of multiple gestation. In: Iffy L, Kaminetsky HA, eds. Principles and practice of obstetrics and perinatology. New York: Wiley, 1981:1183.

Rayburn WF, Lavin JP, Miodovnick M, Varner MW. Multiple gestation: time interval between delivery of the first and second twin. Obstet Gynecol 1984; 63:502.

NUCHAL CORD

JOHN R. DOIG, B.Sc., M.B., Ch.B., M.R.C.O.G., F.R.N.Z.C.O.G.

Nuchal cord entanglement is the term utilized to describe the obstetric complication in which single or multiple loops of umbilical cord become entwined around the fetal neck. Although the diagnosis of nuchal cord is confirmed only at delivery, a presumptive diagnosis is often made during a labor monitored by continuous electronic fetal heart rate recording and may also be suggested antenatally during antepartum nonstress cardiotocographic testing.

INCIDENCE

Single nuchal cords are found in about 25 percent of deliveries, double loops occur in 2.5 percent, and three or more loops in only about 0.5 percent of all births. *The predisposing factor for nuchal cord entanglement is umbilical cord elongation*, in association with such factors as polyhydramnios, maternal uterine laxity, multiparity, small fetal size, and male fetal gender. In general, the longer the cord length, the more numerous the coils. *Conversely, when nuchal entanglement occurs, the shorter the cord, the greater the likelihood that the loops will be tightly entwined*, resulting in fetal distress in labor.

DIAGNOSIS

Since the possibility of a nuchal cord complication is suggested by cardiotocographic demonstration of variable decelerations of the fetal heart, either antenatally or more commonly during intrapartum continuous fetal heart rate recording, the practicing obstetrician must be fully cognizant of the features diagnostic of variable deceleration, understand the pathogenesis of the pattern, and recognize degrees of severity. Extensive experimental animal research, backed up by human findings, has clearly confirmed that *variable fetal heart decelerations are caused by umbilical cord compression or occlusion* and can therefore be produced by cord entanglement around the fetal neck or other body parts or, possibly, transiently compressed between the fetus and uterine wall, especially during uterine contractions. Variable decelerations are characterized by a sudden deceleration phase and a similarly rapid recovery of the heart rate following the nadir of the deceleration. The *nadir generally shows evidence of increased beat to beat variability*, reflecting hyperfunction of the autonomic nervous system. The *deceleration may often be preceded and followed by acceleration "shoulders,"* which are due to differential compression of the umbilical vein, causing a decrease in venous return from the placenta with compensatory fetal tachycardia. With increasing contraction pressure a marked increase in total peripheral resistance occurs, and the end-diastolic pressure in the aorta is similarly markedly elevated; a rapid

increase in baroreceptor activity results, causing vagal nerve stimulation and a profound transient bradycardia, which is relieved by the waning of contraction. As the contraction pressure is reduced, the umbilical vein remains transiently compressed, accounting for the following acceleration "shoulder." Recent evidence from Fienstein and colleagues has reported that *real-time ultrasound scanning may confirm the presumptive diagnosis* and alter management decisions, particularly when positional change does not provide an improvement in fetal heart rate pattern.

MANAGEMENT IN THE FIRST STAGE OF LABOR

Management decisions following a presumptive diagnosis of nuchal cord entanglement are based on the recognition of degree of severity of variable deceleration and awareness that increasing severity is related to the possibility of fetal acidemia, fetal distress, and low Apgar scores, and in rare instances may cause intrapartum and neonatal morbidity or mortality. *Mild variable decelerations* are transient, reflex-mediated responses, are seen in conjunction with baseline fetal heart rates, and last less than 30 seconds. The nadir of deceleration does not fall below 90 beats per minute. Such a pattern does not indicate a need for immediate delivery but should encourage the obstetrician to *change maternal position* in order to relieve cord compression and to continue electronic fetal heart recording with a healthy awareness that the mild pattern may herald increasingly severe patterns with increased strength of labor contraction.

Moderate variable deceleration patterns are recognized when the duration of deceleration is greater than 30 seconds but lasts less than 60 seconds and has a nadir below 90 beats per minute but more than 70 beats per minute. This type of pattern is indicative of significant cord compression, i.e., possible tight nuchal cord entanglement, and may presage the development of fetal acidemia with meconium staining of the amniotic fluid and possible baseline bradycardia. Management decisions now must be based on progress in labor and the likelihood of imminent delivery via the vaginal route. A responsible approach is *urgently to transfer the patient* in a peripheral obstetric unit to a hospital where facilities for cesarean section are at hand. In light of a deteriorating fetal heart rate pattern and when delivery is not imminent, measurement of fetal scalp blood pH can provide additional information and allow the clinician to continue monitoring rather than to effect delivery. A scalp pH of greater than 7.25 means normal labor can continue, whereas a pH in the range of 7.2 to 7.25 suggests some degree of compromise and a need for intensive observation and resampling within 30 minutes, particularly if the deceleration pattern continues. Conversely, a scalp pH of less than 7.19 is indicative of fetal acidemia and warrants immediate delivery by the most appropriate procedure.

Severe variable decelerations are described when the duration of deceleration is 60 seconds or more and when the nadir of deceleration is less than 70 beats per minute. This type of pattern usually coexists with an alteration in baseline fetal heart rate (generally a baseline bradycardia) and with fetal acidemia. If the patient is in the second stage

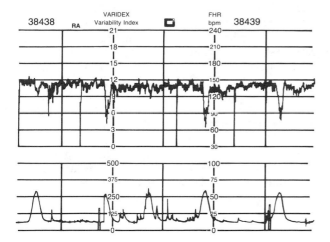

Figure 1 Mild variable decelerations.

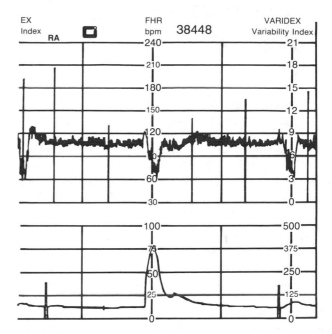

Figure 2 Moderate variable decelerations.

of labor, the infant may be delivered by forceps or vacuum extraction. If she is in the first stage, and delivery is not imminent, cesarean section is indicated as the optimal delivery mode. In conjunction with the *need for operative delivery*, a pediatrician is requested to attend at the delivery to undertake resuscitation of the fetus.

MANAGEMENT OF NUCHAL CORD AT DELIVERY

When loose nuchal cord entanglement is demonstrated during delivery of the fetal head and neck, cord compression may be relieved by slipping the encircling coil over the fetal head. *If, however, the nuchal cord entanglement is tight, the clinician must clamp the cord twice as soon as possible and then cut it between the clamps*, allowing the entangled cord to be unraveled. Following this release, the delivery can proceed normally. In the accompanying illustrations (Figs. 1, 2, and 3) a deteriorating fetal heart rate pattern is shown, and increasing severity of variable deceleration is obvious. At delivery by midcavity forceps, two tight loops of cord were entwined around the fetal neck. These were cut and disentangled prior to completion of the delivery. The 3,570-g female infant had passed thick meconium into the amniotic fluid prior to delivery, reflecting fetal distress. Although her 1-minute Apgar score was only 2, a rapid recovery ensued, with respiration being established at 2 minutes, and a 5-minute Apgar score of 9 was recorded. No evidence of neurologic morbidity was detected during the neonatal course or subsequent development.

Shepherd and coworkers have shown that tight nuchal cord entanglement is associated with an *increased likelihood of neonatal anemia* and, rarely, hypotension. It is therefore recommended that in such cases a blood sample should be taken early in the neonatal period for hemoglobin estimation and determination of hematocrit, and appropriate transfusion given if severe depletion is confirmed.

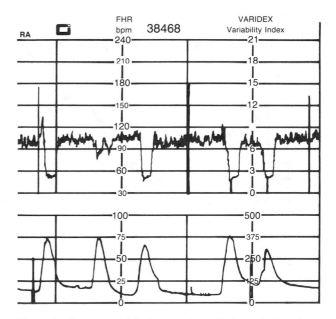

Figure 3 Severe variable decelerations. Tight nuchal cord entanglement. Delivery was by midcavity forceps.

SUGGESTED READING

Feinstein SJ, Lodeiro JG, Vintzileas AM, et al. Intrapartum ultrasonic diagnosis of nuchal cord as a decisive factor in management. Am J Obstet Gynecol 1985; 153:308–309.

Shepherd AJ, Richardson CJ, Brown JP. Nuchal cord as a cause of neonatal anemia. Am J Dis Child 1985; 139:71–73.

PLACENTA PREVIA

RICHARD K. SILVER, M.D.

The perinatal outcome in patients with placenta previa is directly correlated with gestational age at the time of delivery. The focus of contemporary management involves avoiding preterm birth in order to minimize neonatal morbidity without incurring maternal complications. Whereas this may be more readily accomplished in patients with asymptomatic placenta previa, a more aggressive approach is required in patients with recurrent episodes of significant hemorrhage. The components of aggressive expectant management include (1) liberal blood replacement to maintain normal circulating blood volume (hemoglobin ≥ 10 g); (2) parenteral and oral tocolysis to treat concomitant preterm uterine activity; (3) assessment of amniotic fluid phospholipid profile prior to elective delivery; and (4) liberal hospitalization for symptomatic patients, reserving outpatient management for stable patients after prolonged observation. Using this approach, significant delay in delivery can be achieved

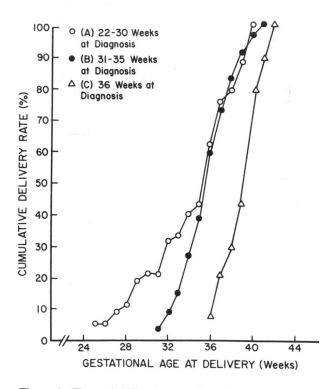

CUMULATIVE DELIVERY RATE BY GESTATIONAL AGE AT DIAGNOSIS

Figure 1 The probability that a patient managed expectantly with placenta previa will deliver when diagnosed (A) before 30 weeks' gestation, (B) between 31 and 35 weeks' gestation, and (C) beyond 36 weeks' gestation. (From Silver RK, Depp R, Sabbagha RE, et al. Placenta previa: aggressive expectant management. Am J Obstet Gynecol 1984; 150:15.)

(Fig. 1), leading to a preterm delivery rate approaching that of uncomplicated, singleton pregnancies (Fig. 2).

As with other pregnancy complications, accurate gestational age assignment is critical in patients with placenta previa. Unfortunately, most symptomatic patients with placenta previas present beyond the first half of pregnancy (the best period for most accurate ultrasound assessment). Therefore, assignment of gestational age in retrospect must employ all available parameters when early ultrasound dating has not been previously obtained. Moreover, unless definitive gestational age assignment is available (e.g., crown-rump length or documented date of conception), elective delivery should be undertaken only after obtaining a mature phospholipid profile from the amniotic fluid.

LOCALIZATION OF THE PLACENTA

With current ultrasound techniques, placental localization is easily accomplished in the majority of cases. Although the diagnosis of a central placenta previa is straightforward, identifying the edge of a marginal or partial previa may be problematic, especially if placental implantation is posterior. Apart from the routine approaches used to maximize visualization of the lower segment (e.g., ensuring a full maternal bladder and using both linear array and sector transducers as appropriate), other maneuvers and observations may be helpful. If the presenting fetal pole obscures the placental edge, manual elevation of the head or breech while scanning may solve this problem. In addition, an increased distance noted between the fetal pole and either the bladder-uterine wall (anterior previa) or sacral promontory (posterior previa) may be suggestive of the diagnosis. Previas are more often associated with malpresentations, especially transverse or oblique lines. Finally, if significant placental tissue is located in the uterine fundus, the diagnosis of placenta previa is less likely.

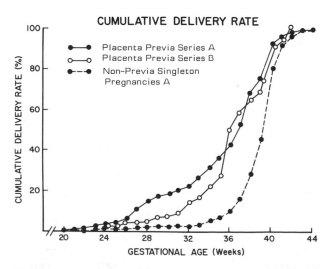

CUMULATIVE DELIVERY RATE

Figure 2 Cumulative delivery rate comparing nonprevia and previa patients managed expectantly. (From Silver RK, Depp R, Sabbagha RE, et al. Placenta previa: aggressive expectant management. Am J Obstet Gynecol 1984; 150:15.)

TABLE 1 Impact of Type of Placenta Previa on the Number and Significance of Hemorrhagic Episodes*

Previa Type	Significant Bleeding Episodes†	Drop in Hemoglobin		
		1 g	2 g	3 g
Total	29	22 (76%)	5 (17%)	2 (7%)
Partial	20	13 (65%)	5 (25%)	2 (10%)
Marginal	12	10 (83%)	2 (17%)	—

* From 91 cases of placenta previa; Silver RK, Depp R, Sabbagha RE, et al. Placenta previa: aggressive expectant management. Am J Obstet Gynecol 1984; 150:15.
† Drop in hemoglobin of at least 1 g from prehemorrhage value.

In an effort to correlate clinical outcome with the degree of placenta previa, attention has been directed to how much of the placenta covers the cervical os. Patients with total previa may have more severe or recurrent bleeding when compared with those with marginal or partial placentation, but there are many exceptions to this relationship (Table 1). As such, the ability to manage a given case expectantly should not be predicated on the specific placental type. Instead, it is appropriate to consider any low implantation with bleeding as a previa, in the absence of signs or symptoms of placental abruption. Since even low-lying placentas can require transfusion and emergent delivery, this simplified definition allows for more uniform management of these patients.

When placental localization is problematic (secondary to obesity or posterior implantation), alternative diagnostic methods may be helpful. One such approach uses real-time sector scanning through the maternal perineum rather than the abdomen. The advantages of this perineal scan include the fact that only routine ultrasound equipment is required, and better visualization of the endocervical canal and lower uterine segment may be obtained. Alternatively, transvaginal ultrasound probes can also provide views of the lower uterine segment and do not rely on the maternal bladder as an interface. Although this approach may be useful in defining placental location, care must be taken to introduce the transducer only into the vaginal vault and not into the cervix. Because the risks of transvaginal scanning may be equivalent to those of digital examination, prior experience with this approach is recommended before its use with placenta previa patients. If ultrasound techniques are insufficient, the application of magnetic resonance imaging (MRI) has been accomplished successfully in patients with placenta previa. This approach provides excellent resolution of static structures and may be suitable for the stable patient in whom the diagnosis is in question. Increased experience with MRI during pregnancy will undoubtedly increase the application of this technique for placental study.

As ultrasound scanning during pregnancy has increased, the diagnosis of placenta previa is often made in the asymptomatic patient during studies performed for other indications (e.g., gestational age assessment). It appears that a low implanted placenta in the midtrimester may persist as a previa at delivery in only 5 percent of patients. This phenomenon of placental migration may relate to the development of the lower uterine segment in the third trimester, coupled with atrophy of the distal portion of the placenta. In contrast, about one-third of the asymptomatic previas diagnosed beyond 30 weeks' gestation persist and may be associated with bleeding later in pregnancy. Furthermore, there are data to suggest that even the midtrimester placenta previas that resolve may be associated with adverse perinatal outcome, including suboptimal intrauterine growth and abruption. These facts underscore the importance of longitudinal follow-up of these patients with repeat ultrasound evaluation to confirm the placental site and evaluate fetal growth.

MATERNAL TRANSFUSION

Notwithstanding the known risks of blood replacement, modern blood banking and maternal transfusion have been instrumental in permitting aggressive management of placenta previa. Maintaining a reasonable hematocrit value and a normal circulating blood volume should be the goals in these patients, since emergent operative intervention may be required at any time and intraoperative hemorrhage may be excessive. In the absence of deteriorating maternal vital signs, transfusion during acute bleeding should be predicated on laboratory changes. The goal should be maintenance of the antepartum hemoglobin level above 10 g per deciliter. Although autologous transfusion and directed donation have been applied successfully during pregnancy, the former is contraindicated in this setting.

Iron deficiency should also be corrected, remembering that a significant delay in reticulocytosis may occur because of the effects of transfusion therapy. Although these goals are somewhat arbitrary, the use of laboratory changes in responding to hemorrhage (after allowing time for hemodynamic equilibration) is superior to reliance upon clinical estimation of blood loss alone.

TREATMENT OF PRETERM UTERINE ACTIVITY

Management of coincident preterm uterine activity in patients with a bleeding placenta previa is controversial. Although some previas are diagnosed incidentally at the onset of preterm labor, many patients present with bleeding and uterine activity simultaneously. Theoretically, the bleeding may either cause uterine irritability or result from changes in the lower segment of the contracting uterus. Tocolytic therapy has been attempted in these patients with some success, even though vaginal bleeding has traditionally been a contraindication to the use of beta-mimetic agents. The decision to institute tocolysis should be based on both the gestational age at diagnosis and the rapidity of blood loss. Pregnancies of less than 32 weeks' gestation may be suitable for tocolysis, even if blood transfusion is required, as long as blood replacement is effective in preserving both the maternal and fetal condition. In this setting, magnesium sulfate may be the preferred tocolytic agent in order to avoid the potential cardiovascular side effects of beta-mimetic therapy. However, the experience with beta-agonists in this setting suggests no increased transfusion requirement or risk of hypovolemic shock when compared with effects on patients receiving magnesium or intravenous hydration alone. The use of tocolytic therapy in selected patients is in keeping with the objective of obtaining a mature fetus at the time of delivery. In patients beyond 32 weeks, tocolysis should only be considered if immature fetal pulmonary status is detected by amniocentesis.

OUTPATIENT MANAGEMENT

Although prolonged hospitalization is the rule in the symptomatic patient, an outpatient approach is safe in properly selected and counseled patients. Criteria for this approach should include (1) at least 72 hours without vaginal bleeding during inpatient observation prior to discharge, (2) stable serial hematocrit values ($\geq$ 35 ml per deciliter), (3) biophysical evidence of fetal well-being (reactive nonstress test or reassuring biophysical profile), (4) patient availability for weekly clinical follow-up and serial ultrasound evaluation (to confirm placental location and assess fetal growth), (5) 24-hour transportation available to the hospital, (6) ability to comply with strict bed rest at home, and (7) patient and family awareness of potential complications. The alternatives to outpatient management would involve either prolonged hospitalization for asymptomatic patients or a stay at a minimal care setting directly adjacent to the hospital facility. Unfortunately, such a situation is currently available in only a limited number of perinatal centers in this country.

DOUBLE SET-UP EXAMINATION AND ROUTE OF DELIVERY

Despite our reliance on ultrasound and other modalities for accurate placental location, there are still selected cases where a traditional "double set-up" examination is appropriate to confirm the diagnosis. Examples of these include patients with the diagnosis of placenta previa who present near term with ruptured membranes and minimal hemorrhage and patients with partial or marginal placentation who have been asymptomatic. Such an examination should be postponed when possible until fetal lung maturity is achieved.

When counseling patients with regard to delivery, it is important to include a discussion of the risks of surgery that are unique to placenta previa in addition to those traditionally cited for cesarean section. The uncommon but real association of placenta previa with an abnormally adherent placenta (e.g., accreta) justifies counseling with regard to possible hysterectomy as treatment for this problem. This association is more common in patients with a prior cesarean section or uterine surgery. Excessive intrapartum hemorrhage may also occur secondary to the implantation site or to relative hypocontractility of the lower uterine segment after placental removal. The 15-methyl derivative of the prostaglandin F series may be particularly useful for either immediate or delayed atony when more conservative measures fail.

POSTDATE PREGNANCY

JAMES A. THORP, M.D.
ROBERT K. CREASY, M.D.

The management of the postdate pregnancy remains a significant and controversial perinatal problem. Most commonly, the postdate pregnancy is defined as that pregnancy advancing 294 days or 42 completed weeks beyond the onset of the last menstrual period. A broad margin of error is inherent in this definition. Since many women have either an irregular or an unknown menstrual history, the diagnosis of postdates is often unclear. In many clinic populations, a first trimester visit from a patient with reliable menstrual history is the exception rather than the rule. Furthermore, a reliable menstrual history does not always reflect accurate conceptual age. Menstrual history, first trimester uterine size, fundal height, auscultation of fetal heart tones, and ultrasound examination cannot date a pregnancy more accurately than within 10 days of actual fetal age. Precise fetal age can be determined only when the time of conception is known. If one uses timed ovulation from basal body temperature charts, only one-third of postdate patients have an accurate diagnosis. The remaining two-thirds of these patients actually have delayed ovulation and are not postdate by actual fetal age.

Depending on the reported study and the criteria used for diagnosis, the incidence of postdate pregnancy ranges from 6 to 14 percent. The introduction of routine obstetric ultrasound examination reduces the incidence to approximately 6 percent. Less than one-third of postdate pregnancies, or approximately 2 percent of all pregnancies, result in infants with postmaturity syndrome. This syndrome, which can only be diagnosed following birth, consists of meconium staining of the infant and fetal membranes, decreased subcutaneous fat, peeling of the skin, and long fingernails. Postmaturity syndrome is thought to be caused by a decrease in uteroplacental perfusion relative to fetal size occurring with advancing gestation. This frequently results in oligohydramnios and some variable degree of chronic hypoxemia.

In the majority of prolonged gestations, the etiology is not well delineated. We are gaining more insight into mechanisms underlying the initiation of normal parturition, and in the future this may provide some clues to the pathophysiology of the postdate pregnancy. Some known associations with postdate pregnancies include anencephaly, fetal adrenal hypoplasia, and placental sulfatase deficiency, but these account for only a few of the cases.

PERINATAL MORBIDITY AND MORTALITY

It is generally accepted that prolonged gestation is associated with an increased incidence of perinatal mortality. Perinatal mortality rates in post-term gravidas are approximately 5 to 7 percent compared with 1 to 2 percent in term gravidas. These rates begin to increase after 42 weeks, double at 43 weeks, and increase by four to six times at 44 weeks compared with term gestations. Morbidity, however, is another important consideration. Fetal heart rate abnormalities, fetal distress, macrosomia, traumatic delivery, meconium aspiration, low Apgar scores, asphyxia, persistent fetal circulation, and neonatal seizures occur with increasing frequency in the postdate pregnancy. In fact, the majority of asphyxiated term-size newborns result from postdate deliveries, even though they make up only 6 percent of term size neonates. Such events have resulted in postmaturity being the single entity most frequently leading to medical-legal difficulties. Studies lowering perinatal mortality rates in the postdate pregnancy have failed to improve rates of perinatal morbidity. It has been pointed out that even the more ambitious combinations of fetal surveillance in the postdate pregnancy fail to predict complicated outcomes. For example, in the postdate pregnancy in which normal twice weekly biophysical profiles are carried out, a one in ten chance of an abnormal outcome still exists.

A growing body of evidence suggests that asphyxia and other complications increase in frequency after 40 weeks' gestation. This is supported by finding linear increases in abnormal contraction stress tests occurring between 40 and 43 weeks. Arias reports significant progressive increases in morbidity after 40 weeks. In his study, the frequency of complications was 5.6 percent between 38 and 40 weeks, 20 percent between 40 and 41

weeks, and 28.5 percent between 42 and 43 weeks' gestation. The cause of this increase in morbidity is partly attributed to a decrease in uteroplacental perfusion, relative to fetal size, occurring after 40 weeks. Macrosomia also contributes to this rise in morbidity. The incidence of macrosomia significantly increases with advancing gestational age. Depending on the definition used and the population studied, there may be a fourfold greater incidence at 43 weeks compared with 38 to 40 weeks of gestation.

MANAGEMENT

The management of the postdate pregnancy continues to be debated in the literature. In order to avoid increased risks of perinatal morbidity and mortality, most authorities agree on induction of labor at 42 weeks' gestation when a ripe cervix is present. However, the management of postdate pregnancy with an unripe cervix is controversial. There are only a few truly randomized, prospective trials comparing intervention at 42 weeks versus expectant management. Conclusions from these trials are conflicting (Table 1).

It should be noted that each of these studies is designed somewhat differently and therefore comparisons between them are difficult to make. One study includes only patients with unfavorable cervices, and the remaining studies include all patients. Two of the reports used prostaglandin E_2 (PGE_2) for cervical ripening, whereas the others did not. Another pertinent fact is that relatively rare outcomes are being studied, and these require very large sample sizes in order to show significant differences. For example, suppose that induction of labor at 42 weeks actually does decrease the stillbirth rate from 3 per 1,000 to 1 per 1,000. In order to have a 90 percent chance of detecting this difference, a sample of 18,500 patients would be required (alpha = 0.05). Until a study of this magnitude is performed, the ideal management of the postdate pregnancy will not be known.

There has been only one prospective, randomized trial in patients with unfavorable cervices, comparing induction (after PGE_2 cervical ripening) at 42 weeks versus expectant management. Forty-two patients received 3 mg of PGE_2 gel intravaginally, and 110 patients received 0.5 mg intracervically. There appeared to be no difference in efficacy between the two routes of administration. The patients managed by PGE_2 gel ripening followed by induction at 42 weeks had a significantly lower incidence of cesarean

TABLE 1 Randomized Prospective Studies Assessing Induction at 42 Weeks

	Elective Inductions	Expectant Management	Primary Fetal Surveillance	Conclusions
Dyson, 1987	152	150	Twice weekly nonstress test	Deliver at 42 wk
Augensen, 1987	214	195	Twice weekly nonstress test	Manage expectantly
Witter, 1987	97	103	Estriol/creatinine 2–3 times/wk	Deliver at 42 wk
Cardozo, 1986	195	207	Initial ultrasound, and nonstress test every 48 hr	Manage expectantly

TABLE 2 Comparison of Perinatal Outcome: Induction Versus Expectant Management

Parameter	Elective Induction (N=152)	Expectant Management (N=150)	p Value
Perinatal death (N/%)	0	1/0.7	Not significant
1-minute Apgar < 7(N/%)	17/11.2	32/21.3	<0.02
5-minute Apgar < 7(N/%)	2/1.3	3/2.0	Not significant
Meconium (N/%)	29/19.1	70/46.7	<0.01
Meconium aspiration (N/%)	0	6/4.0	<0.02
Postmaturity syndrome (N/%)	8/5.3	22/14.7	<0.01
Fetal distress as one indication for cesarean section (N/%)	4/2.6	27/18.0	<0.01
Cesarean section (N/%)	22/14.5	41/27.3	<0.01

Adapted from Dyson DC, Miller PD, Armstrong AM. Management of prolonged pregnancy. Induction of labor versus antipartum fetal testing. Am J Obstet Gynecol 1987; 156:928–934.

section. The increased incidence of cesarean section in the expectant management group was due to fetal distress (14 percent in the expectant management group versus 1.3 percent in the induction group; p < 0.01). The induction group also had significantly lower incidences of meconium-stained amniotic fluid, meconium aspiration syndrome, low Apgar scores, and postmaturity syndrome (Table 2). This study suggests that early delivery can significantly decrease perinatal morbidity without increasing cesarean section rates.

Porreco and colleagues have routinely used PGE₂ gel in the management of the postdate pregnancy since 1980 and have experienced low rates of perinatal morbidity, mortality, and cesarean section. A portion of this observational experience has been retrospectively analyzed.

FETAL SURVEILLANCE

If intervention at 42 weeks is elected, criteria supporting the gestational age should be firm. If PGE₂ is not used for cervical ripening of the unfavorable cervix, then an increased risk of cesarean section should be acknowledged. If continuation of the pregnancy is elected, an increased risk of perinatal morbidity and mortality must be considered and appropriate fetal surveillance techniques used. Both biochemical and biophysical monitoring tests have been used for fetal surveillance in the postdate pregnancy. The incidence of false-negative results of these tests is important to consider. Generally, the false-negative rate (sensitivity) is defined as the incidence of antepartum fetal demise occurring within 1 week of a reassuring or normal test. The false-negative rate does not take morbidity into consideration. Biochemical techniques including maternal human placental lactogen and estriol determinations have lost popularity because of poor sensitivity and specificity. Fetal movement charting is inexpensive and helpful; however, it should not be used as the sole method of fetal surveillance in the postdate pregnancy.

One of the most common primary fetal surveillance tests used in postdate pregnancy is the nonstress test. In the largest studies reported, the nonstress test (for all indications) has a false-negative rate of 1.4 per 1,000 when corrected for congenital anomalies. However, in the postdate pregnancy, there is growing concern about the use of weekly nonstress tests as the only means of surveillance. One study reported a 4 percent perinatal mortality rate in postdate patients within a week after a reactive nonstress test. The majority of these false-negative tests consisted of reactive tracings associated with variable or nonspecific decelerations. The contraction stress test and biophysical profile result in lower rates of false-negative results (less than 1 per 1,000). Some authorities recommend their use for primary surveillance in the postdate pregnancy. Numerous combinations of techniques are proposed, including the following: weekly and/or biweekly contraction stress test, biweekly nonstress test, ultrasound estimates of amniotic fluid volume, and weekly and/or biweekly biophysical profiles. The contraction stress test has been achieved by both nipple stimulation or oxytocin infusion, with similar results. Manning has shown that the corrected perinatal mortality is about 10 percent when amniotic fluid volume is reduced. Thus, a surveillance program including an estimate of the amniotic fluid volume seems logical. Nonstress or contraction stress test tracings demonstrating even mild variable decelerations in the postdate pregnancy should be regarded as evidence of umbilical cord vulnerability and an indication for delivery.

SUGGESTED APPROACH

At our institution the management of the postdate pregnancy is individualized. It is important to emphasize that currently there are a wide range of acceptable management plans for the postdate pregnancy. The following plans represent an approach we favor. All patients having well-established dating criteria for 42 weeks and favorable cervical examinations are induced. The preferred method of induction is amniotomy and oxytocin (Pitocin) administration. Prompt amniotomy increases the chances of a successful induction. In addition, it allows an early indication of both the amount and color of the amniotic fluid. The presence of meconium-stained amniotic fluid is assumed to represent fetal distress until proved contrary by electronic fetal heart rate monitoring or fetal scalp sampling.

If the cervical examination is unfavorable and established dating criteria support 42 weeks' gestation, we usually consider cervical ripening with PGE_2. Induction is then performed as described above. We now use a simple preparation made by combining a 20-mg PGE_2 suppository with 60 cc of surgical lubricant. Adequate mixing achieves uniform dispersion, and six 10-ml aliquots (each containing 3.2 mg) are stored frozen in separate syringes. If the fetal heart rate tracing is reassuring and the patient is not experiencing regular contractions, PGE_2 gel is used. The preparation (10 cc of gel containing 3.2 mg of PGE_2) can be placed intravaginally through a straight catheter behind a previously inserted diaphragm. Continuous electronic fetal heart rate monitoring is employed if there is any indication of potential fetal jeopardy. Monitoring may be discontinued in the low-risk patient if the tracing is reassuring for 90 minutes after insertion. Continuous electronic fetal heart rate monitoring is used on all patients during induction. PGE_2 gel may be repeated at 4-hour intervals if excess uterine activity is not present and fetal heart rate monitoring is reassuring.

If dating criteria are uncertain, then expectant management with careful fetal surveillance is indicated. Fetal movement charting is emphasized at each visit, and patients are advised to call immediately in the event that there is a decrease in self-detected fetal activity. Twice weekly surveillance is preferred, with ultrasonography used at least once a week to assess amniotic fluid volume. Thus, the following all represent excellent choices for fetal surveillance in the postdate pregnancy: twice weekly nonstress tests and amniotic fluid volume assessment; twice weekly biophysical profiles; contraction stress testing and biophysical profiles; contraction stress testing and amniotic fluid volume assessment. If amniotic fluid volume is less than 3 cm (vertical measurement without cord), we feel that delivery is probably indicated. Likewise, if there are any decelerations, regardless of the reactivity pattern, delivery should be considered.

Experienced personnel need to be available during labor and delivery. This includes an experienced resuscitation team if fetal distress or meconium staining is present. When meconium is present, the oropharynx is carefully suctioned on the maternal perineum, and the newborn is immediately intubated and suctioned below the cords. As there is an increased risk of macrosomia, the potential for shoulder dystocia should be anticipated.

SUGGESTED READING

Arias F. Predictability of complications associated with prolongation of pregnancy. Obstet Gynecol 1987; 70:101–106.

Augensen K, Bergsjo P, Eikeland T, Carlsen J, Askvik K. Randomised comparison of early versus late induction of labor in post-term pregnancy. Br Med J 1987; 294:1192–1195.

Cardozo L, Fysh J, Pearce M. Prolonged pregnancy: the management debate. Br Med J 1986; 293:1059–1063.

Dyson DC, Miller PD, Armstrong AM. Management of prolonged pregnancy: induction of labor versus antepartum fetal testing. Am J Obstet Gynecol 1987; 156:928–934.

Manning FA, Lange IR, Morrison I, et al. Determination of fetal health methods for antepartum and intrapartum fetal assessment. Curr Probl Ob/Gyn 1983; 1:1.

Miyazaki FS, Miyazaki BA. False reactive nonstress tests in postterm pregnancies. Am J Obstet Gynecol 1981; 140:269.

Turner JE, Burke MS, Porreco RP, Weiss MA. Prostaglandin E_2 in tylose gel for cervical ripening before induction of labor. J Reprod Med 1987; 32:815–821.

Witter FR, Weitz CM. A randomized trial of induction at 42 weeks gestation versus expectant management for postdates pregnancies. Am J Perinatol 1987; 4:206–211.

POSTPARTUM PSYCHOSIS

RODRIGO A. MUÑOZ, M.D.

AN APPROACH TO THERAPY

Postpartum psychosis occurs in about 0.2 percent of women within the first 90 days after delivery. More common disorders are "maternity blues" and nonpsychotic postpartum depressions.

Maternity blues are very transitory episodes of mild depression that occur within the first week after delivery and last only 1 to 2 days.

Twelve percent of pregnant women suffer a nonpsychotic postpartum depression, characterized by dysphoric mood and often loss of sleep, loss of appetite, loss of energy, retardation or agitation, difficulty in thinking and concentrating, loss of interest in their usual pursuits, feelings of guilt, and in some cases, ideas of suicide. These postpartum depressions, as opposed to maternity blues, often require treatment.

Postpartum psychosis is an acute affective psychosis with florid and fluctuating manifestations. Mania and depressive mood may be equally frequent. This disorder is called psychosis because it is accompanied by delusions, hallucinations, or bizarre behavior.

The following pointers help in diagnosis and management:

1. Although most symptoms start shortly after delivery, some patients may have an insidious onset for a period of weeks. One of our patients, for example, gradually became more ill over the 8 weeks following delivery.
2. The duration of illness before it becomes very evident usually is quite minimal. The disorder may be diagnosed within hours of inception.
3. Many patients fluctuate between euphoria and depression. The practitioner may suspect postpartum psychosis in a patient who seems to be unusually happy or sad while drifting toward the opposite state.

4. Patients with postpartum psychosis respond well to treatment. When properly treated, most recover within a few days. This should encourage early identification and treatment.
5. Because many patients suffer the disorder during their first pregnancy and are the ones likely to have a recurrence, proper supervision and follow-up should provide early diagnosis and treatment of recurrent episodes.
6. Close supervision should also be given to women with a previous history of manic depressive illness. In our experience, a large proportion of patients with postpartum psychosis have had a prior episode of depression.

THERAPY

Three major components of therapy for postpartum psychosis are: psychotropic medications, verbal therapies, and milieu therapy.

Psychotropic Medications

Psychotropic medications include antipsychotic medications, lithium or carbamazepine (Tegretol), and antidepressants. These are each discussed separately.

Antipsychotic Medications

Although the list of antipsychotic medications has been gradually increasing, we discuss some of the most common, including chlorpromazine, thioridazine, haloperidol, perphenazine, fluphenazine, and thiothixene (Table 1).

The best strategy is to become very familiar with one drug and use it as the drug of choice. Exceptions to this rule include:

1. If the patient has responded in the past to an antipsychotic drug, use it again.
2. If another family member has had a similar disorder and responded well to an antipsychotic agent, use the same agent.
3. If the patient is allergic to a chosen antipsychotic agent, as revealed by questioning, select another one.
4. If the patient has a prior history of severe side effects after using an antipsychotic agent, consider using one of a different group. This rule is not absolute and has to be applied according to the patient's circumstances. If she has had severe side effects but has responded positively to the medication, judicious use should be considered.

Once an antipsychotic agent has been selected, a test dose should be administered, for example, 5 mg of haloperidol. One may then go on to the dosage proposed in Table 1. Some have suggested rapid tranquilization using frequent intramuscular administration of antipsychotics. Many now believe, however, that this strategy offers no advantages over the regular administration of oral dosages according to the condition of the patient.

Common side effects are sedation and hypotension with thioridazine or chlorpromazine or extrapyramidal effects (tremors, dystonia, rigidity) with most and especially the low-dose (haloperidol, thiothixene, fluphenazine) antipsychotics.

The daily dose of antipsychotic medications is gradually reduced after the patient has been free of symptoms for several days. Most patients with postpartum psychosis do not need long periods of treatment.

Lithium and Carbamazepine

For patients who have manifestations of mania, lithium and carbamazepine are beneficial. Lithium carbonate is usually given in a dosage of 900 mg a day, distributed so that the patient takes it every 12 hours or only once a day at the same hour each day. Carbamazepine is often given in the dosage of 200 mg three times a day. Blood levels for both medications taken regularly permit proper titration.

Other Medications

Extrapyramidal side effects are relieved with antiparkinsonian medication, as shown in Table 2.

Antidepressants

Two different types of antidepressants may be considered for patients who are clearly depressed: (1) monoamine oxidase inhibitors, and (2) tricyclic antidepressants and similar medications, as presented in Table 3.

TABLE 1 Antipsychotic Medications

Name	Dosage (mg/day)	
	Acute	Maintenance
Chlorpromazine	25–800	40–300
Fluphenazine	5–20	1–15
Haloperidol	1–100	1–15
Perphenazine	16–64	8–16
Trifluoperazine	10–60	2–20
Thiothixene	6–100	6–50

TABLE 2 Antiparkinsonian Drugs

Name	Dosage Ranges (mg/day)
Anticholinergic	
Benztropine	2–8
Biperiden	2–6
Diphenhydramine	25–200
Procyclidine	5–15
Trihexyphenidyl	4–15
Dopaminergic	
Amantadine	100–300

TABLE 3 Antidepressants

Class	Name	Dosage (mg/day)
Tricyclic	Amitriptyline	150–300
	Desipramine	150–300
	Doxepin	150–300
	Imipramine	150–300
	Trimipramine	150–300
	Nortriptyline	50–150
	Protriptyline	15–60
Tetracyclic	Amoxapine	150–450
	Maprotiline	150–450
Monoamine oxydase inhibitors	Isocarboxazid	30–50
	Phenelzine	45–90
	Tranylcypromine	30–50

The same observations made for the antipsychotic medications hold for the antidepressants. It is better to start with an antidepressant that the therapist considers his or her medication of choice. Many psychiatrists prefer the older antidepressants, such as amitriptyline and imipramine. They are usually given in progressively larger amounts according to the clinical response. The maximum dose recommended by the *Physicians' Desk Reference* may not be satisfactory. As many as 80 percent of all patients with depression respond to a 250-mg dose over a 6-week trial period. As with the antipsychotics, the antidepressants are reduced and withdrawn after a reasonable period of observation during recovery. Many feel that the medication should be tapered during a period of 6 months after the patient becomes free of symptoms.

PSYCHOTHERAPY

Psychotherapy options include individual therapy, family therapy, and other interventions.

Individual Therapy

We use interpersonal psychotherapy, which is a short-term psychotherapy aimed primarily at reducing symptoms and improving interpersonal functioning. We have found this type of therapy to be very useful in patients suffering a postpartum psychosis. In these patients, interpersonal conflicts are enhanced by the stress associated with pregnancy and delivery as well as by the readjustments expected of them in the puerperium.

Treatment strategy depends on the problem areas and their importance. Four problem areas are grief, interpersonal disputes, role transitions, and interpersonal deficits. Interpersonal disputes and role transitions are often prominent in patients suffering from a postpartum psychosis.

When dealing with interpersonal disputes, the therapy focuses on specific conflicts and their effect. The therapist determines the issues of the conflict, the differences in expectations and values between the patient and significant others, the patient's wishes in her relationships, and the patient's options. Although initially the patient with a postpartum psychosis is not open to more than reassurance, this changes as improvement (often due to antipsychotic medications) allows her to focus on her problems and their solutions. The patient, together with her therapist, explores alternatives, reviews past relationships, and examines repetitive conflicts and their contributing factors. Therapy sessions may be focused on patterns of communication between the patient and other persons, using the therapist as a sounding board.

Role transition is important in the postpartum situation, especially when the psychosis has occurred after the first delivery. The patient may be experiencing a loss of family support, may have trouble managing emotions, may fear her new responsibilities, and may have to learn new skills. This is often accompanied by a loss of self-esteem and a sense of alienation from others.

Family Therapy

Involvement of the husband and other significant persons greatly enhances the patient's opportunities to readjust. This calls for inviting the patient and her husband to formal meetings with the therapist, during which conflicts, expectations, and feelings are explored, giving all ample opportunity to interact. The best results in these interventions are obtained when the therapist has had an opportunity to interview the participants individually and has formulated a strategy for the family.

Milieu Therapy

Although drug therapy and psychotherapy are effective, most patients need a hospital environment for the therapy to be conducted more successfully.

Hospitalization should be considered in the following situations:

1. The patient is agitated, confused, belligerent, or out of touch with her environment.
2. The patient's behavior is unpredictable.
3. The patient has voiced ideas or intent of suicide.
4. A full evaluation cannot be accomplished outside the hospital.
5. There is no support system that would provide close monitoring of therapy at home or in other places away from the hospital.

Psychiatric units today are geared toward providing therapeutic activities such as group psychotherapy, occupational therapy, recreational therapy, and other programs that contribute to rapid progress. The obstetrician is invited to continue to see the patient while she stays in the psychiatric unit. When the patient's condition allows it, many psychiatric facilities permit the infant to stay with the patient.

PREGNANCY-INDUCED HYPERTENSION

JOHN W. GOLDKRAND, M.D.

Hypertensive diseases represent the most common complications of pregnancy (Table 1). Foremost among them is the unique syndrome of pregnancy-induced hypertension–pre-eclampsia, commonly referred to as toxemia of pregnancy. The significance of these disorders relates to an increase in maternal, fetal, and neonatal morbidity and mortality. It is incumbent on the obstetrician, family practitioner, or certified nurse-midwife to identify those patients at risk and to direct alterations in pregnancy surveillance and therapy in order to achieve improvement in pregnancy outcome.

DEFINITIONS

Pregnancy-induced hypertension (PIH) is often used to denote classic pre-eclampsia, whereas others use the presence of proteinuria in pre-eclampsia to distinguish it from PIH. In the present context, PIH includes PIH and pre-eclampsia.

Hypertension constitutes blood pressure higher than 140/90 mm Hg. If it is present before pregnancy or 20 weeks of gestation, it is *chronic hypertension*, whereas if it appears after 20 weeks' gestation, this would define PIH. Some institutions prefer to use mean arterial pressure as the guide for defining PIH.

Mean arterial pressure is defined as diastolic pressure + 1/3 (systolic-diastolic pressure). Values higher than 105 define patients at risk of having PIH.

Early onset of PIH is seen in patients with hydatidiform mole, underlying vascular disease (e.g., lupus erythematosus), undiagnosed chronic hypertension, or chronic medical diseases that predispose to vascular involvement.

PIH—Mild
The following characteristics typify mild PIH:

1. Hypertension
   a. Blood pressure higher than 140/90 mm Hg or

TABLE 1 Classification of Hypertensive Disease*

Pregnancy-Induced Hypertension
   Pre-eclampsia: Mild or severe

Chronic Hypertension Preceding Pregnancy
   With superimposed pre-eclampsia
   Without superimposed pre-eclampsia
   With superimposed eclampsia

* Modified from Committee on Terminology, American College of Obstetricians and Gynecologyists

   b. Systolic blood pressure increased 30 mm Hg or more, or diastolic blood pressure increased 15 mm Hg or more. These are two readings 6 hours apart at rest.
2. Proteinuria: 300 mg or greater for 24 hours, usually 1 to 2+ on dipstick testing.
3. Generalized edema: involving hands and face in addition to the lower extremities. This may be suspected by a weight gain of 5 lb or more in 1 week.

PIH—Severe
The following characteristics typify severe PIH:

1. Blood Pressure 160/100 mm Hg or higher.
2. Proteinuria: 5 g or more in 24-hour collection.
3. Oliguria: usually less than 400 ml per 24 hours or less than 20 ml per hour.
4. Cerebral or visual disturbances: headache, confusion, scotomata, blurred vision, blindness.
5. Other signs: pulmonary edema, epigastric distress, or right upper quadrant pain.

Eclampsia. Eclampsia is defined as PIH with the occurrence of generalized seizures or coma.

Superimposed Pre-eclampsia. Superimposed pre-eclampsia is characterized by the presence of chronic hypertension with the appearance of the additional features of PIH.

PREDISPOSING FACTORS FOR PIH–PRE-ECLAMPSIA/ECLAMPSIA

Predisposing factors for these disorders include: nulliparity, extremes of reproductive age (less than 18 years or more than 35 years), low socioeconomic status, family history of PIH, multiple fetuses, hydramnios, diabetes mellitus, chronic hypertension, and abnormalities of the vascular, endocrine, or metabolic system.

PATHOPHYSIOLOGY

The hallmark of PIH is the altered vascular reactivity to vasoactive substances, notably angiotensin II, and the presence of arteriolar vasospasm. The etiology of PIH remains one of the major unsolved puzzles in maternal-fetal physiology. Although pregnancies are probably predetermined at conception for the occurrence of PIH, the question remains whether this is a fetal, maternal, placental, or shared abnormality. Newer evidence is now available that relates the increased arteriolar sensitivity to angiotensin II to "imbalances" among the prostaglandins: prostacyclin (PGI_2), which originates in the arteriolar endothelium, is a vasodilator and platelet antiaggregator, whereas thromboxane, which is synthesized in the platelets, is a vasoconstrictor and platelet aggregator. Current and future therapy will be directed against those factors that promote vasospasm and platelet aggregation. Vasospasm is responsible not only for the hypertension, but also for the decreased renal blood flow and glomerular filtration rate, which contribute to salt and water retention. This, combined with injury to the vascular endothelium, fosters the occurrence of edema. Additionally, endothelial hyperplasia and fibrin deposition in the renal glomeruli lead to proteinuria. Maternal, fetal, and neonatal morbidity and mortality are directly related to the severity of the blood pressure elevation as well as to the degree of proteinuria. In addition, the adverse effects on the central nervous system, irritability and seizure potential, and the aberrations in liver function tests and coagulation are predicated on the same pathophysiologic disturbances: vasospasm, vascular endothelial injury, salt and water retention, and shift in the balance favoring thromboxane production over prostacyclin.

RECOGNITION AND EVALUATION

Prepregnancy counseling and evaluation should be encouraged in all patients with known hypertension or conditions predisposing to the development of PIH. At that time, baseline studies of maternal physiology, especially renal and metabolic function, should be undertaken. The physician should provide appropriate and informed counseling regarding the risks to the mother (significant PIH, hypertensive crisis, cerebrovascular accidents, renal failure, placental abruption, and coagulopathy) and offspring (intrauterine growth retardation, premature birth, and fetal and neonatal death) of attempting a pregnancy. If needed, medical therapy should be instituted and the patient stabilized prior to conception. A simple rule on our service is "since normal patients have a better outcome than abnormal patients, we would like you to become as close to normal as possible." One must carefully evaluate proposed medications for potential teratogenesis or other adverse effects on the fetus or the course of the pregnancy, and then determine the maternal-fetal benefits of normalizing the patient's condition versus the risks, known or unknown, of the medication itself. This may often require consultation with specialists in maternal-fetal medicine, internal medicine, genetics, nephrology, and endocrinology. In the patient who is already pregnant, a similar baseline evaluation and therapy should be undertaken as soon as possible.

CLINICAL MANAGEMENT

As in all pregnancies, the objective of clinical management is to carry the pregnancy to fetal maturity with minimal risk to the mother or fetus. Delivery remains the definitive therapy for PIH; all other measures serve to control and stabilize the maternal condition until the fetus is mature and the delivery can be effected safely.

When a pregnant patient exhibits hypertension, with or without edema and proteinuria, the diagnosis of PIH must be considered. A process of maternal-fetal evaluation and surveillance should be initiated. If the diagnosis of increased blood pressure is more secure or if the patient exhibits the full PIH–pre-eclampsia syndrome, she should be hospitalized, at bed rest, for initial evaluation and observation as to normalization of blood pressure, decreased weight and proteinuria, and reassurance of fetal well-being.

Further therapy is based on the outcome of this initial hospitalization.

Mild PIH Evaluation

Evaluation for mild PIH includes (1) ultrasound examination (fetal size versus dates, biophysical profile), (2) laboratory tests (hemoglobin and hematocrit, blood urea nitrogen [abnormal > 10 mg per deciliter], and uric acid [> 6 mg per deciliter]), (3) liver function tests (bilirubin, serum glutamic-oxaloacetic transaminase [aspartate aminotransferase], and lactate dehydrogenase), (4) clotting factors (platelets, fibrinogen, prothrombin time-partial thromboplastin time), and (5) 24-hour urine test (creatinine clearance and total protein).

Fetal surveillance should also be carried out and includes: fetal movement charts twice a day, a nonstress test (after 28 weeks) at least once a week, and a contraction stress test to evaluate placental reserve, especially if there are any aberrations in the nonstress test or decreased fetal movement.

Therapy

At Home. For the patient who is at home, in a supportive environment, is reliable, and has minimal disease, the following treatment is appropriate:

1. Strict bed rest;
2. Daily weight checks;
3. Filling out a fetal movement chart twice a day;
4. Office visits one to two times a week or more frequently if an increase in weight or a change in fetal activity occurs. These visits should include a nonstress test, repeat laboratory tests, and ultrasound surveillance;
5. Optional care, including home visiting nurse visits, home blood pressure monitoring, and use of a urine dipstick for protein checks.

Any change in maternal status (return of hypertension, increase in protein concentration, worsening laboratory values, or increased edema) or fetal status (decreased fetal movement, slow or near absence of fetal growth, onset of oligohydramnios, abnormal nonstress test and/or contraction stress test) demands immediate hospitalization.

Hospitalization. Hospitalization is required for the unreliable, noncompliant patient in a nonsupportive environment. It should be mandatory in patients who have PIH superimposed on chronic hypertension or other underlying medical disease. Maternal-fetal surveillance should be repeated as the situation demands. Remember that the response to conservative therapy does not indicate that the PIH is cured but rather that the clinical picture has ameliorated, and the pregnancy can be allowed to continue until there is deterioration in either maternal or fetal condition, at which time delivery must be considered.

Medications

Phenobarbital. Phenobarbital, 30 mg by mouth every 8 hours, is indicated as an analeptic agent and as a sedative to decrease the cerebral contribution to anxiety and catecholamine production in order to encourage the patient to remain at rest.

Antihypertensives. These should be utilized when diastolic blood pressures remain higher than 90 to 100 mm Hg at rest, prolongation of the pregnancy is desired, and the fetus and mother are otherwise stable. The goal of their use is to stabilize blood pressure at 140/90 mm Hg or less.

Beta-blockers. Either atenolol, 50 mg by mouth every 12 hours, or metoprolol, 50 mg by mouth every 12 hours, may be used. The dose may be increased to 100 mg by mouth every 12 hours.

Alpha- and Beta-Blockers. I recommend labetalol, 100 mg by mouth every 12 hours, which may be increased to 1 to 2 g per day.

Arteriolar Dilators. Use hydralazine, 10 mg by mouth every 6 hours, which may be increased to 50 mg by mouth every 6 hours. Combination therapy of a beta-blocker with hydralazine often produces a synergistic effect.

Sympatholytic Agents. I have used alpha-methyldopa, 250 mg by mouth every 12 hours, which may be increased to 250 mg every 8 hours, then every 6 hours up to 2 g per day.

Calcium Channel Blockers. Use nifedipine, 10 mg by mouth every 8 hours, which may be increased to 20 mg by mouth every 6 hours.

It should be emphasized that these same drugs are recommended for use in patients with chronic hypertension in pregnancy for control of their blood pressure. All patients requiring antihypertensive therapy should have a maternal-fetal medicine and/or an internal medicine consultation prior to the initiation of therapy and throughout the course of the pregnancy. The best medical evidence is against any teratogenic or long-lasting adverse effects in the fetus or newborn as a result of maternal therapy with these agents.

Diuretics. These medications are not recommended in the management of mild PIH unless they are necessary for treatment of the underlying medical disease, e.g., organic heart disease or complications of the disease precipitated by pregnancy. There is no evidence that diuretics exert any prophylactic benefit in the prevention of PIH.

SEVERE PRE-ECLAMPSIA

In severe pre-eclampsia, immediate hospitalization with rapid surveillance of the maternal and fetal condition is *mandatory*. Principles of management include (1) stabilizing blood pressure in the range of 140–150/90–100 mm Hg, (2) restoring adequate circulating blood volume and improving urine output, (3) preventing seizures, and (4) establishing fetal well-being.

Therapeutic Modalities

Blood Pressure Control. This includes administering an intravenous bolus of hydralazine 5 to 10 mg, which may be repeated every 30 to 60 minutes as needed. The patient also receives a continuous intravenous drip of hydralazine, 40 mg in 500 ml 5 percent dextrose in 50 percent normal saline (0.08 mg or 80 μg per milliliter), which is administered by infusion pump only. Start at 400 μg per hour equivalent to 5 ml per hour. This may be increased by doubling the infusion rate until the blood pressure is stabilized at a diastolic pressure of approximately 90 to 100 mm Hg.

Seizure Prevention. Give a 4-g bolus of intravenous $MgSO_4 \bullet 7 H_2O$ over 20 minutes followed by 2 g per hour (40 g of magnesium sulfate in 1,000 ml of 5 percent dextrose in water infused at 50 ml per hour) to maintain levels of 5 to 7 mg per deciliter (4 to 6 mEq per liter). Monitor reflexes and respirations (the latter should be higher than 10 to 12 breaths per minute). Calcium gluconate (1 g) should be available for intravenous use for respiratory depression.

Restoration of Effective Circulatory Volume. Use a Foley catheter, maintain urine output at higher than 20 to 30 ml per hour, evaluate specific gravity and protein concentrations hourly, administer intravenous dextrose (5 percent) Ringer's lactate or 5 percent dextrose in half normal saline at 150 ml per hour, and monitor central venous pressure. Central venous pressure monitoring aids in fluid replacement, especially colloid, for volume expansion using albumin either 50 percent in 50 ml or 5 percent in 500 ml.

If the central venous pressure is higher than 10 mm Hg, Swan-Ganz catheterization of the pulmonary artery is indicated to better assess both the left and right sides of the circulation. This permits proper control of fluid therapy and reduces the risk of circulatory overload and congestive heart failure.

Use an arterial line for continuous blood pressure monitoring, intermittent sampling of arterial blood gases, and other laboratory testing.

Continuous electronic fetal monitoring should also be carried out, including a nonstress test and possibly a contraction stress test.

All laboratory tests are drawn on initial evaluation for a baseline: every 4 hours, magnesium level; every 4 to 8 hours, clotting studies, i.e., platelets, fibrinogen, prothrombin time, and partial thromboplastin time. If any coagulopathy appears, these tests may be needed more frequently. Additionally, fibrin split products may be measured. Every 8 to 12 hours, a complete blood count with a differential count (hematocrit and hemoglobin values are utilized to evaluate hemoconcentration), electrolyte determination, blood urea nitrogen and creatinine levels, and uric acid concentration should be performed.

Blood should be available in the blood bank for transfusion.

The repetition of laboratory tests is imperative to evaluate properly the progress of the patient's disease as well as the course of therapy.

Ultrasound evaluation should be performed to determine fetal size and a biophysical profile carried out to evaluate fetal status.

In hypertensive crises, hydralazine should be the first line of therapy. If this is not effective, intravenous diazoxide 100 to 300 mg or intravenous nitroglycerin by infusion pump (100 mg of nitroglycerin added to 500 ml of 5 percent dextrose in water = 0.2 mg per milliliter; start infusion at 1 milliliter per minute). One must have an arterial line in place when using these medications in order to monitor the patient's blood pressure constantly.

Diuretic therapy (intravenous furosemide, 10 to 20 mg initially) is utilized only for fluid overload with impending or overt pulmonary edema. Some workers have suggested that with adequate fluid replacement, diuretics may be utilized transiently to help improve renal medullary blood flow. However, relief of vasospasm and increased vascular volume will result in increased renal blood flow and glomerular filtration rate with increased free water generation, as evidenced by improved urinary output of decreasing specific gravity.

These patients require intensive care that may be provided in the labor and delivery areas if appropriately trained medical and nursing personnel are available, or in an adult intensive care unit. The staff must be alert for the occurrence of placental abruption and the onset of disseminated intravascular coagulopathy, either alone or secondary to an abruption. In addition to a maternal-fetal medicine consultation, internal medicine and anesthesia consultations may be required to manage these patients effectively. Neonatologists should be advised of the maternal and fetal status. If the hospital facilities cannot manage mothers with this degree of disease or an immature fetus, after initial resuscitation and stabilization maternal transport to an appropriate center should be carried out.

Delay in delivery to attempt to enhance fetal pulmonary maturation through the administration of glucocorticoids (betamethasone 12 mg intramuscularly every 12 hours in two doses) is practiced in some centers. This is predicated on the fact that medical management has stabilized the mother sufficiently and the fetus is showing no signs of distress to allow a delay of approximately 48 hours. Neonatology consultation should be obtained to help evaluate fetal status and the anticipated neonatal course.

HELLP SYNDROME

HELLP (hemolysis, elevated liver enzymes, and low platelet count) features the presence of hemolytic anemia (abnormal peripheral smear, increased bilirubin, increased lactate dehydrogenase, decreased haptoglobin), elevated liver function tests (increased bilirubin, increased serum glutamic-oxaloacetic transaminase, increased lactate dehydrogenase), and low platelets (fewer than 100,000 per cubic millimeter) in association with PIH. However, it must not be confused with other conditions such as acute fatty liver of pregnancy, the hemolytic uremic syndrome, or even maternal sepsis. If the HELLP syndrome is identified and the maternal-fetal unit can be stabilized, the use of low-dose aspirin, 65 mg by mouth every day, is being advised by some as a therapeutic modality to attempt to reverse this syndrome when further fetal maturation is desired. This requires careful monitoring by maternal-fetal and hematologic consultation.

DELIVERY

The end point of therapy is delivery of a viable infant who will not require intensive care. When conservative therapy is utilized in mild PIH, delivery should be considered in (1) hospitalized, stable patients by 37 weeks; (2) at-home, stable patients, by term; (3) as previously mentioned, either of these patients with a mature baby if maternal or fetal condition destabilizes; and (4) patients prior to 37 weeks with a mature baby with any worsening in the maternal-fetal status.

Delivery must be carried out in patients with severe PIH and a mature or an immature fetus when stabilization cannot be accomplished.

Vaginal delivery is still the preferred route unless there are obstetric contraindications, i.e., fetal distress or malpresentation. When an unripe cervix is encountered and delivery is desired, the use of prostaglandin gel or Laminaria may enhance the success of oxytocin induction of labor. Patients with PIH, even in the face of intravenous magnesium sulfate therapy, tend to have a smooth labor.

Indications for Cesarean Delivery

There are three major indications for cesarean delivery: (1) Disseminated intravascular coagulopathy without the anticipation of rapid delivery, or the HELLP syndrome with severe thrombocytopenia. Platelets, cryoprecipitate, fresh frozen plasma, and packed red blood cells must be readily available for transfusion if needed before, during, or after the surgery. (2) Deteriorating maternal condition without the anticipation of rapid delivery. (3) Obstetric indications, including failure to progress in labor, fetal distress, malpresentation, and significant placental abruption adversely affecting the mother or fetus.

POST PARTUM

After delivery, management must be supportive until the spontaneous reversal of the pathophysiology of PIH. If severe vasospasm and oliguria persist, intravenous nitroprusside with invasive monitoring will allow proper management of these patients. The beginning of the resolution process is ushered in by the onset of spontaneous diuresis. All measures utilized ante- and intrapartum are continued. Magnesium sulfate is discontinued when diuresis is established, since it becomes increasingly difficult to maintain therapeutic magnesium levels. The kidney is essentially the only route for the clearance of magnesium. Since 25 percent of seizures may occur post partum, patients are placed on phenobarbital, 60 mg intramuscularly, followed by 30 mg by mouth every 8 hours. Antihypertensives are utilized until normalization of the blood pressure occurs, which may require up to several weeks post partum. Invasive monitoring usually may be discontinued when the resolution process is definitely underway.

Laboratory surveillance is continued until postpartum stabilization is achieved.

ECLAMPSIA

This severe complication of PIH may occur either after the development of clinically apparent pre-eclampsia or as the first manifestation of the problem. Eclampsia is signaled by the onset of generalized seizures, which are often associated with urinary and rectal incontinence, postictal obtundation, and, on occasion, coma. It is the abrupt and acute onset that represents a significant threat to the well-being of both mother (hypoxia, acidosis, aspiration) and fetus (hypoxia). Patients may come to the emergency department with seizures or in a coma, at which time a rapid and correct assessment of the etiology must be made. The physician must differentiate these events from epilepsy, acute maternal intracranial hemorrhage secondary to either an aneurysm or other ruptured blood vessel, or acute hypertensive encephalopathy. In addition to the central nervous system, eclampsia represents multisystem involvement, including the cardiovascular, renal, hepatic, and hematologic systems. Evaluation and therapy, therefore, must be directed to all of these systems simultaneously.

Therapeutic Goals

The primary goals of treatment are to (1) stop seizure activity; (2) restore spontaneous respirations, or if necessary, provide mechanical ventilation; (3) provide oxygen to counter the hypoxia (maternal-fetal); (4) prevent maternal injury; (5) treat hypertension to prevent intracranial bleeding; (6) establish and restore fetal well-being; and (7) accomplish delivery after stabilization.

Therapy for seizures should consist of magnesium sulfate given as a 4-g intravenous bolus loading dose followed by 40 g in 1,000 ml 5 percent dextrose in water at 50 ml per hour (2 g per hour). The physician may need to repeat a 2- to 4-g intravenous bolus if seizures recur or continue. The same maternal monitoring and precautions apply as previously discussed. Additionally, diazepam, 10 mg in an intravenous push, may be administered and may be repeated if needed. This drug is helpful in patients with repetitive seizures that are unresponsive to magnesium sulfate. The patient must be carefully observed for the development of respiratory depression.

After cessation of seizures, if the infant is undelivered, the management reverts to that for severe PIH. If seizures are post partum, after the patient is stabilized, oral analeptic agents, i.e., phenytoin or phenobarbital, should be maintained. Neurologic consultation should be obtained to further evaluate other causes of the seizures or possible sequelae. Electroencephalograms may remain abnormal for months after the occurrence of such eclamptic seizures. However, if there is no other etiology for the seizures, these patients should not be at risk for subsequent seizure disorder.

Patients with eclampsia may die secondary to repetitive seizures and hypoxia, intracranial vascular accidents, pulmonary edema, and hypertensive crises. Therefore, accurate and timely therapy must be instituted to prevent increased maternal morbidity and mortality and to preserve the life and well-being of the fetus.

SUGGESTED READING

American College of Obstetricians and Gynecologists. Management of preeclampsia. ACOG Technical Bulletin No. 91, Washington, D.C., February 1986.
Creasy RK, Resnik R. Maternal fetal medicine: principles and practice. Philadelphia: WB Saunders, 1984.
Gabbe SG, Neibyl JR, Simpson JL, eds. Obstetrics—normal and problem pregnancies. New York: Churchill Livingstone, 1986.
Pritchard JA, MacDonald PC, Gant NF, eds. Williams obstetrics. 17th ed. Norwalk, CT: Appleton-Century-Crofts, 1985.
Sullivan JM. Hypertension and pregnancy. Chicago: Year Book Medical Publishers, 1986.

PREMATURE RUPTURE OF THE MEMBRANES

ANTHONY M. VINTZILEOS, M.D.
WINSTON A. CAMPBELL, M.D.
DAVID J. NOCHIMSON, M.D.

Premature rupture of the membranes (PROM) is one of the most common complications of pregnancy. It occurs in approximately 10 percent of all pregnancies and is causally related to increased incidence of perinatal death, fetal distress during labor, and infection (fetal and maternal). There is general agreement that expeditious delivery is mandatory if the patient presents with ruptured membranes and apparent clinical amnionitis. The real problem lies with the patient who has ruptured membranes without clinical infection. In this chapter we discuss the management of this group of patients who present with PROM and no signs of infection or labor.

When PROM occurs at term, the majority of investigators recommend prompt delivery because of an increased incidence of amnionitis with prolonged rupture of the membranes. However, this action may result in an increased incidence of primary cesarean section for failed induction of labor or cephalopelvic disproportion. When PROM occurs in a preterm gestation, the management is even more controversial. In preterm gestations immediate delivery of the fetus carries a significant risk of hyaline membrane disease, which remains the major contributor to neonatal morbidity and mortality; therefore, conservative management has been advocated by the

TABLE 1 Criteria for Scoring Biophysical Variables

Nonstress Test

Score 2 (NST 2): five or more fetal heart rate accelerations of at least 15 beats per minute in amplitude and at least 15 seconds' duration associated with fetal movement in a 20-minute period

Score 1 (NST 1): two to four accelerations of at least 15 beats per minute in amplitude and at least 15 seconds' duration associated with fetal movements in a 20-minute period

Score 0 (NST 0): one or fewer accelerations in a 20-minute period

Fetal Movements

Score 2 (FM 2): at least three gross (trunk and limbs) episodes of fetal movement within 30 minutes (simultaneous limb and trunk movements are counted as a single movement)

Score 1 (FM 1): one or two fetal movements within 30 minutes
Score 0 (FM 0): absence of fetal movements within 30 minutes

Fetal Breathing Movements

Score 2 (FBM 2): at least one episode of fetal breathing of at least 60 seconds' duration within a 30-minute observation period

Score 1 (FBM 1): at least one episode of fetal breathing lasting 30 to 60 seconds within 30 minutes

Score 0 (FBM 0): absence of fetal breathing or breathing lasting less than 30 seconds within 30 minutes

Fetal Tone

Score 2 (FT 2): at least one episode of extension of extremities with return to position of flexion and also one episode of extension of spine with return to position of flexion
Score 1 (FT 1): at least one episode of extension of extremities with return to position of flexion or one episode of extension of spine with return to position of flexion
Score 0 (FT 0): extremities in extension, fetal movements not followed by return to flexion, open hand

Amniotic Fluid Volume

Score 2 (AF 2): fluid evident throughout the uterine cavity; the largest pocket measures 2 cm or more in vertical diameter

Score 1 (AF 1): the largest pocket measures less than 2 cm but more than 1 cm in vertical diameter

Score 0 (AF 0): crowding of fetal small parts; largest pocket measures less than 1 cm in vertical diameter

Placental Grading

Score 2 (PL 2): placental grading 0, 1, or 2

Score 1 (PL 1): placenta posterior difficult to evaluate

Score 0 (PL 0): placental grading 3

NST = nonstress test; FM = fetal movements; FBM = fetal breathing movements; FT = fetal tone; AF = amniotic fluid; PL = placental grading.
  Maximal score 12; minimal score zero.

majority of investigators. However, the conservative approach carries an increased risk of maternal-fetal infection and cord prolapse. Some management protocols advocate the use of amniocentesis to detect not only the fetus with a mature lung profile but also the fetus most likely to develop sepsis. The problems associated with this approach have been the inability to obtain fluid in almost half of these patients, the invasiveness of the procedure, and the lack of strong correlation between the presence of bacteria in the amniotic fluid and fetal sepsis.

INTRODUCTION TO ANTEPARTUM FETAL ASSESSMENT—THE FETAL BIOPHYSICAL PROFILE

Until recently, the antepartum fetal evaluation of patients with PROM has been confined solely to nonstress testing. The contraction stress test is contraindicated and has no place in the antepartum fetal evaluation of these patients because of the theoretical risk of initiating labor. Real-time ultrasonography now permits objective evaluation of multiple fetal activities—fetal movements, breathing, and tone—as well as assessment of the intrauterine environment, i.e., estimation of amniotic fluid volume and placental grading. The combination of these variables (biophysical profile) as a means of antepartum fetal evaluation enhances the ability to identify accurately the compromised fetus. The most important factor in the sensitivity of this testing method is the combination of acute (nonstress test, fetal breathing movements, fetal movements, and fetal tone) and chronic (amniotic fluid volume, placental grading) markers of the fetal condition. This evaluation includes a nonstress test with maximum duration of 40 minutes, followed by real-time scanning. The duration of observation is extended until each ultrasound-monitored biophysical variable meets normal criteria or 30 minutes have elapsed. The fetal biophysical variables are assigned an arbitrary score of 2, 1, or 0 (Table 1). The maximal score is 12 and the minimal 0. A fetal biophysical profile score of 8 or more offers reassurance of fetal well-being, whereas a score of 7 or less is not reassuring. This method of antepartum fetal assessment has been shown to be more accurate than the contraction stress test in identifying the compromised fetus in high-risk patients.

The fetal biophysical profile, as a means of antepartum fetal assessment, was designed to help the clinician ascertain the following: (1) the fetal condition at the time of testing; this judgment is based on the presence or absence of the acute markers of the fetal condition (nonstress test, fetal breathing movements, fetal movements, and fetal tone). The predictive accuracy of each normal biophysical activity is high, but the false-positive rate for each single abnormal variable is greater than 50 percent. The combination of these acute markers has been shown to decrease the false-positive results and to enhance the ability to identify accurately the compromised fetus. (2) The degree of fetal compromise; this judgment is based on the fact that the first manifestations of fetal compromise are nonreactive nonstress testing and absence of breathing. In advanced fetal compromise, the fetal body movements and fetal tone are also abolished. This concept is of significant value in interpreting the data obtained from the fetal biophysical assessment. The presence or absence of the acute markers of the fetal condition allows for the estimation of deterioration of the fetal condition and perhaps determination of the degree of change in fetal status. (3) If there is chronic fetal stress or compromise; this judgment is based on the amniotic fluid volume estimation. (4) Possibility of in utero death due to cord accident; this judg-ment is based on the presence or absence of oligohydramnios and/or variable decelerations during nonstress testing. (5) Increased risk for intrapartum abnormal fetal heart rate patterns and abruptio placentae; this judgment is based on the presence of a grade III placenta.

THE BIOPHYSICAL PROFILE OF THE HEALTHY FETUS FROM 25 TO 44 WEEKS OF GESTATION AND THE EFFECT OF PREMATURE RUPTURE OF THE MEMBRANES

The need for antepartum surveillance frequently involves fetal gestational ages as early as 25 to 26 weeks; therefore, the question of what the biophysical profile of the normal fetus is throughout gestation should be addressed. In addition, many patients present with PROM. The second question to be addressed, therefore, is the effect of rupture of the membranes on the fetal biophysical activities and scoring throughout gestation. These two questions were investigated by our group in a retrospective analysis of 1,151 fetal biophysical profile scores associated with good pregnancy outcomes. In that study, normal fetal biophysical activities and scores were determined throughout gestation from 25 to 44 weeks in patients with intact membranes and compared with profiles and scores of a group of patients with PROM and good pregnancy outcomes. It was found that although the biophysical scoring of the healthy fetus with intact membranes does not change significantly throughout gestation, some of the fetal biophysical variables (nonstress test, fetal breathing movements, amniotic fluid volume, and placental grading) do. Patients with intact membranes were found to have a higher incidence of reactive nonstress testing after 32 weeks, decreased amniotic fluid volume after 40 weeks, and increased incidence of grade III placentas as pregnancy approached term. In this group of patients, an additional interesting finding was decreased fetal breathing after 40 weeks.

PROM was found to be associated with a higher incidence of reactive nonstress testing, absence of fetal breathing, and reduced amniotic fluid volume in most gestational ages; however, the overall biophysical scoring of the healthy fetus was found to be unaltered throughout gestation by the presence of ruptured membranes. In healthy fetuses the incidence of fetal biophysical scoring of 8 or more as well as of mean biophysical scores does not change from 25 to 44 weeks regardless of gestational age and/or status of the membranes. An interesting observation was that the incidence of nonreactive nonstress testing at less than 32 weeks of gestation was only 13.5 percent in the presence of ruptured membranes. This finding means that the clinician should be careful before he or she attributes nonreactivity to prematurity in these very preterm gestations. As we will discuss below, nonreactive nonstress testing in the presence of prematurely ruptured membranes very frequently is an indication of fetal infection.

THE FETAL BIOPHYSICAL PROFILE IN PATIENTS WITH PROM—AN EARLY PREDICTOR OF FETAL INFECTION

A prospective study by our group using serial fetal biophysical assessment in patients who had PROM demonstrated that an abnormal biophysical assessment frequently represents fetal infection. A total of 73 patients who had premature rupture of the membranes and no signs of labor or infection was included in that study. A biophysical profile assessment was performed on hospital admission and was repeated every 24 to 48 hours if patients remained undelivered. The last biophysical assessment before delivery was compared with the outcome of pregnancy as reflected by the development of amnionitis, possible neonatal sepsis, and neonatal sepsis. The clinical diagnosis of amnionitis was made in the presence of two or more of the following criteria: maternal fever higher than 37.8° C, maternal tachycardia (120 beats per minute or more), leukocytosis (white blood cell count 20,000 per cubic millimeter or higher in the absence of prior corticosteroid administration), fetal tachycardia (greater than 160 beats per minute), uterine tenderness, and foul-smelling amniotic fluid. Possible neonatal sepsis was diagnosed in neonates with strong clinical and laboratory evidence of bacterial infection but with negative cultures. Objective criteria included the presence of two or more of the following: white blood cell count less than 5,000 per cubic millimeter, polymorphonuclear leukocyte count less than 1,800 per cubic millimeter, I:T ratio (the ratio of bands to total neutrophil count) greater than 0.2, or positive gastric aspirate for polymorphonuclear leukocytes greater than 5 per high-power field. Neonatal sepsis was diagnosed only in the presence of positive cultures of blood, urine, or cerebrospinal fluid.

Of the 73 patients, 20 were delivered more than 24 hours from the time of the last fetal biophysical assessment. In this group of patients there was no correlation between the fetal biophysical assessment and infection outcome. Subsequently this group was eliminated from further statistical analysis. There were 53 patients who delivered within 24 hours of the final biophysical assessment; in this group of patients a biophysical score of 8 or more was associated with an infection rate (maternal and/or neonatal) of 2.7 percent, and a low biophysical score (7 or less) was associated with an infection rate of 93.7 percent. The first manifestations of impending fetal infection were nonreactive nonstress testing and absence of fetal breathing. Loss of fetal movements and fetal tone were late signs of fetal infection. The best predictor of infection was found to be the biophysical score, whereas of the individual biophysical variables the nonstress test, fetal breathing movements, fetal movements, and fetal tone were found to be important in the above sequence. The relationship between each biophysical variable and infection outcome in these 53 patients is illustrated in Table 2. Infection developed in 16 cases (with one or more diagnoses); the analysis of the fetal biophysical profile in

TABLE 2 Relationship of Each Biophysical Variable to Infection Outcome

Biophysical Variable	No. of Patients	Total Last Tests (%)	Infected		Noninfected	
			No.	(%)	No.	(%)
NST 2	27	50.9	1/27	3.7	26/27	96.2
NST 1	8	15.0	2/8	25.0	6/8	75.0
NST 0	18	33.9	13/18	72.2	5/18	27.7
FBM 2	24	45.2	0/24	0.0	24/24	100.0
FBM 1	3	5.6	0/3	0.0	3/3	100.0
FBM 0	26	49.0	16/26	61.5	10/26	38.4
FM 2	43	81.1	8/43	18.6	35/43	81.3
FM 1	4	7.5	2/4	50.0	2/4	50.0
FM 0	6	11.3	6/6	100.0	0/6	0.0
FT 2	46	86.7	9/46	19.5	37/46	80.4
FT 1	5	9.4	5/5	100.0	0/5	0.0
FT 0	2	3.7	2/2	100.0	0/2	0.0
AF 2	27	50.9	3/27	11.1	24/27	88.8
AF 1	13	24.5	4/13	30.7	9/13	69.2
AF 0	13	24.5	9/13	69.2	4/13	30.7
PL 2	50	94.3	14/50	28.0	36/50	72.0
PL 1	1	1.8	1/1	100.0	0/1	0.0
PL 0	2	3.7	1/2	50.0	1/2	50.0
Total	53		16	30.1	37	69.8

NST = nonstress test; FBM = fetal breathing movements; FM = fetal movements; FT = fetal tone; AF = amniotic fluid; PL = placental grading.

TABLE 3   Analysis of the Biophysical Profile of the 16 Cases with Infection

Case	NST	FBM	FM	FT	AF	PL	Total Score	Diagnosis
1	2	0	2	2	2	2	10	Amnionitis
2	0	0	2	1	1	2	6	Amnionitis
3	0	0	2	2	1	2	7	Possible neonatal sepsis
4	0	0	2	2	0	2	6	Possible neonatal sepsis
5	0	0	2	2	0	2	6	Possible neonatal sepsis
6	0	0	2	2	1	2	7	Amnionitis—Possible neonatal sepsis
7	1	0	0	1	2	2	6	Amnionitis—Possible neonatal sepsis
8	0	0	2	2	0	2	6	Amnionitis—Possible neonatal sepsis
9	0	0	0	1	0	1	2	Amnionitis—Possible neonatal sepsis
10	0	0	1	2	1	2	6	Neonatal sepsis
11	1	0	2	0	2	0	5	Neonatal sepsis
12	0	0	0	0	0	2	2	Neonatal sepsis
13	0	0	0	2	0	2	4	Amnionitis—neonatal sepsis
14	0	0	1	1	0	2	4	Amnionitis—neonatal sepsis
15	0	0	0	2	0	1	3	Amnionitis—neonatal sepsis
16	0	0	0	1	0	2	3	Amnionitis—neonatal sepsis

NST = nonstress test; FMB = fetal breathing movements; FM = fetal movements; FT = fetal tone; AF = amniotic fluid; PL = placental grading.

these 16 cases is illustrated in Table 3. As can be seen when the fetus was compromised (possible neonatal sepsis or neonatal sepsis, cases 3 through 16), the fetal biophysical score was 7 or less in all cases. Since there was no difference in the cord pH between the infected and noninfected cases, the low scores of the infected group cannot be attributed to hypoxia but rather to fetal infection. The decrease in fetal biophysical activities prior to the development of clinical infection makes sense, especially in cases of an ascending infection in which the fetus seems to be the first target.

RELATIONSHIP BETWEEN INDIVIDUAL FETAL BIOPHYSICAL VARIABLES AND INFECTION OUTCOME IN PROM

Oligohydramnios. In patients with PROM, the degree of oligohydramnios, as defined by our criteria (per Table 1), is well correlated with the outcome of pregnancy, as reflected by pregnancy prolongation, intrapartum fetal heart rate patterns consistent with umbilical cord compression, incidence of cesarean section, fetal distress, infection, and perinatal mortality rate. The association between the degree of oligohydramnios and infection outcome in 90 patients who had PROM and no signs of infection or labor has been presented by our group (Table 4). Patients with severe oligohydramnios (largest amniotic fluid pocket less than 1 cm in vertical diameter) had the highest incidence of amnionitis (47.3 percent), possible neonatal sepsis (26.3 percent), and neonatal sepsis (31.5 percent). Based on these findings, it is recommended that patients with PROM and severe oligohydramnios be followed closely with daily fetal biophysical profile determinations.

Nonstress Testing. Since the nonstress test is most frequently used as a primary antepartum fetal surveillance test, its value in evaluating patients with PROM was determined by a retrospective analysis of 127 consecutive patients who presented with PROM and no signs of infection

or labor. These patients had frequent nonstress tests (every 24 to 48 hours) as a part of the fetal biophysical profile assessment. The last nonstress test performed within 48 hours of delivery was used for comparison with pregnancy outcome. The efficacy of the nonstress test in predicting infection outcome according to gestational age groups is illustrated in Table 5. The data were also analyzed according to the longitudinal trend of the nonstress test results (Table 6). Analysis of the longitudinal trend of the nonstress test results showed that patients who had reactive nonstress tests initially but subsequently converted to nonreactive tests developed infection in almost 90 percent of the cases. Based on these data, it is suggested that daily nonstress testing is a useful screening tool for following patients with PROM. The biophysical profile should be utilized as a means of a follow-up of a nonreactive nonstress test because of its better positive predictive value.

Fetal Breathing Movements. The value of the presence or absence of fetal breathing in predicting infection in patients with PROM was determined by a retrospective analysis of 130 patients with PROM and no clinical signs of infection or labor. The last ultrasound examination performed within 48 hours of delivery was used for comparison with infection outcome. The sensitivity and specificity of fetal breathing in predicting infection were 91.6 and 64.8 percent, respectively. The presence of fetal breathing is a good predictor of noninfection outcome (negative predictive value 95.3 percent), whereas its absence does not necessarily indicate impending infection (positive predictive value 50 percent). The efficacy of the fetal breathing in predicting infection is illustrated in Table 7 according to gestation age groups.

THE FETAL BIOPHYSICAL PROFILE VERSUS AMNIOCENTESIS IN PREDICTING INFECTION IN PRETERM PROM

In our institution a comparison between daily fetal biophysical profile determinations and amniocentesis on

TABLE 4 Relationship Between Amniotic Fluid Volume Before Delivery and Infection Outcome

Amniotic Fluid Volume	Patients (n = 90)	Gestational Age (wk) (Mean ± 2 SD)	Chorioamnionitis No.	(%)	Possible neonatal Sepsis No.	(%)	Neonatal Sepsis No.	(%)	Overall Infection* No.	(%)
AF 2	54	32.5 ± 5.1[a]	5/54	9.2[a]	2/54	3.7[a]	1/54	1.8[a]	6/54	11.1[a]
AF 1	17	31.6 ± 6.5[a]	2/17	11.7[ab]	3/17	17.6[ab]	1/17	5.8[ab]	5/17	29.4[ab]
AF 0	19	30.7 ± 7.0[a]	9/19	47.3[b]	5/19	26.3[b]	6/19	31.5[b]	13/19	68.4[b]

* Included are patients who may have more than one diagnosis.
Proportions (or means) with different superscripted letters are significantly different (p ≤ 0.05):
  a and b = Statistically significant (p < 0.05).
  a and b = Statistically not significant (p > 0.05).
  b and b = Statistically not significant (p > 0.05).
  a and ab = Statistically not significant (p > 0.05).
  b and ab = Statistically not significant (p > 0.05).

TABLE 5 Efficacy of Nonstress Test in Prediction of Infection According to Gestational Age Groups

Gestational Age	Sensitivity (%)	Specificity (%)	Positive Predictive Value (%)	Negative Predictive Value (%)
≤ 32 wk	76.1	58.8	61.5	80.0
> 32 wk	81.8	95.0	75.0	96.6
Entire group (25–41 wk)	78.1	86.3	65.7	92.1

TABLE 6 Longitudinal Trend of the Nonstress Test Results

No. of Patients	Initial Test	Final Test	Infection
19	Reactive	Nonreactive	17 (90%)
5	Nonreactive	Nonreactive	4 (80%)
43	Reactive	Reactive	2 (4.6%)
4	Nonreactive	Reactive	0 (0.0%)
42	Reactive (only one test)	—	3 (7.1%)
14	Nonreactive (only one test)	—	6 (42.8%)
Total = 127			32 (25.1%)

TABLE 7 Efficacy of Fetal Breathing to Predict Infection According to Gestational Age Groups

Gestational Age	Sensitivity (%)	Specificity (%)	Positive Predictive Value (%)	Negative Predictive Value (%)
≤ 30 wk	88.8	45.0	59.2	81.8
> 30 wk	94.4	70.2	43.5	98.1
Entire group (25–41 wk)	91.6	64.8	50.0	95.3

admission (for Gram's stain and culture) was carried out in 58 patients with preterm PROM and no apparent infection or labor. This study was not designed to compare two different tests but to compare two different management protocols. All 58 patients had both a fetal biophysical profile assessment and an amniocentesis performed on admission. The included gestational ages were between 25 and 34 weeks. The fetal biophysical profile determina-

tions were repeated every 24 hours if patients remained undelivered. In addition to the usual indications for delivery, the presence of bacteria on Gram's stain, positive culture results (aerobic/anaerobic), or a persistently low biophysical score (7 or less on two examinations 2 hours apart in the presence of a nonreactive nonstress test and absence of fetal breathing) were also considered indications for delivery. The final fetal biophysical profile assessment and the amniocentesis results on admission (Gram's stain and culture) were compared with the outcome of pregnancy as reflected by the development of amnionitis, possible neonatal sepsis, and neonatal sepsis. A total of 15 patients became infected. The diagnoses in these 15 patients were amnionitis alone (two cases) and amnionitis associated with possible neonatal sepsis or neonatal sepsis (13 cases). Twelve of these 13 cases were associated with a low biophysical score (≤ 7). In the two cases in which amnionitis alone was the diagnosis, the biophysical scores were reassuring. These observations suggest that fetal infection is responsible for the low biophysical activities, whereas maternal infection (amnionitis) without fetal infection may very well be associated with normal scores. The sensitivity, specificity, positive predictive value, and negative predictive value of the biophysical profile scoring were 80, 97.6, 92.3, and 93.3 percent, respectively. The sensitivity, specificity, positive predictive value, and negative predictive value of the Gram's stain were 60, 81.3, 52.9, and 85.3 percent, respectively. The sensitivity, specificity, positive predictive value, and negative predictive value of the amniotic fluid culture were 60, 86, 60, and 86 percent, respectively. These data suggest that daily fetal biophysical assessment is superior to amniocentesis on admission in selecting those patients who are candidates for fetal infection and therefore in need of prompt delivery. At our institution the fetal biophysical profile has replaced amniocentesis because it is simple, noninvasive, and applicable to all patients with PROM; in addition, it can be repeated frequently (daily) and is more efficacious in predicting infection outcome, especially when the fetus is compromised. The disadvantages of using amniocentesis are the inability to obtain fluid in all patients, the impracticality of frequent taps, the invasiveness and inherent risks of the procedure, and the information obtained, which mainly pertains to the presence or absence of bacteria in the amniotic fluid and does not necessarily reflect fetal status.

THE USE OF DAILY FETAL BIOPHYSICAL PROFILES IMPROVES PREGNANCY OUTCOME IN PROM

The protocol used at the University of Connecticut Health Center for following patients with PROM is based on daily fetal biophysical profile determinations and is illustrated in Figure 1. The efficacy of this protocol in terms of improving pregnancy outcome was prospectively evaluated in patients with PROM and no clinical signs of infection or labor. The study group consisted of 73 patients with PROM who were managed with daily biophysical assessment during the period of August 1, 1985 through

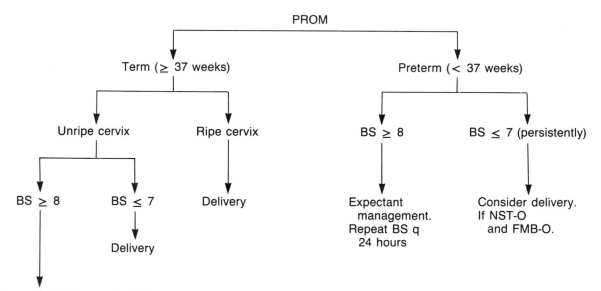

Figure 1 Protocol for management of premature rupture of the membranes. BS = biophysical score; NST-0 = nonreactive nonstress test; FBM-0 = fetal breathing absent; SOL = spontaneous onset of labor. (Reprinted with permission from Vintzileos AM, Campbell WA, Nochimson DJ, et al. The fetal biophysical profile in patients with premature rupture of the membranes—an early predictor of fetal infection. Am J Obstet Gynecol 1985; 152:510–516.)

November 15, 1986. The pregnancy outcome of this group was compared with the outcome of a previous (historical control) group (73 patients) with PROM who were managed expectantly without using the fetal biophysical assessment for management (period of July 1, 1983 through June 30, 1984). The indications for delivery were the same in both groups. In the study group, an additional indication for delivery was an abnormal biophysical assessment (biophysical score of 7 or less on two examinations 2 hours apart in the presence of a nonreactive nonstress test and absence of fetal breathing). Infection outcome—maternal as well as neonatal—and low 5-minute Apgar scores were significantly less in the study than in the control group. The percentage of patients who developed infection in the study group (10.9 percent) was significantly less than in the control group (30.1 percent). This represents a reduction in our infection rate by almost two-thirds. The incidences of possible neonatal sepsis and neonatal sepsis were also lower in the study group as compared with the control group (5.4 percent versus 13.6 percent and 1.3 percent versus 9.5 percent), but possibly because of the small numbers this did not reach statistical significance. However, when possible neonatal sepsis and neonatal sepsis were considered together, the overall neonatal infection rate was significantly lower in the study group (6.7 percent versus 23.2 percent). Maternal amnionitis was reduced from 20.5 percent to 5.4 percent.

A prospective, randomized study would be the ideal design to address the question of whether or not management of PROM with daily fetal biophysical assessment improves pregnancy outcome. Such a study, although desirable, was viewed as ethically unacceptable to all maternal-fetal medicine subspecialists and neonatologists at our institution. Therefore, we used a historical control group for comparison. The similarity, however, between the historical and study groups permitted a meaningful clinical comparison, since both groups consisted of consecutive patients who were studied prospectively and managed in a similar manner other than the indications for delivery.

Our protocol for following patients with PROM takes into consideration the condition of the fetus before deciding on the optimal plan of management. PROM is such a common event in perinatal medicine that it is surprising to find a tremendous diversity of opinion regarding its proper management. It is well recognized that no single management strategy has yet emerged as superior to all others. It is our opinion that this is simply the result of formulating protocols of management without considering the condition of the fetus. Our experience suggests that the fetus is the final arbiter, and any protocol must include the condition of the fetus before deciding on the optimal plan of management. We believe this approach improves pregnancy outcome by reducing the incidence of maternal as well as neonatal infection.

SUGGESTED READING

Vintzileos AM, Campbell WA, Ingardia CJ, et al. The fetal biophysical profile and its predictive value. Obstet Gynecol 1983; 62:271.

Vintzileos AM, Campbell WA, Nochimson DJ, et al. The fetal biophysical profile in patients with premature rupture of the membranes—an early predictor of fetal infection. Am J Obstet Gynecol 1985; 152:510.

Vintzileos AM, Campbell WA, Nochimson DJ, et al. Degree of oligohydramnios and pregnancy outcome in patients with premature rupture of the membranes. Obstet Gynecol 1985; 66:162.

Vintzileos AM, Campbell WA, Nochimson DJ, et al. The use of the nonstress test in patients with premature rupture of the membranes. Am J Obstet Gynecol 1986; 155:149.

Vintzileos AM, Campbell WA, Nochimson DJ, et al. Fetal breathing as a predictor of infection in premature rupture of the membranes. Obstet Gynecol 1986; 67:813.

Vintzileos AM, Campbell WA, Nochimson DJ, et al. Fetal biophysical profile versus amniocentesis in predicting infection in preterm premature rupture of the membranes. Obstet Gynecol 1986; 68:488.

Vintzileos AM, Feinstein SJ, Lodeiro JG, et al. Fetal biophysical profile and the effect of premature rupture of the membranes. Obstet Gynecol 1986; 67:818.

SHOULDER DYSTOCIA

DAVID B. ACKER, M.D.
EMANUEL A. FRIEDMAN, M.D., Sc.D.

Maternal expulsive efforts plus gentle downward traction on the fetal head usually result in descent of the anterior fetal shoulder under the symphysis pubis. When this occurs, it is nearly always followed by rapid delivery. Failure of the shoulders to be delivered by these forces after the baby's head has exited from the pelvis constitutes shoulder dystocia. It is an obstetric emergency requiring rapid and deft, but not hasty and excessively forceful, maneuvers to resolve the mechanical problem of impaction of the fetal shoulders above the maternal pelvic inlet. Unless it can be resolved promptly, the fetus will be asphyxiated; if it is not resolved skillfully, the fetus or the gravida will be traumatized.

Entrance of the shoulders into the true pelvis is influenced by their size, flexibility, and position in relation to the inlet of the pelvis. Conditions that predispose to large fetuses (such as maternal obesity, excessive weight gain, previous large babies, postmaturity, and high parity), or decreased bisacromial flexibility (as is seen in the macrosomic fetus of a diabetic gravida) is associated with shoulder dystocia. Abnormalities of the second stage of labor may also presage this problem, including precipitate, protracted, or arrested descent. Operative vaginal delivery from the midpelvis may also result in shoulder dystocia, perhaps because the fetal shoulders have not been given ample opportunity to accommodate properly to the pelvic inlet.

INCIDENCE

The incidence of shoulder dystocia is usually reported to be less than 1 percent, but it varies with the population being evaluated. At our institution, 2.1 percent of term pregnancies were diagnosed as being associated with shoulder dystocia. Contrary to expectations, the condition occurred across the range of fetal weights, although it was obviously much more common among gravidas delivering large babies. Although the relative incidence in small to average size infants was low, we found almost one-half of the total shoulder dystocias among this group. Moreover, fetuses of diabetic mothers experienced shoulder dystocia more frequently than those of nondiabetic gravidas, even when birth weight differences were taken into account. Postdate pregnancies resulting in the birth of a macrosomic neonate (4,500+ g) were found to have a particularly high incidence of shoulder dystocia, but the rate for smaller post-term infants did not differ from that of term infants with similar birth weights.

Among nondiabetic gravidas who delivered large infants (4,500+ g), shoulder dystocia commonly followed arrest disorders of labor, but this relationship was not as clear-cut among those carrying smaller infants except when the arrest pattern was followed by forceps delivery. In general, however, no other labor pattern was sufficiently predictive to be clinically useful, and none could be considered protective in the sense that shoulder dystocia could not occur subsequently. This means one must be alert to the possibility of shoulder dystocia at all times. It is especially worth noting that electively terminating the second stage of labor by midforceps has been reported to be associated with a particularly high incidence of shoulder dystocia.

PREVENTION

Ideally the best management for shoulder dystocia would be to prevent it entirely, but this is not feasible because it cannot be predicted in most cases. Nevertheless, certain preventive actions have been advocated to reduce its incidence. These measures include avoiding instrumental intervention for midpelvic delivery, if possible, and undertaking cesarean section for the delivery of a large infant. Neither of these approaches is fully accepted or without controversy. However, both deserve consideration in the interest of averting a potentially serious problem.

Avoiding Unnecessary Operative Vaginal Delivery

Labor need not be arbitrarily terminated by forceps delivery or vacuum extraction after 2 hours of second stage activity without some pressing indication. A complete discussion of current management of the second stage of labor is beyond the scope of this chapter, but there are often more acceptable alternatives to immediate delivery. Evaluate the fetal status to ensure well-being and the cephalopelvic relationships to rule out bone dystocia. In the absence of any documentable reason to effect delivery, give serious consideration to allowing conduction anesthesia to abate, aug-

menting ineffectual uterine contractions with oxytocin and providing continued support, encouragement, and rest. By temporizing in this way, one gives the patient the opportunity to continue the labor process. The passage of time permits the fetus to descend and accommodate better to the pelvis. A less traumatic delivery may ensue. Alternatively, insurmountable cephalopelvic disproportion may declare itself by the development of a pattern of arrest of descent coupled with impaction of the fetal presenting part in the pelvis. In the former instance, it is unlikely that shoulder dystocia will occur (but it may, of course); in the latter, it will have been averted.

Cesarean Section for Macrosomic Infants of Diabetic Gravidas

Advances in the care of the diabetic gravida have led to significant decreases in maternal and fetal mortality and morbidity. Attention is now turning toward avoidance of birth trauma. This applies especially to the delivery of the large infants so common among these cases. Given the fact that diabetic gravidas are at such high risk for shoulder dystocia, one must be especially attentive to the need to maintain strict dietary and insulin control and to monitor them carefully for fetal growth and development. As a guide, if the fetus is determined to be in excess of 4,000 g, cesarean section seems reasonable and appropriate. The estimate of fetal weight should be based on the most accurate measurement techniques available, recognizing that estimates based on physical examination are notoriously poor. Notwithstanding the fact that even the more accurate and objective technique of ultrasonography is still rather imperfect, a growing number of authorities are recommending that diabetic mothers carrying fetuses weighing 4,000 g or more should be delivered by the abdominal route. There appears to be adequate support in the form of the balance of risk to benefit to justify this practice.

Cesarean Section for Very Large Infants of Nondiabetic Gravidas

Some have begun to advocate abdominal delivery for fetuses of nondiabetic gravidas whose estimated weight is 5,000 g or more (11+ lb). Even if fetal weight could be estimated accurately, the absolute number of such infants is small. In our experience, not only is it rare to encounter an infant of this size, but ultrasonographic fetal measurements are quite inaccurate in correctly identifying them. At the same time, most fetuses estimated by this means to be over 5,000 g later prove to be smaller.

There are also centers at which abdominal delivery is being done for large fetuses where the cut-off point for selection is as low as 4,500 g. This approach does not yet appear to be warranted. At these marginal levels, the inherent inaccuracy of all ultrasonographic methods makes it difficult to know in any given case whether one is actually dealing with a large fetus. The birth weight may turn out to be relatively low. Until our ability to determine fetal weight becomes more reliable, therefore, it does not seem appropriate to recommend cesarean birth based solely on estimated fetal weight, imposing real surgical and anesthetic risks to the mother to achieve the dubious benefit of avoiding shoulder dystocia in these cases.

ANTICIPATORY PREPARATION

Shoulder dystocia cannot be prevented, but it can and must be anticipated. Identify the patient at risk on the basis of her past medical and obstetric history (diabetes mellitus, prior large baby, grand multiparity), antepartum course (excessive weight gain), physical status (obesity, large fundal measurement, large fetus), and intrapartum problem (disorder of labor progression). This information should serve to alert the clinician to the likelihood that shoulder dystocia will develop. It should prompt a series of preparatory actions, such as mobilizing needed personnel for anesthesia, delivery, and resuscitation, and undertaking certain preliminary measures to facilitate efficient management of shoulder dystocia, if it occurs.

Anesthesia

Because some of the manipulations necessary to resolve shoulder dystocia cannot be done without adequate general anesthesia, it is critical to have a competent anesthetist present, if at all possible. It is apparent that shoulder dystocia can develop without any forewarning, making this prerequisite difficult to fulfill unless full-time anesthesia services are available. Physicians practicing at institutions where an anesthetist is only available on-call are well advised to be doubly watchful for signs suggesting the possibility that shoulder dystocia will develop and to summon the anesthetist as far in advance as feasible to ensure his or her presence at the delivery.

Obstetric Assistance

If for any reason the clinician lacks experience, technical skills, or confidence in his or her ability to deal effectively with shoulder dystocia, a competent senior consultant should be requested to be in attendance in the delivery room. This means the consultant should actually participate in the delivery, already fully scrubbed and ready to proceed with the critical maneuvers for disimpacting a shoulder dystocia if one is encountered. To wait to scrub in until the crisis is recognized risks delay and untoward results. It follows logically that one should not expect an inexperienced and unsupervised resident physician to deliver a patient who is known to be at risk for shoulder dystocia. It is mandatory that every resident in training be fully educated about the steps that have to be taken whenever this emergency situation occurs.

Resuscitation Team

Asphyxia is a common event in shoulder dystocia cases. It results from the delay between delivery of the head and the rest of the fetus, during which time there may be interruption of oxygenation. Among infants delivered vaginally under circumstances of shoulder dystocia at our hospital, more than half were depressed at birth as evidenced by low Apgar scores. Most were readily resuscitated and recovered rapidly without apparent adverse effects, but many needed aggressive and intensive resuscitation. Some even required prolonged ventilation and life-support measures. Because the obstetrician's attention is of necessity directed to the parturient, other personnel capable of providing expert neonatal resuscitation must be summoned to be in attendance prior to the delivery.

Preliminary Delivery Measures

Anticipate the need for a large episiotomy by giving a pudendal block or infiltrating the perineum with a local anesthetic solution prior to the delivery of the fetal head. A prophylactic episiotomy does not need to be performed in most cases, but all instruments should be readily available so that it can be done at once. However, since it will be difficult to cut the episiotomy once the fetal head is delivered, one should at least weigh the benefits of an episiotomy in advance if it is likely that shoulder dystocia will develop. Ensure against bladder distention by catheterization, if needed, before proceeding with the delivery. This will avoid bladder trauma that may occur during the maneuvers done to resolve the shoulder problem and maximize available room to accomplish those maneuvers.

Position the Patient

Deliver the parturient on a delivery table or bed suitable for facilitating performance of the various maneuvers that will be necessary. Although some advocate placing her in a squatting or prone knee-chest position, most obstetricians will find it best to resolve the shoulder dystocia with the patient in the traditional lithotomy position. It is essential for the table to be equipped to enable one to immobilize the patient and abduct her thighs, thereby allowing the attendant to gain access to the perineum for purposes of carrying out the series of examinations and procedures required to expedite the delivery.

Review the Maneuvers

While awaiting the delivery of the fetal head, review the steps that will have to be taken if the shoulders become impacted. It cannot be stressed too frequently that excessive downward traction on the fetal head must be avoided. There can be no justification for persisting in this step and applying increasingly greater force to try to stem the anterior shoulder under the symphysis pubis. If it is clear that the shoulder is impacted, it is far preferable to proceed with other corrective maneuvers (see further on). The exercise involved in reviewing the sequence of steps is especially useful for allaying one's anxiety and perhaps preventing the understandable panic that can arise if shoulder dystocia is encountered unexpectedly. It is especially beneficial to undertake such formal drills with nursing and resident personnel.

TREATMENT

The diagnosis of shoulder dystocia is usually obvious when it occurs. The fetal head is delivered and is immediately pulled tightly back against the perineum. The introitus firmly surrounds an apparently immobile fetal head. Gentle downward traction on the head fails to budge the anterior shoulder. Once shoulder dystocia is diagnosed, stop any further traction on the head and undertake other more appropriate measures instead.

Episiotomy

If it has not already been made, cut a large episiotomy incision. We prefer a mediolateral episiotomy, although some advocate a perineotomy with deliberate incision into the anal sphincter and rectal mucosa to provide maximal room for the procedure to follow. A deep episiotomy is important to permit introduction of a hand into the vagina alongside the fetus, providing access to the fetal shoulders and thorax. An episiotomy also helps to avoid traumatic lacerations of maternal tissues, especially of the rectum.

Hyperflex Maternal Thighs (McRobert's Maneuver)

As a first step aimed at resolving the shoulder dystocia, assistants (one on either side) should hyperflex the parturient's thighs strongly (but not painfully) up against her abdomen. This is done while another attendant simultaneously exerts moderate suprapubic (not fundal) pressure. The objective here is to increase the pelvic outlet dimensions, rotating the pubic symphysis above the impacted anterior shoulder, and to apply downward force on the anterior fetal shoulder. The obstetrician should then again exert gentle downward traction on the fetal head, taking care that the force used is no greater than with a normal delivery.

Rotate Anterior Shoulder

If hyperflexion fails, anesthesia is needed to permit internal manipulation. The obstetrician should insert his or her hand into the vagina to attempt to push the anterior shoulder into an oblique diameter. Use the right hand for a fetus in left occiput transverse position (or the left hand for right occiput transverse). With the thumb up and the palm against the fetal occiput and upper back, the anterior shoulder can be advanced counterclockwise toward the fetal chest (clockwise for the right occiput transverse). Once the rotation has been achieved, again try suprapubic pressure and gentle downward traction to deliver the anterior shoulder. Failure at this point generally means more aggressive action is needed.

Deliver Posterior Shoulder

The next step involves an attempt to deliver the posterior fetal shoulder over the perineum posteriorly. Be-cause it is uncommon for the posterior shoulder to be impacted above the sacral promontory, it is generally quite accessible. If the left shoulder is located posteriorly, the obstetrician inserts the left hand into the vagina (or the right hand for a right posterior shoulder) between the posterior shoulder and the vagina. The shoulder is grasped between the thumb and the opposing fingers (or if the axilla is easily accessible, a finger may be hooked under it) and the posterior shoulder is delivered by traction. If this is accomplished, the anterior shoulder should be promptly deliverable by once again exerting gentle downward traction on the fetal head. Axillary traction can damage structures in this region by blunt trauma.

An alternative method for delivering the posterior shoulder involves inserting one's hand even farther into the vagina to find the posteriorly located fetal upper extremity and to follow it along until one can grasp the forearm and sweep it anteriorly across the fetal thorax. The arm can generally then be gently extracted out of the pelvis. Once this is done, the anterior shoulder should be readily deliverable by applying downward traction on the fetal head. This procedure is not uncommonly associated with fractures of one or more of the long bones of the arm.

Corkscrew (Woods) Maneuver

Another effective means for correcting impacted shoulders employs a corkscrew principle by which the posterior shoulder is brought anteriorly while being advanced caudally, thereby bringing it under the pubic symphysis and allowing delivery to be accomplished in a satisfactory manner. For this approach to be feasible, the posterior shoulder must be located deep in the hollow of the sacrum. Place two or more fingertips posteriorly against the back of the posterior shoulder at the scapula and exert sufficient rotational force to bring the posterior shoulder a full 180 degrees anteriorly. Use the right hand for a left occiput transverse position to rotate clockwise or the left hand for a right occiput transverse fetus to rotate counterclockwise. From this point, the rest of the delivery should proceed uneventfully. If this maneuver has not yet achieved its objective, one can reinsert the other hand behind the current posterior shoulder (the former impacted anterior shoulder) and rotate the fetus 180 degrees in the opposite direction.

Cut the Clavicle

In nearly every instance of shoulder dystocia, it should be possible to accomplish the delivery with one or more of the aforementioned procedures. It is very rarely necessary to consider purposely cutting the fetal clavicle to reduce the size of the shoulder girdle. It is very difficult to fracture a clavicle with one's fingers because the bones of the macrosomic infants who develop shoulder dystocia tend to be so well calcified. It is preferable, therefore, to use bandage scissors to cut the midsection of the anterior clavicle or a Kocher's clamp to snap it, bearing in mind the need to avoid injuring the lung lying beneath.

Reposit the Head

We have no experience with the recently described maneuver of repositing the delivered fetal head back into the uterus and then delivering the fetus by cesarean section. Although it is worthy of mention for completeness, we feel that clinicians should concentrate on the more time-tested and potentially less harmful maneuvers we have described above until wider experience is gained with this innovation to prove its clinical value.

SYSTEMIC LUPUS ERYTHEMATOSUS IN PREGNANCY

MICHAEL D. LOCKSHIN, M.D., F.A.C.P.

Pregnancy in patients with systemic lupus erythematosus (SLE) is often difficult for both the infant and the mother. In the past 5 years, several medical centers in many countries have studied the problem and have, without unanimity, concluded that

1. SLE does not regularly exacerbate during pregnancy. However, pregnancy-associated thrombocytopenia and pregnancy-induced hypertension (toxemia) resemble active SLE and commonly occur.
2. The lupus anticoagulant and the antibody to cardiolipin are closely related but not identical. Both maternal antiphospholipid antibody (anticardiolipin antibody) and the lupus anticoagulant are closely associated with recurrent midpregnancy placental insufficiency and fetal death; live-born infants of mothers with these antibodies are frequently growth-retarded. A false-positive test for syphilis is not a proxy for these assays.
3. Maternal anti-Ro (SSA) antibody is associated with neonatal lupus.
4. The major fetal risk is in utero fetal death or prematurity. Except for the rare neonatal lupus, no other special problems characterize the newborns of SLE patients.

The conclusions reported in the present paper reflect the author's experience with over 100 prospectively followed pregnant patients with SLE. The focus of this paper is on late pregnancy and early newborn events.

IDENTIFYING THE ANTICARDIOLIPIN/LUPUS ANTICOAGULANT (ANTIPHOSPHOLIPID ANTIBODY) SYNDROME

Approximately one-third of mothers with SLE have antiphospholipid antibody. Historical clues to the presence of these antibodies include venous or arterial thrombosis, thrombocytopenia, and a biologic false-positive test for syphilis. Absence of these clues does not exclude the diagnosis.

Approximately two-thirds of mothers with high-titer IgG or IgM antiphospholipid antibody (about one-fifth of all SLE patients) experience pregnancy complications in the following sequence: pregnancy is normal until 15 to 25 weeks; then antepartum fetal heart rate testing (performed weekly in our hospital from 20 to 25 weeks on) first is normal, then shows nonreactivity, then contraction-related bradycardia, and then spontaneous bradycardia. Contraction-related bradycardia gives an approximately 2-week warning of impending fetal death. Fetal growth slows, amniotic fluids resorbs, and either delivery is accomplished or the fetus dies. Women who do not have anticardiolipin antibody or the lupus anticoagulant rarely suffer from this syndrome.

Anticardiolipin antibody is usually identifiable on the patient's first visit and rarely changes in titer during pregnancy. The lupus anticoagulant may or may not be present initially. It often fluctuates in titer during pregnancy. The majority of women with anticardiolipin antibody become mildly thrombocytopenic during pregnancy. Biophysical profiling of the infant may give added prognostic information, but quantitative estriol, beta-human chorionic gonadotropin, prolactin, or other hormone determinations have not been specific enough to give additional predictive information in these patients, nor have placental sonography, uterine artery blood flow, or other measures of fetal health.

The placentas of these pregnancies tend to be very small relative to fetal size. Unlike other investigators, we have not been impressed with evidence of placental infarction. What distinguishes the one-third of women with high titer antiphospholipid antibody who experience untroubled pregnancies from the two-thirds who suffer placental insufficiency and/or fetal death is currently unknown.

DISTINGUISHING TOXEMIA FROM LUPUS EXACERBATION

It is difficult to decide what to do when a pregnant lupus patient develops new proteinuria or an increase in previously stable proteinuria. Although some authorities feel differently, we feel that serum complement levels or platelet counts do not distinguished toxemia from lupus nephritis. Hypertension and edema occur variably. If a patient has clear-cut evidence of other organ systems exacerbation (joints, serosal surfaces, fever, neurologic disease, vasculitis, or unequivocal rash), erythrocyte casts in fresh urine, or rising anti-DNA antibody titer, we diagnose lupus exacerbation. Rash and arthritis may not provide conclusive evidence of lupus exacerbation, since facial blush and palmar erythema are often prominent in pregnant lupus patients in remission, and (bland) knee effusions are common in patients on corticosteroid therapy. Sometimes only rapid recovery after delivery permits a retrospective diagnosis of toxemia.

PREDICTING AND IDENTIFYING NEONATAL LUPUS

Approximately one-third of patients with SLE have antibody to the Ro (SSA), La (SSB), or RNP antigens. Patients who have these antibodies cannot be distinguished from those who do not with confidence, except by specific testing. Of patients with anti-Ro and anti-La antibodies, as many as one-fourth deliver a child with one or more elements of the neonatal lupus syndrome, as does a rare patient with anti-RNP. The most common manifestation of neonatal lupus is a photosensitive macular rash on the face, trunk, and proximal extremities. The rash usually develops in the first few days of extrauterine life, especially if phototherapy is used for jaundice or if the baby is taken into the sunshine. It may appear any time during the first 3 months and usually disappears spontaneously, generally without scarring, by 6 months of age. Skin biopsy is diagnostic, but clinical examination by an experienced clinician, when a relevant autoantibody is present (in either mother or child), is adequate to make the diagnosis. Thrombocytopenia and anemia also occur and are usually mild. The rarest but most serious manifestation of neonatal lupus is carditis. It occurs in less than 3 percent of patients with anti-Ro antibody. Findings include in utero congenital complete heart block, diminished ventricular function and enlarging heart (congestive heart failure), pericardial effusion, and possibly death from cardiac failure. Dizygotic twins are usually discordant for neonatal lupus.

THE MOTHER WITH AUTOANTIBODIES BUT WITHOUT SLE

Most published studies have focused on pregnancies of women selected for SLE. Occasionally women are identified, often on the basis of a history of prior fetal losses or of delivery of a child with neonatal lupus, who do not fulfill clinical criteria to substantiate a diagnosis of SLE but who have either antiphospholipid antibody or anti-Ro antibody. These women appear to have the same fetal risks as do women with SLE, but they do not suffer the same likelihood of lupus exacerbation or toxemia.

TREATMENT OF THE MOTHER

The mother with active SLE must be treated for it. Treatment should be directed by the patient's rheumatologist, in concert with her obstetrician, since control of SLE is mandatory.

Prednisone can safely be given during pregnancy. We do not use corticosteroids other than prednisone unless treatment of the fetus is a goal. Since prednisone increases blood pressure and induces diabetes, lower doses and shorter courses of treatment than would be used if the patient were not pregnant may be indicated, but a high enough dose to control disease manifestations should still be prescribed.

We also use aspirin (80 mg per day) for its anticoagulant effect. Aspirin often ameliorates mild thrombocytopenia and is said to be prophylactic against toxemia. In our hospital we avoid other nonsteroidal anti-inflammatory drugs, hydroxychloroquine, and immunosuppressive agents, largely because of lack of substantial experience verifying safety. Other institutions have supported the use of azathioprine during pregnancy. Rarely, we have used intravenous gamma globulin to treat severe thrombocytopenia, but the protein load is formidable; it may induce hypertension or congestive heart failure in the mother, and the administered IgG will reach the fetus.

For treating hypertension in pregnancy we have felt comfortable using methyldopa, labetalol, hydralazine, nifedipine, and magnesium sulfate.

For management of tocolysis we have used ritodrine. In three of our patients with lupus rash, the rash exacerbated concurrently with the initiation of ritodrine. Whether or not this was a coincidence is unknown at this time. This has not occurred in other institutions.

Occasionally, pregnant women with SLE have had prior total hip replacements for osteonecrosis. Ligament loosening in late pregnancy may contribute to dislocation of the prosthesis; manipulation of the leg during delivery by staff that is unaware of the special problems of artificial joints may similarly threaten the stability of the prosthesis. Prophylactic antibiotic therapy, similar to that given for cardiac valvular disease, is indicated for "dirty" manipulations and operative procedures.

TREATMENT OF THE UNBORN INFANT

There is no clearly established protocol for treatment of the infant threatened either with placental insufficiency or with neonatal lupus. The recommendations that follow are guesses based on experience and should be viewed as such.

Since many patients with anti-Ro or anticardiolipin antibodies have uncomplicated pregnancies, there is not current justification for prophylactic treatment of an SLE patient prior to conception, regardless of her antibody status, nor is there justification for prophylactic treatment of any primigravida while pregnant. (The occurrence of a lupus-related, clinical indication does merit treatment.) If a women has had several midpregnancy fetal losses and does have high titer antiphospholipid antibody, anticipatory treatment with corticosteroid and aspirin may offer benefit. We have found no additional success and in fact more complications when the dose of prednisone exceeded 30 mg per day; we routinely use 80 mg per day of aspirin in patients with antiphospholipid antibody, and we initiate treatment usually by week 12. We have used subcutaneous heparin only in women with a history of prior thromboses. We attempt to taper prednisone by late pregnancy (after 30 weeks), generally staying at 5 to 10 mg per day until delivery. We use "stress" steroid for delivery for patients taking corticosteroid but do not otherwise prophylactically treat patients. If premature delivery seems likely, we switch to betamethasone or dexamethasone for fetal pulmonary indications.

Because neonatal lupus is uncommon and carditis is rare, we do not recommend prophylactic treatment for women with anti-Ro or anti-La antibodies. No large experience has accumulated for the child with identified in utero carditis. Many children have been born with heart block but otherwise normal cardiac function and have grown normally; thus heart block per se is not necessarily an indication for treatment. Reversal of heart block with treatment has not yet been reported.

We monitor pregnancies of women with anti-Ro antibody with fetal echocardiography and antepartum fetal heart rate testing. If pericardial effusion, increasing cardiac size, or other signs of ventricular dysfunction are apparent, in utero treatments of the infant can be considered. Various treatments have been tried, but whether they have been demonstrated to be helpful is arguable. Treatments include administering to the mother corticosteroid that will cross the placenta (dexamethasone or betamethasone), plasmapheresis, and early delivery. All procedures add risk to the mother as well as to the baby; unpublished treatment failures are more common than published claims of good effect. We prefer to administer 9 mg of dexamethasone daily to the mother and to deliver a child who is more than 30 weeks' gestation and who has documented fetal lung maturity by amniocentesis, but we make no claim that this recommendation has value.

CESARIAN SECTION

In our hospital cesarian section rate in SLE patients is high. Reasons do not differ from those for other sick patients. Fetal distress is the major indication, although maternal thrombocytopenia, rapidly advancing preeclampsia, cord complications, breech presentations, prior cesarian sections, and failure of labor to progress probably occur in expected frequencies.

TREATMENT OF THE NEWBORN

From a rheumatologist's point of view, the most important treatment of the newborn is reassuring the parents and staying the hand of the neonatologist. The rashes and thrombocytopenias are mild, do not indicate septicemia, and resolve spontaneously. On occasion, in severe cases (reported by others), corticosteroid treatment of the infant has been recommended, as well as standard cardiotonic measures, for the infant with carditis with or without

heart block. If an infant develops a rash while under phototherapy, individual priorities between risk of kernicterus and risk of neonatal lupus need to be defined. In most cases phototherapy can be discontinued.

PROBLEMS OF PREMATURITY

Prematurity is extremely common, especially in children of mothers with antiphospholipid antibody. We have seen the usual problems of respiratory distress and brain hemorrhage (with subsequent cerebral palsy) and an occasional patient with Wilson/Mikity syndrome and malnutrition. The frequencies do not appear to be excessive for growth-retarded, weight-matched infants of non-SLE mothers. We have not encountered adrenal insufficiency or neonatal lupus cardiac disease developing after birth, nor have we seen pulmonary hypertension from premature closure of the ductus arteriosus in aspirin-treated patients.

LONG-TERM PROGNOSIS FOR THE MOTHER AND THE CHILD

Nothing about pregnancy protects the mother from further ravages of SLE. Both prognoses and surveillance should anticipate continued disease activity, independent of the fact of pregnancy. Long-term renal prognosis may be worsened by toxemia, and other pregnancy complications may add their own morbidities to those of SLE.

Long-term outcome of children with neonatal lupus is unknown. Since neonatal lupus is not thought to be a new disease, and since prior reports of congenital heart block have not noted an unusual frequency of subsequent SLE, the predominant assumption is that infants (without heart disease) will have normal lives. Occasional infants with neonatal lupus have developed SLE after adolescence. Whether these represent an appropriate frequency, since SLE has approximately a 1 percent familial incidence, or are the first published indicators that neonatal lupus is likely to recur as SLE is completely unknown at this time.

This is written from the point of view of a rheumatologist, but I am deeply indebted to my colleagues, Dr. Maurice Druzin (Obstetrics) and Drs. Peter Auld and Alfred Krauss (Neonatology), whose active participation in the care of these patients was always essential.

SUGGESTED READING

Lockshin MD. Lupus pregnancy. Clin Rheum Dis 1985; 11:611–632.
Lockshin MD, Qamar T, Druzin ML. Hazards of lupus pregnancy. J Rheumatol 1987; 14(Suppl 13):214–217.
Watson RM, Lane AT, Barnett NK, et al. Neonatal lupus erythematosus: a clinical, serological and immunogenetic study with review of the literature. Medicine 1984; 63:362–378.

THYROTOXICOSIS IN PREGNANCY

GREGORY P. BECKS, M.D., FRCPC
GERARD N. BURROW, M.D.

Because of unique maternal and fetal considerations, the presence of thyrotoxicosis complicates the management of both pregnancy and the postpartum period. The diagnosis and treatment of thyrotoxicosis in females at risk for pregnancy also warrant special consideration.

Hyperthyroidism is most commonly caused by Graves' disease, affecting up to 1 percent of the general population, and occurs in approximately 0.2 percent, or one in 500, of pregnancies. Hydatidiform mole and trophoblastic tumors are much rarer causes of thyrotoxicosis during pregnancy. Hyperthyroidism in the postpartum period may be due to a relapse of Graves's disease but more often is secondary to painless lymphocytic thyroiditis, which characteristically results in transient thyrotoxicosis followed by a hypothyroid phase with eventual return of normal thyroid function.

THYROTOXICOSIS IN YOUNGER FEMALES

Thyrotoxicosis in younger females and during the childbearing years deserves special consideration with respect to diagnosis and long-term management. Prior to the use of radioactive iodine for determination of thyroid iodine uptake or for the treatment of hyperthyroidism, pregnancy should be excluded by sensitive beta human chorionic gonadotropin measurement, since iodide freely crosses the placenta and is concentrated in the fetal thyroid gland after 10 weeks' gestation. Although it is controversial, to date clear evidence is lacking that young females treated with radioactive iodine subsequently bear children with increased physical or developmental abnormalities. Treatment of hyperthyroidism with radioactive iodine or antithyroid drugs, thionamides, should be based on an informed decision of the patient. Pregnancy may be delayed 6 months following ^{131}I thyroid ablation for thyrotoxicosis or until after a full-length course, 1 to 2 years, of antithyroid drug therapy. This strategy increases the likelihood of a lasting remission so as to avoid an early relapse of thyrotoxicosis in the first trimester of pregnancy. Patients are advised to used adequate contraception in the interim period. If pregnancy does occur inadvertently, there is no great cause for concern. In the case of antithyroid drug therapy, the lowest dose that maintains remission would be continued during pregnancy. Surgery for treatment of thyrotoxicosis in younger females is still a consideration, but it is infrequently used at present and still requires medical control of thyrotoxicosis preoperatively. From another perspective, the possible effects of thyrotoxicosis on fertility are of interest. Severe, untreated hyperthyroidism may be associated with oligomenorrhea or amenorrhea, high serum luteinizing hormone (LH) levels, and decreased pulsatile LH release. On the other hand, there is no good evidence that fertility is significantly impaired in mild to moderate thyrotoxicosis and only a suggestion that fetal loss or congenital abnormalities are increased by maternal thyrotoxicosis in the first trimester.

THYROTOXICOSIS DURING PREGNANCY

We are mainly concerned with thyrotoxicosis that presents or is first recognized during pregnancy. In the first instance, the clinical diagnosis is often difficult to make because normal pregnant women may manifest heat intolerance, sweating, increased warmth, anxiety, hyperdynamic circulation, and even slight thyroid enlargement, which overlap with the signs and symptoms of thyrotoxicosis. Eye changes of Graves' disease or pretibial myxedema, when present, aids in the diagnosis, and a resting heart rate greater than 100 beats per minute (onycholysis) would not be expected in normal pregnancy. Normal pregnancy is a euthyroid state, despite increased thyroidal iodide uptake and basal metabolic rate and slight thyroid enlargement with histologic follicular hyperplasia.

The laboratory confirmation of thyrotoxicosis, straightforward in nonpregnant individuals, is more complex in pregnancy. Increased thyroxine binding globulin during pregnancy results in increased total serum thyroxine (T_4) and triiodothyronine (T_3). T_3 resin uptake (T_3U), an inverse measurement of free binding sites on thyroxine binding globulin, is decreased. When thyrotoxicosis is present in pregnancy, the serum T_4 is usually over 200 nmol per liter (16 μg per deciliter), and T_3U is inappropriately normal. If the patient is clinically thyrotoxic but the T_4 is normal for pregnancy, T_3 toxicosis should be considered. Free thyroid hormone assays are now generally available. The gold standard remains free T_4 (FT_4), measured by equilibrium dialysis or by sensitive radioimmunoassay after ultrafiltration of serum. More recently, using nonequilibrium dialysis techniques, one-stage or two-stage radioimmunoassays have become available to measure FT_4 and free T_3 (FT_3) in untreated serum samples. Free thyroid hormones may increase in pregnancy in the first trimester, due to thyrotropic effects of human chorionic gonadotropin, and levels have been elevated above normal in some but not all studies. Later in pregnancy, free hormone levels return to normal values. In some cases slightly low levels of FT_4 have been found in the third trimester, possibly due to lower albumin levels at this stage, which affect some assays. Recently the low FT_4 level has also been explained as an adaptation in the mother to upregulated thyroid hormone T_4 receptors induced by the hyperestrogenic state.

When thyrotoxicosis is present in pregnancy, FT_4 and FT_3 levels can be expected to be elevated. Thyroid-stimulating hormone (TSH) can now be measured by sensitive immunometric assays that distinguish between a normal range for TSH in euthyroid individuals and suppressed or undetectable TSH values in hyperthyroidism. Since TSH secretion and dynamics are normal in pregnancy, suppressed TSH values can be expected with thyrotoxicosis during pregnancy. The sensitive TSH assay should obviate the need for thyrotropin-releasing hormone testing. This has not been sanctioned for use in pregnancy, because thyrotropin-releasing hormone readily crosses the placenta.

Hyperthyroidism in the mother during the pregnancy is associated with an increased incidence of low birth weight infants and a trend toward increased neonatal mortality. Thyrotoxicosis can develop in the fetus as a result of transplacental passage of maternal thyroid-stimulating immunoglobulin, of the IgG class, although this more often manifests in the neonatal period, perhaps because the mother is treated during pregnancy with antithyroid medication. Treatment of maternal thyrotoxicosis has the potential to cause fetal hypothyroidism and goiter. Hyperthyroidism has been associated with hyperemesis gravidarum in the mother. There is an increased risk of thyroid storm during labor and delivery if thyrotoxicosis has not been adequately controlled. Pregnancy can also affect the course of thyrotoxicosis caused by Graves' disease.

The immunosuppressive effects of pregnancy (probably due to fetal to maternal transfer of immunosuppressive factors and recently characterized by a reduced maternal helper to suppressor T-cell ratio in normal pregnancy and in Graves' disease in pregnancy) often produce a degree of remission of hyperthyroidism in the second and third trimesters, making the disease easier to control. Relapse can occur in the postpartum period associated with the rebound of the immunologic parameters to the prepregnancy state.

TREATMENT

Once a diagnosis of thyrotoxicosis in pregnancy has been established, the priority is to gain control of the mother's disease. Pregnant women tolerate mild to moderate degrees of thyrotoxicosis reasonably well, and one can usually afford to wait until the diagnosis is confirmed. The treatment of choice is antithyroid drugs, thionamides, either propylthiouracil, or methimazole. Propylthiouracil has been the preferred drug because it has lower placental transfer and, therefore, theoretically less chance for producing fetal hypothyroidism, and methimazole has been associated with the scalp defect, aplasia cutis. Although recent studies suggest there is little difference between the two drugs, we still prefer propylthiouracil. It does have the additional advantage of mild inhibition of iodothyronine 5′ deiodinase, decreasing T_3 production from T_4. We start propylthiouracil in divided doses, 100 mg every 8 hours, and this usually brings the mother's thyrotoxicosis under control over several weeks. Following thyroid function tests at monthly intervals thereafter, the dose is gradually reduced to maintenance levels of 100 mg daily or less. Thyroid hormone should be maintained at high normal levels during pregnancy. When hyperthyroidism is severe, high propylthiouracil doses of 150 to 200 mg every 8 hours may be required initially, and additional therapy should be considered to more rapidly control thyroid hormone levels and their peripheral effects. The thyrotoxicosis needs to be controlled even if this requires initial doses of propylthiouracil above 600 mg daily. If the mother is fol-

lowed closely, the fetus does not appear to be at greater risk because of the high dose of antithyroid drug required. Beta-adrenergic blocking drugs, notably propranolol, can be used safely for short periods of time in pregnancy and may be useful in controlling peripheral beta-adrenergic manifestations of thyrotoxicosis, such as tremor and tachycardia. The usual dose is 40 mg orally every 6 hours. Long-term use of beta-blockers is not recommended because problems have been encountered with intrauterine growth retardation, fetal bradycardia, impaired responses to hypoxia, and neonatal hypoglycemia. Selective beta-blockers have not been extensively evaluated for thyrotoxicosis in pregnancy. Excess iodide, in milligram quantities, can acutely block release of thyroid hormones from the thyroid gland and transiently inhibit thyroid hormone synthesis. Iodide, such as Lugol's iodine or potassium iodide, can be used for short periods of time, in conjunction with beta-blockers, to control thyrotoxicosis while propylthiouracil takes effect. Because of the avidity of fetal thyroid tissue for iodide, which readily crosses the placenta, there is an increased risk of iodide-induced goiter, which can cause respiratory obstruction and dystocia. This precludes any long-term iodide administration in pregnancy. At present, there are no recommendations for the use of ipodate (Oragrafin) or iopanoic acid (Telepaque), iodinated oral cholecystography dyes, in pregnancy. Ipodate, a potent inhibitor of T_4 to T_3 conversion in peripheral tissues, has been used for long-term treatment of thyrotoxicosis in nonpregnant patients, but there are reports of tachyphylaxis.

Maternal hypothyroidism should be avoided, and appropriate monitoring of thyroid function tests for elevation of TSH or decreased total or FT_4 is required. Any biochemical evidence of maternal hypothyroidism requires a reduction in propylthiouracil dose and administration of physiologic replacement doses of levothyroxine, 1.5 μg per kilogram per day. At this replacement dose there is little effect on fetal thyroid hormone levels because of limited transplacental passage of thyroid hormones and there is no rationale for routine thyroxine supplementation in mothers taking propylthiouracil. Thionamides do cross the placenta, and there is a risk of fetal hypothyroidism and goiter. This is more than a simple dose-related phenomenon. Recent evidence suggests there is a good correlation of the fetal cord FT_4 index with the area under the curve for propylthiouracil serum levels, measured by radioimmunoassay after an oral dose of propylthiouracil. The fetal thyroid secretes mainly T_4, but only after 10 weeks' gestation, and the requirement for fetal thyroid hormones in earlier fetal growth and development is unclear. Maternal thyroid hormones probably contribute little to fetal thyroid hormone levels. Maternal iodide crosses the placenta and is the substrate for fetal thyroid hormone synthesis. When there is severe fetal hypothyroidism during the second and third trimesters, this can be manifested by delayed skeletal maturation, hypotonia, and respiratory depression at birth along with low T_4 and elevated TSH levels in cord serum. Growth and development may subsequently be normal with prompt treatment of hypothyroidism beginning early in the neonatal period. There is no practical way to routinely test for fetal hypothyroidism in utero, but in the case of mothers taking propylthiouracil, any neonatal hypothyroidism is usually transient. When thionamides are used in the lowest dose necessary to maintain control of maternal thyrotoxicosis, the risk of fetal or neonatal hypothyroidism and goiter is minimal. Goiters tend to be small and nonobstructive, unlike those associated with iodide excess. Follow-up of children of mothers treated with propylthiouracil in pregnancy has shown essentially normal growth and development.

The usual side effects of antithyroid drugs also occur in pregnancy. Patients should be alerted to report symptoms such as skin rash, fever, or sore throat when taking thioamides. Minor skin rashes may resolve with continued treatment or by switching to another agent. Serious complications like vasculitis, granulocytopenia, or agranulocytosis, probably immune-mediated, are associated with a high degree of cross-reactivity between propylthiouracil and methinazole, so thionamides as a group are contraindicated with these complications. Thyroid surgery is an alternative therapy. The other indication for surgery is failure to control the disease medically, which is usually due to poor patient compliance. Since the risks of anesthesia and the surgical complications such as recurrent laryngeal nerve damage and hypoparathyroidism are small, subtotal thyroidectomy is an acceptable alternative treatment for thyrotoxicosis in pregnancy. The usual advice has been to delay necessary surgery until the second trimester to reduce the risk of spontaneous abortion, but this is probably unnecessary. Thyrotoxicosis needs to be adequately controlled prior to induction of anesthesia to reduce the risk of thyroid storm. This is usually achieved with short-term use of oral propranolol and iodide, as discussed above. Ipodate or dexamethasone might be added to block T_4 to T_3 conversion in peripheral tissues. After surgery, thyroid hormone concentrations and TSH levels should be monitored regularly and levothyroxine administered if there is evidence of hypothyroidism.

Use of radioiodine for diagnosis or treatment of thyrotoxicosis is contraindicated in pregnancy. Occasionally, it has been inadvertently administered in early pregnancy. A scanning dose of radioiodine is of little consequence in terms of radiation dose to the thyroid, gonadal, or fetal whole body dose. A therapeutic dose can deliver significant whole body radiation (5 rads), as well as gonadal radiation, and may cause fetal hypothyroidism after 10 weeks' gestation, although this is not a universal finding. Therapeutic abortion is an option. Alternatively, propylthiouracil can be administered for 1 week to block iodide recycling in the fetal thyroid; the neonate should be evaluated carefully for hypothyroidism and appropriate treatment should be initiated if indicated. Several cases have been reported in which the fetus was treated in utero with intramuscular T_4 injections or injection of thyroxine into the amniotic fluid and then was euthyroid at birth, but this was experimental. Reported adverse effects of in utero radiation on subsequent growth and development have generally been associated with whole body exposure in excess of 50 rads, about ten times that received with radioiodine.

Thyroid storm is an endocrine emergency. The outcome may be doubly disastrous in pregnancy. If thyrotoxicosis is poorly controlled or unrecognized, the risk of thyroid storm is increased with the onset of labor, cesarean section, or infection. Marked fever, tachycardia, prostration, and volume depletion occur. Immediate treatment is required, superseding laboratory confirmation. The following should be administered: propylthiouracil 300 mg every 6 hours, propranolol 40 mg by mouth every 6 hours or 1 to 2 mg intravenously initially, sodium iodide 1 g intravenously, and dexamethasone 2 mg orally every 6 hours. This regimen reduces thyroid hormone synthesis and secretion and peripheral deiodination of T_4 to T_3. Isotonic intravenous fluids should be infused, and cooling may be required for hyperthermia.

FETAL AND NEONATAL THYROTOXICOSIS

The pathogenesis of hyperthyroidism in Graves' disease is thought to involve IgG antibodies that stimulate thyroid function and growth through the TSH receptor. These antibodies cross the placenta during the second and third trimesters and the fetus is at risk for thyrotoxicosis. This is actually less common than transient neonatal thyrotoxicosis, which is seen in about 2 percent of pregnancies associated with maternal Graves' disease. The risk is correlated with the titer of maternal thyroid–stimulating immunoglobulins, and pregnancy is one situation in which these assays are clinically useful. A good correlation has also been found between maternal FT_4 and umbilical cord FT_4 at delivery in Graves' disease in pregnancy. It should be noted that the mother need not have active thyrotoxicosis, only the appropriate antibodies that access the fetal circulation. Such a situation exists when Graves' thyrotoxicosis has been previously treated with radioiodine or partial thyroidectomy. Thionamides administered to the mother also treat fetal thyrotoxicosis concomitantly. Clues to fetal thyrotoxicosis are the presence of maternal thyroid–stimulating antibodies and a fetal heart rate over 160 beats per minute. Goiter, growth retardation, advanced bone age, and craniosynostosis may be seen as a result of fetal hyperthyroidism. Treatment involves administration of 50 to 100 mg of propylthiouracil daily to the mother plus thyroxine if she becomes hypothyroid. Effects from maternal thionamides also dissipate quickly after birth, and the neonate may become thyrotoxic during the first several days. Symptoms are nonspecific, including tachycardia, irritability, poor feeding, failure to thrive, and prolonged jaundice. A small goiter and exophthalmos may be present. Mortality is high if cardiac failure develops. Propranolol 2 mg per kilogram per day is the mainstay of therapy, and antithyroid drugs, iodide, and dexamethansone may be added in appropriate pediatric doses, depending on disease severity. Sodium ipodate has recently been used successfully in the treatment of neonatal thyrotoxicosis. Radioiodine is contraindicated since thyrotoxicosis is usually transient, lasting up to 6 weeks, because of clearance of the maternal antibodies. Delayed-onset neonatal thyrotoxicosis has been attributed to the concomitant presence of high-affinity thyroid-blocking antibodies and chronic neonatal thyrotoxicosis lasting over 1 year to the persistent effect of thyroid-stimulating antibodies. Some of these chronic cases probably represent early-onset familial juvenile Graves' disease.

POSTPARTUM THYROID DISEASE

There are often postpartum changes in maternal thyroid function. A relapse of Graves' disease can occur following remission in pregnancy. Because of this we do not stop thionamide treatment after delivery but continue a maintenance dose of 50 to 100 mg of propylthiouracil daily and continue to monitor thyroid function tests. An exception may be in women who wish to breastfeed. Propylthiouracil and methimazole are both secreted in breast milk, but methimazole much more so. Full doses of methimazole, 30 mg daily in the mother, could cause neonatal hypothyroidism, but smaller maintenance does of propylthiouracil are not likely to do so. Neonatal thyroid function does have to be monitored. If there is any laboratory evidence of the development of neonatal hypothyroidism, 25 to 50 μg of T_4 can be administered daily to the baby while mothers continue to take antithyroid medication. These areas remain controversial.

More common is transient postpartum thyrotoxicosis. This occurs in up to 5 percent of normal postpartum women and with increased incidence when Hashimoto's thyroiditis is present before pregnancy. About half the women with positive microsomal antibodies before preg-nancy develop postpartum thyroiditis. The mechanism is thought to be a destructive lymphocytic thyroiditis, along with the development of an enhanced immune response postpartum, leading to release of preformed thyroid hormone. Mild thyrotoxicosis appears 3 to 6 months postpartum. A small painless goiter may be present, and thyroid microsomal antibodies are often detected. Iodide uptake is typically low. Treatment is mainly supportive, and oral propranolol is helpful. A variable period of symptomatic hypothyroidism usually follows, with eventual recovery of normal thyroid function. If a decision is made to give levothyroxine during the hypothyroid phase, it should be continued for 6 to 12 months and then stopped, followed by a re-evaluation of thyroid function 4 to 6 weeks later. In some cases the hyperthyroid phase may be absent or missed, and long-term hypothyroidism can persist. At present it seems that this syndrome is a variant of autoimmune thyroid disease, probably Hashimoto's thyroiditis, even when it manifests in apparently normal women. We would recommend screening for thyroid antibodies in early pregnancy to identify those at increased risk of this disorder.

SUGGESTED READING

Burrow GN. The management of thyrotoxicosis in pregnancy. N Engl J Med 1985; 313:562–565.

Fisher DA. Neonatal thyroid disease in the offspring of women with autoimmune thyroid disease. In: Oppenheimer JH, ed. Thyroid today. Deerfield, IL: Flint Laboratories Inc, vol IX, no 4:1–7.

UTERINE RUPTURE

ROBERT D. EDEN, M.D.
RICHARD A. PIRCON, M.D.

Uterine rupture is an uncommon obstetric event, but is associated with a significant risk of maternal morbidity and mortality. In fact, approximately 5 percent of maternal deaths in the United States can be attributed to uterine rupture. The incidence of maternal mortality from uterine rupture ranges from 4 to 20 percent, whereas perinatal mortality is approximately 40 percent. Nevertheless, the maternal and perinatal mortality associated with uterine rupture may be avoided by early recognition and timely surgery.

DEFINITION

Although uterine rupture has not been uniformly defined, it is important to distinguish between uterine rupture and uterine dehiscence. Anatomically, uterine dehiscence represents a defect in the uterine wall that does not extend through the entire uterus and peritoneal cover-ing. In contrast, uterine rupture refers to a defect that extends through the entire uterine wall and enters the peritoneal cavity. Clinically, a uterine dehiscence describes *any* defect of the uterine wall, whereas a uterine rupture is a dehiscence that requires surgical intervention.

INCIDENCE AND ETIOLOGY

The incidence of uterine rupture is approximately one per 1,400 deliveries. The diagnosis is made with equal frequency before delivery or in the immediate postpartum period. Uterine rupture is most commonly associated with advanced maternal age, multiparity, and obesity, although there are other associated conditions (Table 1). Historically, a previous cesarean section was noted in a significant percentage of women experiencing uterine rupture. However, a recent, retrospective half-century investigation revealed that a previous cesarean section was found in only 20 percent of cases of uterine ruptures. Surprisingly, in the majority of cases uterine rupture occurred following midforceps delivery, breech presentation and extraction, injudicious use of oxytocins, and prolonged labor.

Fekins classified uterine rupture as being spontaneous or traumatic. Spontaneous uterine rupture is usually associated with previous uterine surgery, including myo-

TABLE 1 Conditions Associated with Uterine Rupture

    I.   Traumatic rupture
         A. Instrumental
              1. Uterine sound or curet
              2. Manual removal of placenta
              3. Various tools for induction of abortion
         B. Violence: direct or indirect
         C. Obstetric
              1. Oxytocins, forceps (low, mid, failed), breech
                 extraction
              2. Intrauterine manipulation: internal version, for-
                 ceps rotation, shoulder dystocia
              3. Fundal pressure
              4. Craniotomy (hydrocephalus)
              5. Neglect: cephalopelvic disproportion, transverse
                 lie
    II. Spontaneous (prior to or during labor) rupture
         A. Previous uterine surgery
              1. Cesarean section (low segment vs classic in-
                 cision)
              2. Myomectomy
              3. Salpingectomy
              4. Ventrofixation
              5. Curettage or manual removal of the placenta
         B. No previous surgery
              1. Congenital uterine abnormality
              2. Cornual pregnancy
              3. Hydatidiform mole or chorioadenoma destruens
              4. Placenta percreta
              5. Abruptio placentae
              6. Grand multiparity
              7. No apparent cause

TABLE 2 Symptoms, Signs, and Diagnostic Tests of
Uterine Rupture

    Symptoms
        Suprapubic pain
        Abdominal pain
        "Shearing" sensation

    Physical Findings
        Cessation of uterine contractions
        Palpable fetal parts
        Uterine tenderness
        Recession of presenting part
        Hemorrhagic shock

    Diagnostic Tests
        Urinalysis for hematuria
        X-ray film of abdomen and pelvis
        Culdocentesis

mectomy and cesarean section, but it is also associated with grand multiparity, abruptio placentae, placenta previa, cephalopelvic disproportion; moreover, in recent years, there have been reports of uterine rupture with the use of prostaglandins in the second and early third trimester.

The current practice of encouraging vaginal birth after the patient has had a cesarean section has generated a great deal of interest regarding the incidence of uterine rupture in previous cesarean section patients. Fortunately, *the incidence and timing of uterine rupture are dependent upon the type of previous uterine scar that is present.* The incidence of rupture is 0.5 percent following a previous low segment transverse uterine scar, and 2 percent following a classic or vertical uterine scar. Furthermore, *a significant percentage of vertical scars rupture prior to the onset of labor.*

PRESENTING SIGNS AND SYMPTOMS

The patient experiencing a uterine rupture classically describes her pain as "shearing" in nature. In addition, there is commonly a cessation of uterine contractions, loss of fetal heart tones, and the onset of vaginal bleeding (Table 2). Unfortunately, this "classic" clinical presentation occurs in only a minority of patients. Many variables determine the patient's presenting symptoms, including the nature of the rupture (spontaneous or traumatic), the degree of blood loss, the degree of intraperitoneal bleeding, and the presence of fetal or placental extrusion. Spontaneous rupture of an unscarred uterus is usually associated

with a greater magnitude of pain than that experienced following rupture of a previous cesarean section scar. This observation may be related to the decreased vascularity associated with a previous uterine scar. This hypothesis is supported by the finding of a smaller amount of blood loss and intraperitoneal bleeding in patients with a previous cesarean section scar.

Fetal heart rate monitoring and intrauterine pressure measurement can assist in diagnosing uterine rupture. Extrusion of the placenta through the uterine scar may result in the appearance of late decelerations due to the development of placental insufficiency. Extrusion of the umbilical cord through the uterine defect may result in the appearance of variable decelerations caused by cord compression. Abdominal palpation of the fetus and hematuria should also alert the clinician to the possibility of uterine rupture.

Hemorrhagic shock is commonly associated with uterine rupture when it is complicated by significant blood loss and intrapartum bleeding. Shock most frequently occurs with the rupture of the unscarred uterus.

The differential diagnosis of uterine rupture includes abruptio placentae. Uterine rupture may be differentiated from abruptio placentae with the assistance of several diagnostic modalities. Culdocentesis may reveal intraperitoneal bleeding, and pelvic and abdominal x-ray films may demonstrate free intraperitoneal air, both of which are associated with uterine rupture. Nevertheless, abruptio placentae and uterine rupture can be indistinguishable and may even occur simultaneously. In one study, abruptio placentae was found to be present in 18 percent of uterine ruptures. Because of the association of abruptio placentae with uterine rupture, oxytocin infusion may be hazardous in patients demonstrating evidence of mild placental abruption. However, the use of oxytocin may be indicated in the absence of fetal distress, since uterine activity can be closely monitored by the intrauterine pressure catheter.

TREATMENT

Once the diagnosis of uterine rupture is made, immediate surgical intervention is mandatory. A delay in

TABLE 3 Treatment of Uterine Rupture

I. Preoperative management
   A. Fluid resuscitation
   B. Laboratory evaluation
      1. Blood count
      2. Coagulation studies
   C. Blood products
      1. O negative whole blood prior to availability of cross-matched blood
      2. Cross-matched packed red blood cells
      3. Cross-matched fresh frozen plasma
II. Surgery (see Table 4)
   A. Hysterectomy
   B. Surgical repair of defect
III. Postoperative management
   A. Fluid status
      1. Renal output
      2. Central venous pressure or pulmonary capillary wedge pressure
   B. Coagulation profile
   C. Prophylactic antibiotics

TABLE 4 Factors Affecting Choice of Procedure at Laparotomy

Hemodynamic status of patient
Scarred vs unscarred uterus
Location of rupture
Extent of uterine rupture
Desire for future childbearing
Risk of subsequent uterine rupture after simple repair

definitive surgery is associated with an increase in maternal and perinatal morbidity and mortality. Preoperative management should include aggressive fluid resuscitation (Table 3). The use of a central venous catheter is recommended. When the patient is hemodynamically compromised, blood products should be made available. Transfusion of uncross-matched O negative, whole blood may be required before cross-matched blood can be made available. Laboratory evaluation should include serial electrolytes, blood counts, and coagulation studies, since most maternal deaths are associated with abruptio placentae and the presence of a coagulation disorder.

Total abdominal hysterectomy is usually indicated for the definitive treatment of uterine rupture. However, the surgical procedure performed should be tailored to the specific clinical situation, since not all uterine ruptures require hysterectomy (Table 4). Peripartum hysterectomy involves several technical considerations. Because of the increased likelihood of significant hemorrhage during hysterectomy in the peripartum period, double clamping and delayed ligation of the engorged adnexal pedicles are recommended. Furthermore, the major vascular pedicles should be ligated twice. Bladder flap development can be difficult because of the scarring associated with previous cesarean section and the likelihood of significant hemorrhage. This is best accomplished by midline, sharp dissection using Metzenbaum's scissors. Lateral dissection can result in injury to the venous plexus of Santorini. Initial closure of the uterine defect prior to performing the hysterectomy is usually unnecessary, unless excessive bleeding is encountered. Usually mild to moderate bleed-ing can be temporarily controlled by clamping. Hypogastric artery ligation may also assist in minimizing blood loss. The urinary tract should be examined thoroughly, especially the bladder and ureters, since laceration of the bladder occurs in approximately 10 percent of cases.

Postoperatively, the patient must be monitored closely because acute blood loss can result in renal damage. Fluid intake and urine output should be closely watched as well as urine electrolytes and creatinine level. A central venous catheter may assist in the evaluation of oliguria. Since hypoxia and blood loss are associated with intravascular coagulation, coagulation studies, including fibrinogen, fibrin split products, and platelet count, should be monitored. The patient should receive prophylactic antibiotics because of the increased risk of infection associated with surgical treatment of uterine rupture. A broad-spectrum antibiotic is usually adequate for prophylaxis.

SUGGESTED READING

Chestnut D, Eden RD, Gall SA, Parker RT. Peripartum hysterectomy: a review of cesarean and postpartum hysterectomy. Obstet Gynecol 1985; 65:365.

Claman P, Carpenter RJ, Reiter A. Uterine rupture with the use of vaginal prostaglandin E_2 for induction of labor. Am J Obstet Gynecol 1984; 150:889–890.

Eden RD, Parker RT, Gall SA. Rupture of the pregnant uterus: a 53 year review. Obstet Gynecol 1986; 68:671–674.

Golan A, Sandbank O, Rubin A. Rupture of the pregnant uterus. Obstet Gynecol 1980; 56:549–554.

Paul RH, Phelan JP, Yeh S. Trial of labor in the patient with a prior cesarean birth. Am J Obstet Gynecol 1985; 151:297–304.

Plauche WC, Almen WV, Mueller R. Catastrophic uterine rupture. Obstet Gynecol 1984; 64:792–797.

Plauche WE, Guich FG, Bourgeois MO. Hysterectomy at the time of cesarean section: analysis of 108 cases. Obstet Gynecol 1981; 58:459–464.

Sawyer MM, Lipshitz J, Anderson G, Dilts P. Third trimester uterine rupture associated with vaginal prostaglandin E_2. Am J Obstet Gynecol 1981; 140:710–711.

Schrinsky DC, Benson RC. Rupture of the pregnant uterus: a review. Obstet Gynecol Survey 1978; 33:217–232.

Sheth SS. Results of treatment of rupture of the uterus by suturing. Obstet Gynecol 1968; 75:55–58.

CHORIONIC VILLUS SAMPLING

JOHN M. BISSONNETTE, M.D.
SUSAN OLSON, Ph.D.

Prenatal diagnosis, achieved by obtaining fetal tissue for chromosomal, biochemical, or DNA studies, is an established practice in medical genetics. Prior to 5 years ago fetal cells were obtained by transabdominal amniocentesis beginning at the 15th to 16th week from the last menstrual period. More recently, techniques have been devised to obtain trophoblast biopsies or, as they are more commonly known, chorionic villus samples (CVS), between the 9th and 11th weeks of gestation. The ability to diagnose severe congenital diseases at a significantly earlier time in pregnancy has obvious psychological and obstetric advantages. In families with a high likelihood of an affected pregnancy, such as autosomal recessive or sex-linked disorders, the ability to obtain reassurance that the present pregnancy is unaffected at an early date is a distinct advantage. Considerable clinical and laboratory experience has been obtained with this new technique, and at least three institutions have reported on their first 1,000 cases. Nonetheless, there remain a number of important questions that are only partially resolved. These include the procedure-related risk of abortion and the implications of chromosomal mosaicism seen in the cultured trophoblast tissue.

INDICATIONS

The indications for CVS are similar to those for amniocentesis in the second trimester. In addition to advanced maternal age, these include previous chromosomal abnormalities and biochemical disorders such as Tay-Sachs disease and the Lesch-Nyhan syndrome. CVS is especially well suited for disorders that can be determined by means of DNA probes and restriction enzymes. The thalassemias, sickle cell disease, hemophilia A, Duchenne's muscular dystrophy, and cystic fibrosis are among the more common disorders that can potentially be detected using these approaches. Neural tube defects, which depend on elevated amniotic fluid alpha-fetoprotein concentrations and the presence of acetylcholinesterase to indicate an ultrasound

examination for their diagnosis, are not detected by CVS.

METHODS

Four methods have been described for obtaining CVS in the first trimester. Of these, the use of a flexible catheter introduced transcervically under ultrasonographic visualization is the most commonly used.

Prior to the day scheduled for the procedure, cervical samples are cultured. If detected, treatment is given for B-hemolytic *Streptococcus, Neisseria gonorrhoeae, Chlamydia trachomatis* and other significant pathogens prior to the procedure. Material for herpes simplex cultures is obtained in patients with a previous history of genital herpes and in those whose partners have such a history. CVS is an outpatient procedure, and no preoperative preparation is used. The patient arrives for the procedure with a full bladder. The initial evaluation consists of a careful ultrasonographic study. The 5 MHz sector scanner is the preferred transducer for these procedures. The fetal crown rump length is determined to ensure that the gestation is at least 9 weeks and not longer than 12 weeks in duration. (See below for a discussion of pregnancy loss relative to gestational age). Multiple pregnancies are ruled out. The location of the placental formation is established from its typical echogenicity and from visualization of the umbilical cord insertion. At 9 to 12 weeks' gestation, the cord is 2 to 4 mm in diameter. In severely ante- or retroflexed uterine cavities, such that the pathway for the catheter forms an angle of less than 130° with the cervical canal, the procedure is contraindicated. Additional contraindications include vaginitis; vaginal bleeding; multiple pregnancy, in which distinct placentas cannot be determined; and maternal erythrocyte antigen isoimmunization.

The cervix is prepped with povidone-iodine (Betadine). In the majority of cases traction with a tenaculum to straighten the cervical canal is not necessary, and local anesthesia is used only for this eventuality. A polyethylene catheter (length 21 to 28 cm, diameter 1.0 to 2.0 mm) fitted with a malleable wire obturator is inserted into the cervix, and the tip is localized on the real-time ultrasound picture. Under continuous sonographic guidance, the catheter tip is advanced until it lies within the chorion frondosum (Fig. 1). Minimal resistance is felt as the catheter advances. As the guidewire is removed, the catheter is advanced an additional 0.5 cm to ensure that it remains in

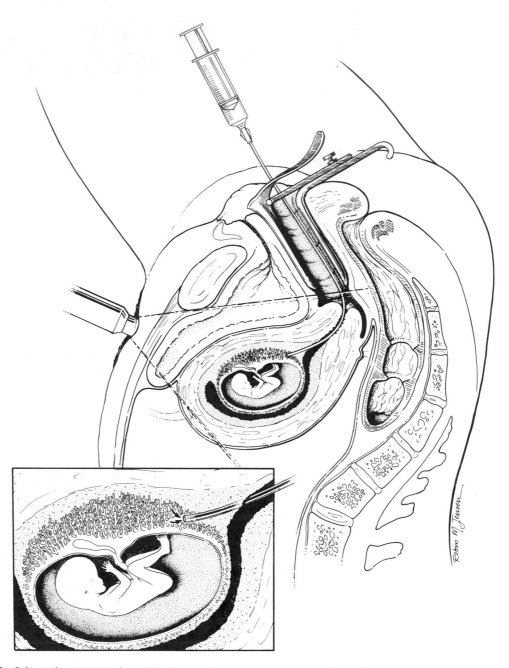

Figure 1 Schematic representation of chorionic villus sampling procedure. *Inset*: Enlarged view of catheter tip depicting aspiration of villi under negative pressure developed by the syringe. See text for further details.

the area of the villi. A 20-ml syringe filled with 5 ml of tissue culture medium is attached to the catheter, and 10-ml negative suction is applied. The suction is maintained as the catheter is withdrawn from the placental site. Suction is stopped when the catheter tip enters the cervical canal, so as to avoid contamination with mucus or blood. The patient may leave shortly after the procedure is completed. No antibiotics are used. Patients who are Rh negative and unsensitized receive 50 μg of anti-D immunoglobulin.

A satisfactory amount of villi (15 to 50 mg wet weight) is usually obtained with a single aspiration. No more than three aspiration attempts are performed. It is important that a fresh catheter be used for each aspiration attempt.

In over 95 percent of cases, the procedure is successful at the first sitting. If it is unsuccessful and the pregnancy is still less than 12 weeks, a second CVS may be attempted 1 week later, or the patient may elect to have amniocentesis.

There are two less commonly used transcervical methods of obtaining chorionic villi. Sonographic guidance is used with a rigid biopsy forceps and alternately a fetoscope is used to obtain a biopsy under direct visualization. CVS can also be performed transabdominally. This method uses ultrasonography, and a 17-gauge or 18-gauge needle is advanced into the placental area. A second biopsy needle (19 or 20 gauge) is advanced 1.5 cm past the tip of the larger needle, and villi are aspirated under negative pressure as described for the transcervical method. The transabdominal approach is useful when uterine position make the cervical route impossible.

CULTURING METHODS

Villi are aspirated into approximately 5 ml of sterile transport medium consisting of GIBCO (HAM) containing 0.5 percent Gentamicin (Garamycin) and 4 percent sodium heparin (1,000 IU per milligram). Following aspiration, the contents of the syringe are emptied into a sterile glass Petri dish containing a sufficient amount of transport medium to allow clear visualization of villi. Villi are evaluated immediately to assess the adequacy of the sample. Healthy, multibranched villi are transferred with sterile forceps from the Petri dish into a transport vial containing medium.

The villi are then placed in a sterile plastic 60-mm Petri dish. Under a dissecting microscope, villi are separated from maternal decidua. At this point, villi may be shipped, DNA may be extracted, or villi may be set up in culture for further chromosomal, biochemical, or DNA analysis. Although chromosome preparations are possible from a direct method, the resulting metaphase spreads are less than optimum. Cultured cells produce longer chromosomes of better quality and allow for further analysis by multiple staining techniques.

In preparing the villi for culture, they are transferred to 5 ml of fresh Chang's medium in a sterile plastic 60-mm Petri dish for an overnight incubation at 37 degrees C, 5 percent carbon dioxide in air. The following day, villi are placed in 3 ml 0.25 percent trypsin (GIBCO) for 1 hour, then transferred to 0.1 percent collagenase (Sigma Type V-S, 410 U per milligram) in 5 ml of Chang's medium for a minimum of 2 hours. At the end of the same day, cells are transferred to tissue culture flasks, maintained with Chang's medium, and harvested according to standard protocol. The average time in culture is approximately 10 days.

For small samples (less than 10 mg wet weight) cells are suspended in 1 ml of Chang's medium and placed in a sterile glass chamber slide. The chamber is flooded the following day with fresh medium (2 ml total volume) and, with sufficient growth, subcultured into plastic flasks. Cultures are then maintained and harvested as above.

For each CVS, 20 G-banded metaphases are analyzed and three karyotypes prepared. Chromosomal diagnosis is made following evaluation of cells from at least two flasks originating from two independent cultures. In cases requiring biochemical testing on cultured cells, analyses are conducted on cells from the same passage as those used for chromosomal studies. Lymphocytes from maternal blood collected at the time of CVS are routinely cultured according to standard methods. Cells are harvested and slides are prepared and held until completion of the CVS study. In the event of a female karyotype or a mixture of male and female cells, maternal and CVS fluorescent chromosome variants are compared to rule out maternal cell contamination.

An additional dilemma is the finding by most centers performing CVS of cases of mosaicism confined to the trophoblast tissue and not representative of the fetal karyotype. Comparison of maternal and CVS chromosome variants have confirmed the fetal origin of the multiple cell lines in many cases. Amniocentesis is generally recommended in an attempt to provide more information for interpreting these results.

COMPLICATIONS

Complications related to CVS can be divided into those that occur prior to 20 weeks' gestation and those that are observed in late pregnancy. In the three largest series reported to date, pregnancy loss prior to 20 weeks is 3.8 percent. This can be compared to an incidence of 2.7 percent in a prospective study of first-trimester pregnancies determined to be normal by an ultrasound examination. In patients age 40 or more with sonographically normal pregnancies, the rate of spontaneous loss is higher. The rate of pregnancy loss after CVS performed prior to 9 weeks and later than 12 weeks is greater than that seen at 9 to 12 weeks. The increased rate of loss before 9 weeks may be due to the fact that there is an increased rate of abortion at that gestational age. However, the rate at 12 weeks or more is considerably above the expected rate and has led to the abandonment of CVS after the end of the 11th week. Although infection is suspected in a number of spontaneous losses after CVS, only a small number of cases of acute chorioamnionitis have occurred. The incidence of septic shock is very low, and in the few cases reported the same catheter was used for a second aspiration attempt. Subsequently, a fresh catheter has been used if more than one transcervical insertion is necessary. Perforation of the amniotic sac during the procedure is also rare. In one series an unexpected increase in the incidence of severe oligohydramnios prior to 20 weeks in fetuses without gross anomalies was noted. This finding, which occurred without a clinical history suggestive of membrane rupture, was not commented on in other large series.

In one study ultrasound examinations were carried out 1 to 3 hours after the procedure and again at 10 to 15 days. Intrauterine hematoma, defined as a new hypoechoic area at the sampling site, was seen in 4.3 percent of the cases. Many of these patients experienced vaginal bleeding. In addition, a total of 12 percent of patients reported vaginal bleeding amounting to a mild hemorrhage during the first 2 to 3 days after the procedure in one series, but this degree of bleeding was not mentioned in others.

CVS does not appear to be associated with an increased incidence of complications in the second half of pregnancy. Congenital anomalies occurring in the infants of such mothers are not greater than expected. The incidence of premature labor, premature rupture of the membranes, abruptio placentae, placenta previa, placenta accreta, and intrauterine growth retardation has been reported to be no greater after CVS.

Thus, while the CVS procedure is still undergoing evaluation, its overall obstetric safety seems established. We currently counsel patients that the rate of spontaneous abortion is approximately 1.0 percent higher than if the procedure had not been undertaken but that otherwise the pregnancy would be expected to proceed as expected.

SUGGESTED READING

Brambati B, Oldrini A, Ferrazzi E, Lanzani A. Chorionic villus sampling: an analysis of the obstetric experience of 1000 cases. Prenat Diagn 1987; 7:157–169.

Hogge WA, Schonberg SA, Golbus MS, Chorionic villus sampling: Experience of the first 1000 cases. Am J Obstet Gynecol 1986; 154: 1249–1252.

Jackson L. Prenatal genetic diagnosis by chorionic villus sampling (CVS). Semin Perinatol 1985; 9:209–218.

Liu DTY, Jeavons B, Preston C, Preston D. A prospective study of spontaneous miscarriage in ultrasonically normal pregnancies and relevance to chorionic villus sampling. Prenat Diagn 1987; 7:223–227.

Olson S, Buckmaster J, Bissonnette J, Magenis E. Comparison of maternal and fetal chromosome heteromorphisms to monitor maternal cell contamination in chorionic villus samples. Prenat Diagn 1987; 7:413–417.

EXTERNAL CEPHALIC VERSION

JAMES R. SHIELDS, M.D.
BARRY S. SCHIFRIN, M.D.

The fetus is in a breech presentation in approximately 3 to 4 percent of all term deliveries. Although the etiology is often obscure, uterine anomalies, multiple gestation, placenta previa, and polyhydramnios all predispose to breech presentation. Before term, prematurity itself predisposes to this type of presentation. Prior to 28 weeks, approximately 25 percent of fetuses present as breech.

Compared with the vertex presentation, breech presentation results in greater perinatal mortality and morbidity. For the term breech infant delivered vaginally, the mortality remains three to four times greater than that for the vertex infant. Morbidity is also increased despite attempts to reduce the risks of vaginal delivery by highly selective protocols. In addition, long-term follow-up of breech presentations has revealed a high incidence of neurologic damage undetected in the perinatal period. These untoward statistics prevail even when the higher incidence of congenital anomalies and preterm births associated with breech presentation are excluded. The corrected excessive mortality and morbidity of the breech births appear related to the risks of asphyxia from prolapsed cord, delay in delivery of the aftercoming head, and trauma to the spine and the unmolded, aftercoming head. Otherwise stated, breech presentations delivered by cesarean section do as well as if not better than vertex presentations delivered vaginally. Based on these data, two approaches have evolved concerning the management of the term breech: routine cesarean section and the careful selection of patients who fulfill criteria for a safe vaginal delivery. Both approaches result in a high cesarean section rate, and neither addresses the fundamental problem—the incidence of the breech presentation at term.

External cephalic version under tocolysis offers an alternative to both routine cesarean section with its inherently high rate of maternal morbidity and selective vaginal delivery with its inherently higher rate of perinatal morbidity and mortality. Many authors have advocated external cephalic version as a simple and safe way to reduce the incidence of breech presentation at term. Several recent controlled trials have indeed demonstrated that the use of external cephalic version in selected term breech fetuses results in a lower incidence of cesarean section for breech presentation, with minimal or no risk to the fetus.

PATIENT SELECTION

Candidates for external cephalic version must have a gestational age of at least 37 weeks. Attempts at version prior to 37 weeks are frequently successful but are associated with an inordinately high rate of reversion back to the breech presentation. Moreover, if complications arise and delivery becomes necessary, prematurity is an added risk factor. Multiple gestation, hypertension, intrauterine growth retardation, uteroplacental insufficiency, placenta previa, previous uterine surgery, uterine anomalies, oligohydramnios, ruptured membranes, third trimester vaginal bleeding, and Rh sensitization are all contraindications to version. Unsensitized Rh-negative patients are usually not excluded as candidates. Patients with a maternal contraindication to the use of intravenous tocolytics (cardiac or thyroid disease, diabetes) may be excluded.

THE VERSION PROCEDURE

We perform external cephalic version in a hospital outpatient setting that allows immediate cesarean delivery if necessary. Once a patient fulfills the criteria set forth above, a detailed real-time ultrasound examination is performed in order to (1) confirm the breech presentation, (2) ensure adequate amniotic fluid volume, and (3) rule out fetal or uterine anomalies or placenta previa. If the patient is Rh negative, a sample of maternal blood is drawn for Kleihauer-Betke analysis. The patient is then placed supine with left tilt or left uterine displacement, and a nonstress test is performed. Version is considered only if the test is reactive. A tocolytic agent (ritodrine hydrochloride or terbutaline sulfate) is administered for 15 to 30 minutes prior to the version attempt. Although some investigators have not utilized tocolytics, tocolysis appears to reduce the force required for version and minimizes trauma to the uteroplacental unit. Although the success rates are not significantly different, the incidence of fetal-maternal hemorrhage with tocolysis (5.6 percent) appears lower than the incidence without it (28 percent).

The version attempt consists of a transabdominal elevation of the breech with subsequent "rolling" of the fetus until it is head-down in the pelvis. The direction of the roll, forward or backward, depends on the lie of the fetus. If the fetal head and spine are on opposite sides of the midline, a forward roll is attempted. If they are on the same side, a backward roll is attempted. If the initial attempt in one direction fails, the other direction is attempted. The fetal heart rate is monitored with ultrasound during the procedure, and, if decelerations or bradycardia develop, the attempt is stopped and the fetus is reverted to the breech presentation. Successful or unsuccessful version is confirmed with ultrasound. After the attempt, whether successful or not, the patient must have (1) a reactive nonstress test, (2) no evidence of labor, and (3) no vaginal bleeding before she is discharged home. If the patient is Rh negative, a repeat Kleihauer-Betke analysis is obtained 24 hours later, and, if indicated, the patient is given Rh-immune globulin. Other protocols routinely administer Rh-immune globulin to all unsensitized Rh-negative patients immediately following the version attempt.

EFFICACY

Success rates vary from 41 to 78 percent. In contrast, the rate of spontaneous cephalic version is significantly lower (12 to 17 percent) and decreases further with advancing gestation. With successful version, the risk of reversion to breech is small (0 to 3 percent). Of those patients in whom version is unsuccessful, 91 to 100 percent present in labor with a breech. Nulliparity, obesity, and especially, engagement of the breech in the pelvis, compromise successful version. Nulliparous patients experience a success rate of 62 percent versus 91 to 95 percent for the multiparous patient. The effect of placental location on success is controversial. Although anterior and lateral placentas have been associated with lower success rates, Morrison and associates demonstrated no difference in success rates between those with anterior and those with posterior placentas.

Successful breech version dramatically reduces the incidence of breech presentation in labor and cesarean section. After adopting a policy of breech version, Morrison and coworkers demonstrated a significant decrease in the incidence of breech presentation at term from 4.6 to 2.8 percent and a concomitant decrease in the cesarean section rate for this indication. In general, a liberal policy of external cephalic version reduces the cesarean section rate by about two-thirds—from 46 to 80 percent in those without version to 10 to 32 percent in those receiving version. Some authors suggest that despite the improvement in section rates with version, it is still increased in patients with successful version.

COMPLICATIONS

Earlier studies have associated breech version with premature labor, bleeding, uterine rupture, placental separation, umbilical cord accidents, injuries including Erb's palsy, fractures, and fetal distress. Most of these studies depict versions done earlier in pregnancy and antedate the use of contemporary surveillance techniques. Utilizing proper patient selection, nonstress testing, ultrasound assessment of amniotic fluid volume, placental location and fetal growth, and judicious manipulation with constant surveillance of the fetal heart rate, most investigators have failed to demonstrate any significant fetal or maternal complications. One study even demonstrated a better neonatal outcome in the version group, but this was related to the relatively high incidence of vaginal breech delivery in the control group (42 percent).

Of the three fetal deaths reported in the recent study by Kasule and coworkers, one was related to cord prolapse in a vertex presentation, another was due to intrapartum anoxia in a vertex presentation, and the third occurred in an infant with Down syndrome. It seems unreasonable to attribute these deaths directly to the version procedure. Furthermore, the authors do not mention whether or not the patients in the study group had reactive nonstress tests both before and after the procedure.

Although fetal heart rate decelerations during the version procedure appear in up to 40 percent of version attempts, all investigators have found them to be transient, with little demonstrable adverse effect on the fetus. Phelan and associates reported fetal heart rate changes in 39 percent of patients undergoing version. More than 95 percent of these changes represented either bradycardia or deceleration, whereas the others represented tachycardia or a sine wave pattern. All of the changes were transient and had no relationship to the fetal outcome. Of interest is that these changes occurred more frequently in nonanterior placentas (40 percent) compared with anterior ones (20 percent). Decreased heart rate variability also occurred more frequently after version, but again, this represented a transient change unrelated to fetal outcome.

SUGGESTED READING

Brenner WE, Bruce RD, Hendricks CH. The characteristics and perils of breech presentation. Am J Obstet Gynecol 1974; 118:700.

Dyson DC, Ferguson JE, Hensleigh P. Antepartum external cephalic version under tocolysis. Obstet Gynecol 1986; 67:63.

Kasule J, Chimbira THK, Brown IM. Controlled trial of external cephalic version. Br J Obstet Gynecol 1985; 92:14.

Morrison JC, Myatt RE, Martin JN, et al. External cephalic version of the breech presentation under tocolysis. Am J Obstet Gynecol 1986; 154:900.

Phelan JP, Stine LE, Mueller E, et al. Observations of fetal heart rate characteristics related to external cephalic version and tocolysis. Am J Obstet Gynecol 1984; 149:658.

Shields JR, Medearis AL. Fetal malpresentations. In: Hacker NF, Moore JG, eds. Essentials of obstetrics and gynecology. Philadelphia: WB Saunders, 1986:171.

Van Dorsten JP, Schifrin BS, Wallace RL. Randomized control trial of external cephalic version with tocolysis in late pregnancy. Am J Obstet Gynecol 1981; 141:417.

FETAL BLOOD SAMPLING

FERNAND DAFFOS, M.D.

Since 1973 fetal blood has been sampled by the use of two different techniques: (1) *placentocentesis*, which allows exceptionally pure fetal blood to be taken but which results in a high rate of fetal loss, and (2) *fetoscopy*, which is an invasive procedure requiring hospitalization of the patient, that can be performed only during a limited period of pregnancy, cannot be repeated, and has many technical difficulties (e.g., tinted amniotic fluid).

We combined the simplicity of the placentocentesis with the efficiency of fetoscopy in a new procedure for fetal blood sampling (FBS) performed on an outpatient basis under local anesthesia. *FBS can easily be repeated many times from 17 weeks until the end of the pregnancy.* It allows pure fetal blood to be obtained routinely without apparent harm to the fetus. This procedure of FBS under ultrasound control has rapidly expanded the study of human fetal biology, the clinical applications in prenatal diagnosis, the establishment of reference ranges for biologic measurements, and the assessment of fetal welfare on objective, biologic criteria. The possibility of obtaining fetal blood without fetal risk during pregnancy allows us to consider the fetus as a separate patient. We can make a precise diagnosis and perform specific therapies. This opens the door to real fetal medicine.

TECHNIQUE

The umbilical cord insertion into the placenta is located with a real-time ultrasound scanner (sector or linear curved). The transducer is then kept strictly immobile and under aseptic conditions, and a local anesthetic in the form of 1 percent lidocaine (Xylocaine) is injected into the abdominal wall at the puncture site. No maternal sedation is given before or after the procedure. A 20-gauge spinal needle, 9 cm long, is primed with a 3.8 percent sodium citrate solution in a 2-ml disposable syringe and introduced into the plane of the ultrasound sector near the transducer. The needle tip emits a clearly visible echo that is followed on the screen toward the insertion of the cord. The cord is punctured at about 1 cm from its placental insertion (Fig. 1). According to placental position, access to the cord is gained either through the amniotic cavity or directly without penetrating the amniotic cavity (Fig. 2).

Immediately after the first drop of blood is obtained, the syringe is replaced with a dry one. According to the stage of gestation, 2 to 4 ml of blood is gently aspirated, and aliquots are transferred into special tubes containing appropriate anticoagulant. The needle is withdrawn, the duration of the bleeding from the puncture point (which is clearly visible on the screen when the procedure is transamniotic) is measured, and the fetal heart rate is recorded for several minutes.

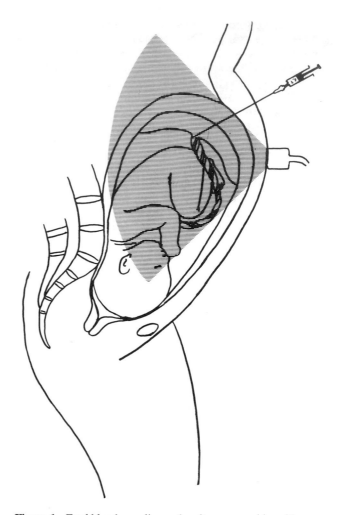

Figure 1 Fetal blood sampling under ultrasonographic guidance.

The procedure is always registered on a videotape, which allows a control afterward of the duration of the different phases and the reactions of the fetuses. One hour after the procedure, ultrasound examination is performed in each case to monitor the well-being of the fetus and the presence or absence of hematoma at the puncture site.

Assessment of the purity of the samples must be included in the technique of the procedure itself. The first step in establishing reference values and ensuring the accuracy of diagnosis is to be sure that the fetal blood sample is not contaminated.

Using our technique, *contamination can occur in maternal blood, amniotic fluid, or sodium citrate.* The overall incidence of contamination in our experience is small (1.2 percent), but the problem must be viewed in relation to the disorder under investigation and the importance of each type of contamination.

We believe that for absolute assurance that there is no contamination, all the following tests need to be performed.

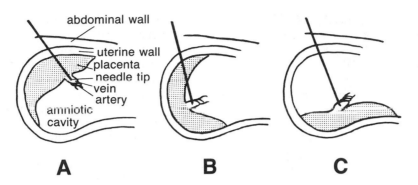

Figure 2 Cord access according to the placental position.

1. Hematologic indices are determined with a Coulter Counter S Plus II. The distribution volumes of leukocytes, erythrocytes, and platelets are recorded (see Fig. 2).
2. The Kleihauer-Betke test is performed using the Boehringer kit.
3. Smears are obtained and stained with the May-GrünwaldGiemsa stain (for the differential count).
4. Anti-I and anti-i cold agglutinins (against red blood cell antigens) are used in appropriate dilution.
5. The beta-subunit of human chorionic gonadotropin is determined in fetal serum.
6. Coagulation factors II and V are measured with a single-stage method.

The percentage of each type of contamination detectable by these methods is summarized in Table 1.

RESULTS

We have performed 1,560 FBSs using this technique between 17 and 41 weeks of amenorrhea in 1,400 pregnancies (Fig. 3). In 50 cases, multiple FBSs were performed during the same pregnancy (between two and six times) to confirm an unreliable diagnosis, to follow the changes in biologic parameters in a fetal disorder (e.g., thrombocytopenia, infection), or for fetal intravascular therapy. Of 11 twin pregnancies, in nine both fetuses were sampled (it was not necessary for two cases after fetal sexing). FBS was successful with a single abdominal insertion in 96.8 percent of cases. In 3.2 percent a second attempt several minutes or several days afterward was re-

TABLE 1 Percentage of Contamination by Each Method of Assessing Sample Purity

	Amniotic Fluid	Maternal Blood	Sodium Citrate
Hematologic indices	20	>5	20
Smear (Giemsa)	10	10	NC
Kleihauer's test	NC*	0.5	NC
Red blood cell antigens	NC	5	NC
Human chorionic gonadotropin	1	0.2	NC
Coagulation factors (V, II)	>0.1	30	10–50

* NC = noncontributory.

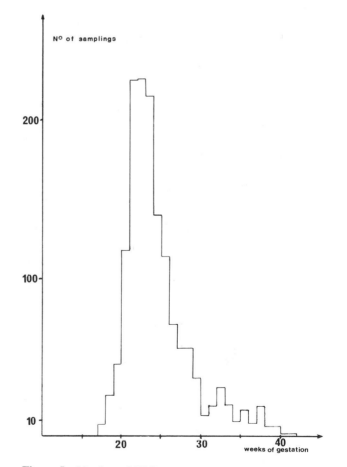

Figure 3 Number of FBSs according to weeks of gestation.

quired either because of contamination of the sample or because contamination did not allow us to arrive at a reliable diagnosis. In four cases FBS was not successful, despite two attempts to obtain pure fetal blood.

The duration of the procedure is usually short—less than 10 minutes in 92 percent of cases. However, certain situations make the sampling more difficult:

Maternal Obesity. In these cases we must use longer needles (15 cm) that are more flexible and thus less maneuverable. More important, the echographic image is of poorer quality and reduces visualization of the cord insertion.

Sonographic Quality. It is necessary to use high-resolution ultrasonography because the quality is an essential factor in the simplification and success of the technique.

Fetal Mobility. Excessive fetal movements can occasionally block access to the cord. Usually the problem may be overcome with a little patience.

Other Problems. Other problems may also be encountered. In cases of polyhydramnios it may be necessary to drain a large quantity of amniotic fluid before being able to reach the cord insertion. Oligohydramnios results in a poor quality ultrasound picture, but in these cases the cord is less mobile and may be punctured along its length. In the case of a posterior placental insertion the fetus may be an obstacle to accessing the cord. Under these circumstances, the fetus either may move spontaneously or may need external manipulation. In some cases the maternal bladder may need to be very full for good access, but more often we find that the bladder is overfull and obscures access to the cord insertion. Maternal position may occasionally need to be varied to provide better access.

In rare instances it has not been possible to have an adequate view of the cord insertion and the needle has been inserted near the abdominal insertion (the other fixation point) or in exceptional circumstances on a loop of cord against the uterine wall.

The results of pregnancies that have been allowed to continue after FBS are summarized in Table 2. The percentage of delivery at term is 94.1 percent, comparable with our normal obstetric population. The percentage of delivery before 37 weeks is 4 percent and of deliveries under 28 weeks is 0.7 percent. We have experienced 18 fetal deaths (1.2 percent), but the majority were not directly associated with the FBS procedure—e.g., severe intrauter-

ine growth retardation present at time of FBS, retroplacental hematoma, or mechanical cord accident. Only four fetal deaths were directly associated with the FBS. Three of these deaths occurred after FBS performed between 18 and 20 weeks' gestation. Immediately after FBS these fetuses had prolonged episodes of bradycardia and died within 24 hours. In one case a fetus with Glanzmann's thrombasthenia (classic form) died of exsanguination from the umbilical puncture site. This is the only case of fetal hemorrhage in our series. In all the other cases, visible bleeding after removal of the needle after FBS has been performed transamniotically is usually absent (60 percent) or of very short duration: less than 1 minute in 22 percent of cases and less than 2 minutes in 6 percent. In 2 percent of cases there has been bleeding from 2 to 6 minutes without apparent fetal consequences.

Fetal bradycardia was noted in 8 percent of cases immediately following FBS. The duration was less than 1 minute in 5.8 percent, from 1 to 2 minutes in 1 percent, and from 2 to 6 minutes in 0.2 percent of cases. We have not noticed any relationship between the duration of bleeding and the presence of fetal bradycardia.

INDICATIONS

In the 1970s and early 1980s, prenatal diagnosis was the only indication for sampling of fetal blood. FBS under ultrasound guidance has been shown to be simple, with minimal risks, and it can be repeated during the last two trimesters of pregnancy. Thus, the technique expands the field of biologic exploration of the fetus. We are able to establish biologic reference values in relation to the gestation of the pregnancy and to be aware of the effects of antenatal maternal therapy. In utero therapy allows us to completely modify our management of acquired fetal disorders and intrauterine growth retardation.

Prenatal Diagnosis

The indications for prenatal diagnosis are summarized in Table 3. In this context it is not possible to detail the diagnostic tests that we performed for each indication.

The traditional indications for prenatal diagnosis of hereditary disorders during the second trimester have been enlarged considerably as a result of infectious disease acquired during pregnancy and of chromosomal analysis in the third trimester in those fetuses manifesting malformations on ultrasound examination.

Fetal Biology

The large numbers of FBS we perform for prenatal diagnosis of congenital toxoplasmosis and the numbers of healthy fetuses in this population allow us to retrospectively establish normal values for biologic variables in the fetuses in relation to gestation. In this way the normal values for fetal hematologic indices, hemostasis, biochemistry, immunology, endocrinology, and acid base status have been established (Table 4). These normal values have been established along two specific directions: (1) to

TABLE 2 Follow-Up of 963 Completely Documented Pregnancies After FBS

• Full-term delivery	94.1 %
• Premature delivery (from 28 to 37 wks)	4 %
• Spontaneous abortion (born before 28 wks)	0.7 %
• In utero deaths (total)	1.2%
(related to the procedure)	0.4%

TABLE 3 Indications for Prenatal Diagnosis

Indications	No. of Samplings
Infectious Diseases	
Toxoplasmosis	1,005
Rubella	85
Others (cytomegalovirus, varicella, herpes)	23
Hemoglobinopathies	
Thalassemia	21
Sickle cell	
Others	
Karyotyping	115
Coagulopathies	
Hemophilia	95
Others (deficiencies of factors V, VII, XIII, Von Willebrand's disease, Glanzmann's disease)	10
Metabolic Disorders	
Alpha$_1$-antitrypsin deficiency	12
Pyruvate kinase deficiency	
Hypercholesterolemia	
Miscellaneous	15
	1,381

permit a reliable prenatal diagnosis by a comparison between the values in the normal and the affected fetus; (2) to have a more complete understanding of the problems of fetal growth and its abnormalities. For this reason we have established normal values for fetal growth factors (somatomedins, thymidine activity), biologic parameters

TABLE 4 Reference Values in Fetal Biology

Hematology
Red blood cells, white blood cells, platelet counts, differential count, hemoglobin, hematocrit, mean corpuscular volume, ferritin, red blood cell antigens, platelet antigens, platelet glycoproteins, hemoglobin electrophoresis, triose phosphate isomerase

Hemostasis
Factors = IIc, IIAg, Vc, VIIc, VIIIc, VIIIRag, IXc, IXAg, Xc, XIIIc, fibrinogen, antithrombin III, heparin cofactor II, protein C, plasminogen, fibronectin, alpha$_2$-macroglobulin, alpha$_1$-antitrypsin

Biochemistry
Total proteins, albumin, γGT, cholesterol, triglycerides, bilirubin, uric acid, glucose, creatinine, calcium, phosphorus, alkaline phosphatase, creatine kinase, alpha-fetoprotein, alpha-interferon, free amino acids

Immunology
Total IgM, Lymphocyte subpopulations = T_{11}, T_3, T_4, T_8, B_1, B_4, BL_{14}, E 135, natural killer activity

Endocrinology
Cortisol, cortisone, dehydroepiandrosterone sulfate, somatomedin C, thymidine activity, transferrin, insulin-like growth factors I and II, thyroid-stimulating hormone

Acid-Base Status
pH, Po_2, Pco_2, HCO_3^-, base excess, lactate

implicated in fetal nutrition (amino acids), and tests of fetal anoxia (e.g., acid-base balance, lactic acid).

Fetal Welfare Surveillance

In the next few years FBS will become a complementary examination in the surveillance of fetal well-being (Table 5). In our department we regularly perform FBS in certain cases of disorders acquired during the pregnancy or where the change in parameters of fetal biologic variables is important to outcome.

Fetal Infectious Disorders. When congenital toxoplasmosis infection is confirmed in the fetus, we follow the course of the disease with nonspecific biologic parameters of infection (Fig. 4) and treat the fetus (by maternal intermediary).

Fetal Anemias. The most frequently occurring fetal anemias are caused by alloimmunization with anti-D antibodies. The direct transfusion of red cell concentrate into the fetal circulation considerably improves the prognosis in severe cases, in particular those with hydrops.

Fetal Thrombocytopenia. On several occasions we have given in utero platelet transfusions before delivery in fetuses with severe thrombocytopenia secondary to alloimmunization in the PLA 1 system. This possible therapy encouraged us to develop a management plan to avoid neonatal bleeding complications (Fig. 5)

In cases of idiopathic thrombocytopenic purpura, it is well established that there is no association between maternal antiplatelet antibody levels, the maternal platelet level, and the degree to which the fetus is affected. In several cases we have found this same dissociation in utero on FBS and have been able to determine the mode of delivery by the true fetal status. In the future it will be interesting to study the efficacy of maternal therapies on fetal platelet levels.

Growth Retardation The complete elucidation of the etiology of intrauterine growth retardation will require

TABLE 5 Indications for FBS in Assessment of Fetal Well-Being and Fetal Therapy

Nonspecific Signs of Fetal Infection	7
Toxoplasmosis	
Rubella	
Anemia	
Rhesus alloimmunization	23
Red blood transfusions*	20
Thrombocytopenia	
Idiopathic thrombocytopenia	15
Alloimmune thrombocytopenia	10
Platelet transfusions*	7
Anoxia	
Intrauterine growth retardation	32
Intravascular Coagulopathy	
Eclampsia	1
Other Fetal Therapy	4
Curare, digitoxin	
Total No of Sample	119

* Treatment performed.

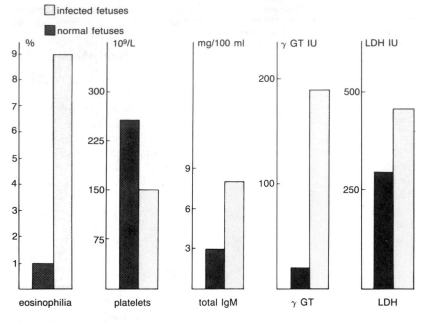

Figure 4 Nonspecific biologic parameters of fetal toxoplasmosis infection.

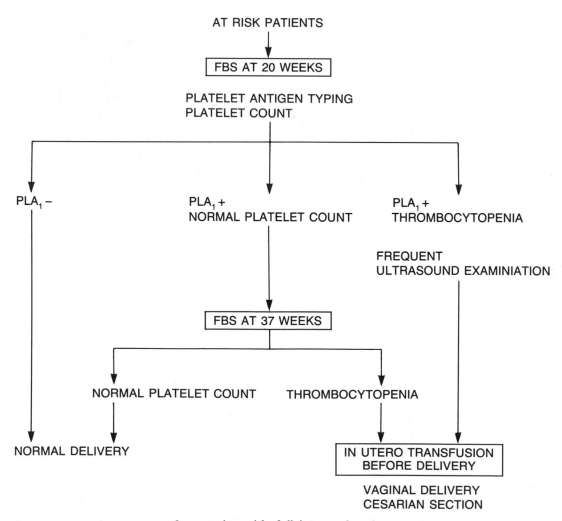

Figure 5 Prenatal management of pregnancies at risk of alloimmune thrombocytopenia.

many years of study. In contrast, the immediate short-term prognosis may be better appreciated by the study of fetal biology. Chronic fetal hypoxia can be assessed by the examination of hematologic indices and impending decompensation may be shown by the pH level in utero. For several months we have been using FBS in association with other classic parameters of fetal welfare (ultrasonography, Manning's score, Doppler examination), and the results seem very promising for the future.

Antenatal Pharmacology and Fetal Therapy

With FBS it is also possible to measure simultaneous maternal and fetal levels of substances and hence their transplacental passage. It is equally easy to study the effect of maternal medication on the fetal biology. For example, we have shown that a single oral dose of 100 mg aspirin by the mother completely inhibits fetal platelet aggregation by arachidonic acid.

INTRAUTERINE TRANSFUSION

VANESSA A. BARSS, M.D.
MICHAEL F. GREENE, M.D.
FREDRIC D. FRIGOLETTO Jr., M.D.

Therapeutic options in severe fetal isoimmune hemolytic disease are limited. It has been suggested that promethazine therapy is helpful in ameliorating the severity of hemolysis by modifying phagocyte function. Others, however, have not had clinical success with this therapy and question its efficacy. There are no controlled trials to prove the efficacy of promethazine. Plasmapheresis to remove the IgG fraction of the maternal blood has been performed. However, to achieve even minimal reductions in maternal antibody titer requires massive volume apheresis at very frequent intervals. This is difficult logistically, is very expensive, and carries with it the potential for maternal infection and electrolyte disturbance. Here too, there is no convincing proof of efficacy. Initial promising reports of desensitization of $Rh_0(D)$-sensitized women by oral treatment with Rh-positive erythrocyte ghosts have not been confirmed. Corticosteroids have not been useful in decreasing the severity of the fetal anemia, although they may transiently affect amniotic bilirubin levels. Preliminary studies using high-dose intravenous immune serum globulin are currently under way. This therapy has been beneficial in patients with immune thrombocytopenia and may have similar effects in those with isoimmune hemolytic disease. Although the mechanism of action is not clearly defined, it may work by feedback inhibition of antibody synthesis, reticuloendothelial Fc receptor blockade, and/or blockade of Fc-mediated antibody transport across the placenta. This leaves only two effective modes of therapy, early delivery with exchange transfusion in the nursery, and intrauterine transfusion. Improvements in neonatal intensive care in the past 10 to 15 years have enabled neonatologists to handle younger and sicker newborns more confidently than ever before. This has permitted the more liberal concomitant use of early delivery in the management of isoimmune hemolytic disease. This approach, however, is not without its own morbidity and mortality. Some fetuses are severely affected at early gestational ages and thus become poor risks for delivery; for these, intrauterine trans-

fusion remains the best option. Since 1983, when Daffos described a relatively safe and uncomplicated technique for ultrasound-guided percutaneous umbilical blood sampling, the diagnosis and management of erythroblastosis fetalis have become less empirical and more successful.

THE INDICATION

As with any surgical procedure, the most important part is deciding which patients will benefit from it and which would do well without it. All pregnant patients are screened at their first prenatal visits for the presence of irregular antibodies that are capable of causing severe isoimmune hemolytic disease. When a patient with such an antibody has been identified, the titer is quantitated every 2 to 4 weeks. The quantitation of the titer should be done either in albumin or by the indirect Coombs' test so that IgG, which crosses the placenta, and not IgM is measured. A patient requires further evaluation when her titer exceeds the value of that laboratory's "critical titer." The critical titer is that value below which no stillbirths or severely affected fetuses have been seen. It is important to emphasize that owing to differences in technique and reagents, the critical titer is laboratory-specific and cannot be generalized from one laboratory to another. Furthermore, to establish the critical titer value at a laboratory requires an extensive and careful follow-up of patients within that laboratory. Once a patient's titer has exceeded the critical titer, it is important to determine the blood type and zygosity of the father of the baby and to consider percutaneous umbilical blood sampling for determination of fetal blood type. If the father is heterozygous for the sensitizing antigen, percutaneous umbilical blood sampling should be offered because there is a 50 percent chance that the fetus' reaction will be negative and will not require further work-up or specialized management. If the fetal blood sampling is positive or if the father is homozygous for the sensitizing antigen, serial assessments of the severity of fetal anemia should be made. This can be determined either by amniocentesis or by percutaneous umbilical blood sampling for the fetal cord hematocrit. Percutaneous umbilical blood sampling is more difficult than amniocentesis, it requires an ultrasonographer and a perinatologist with expertise in the procedure, and carries a procedure-related mortality of 0.2 to 1 percent. However, one can obtain exact information about fetal blood type, hematocrit, or other hematologic indices. Amniocentesis is an easier and safer procedure but provides less accurate information on the fetal status. When amniocentesis is performed, amniotic fluid bilirubin is measured spectrophotometrically as the ΔOD_{450} according to the method of Liley. The value is then interpreted with the aid of Liley's three-zone chart. The first amniocentesis should be performed at 20 to 22 weeks or whenever the critical titer is reached thereafter.

A patient whose ΔOD_{450} falls into the lowest zone needs nothing more than a repeat ΔOD_{450} 2 weeks following the initial determination. If this second point determines a line that is pointing down and paralleling the normal fall in ΔOD_{450}, subsequent amniocenteses may be performed at 3-week intervals. Within the middle zone, there can be both severely affected and unaffected fetuses. The frequency of repeat amniocentesis is determined by how high in the midzone the values are and their trend with time. If they are in the lower half of the midzone and their trend is downward parallel to the curve, studies could be repeated at 1- to 2-week intervals. Values that are high in the midzone and rising must be repeated at 1-week intervals. When the ΔOD_{450} gets up to 80 percent of the midzone, blood sampling is indicated to distinguish which fetuses are severely anemic, i.e., hematocrit value less than or equal to 25 ml per deciliter, and now require transfusion or delivery. Nicolaides and Rodeck and colleagues have shown that the human fetus begins to show elevated lactate concentrations when the hematocrit level falls below 25 ml per deciliter and is at high risk for developing hydrops at hematocrit levels below 15 ml per deciliter. In general, we prefer to follow pregnancies complicated by isoimmunization with serial amniocenteses, reserving percutaneous umbilical blood sampling for the following situations: (1) to determine fetal blood type if the father of the baby is heterozygous; (2) to determine fetal hematocrit if the ΔOD_{450} is at least 80 percent up in the midzone; (3) to follow fetal hematocrit after intrauterine transfusions have been undertaken; and (4) occasionally to ascertain fetal hematocrit between 20 and 26 weeks when the Liley curve is slightly less reliable.

As long as the ΔOD_{450} remains below high zone 2, the pregnancy may continue until 36 to 40 weeks. Decisions regarding timing of delivery must be individualized and should take into account the level of the ΔOD_{450}, pulmonary maturity, and cervical ripening. In the more severe cases, decisions regarding delivery versus intrauterine transfusions depend on a number of factors. As long as the fetal hematocrit is 25 ml per deciliter or higher, we feel that the fetus benefits from further in utero growth and maturation. These fetuses should be followed with weekly nonstress tests and ultrasound examinations weekly or every other week, with delivery planned at 36 weeks or later when pulmonary maturity is documented. When the hematocrit is less than 25 ml per deciliter, delivery is usually indicated if the fetus is older than or equal to 32 weeks and has pulmonary maturity. In selected cases we may choose to perform an additional transfusion or allow the fetus to remain in utero longer to permit further growth or maturation. This decision takes into account ease of procedure, degree of lung

maturity, placental location, fetal size, cervical ripeness and patient compliance. If the fetus is less than 32 weeks old or the lungs are immature, intrauterine fetal transfusion is indicated. All hydropic fetuses receive transfusions directly into the umbilical vein because of the improved survival with this technique. In nonhydropic fetuses, intravascular transfusion is not clearly more successful than intraperitoneal transfusion; therefore, we choose the procedure that is technically easier, taking into account placental location, cord insertion site, and fetal position.

PERCUTANEOUS UMBILICAL BLOOD SAMPLING PROCEDURE

When the patient arrives in the ultrasound suite, a routine sonogram is performed with special attention directed to the placental location and cord insertion site. After a 10 × 10 cm area of the maternal abdomen is prepared with povidone-iodine, a 22-gauge spinal needle is inserted into the umbilical vein near the cord insertion site by the obstetrician. An ultrasonographer holding the real-time ultrasound transducer guides the obstetrician during the entire procedure. Ideally, if the placenta is anterior, the needle can be directed into the umbilical vein without entering the amniotic fluid cavity. If the cord insertion site is not accessible, the needle is directed at the free loop of cord that can be stabilized against the uterine wall. In over 90 percent of patients, the cord is entered on the first attempt.

After the first few drops of aspirated blood are discarded, the required volume of blood is aspirated into a clean syringe and placed into appropriate specimen tubes. We do not routinely use heparinized needles or syringes and have not had problems with clotted specimens if the aspirated blood is placed immediately into tubes containing anticoagulant. Fetal blood type is confirmed by a Betke-Kleihauer test or cell sizing. After the needle is withdrawn, the cord is observed for bleeding, and fetal heart rate is monitored sonographically for several minutes. When the ultrasonographer is satisfied that no bleeding from the cord is occurring and the fetal heart rate is normal, the patient is sent home. No maternal premedication, antibiotics, tocolytic drugs, or intravenous lines are used for the procedure. The ultrasound transducer is not made sterile, as it does not encroach on the povidone-iodine–treated area of the maternal abdomen.

INTRAPERITONEAL TRANSFUSION PROCEDURE

All transfusions are performed as outpatient procedures. The blood bank is notified promptly when intrauterine transfusion has been chosen as the appropriate mode of therapy for a patient. A 20-ml specimen of the patient's blood is forwarded to the blood bank at least 4 hours prior to the planned transfusion. All maternal antibodies directed against blood group antigens are characterized. A donor is then sought who is type O, Rh-negative, and negative for as many other important antigens (e.g., Kell, Duffy, Kidd) as possible. A unit or partial unit, depending on the amount needed for the intrauterine transfusion, is drawn from the donor as close to the time when it is actually to be infused as is practically possible. Generally this is the same day or the night before. The red blood cells are then packed according to the standard procedure in the blood bank to a hematocrit of approximately 85 ml per deciliter. The final step in preparing the blood for transfusion is to irradiate it to destroy the white blood cells and eliminate the possibility of chimerism and graft-versus-host disease.

The transfusion procedure is performed in the ultrasound suite under continuous guidance from a real-time sector scanner. Initially, the ultrasonographer and obstetrician spend a few minutes becoming thoroughly familiar with the position of the fetus and placenta. Safe completion of the procedure requires that the needle insertion site be chosen with consideration for several fetal and maternal anatomic constraints. The cells must be transfused into the fetal peritoneal cavity while avoiding trauma to the fetal kidneys, liver, and spleen and to the umbilical vein. The fetal liver is always enlarged in these cases owing to extensive extramedullary erythropoiesis. The optimal fetal position would be for the fetus to be supine, presenting its entire anterior abdominal wall. In practice, one is rarely this fortunate. If the fetus is lying on either side, this is usually acceptable as long as the fetus does not turn toward the prone position, thereby presenting the kidneys. If the fetus is prone and cannot be prodded to change position, it is best to come back in an hour or so and try again. Maternal anatomy must also be considered. A needle must not be inserted so far lateral as to endanger the inferior epigastric vessels or the uterine vessels or perforate the intestines. With these considerations in mind, every effort should be made to choose a needle insertion site with as short a path to the fetus as possible and one that will allow penetration of the fetal skin surface at as close to a 90-degree angle as possible. Attempts to pierce the fetal abdominal wall at very oblique angles often result in the needle's glancing off and pushing the fetus aside.

Once the needle insertion site has been chosen, the ultrasonographer chooses the position from which he or she can best guide and monitor the procedure. This is usually approximately 4 cm from the needle and from the fetal anterior abdominal wall side. The maternal abdomen is then generously prepared with iodine solution and a sterile field established. With direct ultrasound guidance, a 20-gauge spinal needle is introduced into the fetal peritoneal cavity. The hub of the needle is then connected to extension tubing, which connects to both the 10-ml syringe and the unit of packed red blood cells via a three-way stopcock. Using this closed system, blood can be withdrawn from the unit into the syringe and then manually infused into the fetus in 10-ml aliquots.

The volume of blood to be infused is determined by the equation: volume $= ($weeks' gestation $- 20) \times 10$. The infusion rate should be determined by what is comfortable for the person manipulating the syringe. During the transfusion, the fetal heart rate should be monitored by the ultrasonographer. The transfusion should be stopped if bradycardia occurs and, if possible, some blood should be withdrawn until a normal fetal heart rate is obtained.

INTRAVASCULAR TRANSFUSION PROCEDURE

If an intravascular transfusion is planned, a rolled towel is placed under the right side of the patient to levorotate the uterus and prevent supine hypotension if the procedure is lengthy. After using sterile technique to prepare the maternal abdomen, a 22-gauge spinal needle is inserted into the umbilical vein near the cord insertion site by the obstetrician under ultrasound guidance. After a blood specimen is aspirated for determination of fetal hematocrit, the intravascular transfusion is performed. The volume of blood to be infused is calculated according to the method of Rodeck:

$$\text{Volume of blood transfused} = \frac{\text{Fetal/Placental blood volume (Desired HCT} - \text{Actual HCT)}}{\text{HCT of packed red blood cells}}$$

The desired final hematocrit is generally between 40 and 45 ml per deciliter. The hematocrit of the packed red blood cells is usually between 85 and 90 ml per deciliter. Blood is aspirated into a 10-ml syringe from a unit of washed, radiated, antigen-negative, packed red blood cells via a three-way stopcock and injected into the fetus through the extension tubing. This closed set-up minimizes both the risk of dislodging the spinal needle and that of bacterial contamination. During the procedure, the ultrasonographer monitors the flow of transfused blood into the umbilical vein, which can be directly observed, and intermittently checks the fetal heart rate by observation of the fetal heart, pulsation of the umbilical artery, or Doppler study. At the end of the transfusion, another specimen is obtained to determine the post-transfusion hematocrit. On occasion we have found it necessary to paralyze an active fetus who is obscuring the cord insertion site. Pancuronium (0.5 mg) may be given directly to the fetus either intramuscularly or intravascularly via the umbilical vein to arrest fetal movement temporarily. The patient is sent home at the end of the procedure. Subsequent patient follow-up is at the discretion of the obstetrician and includes weekly or every other week ultrasound surveillance, weekly nonstress testing, and percutaneous fetal umbilical blood sampling to determine fetal hematocrit.

The first two intrauterine transfusions are performed 1 week apart. Subsequent transfusions are necessary at 1- to 4-week intervals with the timing individualized case by case.

COMPLICATIONS OF INTRAUTERINE TRANSFUSION

Cramping and pain when the spinal needle is inserted are the most common complications of intrauterine transfusion. This usually resolves promptly on removal of the needle. We have never observed cramping to develop into premature labor. Amniotic fluid leakage is a rare complication. When the procedure is done under direct ultrasound guidance and using a 22-gauge spinal needle instead of the old catheter method, the incidence of fetal trauma markedly diminishes. However, there is still a 2 to 5 percent incidence of fetal death during or after the procedure. Since many of these fetuses are gravely ill at the time of transfusion and might well have died within a short time without transfusion, some of these deaths probably are not procedure-related. Procedure-induced fetal death can be caused by fetal sepsis from bacterial contamination during the invasive procedure. This has been reported on several occasions and in some centers prophylactic antibiotics are used. Fetal death from exsanguination is also possible despite continuous ultrasound guidance. We lost one fetus when this procedure was performed through an anterior placenta when a fetal placental surface vessel was punctured. In the presence of hepatosplenomegaly, it is possible to puncture intra-abdominal fetal vessels or vascular organs during an intraperitoneal transfusion. Last, if an excessive quantity of blood is transfused into the fetal peritoneal cavity, it is possible to raise the intraperitoneal pressure above the umbilical vein pressure and severely compromise return from the placenta. This has been attributed as a cause of death in an animal model. The risk of septic or traumatic complications increases if multiple needle insertions are required. All procedures should be performed in the proximity of a delivery room so that if complications arise during the procedure in a fetus of viable gestational age, rapid access to a labor and delivery unit to permit emergency delivery of the fetus is an option.

The ability to sample fetal blood and perform intravascular fetal transfusions percutaneously represents a major advance in the diagnosis and therapy of erythroblastosis fetalis. Knowledge of fetal blood type and hematocrit has allowed treatment to be individualized to the specific needs of the patient rather than empirical therapy based on inexact correlations between amniotic fluid bilirubin levels and fetal hematocrit. The ability to transfuse blood directly into the vascular system of the very compromised hydropic fetus has proved to be lifesaving in these patients. We feel that fetuses with mild disease can be followed adequately with ultrasound and amniocentesis. In the patient with more severe disease, invasive umbilical vein procedures are useful. There are no data at present that would allow one to conclude that the intravascular route is superior in the fetus who is not hydropic or in the fetus who has resolved hydrops and is receiving a subsequent transfusion. In this situation, we feel that the technically more feasible route is the procedure of choice.

SUGGESTED READING

Barss VA, Benacerraf BR, Frigoletto FD, et al. Management of isoimmunized pregnancy by use of intravascular techniques. Am J Obstet Gynecol 1988; 159:932–937.

Frigoletto FD, Umansky I, Birnholz J, et al. Intrauterine fetal transfusion in 365 fetuses during fifteen years. Am J Obstet Gynecol 1981; 139:781.

Rodeck CH, Nicolaides KH, Warsof SL, et al. The management of severe rhesus isoimmunization by fetoscopic intravascular transfusions. Am J Obstet Gynecol 1984; 150:769–774.

Soothill PW, Nicolaides KH, Rodeck CH, et al. Relationship of fetal hemoglobin and oxygen content to lactate concentration in Rh isoimmunized pregnancies. Obstet Gynecol 1987; 69:268.

REGIONAL ANESTHESIA

RICHARD B. CLARK, M.D.

Regional (conduction) anesthesia for labor and delivery usually provides an awake, alert mother who can consciously participate in the birth process and who usually brings forth an active infant, unaffected by medication. Regional anesthesia avoids the maternal and neonatal hazards associated with heavy maternal medication or general anesthesia, yet simulates the alertness that is the touchstone of natural childbirth. Despite its occasional technical complications, it enjoys an enormous popularity because of these attributes. Regional anesthesia used during obstetrics usually includes spinal, epidural, caudal, paracervical, and pudendal anesthesia. Although several types of regional anesthesia are utilized for cesarean section, this chapter is limited to regional anesthesia for vaginal delivery.

SPINAL ANESTHESIA

Spinal anesthesia is achieved by injecting a local anesthetic into the cerebrospinal fluid, where the anesthetic action is on the spinal cord and on the nerve roots. Tetracaine (Pontocaine) (4 mg) is the local anesthetic usually employed, and it is mixed with 10 percent dextrose to render the solution heavier than spinal fluid (hyperbaric). Lumbar puncture is achieved below the second lumbar vertebra, to avoid injury to the spinal cord.

Since the spinal anesthetic solution is hyperbaric, the position of the patient is important in determining the eventual level of anesthesia. As spinal anesthesia for obstetrics is commonly injected in the sitting position, the local anesthetic-dextrose mixture gravitates downward. If the patient remains in the sitting position for several minutes after injection, a saddle block results (anesthesia confined to the perineum). If the patient lies flat soon after injection (45 seconds), a higher level of anesthesia (low spinal anesthesia is up to the tenth thoracic dermatome) ensues. The latter is usually preferable, as it results in complete pain relief. Occasionally true saddle block is indicated so that the patient can push more effectively, although it does not provide complete pain relief.

Spinal anesthesia for vaginal delivery, whether saddle or low spinal, is administered in the delivery room, when delivery is imminent. This is one disadvantage when compared with lumbar epidural anesthesia, which can be given in the labor room; the other disadvantage is the possibility of postspinal headache.

The potent drugs used in anesthesiology and the physiologic changes that they cause can lead to potentially dangerous situations. Spinal anesthesia is no exception. Hypotension, respiratory arrest, neurologic damage, and postspinal headache are all potential sequelae. Because the pregnant uterus occludes the inferior vena cava, accentuating the fall in blood pressure often occurring from spinal-induced vasodilatation, arterial hypotension must be aggressively anticipated and rapidly treated. Therapy is composed of left uterine displacement, crystalloid infusion (1 to 2 L), and the intravenous injection of 10 to 15 mg of ephedrine. Respiratory insufficiency or arrest is treated with oxygen, and artificial ventilation of the lungs with bag and mask, anesthesia machine, or (as a last resort) mouth-to-mouth resuscitation. These complications are more likely to occur when spinal anesthesia is given for cesarean section rather than for vaginal delivery, because of the higher levels required. Neurologic sequelae (transverse myelitis, arachnoiditis, cauda equina syndrome, and isolated nerve palsy) are almost unheard of when time-tested methods and drugs are used in normal patients, but the possibility still exists. Spinal headache can occur after any dural puncture (diagnostic lumbar puncture, spinal anesthesia, myelogram); the incidence is directly related to the size of the needle. Treatment is bed rest, analgesics, intravenous fluids, intravenous caffeine (not my own practice), and epidural blood patch.

Spinal anesthesia, per se, has virtually no effect on the fetus or neonate. If there has been a maternal complication, such as hypotension or hypoxia, the infant can be profoundly affected. Local anesthetic levels from spinal anesthesia high enough to detect are found in the infant but never reach clinically significant levels.

EPIDURAL ANESTHESIA

Epidural anesthesia is achieved by injecting a local anesthetic into the epidural (synonymous with peridural) space. The local anesthetic affects the nerve roots as they leave their dural sleeves. The "loss of resistance" technique is commonly used for locating the epidural space (Fig. 1). It is usually performed in the lumbar area. A plastic catheter is frequently inserted into the epidural space so that local anesthetics may continue to be injected, prolonging the block. Epidural anesthesia is usually instituted when the active phase of labor has begun, i.e., 6 cm in the primipara and 4 cm in the multipara. Thus, anesthesia for labor as well as delivery is possible. The epidural is well suited to "segmental" administration, in which only a small amount of local anesthetic is injected periodically, enough to produce a segmental distribution (T10 to L5). This results in a lower total dose of drug, less hypotension, and a labor relatively free from the occasionally retardant effects of epidural anesthesia. Complications of epidural anesthesia occasionally include hypotension and respiratory arrest, treated just as when they occur with spinal anesthesia. Toxic reactions to local anesthetic drugs can occur when they are used for epidural blocks, and they are treated symptomatically—diazepam or barbiturate for seizures, positive-pressure oxygen for hypoventilation, and fluids and ephedrine for hypotension. Since large quantities of local anesthetics may be used, the possibility of a drug reaction is much higher

than with spinal anesthesia. These reactions are best avoided by aspirating before injection, using a test dose including epinephrine, and giving incremental doses of drug. Neurologic complications are as rare as with spinal anesthesia.

Three local anesthetics are commonly used for lumbar epidural anesthesia in obstetrics: lidocaine (Xylocaine), bupivacaine (Marcaine), and chloroprocaine (Nesacaine). Each has its advantages and disadvantages, durations of action, and maternal and neonatal effects (Table 1). Chloroprocaine is the shortest in duration (because of its rapid metabolism), and in a sense the safest in regard to systemic toxicity. Bupivacaine is longer lasting, particularly in the 0.5 percent concentration, but it is more likely to produce maternal toxicity, especially when given intravascularly. Lidocaine is a good compromise, has a good safety record, and is usually our choice.

The three local anesthetics used, unless given in overdose or intravascularly, have little maternal toxic effect. Some comments are in order regarding their neonatal effect. All freely pass the placenta but have no neonatal effect unless blood levels are high. Bupivacaine probably passes less than the others because of its high affinity for maternal plasma protein. Chloroprocaine passes readily but is rapidly metabolized by maternal and fetal plasma enzymes. Lidocaine was suspected of causing some neonatal effects, as determined by neurobehavioral tests, but this has been discounted. None of the local anesthetics given in reasonable doses seem to have neonatal effects. Because of the low doses used with segmental anesthesia, overdosing is rare. For a further discussion of this area, see Shnider and Levinson.

Epidural anesthesia is considered the technique of choice for prematurity. Not only does it reduce the amount

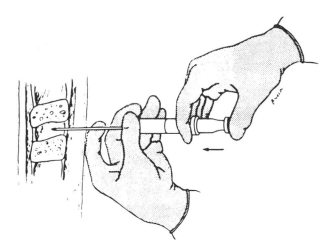

Figure 1 Loss of resistance technique for identifying epidural space. The needle is placed in the interspinous ligament, and resistance to pressure on the plunger of the syringe is determined. The needle is stabilized with the left hand, while the thumb of the right hand applies intermittent pressure to the plunger. (From Shnider SM, Levinson G. Anesthesia for obstetrics. 2nd ed. Baltimore: Williams & Wilkins, 1987:115. Used with the permission of the authors and publisher.)

TABLE 1 Advantages and Disadvantages of Several Local Anesthetics Used in Epidural Anesthesia

Drug	Comments
Lidocaine	Moderately long-acting (1–2 hours) Good safety record Neonatal effects only in overdose
Bupivacaine	Longer acting (1–3 hours) Definitely cardiotoxic with unintentional intravascular injection Little placental transfer Little effect on labor No demonstrated neonatal effect
Chloroprocaine	Short acting (30 minutes to 1 hour) Safest in terms of maternal systemic toxicity Rare neurologic complications Little placental transfer Rapid metabolism No neonatal effect

of narcotic drugs required for labor but it also is thought to reduce trauma to the soft fetal head because it contributes to perineal relaxation. The use of epidural anesthesia in pre-eclampsia is controversial. Because of the contracted blood volume occurring in this disease, use of this block can rapidly lead to maternal hypotension. Since this is well known, the infusion of a balanced salt solution before the block is instituted can avoid this problem. Epidural anesthesia is the technique of choice at our institution for both vaginal and abdominal delivery of patients with pre-eclampsia, but this is predicated on liberal fluid infusion, aggressive monitoring, and vigorous treatment of abnormalities in cardiovascular parameters. Labor in the pregnant diabetic has long been known to be well managed by epidural anesthesia. Last, the use of epidural block in breech presentation or multiple gestation for which vaginal delivery is planned is *not* usually recommended. There may be some interference with labor by the regional anesthetics, so we usually utilize low doses of narcotics and tranquilizers for labor analgesia. Pudendal block and analgesic concentrations of nitrous oxide are utilized for delivery. If uterine relaxation is necessary for release of the trapped fetal head or for version and extraction, deep general halothane anesthesia with endotracheal intubation is recommended.

CAUDAL ANESTHESIA

Caudal anesthesia is performed by injecting a local anesthetic through the sacral hiatus, into the caudal canal. This canal is a continuation of the spinal canal, so that in effect the technique is a peridural block, as in lumbar epidural anesthesia. The block may be a single injection or continuous, like epidural. Segmental anesthesia cannot be performed, however. Caudal anesthesia is instituted when labor is well established. During the 1940s and 1950s it was considered the premier obstetric anesthetic, but by 1960 it was perceived that lumbar epidural anesthesia was superior. Since then epidural anesthesia has achieved dominance. Caudal anesthesia is more painful than epidural, more difficult, and higher doses of drug are utilized. There is some risk of needle misplacement and injection into the fetal head. It is rarely used now for obstetric anesthesia, but caudal block remains very useful for rectal surgery.

PARACERVICAL ANESTHESIA

Injection of a local anesthetic on either side of the cervix, into Frankenhäuser's ganglion, interrupts the pain paths from the uterus to the spinal cord. This is a paracervical block, and anesthesia of the uterus and cervix ensues. It is simple, safe for the mother, and effective. It achieved some popularity in the 1960s, but the high incidence of fetal bradycardia deterred many from its use. This complication has been shown to be true fetal distress, is probably caused by intoxication of the fetus by local anesthetic drug, and has caused this block to fall into disfavor for obstetrics.

PUDENDAL BLOCK

Pudendal anesthesia has long been a mainstay of obstetric practice. It is easily done, safe for the mother (unless there is intravascular injection), and provides perineal anesthesia, which may be adequate for multiparous births. Blood levels of local anesthetic are apparent in mother and neonate but are clinically insignificant. This block undoubtedly will remain a part of medical practice for years because of its simplicity.

SUGGESTED READING

Shnider SM, Levinson G. Anesthesia for obstetrics. 2nd ed. Baltimore: Williams & Wilkins, 1987.

THERAPEUTIC ABORTION

LINDSAY S. ALGER, M.D., F.A.C.O.G.

Obstetric convention divides pregnancy into three equal parts. For many years pregnancy termination methodologies were artificially separated into first and second trimester techniques. However, the difficulty and complication rates associated with any technique actually form a continuum, rising steadily with advancing gestation.

Prior to 16 weeks' gestation, vacuum aspiration, modified to allow extraction maneuvers during the early second trimester, is the procedure of choice. A termination that could be performed during this interval should never be delayed until later in the second trimester in order to facilitate instillation techniques. After 16 weeks, dilation and evacuation (D&E), intravaginal prostaglandin administration, or intra-amniotic instillation methods may be used, depending upon the operator's experience and skill and the patient's history.

INITIAL EVALUATION

The patient can generally be evaluated during a single outpatient visit. In addition to completing the history and physical examination, cervical culture samples for gonorrhea and chlamydia infection are taken. *Chlamydia* is the pathogen most frequently isolated and is associated with postoperative pelvic infection. Alternatively, cultures may be obtained at the time of the procedure; this requires scrupulous follow-up of results and the ability to contact the patient should they prove positive. A complete blood count, blood typing, and antibody screen are performed within 48 hours of the procedure. Additional studies may be indicated on the basis of medical history or patient age. Sonographic confirmation of gestational age is helpful in the second trimester, particularly if the patient is extremely obese, there is a discrepancy between the fetal size and dates, or the fundal height is near the umbilicus. The patient is counseled, the procedure explained, the operative permit signed, and preoperative instructions given. If the procedure is performed the following day, Laminaria can be inserted at this same visit to provide atraumatic cervical dilation.

DILATION AND EVACUATION BEFORE 16 WEEKS' GESTATION

The primary advantage of D&E (or suction curettage) is that in experienced hands it is associated with less morbidity and mortality than any other procedure, particularly during the first 16 weeks of gestation. There are fewer psychological ramifications and, because it is performed on an outpatient basis, it is cost-effective. There are no absolute contraindications to a D&E, since pregnancy and term delivery expose the patient to even greater risks. However, patients with heart disease, hypertension, or other medical problems should not have abortions in a non-hospital setting.

Technique

After first voiding, the patient is placed on the table in the dorsal lithotomy position and a pelvic examination is performed to confirm the size, position, and degree of flexion of the uterus. Catheterization is unnecessary and predisposes the patient to iatrogenic urinary tract infection. A Graves' speculum is introduced and the vagina prepared with an antiseptic solution. Local anesthesia is preferred. Use of general anesthesia is associated with a two- to fourfold increased risk of death as well as increased rates of hemorrhage, uterine perforation, and cervical laceration.

One ml of 1 percent chloroprocaine is injected into the cervix at the 12 o'clock position and a tenaculum placed at this site. A paracervical block using a total of 10 to 12 ml of 1 percent chloroprocaine is placed in increments at 3, 5, 7, and 9 o'clock. If poor patient cooperation necessitates general anesthesia, a paracervical block may still facilitate cervical dilation, particularly in the nulliparous woman. However, the use of Laminaria should eliminate the need for mechanical dilation. Fentanyl, 1 to 2 ml, administered intravenously over 2 minutes, reduces patient anxiety and alleviates discomfort from uterine cramping. The addition of atropine, 0.4 mg, prevents vasovagal symptoms.

Prior to 8 weeks' gestation, a No. 6 flexible suction catheter can be used. Its introduction may not require cervical dilation in the parous woman. Between 8 and 15 weeks, the catheter size is selected to correspond to the number of weeks' duration of the pregnancy. The use of Laminaria minimizes or more often eliminates the need for mechanical dilation of the cervix. If necessary, a suitable tapered dilator (e.g., Pratt's dilators) is used to dilate the endocervix to the same or slightly larger diameter as the chosen catheter. Placing a small amount of sterile lubricant on the tip may facilitate introduction of the catheter.

The uterus is not sounded, to avoid possible perforation. While applying cervical traction to straighten the uterine axis, the catheter is gently introduced until it just meets the top of the fundus. The hose is then connected, the vent closed, and suction applied. The catheter is withdrawn slowly as it is rotated back and forth through 360 degrees so that all surfaces are curetted. Suction is vented open each time the cannula is reinserted into the fundus. Rapid in and out movements are avoided while suction is applied.

With larger gestations the suction apparatus frequently becomes clogged with tissue. At this point an ovum or Sopher's forceps is introduced into the lower uterine segment to remove large obstructing fragments that have been brought down by the suction. It may be necessary to crush the fetal calvarium before it can be successfully removed. Rotating the forceps as it is withdrawn decreases the chance of cervical laceration. Once it appears that no further tissue remains within the uterine cavity, a sharp curettage is performed using the largest size curette the cervix will accept until the characteristic gritty resistance is felt. The suction catheter is introduced a final time, and the uterine walls can be felt to contract down around the tip. A final bimanual examination with uterine massage decreases postoperative uterine bleeding and verifies the absence of pelvic pathology.

In general, oxytocin is not required when the procedure is performed under local anesthesia. With the removal of the amniotic fluid the uterus tends to contract down, closing off the venous sinuses and decreasing the chances of perforation. Excessive uterine contractility may make it difficult to remove second-trimester fetal parts. However, if bleeding is brisk, oxytocin may decrease operative blood loss and increase accessibility of the products of conception, especially for procedures performed under general anesthesia. Uterine insensitivity at these gestations requires relatively high doses of oxytocin.

The uterine contents are now inspected to ensure that all major fetal parts are present. When terminating pregnancies of less than 8 weeks' gestation, fetal parts are not readily identified. To ensure that the conceptus has not been missed, the uterine contents can be floated in a basin containing saline. The characteristic frond-like appearance of villi may then be appreciated.

The patient is observed for 1 hour (2 or more hours after general anesthesia) and is then discharged accompanied by an adult. She is instructed to take her temperature twice a day for 5 days and to allow nothing per vagina for 2 weeks. If the patient has a temperature higher than 100° F, she must contact a physician. Acetaminophen is usually sufficient to treat postoperative discomfort. In the absence of hypertension, the patient is given a prescription for a six-dose methylergonovine maleate (Methergine, 0.2 mg) series. Antibiotics are not administered routinely because of possible associated minor complications, the potential for the emergence of resistant organisms, and cost factors. If the patient has a history of previous pelvic infection, evidence of cervicitis or limited access to medical care, a 3-day course of tetracycline initiated the day prior to the procedure may be considered. This should be sufficient to provide coverage for *Chlamydia* pending culture results in a high-risk population.

Laminaria. Cervical trauma or laceration is largely avoidable with the use of Laminaria tents. Although nulliparous patients can benefit from their use at any gestation, they are used routinely in all patients at 10 weeks or more of pregnancy. A single small or medium-size Laminaria is sufficient until 13 weeks' gestation. For larger gestations, two or more Laminaria are introduced side by side, taking care to ensure that the tips extend beyond the internal cervical os. A 4 × 4 in. sponge is used to hold them in place. Maximal dilation is achieved when these are inserted the day before the procedure, allowing 16 to 18 hours to elapse, but some benefit can be obtained within 4 hours of insertion. The recent development of synthetic tents may allow more rapid dilation using fewer tents of larger size. By placing a synthetic tent intracervically in the morning, adequate dilation can be achieved in approximately 4 hours, permitting completion of the procedure later the same day.

COMPLICATIONS

Hemorrhage, retained products of conception, infection, cervical laceration, anesthesia complications, uterine perforation, and, rarely, other visceral injury can occur.

Perforations made with a cervical dilator or small curette do not necessarily require operative treatment. The procedure may be completed cautiously and the patient observed postoperatively for evidence of intra-abdominal bleeding. When perforation is first recognized after the suction apparatus or grasping forceps has been used, laparoscopy is generally indicated. This enables the operator to assess the extent of injury and to complete the procedure under direct visualization. However, bowel injury cannot be definitely ruled out. The more advanced the gestation the larger the instruments used and the greater the likelihood of significant damage. Laparoscopy is usually inadequate in the second trimester and surgical exploration is required. If abdominal contents can be identified in the evacuated products, the operator should proceed directly to laparotomy.

TERMINATION OF PREGNANCY AFTER 16 WEEKS' GESTATION

Dilation and evacuation procedures may be performed throughout the second trimester with an associated morbidity and mortality that compares favorably with alternative techniques. Hospitalization time is reduced. The patient also generally experiences less discomfort and psychological distress, although when it is performed under local anesthesia the patient may be uncomfortably aware of the nature of the procedure.

The technique is modified to accommodate the larger fetus. Two sets of Laminaria should be used for late second-trimester terminations. The second set is inserted 8 to 24 hours after placing the initial tents. Although greater cervical dilation will be achieved when the first set is removed prior to placement of the second, it is frequently effective and more convenient to simply slide in new Laminaria next to the old ones. The amniotic fluid is completely aspirated before attempting to remove the remaining uterine contents, decreasing the possibility of perforation or amniotic fluid embolism. Specially designed instruments such as Bierer's forceps and an open-sided speculum may facilitate extraction of fetal parts. The forceps are not inserted beyond the lower uterine segment. When possible, the procedure can be performed under direct ultrasonographic visualization, reducing operating time and ensuring that no fetal parts remain within the uterine cavity. Investigators are currently exploring the use of intracervical vasopressin or surgical Pituitrin injection to minimize operative blood loss.

The disadvantage of D&E after 16 weeks' gestation is that until the operator becomes sufficiently experienced, there is an increased risk of hemorrhage, cervical laceration, uterine perforation, and maternal visceral injury. When it is performed under general anesthesia, there are the attendant anesthesia risks. Not inconsequentially, these procedures shift the emotional burden of late pregnancy termination from the patient to the physician and staff.

Prostaglandin Vaginal Suppositories

The use of intravaginal prostaglandin E_2 (PGE_2) suppositories provides a satisfactory alternative. Patients find the delivery route preferable to intra-amniotic instillation techniques; side effects are comparable, and the risk of serious morbidity is reduced. The interval to abortion averages 12 hours, and a 24-hour hospitalization is generally all that is required. Unlike in D&E or instillation procedures, Laminaria are not required (although they may decrease the time interval to delivery slightly). The local application of PGE_2 has a cervical ripening effect that facilitates dilation and reduces the risk of cervical laceration.

TECHNIQUE

An intravenous catheter is placed, and the patient's oral intake is limited to ice chips. The patient is premedicated with prochlorperazine (Compazine), 10 mg intramuscularly, and diphenoxylate hydrochloride with atropine sulfate (Lomotil), two tablets by mouth, which reduce the side effects of nausea and diarrhea to acceptable levels. These medications are repeated every 6 hours as necessary. A 20-mg PGE_2 suppository is introduced into the posterior vaginal fornix such that it lies against the cervix. Ambulation is discouraged for 1 hour after insertion. Subsequent suppositories are introduced every 3 to 4 hours, depending upon uterine contractility. Meperidine hydrochloride (Demerol), 50 to 75 mg, is administered intramuscularly, as necessary, to provide analgesia. Transient pyrexia frequently occurs but is self-limited reverting to pretreatment levels within 2 to 6 hours after administration is discontinued. Treatment is usually unnecessary if the patient is well hydrated. Once membrane rupture has occurred, it may be difficult to prevent washout of the medication. In the presence of adequate cervical ripening, a high-dose oxytocin infusion is therefore added using a physiologic saline solution starting at 100 mU per minute and increasing to 400 mU per minute as uterine response indicates.

With advanced gestations, the potential for delivery of a live-born fetus exists. This risk can be reduced substantially by instructing the patient not to bear down when she first senses rectal pressure and to wait until after she has been examined. The delay is usually sufficient to obviate the possibility of a live-born fetus for pregnancies of less than 20 weeks' duration. However, instillation techniques that ensure in utero fetal death may be preferable at 24 weeks' gestation.

The placenta is usually delivered spontaneously within 2 hours of fetal expulsion. During this period, administering an oxytocin infusion and asking the patient intermittently to bear down while sitting or squatting may hasten the process. After 2 hours the likelihood of infection or unacceptable blood loss rises, and the patient should be taken to the treatment room to expedite placental removal. Frequently, the placenta may be teased out intact using a ringed forceps. Any possible retained tissue should be removed with a large curette using intravenous fentanyl and, if necessary, a paracervical block for anesthesia. This should not require the use of an operating room or general anesthesia. When possible, a digital exploration of the uterine cavity while using the other hand abdominally to bring the fundus within reach completes the procedure.

PGE_2 suppositories should be used with caution in patients with a history of asthma, cardiovascular disease, history of a previous cesarean section, or renal or hepatic disease. They are contraindicated in the presence of active disease. However, if the patient becomes acutely symptomatic the suppository can be retrieved, an advantage over instillation techniques.

INTRA-AMNIOTIC INSTILLATION TECHNIQUES

Intra-amniotic infusion of hypertonic solutions such as saline or urea or of uterotonic agents such as prostaglandin $F_{2\alpha}$ is still the most commonly used technique for performing midtrimester abortions after 16 weeks' gestation in this country. However, it is invasive, requires Laminaria insertion, may require a repeat instillation, and can result in serious complications. Saline injection, on rare occasion, may cause uterine necrosis, coagulopathy, or maternal death. Instillation techniques are unlikely to succeed where PGE_2 suppositories have failed. Urea with $PGF_{2\alpha}$ has fewer serious complications associated with its use. It is most useful when it is necessary to terminate a pregnancy late in the second trimester due to fetal genetic or developmental abnormalities. It allows delivery of an intact fetus that permits confirmational studies while ensuring intrauterine demise prior to delivery. Since $PGF_{2\alpha}$ is no longer commercially available, other prostaglandins, e.g., carboprost tromethamine, must be substituted.

The Rh-Negative Patient

The D antigen is present in fetal tissue as early as the 40th day of gestation. Therefore, Rh_0 (D) immune globulin is administered postoperatively to all unsensitized Rh-negative patients prior to discharge. For pregnancies of 12 weeks' duration or less, 50 μg is used. Following second trimester procedures, 300 μg is recommended.

CONTRACEPTION

Oral contraception, when selected, is commenced 1 week following first-trimester and 2 weeks following mid-second-trimester procedures. Although it is a theoretical possibility, this early resumption does not appear to place the patient at major risk of developing thromboembolic disease.

VACUUM EXTRACTION

REIJO PUNNONEN, M.D.

The first successful vacuum extraction was performed by James Young Simpson in 1849. During the following 100 years, various models of extractors were constructed, but it was only in 1954 that the suction device introduced by Tage Malmström in Sweden was widely adopted in obstetric practice. The vacuum extractor gained popularity in many European countries but not in the United States. In certain centers around the world, the vacuum extractor has almost completely replaced the forceps.

EQUIPMENT

In Malmström's vacuum extractor, the metal suction cups are available in three sizes—40, 50, and 60 mm in diameter. The traction force is applied on the cup with a metal chain, which is passed through a rubber tube and terminates in a metal handle. The chain is fixed to the suction cup with a bottom plate and to the traction handle with a metal pin that passes through the chain. The apparatus is completed by a glass container connected to an electric suction pump.

The most popular vacuum extractor in use in the United States is the soft silicone device, which is considered less traumatic and easier to use than the old Malmström extractor. On the other hand, the traction force of this device is less than that of the metal cup. The fundamental operating principles of both devices are the same.

INDICATIONS

The primary indications for use of vacuum extraction is to a large extent identical to that for application of the forceps: to expedite delivery when progress has failed. In some situations, however, one of these instruments may be more helpful than the other. The main indications for vacuum extraction are as follows:

1. *Delay of the second stage of labor.* The most important causes of dysfunctional labor during the second stage are insufficient uterine contractions, cephalopelvic disproportion, and fetal malpresentation or malrotation. The vacuum extractor is a suitable instrument for delivery of a fetus in occiput posterior or occiput transverse position if there is no fetopelvic disproportion, the cervix is completely dilated, and the fetal head is fully engaged. If even a slight cephalopelvic disproportion is suspected, the use of strong traction force must be avoided.

2. *Fetal asphyxia during the second stage of labor.* The relatively long time needed to form the "chignon" places a limitation on the use of the Malmström extractor in acute fetal distress or asphyxia. In such cases, the silicone cup and especially the forceps may be more suitable.

3. *Maternal diseases* that may restrict expulsive efforts (certain cardiovascular, pulmonary, and neurologic diseases) or in which powerful pushing may be harmful or even dangerous for the mother (e.g., severe toxemia). Epidural anesthesia may also be a relatively common cause of the mother's inability to push during the second stage of labor.

The use of vacuum extraction has been advocated during the first stage of labor when the presenting part is in a high position and the cervix is not fully dilated. In general, however, this situation is no longer considered an indication for vacuum extraction.

The conditions for vacuum extraction are as follows:

1. The amniotic membranes are ruptured.
2. The cervix is completely dilated.
3. The possibility of cephalopelvic disproportion is ruled out.
4. The presenting part is vertex and engaged.
5. The possibility of significant deflection has been ruled out.
6. A major degree of fetal prematurity has been excluded.

Some deviations from these rules may be possible. The second twin, for instance, can be delivered by vacuum extractor even if the cervix is not completely dilated or the fetal head is unengaged. In this situation, a relatively small amount of suction is usually needed. In experienced hands a fetus with a fully engaged head with a thin rim of surrounding cervix may be delivered by vacuum extraction.

TECHNIQUE

The mother is placed in the lithotomy position. The bladder must be empty; catheterization is performed if needed. A pelvic examination is performed to rule out cephalopelvic disproportion and to determine the degree of cervical dilatation and the level and position of the head. Anesthesia is provided; usually local anesthesia is sufficient.

With the Malmström extractor, the largest possible cup should be used, as the traction force applied is proportional to the size of the cup. The cup is pressed strongly backward against the perineum and introduced into the vagina. The silicone cup is soft and can easily be folded and inserted through the vaginal introitus. The cup should be placed as near to the small fontanelle as possible, as this area offers the best conditions for attachment. Running a finger around the edge of the cup ensures that no maternal tissue is included in the cup.

When the Malmström extractor is used the vacuum pressure has usually been 0.7 to 0.8 atm. To provide a greater traction force or an extreme oblique traction for the correction of fetal malpresentation or malposition, the vacuum can be increased temporarily to 0.9 atm. However, the suction cup should be used with as low a vacuum as possible and for a relatively short period of time, since a high vacuum and a heavy traction force sometimes lead to a subgaleal hematoma. A well-formed artificial caput succedaneum filling the cup completely is essential to secure its adherence. The caput should be developed slowly by gradually increasing the vacuum by approximately 0.2 atm at 2-minute intervals. Thus a period of 5 to 10 minutes is needed for perfect adaptation between the scalp and the traction cup. This procedure is very important, and many failures with the Malmström extractor are due to the fact that the time for the procedure has been too short. On the other hand, in cases of fetal distress with a fully engaged head the time has been successfully shortened, with an immediate vacuum pressure of 0.7 atm followed directly by traction.

After creating a vacuum pressure of 0.2 to 0.4 atm, the position of the cup is rechecked. When the head follows with a slight traction, episiotomy has usually been performed but is not necessary in all cases. Traction is applied only during uterine contractions and while the patient is producing expulsive efforts. If the uterine contractions are insufficient, an intravenous infusion of oxytocin is given. It is important that the traction be directed in such a way that the fetal head follows the axis of the pelvis. During traction the examiner's left hand presses the suction cup and the fetal head backwards. This produces a resulting force in the direction of the pelvic axis made up of the driving force of the uterus, the traction force, and the posterior pressure of the head. This cooperation between the right tracting hand and the left posteriorly pressing hand is very important. The left hand must have permanent contact with the traction cup and the fetal head not only in order to exert posterior pressure but also to be able to follow the movements of the head and to correct any tendency of the cup to detach. After the child is delivered, the vacuum is released and the suction cup is detached. The total extraction time is usually 10 to 15 minutes. The suction cup should be applied to the fetal scalp for no longer than 30 minutes. If delivery does not occur within this period, another solution to the problem must be sought.

Using the soft silicone cup, the full vacuum can be created quickly and without interruption. Since this cup fits the fetal head irrespective of its size and shape, it is not necessary to wait for the development of a chignon. With the silicone cup the maximal vacuum pressure is 0.7–0.8 atm. Between uterine contractions the negative pressure can be reduced to a minimum and increased again immediately before the next traction.

The obstetrician using this technique also needs practice in the delivery of the infant's shoulders. Without experience with vacuum extraction and forceps deliveries, delivery of the shoulders may present difficulties in emergency, such as shoulder dystocia.

FAILURE

The most frequent complication of vacuum extraction is the detachment of the cup. This is usually due to the user's lack of experience with the instrument. Traction in the wrong direction, so that the angle of traction does not conform to the axis of the pelvis, is a common cause of detachment. Malposition or malpresentation of the fetus and weak uterine contractions as well as traction that is not synchronized with contractions may contribute to detachment. Another important cause of detachment of the cup is an undiagnosed fetopelvic disproportion. On the other hand, in such cases the detachment also serves as a safety valve, unlike the forceps, which allow unlimited force of traction. When the suction cup has been detached twice, reapplication is not longer indicated. Failure with the suction cup is not an indication for forceps but is always an indication for reevaluation of whether vaginal delivery is possible at all. In this situation, experience and deliberation are needed and the obstetric situation as a whole must be taken into account. Usually in such cases cesarean section is the best way of terminating the pregnancy.

MATERNAL COMPLICATIONS

Maternal complications consists mainly of vaginal and cervical tears, which are usually of minor clinical importance. In our recent comparative study with vacuum extractor and low forceps, severe birth canal traumas were uncommon and their frequency of occurrence was the same in vacuum and forceps deliveries. There were also no statistical differences between the vacuum and forceps groups as to extent of bleeding, fever, or length of hospital stay.

Unlike the forceps, a vacuum extractor does not encroach on the space in the birth canal and does not fix the head in a certain position. Usually a significantly lower maternal morbidity has been found after vacuum extraction than after forceps delivery. All our low forceps deliveries were performed without general anesthesia, which may have increased the gentleness of the procedure.

NEONATAL COMPLICATIONS

In all cases of Malmström extractor use, a pronounced artificial caput succedaneum develops; it usually disappears, however, in 1 to 2 days. In a review article, it was reported that a scalp abrasion or laceration occurred in 13 percent, cephalohematoma in 6 percent and intracranial hemorrhage in 0.35 percent of the infants born by vacuum extraction. In our study cephalohematomas and scalp lesions were significantly more common after vacuum extraction than in low forceps delivery, as was neonatal jaundice and clavicular fracture. Cerebral hemorrhage was diagnosed in two infants born by vacuum extraction but did not occur in the forceps deliveries. One infant had a cranial fracture, and in this case the vacuum extractor had been removed three times. Other neonatal complications were rare, and their incidence did not differ between the two groups. In this study fetal distress and protracted labor were equally common in vacuum and forceps groups. Neither the presentation and station of the fetal head at the start of extraction nor the length of the second stage of labor differed between the two groups. Forceps deliveries, however, were performed by a specialist more often than the vacuum extractions.

Different methods of instrumental delivery were compared by the electronic measurement of compression and traction during delivery. With the exception of when vacuum extraction was used, the overall duration of compression on the fetal head was less marked for instrumental than for normal delivery because of the shorter delivery times. With vacuum extraction the overall traction forces were significantly greater than those associated with any of the forceps methods used. In another study, however, it was concluded that the use of vacuum extraction during the second stage of labor lessened fetal depression. Comparison of the results of vacuum extraction and forceps delivery is very difficult, since many factors in addition to the delivery instrument may have contributed to the differences in the results of series.

Vacuum extractor and forceps have their respective places in the obstetric practice. Obstetricians must know the advantages and limitations of both of these instruments.

SUGGESTED READING

Greis JB, Bieniarz J, Scommegna A. Comparison of maternal and fetal effects of vacuum extraction with forceps or cesarean deliveries. Obstet Gynecol 1981; 57:571.

Katz Z, Lancet M, Dgani R, et al. The beneficial effect of vacuum extraction on the fetus. Acta Obstet Gynecol Scand 1982; 61:337.

Malmström T. Vacuum extractor—an obstetrical instrument. Acta Obstet Gynecol Scand 1954; Suppl 4:33.

Malmström T, Jansson I. Use of the vacuum extractor. In: Wulff GJL, ed. Clinical obstetrics and gynecology, forceps delivery. New York: Harper & Row, 1965:893.

Moolgaoker AS, Ahamed SO, Payne PR. A comparison of different methods of instrumental delivery based on electronic measurements of compression and traction. Obstet Gynecol 1979; 54:299.

Plauché WC. Fetal cranial injuries related to delivery with the Malmström vacuum extractor. Obstet Gynecol 1979; 53:750.

Punnonen R, Aro P, Kuukankorpi A, Pystynen P. Fetal and maternal effects of forceps and vacuum extraction. Br J Obstet Gynecol 1986; 93:1132.

Simpson JY. On a suction-tractor, or new mechanical power, as a substitute for the forceps in tedious labours. Edinburgh Monthly J Med Sci 1849; 32:556.

Sjöstedt JE. The vacuum extractor and forceps in obstetrics: a clinical study. Acta Obstet Gynecol Scand 1967; 46 Suppl 10:1–208.

BABIES DOE: PROBLEMS OF SEVERELY HANDICAPPED NEWBORN INFANTS

H. GORDON GREEN, M.D., M.P.H., F.A.A.P.

Although the nomenclature is relatively recent, the term "Babies Doe" does not refer to a new phenomenon. Physicians, midwives, nurses, and especially parents have been dealing with the problems of severely ill and handicapped newborn infants since the dawn of humanity.

In our society, the healing professions infrequently (and very privately) have allowed death to occur for severely damaged infants without active interference, even though a major tenet of our acknowledged medical tradition calls for making every effort to save an infant's life.

Such private decisions and processes are becoming rarer. The days of the independent, authoritarian, judgmental, and all-knowing physician have passed. Complexities of medical technology and knowledge, including the development of institutional newborn intensive care; constraints imposed by statutes, regulations, and interpretations; and a medically sophisticated population that increasingly demands a partner rather than a paternal relationship with professional caregivers, mandate a broader base for decision making. However knowledgeable one's personal or professional opinion, it remains just that, an opinion, to be considered in the context of the infant's total situation.

BACKGROUND

Following the well-publicized birth and subsequent withholding of corrective surgery for a child with Down syndrome and esophageal atresia in 1982, the United States Department of Health and Human Services acted under authority of Section 504 of the Rehabilitation Act of 1973 to investigate reports of alleged discriminatory failure to care for handicapped infants. The agency adopted a set of rules, since revised, to ensure that physicians and hospitals would not withhold treatment for seriously mentally and physically handicapped newborns. Subsequent developments have included the establishment of *infant care review committees* and *bioethics committees* at many institutions. Decisions regarding care of these babies are now scrutinized, both before and after the fact, and health care professionals who practice in these institutions have varying degrees of obligation to consult with and to involve others in decisions regarding patient management. Considerations have extended from the merely medical to include the ethical, legal, economic, and social aspects of each case. State-specific and institution-specific procedures have been developed to address the concerns of legislators, jurists, child advocacy groups, and others. It is within this context that contemporary management of these challenging cases must be carried out.

It is important to keep in mind, from initial diagnosis to resolution of the situation, the practices and procedures that are currently accepted as standard in the larger community. No matter how good the medical care provided, a lack of regard for others who may be procedurally involved (e.g., family members, hospital administrators, hospital chaplains, and bioethics committees) will almost certainly result in later problems that can consume vast amounts of time, energy, and emotional involvement. Under these circumstances, it is helpful to have a high degree of unanimity among the medical and nursing staff. Prescribed procedures must not be allowed to inhibit the provision of medical care as determined by the appropriate medical professionals. Some accommodation to bureaucratic procedures may be necessary, but it should supplement and not supplant clinical training, knowledge, and experience.

Difficult medical decisions must be made with full consideration given to both technical expertise and informed consent. There should be involvement of hospital staff, the patient's family and others as appropriate. An honest, sympathetic, and caring attitude should be in evidence at all times. As Waller and his associates have noted, in addition to the realistic presentation of the problems and their possible outcomes, there should be the promise of continued communication and therapeutic commitment, even in the most hopeless of cases. At no time should family members or staff feel that either care or caring is being withdrawn. When support for the patient is no longer possible or appropriate, support for the family (and sometimes the hospital staff) must continue to the end, and beyond.

MANAGEMENT PROCESSES

Management of severely ill or handicapped newborn infants must begin with an accurate and realistic *assessment* of medical and other problems. Observation of any defect in the neonate should result in close examination for other problems, since the existence of one malformation is often accompanied by other structural or functional abnormalities. A complete and accurate diagnosis is necessary for adequate prognosis. The systematic review of the infant should be documented fully, so that changes in his or her condition may be noted subsequently.

Such assessment may call for participation by other knowledgeable persons: medical consultants, nursing staff, and others with training and experience in making medical judgments. Inaccurate prognoses are major hindrances to satisfactory resolution of a basically unsatisfactory situation. Stevenson and coworkers have stated that "Difficult treatment decisions are often based on incomplete information or new diagnostic procedures, the meaning of which is not well understood." Thus the prognosis must frequently be guarded. Neither the patient's family nor the hospital staff is well served by faulty projections, either unduly pessimistic or overly optimistic ones. Encouraging maintenance of hope must be balanced against raising unrealistic expectations. Caregivers must retain the option to say, "We don't know."

Furthermore, the assessment may be a time-consuming process that is ongoing and dynamic rather than a one-time event. The true situation involving a given infant may unfold only gradually, over days or even months. It is important not to be locked in to a specific plan that later becomes untenable.

It is helpful to generate a problem list, which then should stimulate a comprehensive management plan that addresses each item on the list. Planning should be as thorough and inclusive as possible, involving consultants, institutions, and agencies, as appropriate. It is important, too, to maintain flexibility in the planning aspect to account for additional information, changing conditions, and revisions in case management options.

Participation by the baby's family should begin with the initial assessment and continue throughout resolution. When practical, one individual on the health care team may be designated to be the major source of family information. Any apparent conflicts or discrepancies in communications regarding the child's current condition and future plans often result in confusion and additional stress on family and friends. Slight differences in information tend to be greatly amplified and take on unjustified importance. These should be resolved, if possible, or the different options presented in a balanced, sensitive fashion with a minimum of jargon. Attending physicians must be aware that nurses often fulfill the de facto role of communicator and source, as a result of their constant presence in the nursery and the sometimes more frequent opportunity for parent contact.

To the extent that medical and nursing staff can present a uniformly supported program of action in relation to the infant's condition, the family will be inclined to develop confidence that care is being provided appropriately. It is important to develop consensus, when possible, among hospital staff. Any friction among the staff may result in situations that erode the sense of teamwork that is necessary for effective functioning of the unit on behalf of patients. Although all members may not necessarily agree, and matters of life and death are subject to strong ethical and moral pressures, the extent to which members of the health team can support each other in caring for these difficult cases is helpful in managing both the immediate case and all future cases with which they may be involved as a team.

The key to developing the infant care team (or perhaps any team) is *mutual respect*. No member should be allowed to express disdain for the feelings or opinions of others. The sensitivity of issues related to care of severely ill or defective newborns requires that extensive efforts be made to ensure that expressions of concern on the part of all involved are heard and given full consideration.

In these most difficult of family counseling sessions, one process that hospital staff have found helpful is the so-called "third person" technique. This allows presentation of materials and options that may be difficult to accept if placed on the basis of "we" or "you." For example, parents might be told that "Some families faced with this (type of problem) have felt that the chances of a child's surviving are so small that they have chosen to accept that any intervention would merely prolong the baby's dying. This was a difficult decision for them, but after the ordeal was over, they took some comfort from the fact that the child did not suffer for long." This allows the parents to express their concurrence or nonconcurrence with the information or option presented, in a less personal fashion, and allows the counselor to go on to deal with the feelings expressed. The counselor must be sensitive to subtleties and ambivalence in these interactions.

PARENTS: SEEKING PARENTS, SEEKING CONTROL

Some parents under the stress of a sick infant look for someone else to assume authority and to assume responsibility for decision making. If the physician does not fill this need, they may turn to other hospital staff, to religious leaders, to more assertive family or friends, or even to an article in a magazine for direction. It is important to maintain sensitivity to this need of distraught parents, so that inappropriate information may be countered by the best and most authoritative medical opinion available under these circumstances. A noncommittal recitation of options will leave these parents floundering. A more directive approach and the offering of detailed, specific recommendations may be helpful to such parents, who at this time of great stress in their lives actually need parenting themselves. Other resources (family, respected friends, clergy) then may be called on to bolster their confidence in their ability to deal with the challenges associated with parenting a severely ill infant. Reinforcement by consensus is often helpful in refocusing on the critical issues.

On the other hand, some parents (or one of the parents) may assume the role of absolute decision maker, rejecting authority and informed opinion. The best educational and informational efforts of professionals may go unheard as the sometimes desperate parents seek to assert control over their own lives and the life of their ill newborn child. In these cases, the child becomes a thing (property) over which parents struggle with medical authority and even with each other. Here, the directive approach may be counterproductive. A professional attitude of guidance and focus is less likely to foster resistance. The more secure physicians and nurses may, within limits and without compromising medical care standards, allow themselves to be manipulated for a period of time as parents adjust to the realities of the situation. Extensive efforts must be made to reach each parent, to understand the grief, rage, denial, fear, and ultimate sadness that provoke irrational actions and even hostility. The parent becomes a patient to be treated concurrently with the infant. An understanding of the need to control will allow health professionals to make extra efforts to channel the parent's energies toward a more productive effort. Again, involvement of others in sharing the burden may be critical to successful management. Respected friends, clergy, psychiatrists, medical social workers, and others may offer avenues of approach to parents who have lost effective communications with health professionals in the nursery.

It is important to keep in mind that the medical problems of the infant are not the only problems. Great stress is placed on the parents and even on the extended family. It may be helpful to acknowledge this fact early in the management process, pointing out to both parents that a severely ill infant's difficulties may create family stress; this may lead to problems between the parents, or it may draw them closer together. Articulating this unspoken fear sometimes makes it possible for them to deal with the prospect constructively. Such frank acknowledgment may lead to a renewed commitment, to a bonding between the parents, to a determination to "see this thing through together."

It is also worthwhile to acknowledge the need for external support at a time of fear, uncertainty, and grief. In attempts to be strong, one or both parents may resist outside counseling or help. The staff should recognize this denial of need for what it is. Guided discussion may lead to understanding and make it acceptable for anxious parents to seek support from community and religious groups, family, and friends. Support groups of other parents who have faced similar situations (e.g., trisomy groups, neural tube defect groups) may help to assure the family that their feelings are not unique but are appropriate and quite normal under the circumstances. It is helpful for parents to know that seeking such help is sanctioned by medical authority and is proper and even routine in these circumstances. It is not to be interpreted as a sign of weakness or an inability to cope.

CONTINUATION OR DISCONTINUATION OF THERAPY

The health care team has a duty to serve as an advocate for patients and their needs. In interacting with parents, administrators, third-party payers, and others, only the health professionals attending the infant must put the patient's interest above all else. The matter of clinical management of these complex and challenging cases is difficult, but a clear perspective on behalf of the patient is helpful in clearing the way through the thicket.

Discontinuation of intensive intervention for neonates who will never experience meaningful life is possible. The criterion for nontreatment or withdrawal of treatment should be the virtual certainty of death or lack of potential for a meaningful life. Of course, this latter concept is subject to interpretation. Even when intensive therapy is discontinued, however, it is important to maintain *care* until the situation is resolved.

The Ethics Committee of the Child Neurology Society has reported that it cannot specify valid criteria for determining brain death in newborn babies. A subsequent Task Force on Brain Death in Children concluded that, for babies under 6 months of age, there is *insufficient information for documenting the reliability of criteria for brain death*. Even more difficult is the *persistent vegetative state*, which is characterized by the presence of brainstem functions and the absence of cerebral functions. This is difficult to recognize in infants because of their immaturity and limited number of normal responses.

Coulter has reviewed the steps in resolving neurologic uncertainty regarding an infant's diagnosis and prognosis. The first step is to determine whether brain death is present. If the cause of the neurologic condition is known, there is no clinical evidence of any cerebral or brainstem function, and arteriography shows no evidence of intracranial blood flow, then the physician may discuss the possibility of organ donation with the family. Infants with brain death are medically and legally dead. Death may be declared but life support maintained until organ removal is completed. If organ transplantation is not contemplated, there is no reason to maintain life support.

If brain death cannot be diagnosed, one must next assess the extent and severity of illness or injury by the appropriate consultation and testing.

The third step is perhaps the most difficult, since it consists solely of hopeful expectancy. A clearer prognosis may become evident with the passage of time. Some infants with severe damage die. Others enter a vegetative state, whereas still others survive with varying degrees of mental and physical disability. It is therefore reasonable to maintain life support for several months after the onset of coma, to see whether the child will recover consciousness or enter the vegetative state. As long as diagnostic or prognostic uncertainty exists, one should wait, obtain more information, reconsider periodically (with appropriate consultation, including family and institutional bioethics committees), and err on the side of continued treatment. Infants who are not in a vegetative state and who are likely to survive, either with or without disability, should receive all appropriate medical treatment, since the outcome may be better than anticipated.

SUGGESTED READING

Coulter DL. Neurologic uncertainty in newborn intensive care. N Engl J Med 1987; 346:840–844.

Green HG. Caring and communicating: observations on 19 Baby Doe patients. Am J Dis Child 1985; 139:1082–1085.

Johnson DE, Thompson TR, Aroskar M, et al. 'Baby Doe' rules: there are alternatives. Am J Dis Child 1984; 138:523–529.

Stevenson DK, Ariagno RL, Kutner JS, et al. The 'Baby Doe' rule. JAMA 1986; 255:1909–1912.

Waller DA, Todres ID, Cassem NH, et al. Coping with poor prognosis in the pediatric intensive care unit: the Cassandra prophecy. Am J Dis Child 1979; 133:1121–1125.

BONDING AND ATTACHMENT

PAUL M. TAYLOR, M.D.

Secure reciprocal attachment between a child and his or her primary caregiver is necessary if the child is to achieve optimal social, emotional, and cognitive development. The primary caregiver and primary attachment figure is usually the mother (and will be assumed to be so in this chapter), although the father may play either of these roles or share them equally with the mother. Read "mother and/or father" for "mother" in much of what follows.

The terms "attachment" and "bonding" are used interchangeably by some authors, but I consider the mother's bonding experience to be one brief phase in the development of the enduring reciprocal emotional relationship between mother and child known as attachment. The mother's attachment to the infant begins at quickening or before; we infer this because mothers grieve for infants who die before birth; and grief does not occur without attachment. Maternal investment in the fetus usually grows throughout pregnancy and then usually increases abruptly on contact with the baby at birth. I reserve the term "bonding" for the mother's emotional response to the baby during their first contact. The infant contributes progressively more to the reciprocal attachment with the mother during the first year, and by the end of that year the quality of their relationship is generally considered to be set.

This discussion deals with how hospital caregivers may foster mother-infant attachment. For uncomplicated full-term deliveries, the main focus is on tactics and models of care that should facilitate the bonding experience. For infants who require intensive care, as typified by the premature infant, consideration is given to overcoming impediments to growth and expansion of the attachment to the infant that the mother has developed before birth.

THE HEALTHY INFANT

During Pregnancy. A late prenatal interview with the mother and father provides the pediatrician with information that may influence his or her care of the newborn and relationship with the parents. Among many other things, behaviors, fantasies, and thoughts indicating attachment to the infant are documented. The parents' active involvement with the fetus is indicated by "nesting" behaviors, which include preparation of the baby's quarters and purchasing clothes and equipment, expectations about gender, appearance, and temperament, and selection of names or narrowing down of list of names. Absence of these behaviors and thoughts is uncommon and requires a search for stressful life events or emotional disturbance sufficient to inhibit investment in the fetus. Such parents may benefit from psychological or psychiatric counseling and support and certainly require special attention and close monitoring after the baby is born.

During the Hospital Stay. Parents are better prepared to enjoy the bonding experience with their newborn infant if stress during labor and delivery is minimized. Mothers report that attempts to adapt to three social and physical environments in quick succession as they move from labor room to delivery room to recovery room distract them from the important work at hand. Stress is built into the traditional labor/delivery/recovery birthing system. It is archaic and should be abandoned. Labor, delivery, and recovery in a single "birthing" room avoids the disruptive moves that define the traditional system. The logical extension of the birthing room concept is to utilize the birthing room as the postpartum room. Single unit maternity care, in which the entire stay takes place in one room, is in successful operation in a growing number of hospitals in this country. It offers the ultimate hospital environment for facilitating early parent-infant contact and flexible rooming-in.

Immediately After Delivery. The healthy mother who has delivered at term with little or no medication and her healthy infant usually interact energetically during contact following delivery. Both are especially alert for about an hour and indeed appear primed for the rich interaction that features mutual visual regard and the infant's responses to the mother's voice, stroking, cuddling, and being put to the breast. This pattern of mother-newborn behavior is predictable and is recalled by mothers with great pleasure and satisfaction. For these and other reasons it has been proposed that extended early contact permanently enhances the quality of the mother-infant relationship. Although clinical trials do not support that hypothesis, I advocate extended contact between mother, father, and infant immediately after delivery, preferably in the privacy of a birthing room. This is a peak emotional experience for the parents. They are drawn to the infant by his or her appearance and behavior and are relieved, as they count fingers and toes, that theirs is the expected healthy baby, not the feared sick or malformed baby. Their observations are reinforced by the physician who examines the infant in their presence and finds him or her normal. I suspect that parents who have extended early contact with the infant are quicker to accept the infant in their arms in place of the infant each had fantasized during pregnancy—an important step in the attachment process.

Parents who have what I consider to be an optimal birth experience—natural delivery in a birthing room followed by extended contact with the baby and flexible-rooming-in—may experience intangible, if temporary, gains in family relationships. Some parents are convinced that extended early contact between mother and newborn baby is *essential* to their developing a healthy, adaptive relationship. Lay publications have presented that unproven notion repeatedly and effectively.

Perhaps one-quarter of families cannot enjoy an ideal birthing experience because of cesarean section delivery, prematurity, or other complications of the infant or the mother. These parents may worry that brief separation from the infant at birth has permanently constrained the quality of their relationship with the child. I regularly elicit parents' feeling about the other than planned delivery, and if they express concern, seek to assure them that the absence of early contact with the infant will not adversely affect their relationship with him or her or the child's development. I remind these mothers and fathers that separation of infants and parents at birth was the rule when they were born and that most children of their generation, adopted children, and premature infants and their parents have developed secure attachments. In other words, I attempt to erase a prophecy that may be self-fulfilling.

Given similar birthing experiences, not all mothers follow the same time course in feeling and demonstrating affection for the new baby. A delay of up to several days may occur before emotionally healthy mothers experience feelings of affection for the new infant; this has been termed maternal lag. Mismatches between the real and fantasized infant's gender, appearance, and temperament may contribute to the delay. During the lag period these mothers are usually aware of violating not only the caregivers' but also their own expectations that they should feel instant and rapturous affection for their infant.

Most mothers who are days slow in becoming enthusiastic about their infants eventually do develop secure and adaptive relationships with them. Until the mother begins to show investment in her infant, however, her behavior must raise the suspicion of possible stress within the family or of psychosis or depression. Close monitoring of her behavior and feelings toward and thoughts about the baby is thus essential. It is important that all caregivers carry out this monitoring discretely and sensitively and that they remain nonjudgmental and especially supportive of the mother.

THE INFANT SEPARATED FROM PARENTS

Brief Separation. Some 5 to 10 percent of full-term and larger premature infants are separated from their parents at birth for a few hours to a few days for observation and assessment. Although they are denied the experience of intense early contact, these parents generally accept their infants enthusiastically and comfortably when reunited with them. Their reassuring behavior with the baby should not be taken as evidence that they do not require special attention, however. A few hours of respiratory grunting or a low Dextrostix examination in an otherwise healthy full-term infant is medically trivial and yet may distress parents and cause them persistent anxiety about the infant. It is important to explain to the parents that the infant's problem was minor and is fully resolved. That message is delivered only after learning their perceptions and concerns about their baby and is followed by determining whether the parents heard the report accurately. A thorough physical examination of the infant in the parents' presence (where I feel *all* infant physicals should be done) goes a long way toward allaying their residual concerns. They may also be worried about the effects of early separation from the infant, as mentioned above, and this, too, should be addressed. The event should be reviewed at the first office visit to be sure that the mother and father have it in proper perspective and that they have no new questions about its effect on the infant.

Longer Separation. Prematures constitute the bulk of those infants who are kept in the hospital from birth. Retrospective studies show significant over-representation of premature infants in populations of infants who were abused or neglected or who failed to thrive without organic disease. With all their limitations, these data suggest that the quality of parent and premature infant attachment is at risk. Many effects of bearing and rearing a premature baby could contribute to an increased incidence of gross parenting failure—e.g., guilt; low self-esteem; physical, emotional, and financial stress; worry about the infant's health and potential; and relatively unrewarding social responses from the baby, at least early on. Discussion here is limited to facets of parents' experiences in the nursery that we can affect, in order to foster growth of their attachment to the infant.

Support for the parents of premature infants and the promoting of attachment are intertwined. Both tasks require awareness of the general reactions of parents to the birth of a premature baby and sensitivity to idiosyncratic expressions of their response to that crisis.

Mothers and fathers usually react to the birth of a preterm (often sick) infant with shock, denial, preoccupation with the baby's vulnerability, guilt, depression, and anger. These are reactions of grief, both for the loss of the expected healthy mature infant and in anticipation of the loss of their premature newborn. In addition, mothers experience a loss of self-esteem at having failed to carry the infant to term. We must also acknowledge that parents of premature infants are premature parents. I take it as a matter of course that the third trimester must be important for the psychological preparation for parenthood, probably especially so for the firstborn, just as it is for the infant's growth and development. We await systematic studies of how parents of premature infants compensate for the loss of this portion of the psychological adaptation to pregnancy.

Our overall goal is to promote growth of the attachment to the infant that the mother began to develop before birth. To reach that goal we must accomplish three specific tasks. We must intervene in a crisis to support the parents through the period of initial shock. We must also facilitate parents' dealing with their burdensome and threatening emotions. This is an ongoing effort, as is the process of encouraging the parents' direct and active involvement with the infant. Pediatricians, nurses and social workers operate as a team to accomplish these tasks.

CRISIS INTERVENTION AND COMMUNICATION

Parents can begin to cope with the crisis of the unexpected birth of a small, sick infant only after overcoming their perfectly natural denial of the situation. This requires that they be given sufficient information to acquire a cognitive grasp of the infant's condition and prognosis and a general idea of management plans and options.

The physician and parents are usually strangers, so that the pediatrician is starting from scratch, without the important background information a prenatal interview would have provided. In this situation, I start with three questions: (1) What have you heard about your baby? (2) Have you been in or visited an intensive care unit of any kind before? (3) Have you or others you know had any experience with sick babies?

The first question gets at what the parents know or think they know about their infant's condition. Knowledge of the parents' perceptions of the situation is the key to fruitful communication. A recital delivered in ignorance of their perceptions often fails to address specific concerns or correct misperceptions and may actually do more harm than good. The second and third questions tap direct or vicarious experiences with seriously ill patients, particularly infants, that may affect parents' perceptions of their infant's prognosis. For example, a parent whose father died in an intensive care unit while on a ventilator during treatment for silicosis will have that experience very much in mind as he watches his son being treated with artificial ventilation for hyaline membrane disease.

I follow these basic guidelines when talking with parents:

1. Stick to a few simple vital facts about the baby's condition. Stressed parents are easily overloaded with information.
2. No matter how intelligent or sophisticated the parents are, assume that they have heard the information incorrectly or not at all in their state of shock. Check that out by whatever ploy comes naturally—e.g., by asking them what they will tell their relatives about the baby's condition. Correct their perceptions as needed. Commence each conversation by determining the parents' perceptions of the infant's condition and what they have heard others tell them about him or her.
3. Avoid vivid modifiers. Stressed parents are in a state of heightened awareness in which terms such as "desperately sick" or "recovery would be miraculous" may be retained forever. This may cause anxiety about the child long after recovery and lead to that neurotic overprotection of the child which has been termed the "vulnerable child syndrome". The term "very sick," or perhaps even "sick," will do and yet will not compromise honesty.

PARENTS' FEELINGS

Parents have intense emotional responses to the birth of a preterm, often sick, infant and, as noted earlier, these best fit the category of grief reactions. Paradoxically, these very reactions that imply attachment to the infant may also inhibit the further development of attachment. Caregivers have a responsibility to assist parents in working through these expected feelings.

We must respect and accept the pace at which parents resolve these reactions to the preterm infant. That pace depends on many factors, including the infant's progress, the parents' prior experiences, education, intelligence, maturity, and emotional and temperamental make-up, and the extent to which they are mutually supportive and supported by family, friends, clergy, and hospital caregivers. It follows that we must get to know a good deal about individual parents in order to work effectively with them. Parents rarely fully trust the caregiver who cannot address them as individuals.

Parents often think that their overwhelming emotions are unique to them. Knowledge that their reactions are shared by almost all mothers and fathers of premature infants reassures them that they are not losing control of themselves and that their threatening, even incapacitating, emotional state is not permanent. Depression, guilt, and preoccupation with the infant are easy enough to spot and discuss. Anger, on the other hand, is infrequently expressed or even commented on by parents, and yet it is almost universal; when repressed, it contributes to depression. When the time seems right, I mention that many parents like themselves feel angry at what is happening, in order to legitimatize their discussion or expression of feelings of rage. This often helps.

INVOLVING PARENTS WITH PREMATURE INFANTS

Parents want to be with sick infants and most can be, even with increasing numbers of high-risk deliveries being performed in perinatal centers. Mothers become very anxious and depressed when newborn infants are transferred from the hospital in which they were born to perinatal centers; fathers' reports of visits to the infant, even when accompanied by pictures, do little to relieve their misery. We have had considerable experience, all positive, with prompt transfer of mothers from the hospital of birth to the perinatal center so that they can be near their sick infants.

Parents usually feel helpless and useless, if not underfoot, during their premature infant's first critical days in the neonatal intensive care unit. They get scant satisfaction from being welcome except during rounds and crisis situations and being permitted to touch the baby as long as they do not dislodge tubes or wires.

Several simple assignments provide parents with a sense of beginning to participate in the infant's care. For example, requesting mothers to pump their breasts sends the message that we expect the infant to survive and that he or she will soon need her milk for nutrition. Most parents can, with supervision, provide basic care such as diapering and tube feeding to critically ill, respirator-bound infants and gain a sense of being of real value to them. We can further their sense of usefulness to the baby by asking their assessment of his or her responses to environmental stimuli such as noise, light, and touch, so that the combinations the infant prefers can be provided and those he or she dislikes can be avoided.

Opportunities for parents to interact with and care for the infant escalate with improvement. Nurses should regularly solicit parents' input when devising care plans. Their observations should ideally form the basis for caregiving, contingent on the baby's behavioral cues, responses, and preferences. Examples include tailoring feedings and environmental and social stimulation to the infant's sleep-wake cycles and to his or her responses to caregiving activities. Having mothers take the lead in planning and refining important aspects of the convalescent infant's care enhances their sense of control and feeling of involvement with and attachment to the baby.

Ideally the mother should take increasing responsibility for planning and providing the infant's care as discharge time nears in preparation for the full responsibility she will assume when the infant goes home. Practically, however, traditional step-down or convalescent nurseries contiguous to neonatal intensive care units have neither enough nursing staff nor space to permit mothers and fathers to become comfortable with the full range of parenting activities. Until recently the best we could provide for parents before the baby's discharge was a day and a night caring for the infant alone in the "nesting room" next to the nursery.

The Transitional Infant Care Home

For the past several years we have offered parents the option of transferring their infant to a Transitional Infant Care Home for the days or weeks before taking him or her home. This large three-story house contains a spacious eight-bed nursery and separate ample rooms in which parents can care for the infant, cook, eat, take care of their other children, and sleep. The Home is staffed by selected nurses with neonatal intensive care unit and convalescent nursery experience and supervised by pediatricians who make rounds there daily. It is equipped and staffed to accept infants ranging from prematures convalescing uneventfully to those with chronic respiratory, central nervous system, or gastrointestinal problems. Parents have enthusiastically accepted this pleasant, "low-tech" facility and respond well to the staff's emphasis on promoting parents' caretaking skills and comfort with their infants. The Home accomplishes these goals and strengthens parents' relationships with their at-risk infants in the process.

IT TAKES TIME

The hours nurses, social workers, and physicians devote to supporting, informing, and counseling parents are not precisely countless, yet it is fair to say that we lose count of them during the premature infant's hospital stay. As a rule of thumb, I think that pediatricians should plan to spend as much time talking with parents as they spend providing or supervising the infant's medical care. A lot of time indeed, but if it contributes to the development of secure parent-infant attachment, it is time well spent.

COMPUTERIZED DATA BASES ON PERSONAL COMPUTERS

NEIL N. FINER, M.D., FRCPC

Although there have been numerous advances in perinatal medicine over the past 30 years, including the development of neonatal and perinatal intensive care units, our need to catalog patient demographic data, treatment, costs, and outcomes has not changed. Indeed, these achievements have led to an even greater requirement for the meticulous prospective audit of perinatal activities. Whereas under ideal circumstances prospective controlled collaborative trials are the mainstay of assessing the risks and benefits of any new form of therapy, prospective ongoing analysis within units of their own activity is often very revealing of trends and becomes the first step toward such controlled trials. All perinatal and neonatal units need to be aware of their year to year mortality and morbidity rates, and it is essential that cost containment, effective billing practices, and staffing requirements be known on a continuing basis. In the past, this has usually required one or several ward clerks or secretaries, and the use of hospital mainframe computers where available. For others, it requires the laborious manual calculation of statistics such as patient through-put, diagnoses, length of stay, and weight-specific mortality for monthly or yearly reporting purposes.

These data needs in perinatal medicine are not dissimilar from those of industry, involving extensive data processing, which led to the development of mainframe multitasking computers and data base management systems to provide a central information bank. Since the development of the original data base management systems (DBMS), which required huge computers and full-time programmers, the last decade has seen the development of personal computers that are far more powerful than the first generations of mainframes. In addition, software manufacturers have produced DBMS that are as sophisticated and powerful as programs currently running on mainframes. It is, therefore, now possible that the data processing needs of an active perinatal or neonatal unit can easily be met by such a system.

This discussion focuses on the use of the personal computer in data base applications. Institutions with minicomputers or mainframes usually have well-established systems groups in charge of such operations. In this environment, the end user (physician, nurse, or secretary) has little to do with the choice of software programs which are usually limited by the hardware, its design, implementation, or modification. In addition, the mainframe data base tends to be very technically oriented, thus making it very difficult for the first-time user to design and implement such a program.

The attraction of personal computers lies in their low cost, small size, and their ability to run literally thousands of programs. Although there are hundreds of models of personal-type computers on the market, the most popular have been the IBM, IBM compatibles (also known as "clones"), and the Apple. Because of the broader range of software originally available and the larger choice of competitive models resulting in lower prices, we have chosen to use the IBM-PC-type machines. The Apple Macintosh models are now becoming nearly as attractive and may be more user-friendly.

A data base is essentially a central information bank, and a DBMS is the collection of programs that allows manipulation of this information. This information is placed in data files, which can be considered two-dimensional tables composed of rows and columns. The rows represent records that are the essential units of a data base and in a neonatal or perinatal application would typically represent a single patient (Fig. 1). The columns represent fields that are the characteristics or attributes that you wish to describe for each patient. These fields can be numeric or text values of a specified or unspecified length, logical values, (true or false) or calculated values from the manipulation of other fields (e.g., TotCost = MDCost + HospCost, where MDCost is the total physician charges and HospCost is the total hospital charges). In this circumstance, the program will calculate the value of TotCost after MDCost and HospCost are entered for the patient. Sophisticated DBMS allow for very complex calculated field values such as the use of if...then...else logic. Thus, if hospital costs are $500 per day for the first 10 days and then fall to $300 per day, you may wish to have a field for HospCost that looks at the length of stay field (LOS), and the HospCost field could read as follows: IF LOS < 11 THEN LOS × 500 ELSE 5000 + ([LOS − 10] × 300).

The simplest programs that allow for the collection of data are *file managers*. These are single file systems, are relatively easy to learn to use, and are limited in the number of fields per record, characters per field, and number of records per file. In addition, queries are of the simplest format. The next level of sophistication involves programs that address multiple files, have more extensive search queries and report generators, and allow the creation of multiple indices that speed up searches. The most sophisticated programs, the *relational data base management systems*, offer all the above with the addition of a powerful programming language. This added feature is both the strength and weakness of these DBMS programs. In terms of its strength, the more sophisticated program allows for extensive data manipulation, is able to perform multiple detailed analyses with simple commands on one or more separate but related files (files having a common field), has extensive report-generating capability, and often includes as optional extras a word processor, a graphics package, and a spread sheet. In addition, there are fewer limitations regarding the number of records per file, the number of characters per field, and the system is limited only by the amount of computer storage capacity. In terms of weaknesses, such a program is more difficult to understand, especially for the inexperienced user, and requires a significant period of learning before one can take advantage of the power of the available routines. As the cost of software has decreased, most of these programs are now available for less than $700.

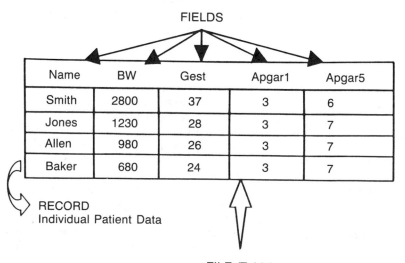

Figure 1 A representation of a table or file in a data base to show the significant components, which include the individual records composed of field entries (values for that patient of the requested item).

With the above information as a background, how does one decide on which program is best suited for one's own needs? Our own experience has suggested that most users tend to purchase the hardware before the software, and this is probably less than optimal. The ideal approach is to plan the data base well in advance on paper, decide on the most suitable software, and then decide on the hardware, which will include the actual computer, hard disk, monitor, and other accessories (see hardware section). The plan should encompass all of the information to be included, the format of this information, and how it will be used. Thus, all of the desired descriptive items should be listed and their data structure and format described, e.g., Mother's Name—(Text), Maternal Age—Years(#), Maternal Transport—Yes/No(Logic), including the actual size (number of characters or numbers) of each field. Perinatal data bases can be very large, with over 100 fields; this fact alone limits the selection of available programs. Since the interests and emphasis of the unit can change from year to year, there should be the option of adding or changing a field at a later date without having to rewrite the data base entirely. If all of the information can logically be placed in a single file, then do so, as multiple files unnecessarily complicate data retrieval, report generation, and data manipulation. On the other hand, if there are reasonably distinct applications and uses of certain of the entries, such as the development of a billing system with accounts receivable, or nursing recertification for specific procedures, then multiple files will speed up the use of these reasonably separate functions and allow for the most compact and efficient patient data base. Keep text entries to a minimum length to reduce storage requirements. In this regard, some of the newer programs actually allow variable length text in a given field and free up the remaining space, whereas most programs assign a specific number of spaces (characters) to every numeric or text field, whether they are filled or not. For example, if you directly enter the patient's final diagnosis, you may have to reserve a field of 124 characters or more for the complicated patient with multiple problems (e.g., prematurity, patent ductus arteriosus, necrotizing enterocolitis, hyaline membrane disease), although the majority of patients may only have one entry. In this circumstance, each record reserves 124 bytes for that field, which will increase the size of the file. *The use of numerical codes for each diagnosis, on the other hand, allows the same information to be entered into a much smaller space* (e.g., 1, 3, 5, 7, 12). This method, however, requires a dictionary of available diagnoses and does not allow for unusual entries.

Considerations such as these should precede the selection of a specific program. Other factors to consider are the ease of use, facilitated by help menus (descriptions of specific aspects of a program function that appear on screen when requested) or by menu-driven systems that allow the user to develop his or her query without having to master the programming language. Adequate documentation (usually too detailed and aimed at the experienced user) is essential. Other factors, such as the amount of computer memory required to run the program (usually 256 kilobytes or more), the ease of creating data entry forms and reports, the kinds of searches that can be performed, and the speed of operation of the program are all important in making a final choice of a DBMS. Because of the frequent need to calculate length of stay or duration of a given treatment, the program should perform calendar mathematics, allowing the calculation of intervals in days from one entered date to another. It is important to be able to add new fields or to change fields without having to re-enter data and to be able to transfer data from other programs that you may be using. Although industry is typically more interested in data security than are medical users, this aspect of programs is, nevertheless, important to consider. For example, if your data base contains entries regarding patient billings, nursing certification, or other information considered to be confidential, you may wish to restrict access to this area of the data base to certain individuals. More important, in our experience, is the ability to allow free access to most of the information so that house staff, nursing, and secretarial staff can obtain the information while restricting their ability to write in new data or to accidentally erase existing information (so easily done). Although there may be many other factors that enter into the decision as to which DBMS program is ideal for your needs, these are some of the more important considerations. The more desirable attributes of a data base program are shown in Figure 2. There are always current reviews of these DBMSs in the computer literature (*PC Magazine*, *PC World*), and these and other reviews should be consulted for a specific objective evaluation of any program before making a final decision.

HARDWARE

The development of personal computer "clones" has led to drastic reductions in price. The introduction of the 80286 processor (e.g., IBM-AT and clones, Compaq 286) has quadrupled speed while maintaining compatibility with existing software, and the more recent 80386 processor provides mainframe performance in a desktop machine. Since it is now possible to purchase a 80286 based machine for under $3,000, such models currently offer the best value. Essential items include a clock, serial and parallel ports, at least 640 kilobytes of RAM (random access memory), and a graphics card. Although it is possible to develop large data bases using floppy disks, (capacity = 360 kilobytes), this is not recommended. The use of floppies is cumbersome, time-consuming, and limits the useful size of your files. Hard disks are now very inexpensive, and we believe that a minimum of 20 megabytes is required for effective DBMS programs. Our own neonatal data base requires approximately 1 megabyte per year, and the programs themselves often require up to 5 megabytes of disk space. Do not forget that all hard disks are not created equal, and DBMSs are disk labor-intensive. Examine the operating characteristics of available units and look for units that automatically park the disk recording heads on a powerdown or after a period of nonuse and have a rapid average access time (= <40 msec). We would further strongly recommend the purchase of an independent medium for back-up (against disk data disasters), such

Neonatal Data Base

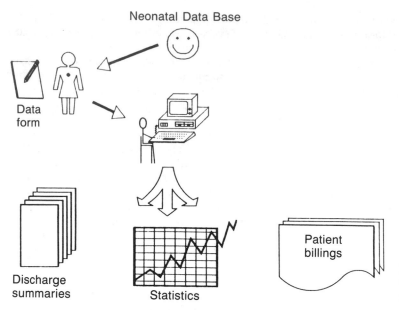

Data form

Discharge summaries

Statistics

Patient billings

Figure 2   A schematic representation of some of the more important features to consider in evaluating DBMSs.

as a tape back-up that can either be installed directly into the computer or be a stand-alone peripheral. Such a device allows quick back-up of very large files and protects your data from being accidentally erased or damaged. In addition, most warranties for computers are short term, and hardware problems are inevitable. As a result, consideration should be given to long-term service contracts.

SOFTWARE

Although it is beyond the scope of this discussion to review in depth all of the available programs, at least three products are widely used, powerful, and similar in price and concept, each with specific unique characteristics that are an advantage in specific situations. These are dBASE III Plus (Ashton-Tate), Knowledge Man (Micro Database Systems), and R:BASE System V (Microrim). Each of these products has a powerful programing language that makes it very flexible but at the same time somewhat formidable for an initial user. Whereas dBASE III Plus allows up to 254 characters per field and 4,000 characters per record, R:Base System V limits fields and records to 4,096 characters, and Knowledge Man allows up to 65,535 characters per field or record. dBASE III Plus allows 128 fields per record, somewhat restrictive for a large single table perinatal data base, compared with 400 for the R:BASE System V and 255 for Knowledge Man. Of these programs, dBASE III Plus appears to be the fastest, R:BASE System V has the most user-friendly and complete menu-driven system, and Knowledge Man has one of the strongest and most sophisticated program languages. All require at least 256 kilobytes of memory, and all should be used with a hard disk. These programs are only a few of those available, but all three are well supported by their manufacturers, undergo frequent updates, have been extensively reviewed in the computer literature, and are powerful and sophisticated enough to handle almost any data base application.

PRACTICAL USE

Now that we have discussed the basics of DBMS programs, it would be appropriate to demonstrate the use of such applications in perinatal medicine (Fig. 3). After you have chosen appropriate software and hardware, designed your data base, and successfully entered patient information, what use can be made of the information? For any given patient, the complete record is essentially a summary of the perinatal course, although in a poorly readable form. Since discharge summaries are a universal requirement, they can be generated by designing a program either within your DBMS program or using a simple basic program. This program will read the relevant fields and essentially "fill in the blanks" on a discharge summary, creating an individual document for each patient. You can add specific comments as desired and make such a report as detailed or brief as is your custom. All of this can be done within a DBMS, or such a report can be imported into your word processing program for any modifications. The advantage of this system is that while in one way or another we all review the chart while dictating a summary, this review differs with the individual, and its result is the summary, which is usually not objective enough to serve as a source for each diagnosis, treatment, or complication. The data base, however serves all of these functions, and the discharge summary is a bonus. If patient or hospital billings are being generated from the unit, the information required for submission of these is usually already available in the data base, or should be, if this is a requirement. In this circumstance, a separate file or table for billing information that contains the appropriate fees for procedures and hospital and physician charges could link with the main patient file and match diagnoses and length of stay with billing charges. The appropriate forms could then be *automatically* produced using the forms generator of the DBMS. Accounts receivable and ledgers are standard functions in the more sophisticated programs.

Data Base Programs

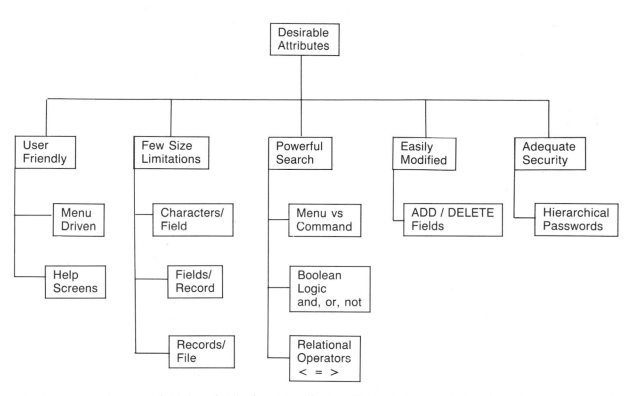

Figure 3 An overview of a neonatal data base that involves data collection using forms that contain the relevant information, usually initially completed by the caretakers. This is then checked and entered into the computer and can subsequently be questioned to produce a variety of reports and statistics.

All perinatal units need to audit their own activity, and yearly or monthly reports of patient through-put, length of stay, mortality, morbidity, and infections are easily produced using such a DBMS. Most of the top-end programs include graphics modules, so that charts and graphs are easily generated from the information in the data base.

As an example the following single-line command in our own data base—"**select name, bw, gest, ivhgr, mvent from bab86 for bw <1000, dead=false, Mvent>10, ivhgr>2, ropgr=0, order by az bw**"—will produce a list. This includes the patient's name, birth weight, gestational age, intraventricular hemorrhagic grade, and length in days of mechanical ventilation sorted in ascending order of birth weight of all infants under 1,000 g birth weight, and who survived, who required mechanical ventilation for more than 10 days, had an intraventricular hemorrhage of grade 3 or higher, and who did not have evidence of retinopathy of prematurity. In addition, the averages for each of these fields is calculated.

Special files can be created that stack several such commands and produce tables of mortality by birth weight or gestation. As can be seen, very detailed queries can be addressed to such a system, and reviewing a unit's ex-perience with a given diagnosis or treatment complication is relatively simple. All of the above obviously depends on having previously appropriately planned your data base and on the relevant information having been accurately entered.

There are a number of recommendations that we would make, based on our experience using personal computers for a number of perinatal applications, the most frequent of which has involved data base management.

1. Always *make copies of your data* on a regular basis. This should be done to floppy disks, to media (tape back-up), or to another hard drive. Once a data base is installed and operational, the information contained is invaluable. Using back-up of floppies as well as to a tape or another hard disk allows you to use your data on another computer in case you experience an equipment failure.
2. *Use an uninterruptable power source*, since voltage surges from unprotected power sources can erase your data, and temporary power losses will erase all data in the memory.
3. Have *as few operators as possible* directly using the

system. Use program security passwords so that intermittent users can query the system but cannot erase or alter the information ("read only" mode).

4. Once you have begun to work with a given program, *avoid the temptation to change* to another. Software development is constantly occurring, and newer tends to look better. This appearance is misleading, and once you have progressed on the learning curve of your particular program, *you will achieve more by pushing your current program to its limits than by starting fresh with a new product*. Any well-established program is frequently updated, and software support is usually only a phone call away.

One of the advantages of using personal computers and proprietary software for perinatal data bases is the ability to develop relatively uniform methods of collecting information that can then be shared between units. It is hoped that such useful sharing of information would form the basis for future collaborative trials to answer important questions regarding patient management.

SUGGESTED READING

Glossbrenner A. How to buy software: the master guide to picking the right program. New York: St. Martin's Press, 1984.
Kruglinski D. Database management systems MS-DOS: evaluating MS-DOS data base software. Berkeley, CA: Osborne McGraw-Hill, 1986.

DIAGNOSIS-RELATED GROUPS

RONALD L. POLAND, M.D.

The Health Care Financing Administration (HCFA) has developed a prospective payment system for reimbursing hospitals for the care of Medicaid and Medicare admissions. This system was designed to provide incentives for cost containment or reduction that are not found in the traditional retrospective cost reimbursement systems. The prospective payment system (PPS) is based on a classification of patients discharged from the hospital known as diagnosis-related groups (DRGs). DRGs are an expansion of 23 medical diagnostic categories (MDCs). MDCs are similar to the classification of medical conditions (primarily by organ system) found in the *Index Medicus*. DRGs are subclassifications of MDCs based on factors such as specific diagnosis, age of the patient, major surgical or diagnostic procedures, and discharge status that modify the length of stay and the average consumption of resources. Of the 470 DRGs, each hospital discharge must be categorized into just one.

HISTORICAL PERSPECTIVE

The DRG system was developed by Fetter, Thompson, and their associates at Yale University in the 1970s as a means of making comparisons of the quality and efficiency of care among hospitals. The Tax Equity and Fiscal Responsibility Act, PL 97-248, was passed in 1982 mandating the development of a prospective payment system. The DRG system was seen as a good model on which to base a prospective payment system, and it had undergone some verification by 1982. The following year PL 98-21 (a Social Security reform bill) was passed. It provided for the implementation of the PPS based on the DRGs developed at Yale. The bill represented a very rapid transformation of theory to law. The adoption of this revolutionary new method of payment for hospital care was motivated by a persistently high rate of inflation in the cost of hospital care for Medicare recipients (18 percent per year from 1979 to 1982) that was three times that of the general inflation rate in the United States. The PPS was piloted by the Health Care Financing Administration in New Jersey, and the DRG classification system was modified and expanded to the present number of categories based on that experience. A prospective payment system based on DRGs has now been implemented widely for Medicare and Medicaid programs.

HOW DRGs ARE USED

Hospital Reimbursement

In general, hospitals are reimbursed with a fixed rate for each discharge categorized under a particular DRG. The formula for determining the price includes the average number of hospital days expected and the average consumption of hospital resources for patients fitting into that DRG. These average statistics have been derived from large data bases primarily amassed by the Medicare system. *Data for perinatal events and for the hospitalization of infants and children were either not included in the planning process or were obtained from smaller data bases.* In addition, each hospital was assigned a predetermined institution-specific cost correction factor established by that hospital's operating expenditures for its mix of DRGs in an index year. This latter correction tends to adjust for area of the country, differences in local wage structures and costs of supplies, type of population served, and other factors that may affect expenditures for care in that hospital. In time, the correction factor will become a regional one instead of a hospital-specific one.

The method of classification of discharges into DRGs is not left entirely to the discretion of the institutions or physicians. The system does not allow institutions to classify their discharges in a subjective or biased manner. When a patient is discharged from the hospital, the diagnoses and procedures are coded on the face sheet using the International Classification of Diseases (ICD). There are more than 12,000 diagnostic codes and 4,000 procedure codes in the ICD. *The ICD codes on the front sheet of the medical record are analyzed by the specialized computer program called a "grouper," which is approved by the payer.* This computer program assigns a single DRG category to the patient's hospitalization based on the ICD codes and other information such as the age of the patient and his or her status at discharge. The DRG, in turn, determines the dollar value that Medicare or Medicaid assigns to that hospitalization.

Reimbursement for patients fitting into a particular DRG is the same whether they develop complications or not: whether they stay in the hospital one day or 100 days; whether they have 10 diagnostic tests or 1,000. This single price per DRG approach to compensation was designed to reward hospitals that minimize the length of hospital stay and the utilization of resources (e.g., services, diagnostic tests) for patients. The resultant savings can contribute to a "profit margin" for the institution but may lead to a gradual reduction in the price of the DRG. *The financial incentives to the hospital to limit expenditures for patient care are supposed to be offset by the ethical behavior of the physicians, by internal and external quality assurance programs, and by the threat of malpractice judgments that might result from inadequate care.*

In the PPS, low-risk short stays such as those associated with a normal vaginal delivery reimburse hospitals with an amount exceeding expenditures, whereas catastrophic illnesses such as extreme prematurity with bronchopulmonary dysplasia represent significant financial burdens for hospitals. The mix of patients and of DRGs determines the overall financial performance of the institution participating in the PPS. Currently, the Medicare system and several state Medicaid programs have adopted a PPS based on DRGs as their method of hospital reimbursement. The individual states have adopted modifications to the original federal proposal designed to correct for deficiencies in the original system, to meet local needs, and to accommodate for local conditions. For example, Michigan expanded the DRG coding system for neonates to pay more to tertiary or regional centers for a particular DRG than is paid to a level I or level II institution. This modification, however, still does not pay for the costs of care in a tertiary children's hospital environment. Others are working on a subclassification that considers a measure of severity. With these modifications, the prediction of actual costs might become more accurate and the variation in costs within a category should become more narrow or discrete.

The PPS does include a mechanism designed to adjust for very unusual or catastrophic illnesses. As previously noted, each DRG is rated using the average length of stay and the average value of resource consumption. In addition, an "outlier" length of stay is computed, which is designed to include the lengths of stay for 94 to 95 percent of patients categorized in that DRG. For example, the original federal proposal allows an average length of stay of 17.9 days for infants weighing less than 1,000 g at birth who survive (DRG No. 386) and an outlier length of stay of 38 days. This assumes that fewer than 5 percent of infants in that DRG will be hospitalized longer than 38 days. Reimbursement for the remaining 4 to 6 percent of patients with lengths of hospital stay beyond the outlier value includes the DRG figure plus 60 percent of the average

daily cost of patient care in the hospital per day for each day of hospitalization beyond the outlier length of stay. In this way, unusual catastrophic illnesses are supposed to be accounted for. However, hospitals that specialize in the care of the very ill or that act as regional centers for tertiary care often serve a population with more than 6 percent of these kinds of patients. Some states have made adjustments for such institutions to maintain regional programs and academic centers with levels of care appropriate to the needs of the region.

The above example demonstrates another problem with the federal proposal. No infant weighing less than 1,000 g at birth is discharged alive from the hospital in less than 18 or 38 days. The "averages" published by the federal government were based on geometric means. The geometric mean is the antilog of the average of the logs of lengths of stay and is always smaller than the arithmetic mean or the simple average. The geometric mean is traditionally used to express serum titers and dose-response data and is an appropriate statistic to use when the distribution of the logs of a measure is normal. There is no justification for the use of the geometric mean for the purpose of estimating the central tendency of lengths of stay except to minimize payments. The State of Michigan Medicaid system has recognized this problem and recalculated its DRG lengths of stay using the arithmetic mean.

Kinds of Data Emanating from the DRG System

Many hospitals that are reimbursed by a PPS such as the one described here have developed systems to track their internal costs for each DRG. The simplest data to collect are the lengths of stay. In addition, many hospitals now compile information about the consumption of all resources, including diagnostic tests, medications, other treatments, and personnel time. They are then able to recognize which DRGs cost the hospital less than the PRS pays ("winners") and which cost more than the reimbursement ("losers"). Such summary information can be tracked by the medical department, by the practice group, or by the individual physician. The hospital can then track cost differences between groups or individuals and identify the components of care that make up the differences in costs. This information might be used, then, to evaluate the utility and effectiveness of higher cost versus the lower cost treatment schemes.

Impact on Hospital Planning

When the leadership of a hospital learns that a particular DRG is always in the loser category regardless of attempts to manage it more efficiently, certain value judgments concerning the policy of the institution may be made. Can the hospital afford to offer services appropriate to that DRG? Can the unreimbursed costs of that DRG be offset adequately by "winner" DRGs or by other income? *Should patients with "loser" diagnoses be redirected to other institutions?* Can the hospital influence modifications in the management of the PPS in that state or continue to participate in the PPS? How can the institution obtain the cooperation of its medical staff in reducing the costs of a DRG or eliminating it from the array of services offered at that institution?

Impact of DRGs on Patient Management

A prospective payment system provides opportunities for physicians to review styles of patient management and the value of the various diagnostic and therapeutic maneuvers that we employ. We can obtain comparisons of resource consumption (including number of hospital days, diagnostic tests, and treatments) between our own practice and that of others in the same environment for patients who are grouped in a single DRG. We can make comparisons of outcomes and evaluate how the results of tests affect the care of patients. When one finds that a particular diagnostic procedure is done routinely in one practice but not in another, the value of that procedure comes into question. It might be shown that outcome is favorably altered by the use of the procedure or that the procedure shortens or improves the diagnostic process. It might also be shown that a routinely ordered procedure is not cost-effective. If retrospective analysis does not provide a clear answer about the utility of certain maneuvers, prospective studies should be undertaken.

In this era of prospective payment systems, students of medicine should always be asked a follow-up question after the common one of "Did you obtain a _____ ?" The appropriate follow-up question for our students and for ourselves should be "Why?" When we order tests, we need to anticipate our response to all possible results. If an abnormal result will lead only to a repeat of the test, since abnormality is not expected and will not be believed, then perhaps we should forego having it done in the first place. *We need to know how often an abnormal result is found in a particular set of circumstances and whether it leads to a modification of the care given.* If the course of treatment will not be altered after the result is known, then the test has no real value. If we spend more time evaluating the need for the tests and procedures we order, we may wind up spending less of the nation's resources for care without compromising the quality of that care.

Hospital Privileges and Employment of Physicians

A logical extension of the uses of the DRG-related data already noted might be the use of such information in the process of medical staff appointments and employment of physicians in a practice environment. If the financial well-being of an institution depends substantially on the efficiency of its medical staff's use of resources, efficiency is an attribute that might be added to the list of a physician's personal qualifications used to decide about staff appointments. If a physician is known to be artful, knowledgeable, ethical, kind, stable, and effective but he or she practices in such a way that the cost per DRG is much above the norm, hospital privileges for that individual might be judged too expensive for a given institution, and HMOs and group practices might hesitate to employ such a physician.

FUTURE DEVELOPMENTS

It is possible that medical insurance carriers other than Medicare and Medicaid may adopt the PPS if it is shown that the goals of the system have been achieved. In addition, a similar system has been proposed for the reimbursement of physicians. Since the current system has been shown to fall short of equity in many areas and the PPS is undergoing extensive modifications as experience with it accumulates, it is possible that the PPS might become yet another boondoggle in the history of health care financing. The whole concept of a PPS based on DRGs may evolve sufficiently to meet the needs and goals of society or it may eventually be supplanted by a system of capitation with its own unique problems. In the meantime, we can take the present opportunity to look at what we do for patients with new eyes, to reevaluate our routines and methods, and to separate the effective from the merely traditional. In this way, we can all contribute to reducing the monetary costs of medical care and other burdens we impose on our patients without compromising the quality and outcomes of our care.

FLUID THERAPY

STEVEN J. WASSNER, M.D., F.A.A.P.

Several methods are available for the determination of fluid therapy in the neonatal period. The method described here utilizes a factorial approach; it is applicable to all age groups and is presented here with modifications for the special anatomy, physiology, and circumstances present during the neonatal period. There is general agreement that requirements for fluid therapy are best described on the basis of caloric needs (per 100 kcal intake). On a practical level, however, fluid orders are most often calculated in the neonatal period per kilogram body weight. Both schemes are noted here.

The factorial method seeks to identify each component of ongoing fluid gain or loss by the infant. The arithmetic sum of all gains and losses equals fluid balance. Let us leave aside for now the question of whether there are situations in which that sum should be positive, negative, or zero. Water is gained by the infant through dietary intake or parenteral therapy. Under normal circumstances there are three sources of water loss: insensible water loss, renal water loss, and stool loss. Other less common sources of water loss include perspiration, nasogastric drainage, or the creation of ileostomies or colostomies. Perspiration is uncommon in early infancy, since the eccrine sweat glands are still immature. The other, nonphysiologic losses are not dealt with here, except to note their occurrence and that, if present, they must be taken into account in the determination of fluid and electrolyte balance.

INSENSIBLE WATER LOSS

Insensible water loss may be divided into two subcategories: water lost by evaporation through the skin and water lost by evaporation through the alveoli. Insensible water loss from the skin serves an important cooling function for the organism. In the basal state, a significant percentage of the heat generated by the body is derived from the function of the four metabolically active organs: the brain, heart, liver, and kidneys. Infants have less body fat and muscle than older children and adults, so that these four organs form a higher percentage of total body weight. A portion of this energy is transferred to water to convert it from a liquid to a vapor. This heat, equal to 0.58 kcal per milliliter of water, is "latent heat of vaporization." Since infants have a higher rate of energy production, they also have higher rates of insensible water loss (per kilogram body weight).

In addition to the presence of higher metabolic rates, insensible water loss through the skin is further increased in newborn infants, particularly those born prematurely (Table 1). When factored for body mass, the surface area of infants is significantly greater than that of adults. This allows evaporation to take place over a much larger relative surface area, so that evaporative losses are relatively greater than those seen in adults. Infants, particularly premature infants, have significantly less subcutaneous fat. This decreases their insulation and increases heat transfer to the epidermis. The skin of the infant is thinner than that of the adult and, in addition, the cornified layer is less developed. All these factors increase the passage of water through the skin and enhance evaporative losses.

Under normal circumstances, water lost through the alveoli may constitute up to one-third of the total insensible water loss. The quantity of water lost by this route is related to temperature and humidity differences between the ambient atmosphere and the alveoli as well as to the infant's minute ventilation. The amount of water lost in this manner may be minimized, or even eliminated, by use of modern respiratory support equipment that is designed to provide temperature-controlled and fully humidified air mixtures.

It is clear that the younger, the more premature, and the more stressed the infant, the higher these losses be-

TABLE 1 Causes of Increased Insensible Water Loss Through the Skin of Newborn Infants

Increased surface area/unit body mass
Decreased subcutaneous fat tissue
Thin epidermis
Increased permeability of the epidermis

TABLE 2 Estimates of Insensible Water Loss at Different Body Weights*

Body Weight (g)	Insensible Water Loss (ml/kg/day)
< 1,000	60–70
1,000–1,250	60–65
1,251–1,500	30–45
1,501–1,750	15–30
1,751–2,000	15–20

* Infants in a thermoneutral environment during the first week of life.

come when measured on a per kilogram basis. Table 2 notes current estimates of insensible water loss for infants of different weights.

STOOL WATER LOSS

Under most circumstances, the amount of water lost through the stool is relatively small. For the first few days of life, until the infant starts stooling on a regular basis, these losses may be negligible. Thereafter, in the absence of diarrhea, stool water losses are in the range of 7 to 10 ml per kilogram or 5 to 7 ml per 100 kcal per day.

RENAL WATER LOSS

The purpose of the kidneys is to maintain the internal milieu for fluid, electrolytes, and metabolic wastes. During gestation, the placenta functions in place of the fetal kidneys, so that electrolyte and osmolar status is normal, even for infants born without kidneys. Immediately after birth, a coordinated series of events occurs that leads to a decrease in renal vascular resistance, an increase in renal blood flow, and an increase in the glomerular filtration rate (GFR). GFR increases throughout infancy, reaching adult values (again factored for size or surface area) only by 18 to 24 months of age. In addition to differences in GFR, there are also significant differences in tubular function between infants and adults. The most important of these involve the ability to concentrate urine, as well as the reabsorption of sodium, bicarbonate, and glucose.

Even premature infants are able to excrete a fully dilute urine. The total amount of water that they can excrete is, however, limited by their lower GFR. Unlike dilution, there is a major difference between the infant and adult in urinary concentration. Whereas normal adults are able to concentrate urine to the range of 1,000 to 1,300 mOsm per kilogram water, it is well established that infants are unable to concentrate their urine beyond 600 to 800 mOsm per kilogram water. In practical terms, this means that an infant must void approximately twice the volume of an adult in order to excrete the same quantity of solute. Although this appears to be a significant disadvantage, it must be remembered that, from an evolutionary point of view, infants were designed to ingest breast milk, a low osmolar formula. Normal infants ingesting this formula have no difficulty excreting water and solute with osmolarities well within their accessible ranges. It is only with the advent of modern technology that more immature, sicker infants are being cared for. It is in these infants that requirements for fluids and nutrition may conflict with the ability of their immature kidneys to excrete both the excess solute and solvent.

Infancy is normally a period of profound anabolism. At no other time of life is a greater proportion of intake utilized for the construction of new tissue. Provision of appropriate dietary intake decreases endogenous catabolism and delivers adequate but not excessive energy, protein, and electrolytes to the peripheral tissues. When this is accomplished, infants produce and must excrete from 12 to 35 mOsm per 100 kcal ingested (10 to 30 mOsm per kilogram body weight). The lower number is more in keeping with anabolic infants receiving breast or "humanized" milk. The higher number is seen in starving infants or those receiving higher protein or electrolyte intakes. Infants receiving parenteral therapy also fall within these two limits. If we attempt to provide enough fluid to ensure that urine osmolality remains in the range of 100 to 300 mOsm per kilogram water, providing 40 to 100 ml per kilogram body weight per day for urinary needs would achieve that goal.

SODIUM BALANCE

Although it is obvious that sodium is the major extracellular cation, it is often not appreciated that approximately 50 percent of total body sodium is sequestered within bone. Therefore, the high growth rates seen in infancy require the maintenance of a positive sodium balance. In the absence of diarrhea, the only significant route for sodium loss is through the kidneys. Whereas children and adults have the ability to adapt to an enormously wide range of sodium intakes, ranging from as little as 1 mEq per day (total) to as high as 500 mEq per day even healthy, full-term infants are limited in their ability to both conserve and to excrete sodium. Premature infants are unable to reabsorb sodium even as efficiently as full-term infants and thus demonstrate abnormally high levels of urinary salt loss. This appears to be due both to a decreased responsiveness of the immature adrenal gland to circulating renin and to a diminished responsiveness of the distal nephron to circulating aldosterone. On the other hand, the relative immaturity of the kidney, coupled with very low GFR rates, limits the absolute quantity of sodium that can be excreted by the infant in the face of an acute salt load. Sodium balance can be maintained in full-term infants by the provision of 1 to 2 mEq of sodium per kilogram per day, whereas premature infants may require as much as 4 mEq per kilogram per day to prevent volume depletion and significant hyponatremia.

SITUATIONS THAT ALTER FLUID BALANCE FROM THE IDEAL

The Transition from Fetal to Neonatal Life

Previous sections have dealt with the components of fluid balance but did not address the question of what the fluid balance should be during different phases of the neonatal period. Birth involves a significant alteration and redistribution of body water within the neonate. Reliable data are available documenting both total body water and extracellular fluid volumes from fetal through adult life. Calculated as a percentage of body weight, total body water is approximately 80 percent at 32 weeks of gestation and 78 percent at term, and it decreases still further to 65 percent of body weight at 1 year of life. This change is due to two major factors. First, there is a decrease in extracellular fluid that occurs primarily within the first week of life. This is responsible for the weight loss seen during this period and is accomplished by renal excretion of the excess extracellular fluid. Full-term infants lose from 5 to 10 percent of their birth weight, whereas premature infants may lose as much as 15 percent of their birth weight within the first week to 10 days of life. This loss is associated with a net negative fluid balance that is both physiologic and necessary. Second, throughout the first year, there is a continuous increase in the percentage of body fat, a tissue that contains very little water.

Heat Transfer To and From the Neonate

As noted above, insensible water loss may be significantly altered by situations that increase the infant's evaporative loss. In addition to the reasons noted in Table 1, water loss is affected by ambient temperature and humidity. The ability to maintain the infant in a thermoneutral environment decreases the need for heat production, thus decreasing insensible water loss. In addition, when this environment is provided by an incubator, humidity may be better maintained and insensible water loss is decreased considerably as opposed to in those infants maintained without incubators. If the temperature of the incubator is allowed to rise beyond that of the thermoneutral zone, the increased heat provided will lead to increased insensible water loss. For low birth weight infants, the use of a heat shield, such as plastic "bubble wrap" inside the incubator, further decreases insensible water loss by decreasing heat loss and creating a microenvironment of higher humidity around the infant. Some severely ill infants benefit from care under radiant heaters. Although this gives better visibility and improved access to the infants, it is at the cost of increased insensible water loss due to increased air movement and the external radiant heat source. Phototherapy is commonly utilized in the care of neonates, and its use is correlated with immaturity. Phototherapy

TABLE 3   Adjustments to Insensible Water Loss*†

Use of an incubator	−50%
Heat shield	−50% in low birth weight infants
Humidification	−30%
Radiant heaters	+50–100%
Phototherapy	+30–50%
Ventilator therapy	−30%

* Basal values are for a full-term infant.
† The adjustments for radiant heaters and phototherapy are additive.

TABLE 4 Estimated Fluid Requirement for Full-Term Infants

	ml/kg	ml/100 kcal
Insensible water loss	15–20	40
Renal water loss	60–90	50–75
Stool water loss*	10	8
Growth*	10–15	12
Water of oxidation	−15	−12

* On day 1 of life, these values should be zero, rising to the stated numbers by day 3.

is associated with increased peripheral blood flow and increased insensible water loss. The need for assisted ventilation is common in the neonatal period. When the inspired air is properly warmed and humidified, insensible water loss through the lungs can be decreased to zero. Table 3 shows the changes in insensible water loss associated with the factors noted above.

CALCULATION OF WATER REQUIREMENTS

With the data presented above, some guidelines can be formulated to assist in the calculation of fluid therapy in the neonatal period. The utility of these guidelines is, however, proportional to the child's maturity. The more premature and/or ill the infant, the less reliable these suggestions become. Adherence to published guidelines can never replace repeated, careful, clinical assessment. Using the factorial method presented above, water balance for full-term infants is calculated in Table 4.

In addition to the assigned values for insensible water loss, urine, and stool water loss, it is necessary to take into account the water of oxidation as well as the water needed as part of the accretion of lean body mass. The term "water of oxidation" reflects the water obtained from oxidative metabolism that produces both H_2O and CO_2. This provides the infant with 12 ml of water per 100 kcal metabolized or 15 ml per kilogram body weight. Full-term infants grow at the rate of approximately 12 to 15 g per kilogram per day. Since the composition of lean body mass is approximately 80 percent water, 10 to 15 ml per kilogram of water is required for growth alone. In accounting for the lack of stool and the expected loss of body weight, 15 to 20 ml per kilogram less should be administered during the first 2 days of life.

Please note that Table 4 refers to the care of full-term neonates. Insensible water loss is increased in premature infants. Estimation of fluid requirements for these smaller infants requires substitution of insensible water loss values listed in Table 2, as modified by the considerations in Table 3, for those noted in Table 4.

ASSOCIATED MEDICAL CONDITIONS

Water balance must never be considered in the abstract but rather as one component of the infant's total care plan. Premature infants are prone to numerous medical conditions that necessitate modification of fluid therapy. Table 5 lists some of the conditions either aggravated by excessive fluid intake or associated with decreased fluid intake.

Clinical improvement in infants suffering from respiratory distress syndrome is preceded by a diuresis, suggesting although not proving that excess pulmonary fluid may be a component of respiratory distress syndrome. Studies have demonstrated that premature infants receiving larger amounts of fluid are more likely to develop clinical evidence of a patent ductus arteriosus as well as to suffer from an increased incidence of necrotizing enterocolitis. Neonates requiring long-term ventilatory support often develop bronchopulmonary dysplasia, a condition likely associated with and aggravated by excessive amounts of interstitial lung fluid. Thus, appropriate management necessitates calculating fluid intake to keep these infants on the "dry side."

Several phenomena may be responsible for the development of severe intravascular dehydration in premature infants. These include conscious attempts to limit fluid intake in these often severely ill infants; a relative inability to conserve both salt and water; and the possibility that the infants' effective intravascular volume may be decreased by diminished cardiac function or the sequestration of fluid within body tissue ("third spacing"). Some of the consequences of the development of dehydration are also noted in Table 5 and include the rapid development of shock with or without renal failure, a coagulopathy that is either generalized or limited to an organ, such as the kidney or brain, and the development of either hyper- or hyponatremia.

The unfortunate frequency of these complications, particularly in the very small premature infant, is a forceful

TABLE 5 Conditions Associated With Excessive or Insufficient Fluid Intake

Excessive Fluid Intake	Insufficient Fluid Intake
Respiratory distress syndrome	Acute renal failure
Intracranial hemorrhage	Shock
Bronchopulmonary dysplasia	Coagulopathy
Necrotizing enterocolitis	Hyper-/hyponatremia
Patent ductus arteriosus	

TABLE 6 Assessment of Fluid Status

Body weight
Blood pressure
Hematocrit
Blood urea nitrogen/creatinine
Urine specific gravity/osmolality
Skin turgor/peripheral perfusion
Pulse
Urine output
Serum sodium
Fractional excretion of sodium

argument against the use of any predetermined scheme for the calculation of fluid therapy. Each infant should have regular, frequent *reassessment* of his or her fluid status, with particular attention paid to signs either of volume overload or of depletion. Table 6 notes some of the measurements that have been found helpful in the assessment of fluid status. The single most important measure of fluid status is the determination of body weight. Since the rate of accretion of lean body mass is well established, any large increase or decrease in body weight over a short time period can be assumed to be due to changes in body water. In the severely ill infant, body weight should be measured every 8 to 12 hours and the results examined for the early detection of significant changes. Elevation of the pulse rate is a relatively early sign of dehydration, whereas adequate blood pressure is frequently maintained by peripheral vasoconstriction until the development of moderate to severe dehydration. Careful re-examination at frequent intervals may document the progression of dehydration by the sequential observation of pale, cool, or even mottled extremities. Urine output and a measure of urine concentration should be routinely monitored in all sick neonates. Urine volumes of between 1 and 4 ml per kilogram per hour are considered adequate. Urine outputs of between 0.5 and 1 ml per kilogram per hour may be acceptable in the face of other, complicating medical conditions, but values of less than 0.5 ml per kilogram per hour represent oliguria, the cause of which must be investigated and prompt treatment attempted. Urine specific gravity, an indirect assessment of the more important measure, urine osmolality, should be determined at regular intervals. In the absence of 2+ or greater urinary glucose or albumin, values of between 1.002 and 1.012 reflect an osmolality of 100 to 300 mOsm per kilogram water. Although urine specific gravities of greater than 1.020 generally reflect concentrated urine, they are uninterpretable in the presence of significant urinary glucose or protein concentrations. In such a case, a direct determination of urinary osmolality is mandatory to assess urine concentration. In sick premature infants in whom the development of volume overload is a concern, even narrower limits of specific gravity urine (1.006 to 1.012) are appropriate.

A sudden change in hematocrit is a clue to the presence of over- or underhydration but must be assessed in the light of the frequent transfusions and blood drawings that occur in these infants. In the same manner, regular determinations of the blood urea nitrogen and creatinine levels are helpful in assessing volume status. Since both blood urea nitrogen and creatinine reflect maternal and not infant renal status at birth, these measurements are most useful when followed sequentially. And because the body attempts to maintain isotonicity, abnormalities in serum sodium concentration most frequently reflect alterations in the content of total body water. Because of the possibility of increased neonatal salt loss, the finding of hyponatremia in the neonatal period must be correlated with an assessment of urinary sodium concentration and the fractional excretion of sodium (FE_{Na}). Calculating FE_{Na} provides a useful tool for assessing the ability of the kidney to conserve salt. The four concentration values needed for the determination of FE_{Na} are serum sodium (S_{Na}), serum creatinine (S_{cr}), urinary sodium (U_{Na}), and urinary creatinine (U_{cr}). The calculation is given below and, by convention, the result is multiplied by 100 so that it reflects the percentage of the sodium filtered by the kidney that is actually excreted.

$$100 \times U_{Na}/S_{Na}/(U_{cr}/S_{cr})$$

Under normal circumstances this is generally less than 1 percent. In infants less than 30 weeks' gestation, FE_{Na} may be as high as 5 percent during the first 3 days of life. Infants born after more than 32 weeks of gestational age have FE_{Na} values at or below 1 percent. In the face of volume depletion, healthy kidneys will conserve sodium and FE_{Na} values will be less than 1 percent. Renal immaturity aside, values over 2.5 to 3 percent most likely reflect recent administration of diuretics, such as furosemide (Lasix) (within 6 hours), or the development of acute renal failure secondary to acute tubular necrosis. Thus, in the face of rising blood urea nitrogen or creatinine levels, declining urine output, or hyponatremia, determination of the FE_{Na} will assist in differentiating hypovolemia with intact renal function from the development of acute tubular necrosis.

Hyponatremia may be associated with either hyponatremic dehydration or the development of water intoxication. The secretion of antidiuretic hormone is controlled by both volume and osmolar stimuli. With the development of moderate to severe dehydration, the volume stimulus predominates, and water is conserved even at the cost of progressive hypo-osmolarity and hyponatremia. Additionally, as noted earlier, premature neonates may be unable to conserve sodium adequately and urinary sodium losses may be inappropriately high. The net effect of these two forces is to promote the development of hyponatremia dehydration. On the other hand, water intoxication may be due either to excess water intake or to the presence of the syndrome of inappropriate release of antidiuretic hormone, a condition known to occur in sick, stressed, premature neonates.

Hypernatremia may be due either to the administration of an excessive salt load or to the provision of too little water. In sick premature neonates, the development of glycosuria is not uncommon, especially when glucose-containing intravenous fluid is given in the high volumes required to maintain fluid balance in such preterm infants. Marked glycosuria can thus be associated with the development of an osmotic diuresis and dehydration. Replacement of these losses with standard intravenous solutions has been associated with excessive salt intake, which infants cannot adequately excrete because of their low GFR. Clearly, therapy of this complication requires an alteration in both the volume and composition of the fluid administered.

IMMUNIZATIONS

BETTY R. VOHR, M.D.
WILLIAM OH, M.D.

The purpose of providing immunizations for the normal and at-risk infant during the first year of life is to prevent the devastating mortality and morbidity associated with diphtheria, tetanus, pertussis (DTP), and poliomyelitis, diseases that were prevalent in the United States prior to the development of immunization procedures for prophylaxis. The specific guidelines, as shown in Table 1, developed by the American Academy of Pediatrics, Committee of Infectious Disease (*The Red Book*), are used by primary care physicians in recommending immunization for normal term infants during the first year of life. These guidelines are based on extensive studies that document an immune response in term infants following current standard immunization procedures. This response offers excellent protection against DTP and poliomyelitis. Studies documenting immunologic responses of high-risk infants, however, are less extensive.

A 1985 study documented a similar effective immunologic response of high-risk low birth weight infants (special care nursery graduates) in response to DTP immunization. The investigators quantitated DTP specific antibodies and showed that 100 percent of preterm infants had evidence of specific antibody production against DTP after the second immunization. These *observations suggest that the American Academy of Pediatrics guidelines for term infants can be applied to low birth weight infants and that DTP immunization need not be delayed* beyond 2 months of age. A study examining the immunization practices of community physicians for graduates of a neonatal intensive care unit revealed a significant delay in the actual administration of DTP immunizations as recommended by the *The Red Book*. Linear regression analysis revealed a significant inverse correlation between birth weight and age of immunization for DTP. Therefore, the smallest, most vulnerable infants were least likely to receive the recommended immunization schedule. In fact, 91 percent of infants with birth weights of less than 1,000 g were not fully immunized at 6 months of age. This failure of the health care system, coupled with the current medico-legal atmosphere of the 1980s and the negative (at times biased) media coverage of the immunization issue, make appropriate immunization of the low birth weight infant an important preventive medicine priority. Pediatricians and parents need to be informed of the most current state of the art and encouraged to follow through with recommended schedules that facilitate the health and welfare of infants.

INFORMED CONSENT: MEDICO-LEGAL ASPECTS

Our nursery has informational and informed consent forms available that are provided by the Rhode Island Department of Health. Prior to immunizing an infant, the form is reviewed with the parents. These forms include descriptions of the three disorders (DTP) and their morbidities and describe the types of side effects from the DTP vaccine, the relative risks of experiencing these side effects, and contraindications to receiving immunizations. The *parents have the opportunity to ask questions and are then asked to sign a request for immunization of their infant. Information regarding the immunization is then forwarded to the infant's primary care physician.*

SPECIAL CARE NURSERY GRADUATES: HIGH-RISK POPULATION FOR COMPLICATIONS FROM DTP IMMUNIZATION

Perhaps one of the reasons there is controversy regarding immunization of the high-risk infant is that pediatricians are now dealing with an entirely new population of infants. As a result of sophisticated medical management, survival of these high-risk infants has increased significantly. For instance, those weighing less than 1,000 g at

TABLE 1 Recommended Schedule for Active Immunization of Normal Infants and Children*

Recommended Age	Vaccine(s)	Comments
2 mo	DTP, OPV[†]	Can be initiated earlier in areas of high endemicity
4 mo	DTP, OPV	2-mo interval desired for OPV to avoid interference
6 mo	DTP, OPV	OPV optional; desirable for areas where polio might be imported, e.g., some areas of the south-western United States

* American Academy of Pediatrics Report of the Committee on Infectious Diseases: The 1986 Red Book. 20th ed. Evanston, IL: American Academy of Pediatrics, 1986.
† DTP = diphtheria, tetanus, pertussis; OPV = oral polio virus vaccine containing attenuated polio virus types 1, 2, and 3.

birth now have a survival rate of 60 to 80 percent. These same low birth weight infants also have a high incidence of intraventricular hemorrhage (30 to 40 percent) and chronic lung disease (20 to 40 percent). Physicians are, therefore, seeing more babies who are smaller and who have had multiple neonatal complications, including sequelae of intraventricular hemorrhage, ventricular dilatation or seizures, and who may have chronic morbidities, such as chronic lung disease, shunted hydrocephalus, cerebral palsy and chronic seizure disorders. These infants are particularly vulnerable to secondary disease, such as pertussis, because of their impaired nutritional status and their minimal pulmonary reserve. Children with chronic lung disease are particularly susceptible to recurrent upper and lower respiratory infections, because of damage to and scarring of their airways. A bout of pertussis in such a vulnerable infant invariably results in prolonged rehospitalization with possible oxygen supplementation and assisted ventilation.

The Centers for Disease Control report that there is a recent increase in the number of cases of reported pertussis. Morbidity and mortality are known to be greatest during the first year of life in full-term normal children. These sequelae occur even more frequently in the at-risk infant.

IMMUNIZATION GUIDELINES

Because of concerns regarding increased morbidity which may be encountered in at-risk infants, the *following guidelines for immunization of neonatal intensive care unit graduates* are offered:

1. The first full dose (0.5 ml) of DTP is administered to all high-risk infants who have attained a chronologic age of 2 months and a weight of 1,800 g or more, provided they are clinically stable, are not on assisted ventilation, and are growing normally.
2. The DTP dose is to be given at least 48 hours prior to discharge in order to observe and record potential local or systemic side effects.
3. The DTP dose should not be given if the infant has evidence of an acute respiratory illness.
4. Informed consent is obtained.

5. The immunization site, dose, and any reactions are recorded in the chart.
6. *The immunization record of dose(s) and date(s) administered is included in the discharge plan and the summary sent to the primary physician.* A regular follow-up program affords an excellent opportunity to assess subsequent immunization schedules and encourage appropriate immunizations, as outlined in Table 1.

CONTRAINDICATIONS

As shown in Table 2, once an infant is stable, there are only three primary contraindications to administering pertussis vaccine. Aside from these serious progressive neurologic disorders, children with primary immune deficiency also should not receive any live virus vaccine. It is obvious from these considerations that there are infants now being discharged who may have multiple morbidities related to low birth weight yet who are valid candidates for the currently recommended immunization schedule. If, however, the infant had a serious systemic complication in response to his or her first DTP dose, as listed in Table 3, subsequent doses should include only DT. It is noteworthy that *the risk of reactions such as encephalitis, shock, and somnolence, is extremely small.*

Mild local and systemic reactions to DTP immunization are identified in approximately 40 to 70 percent of doses administered. Premature infants have not been shown to have a higher incidence of these reactions. Local reactions include erythema and induration, tenderness, a nodule at the site of injection lasting several weeks, abscess at the site of injection, and occasionally a severe local reaction associated with a history of multiple prior boosters. Systemic reactions, which are not uncommon, include a mild to moderate fever (38 to 40.4° C) and mild somnolence, irritability, and malaise. Treatment of mild reactions consists of supportive therapy, including cool compresses to the area, avoiding pressure, treatment of allergic reaction, and antipyretic treatment.

In some cases of prolonged hospitalization, infants may receive all three doses of DTP prior to discharge. Although infants with chronic disease have limited muscle mass, partial dose administration is not advisable, since

TABLE 2 Risk Factors in Neonatal Intensive Care Unit Graduates Affecting Immunization

DTP May Be Administered	DT Should Be Administered
Bronchopulmonary dysplasia	Progressive neurologic disorders
Intraventricular hemorrhage, grades I, II, III, IV	Deteriorating neurologic disorders
Apnea	Seizures—on anticonvulsant therapy
Receives supplemental oxygen	
Neonatal asphyxia	
Very low birth weight	
Neurologic signs: increased or decreased tone*	
Hydrocephalus	
Cerebral palsy	

* If neurologic signs appear to be in the process of changing, may defer to stable period.

TABLE 3 Subsequent Dose—DT Only

Use if first DTP dose was associated with any of the
following:
  Seizure (within 48 hours of vaccine)
  Encephalitis
  Focal neurologic signs
  Collapse or shock
  >3 Hours of excessive somnolence or screaming
  Temperature >40.5° C (≥105° F)
  Systemic allergic reaction
  Thrombocytopenia, hemolytic anemia

it may result in incomplete protection. The anterolateral
aspect of the thigh provides the largest muscle mass and
is the preferred site for intramuscular injection. Infants
who receive three full doses have more than 80 percent
protection from pertussis.

DIPHTHERIA AND TETANUS

Diphtheria antitoxin has rare side effects and offers
greater than 98 percent protection. Tetanus toxin may
produce mild local and systemic reactions and should be
given in the full recommended dose.

POLIOMYELITIS

Prior to the onset of immunization procedures for
poliomyelitis in the 1950s, there were 15,000 cases annually in the United States. In the 1980s, fewer than 10 cases
per year have been reported. Choices for administration
include oral polio vaccine, which is a live attenuated virus,
and intramuscular polio virus, which is an inactivated polio
virus; the former is the method of choice. Serious adverse
effects are extremely rare, and the vaccine offers greater
than 95 percent protection. *To avoid cross-infection with
oral polio vaccine in the nursery, it is initiated after discharge from the hospital.* If the first DTP or DT was given
during hospitalization, the primary physician can administer the oral polio vaccine with the DTP or DT 2
months after the initial dose. *Doses are not reduced for
preterm infants.*

SUGGESTED READING

Bernbaum JC, Daft A, Anolik R, et al. Response of preterm infants to
  diphtheria-tetanus-pertussis immunizations. J Pediatr 1985;
  107:184–188.
Report of the Committee on Infectious Diseases: The 1986 red book.
  20th ed. Evanston, IL: American Academy of Pediatrics, 1986:266.
Vohr BR, Oh W. Age of diphtheria, tetanus, and pertussis immunization of special care nursery graduates. Pediatrics 1986; 77:569–571.

INFANT TRANSPORT

JEFFREY B. HANSON, M.D.
MARY K. BUSER, N.N.P., M.S.
L. JOSEPH BUTTERFIELD, M.D.

Transport of the newborn or child to a regional perinatal or pediatric unit is an essential component of modern
pediatric care. Health planning has integrated the concept
of newborn and pediatric transport into regional pediatric
care plans.

Since the adoption of a policy in support of regional
perinatal care by the American Medical Association House
of Delegates in 1971, strong support of this premise by such
groups as the American Academy of Pediatrics, American College of Obstetricians and Gynecologists, and
American Academy of Family Physicians has flourished.

In the pluralistic health care delivery system of the
United States, many variations on the theme of regional
perinatal and pediatric care have evolved in the past 20
years. Basic to all is the efficient, effective, and safe transport of newborns and children to the appropriate regional
center.

This chapter focuses on the philosophy and the style
of newborn-pediatric transports that are universally relevant. We base these remarks on our experience with a
transport system that dates back to 1965 and that accounted for 1,294 newborn and 539 pediatric transports from

a service region of 500,000 square miles in 1986. Details
of staffing, equipment, and treatment protocols are available in several published references.

PHILOSOPHY

The sole objective of a newborn or pediatric transport system is the delivery of the highest quality of in-
terhospital critical care to that patient.

Transport systems are a mobile extension of the tertiary hospital's resources, including medical, nursing, and
respiratory therapy expertise. Thus, the newborn or pediatric transport system is a key service to the community.
For purposes of this discussion, the word "SERVICE"
can be used as an acronymic agenda: Service, Expertise,
Response, Vicinity, Insight, Competition, and Excellence.

SERVICE

The transport system offers both human and technical services. An important aspect of such a system is the
consultation service; often a consultation leads to a transport or enhances the stabilization process at the local
hospital. The referring physician and hospital staff play
integral roles in this service, as the care provided during
transport is merely a continuation of the care begun in the
referring hospital.

On occasion prenatal consult converts a planned neonatal transport into a maternal transport that has outcome
and economic advantage.

The communication network is a vital piece of the transport system. The credibility of such a system depends not only on the ability to communicate with the referring physician and referral hospital staff but also on the capability of maintaining contact with the transport team during a transport.

The selection and training of personnel are influenced by the unique requirements of each transport system. Variables include length and number of transports, availability of skilled professionals, and expertise of the referring staff.

The appropriate staff configuration for transport continues to be a subject for debate. Currently, teams utilize combinations of physicians, nurse practitioners/clinicians, staff nurses, respiratory therapists, emergency medical technicians, and paramedics.

The final determining factor should be the choice that will provide the best level of care in the most cost-effective manner. The staff must have a solid basis in anatomy, physiology, pathophysiology, treatment modalities, and an understanding of the stresses of their position.

EXPERTISE

The existence of a newborn-pediatric transport system should make available to the region served the latest medical and technological expertise. Representatives from all pediatric subspecialties should be available on a 24-hour basis to assure that state-of-the-art medical care can be activated by a phone call.

Airborne patient transfers, although dramatic, are inadvisable in that the stabilization required can be performed most effectively in a hospital environment. Short cuts may have disastrous effects.

The emphasis should be on providing a level of care during stabilization and transport equivalent to the level of care the child will obtain at the receiving hospital. This implies that the combined expertise of the referring staff and the transport team can provide that level of assessment and care.

RESPONSE

The majority of newborn-pediatric transports are emergencies. An appropriate and timely response without endangering the staff and the patient is a basic principle of a transport system. Newborn patients, with rare exception, are hospitalized with available nursing and physician skills as well as supportive thermoregulation, oxygen therapy, monitoring of vital signs, and intravenous fluids when needed. A newborn transport service functions differently than do most adult trauma systems, which generally subscribe to the philosophy of "swoop and scoop," a philosophy originating in the Korean War via the helicopter that was extended in the Vietnam War.

Such is not the case with neonatal-pediatric transport services, in which the major emphasis is on stabilization of the patient and later transfer. Stabilization should be in process as the transport team is en route, and then it is continued by the team upon arrival. Movement of the patient occurs when the newborn or child is as stable as possible, unless definitive therapy is available only at the tertiary center.

An important component of such a system is frequent communication. Depending on the area served, the response time may be several hours, and this is weather-dependent. Timely phone calls to the referral hospital elicit key information regarding the patient and also give reassurance that the transport team is en route.

Courteous and professional interaction by the transport staff with the referring physician and hospital staff is assumed, although occasionally forgotten in a hectic transport situation. Prompt reports of the follow-up of the patient's outcome to the referring physician and the staff of the hospital of birth complete the transport process. Notations of these reports in the patient's chart are evidence of optimal transport care.

Essential to the success of the transport system is an ongoing evaluation process. Mechanisms should be in place that promote input from and to everyone involved in the transport system. This includes evaluation by the referring physician and staff. Areas requiring regular re-evaluation include communications, response time, patient management, and follow-up. Case review and the use of written and oral feedback can be very valuable in assessing the success of the system.

VICINITY

The response time and the mode of transport depend on the particular newborn-pediatric transport service. Distance, climate, and local geographic factors influence the choice between ground ambulance, helicopter, or fixed wing, turbo prop jet, or Lear jet. Cost analysis of time of transport and staff time is an important process in the selection of a transport mode.

Networking by regional medical centers in a region helps facilitate patient movement to appropriate centers. Decisions are made with regard to availability of beds and staff when one center is overloaded and "shunting" is appropriate.

Occasionally, smaller centers and transport systems can facilitate movement of patients to tertiary centers in a more timely fashion because of their proximity to the patient. The nature of the newborn emergency and the requirements for special expertise must be considered in these decisions, since all transport systems are not equal.

INSIGHT

The newborn-pediatric transport system is an essential link between the physician in practice in a community or regional hospital and the tertiary center. It is that segment of the tertiary center that interacts on a daily basis with one or more medical communities in the region it serves. In addition to providing quality service, the transport system should be ever-sensitive to the general problems and concerns of the referring physicians and staff. These observations can provide a needed loop in planning outreach education programs and special training sessions at the tertiary center.

The transport staff needs to remember that the referring physician not only practices medicine in the community but also lives there. Constructive criticism is healthy and an important part of the interaction between the parties on both ends of a newborn-pediatric transport, but emotional or editorial comments and inappropriate behavior are not acceptable. The newborn-pediatric transport team must not lose sight of the major goal: the delivery of the best medical care possible to the sick newborn or child during transport to a referral hospital. The tertiary and referral hospitals represent a partnership in care.

As soon as appropriate, return transport of the newborn or child to the hospital of origin both reinforces the paradigm of partnership and brings the recovering patients closer to home and family support.

COMPETITION

Medicine in the 1980s has evolved or "devolved" into serious, sometimes deadly, competition for patients. The same can be said for scarce resources and for visibility in the community.

The absence of national standards for newborn and pediatric transport has allowed any system to call itself an emergency transport service. When several transport services are available, the referring physician must exercise judgment as to which service to utilize and consider the level of expertise required after balancing that concern with the desired response time. A judicious selection of a transport service then can be made.

EXCELLENCE

Although standards exist for training, certification, and maintenance of skills for neonatal nurse clinicians, respiratory therapists, and emergency medical technicians, there are no national standards for neonatal and pediatric transport systems.

A certain volume of transports is necessary to maintain skills and efficiency and to justify utilization of costly resources.

A medical director for any emergency transport service should be charged with medical supervision, development, and adaptation of new therapies and should view continuing education as essential. Peer review, outreach education, and exchange of ideas at regional and national meetings are needed at regular intervals.

FUTURE CONSIDERATIONS

No neonatal or pediatric transport system operates in a vacuum; all are subject to present trends of modern medicine. One such disturbing trend is that of "deregionalization". The present atmosphere of competition means that more hospitals opt to be full service in the attempt to obtain contracts with third-party payers. Transport lends itself least well to such an attitude, for consistent activity and volume are necessary for maintenance of competence.

The trend toward treating the sicker patient in the referring hospital, closer to the family, with recently trained physicians and continuing education programs, may contribute to further decreases in utilization of specialty transport services. Also, financial incentives for individual hospitals to keep paying patients may not only decrease utilization of newborn and pediatric transport but may stimulate the development of more small-volume services.

The key question is, What is in the best interest of the newborn, infant, or child when new and duplicative transport systems are proposed?

SUGGESTED READING

Guidelines for perinatal care. American Academy of Pediatrics/American College of Obstetricians and Gynecologists. Chapter 8. Washington, D.C. 1983:195.
Honeyfield PR, Lunka ME, Butterfield LJ. Air transportation of the sick neonate. In: Ferrara and Harin, eds. Emergency transfer of the high-risk infant. St Louis: CV Mosby, 1980:25.
Rogers M. Transportation of the critically ill child. In: Rogers M, ed. Textbook of pediatric intensive care. Baltimore: Williams & Wilkins, 1987:1395.

NURSE CLINICIANS

LAWRENCE J. FENTON, M.D.
TERESA J. REID, R.N./M.S.N.
LAWRENCE R. WELLMAN, M.D.

In 1982, Harper reported that over 60 percent of neonatal units were using neonatal nurse practitioners and over half of these units hired the practitioners to replace pediatric house staff. In 1983, the NAACOG Certification Corporation developed the first certifying examination.

Neonatal nurse practitioners are here to stay and will become increasingly important in the delivery of newborn health care. But, who and what are they, how are they trained, and what do they do?

DEFINITION OF TERMS

As the terms "clinician" and "practitioner" are used in this paper they mean an individual who has had sufficient training to become eligible for the neonatal nurse practitioner/clinician examination given by the NAACOG Certification Corporation. This examination requires a minimum of a 9-month course, including a preceptorship experience. The word clinician is sometimes rather loosely applied to nurses who have had a brief training period in resuscitative physiology and procedures. Courses for this type of technical training may be as short as 4 weeks in some centers and may fulfill the need of a particular intensive care unit for personnel to staff transport teams and delivery rooms and to provide technical back-up in the neonatal intensive care unit. Thus, in the literature the term clinician is often used to describe both the briefly and the more thoroughly trained individual.

In some states and in some hospitals, clinician is used instead of practitioner as the title for a fully trained nurse because practitioner may connote a nurse who intends to enter into private practice. The neonatal nurse practitioner may meet resistance from the medical community, who may not separate the activities of one type of practitioner from another. In other locales the fully trained nurse is called a practitioner and may be certified under the guidelines of a nurse practice act with all the privileges and responsibilities entitled by state law. Frequently, this includes the ability to write prescriptions, make diagnoses, and do procedures without direct supervision by a physician. It often entails contractual arrangements between a supervising physician and the practitioner.

The term "clinical nurse specialist" is used here to denote a nurse practitioner or clinician who has obtained a master's degree in nursing.

In our experience, practitioner is the most appropriate title for the nurse to have, especially if it is officially recognized and comes within a state's Nurse Practitioner Act. This title eliminates any questions of a legal nature, is accepted by third-party payers for the purposes of billing, and enhances the nurse's stature within the hospital, allowing the hospital to reimburse the nurse on a pay scale that is different from the scale for other nurses within the institution.

TRAINING

Currently, there are six formal continuing education programs for neonatal nurse practitioners. All are associated with a medical school or a school of nursing. Requirements for entrance into such programs and the actual contents of the programs are not yet standardized. There may be extremely wide variations in course content and emphasis, but we suspect there are more similarities than differences. The program in South Dakota was begun in 1978 and resulted from a combined effort of the South Dakota State University School of Nursing, the University of South Dakota School of Medicine, and the Sioux Valley Hospital. Our program is offered for continuing education and academic credit through South Dakota State University School of Nursing. The program will eventually be expanded to grant a master's degree. Current admission requirements include a baccalaureate degree in nursing, a minimum of 2 years of nursing experience following graduation, and 1 year's experience in a newborn intensive care unit under the medical direction of a full-time neonatologist. This experience must have occurred within 3 years of the time of application. In addition, the nurse must be currently practicing in a newborn intensive

care nursery under the full-time direction of a neonatologist.

Learning basic physiology, physical examination skills, differential diagnosis, the problem-solving approach, and treatment modalities is often difficult for nurses, because the traditional approach to the disease process in nursing education is very different from that of the physician. Assuming responsibility for numerous procedures and treatments requires a major role reorientation that takes time and maturation. The actual course consists of a 12-week didactic portion, a 6-week applied clinical section, and a 32-week clinical preceptorship. The initial didactic portion integrates the basic sciences and pathophysiology of neonatal diseases with clinical management. Nearly 300 hours of lecture are given during the first 12 weeks, with most of the neonatal physiology being taught by neonatologists. Practical experience and knowledge of procedures, such as endotracheal intubation, placement of a thoracostomy tube, catheterization of umbilical vessels, arterial punctures, and spinal taps, are gained during this time with the use of animal and laboratory models. Periodic examinations are given for evaluation of students during the didactic portion of the course. The didactic portion consists of three modules called the Advanced Natural Science Module, Care of the Neonate Module, and the Psychosocial and Role Orientation Module. Table 1 lists the subjects taught in each module.

After the formal lecture portion of the course, the practitioner students are involved in an intensive clinical experience for 6 weeks in the intensive care nursery. They are jointly supervised by neonatologists, the neonatal clinical nurse specialists, and nurse practitioners in the unit. During this period of time, the practitioner students learn to do initial patient evaluations and manage a case load. Under close supervision by neonatologists and the clinical nurse specialist, they take patient histories, talk with parents, and perform procedures. Daily rounds provide a forum for reviewing patient problems with the neonatologist and an opportunity to discuss and defend patient assessments and management plans. Continuity of care is stressed as the practitioner student gains experience in managing the neonatal patient from admission to discharge.

After the student has completed the applied clinical portion of the course, the preceptorship follows as a continuation of the student's clinical experience under the direct supervision of a neonatologist and the clinical nurse specialist. The student's write-ups, daily progress notes, and presentations are evaluated and critiqued by the neonatologist and clinical nurse specialist. A comprehensive case-oriented final examination is given upon completion of the course. The students are encouraged to take the NAACOG certification examination for neonatal nurse practitioners.

ROLE OF THE PRACTITIONER—HOW WE DO IT

The role of the neonatal nurse practitioners has been as varied as the number of intensive care nurseries that utilize them. Although the practitioner is an experienced

TABLE 1 Curriculum

Advanced Natural Science Module

This module is taught by neonatologists and other M.D. subspecialists. It includes:

Math Review
Introduction to Pharmacology
Basic and Organic Chemistry and Biochemistry
Principles of Human Genetics
Fetal Development
Embryology
Maternal Risk Factors
Placental Physiology
Gas Laws
Introduction to Pulmonary Physiology
Respiratory Diseases in the Newborn

Neonatal Neurology
Introduction to Gastrointestinal Physiology
Liver Function and Disease
Infections and Neonatal Immunology
Feeding and Nutrition in the Neonate
Apnea and Sudden Infant Death Syndrome

Infections in the Newborn
Substance Abuse
Coagulation Problems in the Newborn
X-Ray Interpretation
Neonatal Anemia and Polycythemia
Neonatal Endocrinology
Neonatal Cardiology

Hyperalimentation
Renal Physiology and Renal Disorders
Neonatal Surgery, Pre- and Postoperative
   Management
Perinatal Glucose Homeostasis
Gastrointestinal Diseases
Jaundice in the Newborn
Introduction to Microbiology
Follow-up Care of the High-Risk Neonate
Introduction to Medical Statistics

Care of the Neonate Module

This module is largely taught by clinical nurse specialists and other experienced neonatal nurse practitioners. It includes:

Physical Examination of the Neonate
Thermoregulation
Neonatal Resuscitation and the Management of
   Shock
Interpretation of Blood Gases
Interpretation of Laboratory Data
Nursing Process and Problem Solving
Problem-Oriented Medical Charting
Procedure Labs
   Intubation; needle aspiration of chest; chest
   tube; lumbar puncture; umbilical catheter;
   arterial puncture; bladder tap

Basic Laboratory Terminology
Transitional Period
Care of the Neonate on the Ventilator

Management of Respirators
ECG Interpretation
Administration of Medications
Transport Physiology and Logistics

Psychosocial and Role Orientation Module

This module is taught by a developmental psychologist and master's degree–prepared nurses. It includes:

Interactions Between Mother and Baby
History Taking
Teaching Skills
Role of the Practitioner in Research

Fetal and Neonatal Development
Interviewing Skills
Leadership Training

intensive care nurse who has special training in background physiology and in procedures involving the sick newborn, it is important to understand that the practitioner is not a neonatologist. The training received qualifies the practitioner for many responsibilities, but *only* under the supervision of a neonatologist. Although the precise function of the practitioner within a tertiary-level neonatal intensive care unit may vary, we will describe the typical model for the utilization of the practitioner, which has worked extremely well for our unit, as well as others, throughout the country.

In all appropriate models, the neonatal nurse practitioner should function as an integral part of the health care team. In our nursery, where there are no pediatric house staff members, a nurse practitioner's function is similar to that of the pediatric house officer. There is an extreme-ly close collegial relationship between the neonatologist and the practitioner. All practitioners are required to have passed the NAACOG certifying examination. We utilize 12 practitioners divided into teams, with each team managing a case load of patients from admission to discharge. Each day, during rounds, at least one member from each team is present to examine the patients on their team in order to provide continuity from day to day. This need for continuity has become even more important, as the staff nurses are now utilizing a work schedule in which each nurse works only three 12-hour shifts per week, which tends to interrupt continuity on the staff nurse level. The patient management by the nurse practitioner involves daily examination, assessment, and evaluation of the patient data in order to develop an ongoing care plan. The management and diagnostic plans are always developed in collaboration with the neonatologist and the nursing staff caring for the patient, thus preserving the team concept of patient care.

Nurse practitioners begin the day by receiving a report on their patient case load from staff nurses and practitioners on the previous shift. Following the report, they examine the patients, review the charts and laboratory data, and formulate a plan of care for the next 24 hours. Throughout the process, input is obtained from the primary staff nurse as well as other pertinent ancillary staff (e.g., respiratory and dietary care). During formal rounds, each infant's case is discussed with the attending neonatologist. At this point, the practitioner presents the relevant findings and outlines the plan of care formulated earlier. The plan is then discussed and revised as needed. Once the plan of care has been agreed upon, the practitioner documents this information in the form of a progress note on each patient's chart. Having been delineated, the plan can then be followed throughout the day by both the practitioner and the staff nurses. Part of the educational training has prepared the practitioner to discern variations of laboratory data and physical findings. Continual presence in the intensive care nursery allows the practitioner to assess critical changes in the patient's status and readjust the care plan accordingly. Of course, the neonatologist is always available for consultation if new information is obtained and the plan requires major revision. During the entire process, the practitioner takes direct responsibility for gathering and assessing data, formulating management plans, reassessing outcomes, and revising care plans based on ascertained needs. In this way, the practitioner is an integral part of the ongoing care and provides continuity for the patient. The neonatologist must learn to pay careful attention to the practitioner's suggestions on rounds, because it is truly the practitioner who most intimately knows the patient, the chart, and the course over the last several days.

In our institution, the neonatal nurse practitioner is utilized for all low- to medium-risk deliveries in which a neonatologist is not requested. For example, the rules and regulations of our hospital state that a nurse practitioner and neonatal staff nurse are required at the delivery of all infants born between 35 and 37 weeks' gestation, in any situation in which there is staining of the amniotic fluid or fetal distress, and for all cesarean sections. For more serious problems, such as very significant fetal distress, thick meconium, or babies of less than 35 weeks' gestation, the neonatologist is required to be in the delivery room along with the practitioner and staff nurse. In our experience, the resuscitation team of a neonatologist, neonatal nurse practitioner, and staff nurse is an extremely organized and efficient operation.

The nurse practitioner is the leader of the transport team. Because of his or her educational preparation, the practitioner is equipped to direct emergency resuscitation and perform lifesaving procedures that may require a great deal of independent judgment and expertise. We have found that interpretation of x-ray films is an extremely valuable skill in the field. In addition to clinical expertise, the transport situation frequently demands all of the public relation skills and diplomacy required of an ambassador.

The practitioner should also provide an important leadership role within the intensive care nursery. Because of their additional education, practitioners are respected by the staff nurses and looked to for their increased knowledge and expertise. The practitioner, therefore, becomes a resource person for all members of the team in the intensive care unit. His or her continual presence within the nursery allows easy accessibility to the staff whenever care issues or questions arise. The practitioner may delegate various responsibilities to the staff nurses and may act as a liaison between staff nurses and neonatologists, helping to keep lines of communication open among all nursery staff. He or she should also be a major resource for in-service education and orientation classes for staff nurses within the intensive care nursery. The practitioner may be used to instruct and supervise not only new staff nurses but also house officers and medical students. The practitioner also forms the backbone of outreach education teams to other hospitals in the region, thus improving care as well as ensuring a good referral pattern from outlying hospitals.

Many nurse practitioners have become interested in performing research in the intensive care unit. They are experts in evaluating medical and nursing methodology and techniques utilized within a unit. Their continual presence with the intensive care unit facilitates many research projects by assuring that protocols are appropriately followed.

CHRONIC PATIENTS

In many institutions, the neonatal nurse practitioner may be utilized to care only for the chronic, long-term hospitalized patient. The nurse practitioner in this situation may have a major managerial responsibility for these long-term patients, with daily input from the neonatologist on rounds but very little input during the day either being necessary or desired. This situation is very workable, but its success is highly dependent upon the mind set of the nurse practitioner. Our experience is that most neonatal nurse practitioners are acute care, action-oriented people; their relegation to a chronic care unit may relieve the neonatologist of a great deal of responsibility for time-consuming work and provide a great deal of continuity for these difficult patients, but it may also lead to rapid job dissatisfaction on the part of the nurse practitioner. We feel that is important for the nurse practitioner to follow both the acute and chronic phase of the patient's care in order to maintain clinical skills. On the other hand, some nurse practitioners, especially after they have been in the acute care role for a while, find themselves particularly well-suited to caring for the chronically ill patient and, with their knowledge of acute care and physiologic background, they are superbly prepared to play a prime managerial role in the care of the complex, chronically ill patient. Therefore, a properly selected nurse practitioner who enjoys older children, developmental medicine problems, and closely interrelating with families and nursing staff may find this role ideal. If such an individual is not available, however, we would caution against the use of a practitioner solely in a chronic care role.

INAPPROPRIATE MODELS FOR UTILIZATION OF THE NEONATAL NURSE PRACTITIONER

The proliferation of level II units has led to the utilization of some neonatal nurse practitioners in a care delivery model that may be highly inappropriate. A well-trained nurse practitioner placed in a unit where the supervision is done only by general pediatricians may provide an impetus for that unit to care for sicker babies over a long period of time. In this situation, there is a tendency to utilize the nurse's expertise as if he or she were the neonatologist in a consultative situation. The net result may be that level II centers may decide to deliver higher risk mothers and care for sicker infants for an inappropriate length of time before referral to a level III center. Recent data in the literature would support the notion that mortality may indeed be higher in some level II centers than in level III centers, although the reverse should be true.

We are aware, however, of level II units in which the neonatal nurse practitioner has been most appropriately used. In these hospitals the practitioner has served mostly to stabilize sick infants prior to transport. Although a nurse practitioner may be of great help in smaller hospitals under these circumstances, such a practitioner frequently becomes professionally frustrated because of the inability to utilize the full range of training and knowledge gained in the course. Career satisfaction is therefore threatened.

CURRENT STATUS AND FUTURE OF THE NEONATAL NURSE PRACTITIONER

There is an increasing amount of data to indicate that appropriate models have been highly successful utilizing neonatal nurse practitioners who have been trained in a manner similar to our description. The mortality rate in our unit (in which there are no pediatric house officers) is quite comparable to that of other units that are similar in size and patient population but are more traditionally staffed with house officers. It has been shown that the practitioner provides a highly consistent form of care without fluctuations in morbidity or technical errors that can occur with the influx of new house staff or possibly with very tired house staff who have been without sleep for over 24 hours. Current concepts in pediatric training, along with the increased survival chances of very small babies, have combined to create a permanent place for the neonatal nurse practitioner in the delivery of newborn intensive care.

The continued success of the neonatal nurse practitioner will be highly dependent on the standardization of training programs. Although the current requirements for taking the NAACOG certification examination are an important step in that direction, the content of the course and the experiences required have not yet been spelled out. Some of our practitioner students have taken their preceptorships in units that are totally unfamiliar with neonatal nurse practitioners and do not completely understand the practitioner role and, therefore, the training of the student in these circumstances is frequently not optimal. The preceptorship content and the role of the practitioner student in this situation need to be more carefully structured and standardized.

There is a national trend toward having practitioners acquire a master's degree along with their training. Currently, most "nonpractitioner" neonatal nurses with master's degrees have reasonable backgrounds in many aspects of newborn physiology, educational principles, and administration of neonatal intensive care units but have little hands-on clinical expertise. There are very few master's degree–prepared neonatal nurses who would currently feel comfortable in managing the resuscitation of an 800 g infant who required intubation, placement of a chest tube and an umbilical artery catheter, appropriate interpretation of x-ray studies, and determination of initial ventilator settings. Most continuing education courses, including our own, now require that the entering student have a bachelor's degree. Eventually, the majority of such courses will evolve into master's degree programs and should, therefore, correct what we see as a clinical deficiency in current master's programs. In general, we feel that the trend toward master's degree–prepared practitioners is healthy for the nursing profession and should be encouraged.

SUGGESTED READING

Harper RG, Little GA, Sia CG. The scope of nursing practice in level III neonatal intensive care units. Pediatrics 1982; 70:875.

Martin RG, Fenton LJ, Leonardson G, Reid TJ. Consistency of care in an intensive care nursery staffed by nurse clinicians. Am J Dis Child 1985; 139:169-172.

Wellman LR, Stevens DC, Wilson AL, Fenton LJ. Mortality outcome in a tertiary neonatal intensive care unit utilizing nurse clinicians in place of pediatric housestaff. Pediatr Res 1981; 15:686.

SYMPTOMATIC INBORN ERRORS OF METABOLISM

SAUL W. BRUSILOW, M.D.
DAVID L. VALLE, M.D.
PAMELA ARN, M.D.

The single most important feature of newborn infants who have symptomatic inborn errors of metabolism is their gestational age; it appears that *these diseases are found principally in full-term infants*. There is reason to believe that full-term neonates who have no perinatal risk factors are as likely to have an inborn error of metabolism as sepsis. In the full-term and preterm neonate, nonspecific symptoms such as poor feeding, lethargy, vomiting, respiratory distress, coma, and seizures may indicate any of several common maladies, including sepsis and diseases of the cardiopulmonary, gastrointestinal, and central nervous systems. These same nonspecific symptoms are also the presenting manifestations of a variety of symptomatic inborn errors of metabolism of the newborn. Among the large number of human genetic diseases, only a few are definitely associated with symptoms in the neonate (Table 1). These include four disorders of ureagenesis, defects in branched-chain amino acid metabolism (maple syrup urine disease and isovaleric acidemia), disorders of propionate and methylmalonate metabolism, multiple carboxylase deficiency, glutaric acidemia type II and other electron transport chain diseases, disorders of pyruvate metabolism, galactosemia, type I glycogen storage disease, fructose-1,6-diphosphatase deficiency, nonketotic hyperglycinemia, oxoprolinuria, and acyl CoA dehydrogenase deficiencies. Each of these diseases is rare; however, as a group they constitute an important cause of morbidity in the full-term newborn. Early diagnosis is particularly important, since many of these enzymatic deficiencies are amenable to therapy, provided effective intervention is instituted prior to the onset of irreversible damage of the central nervous system.

Although some of these disorders may be detected by neonatal screening programs, symptoms usually occur before the results of the screening tests are reported. Thus, for these disorders, there is no substitute for the alert and thoughtful physician. In contrast to inborn errors of metabolism with an insidious onset (e.g., phenylketonuria), in which a diagnostic delay of a few days may not be significant, a delay of a few hours in neonates suffering from symptomatic inborn errors of metabolism may have dire consequences. Because the symptoms are nonspecific and overlap with those of other diseases, *we recommend that all sick full-term neonates be considered at risk for one of these disorders*.

Other clues that suggest symptomatic inborn errors of metabolism in the full-term neonate include a family history of neonatal deaths within the same sibship or in male infants on the mother's side of the family. This information should be obtained prospectively so as to identify infants at risk. Lack of such a positive history does not make these disorders less likely, however, since most are inherited as autosomal recessive traits with only a 25 percent risk for each birth in a sibship. Consanguinity increases the likelihood of rare recessive disorders and should also heighten diagnostic suspicion.

The time of onset of symptoms is also an important factor in directing attention to genetic disease. Most infants with symptomatic inborn errors are initially (first 24 hours) symptom-free while toxic substrates (e.g., ammonium, amino acids, keto acids, organic acids, galactose) accumulate. During fetal life these compounds are cleared by the placenta and metabolized by the mother. An exception to this general picture occurs in those diseases in which product deficiencies may be the cause of symptoms, i.e., disorders of pyruvate carboxylase, pyruvate dehydrogenase, and the respiratory electron transport chain. These infants may present in the first few hours after birth with respiratory distress and metabolic acidosis.

We present here our diagnostic (Table 1, Fig. 1) and therapeutic (Tables 2, 3, and 4) approaches to infants suspected of having a symptomatic inborn error of metabolism.

We recommend that all *full-term newborn infants who are sick enough to warrant a blood culture should be evaluated for a genetic disease* by measuring the plasma level of ammonium and amino acids as well as performing qualitative tests for urinary ketones, keto acids, and galactose. Plasma amino acids should be measured by quantitative column chromatography rather than paper chromatography or high-voltage electrophoresis. The results of these tests in symptomatic inborn errors of metabolism of the neonate appear in Table 1. It should be noted that an occasional patient with propionic acidemia or methylmalonic acidemia may not be acidotic or ketotic. Thus, urine organic acids should be measured by gas chromatography–mass spectrometry in all symptomatic hyperglycinemic patients. Occasionally, the presence of thrombocytopenia and neutropenia may suggest isovaleric acidemia, propionic acidemia, methylmalonic acidemia, or multiple carboxylase deficiency.

If hyperammonemia is present, we utilize the diagnostic protocol outlined in Figure 1.

If a nonglucose urinary reducing substance is found, qualitative analysis of urine sugars by thin-layer chromatography and measurement of galactose-1-phosphate-uridyl transferase in erythrocytes should be done. The infant should be placed on a galactose-free formula until a precise diagnosis is made.

The presence of ketone bodies in the urine suggests an organic acidemia or type I glycogen storage disease. Urine organic acids should be evaluated as already described. Additional features of type I glycogen storage disease include hepatomegaly, hypoglycemia after fasting for 3 to 4 hours, and failure to increase blood glucose following parenteral glucagon (0.1 mg per kilogram intramuscularly). The presence of dinitrophenylhydrazine-positive material in the urine in this clinical setting suggests maple syrup urine disease, which can be confirmed by

TABLE 1 Laboratory Evaluation of Infants With Symptomatic Inborn Errors of Metabolism

Disorder	Deficient Enzyme(s)	Acid-Base Status	Anion Gap	Plasma Lactate	Plasma Pyruvate	Plasma Ammonium‡	Plasma* Amino Acids	Urine Dinitrophenylhydrazine	Urine Ketones	Urine Reducing Substances	Urine† Organic Acids	Other
Amino Acid and Organic Acid Disorders												
Carbamylphosphate synthetase deficiency	Carbamylphosphate synthetase I	Respiratory alkalosis	N	N	N	4+	Absent citrulline and low arginine	–	–	–	–	–
Ornithine transcarbamylase deficiency	Ornithine transcarbamylase	Respiratory alkalosis	N	N	N	4+	Absent citrulline and low arginine	–	–	–	–	Increased urine orotic acid
Citrullinemia	Argininosuccinate synthetase	Respiratory alkalosis	N	N	N	4+	Citrulline 50–100 × increased: low arginine	–	–	–	–	Increased urine orotic acid
Argininosuccinic acidemia	Argininosuccinate lyase	Respiratory alkalosis	N	N	N	4+	Argininosuccinate and anhydrides present; citrulline 10–20 × increased; subnormal arginine	–	–	–	–	Increased urine ototic acid
Maple syrup urine disease	Branched chain ketoacid decarboxylase	Metabolic acidosis	N-increased	N	N	N	Leucine, isoleucine, and valine 5–40 × increased; alloisoleucine present	+	+	–	2-Ketoisoproic 2-Ketoisovaleric 2-Keto-3-methyl-valeric	Odor of maple syrup
Isovaleric acidemia	Isovalcryl CoA decarboxylase	Metabolic acidosis	N	N	N	N-2+	N	–	+	–	Isovalerylglycine 3-Hydroxyisovaleric acid	Odor of sweaty feet
Propionic acidemias	Propionyl CoA carboxylase	Metabolic acidosis	N-increased	N	N	N-4+	2–4 × increased glycine	–	+	–	3-Hydroxypropionic acid Methylcitric acid	
Methylmalonic acidemias	Methylmalonyl CoA mutase Adenosylcobalamin synthetic enzymes	Metabolic acidosis	N-increased	N	N	N-4+	2–4 × increased glycine (one form with homocystinuria)	–	+	–	Methylmalonic acid	Some with homocystinuria
Multiple carboxylase deficiency	Holocarboxylase synthetase	Metabolic acidosis	N-increased	N-increased	?	N-2–	?	–	+	–	3-Methylcrotonyl glycine 3-Hydroxyisovaleric acid 3-Hydroxypropionic acid Methylcitrate	Lactic acidosis
Nonketotic hyperglycinemia	Glycine cleavage	N-respiratory	N	N	N	N	3–5 × increased	–	–	–	–	
Glutaric acidemia, type II	Electron transport flavoprotein Electron transport flavoprotein dehydrogenase	N-metabolic acidosis	N	N	N	N-2+	N	–	–	–	Glutaric acid 2-Hydroxyglutaric acid 3-Hydroxyisovaleric acid Methylsuccinic acid Methylmalonic acid	Odor of sweaty feet Some with dysmorphic features

Table continues on following page

TABLE 1 Laboratory Evaluation of Infants With Symptomatic Inborn Errors of Metabolism (Continued)

Disorder	Deficient Enzyme(s)	Acid-Base Status	Anion Gap	Plasma Lactate	Plasma Pyruvate	Plasma Ammonium‡	Plasma* Amino Acids	Urine Dinitrophenylhydrazine	Urine Ketones	Urine Reducing Substances	Urine† Organic Acids	Other
Pyroglutamic acidemia (5-oxoprolinuria)	Glutathione synthetase	Metabolic acidosis	?	N	N	N	N	–	–	–	Pyroglutamic acid	Hyperbilirubinemia
Carbohydrate Disorders												
Galactosemia	Galactose-1-phosphate uridyl-transferase	Hyperchloremic metabolic acidosis	N	N	N	N	N-2-5 increased tyrosine, methionine	–	–	+		Cataracts often not detectable early
Fructose-1,6-diphosphatase deficiency	Fructose-1,6-diphosphatase	Metabolic acidosis	Increased	Increased	Increased	N	N-increased alanine	–	+	–		Hypoglycemia
Type I glycogen storage disease, A and B	IA-Glucose-6-phosphatase IB-Glucose-6-phosphate translocase	Metabolic acidosis	Increased	Increased	Increased	N	N-increased alanine	–	+	–		Hypoglycemia Hypocholesterolemia Hypertriglyceridemia Hyperuricacidemia
Congenital lactic acidoses*	Pyruvate dehydrogenase complex Pyruvate carboxylase Components of electron transport system	Metabolic acidosis	Increased	Increased	Increased	N	Increased alanine	–	–	–	Lactic acid	Hyperpyruvicacidemia Some with dysmorphic features
SCAD	Short-chain acyl CoA dehydrogenase	Metabolic acidosis	Increased	?	?	N-2+	N	–	Usually absent	–	Ethylmalonic acid	Hypoglycemia Hypocarnitinemia
MCAD	Medium chain acyl CoA dehydrogenase	Metabolic acidosis	Increased	?	?	N-2+	N	–	Usually absent	–	Medium-chain dicarboxylic acids and acyl carnitines, hexanoyl glycine, phenylpropionyl glycine, subaryl glycine	Hypoglycemia Hypocarnitinemia
LCAD	Long-chain acyl CoA dehydrogenase	Metabolic acidosis	Increased	?	?	2+	N	–	Usually absent	–	Dicarboxylic acids	Hypoglycemia Hypocarnitinemia
Hydroxymethylglutaryl CoA lyase deficiency	Hydroxymethylglutaryl CoA lyase	Metabolic acidosis	Increased	?	?	2+	N	–	Absent	–	Hydroxymethylglutaric, 3-Methyl-gluconic acids	Hypoglycemia

Abbreviation and symbols: N,normal; –,negative; +,positive; ?,not known; 1+–4+ indicates increasing severity of abnormality; SCAD, short-chain acyl CoA dehydrogenase; MCAD, medium-chain acyl CoA dehydrogenase; LCAD, long-chain acyl CoA dehydrogenase.
* Measured by quantitative column chromatography.
† Measured by gas chromatography–mass spectrometry.
‡ Hyperammonemia is usually associated with hyperglutaminemia.

TABLE 2 Outline of Treatment of Inborn Errors of Urea Synthesis*

Enzyme Deficiency and Treatment	Regimen
Carbamyl phosphate synthetase and ornithine transcarbamylase	
Protein	0.5–0.7 g/kg/day
Essential amino acids	0.5–0.7 g/kg/day
Sodium benzoate	0–250 mg/kg/day
Sodium phenylacetate	250–550 mg/kg/day**
Citrulline	170 mg/kg/day
Argininosuccinic acid synthetase	
Protein	1.5–2.0 g/kg/day
Sodium benzoate	0–250 mg/kg/day
Sodium phenylacetate	250–550 mg/kg/day**
Arginine (free base)	350–700 mg/kg/day
Argininosuccinase	
Protein	1.5–2.0 g/kg/day
Arginine (free base)	350–700 mg/kg/day

* All patients should receive at lest 120 calories per kilogram per day. The calcium salts of benzoate and phenylacetate may be used in place of the sodium salts.

** Sodium phenylbutyrate (600 mg/kg/day) may be substituted for sodium phenylacetate because of the repugnant odor of the latter.

TABLE 3 General Protocol for Diet-Responsive Symptomatic Inborn Errors of Metabolism in the Neonate

1. Discontinue intake of the offending compound(s) and/or its precursor(s).
2. Institute appropriate measures to eliminate toxic metabolite(s) (fluid and electrolyte replenishment, hemo- or peritoneal dialysis).
3. Provide a minimum of 120 cal/kg/day utilizing intravenous and oral nutrition. The oral therapy will require a special formula, perhaps supplemented with the nonprotein containing diet substance MJ80056.*
4. Institute pharmacologic trial of specific vitamin cofactor (see Table 4).
5. As indicated by careful and frequent monitoring of plasma levels, add the minimal required amounts of the essential offending compound(s) to the diet (see Table 4).
6. Adjust the caloric, fluid, and limited offending compounds according to the patient's individual needs as indicated by growth and plasma concentrations.

* Mead Johnson

TABLE 4 Information for the Dietary Treatment of Selected Inborn Errors of Metabolism

Disorder	Substance to be Limited	Estimated Daily Requirement	Special Formulas	Test for Vitamin Response	
				Vitamin	Daily Dose
Maple syrup urine disease	Leucine Isoleucine Valine	75–150 mg/kg 80–100 mg/kg 85–105 mg/kg	MSUD Diet Powder*	Thiamine	10 mg IM or PO
Isovaleric acidemia	Leucine	See above	MSUD Diet Powder*† S-14‡	Biotin	10 mg IM
Propionic acidemias	Isoleucine Valine Methionine Threonine	See above 30 mg/kg 90 mg/kg	OS-1§	Biotin	10 mg IM
Methylmalonic acidemia	Isoleucine Valine Methionine Threonine	See above	OS-1§	Hydroxycobalamin	2 mg IM
Multiple carboxylase deficiency				Biotin	10 mg IM or PO
Galactosemia	Galactose	Not essential	Isomil# Nutramigen*		
Congenital lactic acidosis	Depends on the particular enzyme defect			Thiamine Biotin Lipomade Riboflavin	10 mg IM 20 mg IM 20 mg IM or 100 mg PO 50 mg IM

* Mead Johnson Laboratories.
† Since MSUD Diet Powder lacks all three branch-chain amino acids, it must be supplemented with normal amounts of isoleucine and valine when used for isovaleric acidemia. We also add L-glycine 0.25 g/kg/d to the formula to augment the conjugation of excess isovaleryl CoA to the nontoxic isovalerylglycine.
‡ Wyeth.
§ Milupa.
# Ross Laboratories.

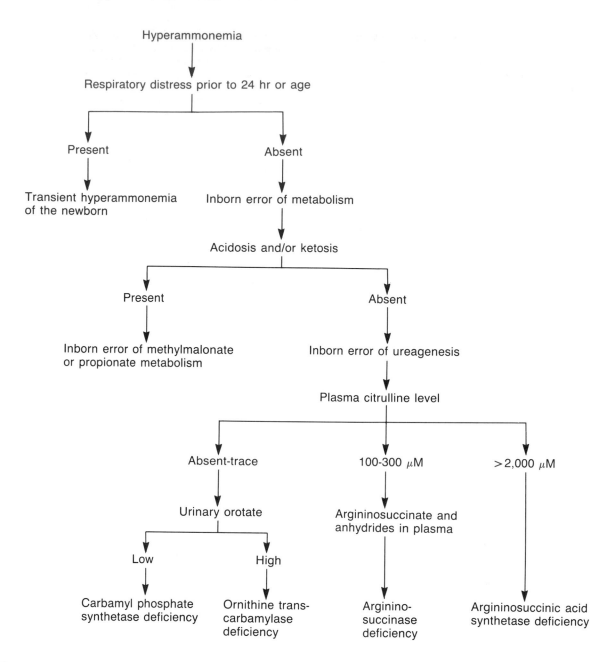

Figure 1 Algorithm for the diagnosis of hyperammonemia of the neonate.

plasma amino acid analysis. The urine and sweat of these patients may also have the characteristic odor of maple syrup.

Acidosis accompanied by an increased anion gap is not uncommon in neonates and is usually a consequence of lactic acidemia secondary to peripheral hypoperfusion and/or hypoxia. However, when tissue hypoxia is not a factor, diagnostic attention should be directed toward evaluating accumulation of organic anions secondary to an inborn error of metabolism (see Table 1).

TREATMENT

Because the metabolites that accumulate in disorders of ureagenesis, in maple syrup urine disease, and in dis-

orders of propionate and methylmalonate metabolism are toxic to the central nervous system, we believe that therapy should be aggressive and, prompt. Thus, any patient with these diseases who is in stage II coma (poor muscle tone, few spontaneous movements, but responsiveness to painful stimuli) or worse is a candidate for immediate hemodialysis, to be followed by appropriate medical therapy. *Hemodialysis is 10 times more effective in removing small molecules than is peritoneal dialysis or arteriovenous hemofiltration.* Although exchange transfusion is effective in removing metabolites bound to plasma proteins (e.g., bilirubin), it is ineffective in removing metabolites that are distributed in total body water.

Treatment of inborn errors of ureagenesis is tailored to the specific defect, as determined by the algorithm shown in Figure 1. Transient hyperammonemia of the newborn is a poorly understood syndrome characterized by low birth weight, respiratory distress within the first 24 hours of life, a positive finding on the chest roentgenogram, and spontaneous resolution. Table 2 describes current therapy for deficiencies of carbamyl phosphate synthetase, ornithine transcarbamylase, argininosuccinic acid synthetase, and argininosuccinase.

Treatment of nonurea cycle symptomatic inborn errors of metabolism in the neonate is outlined in Table 3. Unfortunately, there is no consistently effective therapy for nonketotic hyperglycinemia or for disorders of pyruvate metabolism or the electron transport chain (congenital lactic acidoses). Occasional infants with this latter group of disorders have had improvement when treated with vitamin cofactors for the various enzymes (see Table 4) or with ketogenic diets. For patients with acyl CoA deficiency, prolonged fasting should be avoided. Dietary carnitine supplementation is recommended for these patients by some investigators, but its value is yet to be established.

This work was supported in part by NIH grant HD11134 (SWB). EY02948 (DV), M01-RR0052, GM07471 (PA) of Kettering Family Foundation (SWB), the MA and TA O'Malley Foundation and the March of Dimes Birth Defects Foundation (DV). Dr. Valle is an investigator of the Howard Hughes Medical Institute.

VITAMIN E SUPPLEMENTATION

JAMES A. LEMONS, M.D.

Since its discovery in 1922, vitamin E (alpha-tocopherol) has often been referred to as a treatment in search of a disease. Although the structure and biochemical functions of this vitamin have been elucidated in considerable detail, the role of alpha-tocopherol in the clinical setting has still eluded scientists. Most recently, the potential role of vitamin E in nutrition of the very low birth weight infant has received considerable scrutiny. In spite of extensive investigations, however, the exact function of this "shady lady" of the vitamins remains obscure.

BACKGROUND

Vitamin E or alpha-tocopherol is a fat-soluble vitamin that was first noted for its importance in sustaining pregnancy in rats. Tocopherol, which means child-bearing, is one of the most widely distributed vitamins in foods. Of the eight naturally occurring isomers, alpha-tocopherol possesses the greatest biologic activity and constitutes approximately 90 percent of the tocopherols present in animal tissues. Vitamin E activity, however, is standardized against alpha-tocopherol acetate, an acetate ester that contains by definition one unit of biologic vitamin E activity per milligram. Vitamin E is generally available for supplementation in the neonate as alpha-tocopherol acetate (in Aquasol E and M.V.I. Pediatric).

PHYSIOLOGIC FUNCTIONS

Vitamin E is thought to be the most important endogenous antioxidant present in human tissues. Deficiency states of this vitamin are associated principally with alternations in cellular membrane permeability and fragility, suggesting that alpha-tocopherol may be important in stabilizing the lipid component of the membrane. Lipids and, in particular, polyunsaturated lipids are susceptible to peroxidation by unstable free oxygen radicals and normal byproducts of oxidative metabolism. The lipid peroxides that are formed may be relatively unstable themselves and lead to further spontaneous lipid peroxidation. Vitamin E is thought to inhibit peroxidation of polyunsaturated fats by acting as an antioxidant or reducing agent. Unstable radicals, including lipid peroxides, accept protons from alpha-tocopherol and are converted to water or other stable intermediates. In addition, further experimental evidence suggests that vitamin E is an important structural component of the cellular membrane. Alpha-tocopherol, by way of its methyl side groups, appears to fit within the tertiary structure of the fatty acid residues within the biologic membrane, enabling it to function as a local antioxidant.

NEONATAL STORES AND REQUIREMENTS FOR VITAMIN E

In evaluating vitamin E stores, it is important to remember that alpha-tocopherol is lipid-soluble. It is therefore found in most body tissues in amounts proportional to fat content. At approximately 20 week's gestation, the fetus contains approximately 1 mg of tocopherol, whereas at term the fetus contains approximately 20 mg. As reviewed by Bell, total fetal tocopherol content appears to be linearly related to body weight during human gestation (approximately 5 mg per kilogram weight). In comparison, however, the adult human contains between 50 and 150 mg per kilogram of weight. However, this discrepancy between fetal and adult stores disappears when tocopherol content is corrected for body fat stores. The fetus contains 0.27 mg tocopherol per gram of lipid, whereas the adult male contains 0.25 mg per gram and the adult female 0.46 mg per gram fat.

The relatively constant ratio of tocopherol to total lipid stores may be expected, recognizing the lipid solubility of vitamin E. More specifically, one may anticipate that vitamin E requirements are directly related to polyunsaturated fatty acid content of tissues and diet. Dietary supply of vitamin E should parallel the intake and tissue content of polyunsaturated fatty acids. Other factors that may increase the requirement for vitamin E include exogenous oxidant stresses (such as additional iron supplementation or an oxygen-enriched environment).

Vitamin E status is generally evaluated on the basis of plasma or serum concentrations of tocopherol. In addition, some measure of antioxidant protection (such as the peroxide hemolysis test) has been found to be useful. The method used to quantitate vitamin E in blood is important in that colorimetric techniques measure total tocopherols present, regardless of biologic activity, whereas high-pressure liquid chromatography distinguishes between the alpha and the beta/gamma isomers. This distinction may be important if a significant portion of the vitamin E available to an infant is provided as the gamma rather than the alpha vitamer (as occurs with some intravenous fat preparations). Beta and gamma vitamers possess only 10 percent and 30 percent, respectively, of the biologic activity of alpha-tocopherol acetate.

Results of peroxide-induced hemolysis tests suggest that the majority of babies weighing less than 1,500 g at birth may be vitamin E–deficient. Serum levels of tocopherol are generally less than 0.5 mg per deciliter in these cases. Although many infants with serum levels of less than 0.5 mg per deciliter have adequate stores of vitamin E and normal hemolysis tests, 0.5 mg per deciliter is generally accepted as a reasonable lower limit for tocopherol levels in both adult and neonatal populations. Therefore most clinicians rely upon the plasma-serum concentration of vitamin E to screen for vitamin E deficiency, as this test is readily available in most laboratories compared with the erythrocyte peroxide hemolysis test. Some investigators have recommended relating the concentrations of tocopherol in blood to the amount of circulating lipid, although most experts have not found this to be useful in predicting vitamin E deficiency in the preterm infant.

Although studies have yielded conflicting results, vitamin E appears to be well absorbed from the gastrointestinal tract by most very low birth weight infants. However, efficiency of absorption is variable and may depend upon gestational age, postnatal age, relative fat absorption, and the rate of intestinal hydrolysis of the acetate ester. Enteral preparations of vitamin E are given as alpha-tocopherol acetate, which requires hydrolysis in the intestinal mucosa prior to absorption into the lymphatics and then the blood. Serum levels normally increase in the first 1 to 3 weeks of age to normal adult ranges (greater than 0.5 mg per deciliter) when infants are fed standard formulas or human milk. Intramuscular preparations result in prompter increases in serum levels when water-miscible preparations are used, although this route is not generally employed in the small preterm infant. Intravenous administration of vitamin E also results in predictable levels, depending on the rate and dosage employed. The vitamer generally available for intravenous administration is also alpha-tocopherol acetate, which appears to be hydrolyzed to the free alcohol form in very premature infants without difficulty.

Most investigators have recommended a dietary vitamin E intake of at least 0.4 mg of alpha-tocopherol per gram of polyunsaturated fatty acid. This is supported by the Committee on Nutrition of the American Academy of Pediatrics, which recommends that premature infants receive at least 1.0 IU of vitamin E per gram of linoleic acid (similar to 0.4 mg tocopherol per gram polyunsaturated fatty acid). *Currently available formulas, particularly the formulas developed specifically for the very low birth weight infant, provide ample vitamin E to meet this requirement.* If an infant requires parenteral nutrition, we provide 3 to 6 mg per kilogram per day of vitamin E in the form of alpha-tocopherol acetate (as M.V.I. Pediatric). Additional supplements, given either parenterally or enterally, are not required for the very low birth weight infant in most circumstances.

PROPOSED USES OF SUPPLEMENTAL VITAMIN E IN THE VERY LOW BIRTH WEIGHT INFANT

Vitamin E supplementation in varying amounts has been alleged to (1) prevent hemolytic anemia of prematurity, (2) decrease bilirubin concentrations, (3) reduce the severity of bronchopulmonary dysplasia, (4) reduce the frequency and severity of retinopathy of prematurity, (5) reduce the frequency and severity of intraventricular/parenchymal hemorrhage, and (6) improve survival rates in extremely small infants weighing less than 1 kg at birth. To date, *extensive investigations of vitamin E in each of these areas have failed to uniformly demonstrate benefit of supplemental vitamin E.* In reviewing these studies, it is apparent that investigators may utilize different preparations, dosing schedules, dosing amounts, and patient populations, which preclude exact comparison of results. Nonetheless, routine supplementation of vitamin E beyond what is normally provided in parenteral and enteral nutritional preparations is not recommended at this time.

Vitamin E Deficiency Hemolytic Anemia. Numerous studies have been performed to document whether vitamin E supplementation ameliorates or prevents the anemia normally seen at 6 to 10 weeks of life in the premature infant. A carefully controlled study by Zipursky did not demonstrate any benefit from supplementation of 25 IU of alpha-tocopherol enterally to infants weighing less than 1,500 g during the first 6 weeks of life. Parameters monitored included hemoglobin, hematocrit, erythrocyte peroxide fragility, reticulocyte count, platelet count, vitamin E levels, and red cell morphology. No differences in these parameters were noted between the unsupplemented and supplemented infants.

Jaundice. Conflicting results have been found concerning a possible effect of vitamin E in lowering bilirubin levels during the first days of life. There is no clear-cut evidence that a significant benefit may result for the very low birth weight infant.

Bronchopulmonary Dysplasia. In spite of initial preliminary data suggesting a potential benefit of vitamin E supplementation in preventing lung injury, prospective controlled clinical trials have not demonstrated improved outcome with vitamin E supplementation.

Retinopathy of Prematurity. The role of vitamin E in prevention or amelioration of retinopathy of prematurity has generated considerable controversy in recent years. Several prospective studies have suggested that supplemental vitamin E may decrease the frequency of more severe grades of retinopathy in infants weighing less than 1,500 g at birth. Recommended doses have ranged from 50 to 200 mg per kilogram per day by the oral route with additional parenteral dosing in some instances. The most recent and most carefully designed prospective trial did not detect any improvement in either the incidence or the severity of retinopathy of prematurity with vitamin E supplementation.

Intraventricular Hemorrhage. Controversy persists regarding the possible effect of vitamin E on the frequency and severity of intraventricular hemorrhage in the very low birth weight infant. Several investigations failed to demonstrate an effect, whereas other studies have indicated that intramuscular supplementation with vitamin E during the first 3 days of life may reduce both the frequency and severity of intraventricular and parenchymal hemorrhage in the very low birth weight infant. Additional studies have actually demonstrated a higher frequency of intraventricular hemorrhage in very low birth weight infants when supplemental vitamin E was administered intravenously. It remains uncertain whether vitamin E has an effect on intracranial hemorrhage in the low birth weight infant. If there is a positive effect, it is unclear what formulation, dosage, or schedule of administration should be recommended.

Mortality. Initial reports suggested that the survival rate of infants weighing less than 1 kg at birth was improved with supplemental vitamin E administration. Other studies have failed to confirm this observation.

TOXICITY

If vitamin E were free of risks, then its use in different clinical settings would be reasonable, even if the benefit was only theoretical. However, it is essential that risks be negligible before we utilize vitamin E in other than normal physiologic amounts (as are present in human milk and most formulas). In this regard, a number of side effects have been reported for vitamin E, including local irritation with intramuscular injection; altered platelet metabolism and aggregation; impaired wound healing; hepatomegaly; possible increased risk of intraventricular hemorrhage with intravenous injection; and at higher serum levels (higher than 3.5 mg per deciliter) in the very low birth weight infant, an increased risk of necrotizing enterocolitis and bacterial sepsis. In 1983 a syndrome of hepatotoxicity, hypotension, renal failure, and *death of some preterm infants was associated with the use of an intravenous preparation of vitamin E (E-Ferol)*. The exact cause of the clinical deterioration of these infants has not been identified (i.e., the vitamin E itself versus the emulsifying agent in that particular preparation of vitamin E). Therefore, from a review of available literature, it is apparent that vitamin E is not without potential risk when used as a supplement in the premature infant at doses of 25 to 200 mg per kilogram per day by the oral route. Even at the lower doses of 25 mg per kilogram per day by the enteral route, serum levels may reach potentially toxic levels (higher than 3.5 mg per deciliter).

SPECIFIC CLINICAL ENTITIES

ACUTE RENAL FAILURE

GARY R. LERNER, M.D.
ALAN B. GRUSKIN, M.D.

Acute renal failure (ARF) may be defined as a symptom complex that occurs when body fluid homeostasis is impaired by the rapid loss of renal function. This chapter focuses on the management of ARF in the newborn period and assumes that a working diagnosis of prerenal, intrarenal, or postrenal failure has been established.

MANAGEMENT OF PRERENAL ARF

General supportive management includes maintenance of blood pressure, oxygenation, and extracellular volume. If the baby has developed symptomatic anemia or experienced blood loss, a blood transfusion is indicated. A transfusion of 10 ml per kilogram of packed red blood cells raises the hematocrit by 10.

In volume-depleted neonates differentiation of pre-ARF from intrinsic ARF by means of a fluid challenge is indicated. It may prove useful to have central lines, such as central venous pressure and arterial lines, in place to monitor changes in cardiovascular parameters during the diagnostic or therapeutic fluid administrations.

Treatment of the oliguric neonate begins with an adequate fluid challenge. We recommend giving 15 to 20 ml per kilogram of an electrolyte solution containing sodium in a concentration that exceeds 75 mEq per liter (we usually give normal saline). The fluid challenge is divided into two infusions of 10 ml per kilogram each; each infusion should take no longer than 30 minutes. After each infusion is completed, vital signs, urine output, and so forth are re-evaluated. One should avoid giving potassium- and phosphate-containing solutions. If urine output does not increase, 1 to 3 mg per kilogram of furosemide is given as an intravenous infusion at a rate not to exceed 0.2 mg per kilogram per minute. If urine output again fails to increase, a second dose of furosemide, 3 to 5 mg per kilogram, is given. Some physicians also give mannitol, 0.5 g per kilogram, before the second dose of furosemide. If, after the second dose of furosemide, the urine output fails to exceed 2.0 ml per kilogram per hour, a diagnosis of intrinsic ARF is assumed and further management planned accordingly.

MANAGEMENT OF POSTRENAL ARF

The diagnosis of obstructive uropathy is suspected in the neonate who presents with oliguria/anuria and/or a suprapubic or flank mass. For an obstructive lesion to manifest as ARF, one must assume that the lesion is bilateral or that the patient has only a single kidney. Once the diagnosis of ARF secondary to obstruction has been made, a pediatric urologist should be consulted to relieve the obstructive lesion (e.g., posterior urethral valves, bilateral ureteral obstruction, and so forth). The management of such a patient includes supportive therapy preoperatively. Particularly close attention should be paid to serum chemistries such as potassium, calcium, and sodium levels, as well as the fluid status, in order to maximize the patient's preoperative status. Abnormal chemistries should be corrected before surgery.

A major problem following relief of obstruction is postobstructive diuresis. This is managed by strict attention to the fluid and electrolyte replacement of all urine. Fluid therapy is calculated as insensible water loss (30 ml per kilogram per day for the term infant; 40 to 50 ml per kilogram per day for the preterm infant; these values are increased by an additional 20 to 30 percent if the infant is receiving phototherapy) plus urine replacement. Urine losses are replaced milliliter for milliliter with a solution containing concentrations of NaCl and KCl equal to those measured in the urine (ideally measured 2 to 3 times per day). We prefer to administer this combination of fluids in two bottles with the aid of infusion pumps: one containing water and glucose (only) to replace the insensible water loss and the other for the continuing milliliter for milliliter urine replacement. The two infusions are then piggybacked together if the vein will allow such volume to be given. This strict replacement is continued until the blood urea nitrogen (BUN) and creatinine values stabilize, which may take several days. Subsequently, the kidney is challenged by restricting fluid to see if it can respond appropriately to volumetric stimuli. Blood chemistries, including sodium, potassium, chloride, HCO_3, calcium, phosphate, BUN, and creatinine, are initially checked twice a day, later once daily. Any significant deviations from normal in blood chemistries need to be corrected.

Acidification defects commonly occur during and after this time. Bicarbonate is added to the insensible water replacement as needed to correct acidosis up to a bicarbonate concentration of 20 mEq per liter.

PREOPERATIVE MANAGEMENT OF THE NEONATE WITH ARF UNDERGOING SURGERY

Serum electrolyte, calcium, and phosphate levels should be checked 1 hour before surgery, since these often change abruptly in neonates with ARF. Once blood is drawn, the neonate should continue to receive nothing by mouth. Additionally, the patient should be euvolemic, as hypovolemia before general anesthesia may exacerbate renal hypoperfusion and worsen any existing renal damage. Clues to hypovolemia can be gleaned from central venous pressure readings, arterial blood pressure measurements, pulse rate, and changes in weight.

MANAGEMENT OF INTRINSIC RENAL FAILURE

Aside from the initial fluid management mentioned above (postobstructive diuresis), the therapy for any type of renal failure is similar. Should oliguria or anuria be present, the fluid orders can be written as above; i.e., insensible water loss plus milliliter for milliliter urine replacement. This approach guarantees that the patient will remain euvolemic. Attention to weight, however, is imperative, because initial quantities of water are based only on estimates of water turnover. No weight change over the course of ARF, (which can run for weeks) actually indicates an increase in total body water, if sufficient energy and protein have not been provided. We expect that, unless energy and protein are provided, a weight loss of 1 to 1.5 percent per day should be anticipated.

Nutrition

Three approaches to providing adequate calories are available: (1) high concentration solutions via a central line, (2) dialysis, and (3) peripheral and/or central alimentation in conjunction with continuous arteriovenous hemofiltration (CAVH). Energy requirements during ARF have been met by infusing highly concentrated solutions (50 to 70 percent) of glucose into a central vein. We are unaware, however, of any experience in neonates. Adequate caloric intake will be impeded if the patient is oliguric, since, even with hyperalimentation as practiced in neonates, there are significant fluid requirements. In oliguric or anuric infants, the provision of adequate calories requires that high concentrations (30 to 60 percent) of glucose be given centrally in small volumes, or lesser concentrations of glucose in larger volumes. The latter requires that steps be taken to simultaneously increase water removal by either dialysis or CAVH. The decision to provide normal amounts of energy and/or nutrients is also an indication for dialysis or other means of fluid removal, such as CAVH. CAVH filters are available small enough to be used in the neonate, with some modifications to prevent too abrupt fluid removal. We maximize carbohydrate and fat calories while keeping calories derived from protein at the lower end of normal. Should parenteral therapy be required, essential and nonessential amino acids can be administered to these patients to meet their requirements. Feld reported using a parenteral nitrogen intake in the range of 120 to 240 mg per kilogram per day in his hypercatabolic patients with renal failure.

MANAGEMENT OF ELECTROLYTE DERANGEMENTS

Electrolyte management remains the key to immediate survival. Close attention to potassium balance is important. In the patient with ARF who also may be hypercatabolic because of such complications as infection, starvation, and shock, rapid cell turnover can quickly lead to hyperkalemia. Hyperkalemia is defined as a potassium level of more than 7 mEq per liter and/or electrocardiographic changes such as T-wave tenting and QRS widening. When acute therapy to control hyperkalemia is required, 10 percent calcium gluconate (0.1 to 0.2 ml per kilogram) is given intravenously, slowly, while the heart rate is monitored. If the heart rate decreases, the infusion is either slowed or stopped. The use of calcium counteracts the effect of the potassium on the myocardium. Other methods of palliative therapy include insulin with glucose (intravenous glucose, 0.5 g per kilogram over 1 to 2 hours with 1 unit of insulin per 5 g of glucose), or bicarbonate infusions (2 to 3 mEq per kilogram $NaHCO_3$ over 5 to 10 minutes). Uptake of glucose by the cells induces glycogen synthesis and also increases potassium uptake. The bicarbonate causes potassium to shift intracellularly by raising the blood pH. In either case the effect is only transient, and steps must be taken to enhance potassium removal from the body. Short of dialysis, the only other way to remove potassium from the body is to use an exchange resin, sodium polystyrene sulfonate (Kayexalate), in doses of 0.5 to 1.0 g per kilogram rectally, with 5 ml per kilogram of 10 to 20 percent sorbitol up to 4 to 6 times a day. Care must be used, since there is 4 mEq of sodium per gram of Kayexalate and sodium retention can contribute to fluid overload and congestive heart failure (CHF).

Aberrations of serum sodium levels in either direction occur in ARF. Hyponatremia is usually due to the neonate receiving too much free water in the face of a decreased ability of the kidney to excrete free water properly. This most often occurs because of the use of hypotonic solutions either orally or intravenously to replace extrarenal loss of water and solute. No therapy is needed if the serum sodium is greater than 125 mEq per liter, but if the level falls below 120 or if seizures occur, therapy is instituted. The therapeutic goal is to raise the serum sodium to 125 mEq per liter, which should alleviate the symptoms. The quantity of sodium required can be calculated by the following formula:

Number of mEq Na required = [(desired serum Na– observed serum Na) × body weight (kg) × 0.7)]

Since the total body water of a neonate is higher than that of the older child or adult, the factor 0.7 is substituted for the 0.6 normally used. The rate of rise of serum sodium should not exceed 2 mEq per hour. Once the level of 125 mEq per liter is reached, a slower increase in the serum sodium to values above 130 mEq per liter is planned. In view of the reduced urine output in oliguric renal failure, the use of 3 percent NaCl may be indicated to limit the volume of infused solute. Complications of hypertonic solute infusions in a patient with decreased or absent urine output include volume overload leading to CHF, pulmonary edema, and hypertension. Frequent monitoring of vital signs and weight changes is important during such therapy. It may be necessary to plan for dialysis or CAVH if the hypotonic neonate experiences clinical symptoms of volume overload. If the neonate is receiving solute-free water to replace insensible losses, free water should be withheld until the serum sodium is increased to acceptable levels.

Hyponatremia is more common than hypernatremia. Hypernatremia occurs in neonates when there is excess free water loss, such as in certain instances of obstructive uropathy, or when there is inordinate administration of high-concentration salt solutions in the face of decreased renal function. Therapy requires the limiting of further sodium intake and/or the administration of free water in a volume calculated to decrease the serum sodium to safer levels. Usually this is accomplished by the use of 0.2 or 0.3 NS at a rate calculated to decrease the serum sodium no faster than 1.0 mEq per liter per hour. In addition, the amount of free water needed to help correct the hypernatremia is estimated from the following formula:

$$\text{Deficit (liters) of total body water (TBW)} = \text{present TBW} \times [Na]/140 - 1$$

Free water should never be given alone, as it can cause red cell hemolysis.

Divalent metabolism of calcium and phosphorus is affected by the malfunctioning kidney. Hyperphosphatemia is more common than hypocalcemia. Dietary intake of phosphorus should be limited, and endogenous production of phosphate limited by control of infections and hemolysis. Although the use of aluminum-containing gels has been advocated for the removal of phosphate, we avoid their routine use, because of the risk of aluminum toxicity in the neonate's central nervous system. Dialysis is the only other method of removing phosphate from the body, and peritoneal dialysis is more efficient at its removal than hemodialysis. The risk of maintaining a severely elevated phosphate is that a calcium-phosphorus product above 70 can produce extraskeletal calcifications in muscle, vessels, lung, brain, and heart. Also, hyperphosphatemia leads to a reciprocal decrease in serum calcium levels.

Hypocalcemia is associated with seizures, but is rarely symptomatic in ARF patients because of acidemia causing an increased ionized fraction and the finding of hypoalbuminemia in ARF, which allows for an increased free fraction of calcium. If therapy is necessary, it must be remembered that acidemia should be corrected only after correcting hypocalcemia. The dose of calcium gluconate (10 percent solution) is 50 to 100 mg per kilogram four

to six times per day by slow intravenous infusion, with the patient connected to a cardiac monitor and the infusion either slowed or stopped for decreasing heart rates. If hyperphosphatemia prevents a sustained increase in serum calcium, dialysis is indicated.

HYPERTENSION CONTROL

Because of either intrinsic damage to the kidney or an expanded intravascular volume, hypertension is an important complication of ARF, one that needs to be aggressively managed. Hypertension in a newborn has been defined by the Task Force on Blood Pressure Control as a systolic blood pressure greater than 96 mm Hg, and in an infant in the first month of life as a systolic blood pressure greater than 104 mm Hg. Volume depletion in the absence of an adequate glomerular filtration rate as a mechanism for controlling hypertension usually requires dialysis, or, if time permits, reduction in fluid input, so as to allow a decrease in extracellular volume from insensible and radiant loss. Diuretics are usually ineffective. Table 1 lists recommended doses of antihypertensive agents. Our preferred initial drug is hydralazine in steadily increasing doses. If the hypertension is severe and there is no or little response to increasing doses of hydralazine, we next give diazoxide (1 to 3 mg per kilogram per dose every 20 to 30 minutes), followed by nitroprusside if this regimen is unsuccessful. If an adequate response does not occur in 24 to 48 hours, a beta-blocker is added, followed by methyldopa (Aldomet) and/or an angiotensin converting enzyme inhibitor. Our experience has been that control of extracellular fluid volume is usually more important than antihypertensive therapy in sustaining a lowered blood pressure in ARF.

DIALYSIS

Neonates needing hemodialysis should be referred to centers with appropriate equipment. Fortunately, it is rarely necessary to undertake hemodialysis in neonates with ARF.

Dialysis Indications

The decision to institute dialysis is based on an overall assessment of the patient's clinical status, the degree of chemical imbalance, and the anticipated course. The factors we use to decide to initiate dialysis are listed in

TABLE 1 Antihypertensive Agents

Drug	Dose
Hydralazine	0.1–0.3 mg/kg/dose IV
Furosemide	1–4 mg/kg/day IV, PO
Propranolol	0.5–5 mg/kg/day PO b.i.d.–q.i.d.
Diazoxide	1–3 mg/kg/dose IV q 20–30 min
Nitroprusside	0.5–8 μg/kg/min IV
Captopril	0.1 mg/kg test dose to 5 mg/kg/day

Table 2. Most centers use peritoneal dialysis (PD) because of the need for specialized equipment for performing hemodialysis in neonates. Three components of the dialysis procedure are under the direct control of the physician: the volume of "dwell", the length of dwell, and the composition of the PD fluid. Varying one or more of these factors changes the effectiveness and efficiency of the dialysis procedure. After the acute PD catheter is in place and good drainage has been demonstrated (15 ml per kilogram of infusion volume), we increase the infusion volume to 30 to 50 ml per kilogram per pass to allow for adequate solute and water removal. If it appears that the patient will require PD for more than 2 to 3 days, we have a permanent Tenckhoff catheter placed surgically. This decreases the problems of leakage and infection related to a percutaneous catheter. Dialysis is done on a continuous basis until adequate control of the factors leading to dialysis is obtained. After that, depending on the stabilization of the patient's chemistries and volume status, dialysis is restarted as needed.

Infusion and dwell should take 75 to 80 percent of the total exchange time, with the remainder used for drainage. Our initial exchange time is 30 to 60 minutes. Because of the small volumes required in neonates, a Buretrol is hung in line in order to measure carefully the volume infused during each exchange. The precise volume infused and drained needs to be scrupulously recorded, in order to define the magnitude of water balance, either positive or negative. Neonates often experience positive water balance while undergoing PD. The reasons for this are not entirely clear, but include (1) both a more permeable and a functionally larger peritoneal membrane, which allows the transmembrane osmotic driving force for ultrafiltration to dissipate rapidly, because of the movement of dialysate into the body; and (2) starvation—in malnourished infants glucose moves more rapidly into cells, and thus maintains a larger transmembrane gradient for glucose transport across the peritoneal membrane into the body. Net solute transport in both directions is increased secondary to this leaky membrane phenomenon.

The usual solution used to start dialysis consists of the following: dextrose, 1.5, 2.5, or 4.25 percent; sodium, 132 mEq per liter; calcium, 3.5 mEq per liter; magnesium, 0.5 mEq per liter; chloride, 96 mEq per liter; lactate, 40 mEq per liter. Three mEq per liter of potassium is added to the dialysate if, after dialysis is started, the serum potassium level has fallen to less than 3.0 mEq per liter. The starting glucose concentration is 1.5 percent in the initial exchange. If the patient is severely volume overloaded and/or there is inadequate ultrafiltration, the concentration can be increased to 2.5 or 4.25 percent. Because of the need in many cases to use solutions with higher glucose concentrations, these patients may become hyperglycemic. In our experience, this occurs more often in neonates than in older children on PD, most likely because of the different characteristics of their peritoneal membrane. This underscores the need to monitor blood sugar levels carefully. If the blood sugar increases to values greater than 250 mg per deciliter, consideration should be given either to reducing the dialysate glucose concentration or adding insulin (1 to 2 units Regular per liter) to the dialysate, if the patient cannot tolerate the anticipated decrease in ultrafiltration. Bicarbonate can be substituted for acetate if the patient has organic acidemia or lactate acidosis, in which case our pharmacy mixes the solution.

CONTINUOUS ARTERIOVENOUS HEMOFILTRATION (CAVH)

Because of the high caloric needs of neonates in general and catabolic, sick neonates in particular, the need for calories can be regarded as a need for dialysis. The great amount of fluids needed to supply sufficient calories for maintaining homeostasis and growth makes the need for adequate fluid removal critical. Some institutions have begun to employ CAVH in neonates who do not need intensive dialysis, but who do require ongoing fluid removal.

CAVH has the advantage that a hemodialysis machine is not needed. The devices have a high ultrafiltration coefficient that allows much more fluid removal per unit of pressure than seen with a traditional dialyzer. In fact, the ability to remove fluid is so high that a pump is sometimes required to apply counterpressure in order to decrease the rate of fluid removal.

The high ultrafiltration coefficient of the membranes used in CAVH allows for fluid removal even while using only the patient's own cardiac output. Special neonatal cartridges are available that take into account the small circulating volume of these patients and still allow for adequate ultrafiltration. An advantage of CAVH is the ability to achieve this control without the need for a hemodialysis machine or purified water. The use of CAVH requires systemic heparinization to avoid clotting of the CAVH cartridge. This cannot be taken lightly, in view of the fact that in sick, stressed neonates one must always be aware of the risk of significant intracranial bleeds. Needless to say, the intense monitoring that is called for

---

TABLE 2   Indications for Dialysis

Hyperkalemia: Persistently greater than 7.0 mEq/L or electrocardiographic changes

Acidosis: Unresponsive to base administration or inability to give more base (NaHCO₃) owing to volume overload, congestive heart failure

Congestive heart failure: Due to volume overload

Hypertension: Most often due to severe volume overload

Hypercatabolism: Rapid rise in BUN; hyperuricemia

Relative Indications

Central nervous system changes: Soft signs of uremia, such as decreased consciousness, myoclonus, asterixis, seizures

Cardiac: Pericarditis, arrhythmias

Abnormal serum sodium concentration

Hyperphosphatemia

in a neonate on dialysis is also a "must" in this mode of therapy (frequent weights, accurate fluid intake and output records, and so forth). The ultrafiltrate generated during CAVH contains fluid and electrolytes in concentrations virtually equal to those in serum, and thus serum chemistries do not change because of the procedure. The physician has the luxury of determining the replacement fluid on the basis of solute removed as well as the ongoing needs of the patient. The procedure by definition can go on continuously for days, allowing for a steady fluid removal. The use of CAVH avoids the stress of frequent peaks and valleys in intravascular space volume on the cardiovascular system.

SUGGESTED READING

Feld LG. Total parenteral nutrition in children with renal insufficiency. In: Lebenthal E, ed. Total parenteral nutrition: indications, utilization, complications, and pathophysiological considerations. New York: Raven Press, 1986:385.

Gruskin AB, Baluarte HJ, Polinsky MS, et al. Therapeutic approach to the child with acute renal failure. In: Strauss J, ed. Acute renal disorders and renal emergencies. Boston: Martinus Nijhoff, 1984:311.

Lieberman KV, Nardi L, Bosch JP. Treatment of acute renal failure in an infant using continuous arteriovenous hemofiltration. J Pediatr 1985; 106:646.

Strauss J, Zilleruelo G, Freundlich M. Neonatal renal functions, fluid and electrolytes in intensive care units. In: Vidyasagar D, Sarnaik AP, eds. Neonatal and pediatric intensive care. Littleton, MA: PSG Publishing, 1985:151.

AIDS: PERINATAL HIV INFECTION

JOHN H. DOSSETT, M.D.

Pediatricians are generally surprised to learn that the burgeoning epidemic of human immunodeficiency virus (HIV) infection has included a large number of infants and children. These babies come to our attention in one of two ways. Some infants with HIV infection are identified because of signs and symptoms (Table 1) suggesting the diagnosis, whereas others are identified because the mother has documented HIV infection or risk factors (Table 2) suggesting that she might be infected with HIV.

HIV is not universally transmitted from infected mothers to their infants, however; only approximately one-half of the babies born to mothers with HIV infection become infected. The majority of these mothers are asymptomatic, their only evidence of HIV infection being their history of high-risk behavior and a positive serologic test. In many instances, the first evidence that a mother has HIV infection is when the infant develops symptoms that are compatible with HIV infection and is found to be antibody-positive. The hope of early diagnosis in infants depends on a careful survey for risk factors in *all* pregnant women. Moreover, it is likely that serologic screening for HIV infection will become a routine part of prenatal care, much like the recommendations for rubella virus screening and hepatitis B virus screening.

TRANSMISSION

Transmission of HIV from infected mothers to their infants may occur in utero, intrapartum, or even through breast milk. Before routine testing of donor blood was instituted, a number of infants and children were infected through transfusions of infected blood or blood products (Table 3). It appears, however, that the great majority of transmissions occur in utero. Even so, the possibility of transmission through breast milk to an infant who was not infected in utero requires that breast-feeding be avoided in babies of mothers who are HIV-positive.

Maternal antibodies from infected mothers are transported to all their children so that even those who are not infected are, typically, antibody-positive by both enzyme-linked immunosorbent assay (ELISA) and Western blot testing. Direct tests for HIV in the blood of infants who are antibody-positive include a culture for HIV or a test

TABLE 1 Clinical Manifestations of HIV Infection in Infants and Children

Lymphadenopathy
Hepatosplenomegaly
Recurrent bacterial and viral infections
Failure to thrive
Chronic or recurrent diarrhea
Oral candidiasis
Opportunistic infections
Encephalopathy
Recurrent fever
Lymphoid interstitial pneumonitis
Parotitis
Hepatitis
Eczematous rash
Nephritis
Cardiomyopathy
Malignancy

TABLE 2 HIV Risk Factors in Women of Childbearing Age

Intravenous drug use
Multiple sexual partners
Sexual partner who has
    infection with HIV
    bisexual practices
    history of intravenous drug use
    hemophilia
Blood transfusions received
    between 1978 and 1985

TABLE 3   Modes of Transmission of HIV to Infants

Intrauterine
Intrapartum
Breast milk (rare)
Transfusions with infected blood or blood products
(rare since July 1985)

for HIV antigens in the plasma. However, these direct tests are neither readily available nor sufficiently reliable for confirmation of HIV infection. Consequently, a confirmed diagnosis of HIV infection in infants who are antibody-positive is commonly dependent on their development of clinical manifestations of infection or on other indirect laboratory tests.

EVALUATION OF HIV-POSITIVE INFANTS

When the appropriate tests are available and sufficiently reliable, all babies born to HIV-positive mothers should have direct tests for HIV antigens in their blood. A positive culture for HIV or demonstration of HIV antigens in the plasma confirms that the infant is infected. However, a negative culture or antigen test does not confirm that the baby has been spared. Most newborns infected with HIV are completely asymptomatic and have no clinical manifestations that are attributable to HIV. If they do have symptoms, they are probably attributable to the general health of the mother, who is likely to have other sexually transmitted diseases and to be a drug and/or alcohol abuser. Concomitant infections may include cytomegalovirus, Epstein-Barr virus, *Toxoplasma gondii*, *Neisseria gonorrhoea*, and *Chlamydia trachomatis*.

Most babies with HIV infection develop typical symptoms. These symptoms, however, are usually not manifest until 4 to 24 months of age. A few babies have clinical symptoms before 1 month of age, but some do not develop symptoms until they are 7 or 8 years old. These symptoms typically include lymphadenopathy, hepatosplenomegaly, failure to thrive, neuromotor delay, diarrhea, skin rashes, recurrent fever, parotitis, lymphoid interstitial pneumonitis, *Pneumocystis carinii* pneumonia, and recurrent episodes of pyogenic bacterial infections. They are also likely to develop opportunistic infections (Table 4). Any combination of these clinical manifestations is a strong indication that the infant has HIV infection.

TABLE 4   Opportunistic Infections in Children With HIV Infection

Pneumocystis carinii pneumonitis
Candida esophagitis
Chronic recurrent herpes simplex infection
Disseminated cytomegalovirus infection
Toxoplasmosis
Mycobacterium infections
Cryptococcosis

Care of the Mother

Women with HIV infection may survive for many years, during which time they may be clinically well, persistently infected, sexually active, and fertile. Many such women have borne two or more infants who were infected with HIV. Consequently, pregnant women with HIV infection should be informed of this risk and strongly encouraged not to become pregnant again. When possible, this counseling should occur prior to delivery so that they can be offered tubal ligations while still in the hospital. If that option is not accepted, they should be provided with reliable oral contraceptives. They should also be counseled regarding the use of condoms and vaginal foams that will reduce the risk of transmitting HIV to their sexual partners.

Care of the Infant

Infants of HIV-infected mothers should be seen by the physician each month, at which time a thorough search should be carried out for clinical signs of HIV infection. The mothers and other caregivers need frequent instruction in the signs of HIV infection, so that they can recognize clinical indicators that may develop between physician visits. Those babies who remain asymptomatic, maintain normal growth and development, and have normal physical examinations should receive routine immunizations. In the absence of clinical manifestations, these babies should have laboratory screening scheduled at approximately 4-month intervals. The tests performed should include repeat HIV antibody testing, complete blood count and differential count, and immunoglobulin levels.

Although the antibody test may remain positive for 12 to 15 months in the infant who is *not* infected, it is appropriate to test these babies at more frequent intervals, so that the parents of those who become negative earlier can be reassured. The complete blood count may reveal lymphopenia as an early indicator of HIV infection.

Hypergammaglobulinemia is the indirect laboratory finding most consistently seen in infants and children with HIV infection. Tests of lymphocyte function and lymphocyte subset ratios (T_4/T_8) are not sufficiently reliable indicators of infection to justify their use as screening tests in asymptomatic babies. By 1 year of age those infants who are not actually infected typically have become antibody-negative and their immunoglobulin levels have remained normal. Infants who are positive by both ELISA and Western blot testing after 1 year are assumed to be infected with HIV, even though they may still be asymptomatic; see the diagnostic algorithm in Figure 1.

ISOLATION OF INFANTS WITH HIV INFECTION

Infants who are suspected of having HIV infection and those who are known to be infected do not need specific isolation. Their caretakers should follow the Universal Precautions published by the Centers for Disease Control. These precautions are applicable to all patients.

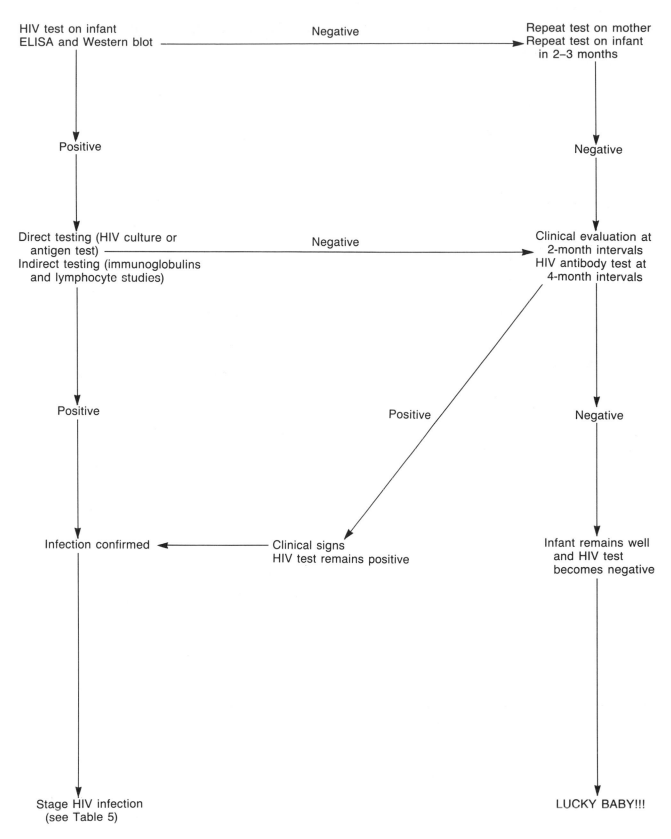

Figure 1 Management of infants born to HIV-positive mothers. Counsel mother regarding further HIV transmissions by avoiding: (1) pregnancy, (2) sharing needles, (3) risky sexual practices.

TABLE 5   Centers for Disease Control Classification of HIV Infection in Children

Class P-0. Indeterminate Infection. Perinatally exposed infants, under 15 months old, who have not met laboratory or clinical criteria for confirmed infection.

Class P-1. Asymptomatic Infection. Children who meet criteria for confirmed infection but who have had no signs or symptoms of HIV infection. They may be subclassified on the basis of immunologic testing.
   Subclass A. Normal immune function.
   Subclass B. One or more common immune abnormalities, such as hypergammaglobulinemia, T_4 lymphopenia, absolute lymphopenia, and decreased T_4/T_8 ratio.
   Subclass C. Not tested.

Class P-2. Symptomatic Infection. Subclasses are based on the type of signs and symptoms present. Patients may be classified in more than one subclass.

   Subclass A. Nonspecific Findings. This includes children with two or more unexplained nonspecific findings that persist for more than 2 months, including fever, failure to thrive, weight loss (10%), hepatomegaly, splenomegaly, generalized lymphadenopathy, parotitis, and diarrhea.

   Subclass B. Progressive Neurologic Disease. This includes children with one or more of the following conditions: (1) loss of developmental milestones or intellectual ability, (2) impaired brain growth, or (3) progressive symmetric motor deficits.

   Subclass C. Lymphoid Interstitial Pneumonitis. Children with a histologically confirmed pneumonitis characterized by diffuse interstitial and peribronchial infiltration of lymphocytes and plasma cells. Other causes of interstitial infiltrates should be excluded, such as tuberculosis, *Pneumocystis carinii*, cytomegalovirus, and other viral or parasitic infections.

   Subclass D. Secondary Infectious Diseases. Children with an infectious disease that is the result of immune deficiency caused by HIV infection.

      Category D-1. Opportunistic infections (see Table 4).
      Category D-2. Recurrent and serious infections with pyogenic bacteria. These include sepsis, meningitis, pneumonia, bone and joint infections, and abscess of an internal organ.
      Category D-3. Other infectious diseases, such as oral candidiasis, two or more episodes of herpes stomatitis, and multidermatomal or disseminated herpes zoster infection.

   Subclass E. Secondary Cancers. Children with cancers known to be related to HIV infection and immune deficiency.

   Subclass F. Other Diseases. This includes children with other conditions possibly due to HIV infection, such as hepatitis, nephritis, cardiopathy, skin diseases, and hematologic disorders.

TREATMENT OF INFANTS AND CHILDREN WITH HIV INFECTION

Treatment of HIV infection and its related diseases is largely empirical and currently unsatisfactory. Intensive research is focused on attempts to alter the course of the primary infection and its complications.

Appropriate treatment of opportunistic and pyogenic infections requires accurate and specific identification of the various microbial organisms. Liberal use of cultures for viruses, bacteria, and fungi is required. Lung biopsy is commonly required to distinguish between *Pneumocystis carinii* pneumonitis, lymphoid interstitial penumonitis, cytomegalovirus pneumonitis, and other agents.

Many children with class P-2 HIV infection (Table 5) are given trimethoprim-sulfamethoxazole in the hope of reducing the risk of *Pneumocystis carinii* pneumonitis and some bacterial infections. If they have oral thrush, they are given oral ketoconazole to prevent *Candida* esophagitis. Monthly infusions of intravenous gamma globulin are given to prevent frequent bacterial infections. Many children with HIV infection have antibody deficiency in spite of their hypergammaglobulinemia. Vigorous attention to maintaining optimal nutrition seems to be beneficial.

HIV-infected children have tolerated live virus vaccines. However, because of their immune deficiency, they should be given inactivated polio vaccine rather than the live oral polio vaccine. Measles, mumps, and rubella vaccines should be given at 15 months, as normally scheduled.

Caring for HIV-infected children and their families is remarkably demanding and requires the committed and combined attention of physicians, nurses, social workers, psychologists, and clergy.

SUGGESTED READING

CDC classification system for human immunodeficiency virus (HIV) infection in children under 13 years of age. MMWR 1987; 36:225–236.
CDC update: Universal precautions for prevention of transmission of human immunodeficiency virus, hepatitis B virus, and other bloodborne pathogens in health-care settings. MMWR 1988; 37:377–388.

APNEA

GEORGE A. LITTLE, M.D.

Apnea is cessation of respiratory air flow. This basic or "gold standard" definition describes an event that can be associated with little or no neuromuscular activity, as in *central* or *diaphragmatic* apnea, or with activity, as in *obstructive* apnea. A *mixed* central and obstructive apnea also occurs in the newborn. Short central apnea (less than 15 sec) is seen at all ages, and *periodic breathing* (three or more respiratory pauses of more than 3 sec with less than 20 sec between pauses) can be normal at all ages and is seen in premature and term newborns.

Pathologic apnea is a respiratory pause that is prolonged (many nurseries use 20 or more seconds as a limit) and/or is associated with cyanosis, abrupt pallor or hypotonia, or bradycardia. *Apnea of prematurity* is pathologic apnea in a premature infant and usually ceases by 37 weeks' gestational age (menstrual dating) but may persist several weeks longer. *Apnea of infancy* occurs in infants who are at term or older at the onset of their apnea but otherwise can have characteristics similar to apnea of prematurity. *ALTE*, or *"apparent life-threatening event,"* is a clinical syndrome that has marked signs of physiologic instability, such as apnea, color change, change in muscle tone, and usually limpness, choking, or gagging, and is frightening to the observer. Numerous disorders, such as seizure or gastroesophageal reflux, can cause ALTE, as can apnea of infancy. The diagnosis of apnea of infancy as a cause of ALTE is one of exclusion.

The term ALTE is a suitable replacement for "near-miss" or "aborted sudden infant death syndrome." Because of the diagnostic implications of the latter terms, and because the hypothesis that apnea is the cause of sudden infant death syndrome has never been proved (or disproved), the ALTE terminology is more appropriate.

EVALUATION

Because apnea can be an early manifestation of numerous life-threatening diseases, the clinician must first and foremost always suspect the worst, especially if an otherwise stable infant begins to manifest pathologic apnea. Apnea can also be an isolated phenomenon occurring without other apparent disease processes.

Diagnosis in the preterm infant can be especially difficult, as approximately 50 percent have periodic breathing and half of these have apnea of prematurity. Apnea in the preterm and to a lesser extent in the term infant can be related to factors such as temperature instability, hypoxemia due to respiratory insufficiency, decreased oxygen-carrying capacity or anemia, obstruction due to position or secretions, and pharyngeal stimulation from tubes or regurgitated feeding. The preterm and term infant may become apneic with sepsis, seizures, patent ductus arteriosus, intracranial pathology including hemorrhage or ischemia, metabolic disorders, and many other conditions.

Thus, evaluation must include environmental or physiologic causes that are amenable to manipulation as well as consideration of disease states. For example, apnea due to problems such as pharyngeal obstruction or regurgitation should be evaluated through review of time of occurrence, as related to feeding, and through discussion with nurses and parents. Diagnostic tests, including invasive procedures such as lumbar puncture as part of an evaluation for sepsis, are undertaken when infection seems possible. It is hard to fault the decision to do a "sepsis work-up" when apnea is documented.

THERAPEUTIC INTERVENTIONS

The dictum of using the least invasive therapy first holds for management of apnea. Unfortunately, there is a tendency to use more invasive techniques without adequately determining whether less invasive interventions, which may be more labor-intensive, will work. This is especially true for the premature infant, in whom pharmacologic or respiratory pressure interventions are often utilized without adequate trial of other techniques.

Changes in Management

A few infants respond to being placed in or returned to a slightly cooler or warmer milieu or removed from a situation with significant radiant heat loss. Babies who manifest apnea after feeding may respond to a change in the feeding schedule or the amount of the food, combined with a positional change. A change of position alone may prevent or decrease apnea when obstruction is a factor.

Sensory Stimulation

Treatment of apnea by tactile stimulation can be effective. Stimulation by touch, gentle flicking of an extremity, or stroking of the chest is much preferred to rapping the incubator or moving the mattress but requires clean hands. Proprioceptive stimulation using devices such as a water mattress attached to a pressure oscillator may also be effective. Premature infants are undoubtedly often excessively stimulated in most nurseries with light, sound, and touch; additional constant proprioceptive stimulation may not be entirely beneficial. Further study is needed.

Oxygen Supplementation and Transfusion

Supplemental oxygen, even at such seemingly insignificant increases over room air as 23 to 24 percent can decrease the incidence of apneic episodes. Blood gases or hemoglobin saturation should be followed. Anemia is a well-recognized cause of apnea, especially in the premature infant, and transfusion can be helpful.

Drug Therapy

Methylxanthines are used extensively in the treatment and prevention of apnea of prematurity and have value in

TABLE 1 Methylxanthine Dosage for Neonatal Apnea*

Agent	Route	Loading Dose	Maintenance	Serum Level
Theophylline	PO	5 mg/kg	1.1 mg/kg q8h	5–10 mg/L
Aminophylline	IV, PO	As above	As above	As above
Caffeine (aqueous caffeine citrate)	IV, PO	20 mg	2.5 mg/kg/day	5–20 mg/L

* There is considerable variability in recommended values in the literature. These values are within the limits of most. Preparations and individual infant metabolisms vary considerably.

other situations, including apnea of infancy and some cases of central hypoventilation. Stimulation of the central nervous system and, specifically, of the respiratory center appears to be their primary mode of action, although increased skeletal muscle tone and decreased diaphragmatic fatigue may contribute.

The pharmacokinetics of xanthine metabolism are complex, and major differences between the neonate and the older child or adult make management of the neonate a challenge. A loading dose is usually used to avoid a delay in achieving therapeutic levels. Half-life in the neonate, although variable, is on the order of several times longer than for the adult. Adults metabolize caffeine to theophylline, but premature infants are not as easily able to do so and most caffeine is excreted unchanged. In addition, there is evidence that premature neonates metabolize theophylline to caffeine. Some clinicians suggest that caffeine is the more appropriate agent. Monitoring of clinical status and blood level is important. Table 1 contains prescription information. Most of our experience is with theophylline, and we utilize the dosages mentioned there.

We feel that the best plan is a finite period of medication of from 7 to 14 days, depending on age at time of initial use. A trial without medication then follows. In fact, we tend to use theophylline until the infant is approximately 34 weeks old and/or weighs 1,800 g. We do not taper the medication.

Clinicians may underestimate the broad systemic effects of xanthines, which include possible alterations in cerebral blood flow, increased urine output and sodium excretion, and alterations in metabolism, including increased blood glucose and oxygen consumption. Furthermore, in spite of close monitoring of dosage and blood levels, tachycardia, jitteriness and vomiting continue to occur as complications of theophylline use. Less common possible complications include abdominal distention, leading one to consider necrotizing enterocolitis, and convulsions, especially in infants with intracranial abnormalities. We have had the experience of receiving spontaneous comments from mothers that their babies' affectual state changed when theophylline was discontinued; they became less active and changed their feeding patterns.

We try not to discharge babies home on methylxanthines. There is a place, however, for prolonged use at home, especially in infants with apnea of infancy. See also the section on monitoring for discussion of theophylline to facilitate discharge and the use of monitors.

Doxapram has received attention because of its central stimulation and effect on peripheral chemoreceptors. Its use in infants and premature neonates is not extensively reported, however, and additional studies are needed.

Continuous Positive Airway Pressure

An increase in airway/alveolar pressure above atmospheric in the form of continuous positive or distending airway pressure (CPAP or CDAP) is a useful therapeutic modality. Relatively small increases in pressure, such as 3 to 4 cm H_2O, can be applied via nasal prongs or a nasopharyngeal tube. Face masks and sealed enclosures have been used, but there are appropriate concerns about constricting material being placed around the head; alteration in blood flow and intracranial hemorrhage are possible complications. In our experience, nasal CPAP is effective but requires special attention and understanding by the nursery staff. Nasal prongs can be difficult to keep in place. It is not necessary to continue CPAP during a feeding, bath, or other care when a nurse is handling the baby. Some infants seem to have increased abdominal distention when the prongs are in place. One can debate whether CPAP or drug therapy is more invasive. At present we use medication before attempting CPAP in most infants; certainly, nasal prongs are less invasive than endotracheal intubation.

Positive Pressure Ventilation

Severe apnea that is not responsive to other interventions and requires intubation and intermittent positive pressure ventilation is usually not an isolated phenomenon but is associated with a disease process. Most intensive care nurseries are heavily involved with treatment of chronic pulmonary insufficiency associated with respiratory distress syndrome, intracranial pathology, and other problems. The very low birth weight premature infant and a few large prematures without other specific problems may manifest severe apnea of prematurity that requires positive pressure ventilation. The infant with an occasional isolated event may be treated with bag and mask ventilation, but repeated episodes require intubation and a mechanical ventilator.

In treatment of the isolated event requiring positive pressure ventilation, an inspired oxygen concentration *equal to that inhaled prior to onset* should be used. Higher levels are not necessary unless there is evidence of persistent hypoxia. The inexperienced nurse or physician may attach a bag to 100 percent oxygen, thereby hyperoxygenating the infant.

Management should be directed toward minimizing the time on the ventilator as much as possible. This includes both the breaths per minute and the total time of intubation. Some infants do well with less than 10 breaths per minute and a few centimeters of H_2O CPAP. Some very low birth weight babies with poor nutritional status and apnea seem to respond to a period of aggressive assisted ventilation, during which their *nutritional intake is maximized and the energy expenditure associated with respiration is minimized.*

MONITORS

Monitors have an important role in the detection and management of apnea. Impedance-based devices measure change in impedance across two points, usually on the lateral chest walls. They are extensively used and are effective, but they have important limitations that should be recognized by all personnel. The motion of the heart changes impedance whether or not respiratory motion is present. Because of the need to compensate for factors such as cardiac artifact, there are false-positive and false-negative report rates.

Some physicians feel that cardiac rate monitoring alone is sufficient, and monitors for this function are relatively simple and inexpensive. Most authorities measure respiratory activity, and there are a number of devices available, including mattresses sensitive to motion and thermistors that detect air flow. Monitors that follow the status of blood oxygen concentration, such as transcutaneous oxygen devices, or saturation, such as oximeters, are in use. *The rapid response time of oximeters and their ease of application has led to their increased use in our nursery for many problems, including apnea.*

In our nursery, respiratory function, or lack thereof, is not followed alone. Cardiac rate is also monitored. Apnea-associated bradycardias, or "As and Bs," are detected with devices set to sound an alarm at a heart rate such as 100 to 110 beats per minute in the preterm or 80 beats per minute in the term infant. Respiration is followed with alarm delays commonly set at 15 or 20 sec.

The so-called pneumogram or two-channel (cardiac and respiratory) hard copy impedance monitor receives little use in our nursery as an apnea risk assessment tool, as we agree with authorities who feel its effectiveness remains undocumented. It does have a role in monitoring of methylxanthine therapy at some centers.

The decision to discontinue monitoring is based on clinical information. The fact that over 90 percent of deaths from sudden infant death syndrome occur by 28 postnatal weeks can be taken into consideration, while remembering that sudden infant death syndrome is not related to a specific factor, such as the presence of a tracheostomy or bronchopulmonary dysplasia. Those entities are associated with sudden death and not sudden infant death syndrome. Most clinicians prefer to see an interval of 5 to 7 days without a documented apneic incident prior to discharge of the infant from the hospital, although shorter intervals might be appropriate in well-defined situations. As mentioned, *the efficacy of the pneumogram as a risk assessment tool* prior to monitoring *is unproved* and cannot be relied on in the decision to discontinue. Discontinuation of home monitoring is also dependent on the clinical situation, and parents should play an active role in the decision.

Home Monitoring and Discharge

A very few infants with apnea of prematurity have persistent apnea when they are otherwise ready for discharge by having demonstrated temperature stability in the room environment and a good weight gain on all oral feedings. A consensus panel has concluded that resolved apnea of prematurity is not an indication for home monitoring and that pneumograms should not be used as a risk screening tool in the premature population. We agree.

The pressure to scrutinize and decrease length of stay, along with the desire to get new babies home as soon as possible, has led to the use of home monitors for infants with persistent apnea of prematurity. Some authorities have used methylxanthines with or without monitoring to expedite discharge. Our practice is to minimize the use of medication and home monitors as we feel that (1) there is no indication that in asymptomatic premature neonates they should be used for resolved apnea of prematurity, (2) many prematures of 32 to 36 weeks' total age spontaneously stop manifesting apnea soon, and (3) there are very significant real and negative effects of medication and home monitors, including family stress and cost. There are, however, definite cases where home monitoring is indicated, and we prescribe it, complete with support system. The risk of apnea in these situations is usually associated with a specific problem, such as a previous ALTE (perhaps due to apnea of immaturity), bronchopulmonary dysplasia, or the presence of a tracheostomy.

SUGGESTED READING

Infantile apnea and home monitoring, report of a consensus development conference, Sept. 29 to Oct. 1, 1986. Bethesda, MD: NIH Publication No. 87–2905, 1987; summary in Pediatrics 79:292.
Kattwinkle J. Neonatal apnea: pathogenesis and therapy. J Pediatr 1977; 90:342.

APPARENT LIFE-THREATENING EVENTS

JOHN G. BROOKS, M.D.

Over the past two decades there has been increased attention in both the scientific and lay communities to the diverse group of infants who have demonstrated frightening episodes of apnea and/or color change. These episodes can occur during sleep, quiet or active wakefulness, or feeding. They are most commonly described as some combination of apnea (central or occasionally obstructive), color change (usually cyanotic or pallid, but occasionally erythematous or plethoric), marked change in muscle tone (usually marked limpness), or choking or gagging. In the majority of cases the observer felt that the episode was actually or potentially life-threatening or, in some cases, that the infant had actually died. This concern is the common theme among this heterogeneous infant population. The term "apparent life-threatening event" (ALTE) describes the chief complaint that brings these patients to medical attention. These infants have previously been referred to as "near-miss for sudden infant death syndrome" or "aborted crib death," but these terms imply a misleadingly close relationship between these alarming episodes and subsequent death from sudden infant death syndrome. A variety of identifiable diseases or conditions can cause such episodes, and all these infants should be evaluated for the presence of any treatable causes. In many cases, however, despite extensive work-up, no specific cause can be identified. If such an unexplained spell is associated with apnea, this is referred to as apnea of infancy (i.e., idiopathic ALTE).

Sudden infant death syndrome is defined as "the sudden death of any infant or young child that is unexpected by history, and in which a thorough postmortem examination fails to demonstrate an adequate cause for death." An autopsy must be performed before the diagnosis of sudden infant death syndrome can be established, since this is the only way definitively to rule out other causes of sudden unexpected death of infants such as meningitis, intracranial hemorrhage, myocarditis, or overwhelming infection.

RELATIONSHIP OF APPARENT LIFE-THREATENING EVENT TO SUDDEN INFANT DEATH SYNDROME

In 1972, Steinschneider reported that two of five infants with documented sleep apnea subsequently died of apparent sudden infant death syndrome. Over the intervening time, several histologic tissue differences have been found in groups of sudden infant death syndrome victims when compared with samples from controls. These tissue markers, most of which are found in about 50 or 60 percent of sudden infant death syndrome victims and are therefore of no help in diagnosing this syndrome, are

extramedullary hematopoiesis, increased periadrenal brown fat, and brainstem gliosis. It has been proposed that these histologic differences could be explained by recurrent episodes of hypoxemia prior to death in infants who subsequently succumb to sudden infant death syndrome. These histologic changes are compatible with this hypothesis but do not prove it.

The incidence of sudden infant death syndrome in the ALTE population is about 10- to 30-fold increased compared with that of the general population. ALTE subgroups with a significantly higher risk of sudden, unexpected death have been identified. Infants whose initial episode occurs during sleep and is perceived to require mouth-to-mouth resuscitation have a subsequent *mortality of about 10 percent DESPITE the prescription of a home monitor* in most cases. If these same infants have a subsequent severe spell requiring resuscitation or vigorous stimulation, their risk of sudden death can increase to 30 percent or more. Such infants are rare. The incidence of sudden infant death syndrome in the general population is approximately 0.15 percent. *Less than 5 percent of sudden infant death syndrome victims, however, have been noted to experience ALTE prior to their death.* The incidence of ALTE in the general population is about 2 to 3 percent. Thus, most sudden infant death syndrome victims do not come from the ALTE population.

ETIOLOGIES OF APPARENT LIFE-THREATENING EVENTS

The wide variety of specific diagnoses that can be present with apparent life-threatening events can be considered in three categories: "normal," acute infection, or chronic condition. Table 1 summarizes the most common etiologies. In approximately 50 percent of cases, no specific diagnosis is identified. Of the remaining cases, the most common diagnoses are seizure disorder, infection, and laryngeal chemoreceptor apnea related to dysfunction of the upper gastrointestinal tract (e.g., pharyngeal incoordination or gastroesophageal reflux).

MANAGEMENT

The first question that must be considered when one is confronted with an ALTE infant in person or by phone is whether the infant's life is immediately in danger. The

TABLE 1 Causes of Apparent Life-Threatening Events in Infants

Chalasia—laryngeal chemoreceptor apnea
Seizure disorder
Infection (e.g., respiratory syncytial virus, pertussis, or sepsis)
Upper airway obstruction
Cardiac disease
Breath-holding
Anemia
Central hypoventilation syndromes
Central nervous system tumors

second question is whether something abnormal definitely occurred or whether this was the observer's overreaction to a normal event. Unless one is convinced that nothing abnormal happened, or unless the episode occurred days or weeks earlier, hospitalization of the infant is indicated for observation, intervention if necessary, and evaluation and counseling. The general purposes of the evaluation are threefold: (1) try to observe spells if they recur; (2) look for direct or indirect signs of recurrent hypoxemia or hypoventilation; and (3) perform a workup for identifiable, treatable disease.

A careful history and physical examination are of utmost importance in this evaluation. History of the presenting episode should include answers to questions about the infant's state of consciousness before, during, and after the spell, duration of the spell, color change, muscle tone, movements, respiratory efforts during the episode, resuscitation and response to this intervention, relation to feeding, associated choking, and any other associated symptoms (e.g., mild upper respiratory tract infection). The past history should include evidence of any previous ALTEs, abnormal breathing patterns (e.g., excessive snoring), feeding problems, other medical problems, and family history of apnea or infant deaths or other cardiopulmonary problems. A careful physical examination should be performed, with particular attention to a careful neurologic examination, to heart sounds (e.g., increased pulmonic component of the second heart sound indicating pulmonary hypertension), and to any evidence of airway obstruction. The infant's breathing pattern during sleep should be observed and he or she should be watched during a feeding.

If the history and physical examination suggest a specific diagnosis, appropriate laboratory and other tests should be performed. *In the absence of such direction, extensive testing is rarely very fruitful.* A serum bicarbonate measurement obtained as soon after the episode as possible (such as in the Emergency Room) can be very helpful if it demonstrates a metabolic acidosis, as objective confirmation of the caretaker's report of a significant ALTE. Other minimal evaluation includes a complete blood count with differential to look for evidence of significant anemia or suggestion of sepsis or lymphocytosis (suggesting pertussis) and continuous cardiorespiratory monitoring during the hospitalization.

No test can predict the risk of subsequent death in these infants. Use of pneumograms (hard copy recordings of 12 to 24 hours of cardiorespiratory pattern) for this purpose is inappropriate, since there are *no data to suggest that abnormal amounts of periodic breathing or prolonged respiratory pauses noted on a pneumogram identify high-risk infants.* In fact, infants who have been tested and subsequently succumbed to sudden infant death syndrome have not demonstrated these abnormalities any more frequently than survivors. A pneumogram or some other hard copy recording of cardiorespiratory patterns surrounding a monitor alarm may be useful in distinguishing real from artifactual alarms, both in the hospital and at home. Although there is information about the 95 percent confidence limits of the amount of periodic breathing and var-

ious other parameters of respiratory instability, there is no indication that infants who demonstrate patterns that exceed these "normal" limits are at increased risk of sudden unexpected death. For this reason *it is inappropriate to use pneumogram recordings as the basis for the decision about whether to start or discontinue a home monitor.* Likewise, risk of subsequent death cannot be predicted by pneumograms, so it is inappropriate to use them as screening devices in either symptomatic or asymptomatic populations.

In occasional ALTE patients, if significant obstructive apnea, chronic hypoventilation, or apneic seizures are likely, more extensive, physiologic testing as provided by polysomnography may be considered, but this is rarely necessary.

There are several different approaches for evaluation of and intervention for ALTE infants. One approach advocates more extensive initial in-hospital evaluation and less widespread use of home monitors. The alternate approach, appropriate for the majority of infants in whom no treatable diagnosis is identified and serious spells do no recur during hospitalization, involves a brief hospitalization (36 to 48 hours), minimal laboratory evaluation (see above), and discharge with a home monitor. The monitor serves both as an intervention and as the next diagnostic test. Particularly when minimal laboratory evaluation was performed initially, infants who experience recurrent significant alarms are likely to require rehospitalization for further evaluation (e.g., electroencephalogram, electrocardiogram chest x-ray examination).

The recent federally sponsored *Consensus Conference on Infantile Apnea and Home Monitoring divided all infants into three groups with regard to the appropriateness of home monitoring.* ALTE infants for whom cardiorespiratory monitoring or an alternative therapy is indicated are those who have experienced a severe ALTE perceived to require mouth-to-mouth resuscitation or vigorous stimulation. The second group, those for whom cardiorespiratory monitoring is not medically indicated, includes normal, asymptomatic infants who have not experienced an ALTE and who are not in any population group at increased risk of sudden infant death syndrome. For the third group, those with less severe ALTEs the decision about monitoring should be made on a case by case basis after consideration with the family of the potential benefits, uncertainties, and psychosocial burdens. No family in this group should be pressured to use a monitor against its wishes. ALTE infants are also more likely to be monitored if they have a family history of sudden infant death syndrome or severe ALTEs have occurred in siblings, if they have recurrent ALTEs requiring intervention, or if they have a convincing history of significant, prolonged apnea with associated definite changes in color or tone or both.

Decisions about duration of home monitoring must be individualized, but the National Institutes of Health Consensus Conference *recommends monitor discontinuation when infants have been free of significant episodes for 2 to 3 months.* It is also preferable to have such infants demonstrate their ability to tolerate stress, such as an infection, without alarms prior to discontinuing the monitor. Decisions about monitor discontinuation should not be based on nor should they require normal pneumograms for the reasons mentioned above. Although home monitors certainly can provide some reassurance to the family, and it is highly likely that they alert some caretakers to potentially fatal episodes that are successfully interrupted, there are also important adverse consequences of their use. These include sleep disruption for the infant and the parents due to false alarms, interference with normal parent-infant relationships, and decreased mobility of the caretaking parent. At least several dozen infants have died despite the prescription of home monitors, some because the monitor failed or was not being used properly and some despite an apparently proper resuscitation attempt.

Prior to discharging an infant from the hospital with a home monitor, the caretakers must be fully instructed in infant resuscitation, monitor use, and trouble-shooting and must demonstrate these skills satisfactorily. In addition, the reasons for monitoring and its intended duration must be fully discussed, as well as its potential adverse consequences. Finally, reasonable alarm settings should be established—usually a respiratory pause of 20 seconds and a heart rate of 70 beats per minute for a young infant. Lower heart rate settings are appropriate for older infants. A record of all alarms, the infant's appearance at the time, and the intervention necessary must be kept by the caretakers. They should be instructed as to what type of episodes to report immediately or within 12 hours to the health care providers. There must be continuous ready availability of medical and technical support to the family by phone and, if necessary, in person. Resources for psychosocial support should also be available to the family at their discretion. It is helpful to provide the families with a list of key emergency telephone numbers.

Pharmacologic therapy may occasionally be appropriate for infants with ALTEs if there is significant evidence of a seizure disorder or alternatively a suggestion of a chronically weak or immature respiratory drive. Respiratory stimulants, particularly methylxanthines, are used in the latter situation, whereas anticonvulsants are appropriate for suspected seizures. These medications are usually initiated in the hospital, since some anticonvulsants may exacerbate symptoms in patients with inadequate respiratory drive, and conversely, respiratory stimulants may exacerbate seizure disorders.

It is appropriate to be very optimistic with families by suggesting that ALTEs are, in most cases, a developmental problem that will clear completely as the infant grows, usually over a period of weeks or months. In fact, the majority of infants do not have recurrent severe ALTEs. The families should also be reminded that most infants with ALTEs do not die of sudden infant death syndrome and that most sudden infant death syndrome infants have never experienced ALTEs.

SUGGESTED READING

American Academy of Pediatrics Task Force on Prolonged Apnea. Prolonged Infantile Apnea: 1985. Pediatrics 1985; 76:129–131.
National Institutes of Health Consensus Development Conference on Infantile Apnea and Home Monitoring, September 29–October 1, 1986: Consensus Statement. Pediatrics 1987; 79:292–299.
Oren J, et al. Identification of high-risk group for sudden infant death syndrome among infants who were resuscitated for sleep apnea. Pediatrics 1986; 77:495–499.
Ward SLD, et al. Sudden infant death syndrome in infants evaluated by apnea programs in California. Pediatrics 1986; 77:451–455.

BREAST-FEEDING JAUNDICE

ANDRÉ D. LASCARI, M.D.

The distinctions between early-onset (third to fourth day) and late-onset (fifth to fifteenth day) breast-feeding jaundice have been reviewed recently. Although the treatment of the two types is similar, there are several differences.

EARLY ONSET

The most effective treatment of the early-onset form is prevention. Although other factors also may be involved, the frequency of human milk feedings and the adequacy of caloric intake have been shown to be related to increased bilirubin levels on the third and fourth days of life. Frequent feedings may stimulate gut motility, thereby decreasing the enteric absorption of bilirubin. Breast-fed infants receive fewer calories than formula-fed infants, and there-

fore decreased caloric intake may also be a factor in jaundice, since starvation increases enteric bilirubin absorption, as demonstrated in animal studies.

Thus, the recommendation to encourage mothers to nurse as frequently as possible, particularly if neonatal bilirubin levels are rising, has a scientific basis. Gartner has recommended nursing at an average interval of 2 hours, although this may not always be easily achieved. Feeding dextrose in water or water supplementation should be avoided because it does not reduce serum bilirubin levels. If supplementation cannot be avoided, formula would be the best choice.

All nursing infants should be carefully followed for increasing jaundice, as the frequency of early-onset breast-feeding jaundice may be as high as 25 percent. Daily outpatient bilirubin determinations from the third day of life may therefore be indicated in nursing infants with rising bilirubin levels. If the bilirubin levels are increasing, the importance of frequent feedings can again be emphasized with the mother. Daily bilirubin determinations in such infants allow the physician to know when the levels approach 15 to 17 mg per deciliter rather than suddenly finding a very jaundiced infant with a level of 20 mg per deciliter or higher. Osborn has recommended daily outpatient bilirubin determinations when total bilirubin levels are higher than or equal to 9 mg per deciliter at more than or equal to 36 hours; higher than 10 mg per deciliter at more than 48 hours; and higher than or equal to 11 mg per deciliter at more than or equal to 72 hours until the levels stabilize or intervention is necessary.

When the levels of indirect bilirubin reach 15 mg per deciliter, investigations such as direct bilirubin concentration, blood type, direct and indirect Coombs' test, complete blood cell count, reticulocyte count, and smear for red cell morphology are indicated. It should be emphasized that infants with early-onset or late-onset breast-feeding jaundice are healthy and the physical examination (other than jaundice) and the above laboratory tests are normal.

If the indirect bilirubin levels continue to rise in the range of 15 to 17 mg per deciliter, it may then be the appropriate time to temporarily discontinue breast-feeding for 24 to 48 hours as an outpatient diagnostic test. Formula should be given every 2 hours, and the increasing bilirubin level usually stabilizes and then decreases by several milligrams per deciliter. The diagnosis is then confirmed, and breast-feeding may be resumed.

Some physicians wait until the level reaches 20 mg per deciliter before interrupting nursing. This is perfectly satisfactory, although often when bilirubin does reach this level anxieties run high and the infant may be admitted to the hospital, many unnecessary laboratory tests may be done, and phototherapy is often instituted. This adds a second variable to interruption of nursing so that when the subsequent decrease in bilirubin level occurs, it cannot be ascertained whether it was the formula feeding or the phototherapy that resulted in the decreased levels. The diagnostic value of interruption of nursing is then lost, although the probability is still very high that the hyperbilirubinemia was related to breast-feeding.

When nursing is interrupted it is very important to emphasize to the mother that this is temporary and that there is nothing wrong with her milk. Instructions should be given to the mother to manually express her milk, and breast pumps may be provided if desired. Although many physicians feel that interruption of breast-feeding for 24 to 48 hours may interfere with its resumption, studies have not shown this to be true.

If the bilirubin level exceeds 20 mg per deciliter and is in the 21 to 22 mg per deciliter range, I would interrupt nursing, feed formula every 2 hours, and institute phototherapy. Although no infant has ever been reported to develop kernicterus with early-onset or late-onset breast-feeding jaundice, there are no studies to show that it cannot occur. Therefore, for medical and legal reasons many physicians would consider exchange transfusion when the levels exceed 20 mg per deciliter and particularly when they rise to the 22 to 25 mg per deciliter range. Others, however, feel that the entity is completely benign and would not do an exchange transfusion, thereby avoiding the small but definite risk of the procedure. Fortunately, bilirubin levels in the 22 to 25 mg per deciliter range are

rare in jaundice associated with breast-feeding, and other etiologies should be considered when levels are in that range.

The response to phototherapy in infants with breast-milk jaundice is similar to that seen with interruption of nursing in terms of the decrease of bilirubin concentrations. It is important to ensure adequate caloric intake during phototherapy, since it appears to be relatively ineffective in the presence of a low calorie intake.

LATE ONSET

The etiology of the late-onset (fifth to fifteenth day) form of jaundice that may occur in 30 percent of nursing infants has been attributed to various substances in the mother's milk, including pregnane 3-α-20-β-diol, to elevated levels of lipoprotein lipase and nonesterfied long-chain fatty acids, and more recently to β-glucuronidase. The mechanism has been attributed to the inhibition of bilirubin conjugation by glucuronyl transferase or the increased absorption of bilirubin from the gastrointestinal tract. Studies have not been reported as to the possible effects of the frequency of feedings and caloric intake on the late-onset form.

Management of the late-onset form consists of interruption of nursing as an outpatient test as outlined for the early-onset type. I would elect to do the test at a higher bilirubin level (18 mg per deciliter), since the infant with this type of jaundice is more mature (10 to 15 days) at the time of the peak level and perhaps less susceptible to the remote chance of developing kernicterus in the event that the bilirubin level continues to rise. With temporary (24 to 28 hours) interruption of nursing and institution of formula feeding, the bilirubin concentration may decrease in the late-onset type by as much as 50 percent in 1 to 3 days. When nursing is resumed, the bilirubin levels may rise slightly for several days, then level off and gradually decline, but they may not return to normal until 3 to 12 weeks of age.

An alternative to complete interruption of nursing is a trial of alternating breast-feeding and formula feeding or heating the expressed milk. If alternating nursing and formula feeding is not effective, then complete interruption of nursing would be necessary.

SUGGESTED READING

Amato M, Von Muralt G. New clinical findings in breast milk jaundice. J Pediatr 1987; 110:329–330.

Gartner LM. Jaundice in the breast-fed infant. In: Counseling the mother on breast-feeding. Roundtable Report. Columbus, Ohio: Ross Laboratories, 1980.

Gartner LM. Breast milk jaundice. In: Hyperbilirubinemia in the newborn. Report of the 85th Ross Conference on Pediatric Research. Columbus, Ohio: Ross Laboratories, 1983.

Gourley GR, Arend RA. β-Glucuronidase and hyperbilirubinemia in breast-fed and formula-fed babies. Lancet 1986; Vol I:644–646.

Lascari AD. "Early" breast-feeding jaundice: clinical significance. J Pediatr 1986; 108:156–158.

Maisels MJ, Gifford K. Normal serum bilirubin levels in the newborn and the effect of breast-feeding. Pediatrics 1986; 78:837–843.
Nicoll A, Ginsburg R, Tripp JH. Supplementary feeding and jaundice in newborns. Acta Pediatr Scand 1982; 71:759–761.

Osborn LM, Bolus R. Breast feeding and jaundice in the first week of life. J Fam Pract 1985; 20:475–480.
Wu PK, Hodgman JE, Kirkpatrick BV, et al. Metabolic aspects of phototherapy. Pediatrics 1985; 75 (Suppl):427–433.

BRONCHOPULMONARY DYSPLASIA

GORDON B. AVERY, M.D., Ph.D.

Bronchopulmonary dysplasia (BPD) is the result of primary lung disease and of well-intentioned therapy. It represents severe injury to the lung, which fortunately has significant powers of growth and regeneration. As it is a complication rather than a primary disease, attention must be given to prevention rather than merely to management.

ANALOGIES

BPD is like an internal burn of the lining layer of the lung. As such there is disruption of the integrity of respiratory epithelium, local inflammatory reaction, exudation of fluids and proteins, chance of opportunistic infection, and healing with varying amounts of scarring and subsequent disordered growth.

A BPD patient is like a child with both cystic fibrosis and asthma. As such there is excess and poorly cleared mucus, chronic, indolent pulmonary infection with periodic flare-ups, emphysema, gas trapping, abnormalities of ventilation-perfusion matching, and periodic episodes of bronchospasm.

A BPD patient is like an infant with failure to thrive. As such there is evidence of maternal deprivation and hospitalism, a tendency towards depression and withdrawal, delayed developmental progress, sensitivity to environmental conditions, especially overstimulation, and a tendency toward poor feeding and growth.

PREVENTION

Prevention is obviously a prime aspect of reducing BPD morbidity and mortality. Problems contributing to BPD are listed in Table 1, together with measures that help to minimize their impact. Intubation, ventilation, oxygen therapy, and positive airway pressure are necessary features of therapy in many sick newborns but should be sharply limited if chronic lung disease is to be reduced. Obviously, the unstable infant in the acute phase requires more liberal use of these measures. Pulmonary interstitial emphysema represents disruption of lung architecture and is a harbinger of BPD. Hence early pulmonary interstitial emphysema should be taken seriously and every effort should be made to reduce barotrauma. High-frequency ventilation may not be a panacea for respiratory support, but it currently appears to be especially useful in pulmonary interstitial emphysema because of reducing tidal volume and peak airway pressures.

PATENT DUCTUS ARTERIOSUS

BPD is primarily a disease of very low birth weight infants, and these babies have a high incidence of symptomatic patent ductus anteriosus, manifesting at 3 to 5 days of life as bounding pulses, congested lung fields, and hyperactive precordium, with or without murmur and cardiac enlargement. The increased pulmonary circulation reduces lung compliance and often delays weaning from the respirator. Accordingly, we recommend a trial of indomethacin, given as three intravenous doses of 0.2 mg per kilogram at 8-hour intervals. Contraindications are necrotizing enterocolitis, bleeding problems, thrombocytopenia, or severely curtailed renal function. A mild, transient reduction in urine output, with a rise in blood

TABLE 1 Prevention of Bronchopulmonary Dysplasia

Problem	Prevention
Oxygen toxicity	Keep PaO_2 at 50–70 torr
	Wean rapidly by $TcPO_2$ or pulse oximeter
Barotrauma	Avoid overventilation
	Allow $PaCO_2$ to reach 50–65 if stable and pH > 7.25
Pulmonary interstitial emphysema	Avoid high peak pressures unless chest not moving
	High-frequency ventilation for pulmonary interstitial emphysema
Chronic intubation	Liberal use of continuous positive airway pressure
	Aggressive weaning after initial acute period
	Extubate from intermittent mandatory ventilation of 10–13 breaths per minute if good respiratory effort
	Racemic epinephrine, sigh bagging for postextubation stridor, atelectasis
Secondary infection	Work-up and treat for infection if unexpected glucose intolerance, purulent tracheal aspirate, or signs of systemic sepsis
Patent ductus arteriosus	Indomethacin or ligation of symptomatic patent ductus arteriosus by 4–8 days
Inadequate central respiratory drive	Correct metabolic alkalosis
	Consider theophylline or caffeine
	Allow moderate rise of $PaCO_2$ (50–65 torr)

urea nitrogen and creatinine levels, is tolerable. In the approximately 30 percent of babies who fail to respond to indomethacin, surgical ligation is preferable to prolonged respirator dependency.

RESPIRATORY DRIVE

Inadequate respiratory effort may arise from many factors: immaturity of the respiratory centers, imbalance between stiff lungs and weak muscles, debilitating malnutrition and disease, brain injury from hypoxic-ischemic encephalopathy or hemorrhage, or unrecognized metabolic alkalosis. The net result is prolonged mechanical ventilation with increased likelihood of BPD. Prudent measures include vigorous treatment of intercurrent illnesses, correction of low serum chloride values, vigorous nutritional support, and normalization of any metabolic abnormalities. Despite these measures, many babies allow the respirator to carry some of the load and remain on intermittent mandatory ventilation settings of 10 to 20 breaths per minute. In such circumstances, theophylline or caffeine treatment seems justified to increase central respiratory drive, even though apneic spells as such have not been noted. We favor theophylline, adjusted to yield blood levels of 10 to 15 μg per milliliter, because this drug apparently increases diaphragmatic contractility and may provide useful bronchodilation in some patients.

WEANING

Although weaning from the ventilator is opportunistic, some general principles can be offered. First, *ventilator settings and blood gas readings must be displayed at the bedside in a form that permits easy trend analysis.* Thus a flow sheet with settings and gases arranged in columns, with a time of entry with each row, allows scanning a column to sweep all the PaO_2 or $PaCO_2$ values for a shift or for a day. Responses to the blood gas report (altered settings) can be a final item in the row and can be signed as a respiratory order. This allows a broader perspective in tracking the infant's response to ventilatory management and avoids the tendency to react to each gas reading as an isolated entity. Another useful tool is a respiratory care plan that is updated at the beginning of each shift. The plan should be written in enough detail to specify tolerable limits for pH, PaO_2 and $PaCO_2$, and priorities for weaning. In many centers this care plan can be followed by nurses or respiratory therapists without requiring a physician's notice of each minor change in ventilator settings or FIO_2.

Oxygen dependency and need for ventilatory support are interrelated but separate considerations. Oxygen need is influenced by right-to-left shunts (perfused but unventilated lung tissue, pulmonary hypertension), diffusion barriers, and oxygen-carrying capacity (hemoglobin level). Need for ventilatory support is measured by $PaCO_2$ and is influenced by central respiratory drive, efficiency of respiratory apparatus (intercostal muscles, diaphragm, chest cage), lung compliance and airways resistance, and wasted ventilation due to dead space and ventilation-perfusion imbalance. Thus, weaning FIO_2 and weaning

ventilation may be out of synchrony in individual patients.

Oxygen support can be given as continuous positive airway pressure or hood oxygen, independently of the ventilator. Weaning from the ventilator is therefore a matter of establishing independent respiration of sufficient degree and reliability to keep pace with CO_2 production. The infant is typically laboring under the simultaneous handicaps of diminished CO_2 responsiveness, inefficient respiratory apparatus, and stiff lungs. If "normal" $PaCO_2$ values are taken as the requirement for lowering respirator settings, the baby may rest and allow the ventilator to carry him or her while chronic lung injury gradually increases this dependence. It is therefore prudent to *allow the $PaCO_2$ to rise moderately provided oxygenation is adequate and pH is higher than 7.25.* This increases respiratory drive and gives some opportunity for reducing support. Loading with theophylline may also increase central respiratory drive.

Two prime variables control ventilation: rate and depth. Weaning can be accomplished by reducing either rate or peak pressure, which in turn reduces tidal volume. As the lung improves and pulmonary compliance increases, the same peak pressure causes ever greater chest excursions. When the chest excursion is substantial, weaning peak pressure minimizes barotrauma. When chest excursions and breath sounds are minimal, rate should be weaned instead. *A positive care plan* ("wean peak pressure by 1 cm H_2O every 2 hours unless $PaCO_2 > 55$") *produces more tapering than a static care plan* ("keep $PaCO_2$ at 45 to 55"). Expiratory time is important because it provides intervals in which the infant can breathe. Reducing rate and inspiratory time thus encourages spontaneous respirations. Expiratory pressure helps determine the resting lung volume and can be increased to fight atelectasis or decreased to avoid hyperinflation.

Extubation is attempted when sustained independent respiration seems likely. For a premature infant with hyaline membrane disease, this might be when the FIO_2 is less than 0.4, intermittent mandatory ventilation is 10 breaths per minute, spontaneous respiration is adequate, and blood gas levels are acceptable. Racemic epinephrine given by aerosol, 0.25 mg per milliliter, may minimize stridor. Nasal continuous positive airway pressure and periodic brief bagging with inflation hold (sigh) may be helpful in combating postextubation atelectasis.

DIURETICS

Diuretics are frequently used in BPD. A number of studies have demonstrated transient improvement in lung function after brisk diuresis with furosemide, and most clinicians have observed this phenomenon. Empirically, any extra fluid appears to wind up in the lungs and to complicate pulmonary function. Explanations vary, but the limited compliance of the neonatal left ventricle makes left ventricular failure more likely, with back-up of fluid in the lungs. Oxygen toxicity, pulmonary infection, and pulmonary hypertension may increase capillary permeability. The formation of fetal lung fluid, which normally ceases at birth, may continue as part of the pathophysiology of BPD. In any event, diuretics are a useful adjunct to BPD management, and furosemide is particularly helpful, perhaps because it has some local action in the lung and can function as a prostaglandin antagonist. An important caveat is that prolonged furosemide use causes depletion of chloride, potassium, and sodium, resulting in metabolic alkalosis, blunted CO_2 responsiveness, and growth failure. It is *advisable to give the patient periodic respites from loop diuretics and to correct electrolyte deficiencies with particular attention to chloride.* Our policy is to give potassium chloride until the potassium rises, sodium chloride until the sodium rises, and if needed, ammonium chloride until the chloride rises.

BRONCHOSPASM

Disordered growth of the injured lung (BPD) has been shown to include underdevelopment of terminal airways and increased bronchial smooth muscle. Problems of airways resistance are a common feature of advanced BPD and increase the work of breathing. Manifestations include air trapping, areas of high ventilation-perfusion with wasted ventilation, and episodes of "tightness" with labored breathing, poor chest movement, and diminished breath sounds. Bronchodilators are sometimes helpful, but response is variable. In some instances one bronchodilator works when another is unsuccessful. A frequent complication is overstimulation, with restlessness and tachycardia. We try various medications to determine the infant's individual response, attempting to keep the heart rate below 200 beats per minute. One should be aware of the possibility that various beta agonists result in cumulative toxicity.

NUTRITION

Nutritional support is a vital element in care of patients with BPD. The work of breathing confers additional caloric demands. Growth is needed to provide additional bulk and strength to respiratory muscles and new lung tissue that offsets damaged lung. Yet nutrition is extremely difficult in the face of chronic lung disease. Wet lungs lead to use of diuretics and fluid restriction. This limits caloric intake or requires extraconcentrated feedings, whether intravenous or enteric. Rapid respirations interfere with the infant's ability to take oral feedings. Acidosis, hypochloremia, recurrent infection, and steroids or other drugs may interfere with growth. Our policy is to pursue nutritional support vigorously regardless of the infant's other circumstances. A growth target should be established and regularly monitored. The actual as opposed to the intended intake should be charted. It is often necessary to provide 150 cal per kilogram per day orally (115 cal per kilogram intravenously) to achieve sustained growth. In some infants with intractable disease who must go home on oxygen, a gastrostomy may be considered.

MONITORING

Monitoring of these chronically ill infants has many dimensions. Pulmonary management requires periodic chest x-ray examinations, blood gas determinations, chest auscultation, and often dynamic monitoring of pulse, respiratory rate, blood pressure, transcutaneous oxygen, and CO_2 or pulse oximetry. Nutritional monitoring includes body measurements, electrolytes, blood chemistries (including proteins), and observation of gastric emptying and abdominal girth. Fluid balance requires daily weight measurements, urine output, and specific gravity. Drug therapy is frequently multiple, and the physician must be aware of possible interference among drugs and the cumulative toxicity of their use over time. Drug level measurements are imperative with agents such as theophylline and gentamicin.

TRANSFUSION

With marginal lung function, ventilation-perfusion imbalance, and, in some patients, cor pulmonale, blood oxygen-carrying capacity must be kept optimal. Thus, judicious transfusion with washed, packed red cells to keep the hematocrit at 36 to 45 ml per deciliter seems prudent.

STEROIDS

Steroids are not helpful in treating acute neonatal lung disease or in managing long-established chronic lung disease with severe disruption of lung architecture. However, several studies suggest that certain infants gain a functional advantage from steroid treatment that may allow weaning from the ventilator of otherwise ventilator-fast infants with early BPD. This "window of opportunity" is defined by the following criteria:

1. *Postnatal age 2 to 6 weeks*
2. *Stalled on the ventilator*; no progress for 5 days
3. Absence of complications: sepsis, patent ductus arteriosus, pneumothorax
4. X-ray film changes of early BPD.

Such infants may receive a trial of intravenous dexamethasone, 0.25 mg per kilogram every 12 hours, for 3 days. A positive response is weaning from the respirator in this time or a substantial reduction in FiO_2 and respirator settings. If it is unsuccessful, the dexamethasone can be abruptly discontinued without adrenal suppression. If it is successful, tapering the drug over about a month is accomplished by the following regimen (divided doses): 0.5 mg per kilogram for 3 days; 0.3 mg per kilogram for 3 days; then reduction every 3 days by 10 percent (0.03 mg) until the dose is 0.1 mg per kilogram; then 0.1 mg per kilogram every other day for 1 week; then discontinue entirely. A report of this regimen has been published.

It should be emphasized that the precise indications and complications of the steroid treatment of early BPD remain to be worked out. Potential complications include sepsis, glucose intolerance, hypertension, and adrenal suppression.

SECONDARY INFECTION

Low-grade pulmonary infection is difficult to confirm or rule out. Tracheitis may be suspected if there is a puru-

TABLE 2 Drug Therapy

Drug	Dosage	Indication
Furosemide (Lasix)	1–3 mg/kg IV, IM, or po, repeat q6–8h as needed	Preferred diuretic Sudden weight gain, pulmonary edema
Ethacrynic acid	1 mg/kg IV or po, repeat q8–12h as needed	Diuretic, when refractory to furosemide
Bumetanide (Bumex)	0.02–0.1 mg/kg IV, IM or po q12h	Diuretic, when refractory to furosemide
Spironolactone, hydrochlorothiazide (Aldactazide)	0.8–1.6 mg/kg po q12h (as spironolactone)	Diuretic, convalescence or refractory to furosemide
Digoxin	0.025–0.04 mg/kg total digitalizing dose	Heart failure; occasional cor pulmonale
Dexamethasone (Decadron)	0.25 mg/kg IV q12h × 6; then 0.15 mg q12h × 6; then decrease 10% q3d	Early BPD stuck on the respirator; see text
Chloral hydrate	25 mg/kg po or pr	Sedation with minimal respiratory depression
Indomethacin (Indocin)	0.2 mg/kg IV q8h × 3	Functionally significant patent ductus arteriosus
Caffeine citrate	20 mg/kg IV or po loading; maintenance ~2.5 mg/kg, monitor levels	Apnea; respiratory stimulation
Aminophylline (theophylline)	5 mg/kg loading, ~2 mg/kg maintenance, monitor levels	Respiratory stimulation, bronchodilation
Metaproterenol (Metaprel)	Aerosol, 0.1 mg	Bronchodilation
Atropine	Aerosol, 1 mg	Bronchodilation
Terbutaline	Aerosol, 0.1 mg	Bronchodilation
Epinephrine	Aerosol 0.25 mg/ml	Postextubation stridor or bronchospasm

lent tracheal aspirate with many polymorphonuclear leukocytes containing intracellular bacteria and a culture revealing a likely pathogen such as *Staphylococcus aureus*. Septic symptoms appearing abruptly, together with pulmonary infiltrates, may represent acute superimposed pneumonia. For the most part, prolonged and uncritical use of antibiotics should be avoided because of the emergence of resistant strains and particularly the danger of systemic fungal infection. The role of indolent, atypical pulmonary infections such as with *Chlamydia* or *Pneumocystis* is unknown. Occasionally we have treated patients with such infections empirically with erythromycin or trimethoprim-sulfamethoxazole (Bactrim) in an unusually unresponsive case, and occasionally it has seemed to help.

ENVIRONMENT

The environment of the usual intensive care nursery is poorly adapted to the needs of the older infant with protracted BPD. The baby needs a few sensitive, relatively constant caretakers. He or she needs interventions to be clustered and balanced by periods of quiet and rest. Painful interventions need to be offset by pleasant contacts with adult caretakers. The child becomes easily disturbed by stimuli, whether they be noise, light, or touch. The result can be either a protective withdrawal or a wild, unfocused, stimulus-driven response that ends in a frantic attack of bronchospasm and air hunger. Yet these same infants also need substantial respiratory support and the expertise typically found in intensive care nurseries. When there are several such babies under care, they can sometimes be clustered in a quiet corner of the nursery. The answer is often teaching the essentials of care to the parents and arranging home care with nursing, respiratory therapy, and social services support.

SUPPORT OF THE FAMILY

Being the parent of a child with BPD is a long, wearing vigil. Anxiety about the mere fact of survival is gradually replaced by anxiety about how the demands of this strenuous illness can be met. Typically there is a roller coaster disease course that keeps parents off balance and uncertain of what to believe. The long-range quality of life for the child is another major anxiety. Small wonder that parents sometimes strike out in anger and frustration. There are no tricks or shortcuts for dealing with the parents of BPD babies. Members of the medical team must show that they respect and care about the baby and demonstrate that they are doing their best. They must tell the truth, even about unpleasant complications. They must allow the parents to ventilate. They must keep sight of the big picture even while dealing with all the small details. And they must keep their own frustrations under control.

PROGNOSIS AND OUTCOME

About 25 to 35 percent of infants with severe BPD die. Hospitalizations are long, often lasting 3 to 5 months. During the infant's first year of life there are frequent hospital readmissions, often for respiratory infections. After the first year, growth of new lung begins to balance the disease tissue, and function improves. Subtle functional changes can still be detected during preschool years, but the chest x-ray film usually becomes normal. On a day-to-day basis, most survivors develop surprisingly good lung function and are not respiratory cripples. About 25 percent of the survivors have significant neurodevelopmental handicaps, but many are perfectly normal.

SUGGESTED READING

Avery GB, Fletcher AB, et al. Controlled trial of dexamethasone in respirator-dependent infants with bronchopulmonary dysplasia. Pediatrics 1985; 75:106–111.

CHLAMYDIAL INFECTIONS

LILLIAN R. BLACKMON, M.D.

During the last decade, *Chlamydia trachomatis* has come to be recognized as a significant pathogen with a high infectivity in the neonate. The organism shares with viruses the characteristic of being an obligate intracellular parasite, but like bacteria, has a cell wall, multiplies by binary fission, contains both DNA and RNA, and can be inactivated by several antimicrobial agents. In the human, invasion occurs across mucus membranes; the conjunctiva, the upper airway, and the genital tract in specific have been identified as portals of entry, hence the occurrence of congenitally acquired infection in the infant. In the adult, transmission is believed to be venereal, and recent evidence suggests a respiratory route of transmission in the young child.

Several population surveys have reported 5 to 20 percent of pregnant women with positive cervical cultures. Infection is more common in adolescents and women of lower socioeconomic class. In one study, 67 percent of infants born to infected mothers developed evidence of infection.

ETIOLOGY

In infants, infections involve primarily the mucus membranes that are exposed during the birth process: the conjunctiva, upper airway, and lower respiratory tract. Chlamydial conjunctivitis, formerly labeled inclusion blennorrhea, has been known for decades. It is the most common chlamydial infection in infancy. The incubation period is 5 to 21 days, with greatest occurrence taking place at 8 to 12 days. Clinical signs vary from minimal to severe inflammation, with edema of lids, chemosis, hyperemia of the palpebral conjunctivae, and copious yellow exudate; more commonly, symptoms are mild and gradual in progression. If untreated, signs of inflammation and discharge may persist for weeks with gradual resolution. Infrequently, conjunctival scarring and micropannus formation have been seen. Chlamydial conjunctivitis can be differentiated clinically from the other causes of conjunctivitis in the neonate by the time of onset (after the first week of life) and by the clinical presentation (mild symptoms) though definitive staining and cultures should be obtained. Recently, a direct immunofluorescent monoclonal antibody stain technique for rapid diagnosis has been reported.

To demonstrate the intracytoplasmic inclusions of *Chlamydia*, it is necessary to obtain conjunctival epithelial cells by scraping rather than smearing the exudate. With the Giemsa stain, they appear as large, round, intensely basophilic bodies within the cytoplasm. Immunofluorescent staining and electron microscopy techniques have also been previously described. Special tissue culture techniques are required for laboratory propagation, using McCoy cells with arrest of cell division before inoculation.

CHLAMYDIAL PNEUMONIA

A syndrome of afebrile pneumonitis occurring in early infancy (at 2 to 13 weeks of age) is now recognized as a clinical manifestation of chlamydial infection in infancy. As many as 50 percent of infants have a history of conjunctivitis before the onset of respiratory symptoms. The clinical presentation includes nasal congestion with little discharge, tachypnea, and staccato coughing, which is at times paroxysmal. Physical findings are of a mild to moderately ill infant usually not in marked distress, afebrile, with diffuse, most often bilateral, crepitant rales. The onset is gradual, and the course of the untreated disease is prolonged over several weeks. Wheezing and prolongation of expiration is said to occur in 15 to 20 percent of patients. No deaths due to chlamydial pneumonia have been reported.

In one series in which multiple pathogens were sought, combined infections with cytomegalovirus, *Ureaplasma urealyticum*, and *Pneumocystis carinii* were reported in 26 percent of infants. The only clinically distinguishing feature was that infants with combined infection tended to be more ill, having recurrent apnea and significant respiratory failure requiring oxygen and ventilatory assistance. Tipple et al reported abnormal middle ear findings consisting of opaque, pearly white, sometimes bulging, tympanic membranes, diffuse light reflex, and poorly seen short process in 59 percent of chlamydia-positive infants presenting with pneumonitis. Myringotomy consistently yielded a gelatinous aspirate.

The radiographic findings most commonly seen are of diffuse interstitial infiltrates with hyperinflation. Patchy areas of density, either infiltrate or subsegmental atelectasis, can be seen and correlate poorly with the clinical findings. Eosinophilia of greater than 300 per cubic millimeter and nonspecific elevation of immunoglobulins IgA and IgM are the only laboratory findings seen consistently. A rise in titer of specific antibodies can be demonstrated both in serum and in tears or nasopharyngeal secretions by a variety of techniques. Abnormalities in blood gases (usually only a mild oxygenation deficit) do occur.

There are reported instances of chlamydial pneumonia occurring late (4 to 8 weeks postnatally) in preterm infants. The onset is described as insidious, with significant respiratory failure being a frequent feature. Furthermore, the course of the disease is prolonged in some cases, resulting in chronic lung disease.

Confirmation of *Chlamydia* as the etiologic agent is possible by Giemsa stain of nasopharyngeal secretions obtained by swabbing or catheter aspiration, by tissue culture of the same, by a rise in antibody titer, or by culture from lung biopsy.

Other clinical disease in infancy associated with *Chlamydia* has not been clearly defined. Obstructive rhinitis with chronic low-grade discharge and failure to thrive has been seen in our clinic concomitantly with a positive nasopharyngeal culture. Symptomatic improvement has occurred with antibiotic treatment.

MANAGEMENT

The usual treatment for chlamydial conjunctivitis has been sulfacetamide ophthalmic preparations administered for 10 to 14 days. Tetracycline ointment has also been used. Relapse and recurrence are frequent with topical management. Whether the failure arises from inadequate applica-

tion, antimicrobial failure, or reinfection from the nasopharynx via the nasolacrimal drainage system is not clear. After 3 weeks of oral erythromycin therapy, eradication from both conjunctiva and nasopharynx occurs. When initiating therapy for conjunctivitis, one must weigh the affordability of topical treatment, with its possible risk of relapse or recurrence and of unrecognized nasopharyngeal colonization, against the more costly oral therapy, which may not be necessary if nasopharyngeal colonization is not present. The availability of diagnostic staining and culture techniques also enters into the management decision.

It is clear that nasopharyngeal infection is associated with a higher likelihood of pneumonia. In the largest prospective series reported, 17 percent of infants with positive nasopharyngeal culture went on to develop the clinical syndrome of afebrile pneumonitis. Because conjunctival infection occurring during the first 2 weeks of life was associated with nasopharyngeal infection in only four of 14 infants in that series, an initial course of topical treatment may be appropriate for infants younger than 2 weeks of age, followed by oral erythromycin if there is relapse or failure. After the age of 2 weeks, oral therapy either with or without culture confirmation should be used as concurrent infections become more frequent. Oral therapy is probably indicated in preterm infants at known risk—i.e., those with positive maternal cervical culture or conjunctivitis—because of the apparently more severe course of chlamydial pneumonia in these infants.

Treatment of the afebrile pneumonitis syndrome is both supportive and antimicrobial specific. Although apnea and significant respiratory failure occur in less than 25 percent of infants, hospitalization for at least 5 to 7 days of observation and antibiotic treatment is justifiable if either is present, because of the severity of consequences that could result. Reduction in symptoms has been reported with both erythromycin and sulfisoxazole within this 5- to 7-day period. A total of 14 days of antibiotic therapy is recommended. Supportive care consists of parenteral fluids, chest physiotherapy, cardiorespiratory monitoring, and oxygen as required. Recurrent apnea or hypercarbia necessitates ventilatory assistance. Multiple etiologic agents should be suspected with a more severe clinical course.

Oral erythromycin or sulfisoxazole treatment can be used on an outpatient basis for upper respiratory tract illness caused by *Chlamydia*.

CHLAMYDIAL CERVICAL INFECTION

The role of chlamydial cervical infection in pregnancy as a significant cause of poor pregnancy outcome has been studied by several groups. One group has reported an increased incidence of stillbirths and neonatal deaths in chlamydia culture–positive women. A recent study at the University of Maryland found chlamydial cervicitis to have a significant etiologic role in preterm premature rupture of membranes. A prospective investigation of cervical infections caused by multiple pathogens (*Mycoplasma hominis*, *Chlamydia trachomatis*, and *Ureaplasma urealyticum*) by another group found an increase in infants with low birth weight and premature rupture of membranes (PROM) only in the subset of women who were both cervical culture–positive for *Chlamydia* and IgM seropositive. This suggests that a primary cervical infection with *Chlamydia* is more likely to affect pregnancy outcome than a chronic one. There has also been high incidence of multiple infection. A prospective clinical trial of early diagnosis and treatment of chlamydial cervicitis to prevent PROM is currently underway at our institution.

Alteration of current approaches to prevention of neonatal ophthalmia also remains an issue. A report suggesting a progression from conjunctival to nasopharyngeal infection over the first 2 weeks of life would support the use of an antichlamydial agent in neonatal ophthalmia prophylaxis. The instillation of silver nitrate solution into the conjunctival sac does not prevent invasion of chlamydia, nor does topical tetracycline hydrochloride or a single intramuscular injection of penicillin G at birth. One study reported a single application of erythromycin ointment at birth to have a beneficial effect in preventing conjunctivitis but not in preventing nasopharyngeal infection or pneumonia. A full course of oral therapy is necessary for the latter. However, the cost and inconvenience of this approach precludes its widespread usage for prophylaxis.

CHRONIC CHOLESTASIS

DONALD A. NOVAK, M.D.
WILLIAM F. BALISTRERI, M.D.

Infants with hepatobiliary dysfunction, regardless of etiology, are at risk for developing clinical sequelae from prolonged cholestasis. These complications are due directly or indirectly to diminished bile flow. Substances normally excreted into bile, such as bile acids, bilirubin, and cholesterol, are retained in the liver and are subsequently regurgitated into the serum and tissues. Bile acid concentrations in the intestinal lumen may fall, resulting in malabsorption of long-chain triglycerides and fat-soluble vitamins. Impairment of hepatic function may alter nutrient utilization as well as cause myriad other endocrinologic and metabolic aberrations.

Neonatal cholestasis (prolonged conjugated hyperbilirubinemia) can be the initial manifestation of a wide variety of diseases, including anatomic abnormalities (both intra- and extrahepatic), metabolic disorders, and infectious and toxic hepatitides (see Table 2). Differentiation between these disorders is essential, as specific treatment may be available and its delay may have tragic consequences. For example, *early diagnosis of biliary atresia is the initial step toward maximizing the success rate for surgical amelioration*. Diagnosis begins with assessment of historical features, such as direct query regarding a history of maternal exposure to infectious agents, a family history of cholestasis, and a feeding history for the infant. Clinical features aiding in discrimination include sex (neonatal hepatitis occurs more frequently in males, whereas biliary atresia occurs with greater frequency in females), the presence or absence of other congenital anomalies (as seen in extrahepatic biliary atresia), and stool pigmentation, the consistent absence of which would suggest biliary obstruction. Laboratory examination should begin with measurement of the total and the direct reacting fractions of serum bilirubin. In "physiologic" hyperbilirubinemia, breast-milk jaundice, Rh and ABO incompatibility, and the less commonly encountered Gilbert's and Crigler-Najjar syndromes, there is primarily an elevation (greater than 80 percent) of unconjugated bilirubin. *Cholestasis is present if the conjugated fraction constitutes more than 20 percent of the total bilirubin* in a jaundiced infant. Additional diagnostic approaches may be found in Table 1.

Discussion of diagnostic modalities is beyond the scope of this article; however, a few words of caution are in order. Alpha$_1$-antitrypsin deficiency is best diagnosed by determination of alpha$_1$-antitrypsin phenotype, as serum concentration alone may not accurately reflect the deficiency (PiZZ) state. Reducing substances may not be present in the urine of the patient with galactosemia who is receiving a diet deficient in galactose or if vomiting is significant. A specific assay of galactose-1-phosphate uridyl transferase in red blood cells is available and reliable, provided that the infant has not recently received blood transfusions. Elevated serum concentrations of tyrosine and methionine may be noted in liver disease of any etiology and are therefore not specific for tyrosinemia. The detec-

TABLE 1 Initial Work-Up of the Neonate With Suspected Cholestasis

1. Fractionated serum bilirubin and serum bile acid determinations
2. Index of hepatic synthetic function (prothrombin time)
3. Examination of stool color
4. Cultures (blood, urine, spinal fluid)
5. HB$_s$Ag, toxoplasmosis, rubella, cytomegalovirus, and herpes simplex (TORCH) and veneral disease research laboratory (VDRL) titers
6. Alpha$_1$-antitrypsin phenotype
7. Metabolic screen (urine/serum amino acids, urine reducing substances)
8. Thyroxine and thyroid-stimulating hormone
9. Sweat chloride test
10. Ultrasound examination
11. Duodenal intubation for bilirubin content
12. Hepatobiliary scintigraphy
13. Liver biopsy

TABLE 2 The Differential Diagnosis of Neonatal Cholestasis

I. Extrahepatic disorders
   A. Biliary atresia
   B. Biliary hypoplasia
   C. Bile duct stenosis
   D. Anomalies of choledochal-pancreatico-ductal junction
   E. Spontaneous perforation of bile duct
   F. Mass (neoplasia, stone)
   G. Bile/mucus plug

II. Intrahepatic disorders
   A. Idiopathic
     1. Idiopathic neonatal hepatitis
     2. Intrahepatic cholestasis, persistent
       a. Arteriohepatic dysplasia (Alagille's syndrome)
       b. Byler's disease (severe intrahepatic cholestasis with progressive hepatocellular disease)
       c. Trihydroxycoprostanic acidemia (defective bile acid metabolism and cholestasis)
       d. Zellweger's syndrome (cerebrohepatorenal syndrome)
       e. Nonsyndromic paucity of intrahepatic ducts (apparent absence of bile ductules)
     3. Intrahepatic cholestasis, recurrent (syndromic?)
       a. Familial benign recurrent cholestasis
       b. Hereditary cholestasis with lymphedema (Aagenaes)

   B. Anatomic
     1. Congenital hepatic fibrosis/infantile polycystic disease
     2. Caroli's disease (cystic dilation of intrahepatic ducts)

   C. Metabolic disorders
     1. Disorders of amino acid metabolism
       a. Tyrosinemia
     2. Disorders of lipid metabolism
       a. Wolman's disease
       b. Niemann-Pick disease
       c. Gaucher's disease
     3. Disorders of carbohydrate metabolism
       a. Galactosemia
       b. Fructosemia
       c. Glycogenosis IV
     4. Metabolic disease in which defect is uncharacterized
       a. Alpha$_1$-antitrypsin deficiency
       b. Cystic fibrosis
       c. Idiopathic hypopituitarism
       d. Hypothyroidism
       e. Neonatal iron storage disease
       f. Infantile copper overload
       g. Familial erythrophagocytic lymphohistiocytosis

   D. Hepatitis
     1. Infectious
       a. Cytomegalovirus
       b. Hepatitis B virus (? non-A, non-B virus)
       c. Rubella virus
       d. Reovirus type 3
       e. Herpesvirus
       f. Varicella virus
       g. Coxsackievirus
       h. Echovirus
       i. Toxoplasmosis
       j. Syphilis
       k. Tuberculosis
       l. Listeriosis
     2. Toxic
       a. Cholestasis associated with parenteral nutrition
       b. Sepsis with possible endotoxemia (urinary tract infection, gastroenteritis)

   E. Genetic/chromosomal
     1. Trisomy E
     2. Down syndrome
     3. Donohue's syndrome (leprechaunism)

   F. Miscellaneous
     1. Histiocytosis X
     2. Shock/hypoperfusion
     3. Intestinal obstruction
     4. Polysplenia syndrome

Modified from Balistreri WF. Neonatal cholestasis: medical progress. J Pediatr 1985; 106:171.

tion of specific metabolites reflecting altered pathways of tyrosine degradation (e.g., succinylacetone) provides a more specific diagnosis of tyrosinemia. Parenteral nutrition–related cholestasis may be the most commonly encountered cause of neonatal cholestasis. It is essential, however, that in the infant with suspected parenteral nutrition–related cholestasis other treatable entities be ruled out prior to accepting the diagnosis. Parenteral nutrition–related liver disease is typically noted in low birth weight infants with a myriad of other risk factors for hepatic disease, including multiple transfusions and drugs as well as a history of asphyxia. Metabolic, infectious, and anatomic etiologies, as indicated in Table 2, must first be considered, as must the possibility of parenteral nutrition-related cholelithiasis.

Although the cholestatic neonate is unique and the list of potential underlying etiologies is large and diverse, the end point of each syndrome is similar, resulting in the well-known clinical consequences of prolonged cholestasis. Therapy is aimed at limiting discomfort, avoiding complications as much as possible, and maximizing growth with a final goal, in many cases, of liver transplantation.

NUTRITION

Chronic hepatobiliary dysfunction may have a limiting effect on nutrition and growth. As noted earlier, fat malabsorption is common and is related to diminished concentrations of bile acids in the intestinal lumen. Administered medications, such as cholestyramine, may further compromise fat absorption. The seriously ill neonate who develops cholestasis while receiving parenteral nutrition may sustain further compromise in nutritional status through well-intended reductions in parenteral calories in an attempt to ameliorate liver disease. Anorexia, either secondary to the presence of infection or related to a specific nutrient deficiency (i.e., zinc), is often seen. Organomegaly and ascites may cause visceral compression, which result in early satiety and gastroesophageal reflux with esophagitis. Hepatic dysfunction and disordered hepatic metabolism may affect nutrient homeostasis. Adults with cirrhosis have been noted to demonstrate glucose intolerance and insulin resistance. Serum levels of branched chain amino acids (valine, leucine, and isoleucine) are often diminished in chronic liver disease, in conjunction with increased levels of the aromatic amino acids (tyrosine, phenylalanine, and methionine). The end result of these alterations is unknown; however, it is likely that they have adverse metabolic and nutritional effects. Regardless of the etiology of cholestasis, it is imperative that appropriate, adequate nutrition (i.e., energy, specific nutrients) be given.

The initial steps in the nutritional management of the patient with chronic cholestasis are to obtain accurate measurement of current nutritional status and to document current hepatic synthetic capabilities (i.e., albumin, prothrombin time, partial thromboplastin time), which may, if inadequate, limit growth despite administration of adequate nutrition. Height, weight, and skin fold measurements also are of use; however, weight may be falsely elevated because of fluid retention. Caloric needs may be estimated through the use of indirect calorimetry, a noninvasive method in which determination of oxygen consumption and carbon dioxide production allows inference of resting energy expenditure. Fat malabsorption can be quantitated and the presence or absence of specific vitamin deficiencies (A, D, E, K) inferred through serum levels.

The goal of the nutritional management of the patient with chronic cholestasis is to maximize growth. Supplements containing medium-chain triglycerides as a substitute for dietary long-chain triglycerides help to maximize fat absorption. Medium-chain triglyceride–containing formulas such as Portagen or Pregestimil may be of use to ensure that adequate protein, fat, and carbohydrate calories are provided. The use of medium-chain triglycerides allows more efficient fat absorption, since their absorption is less dependent on intraluminal bile acid concentration; however, deficiency of essential fatty acids (e.g., linoleic acid) must be avoided. Essential fatty acids must constitute 2 to 3 percent of the infant's total caloric intake. Pregestimil has a much larger proportion of calories derived from linoleic acid than does Portagen, thus reducing the risk of essential fatty acid deficiency. Breast milk, although superior to formulas which do not contain medium-chain triglycerides, may be ineffective in growth promotion in the cholestatic infant. The breast-fed infant with hepatobiliary disease may thus require supplementation with formula containing medium-chain triglycerides. Replacement of micronutrients such as calcium, phosphate, and zinc and supplementation with fat-soluble vitamins are essential, regardless of the formula utilized. Use of newer methods of enteral feeding will help meet all of these requirements. *Of particular benefit may be the administration of formula through soft No. 5 to No. 8 French nasogastric catheters in intermittent, continuous, or nocturnal fashion.* This technique allows the administration of an adequate balanced diet in a safe, efficient, and cost-effective manner that is without the risks and complications of parenteral nutrition. Regardless of the manner in which feedings are administered, however, salt restriction may be necessary, especially in the presence of ascites. In addition, protein restriction may be required because of encephalopathy. It must be reiterated, however, that in the presence of limited hepatic synthetic function, growth may not occur, despite administration of adequate calories and nitrogen.

Fat-soluble vitamin deficiencies, as seen in chronic cholestasis, are often associated with specific symptoms. Hypoprothrombinemia may be present in the infant with cholestasis; thus vitamin K (2.5 to 5.0 mg intramuscularly) should be given early in the evaluation of any cholestatic infant and continued throughout the course of the disease. It is hoped that this regimen will prevent catastrophic spontaneous bleeding such as intracranial hemorrhage. Deficiency of vitamin E, common in chronic cholestasis, is responsible for a progressive neuromuscular syndrome, characterized by loss of myelinated axons of peripheral nerves and degeneration of spinal cord posterior columns. Vitamin E–deficient patients have low

TABLE 3 Suggested Medical Management of the Nutritional Consequences of Persistent Cholestasis

Effect	Management
1. Malabsorption of dietary long-chain triglycerides	Replace with dietary formula or supplement containing medium-chain triglycerides • Adequate protein (vegetable protein) = 2–3 g/kg/day • Adequate calories (complex starch)
2. Fat-soluble vitamin deficiency Vitamin A (night blindness, thick skin)	Replace with *5,000–15,000 IU/day*, as in Aquasol A
Vitamin E (neuromuscular degeneration)	Replace with *50–400 IU/day*, as in oral D-α-tocopherol (may require parenteral administration)
Vitamin D (metabolic bone disease)	Replace with *5,000–8,000 IU/day of vitamin D_2* or 3–5 μg/kg/day of 25-hydroxycholecalciferol
Vitamin K (hypoprothrombin-cmia)	Replace with 2.5–5.0 mg every other day as water-soluble derivative of menadione
3. Micronutrient deficiency	• Calcium/phosphate/zinc supplementation
4. Deficiency of water-soluble vitamins	• Supplement with twice the recommended daily allowance

serum vitamin E concentrations as well as a low ratio of serum vitamin E to total serum lipids (defined as less than 0.6 mg per gram for children under 12 and less than 0.8 mg per gram for older patients). Administration of high oral doses of vitamin E may be required to prevent deficiency (Table 3). After a therapeutic trial of oral vitamin E, serum levels should be measured. Patients with an inadequate response should be given vitamin E (DL-alpha-tocopherol) intramuscularly, typically in doses of 0.8 to 2.0 IU per kilogram per day. Unfortunately, as of this writing, vitamin E for intramuscular injection remains an investigational product. Cholestatic patients may also develop vitamin D deficiency. Malabsorption may cause low serum vitamin D levels or, if levels are normal, functional deficiency may occur because of diminished hepatic hydroxylation. Clinically evident metabolic bone disease (rickets or osteoporosis) may occur; thus vitamin D supplements must be given. Deficiency of vitamin A has also been noted to occur in chronic cholestasis, and therefore it is essential to monitor vitamin A status and to increase supplementation when levels are low. It is also possible that water-soluble vitamin deficiencies may occur; this has been noted in adults with cirrhosis. Finally, mineral balance is often altered. Excessive accumulations of the toxic compound copper may be noted in chronic liver disease. Magnesium, potassium, phosphorus, and calcium balance may be altered as well. Low levels of serum iron, associated with decreased transferrin synthesis and blood loss, are described. Careful initial attention to and continued re-evaluation of the patient's nutritional status are required, as adequate nutrition may allow the patient time for hepatic regeneration. If hepatic transplantation becomes a necessity, the success rate and the degree of organ availability increase significantly with attainment of adequate infant size (> 10 kg).

PRURITUS

The pruritus associated with chronic cholestasis is infrequently noted in the neonatal period but may become a problem before the end of the first year. The etiology of cholestatic pruritus is unknown. Although it has long been felt to be secondary to retained bile acids, little correlation has been found between the degree of pruritus and skin or serum bile acid levels. It is possible that pruritus may result from unusual physiochemical forms of bile acids. Partial relief has been achieved through the use of the choleretic agent, phenobarbital, as well as with the use of cholestyramine, a bile acid–binding resin. Cholestyramine is efficacious in the treatment of pruritus, but unfortunately the resin is unpalatable and difficult to administer to infants and children. Side effects of cholestyramine include constipation, hyperchloremia, and exacerbation of fat-soluble vitamin deficiency. Phenobarbital (3 to 5 mg per kilogram per day) may be useful in patients with some degree of residual bile duct patency. Side effects of phenobarbital included initial sedation, paradoxical hyperexcitability, and addiction. In addition, metabolism of other concomitantly administered drugs may be altered. Both phenobarbital and cholestyramine may require 2 to 4 weeks to produce the desired effects. Therapy with ultraviolet light (UV-B) has also proved useful. Plasma perfusion and carbamazepine (Tegretol) therapy have been successfully utilized in adults; however, their usefulness in the pediatric population remains to be established.

ASCITES

Ascites is a common problem in patients with chronic liver disease and portal hypertension. Although the etiology of ascites remains uncertain, several factors are probably important: (1) increased lymphatic flow secondary to portal hypertension may lead to peritoneal fluid collection; (2) hypoalbuminemia, although not critical to ascites formation, may contribute to it; (3) renal retention of sodium and water seen in chronic liver disease contributes to the already elevated pressure in the splanchnic circulation, again with ascites as the end result. The last factor may be the most important. Treatment of ascites is a challenging problem. Therapy is aimed at addressing the altered renal handling of salt and water seen in liver disease and typically includes a limitation of dietary sodium intake to 1 to 2 mEq per kilogram per day. Administration of Portagen or Pregestimil in the amount of 180 ml per kilogram per day results in a sodium intake of approximately 2.5 mEq per kilogram per day. Increased calories may be provided while keeping salt and fluids stable by the addition of medium-chain triglycerides and/or glucose polymers to formula, thereby increasing the caloric density. The addition of glucose polymers does, however, increase formula osmolality, leading to potential delayed gastric emptying and/or diarrhea. Modification of formulas should be performed only if volume and/or salt intolerance is demonstrated. The maximum tolerable caloric density is approximately 30 calories per ounce; caloric density should be tailored to the individual patient. Fortunately, fluid restriction is generally not required in patients with adequate urine output in whom hyponatremia is absent. When diuresis is required, the aldosterone inhibitor, spironolactone (Aldactone), 2 to 3 mg per kilogram per day (the dose may be doubled if the response is inadequate), may be clinically useful. It offers the advantage of potassium sparing. Response to spironolactone administration typically occurs within 70 to 96 hours; this may be monitored by observation of the urine sodium: potassium ratio. If response remains inadequate, i.e., a Na^+/K^+ ratio of less than 1, an additional diuretic (thiazides, furosemide, or ethacrynic acid) may be added. Complications of diuretic therapy include hypokalemia, hyponatremia, and, less frequently, azotemia and encephalopathy. Measurement of serum and urine electrolyte concentrations as well as of serum creatinine levels is part of careful follow-up. Paracentesis, except as a diagnostic measure, is not indicated.

VARICEAL HEMORRHAGE

The presence of portal hypertension in the infant with hepatobiliary disease may be associated with the development of esophageal varices and subsequent variceal hemorrhage. Treatment of this complication in the perinatal period is difficult. Initial management must include differentiation of variceal bleeding from other causes, generally via flexible endoscopy. Lavage of the stomach, typically with saline, is then performed through a large-bore nasogastric tube. Volume replacement is given, using care to avoid overadministration of sodium or of volume, which might worsen variceal hemorrhage. Hematocrit values must be monitored and, if needed, supplemented with transfusion of red blood cells, while at-

tention to platelet counts and clotting factors must also be maintained. *Most episodes of bleeding subside with conservative management.* Intravenously administered vasopressin may be given as a bolus of 0.3 U per kilogram (maximum of 20 U), diluted in 2 ml per kilogram of a 5 percent dextrose solution and delivered over 10 to 20 minutes. Subsequently, a continuous infusion of 0.2 to 0.4 U per 1.73 m² per minute may be utilized for 12 to 24 hours, as required for recalcitrant bleeding. Efficacy in the perinatal period is not, however, well established, and side effects are common. Other methods of hemorrhage control, such as tamponade with a Sengstaken-Blakemore tube or sclerotherapy, may be limited by patient size. Surgical shunting procedures are technically difficult in small children, carry a high mortality if done on an emergency basis, and make future hepatic transplantation difficult.

SPECIFIC MANAGEMENT OF CHOLESTATIC SYNDROMES

Symptomatic therapy of the clinical manifestations of cholestasis is indicated in all cholestatic patients. In addition, certain patients, afflicted by defined syndromes, require specific and in some cases immediate intervention.

Lesions Amenable to Surgery

Surgical correction or amelioration is indicated in biliary atresia, bile duct stenosis, spontaneous perforation of the bile duct, annular pancreas, and choledochal cyst. The treatment of choice for choledochal cyst is excision of the cyst and Roux-en-Y choledochojejunostomy. Postoperative management must include prompt recognition and vigorous treatment of episodes of cholangitis. In addition, retained cystic tissue poses a risk for the development of carcinoma. Surgical therapy of biliary atresia traditionally consists of the hepatoportoenterostomy procedure of Kasai, which attempts to establish biliary drainage via excision of obliterated extrahepatic ducts with apposition of the resected surface of the porta hepatis to bowel mucosa. Although it is not curative, the procedure may allow sufficient growth of the patient to facilitate hepatic transplantation. Prognosis is affected by age at operation, with *success rates of 90 percent in patients under 2 months of age, dropping to less than 20 percent in patients over 90 days of age.* Also important is the size of the residual ductal lumen encountered at surgery; those with diameters of greater than 150 μ are associated with a better prognosis. Most posthepatoportoenterostomy patients have residual, perhaps progressive, hepatic disease and require transplantation at a later date.

Metabolic Diseases of the Liver

Specific therapy of metabolic diseases of the liver is, in some cases, available. Galactosemia is a nutritional toxicity syndrome in which deficiency of galactose-1-phosphate uridyl transferase allows accumulation of injurious concentrations of galactose-1-phosphate and galactitol. Deficiency of galactokinase does not cause liver disease. Treatment involves the early removal of all dietary galactose. Useful formulae have been Pregestimil and Nutramigen, which contain only very small amounts of galactose that are not of therapeutic importance. Soy formulae, which have galactose in unavailable form, may also be used. Removal of galactose from the diet dramatically reduces cholestasis; this restriction is necessary throughout life. It is of note that the patient with untreated galactosemia has a high incidence of *Escherichia coli* sepsis.

Hereditary fructose intolerance caused by deficiency of fructose-1-phosphate aldolase may manifest in infancy with hepatic dysfunction. Symptoms typically begin at weaning from breast milk, with the use of sucrose-containing formulas, or when supplementation with fructose-containing foods begins. Treatment consists of a strict fructose-free diet. With strict compliance, life expectancy is apparently normal.

Tyrosinemia may also appear in the neonatal period. In the acute form of neonatal tyrosinemia, death typically occurs from hepatic failure within the first year of life. Diets low in phenylalanine, methionine, and tyrosine have been used but do not appear to reverse liver disease or to prolong life in the acute form of tyrosinemia. Control of diet may be of benefit in chronic disease.

Infectious Causes of Cholestasis

Urinary tract infection secondary to *Escherichia coli* is an important cause of neonatal cholestasis and must be ruled out. Eradication of the infecting organism reverses cholestasis. Similarly, specific treatment for syphilis, *listeria* infection, and tuberculosis is available. Therapy for hepatitis B (probably an uncommon cause of neonatal cholestasis) is preventive, with the hepatitis B vaccine. Prepartum screening of women in high-risk groups is therefore recommended. *High-titer hepatitis B immune globulin (0.5 cc) should be administered to the infant at risk within 12 hours of birth.* Hepatitis B vaccine should then be given within the first 3 days of life at a site distinct from the site of hepatitis B immune globulin administration. Second and third doses of the vaccine may be given at 1 and 6 months.

Miscellaneous

Endocrinopathies, such as hypothyroidism and pan-hypopituitarism, may cause cholestasis. Correction occurs with treatment of the underlying endocrinologic problem. Cholestasis associated with parenteral nutrition, occurring largely in sick premature infants requiring parenteral nutrition as a primary source of calories and nitrogen, is a limiting factor in the use of parenteral nutrition. *Total parenteral nutrition-associated cholestasis generally has an insidious onset, typically presenting with progressive jaundice and hepatosplenomegaly. The etiology of this disorder remains unclear*; however, attention has focused on excessive administration of toxic amino acids or metabolites, such as tryptophan, versus deficiencies of other essential factors, such as taurine. Treatment is empiric, but it is of primary importance that adequate nutrition be maintained. If possible, *enteral nutrition should be initiated to decrease the amount of parenteral nutrition necessary, as well as to stimulate enteric hormone secretion*, which may have a trophic effect on hepatobiliary function. Other potentially beneficial modalities, such as cyclic administration of hyperalimentation and alterations in amino acid composition, require further investigation in infants.

TRANSPLANTATION

Liver transplantation is a viable alternative for patients with chronic cholestasis and subsequent end-stage liver disease. This alternative must be strongly considered for patients in whom the risks of complications from liver disease outweigh the risks of surgery. Transplantation may offer an important life-prolonging alternative to the patient with chronic liver disease due to, among other causes, alpha-1-antitrypsin deficiency and tyrosinemia. Contraindications to transplant include severe cardiopulmonary disease, metastatic cancer, and acquired immunodeficiency syndrome. Currently, with the use of cyclosporine A and other new selective immunosuppressive agents, *survival rates in the pediatric age group are over 75 percent*. A limiting factor, however, continues to be availability of size-matched donor organs, especially in patients weighing less than 10 kg. Adequate public education and efficient organ procurement networks will help to alleviate this problem.

CIRCUMCISION

THOMAS V.N. BALLANTINE, M.D., F.A.C.S.

Circumcision has a long and strange history. The literature reveals that for most couples, the request for circumcision arises from their cultural historical bias.

Because of the frequency of circumcision in our community, it has been our educational policy to teach the pediatric resident rotating on pediatric surgery two techniques for circumcision: (1) the Gomco clamp, and (2) the disposable ligature (Plastibell). Since many pediatricians now do not recommend or are not in favor of circumcision, the operation has become a surgical issue.

When we are notified that a family desires their newborn male child to be circumcised, we first inquire whether the pediatrician has discussed the operation with the family. In most instances, the primary doctor has stated, "We generally advise against circumcision, but the pediatric surgeon will discuss it with you."

The family is asked what they feel the indications for circumcision are. Answers vary. The family is informed that the procedure has now been deemed an unnecessary one for most boys and many insurance companies no longer pay for the procedure. In an understanding and nonthreatening manner, the family is given a historical perspective, pointing out that ritual circumcision was an important part of early Jewish tradition. They are told that in the 20th century, there are no indications for circumcision on the basis of cleanliness. Furthermore, they are told that some authors have stated that the reason for the high circumcision rate in the United States is based on the fact that it may generate a professional service fee for the obstetrician, pediatrician, or surgeon attending the baby. They are also informed that as with any operation, there is always a risk of infection or hemorrhage.

The long-term risks of circumcision are pointed out as either cosmetic or the subsequent development of meatal stenosis; the latter may require a meatotomy, adding the risks of general anesthesia.

If a circumcision is not to be performed, the parents are informed of some data indicating that there may be a higher risk of urinary tract infection in boys who are not circumcised as compared with those who have had the operation. Additionally, the family is told that, while we oppose circumcision, we strongly believe that it should be done by someone competent in performing the procedure and with a good understanding of sterile technique. Accordingly, if the family desires it, the procedure may be undertaken before the infant is discharged from the hospital.

This counseling has not been carried out on a prospective protocol and its effectiveness has not been tested statistically. A report from our neonatal unit, published *before* third-party payers refused reimbursement, suggests that this effort at educating parents of newborns has been fairly ineffective.

If the family elects not to have the infant circumcised, they are advised that no special procedures need to be performed on the foreskin and that, in fact, it remains adherent to the glans until the boy is 3 to 5 years of age. Eventually, the foreskin becomes freely retractile.

If the family elects circumcision for the infant the procedure is carried out, using a bupivacaine hydrochloride (Marcaine) 0.5 percent block of the penile sensory nerve.

The Gomco clamp is generally available in three sizes: 11 mm, 13.5 mm, and 14.5 mm. The institution's central supply facility should provide all three sizes to the operator. The penis and peripubic area are prepared with iodophor and sterilely draped. Since infection is one of the most dreaded complications of this operation, we insist that the operator and the assistant wear a cap, mask, gown, and gloves. The foreskin is reduced using two sterile gauze sponges to retract the prepuce away from the glans and the corona. This may be quite difficult in a small penis, and the operator must be sure that the prepuce is *completely* reduced. If not, an unsatisfactory cosmetic appearance will result. The foreskin is then reduced and the bell is introduced so that it completely covers the glans. Occasionally a small dorsal slit of the foreskin may be required to accommodate the diameter of the Gomco bell. Using two hemostats, the foreskin is passed through the hole in the Gomco anvil and elevated while the lever is affixed to the bell and the bell is tightened against the anvil using the wing nut. It is important that the wing nut be tightened maximally, since the principle of the procedure is to crush the penile skin against the mucosa, assuring normal healing and hemostasis. Redundant foreskin is excised. After 3 minutes of crushing, the Gomco clamp is completely disassembled, with the operator taking care not to disrupt the tissues that have been pressed together. The bell is gently removed from the foreskin and the procedure is terminated with the application of a small amount of antibacterial ointment and a dry sterile dressing. Postoperative care includes a very loose diaper for the child's comfort and a follow-up appointment in 10 days to 2 weeks. The family is cautioned that an inflammatory response will ensue and that, in about 5 days, the penis will look unattractive. If redness is noted on the shaft of the penis, the physician should be contacted immediately.

The advantage to the Gomco clamp technique is that the operator can appreciate the appearance of the penis immediately at the end of the operation.

Our other procedure involves the use of the Plastibell. The foreskin is prepared as indicated above, and the plastic bell is inserted over the glans as described. The foreskin is crushed by a heavy ligature to assure necrosis of the prepuce. The handle of the Plastibell is broken off, and the family is told that the foreskin and the plastic ring will fall off in 7 to 14 days. They are again cautioned to watch for any signs of infection.

CLEFT DISORDERS

WILLIAM P. GRAHAM III, M.D.
RICHARD S. FOX, M.D.

To heal a crooked child, "but what good is it to walk to ask for a job if I cannot speak?" The lament of the child with a cleft. (Herbert C. Cooper, founder of the Lancaster Cleft Palate Clinic, Pennsylvania)

Among the most common of congenital anomalies (1 of 850 live births), cleft lip and palate follow an inherited pattern in many instances. Doubtless this genetic expression is a multifactorial one and not determined by a single gene or simple genetic combination. Whether the occurrence of these defects is facilitated by failure of mesenchymal penetration, mechanical fusion, or a combination of these two aspects influenced genetically is conjectural. The impact of either of these deformities on the development of each other is yet another phenomenon of importance in clefting. Developmentally, central facial fusion occurs earlier than the in utero extension of the head, which clears the tongue away from the palatal shelves, allowing their descent and eventual fusion in a horizontal plane.

For the parents of a child with a cleft, the anguish is often great and the uncertainties of future management disturbing. Few of these problems are solved with a single operative procedure, and often there are certain alterations in growth and development. Consequently, one anticipates a long-term follow-up and the need for periodic reassessment. Absolute timing is not so crucial to repair as the appropriate integration of the surgical efforts and the needs of the child for care by other specialists.

THERAPEUTIC ALTERNATIVES

Successful treatment of cleft disorders has proved most effective with a team approach. Since most of the dramatic therapeutic adventures involve surgery, the surgeon usually nominally heads the team. Others of importance include the pediatrician, neonatologist, otolaryngologist, audiologist, speech pathologist, dentist, prosthodontist, pedodontist, and social service worker.

Occasionally, when the deformities are more severe or the program is more generally oriented (includes other major craniofacial anomalies), the neurosurgeon, ophthalmologist, and the pediatric surgeon contribute, and other craniofacial procedures are done in conjunction with the palatal surgery.

CLASSIFICATION OF CLEFT LIP AND PALATE

Clefting may involve either the lip or palate, be unilateral or bilateral, and present with any conceivable combination of these. The lip elements anterior to the incisive foramen (lip, alveolus, and anterior four teeth) are also referred to as the primary palate or prepalate. The elements of the roof of the mouth and posterior tissues behind the incisive foramen are referred to as the secondary palate or palate. The nostrils, alar cartilages, septum, and nostril bases are variably involved but are not included in the classifying schema.

Most programs adhere to a general timetable for repair, with modifications depending on the appropriateness of growth and development and any associated major medical or surgical problems (Tables 1 and 2). Of paramount concern in the growing child with a cleft palate is the tendency to acquire chronic otitis media due to eustachian sphincter incompetence and frequent retrograde reflux from the pharynx.

A few programs consider lip repair in the immediate perinatal period, stressing the improved scar that is obtained, the lessened psychological impact on the parents, and improved feeding. Waiting a 10- to 12-week* period does allow for some growth, a greater opportunity to educate the parents, and an assurance of good health for the child. With patience, feeding usually is not too great a problem, and many mothers are able to successfully nurse these children, establishing a deep bonding.

CLEFT LIP REPAIR

Although there are many operative procedures for lip repair, two basic techniques are employed by most surgeons today and adapted individually. For the simple unilateral cleft that is not overly wide, the Millard rotation advancement technique is often ideal. For the wider, more deformed unilateral cleft, the Tennison-Randall triangular flap becomes the procedure of choice. Although the rotation advancement repair allegedly permits later revision more readily, in actual practice that is not so, and the experienced surgeon often finds revision, especially for length adjustment, less complicated with a previous triangular flap repair. Very wide clefts are often treated by an initial lip adhesion at 8 to 10 weeks of age and a subsequent definitive repair 6 to 12 weeks later.

Multiple combinations of repair are often necessary to manage bilateral prepalatal defects. Usually repair of these is deferred until 3 months of age. The sides are often repaired separately, employing the same pattern on each side and staging the procedures 6 to 8 weeks apart. This approach is reserved for extra-wide clefts, especially in infants in whom a preliminary lip adhesion procedure was utilized. If it is determined that a dual repair is feasible as a one-stage operation, either a Millard or Manchester type procedure is used.

The alveolar clefts are seldom closed during these early operations and with time may narrow sufficiently to render closure unnecessary. Paramount concerns relative to lip repair are (1) maintenance of a lip-alveolar sulcus, (2) preservation and molding of the dental arch with appropriate positioning of the premaxilla, (3) correcting

---

* Rule of tens: 10 weeks of age, 10 pounds of weight, 10 g of hemoglobin, and a white cell count less than 10,000 per cubic millimeter.

TABLE 1 Sequential Surgical Treatment of Cleft Lip

Procedure	1 Month	3 Months	6–8 Months	10–16 Months	6 Years +
Unilateral lip	Adhesion*	Definitive repair			Scar revision
Unilateral lip and unilateral palate	Adhesion*	Definitive repair and vomer flap		Definitive closure of soft palate	Anterior fistula closure
				Bone graft (alveolar grafts)	
Bilateral lip	Adhesion(s)*	Adhesion(s)*	Unilateral or bilateral lip repair (6 months)	Remaining lip (9 months)	
Bilateral lip (alternatives)		Definitive unilateral lip repair	Definitive second lip repair		
Bilateral lip (alternative)		Bilateral definitive lip repair			
Nasal tip rhinoplasty		Combined with lip surgery			9–16 years; independent procedure
Scar revisions of lip and nose					Usually after puberty, younger if very unsightly
					Bony alveolar augmentation for contour
Rhinoplasty and septoplasty					Usually after puberty

* Optional.

TABLE 2 Sequential Surgical Treatment of Cleft Lip

Procedure	1 Month	3 Months	6 Months	10–16 Months	3–6 Years	6 Years +
Submucosal palatal cleft				Closure and lengthening, possible posterior pharyngeal flap	May delay until certain about velopharyngeal incompetence	
Bilateral palate				Posterior or complete palate repair	Anterior palate, if necessary	
Bilateral lip and palate	Adhesion*	Adhesion*	Definitive unilateral or bilateral lip repair	Definitive repair other side and soft palate	Anterior palate, if necessary	Alveolar bone grafting for stability and orthodontia
(Alternative)		Unilateral lip	Unilateral lip	Soft palate	Anterior palate	
Velopharyngeal incompetence					Posterior pharyngeal flap, superior or inferior based	

Modified from Cooper HK, Harding RL, Krogman WM, et al. Cleft Palate and Cleft Lip: A Team Approach to Clinical Management and Rehabilitation of the Patient. Philadelphia: WB Saunders Co, 1979.
* Optional

without distortion and extensive additional dissection of the nasal deformity, and (4) endeavoring to achieve minimal scarring and natural lip contour. As the child matures, alveolar bone grafting is utilized to achieve premaxillary stability or to provide "bone stock" in the cleft area for migration of teeth by the orthodontist.

CLEFT PALATE REPAIR

Like the lip repair, procedures on the palate are varied and fitted to the individual patient. Although a few surgeons repair the palate at 6 months of age, most wait until the child is 1 year old or older. Before considering palate repair, the competence of the airway is assessed. In children with the Pierre Robin syndrome, neurologic difficulties, retarded development, or a history of airway obstruction, it is best to defer surgery until more growth has occurred.

Some surgeons close the anterior palate first (at times in conjunction with the prepalatal repair) and wait for more growth before proceeding with the soft palate. Others do the reverse, and still others endeavor to close the entire defect in a single step. By and large, it is more appropriate to select a particular operation to suit a specific child than to make the patient "fit" the operation.

Our preference is to close the entire palatal defect in a single step, with or without further lengthening through the addition of a posterior pharyngeal flap. Two basic operative approaches are used, the Wardill-Kilner advancement flap method and the Dorrance horseshoe-shaped flap. For the simple narrow cleft with apparently adequate palate length, the classic Von Langenbek operation is used.

Despite the best closure technique, approximately 25 percent of patients eventually manifest velopharyngeal insufficiency that is not alleviated by speech training. Some time passes before many of these children are recognized. Once it is determined that the child has velopharyngeal incompetence, a secondary procedure on the palate is preferred to speech therapy. Usually either an inferiorly or a superiorly based pharyngeal flap is chosen. For most children, an adenoidectomy should accompany the pharyngoplasty, since placement of the flap precludes their later removal. If the tonsils are inordinately large and the child is very young, it is better to remove them than to risk postoperative airway obstruction.

LONG-TERM MANAGEMENT

For the child with a cleft lip, future orthodontia will be imperative. Occasionally alveolar bone grafting is needed to provide a suitable base for the repositioning of erupting teeth. This is usually done between the ages of 6 and 10 and may be combined with other indicated procedures. At times bone augmentation of the alveolus is needed to enhance upper lip contour.

Even today there is an occasional child whose palatal defect is so large and the residual tissue so deficient that repair is not feasible. For these children a palatal prosthesis with a pharyngeal obturator is a good alternative. The fabrication of these requires the skill of an expert prosthodontist. Adjustments are made periodically to compensate for the child's growth. Close attention is paid to maintaining good dental hygiene, and prompt attention is given to any caries, since the teeth are essential for anchoring the appliance.

As the child matures, consideration is given to correcting any residual nasal deformity. Often septoplasty is needed along with nasal alar alignment, and for children with bilateral prepalatal clefts, columellar lengthening is frequently required. Seldom are these corrections possible before the age of 10 or 11 years. At the same time, any indicated revisions of the lip scars and free vermilion border are also done.

A few children, especially those with severe bilateral clefts or associated anomalies (Crouzon's deformity, Pierre Robin anomalad, Treacher Collins syndrome), have marked deficiencies of growth of certain portions of the face. To ensure facial symmetry and the adequacy of occlusion, craniofacial or maxillofacial surgery is needed. The timing of this procedure varies from infancy to near maturity, depending on the type and severity of the problem. Occasionally, serial procedures are required to keep pace with the rest of the child's facial maturation.

The treatment of the child with the common cleft disorders represents a continuum from birth to full maturity and, at times, beyond. The early treatment involves surgical corrections with periodic observation, assessing the appropriateness of facial growth, speech development, and the quality of hearing as well as the dental status of the patient. When the patient is managed by a team of professionals interested in these children, less cost is incurred by the parents and delays in appropriate treatment are averted. No child fits the mold perfectly, and so the treatment program is flexible enough to allow for individual differences in anatomy, growth, development, and psychology.

Clostridium difficile INFECTION

HIROSHI USHIJIMA, M.D., Ph.D.

The genus *Clostridium* includes anaerobic, spore-forming gram-positive bacilli. Their natural habitat is soil and the intestinal tract of humans and animals. There are approximately 61 species.

Under certain circumstances, some of these saprobes are also human pathogens: *C. tetani*, *C. botulinum*, *C. perfringens*, and *C. difficile* cause tetanus, botulism, gas gangrene, and pseudomembranous colitis, respectively. The pathogenicity of these organisms depends on the release of exotoxins or destructive enzymes.

C. difficile is found in human intestinal microflora and produces an enterotoxin that causes fluid accumulation in the rabbit ileal loop; in addition, it produces an enterotoxin that increases vascular permeability in the rabbit, is lethal to mice, and is a highly active cytotoxin. The former is designated as toxin A or D-1 toxin and the latter as toxin B or D-2 toxin.

EPIDEMIOLOGIC ASPECTS

C. difficile is now widely accepted as the major causative organism of pseudomembranous colitis. The organism can be isolated with great frequency from the stools of patients with pseudomembranous colitis and also from patients receiving antimicrobial therapy who do not have this disease; it is found only rarely in normal adults. Furthermore, *C. difficile* cytotoxin has been demonstrated in the feces of 97 percent of patients with pseudomembranous colitis. Less than 4 percent of adults test positive for *C. difficile*.

In contrast to adults, children commonly harbor *C. difficile* in the intestinal tract (up to 40 percent). Stools from both breast-fed and formula-fed infants between 1 and 45 weeks of age can demonstrate the presence of *C. difficile* by cell culture. Yet, pseudomembranous colitis is even rarer in children than in adults.

Outbreaks of diarrhea associated with *C. difficile* and its toxin in day care centers have been reported. Evidence supports person-to-person spread. Repeated exposure to antibiotics or contact with playmates who are positive by culture may be the cause of an outbreak. In addition, young children are known to practice indiscriminate defecation and lack proper personal hygiene because of their age. Diapering can also be the cause of transmission of *C. difficile*. Thus, environmental contamination is considered to be a significant factor in day care centers. Our experience in the neonatal intensive care unit includes an outbreak of diarrhea associated with *C. difficile* (see farther on).

Major pathogens such as *Shigella*, *Giardia*, rotavirus, adenovirus, and calicivirus cause outbreaks of diarrhea. These pathogens usually invade outside environments.

Clostridium difficile is considered to be a cause of necrotizing enteritis in neonates. However, there are also reports in which *C. difficile* was isolated frequently from healthy neonates. Cytotoxin of *C. difficile* has been detected in feces of symptomatic and asymptomatic infants in a neonatal intensive care unit. It has not been concluded whether or not *C. difficile* toxin is a cause of intestinal infection in neonates.

C. difficile is not unique in its selective colonization of the human intestine during infancy. Other species (e.g., *C. butyricum*) have been shown to occur frequently in infants but only rarely in adults, reflecting fundamental differences in the composition and physicochemical conditions of the intestinal milieu in different age groups. However, *C. difficile* is exceptional in that it exists as a harmless commensal in a considerable proportion of healthy infants but causes symptoms of pseudomembranous colitis in certain patients. The reason for this difference is unknown, and to date most work has concentrated on the pathogenic role of the organism. It is suggested that certain infants are protected from the effects of toxin because, for example, they lack toxin receptors or the means for further processing of the toxin.

DETECTION METHODS

There are several methods for detecting *C. difficile* or *C. difficile* toxin in stool specimens. Sometimes it is important to detect the toxin early because a patient may require rapid effective treatment. The latex agglutination test is a simple and rapid method and may be the most useful in a clinical laboratory. Various detection methods are described below.

Cytotoxic Assay. This toxin assay is performed by inoculation of 25 and 50 μl of a filtered portion of stool supernatant onto a monolayer of HEp-2 cells or other cells. Cells are observed at 24 and 48 hours for actinomorphic changes or any degree of enlarging or rounding, as compared with the negative control. If cytopathic changes are observed, a neutralization assay is performed with high-titer *C. sordellii* or *C. difficile* antitoxin. (These two antitoxins are cross-reactive to *C. difficile* cytotoxin.)

Recently, a commercial system for detecting this toxin was introduced for laboratory testing by Bartels Immunodiagnostic Supplies/Tox-titer microtiter plate system. The conventional cytotoxicity assay does not require a CO_2 incubator and specific microscope. Cytotoxic assay is not specific for only *C. difficile* but also detects toxins of other clostridia.

Latex Agglutination Test. Approximately 0.2 g of feces and 0.2 ml of dilution buffer (0.2 M TRIS-HCl, 0.9 percent NaCl, 0.1 percent bovine serum albumin) in microcentrifugation tubes are mixed and centrifuged at 6,000 g for 10 minutes. Fifty μl of supernatant is mixed with 10 μl of anti-D-1 antisera coated latex (C.D. CHECK D-1 kit from Mitsubishi Chemical Industry, Japan, or Culturette Brand Rapid Latex Test from Marion Laboratories Inc., US) for 3 minutes on a black glass plate, and agglutinations are observed under transmitted light. Pretreatment of supernatant with 2 μl of anti-D-1 antisera for 1 minute is undertaken to check for any false-positive reaction.

Nontoxigenic strains of *C. difficile*, which have no biologic activity, are sometimes antigen-reactive with anti-D-1 toxin. Large amounts of *C. sporogenes* and *C. botulinum* react with anti-D-1–coated latex. Nevertheless, it is useful for clinical examination because, if the latex test is positive, bacteria will be examined by culture method and toxin by cytotoxic assay. The latex agglutination test is useful for emergency treatment.

Enzyme Immunoassay. A sandwich enzyme immunoassay has been developed to detect *C. difficile* toxins A and B in stool specimens. Immune serum to *C. difficile* toxin and nonimmune serum are coated onto polystyrene microtiter plates to act as capture antibodies; toxin A and B. The enzyme-linked immunosorbent assay (ELISA) for toxin B shows cross-reactions with *C. bifermentans* and *C. sordellii* and lacks diagnostic sensitivity in clinical samples. The ELISA for detection of toxin A shows no cross-reaction with other clostridia. Compared with cytotoxin assay, the ELISA for toxin A constitutes a sensitive and specific tool for diagnosis of *C. difficile*–

associated diarrhea and colitis. Monoclonal and specific polyclonal antibodies for immunoassay of *C. difficile* toxin A have been developed. Unfortunately, enzyme immunoassay test kits are not yet available commercially.

Gas Liquid Chromatography. Gas liquid chromatography has been used for the rapid diagnosis of anaerobic infections by detection of short-chain fatty acids in clinical specimens. Isocaproic acid and butyric acid of the metabolic end product of *C. difficile* and other clostridia are detected.

Counterimmunoelectrophoresis. Twenty microliters of undiluted stool filtrate or positive culture filtrated control are applied to the cathodal well, and the same volume of antitoxin is applied to the anodal well of a 1 percent agarose-coated slide. After electrophoresis, the slides are examined for precipitin lines.

Endoscopy. Pseudomembranous findings by colonoscopy indicate *C. difficile* colitis. Even if endoscopic findings are normal, *C. difficile* may still be present. Endoscopic analysis is one of the rapid methods to discover *Clostridium* infection.

Culture Method. Stools are inoculated onto cycloserine-cefoxitin-fructose agar and colistin-nalidixic acid agar. Plates are incubated anaerobically at 35°C and examined after 48 to 72 hours of incubation for characteristic *C. difficile* colonies. All presumptive *C. difficile* organisms are confirmed by biochemical methods, gas-liquid chromatography, and immunologic methods.

Confirming assays for *C. difficile* infection requires detection of bacteria and toxin. Results of toxin assay of the colony following culture usually take more than 1 week. Detection of toxin by enzyme immunoassay, counterimmunophoresis, and, especially, the latex agglutination test, is rapid and useful in clinical medicine. Latex agglutination can be done easily by any physician. Endoscopic examination can detect pseudomembranous lesions directly. Repeated examinations may be necessary during the course of the disease.

In our own study using the latex agglutination test (the C.D. CHECK D-1 kit) in 59 neonates, enterotoxin (D-1) was detected in 13 symptomatic and nine asymptomatic neonates in the intensive care unit between October 1983 and February 1984. Toxin was nearly always found in the stools of some infants in the intensive care unit regardless of whether antibiotics were used. Toxin was not detected in 18 neonates in two newborn nurseries, one of which was located on a different floor of the same hospital and the other in a different hospital. Breast-feeding and vaginal delivery were not associated with high frequencies of toxin detection in the intensive care unit. These findings suggest that nosocomial factors influenced the existence of *C. difficile* and the outbreak of diarrhea associated with *C. difficile* in the intensive care unit.

C. difficile is recovered from almost all latex agglutination–positive stools and is not detected in almost all latex agglutination–negative stools. The method is sensitive to 15 ng per milliliter of enterotoxin and can be especially useful in detecting the colitis and diarrhea associated with antibiotic usage in children and adults, even though *C. difficile* is sometimes found in asymptomatic children (neonates).

SYMPTOMS AND SIGNS

Diarrhea in children caused by antibiotics usually stops within a few days after discontinuation of therapy. The symptoms and signs of pseudomembranous colitis occur within 1 week after the initiation of antibiotics. The disease rarely occurs after antibiotics are discontinued. Fever, abdominal distention, vomiting, and diarrhea (sometimes bloody stool) are seen in pseudomembranous colitis. The condition only rarely progresses to life-threatening dehydration, hypoproteinemia, electrolytic imbalance (hyponatremia, hypokalemia, and hypochloremia), and shock. Fatal signs are toxic megacolon, peritonitis, septicemia, and disseminated intravascular coagulation. Pseudomembranous colitis has been diagnosed in children treated with penicillin, usually ampicillin, cephalosporins, 5-fluorouracil, and clindamycin, although no cases associated with erythromycin treatment have been reported. Although pseudomembranous colitis is rare in neonates, it can be fatal.

TREATMENTS

Vancomycin given orally is an effective treatment for *C. difficile*. When the general condition of a patient is severe or the antibiotics cannot be stopped because of other bacterial infections, vancomycin is the first choice. Vancomycin is hard to absorb from the intestine. Parenterally administered vancomycin does not produce adequate intestinal concentration. Five hundred mg per day to 2 g per day given orally every 6 hours for 5 to 10 days in adults is recommended. In neonates, about 100 mg per day is recommended. Problems include cost and relapse rate (approximately 20 percent) after discontinuation. Retreatment with vancomycin improves the relapse, but repeated relapses occasionally occur. Metronidazole, which is a much less expensive drug, has also been used orally with success and may be especially useful as a parenteral agent for the patient who cannot take oral medication. About 25 to 50 mg per day is recommended.

Anion exchange materials, cholestyramine and colestipol, absorb toxin. Oral intake of these drugs may be useful. In the case of relapse, a 2-week course of vancomycin, followed by a 3- to 4-week course of cholestyramine, may be recommended. Replacing the colonic flora using lactobacilli has been suggested. Anticholinergic drugs (atropine or diphenoxylate) are not recommended because they delay defecation.

Supplementary therapies for hypoproteinemia and electrolyte disorder must be given approximately. Surgery is required infrequently and should be reserved for the severely ill, e.g., those with toxic megacolon with impending perforation.

SUGGESTED READING

Aronsson B, Granstom M, Mollby R, Nord CE. Enzyme immunoassay for detection of *Clostridium difficile* toxin A and B in patients with antibiotic-associated diarrhea and colitis. Eur J Clin Microbiol 1985; 4:102–107.

Kamiya S, Nakamura S, Yamakawa K, Nishida S. Evaluation of a commercially available latex immunoagglutination test kit for detection of *Clostridium difficile* D-1 toxin. Microbiol Immunol 1986; 30:177–181.

Kim K, DuPont HL, Pickering LK. Outbreaks of diarrhea associated with *Clostridium difficile* and its toxin in day-care centers: Evidence of person-to-person spread. J Pediatr 1983; 102:376–382.

Pepersack A, Labbe M, Nonhoff C, Schoutens E. Use of gas-liquid chromatography as a screening test for toxigenic *Clostridium difficile* in diarrheal stools. J Clin Pathol 1983; 36:1233–1236.

Sherertz RJ, Sarubbi FA. The prevalence of *Clostridium difficile* and toxin in a nursery population: A comparison between patients with necrotizing enterocolitis and an asymptomatic group. J Pediatr 1982; 100:435–439.

Sydney M, Finegold W, Lance G, Mulligan ME. Anaerobic infections. Chicago: Year Book Medical Publishers, 1986.

Ushijima H, Shinozaki T, Fujii R. Detection of *Clostridium difficile* enterotoxin in neonates by latex agglutination. Arch Dis Child 1985; 60:252–271.

Wu TC, Fung JC. Evaluation of the usefulness of counterimmunoelectrophoresis for diagnosis of *Clostridium difficile*-associated colitis in clinical specimens. J Clin Microbiol 1983; 17:610–613.

CONGENITAL DIAPHRAGMATIC HERNIA

BRADLEY M. RODGERS, M.D.

Congenital posterolateral diaphragmatic hernia (CDH) remains one of the absolute surgical emergencies in pediatric surgical practice. Despite significant advances in pediatric anesthesia and operative care, the mortality rate associated with this lesion has remained high and relatively unchanged over the past three decades. Bochdalek hernias occur in approximately 1 in 2,200 live births. They occur with equal frequency in males and females. Eighty percent of these hernias involve the left hemidiaphragm, and 20 percent have a peritoneal sac extending into the hemithorax. The mortality rate for all patients with CDH ranges from 40 to 50 percent. Approximately 40 percent of these infants present with respiratory symptoms within the first 24 hours of life, and the mortality rate is 60 to 80 percent.

It is impossible to plan for the operative care of infants with CDH without an understanding of the embryology of pulmonary development and the physiology of the pulmonary vasculature. Lung development begins with the evagination of the lung buds from the primitive gut tube at approximately the fourth week of gestation. The development proceeds with successive generations of bronchial branching, each developing with its own pulmonary artery segment. By the 16th week of gestation, the bronchial branching is complete and further pulmonary development merely involves the growth in the number of alveoli on each terminal bronchiole. This process continues postnatally until the patient is approximately 8 years of age.

Compression of the developing lung bud by herniated abdominal viscera at the 10th to 12th week of gestation, the time when the viscera is returning from the umbilical stalk, creates a maturational arrest at this stage of lung development. The extent of this developmental arrest is more severe on the ipsilateral than on the contralateral lung. The resul-

tant pulmonary hypoplasia is marked by diminished lung weight, diminished numbers of terminal bronchioles and alveoli, and a reduction in the total size of the pulmonary vascular bed, with an increase in the amount of arterial smooth muscle.

The postnatal pulmonary physiology of these infants is reminiscent of that in children with persistent fetal circulation and is manifest by a markedly increased reactivity of the pulmonary vascular bed, resulting in increased vascular resistance. In the normal infant, pulmonary vascular resistance is increased by several common stimuli: hypoxia, acidosis, hypothermia, hypercarbia, and hypocalcemia. The effects of these stimuli on the pulmonary vasculature are often synergistic. For example, the coexistence of acidosis significantly augments the increase in pulmonary vascular resistance seen with hypoxia. In the infant with CDH, the pulmonary vascular bed appears unusually sensitive to all these stimuli. Many of the most critical aspects of the management of these infants involve identifying and correcting these defects to minimize the degree of pulmonary vascular spasm experienced by these infants postoperatively.

INITIAL DIAGNOSIS AND RESUSCITATION

Forty percent of infants with CDH experience severe respiratory distress within the first 24 hours of life. It is these infants who represent the most significant surgical challenge and to whom this chapter is addressed. The presenting manifestations of CDH in these infants include tachypnea and cyanosis. On physical examination, one notes a barrel-shaped chest with a scaphoid abdomen. There are signs of mediastinal shift, with displacement of the trachea in the suprasternal notch to the contralateral side. Auscultation reveals diminished breath sounds bilaterally, most markedly on the ipsilateral side. Bowel sounds (as classically described) within the chest are rarely heard in these infants, and indeed, breath sounds may be transmitted relatively equally across the chest. The diagnosis is confirmed by a portable anteroposterior chest roentgenogram. I find that it is helpful to place a radiopaque nasogastric tube before obtaining these films to identify the position of the stomach. The radiographs demonstrate the presence of bowel gas within one hemithorax and shift of the mediastinal structures. The diagnosis of a Bochdalek's hernia presenting within the first 24 hours of life is not usually difficult to make with a good physical examination and simple chest roentgenogram; more sophisticated radiographic studies are rarely necessary or indicated.

Having established the diagnosis of a CDH, one should immediately plan for the transport of the infant to a medical center that has the appropriate surgical and anesthetic support for correction. The object of the initial resuscitation is to have the infant stabilized and ready for immediate surgical correction upon arrival at the treating center. Even for the infants born within such a center, the initial resuscitation should have this same objective.

These infants should *never* be ventilated with a mask. Mask ventilation forces air into the upper gastrointestinal tract, further distending the stomach and small bowel and causing further pulmonary compression. If assisted ventilation is necessary for these infants, they should be intubated immediately. A nasogastric tube of the largest practical size (No. 10 F.) should be placed into the stomach and frequently irrigated and aspirated to keep the gastrointestinal tract maximally decompressed. If assisted ventilation is not to be used, this tube should be passed through the mouth, leaving the nares unobstructed for breathing. The infant should be nursed in a lateral position with the side of the hernia dependent, to maximize the efficiency of ventilation of the contralateral lung. Body temperature should be closely monitored and maintained within a physiologic range by warm blankets and overhead heaters. An intravenous line should be established early, but extreme caution must be exercised to minimize the volume of crystalloid infusion. The basal crystalloid requirements of these infants should be calculated at 30 cc per kilogram per 24 hours and provided in the form of $D_{10}\frac{1}{4}$/NS. *These infants are extremely sensitive to excess fluid volume, and there is a great tendency to overhydrate them.* The hypoplastic lungs quickly accumulate interstitial fluid with excessive crystalloid replacement, further impairing an already compromised gas exchange. In addition, with a fixed pulmonary vascular resistance, any increase in intravascular volume augments extrapulmonary shunting, causing peripheral hypoxia and acidosis. If possible, an umbilical artery catheter should be inserted and blood gases obtained early during the resuscitation. The presence of acidosis (pH less than 7.20) indicates the need for bicarbonate infusion. If one cannot establish an umbilical artery line, it is imperative that an infant requiring immediate ventilatory support receive 3 cc of sodium bicarbonate.

If mechanical ventilatory support is necessary, one must be extraordinarily cautious to avoid producing a pneumothorax. Both the contralateral and the ipsilateral lungs are hypoplastic and can be easily ruptured with artificial ventilation. After intubation, the infant should be ventilated with a rapid rate (60 to 80 respirations per minute) and low inspiratory pressures (less than 20 to 25 mm Hg). *The infant should be ventilated with 100 percent oxygen from the onset, irrespective of the initial* PaO_2. The use of the transcutaneous oxygen monitor has demonstrated wide fluctuations in PaO_2 in these infants, even under "basal" conditions.

One must absolutely avoid the hypoxic stimulus to increased pulmonary vascular resistance and therefore must accept the risks of the higher PaO_2 that occasionally results from the use of 100 percent oxygen. After intubation and initiation of mechanical ventilation, a portable chest radiograph should be obtained to confirm the position of the endotracheal and nasogastric tubes and to rule out the presence of pneumothorax.

Infants with CDH undergo transport poorly. The accepting institution should provide a physician or skilled transport nurse to travel with these patients. This individual must be skilled in the insertion of chest tubes, as any sudden deterioration in the condition of these infants usually indicates the development of a pneumothorax. If air transport is to be employed, a pressurized cabin should be used to avoid further distention of the abdominal viscera within the chest. To assure absolute gastrointestinal decompression, careful attention to the nasogastric tube must be continued during transport.

OPERATION

The operative management of the infant with congenital Bochdalek's hernia begins at the time of the patient's arrival at the accepting institution. The infant's condition must be thoroughly and rapidly assessed. The critical points of the initial assessment include assuring that there is adequate ventilation with 100 percent oxygen, restricting intravenous fluids with $D_{10}\frac{1}{4}$/NS, maintaining adequate blood glucose levels with intermittent 50 percent dextrose boluses as necessary, and assuring that there is adequate nasogastric decompression. Arterial blood gases should be reassessed immediately upon the patient's arrival, and the pH should be corrected with sodium bicarbonate, if necessary. Blood should be drawn for type and cross-match and for the preparation of fresh-frozen plasma. Vitamin K_1 oxide (1 mg) and broad-spectrum antibiotics (ampicillin, 200 mg per kilogram per 24 hours, and gentamicin, 6 mg per kilogram per 24 hours) should be administered immediately. A central venous catheter for administration of drugs and fluids should be inserted either in the neonatal intensive care unit or immediately upon arrival in the operating room. A cutdown on the right external or internal jugular vein and a 19-gauge (4 Fr) Silastic catheter inserted into the right atrium are used for this purpose. This catheter is large enough to allow measurement of central venous pressure.

The anesthetic management of these infants is critical. Core body temperature must be carefully monitored and maintained with circulating heated water-blankets and overhead warmers. Reduction of body temperature below 36°C cannot be tolerated because of its effects on pulmonary vascular resistance. Ventilation must be maintained with 100 percent oxygen throughout the operation, despite high levels of arterial oxygen tension. *One must resist the temptation to reduce the inspired oxygen concentration in these infants.* Ventilation should be maintained with low inspiratory pressures and rapid rates. The use of positive end-expiratory pressure (PEEP) should be minimized, as reduction of the mean intrathoracic pressure facilitates pulmonary blood flow.

Extreme care must be exercised to minimize the amount of intravenous crystalloid administered to these infants in the operating room. Hypotension (blood pressure below 50 mm Hg systolic) should be treated with intermittent boluses of fresh frozen plasma (10 cc per kilogram) and not with increases in crystalloid administration. Administration of muscle relaxants, in the form of pancuronium bromide (0.1 mg per kilogram every 2 to 4 hours) should be instituted in the operating room and continued throughout the immediate postoperative period. Complete muscle paralysis not only facilitates ventilatory mechanics, but also decreases peripheral oxygen consumption. In addition, pancuronium bromide may directly reduce pulmonary vascular resistance by its histamine-like effect.

I perform the operative correction of CDH through a transverse left upper quadrant abdominal incision. The incision should be placed 2 cm below the left costal margin to preserve a sufficient flap of transversus abdominus muscle to reinforce the diaphragmatic closure, if necessary. The contents of the hernia are carefully reduced, and the entire gastrointestinal tract is inspected for other congenital anomalies. I then carefully inspect the defect for the presence of a hernia sac, which is excised if present. There is usually a small rim of diaphragmatic tissue anteriorly and laterally. Posteriorly, the muscle frequently adheres to Geroda's capsule. Prosthetic material is not usually required for closing these defects, but if it is, a soft Teflon mesh or Gortex fabric is preferable. Marlex material should not be used in this position, since its stiffness may later erode the adjacent bowel. I then close the diaphragm in two layers using interrupted, nonabsorbable suture material. The diaphragm closure may be reinforced with transversus abdominus muscle, rotated back from the costal margin. Before final closure of the diaphragm, a chest tube is placed in the ipsilateral hemithorax. This tube is connected to underwater seal drainage and clamped. A tube gastrostomy is performed, not only for gastrointestinal tract decompression, but also to prevent axial volvulus of the stomach. If the primary abdominal wall closure appears likely to be so tight as to impair ventilation, a ventral hernia should be constructed with Silastic material. This may be removed within the next 10 days and secondary abdominal closure achieved. At the completion of the abdominal procedure, the chest tube is opened briefly to allow evacuation of some of the air within the ipsilateral hemithorax. A right radial arterial catheter is inserted to compare preductal PaO_2 with postductal PaO_2 obtained through the umbilical artery catheter and to estimate extrapulmonary shunt fractions.

POSTOPERATIVE MANAGEMENT

The postoperative phase of the management of these patients is the most critical. This phase is often manifest as a "honeymoon period," during which the patient appears stable for 12 to 24 hours and then deteriorates rapidly. One should be cautious not to relax the intensity of therapy in these infants on the basis of a favorable immediate postoperative course. *The critical period for pulmonary vascular reactivity is the first 72 to 96 hours after surgery.* During this interval, these patients should be maintained on 100

percent oxygen with rapid, low-pressure ventilation. The respiratory management of these infants is best accomplished with a flow-regulated ventilator. The use of a transcutaneous oxygen electrode placed on the upper chest allows constant monitoring of preductal PaO_2. Using this monitor, the inspiratory-expiratory ratio of the ventilator should be decreased in order to decrease mean airway pressure while providing maximum oxygenation. Intravenous fluids should be restricted to a total of 30 ml per kilogram per 24 hours, and the majority of these intravenous fluids should be D20 ("hyperalimentation") to prevent hypoglycemia. One should resist the temptation to increase crystalloid infusion during these first 72 to 96 hours after surgery, despite elevations of urinary specific gravity or decreased total urine volume. Hypotension should be treated with fresh-frozen plasma. The chest tube in the ipsilateral hemithorax should be opened for short intervals every other hour to evacuate the air from the chest slowly. Removing this air too rapidly may cause excessive shift of the mediastinum, with resultant venous compression or excessive expansion of the contralateral lung with rupture and pneumothorax. All infants receive 1 to 2 mg of chlorpromazine hydrochloride (Thorazine) intravenously upon their return to the neonatal intensive care unit and are maintained on pancuronium bromide for as long as they receive ventilation.

One must constantly watch for the development of intrapulmonary or extrapulmonary shunts. A rise in the arterial Pco_2 indicates intrapulmonary shunt and is best treated by an inotropic agent. Reductions in the arterial Po_2 indicate extrapulmonary shunt and are best treated with pulmonary vasodilators. Mild reductions in arterial Po_2 may be successfully treated with repeated doses of Thorazine, but for more significant shunting, tolazoline hydrochloride is required. Tolazoline hydrochloride is an alpha-blocking agent that also appears to have direct relaxant effects on arterial smooth muscle. Initially, a bolus of 1 mg per kilogram is administered, and if a favorable response is achieved, a continuous infusion of 2 mg per kilogram per hour is used. As a powerful alpha-blocking agent, tolazoline hydrochloride is expected to cause a decrease in systemic blood pressure. It may induce gastrointestinal hemorrhage from its histamine-like effect. Dopamine is used for its positive inotropic effect, as well as to reduce systemic vascular resistance and increase renal blood flow. This drug is administered at a rate of 4 μg per kilogram per minute, with adjustments to this rate made on the basis of clinical response. Often, treatment with both of these drugs can be instituted simultaneously in these infants.

During the first 72 to 96 hours postoperatively, one must be cautious not to relax the intensity of this care. It is during this interval that fluctuations in oxygenation or pH can cause marked pulmonary vasospasm and precipitate irreversible shunting. On the fourth postoperative day, if the baby is stable and has good blood gases, the pancuronium bromide is discontinued and the infant is slowly weaned from the ventilator, using the intermittent mandatory ventilation circuit. It is during this interval that the ventral wall hernia is repaired. Oral feedings are instituted once the child has been extubated and antibiotics are discontinued on the seventh postoperative day.

FAMILY

The sudden, intense care necessary in the management of these infants frequently separates the infant from family before either the mother or the father can see their baby. This disruption, along with the very high mortality rate involved with this lesion, create tremendous anxieties for the family members. Frequent and frank discussions with the family should be coordinated through the operating surgeon. The family must be carefully prepared for the "honeymoon period," lest they develop unrealistic expectations at this stage. If the infant survives the repair of the congenital diaphragmatic hernia, the family should be assured that most of these children progress to develop quite acceptable pulmonary function, and that few are limited by inadequate respiratory reserve. Congenital diaphragmatic hernia appears to be an isolated anomaly in most instances, and it is unusual for there to be significant impairment from associated conditions.

FUTURE THERAPIES

Since the first successful repair of a congenital diaphragmatic hernia by Robert Gross in 1946, there has been little improvement in the overall survival of those infants presenting with symptoms during the first 24 hours of life. Newer methods are necessary to improve these statistics. In several centers, extracorporeal membrane oxygenators are currently being employed to provide ventilatory support during the critical postoperative interval. Advances in prenatal diagnosis should allow in utero detection of this defect through ultrasonography and will facilitate transport of the mother to an appropriate surgical center before delivery. Many new drugs for reducing pulmonary vascular resistance in these infants are being explored. The most promising among these drugs appear to be the prostaglandins. The fact that these infants do go through a "honeymoon period" postoperatively indicates that they probably have sufficient alveolar numbers to support respiration. Their subsequent deterioration most likely represents increased pulmonary vascular resistance, which is often irreversible with the medications currently employed. Suggestions have recently been made that infants with CDH may be amenable to intrauterine surgical correction in the future. The task will be to identify in some manner those infants with the most severe pulmonary hypoplasia and the highest postnatal mortality. Subjecting the mother to the risks of intrauterine surgery to correct those infants with less severe pulmonary hypoplasia seems unwarrented at this time.

CONGESTIVE HEART FAILURE

BARBARA L. GEORGE, M.D.

Congestive heart failure (CHF) is the inability of the heart to pump blood in a quantity sufficient to meet the body's demands. This may be due to decreased myocardial function, excessive hemodynamic demands, or both. The signs and symptoms of CHF reflect attempts by the body to compensate for a disordered circulatory state. As these compensatory mechanisms fail, symptoms of circulatory congestion and inadequate cardiac output become increasingly severe.

Our ability to treat neonatal CHF has improved significantly because of advances in our understanding of the factors that regulate cardiac performance. In addition, physicians now have the means to manipulate the loading conditions of the heart independent of, or in association with, efforts directed at increasing the contractility of the myocardium.

Table 1 lists conditions that commonly result in cardiovascular compromise of the neonate. Some of these conditions are not amenable to medical management alone and surgical intervention may be required, with medical therapy aimed only at stabilizing the patient before surgery.

GENERAL INTERVENTIONS

The aims of any therapy for CHF are to improve cardiac function, to increase peripheral perfusion, and to decrease circulatory congestion. In this regard, both general and specific interventions are available (Table 2). The general interventions are designed to make the infant more comfortable and to avoid placing any additional burdens on an already overburdened cardiocirculatory system.

SPECIFIC INTERVENTIONS

Cardiac output is a key reflection of the basic function of the heart to pump sufficient blood to meet the metabolic demands of the body. There are four principal determinants that regulate cardiac output: (1) ventricular preload, (2) afterload, (3) contractility, and (4) heart rate. When one or more of these determinants is disordered, CHF ensues. Optimal therapy for CHF is assured only when the disordered variables are recognized and specifically treated.

Manipulation of Preload

Preload is defined as the diastolic loading condition of the heart and is a function of intravascular blood volume, venous return, and compliance of the ventricles. In the neonate, the liver size is the single most important clini-

TABLE 1 Common Causes and Time of Onset of Heart Failure in Infants

Birth
  Arrhythmias
  Anemia/hyperviscosity syndromes
  Systemic arteriovenous fistulas

Day 1
  Persistent pulmonary hypertension of neonate
  Hypoplastic left heart syndrome
  Valvar regurgitation
  Myocarditis
  Asphyxia, ischemia—myocardial dysfunction
  Metabolic disorders—e.g., hypoglycemia, hypocalcemia
  Sepsis

1st and 2nd Week
  Coarctation/coarctation syndrome
  Aortic stenosis
  Patent ductus arteriosus in premature infants
  Total anomalous pulmonary venous return
  Transposition of great arteries
  Persistent truncus arteriosus
  Anomalous origin of left coronary artery from
    pulmonary artery
  Central nervous system, renal, and endocrine disorders

cal estimate of preload. Although a more accurate measurement of central venous pressure is desirable, it is not necessary in most cases. An infant's liver size changes very rapidly with changes in preload and it serves, therefore, as a good guide to therapy. Preload is usually increased

TABLE 2 Treatment of Congestive Heart Failure

General Interventions
  Rest (occasional sedation)
  Temperature and humidity control
  Oxygen
  Ensure adequate calorie intake–often requires
    150 kcal/kg/day
  Avoid aspiration with semi-Fowler's position, during and
    immediately after feeding
  Treat infection, if present

Specific Interventions
  Preload
    Increase preload by volume infusion
    Decrease preload with diuretics, venodilators

  Afterload reduction
    Facilitate ventricular emptying by reducing wall tension
    Reduce blood viscosity
    Drugs: arteriolar dilators
    Mechanical counterpulsation

  Inotropic stimulation
    Improve physical and metabolic milieu: pH, PaO_2,
      glucose, calcium, magnesium, hemoglobin
    Common drugs: digitalis, catecholamines

  Heart rate
    Control rhythm disturbances with pacing, drugs

  Other
    Mechanical ventilation
    Prostaglandin manipulation

Surgery

in neonates with CHF. Reduction in preload is achieved most commonly by diuretic therapy, usually furosemide (2 to 4 mg per kilogram per day in two divided doses every 12 hours). Sometimes, particularly when a patient has been on chronic diuretic therapy, one or two doses of ethacrynic acid (1 mg per kilogram per dose) may be required; however, this agent should not be used on a chronic basis because of its toxicity.

Occasionally, there may be inadequate preload because of acute or chronic volume losses. Blood losses should be replaced in most cases by a combination of packed red blood cells and fresh frozen plasma; other types of volume depletion associated with cardiocirculatory compromise should be treated with colloid in the form of albumin (10 to 20 ml per kilogram per dose), unless it can be clearly demonstrated that the problem is due to inadequate free-water intake. Under these circumstances, crystalloid replacement is appropriate. When the preload is inadequate, a more direct measurement of central venous pressure may be necessary, particularly if the administration of large volumes of fluid is indicated.

Afterload Reduction

Afterload is the force that opposes ventricular ejection. It is estimated clinically by measuring the blood pressure and assessing the peripheral perfusion. The measurement of toe temperature (or that of the foot in the case of the neonate) can be helpful in the noninvasive evaluation of systemic vascular resistance and peripheral perfusion. This measurement is achieved by attaching a thermistor to the sole of the baby's foot. When myocardial dysfunction is present, the afterload is usually increased as a consequence of the body's compensatory mechanisms. In response to CHF, both the sympathetic and renin-angiotensin systems are activated, which results in peripheral vasoconstriction and increased ventricular afterload. Under these circumstances, cardiac output can usually be improved by the use of afterload reducing agents. Fluctuations in toe temperature, blood pressure, and heart rate provide a clinically useful, noninvasive evaluation of the efficacy of these agents.

For reduction of systemic afterload, nitroprusside is the drug of choice (0.5 to 8 μg per kilogram per minute) for acute intravenous therapy. Blood pressure and heart rate must be closely monitored for signs of excessive effect. These two parameters, in association with toe temperature, should be monitored to evaluate efficacy and the need for dosage adjustment. Thiocyanate and cyanide levels should be obtained if the drug is used for more than 6 hours at a dose equal to or greater than 3 μg per kilogram per minute. These levels should also be monitored if the drug is administered for more than 24 hours, regardless of dosage.

In the neonate, the most commonly used agent for chronic afterload reduction is captopril. The starting dose is 0.1 mg per kilogram given every 8 to 12 hours. The dosage of captopril is gradually increased until the desired effect is achieved without adverse side effects. In newborns, it is unusual to require more than 0.4 mg per kilogram per dose every 6 to 8 hours. Captopril-induced hypotension may be treated with volume, or vasoconstrictors if necessary (e.g., phenylephrine). Hydralazine (1 to 4 mg per kilogram per day in 3 to 4 divided doses) has also been used for reduction of chronic afterload. However, there appear to be significantly more side effects associated with this drug than with captopril.

Reduction of pulmonary artery pressures results in reduction of right ventricular afterload. The ability to produce pulmonary vasodilatation without systemic dilatation would be extremely useful in some forms of neonatal CHF, but unfortunately there are no specific pulmonary vasodilators. Recently, however, increasing experience has been accruing with continuous intravenous infusion of nitroglycerin (an agent known to reduce preload in children and adults). It was first used in adults and is now being given to infants and neonates. The dosage remains to be established for neonates; however, a starting intravenous dose of 0.5 μg per kilogram per minute and a maintenance dose of 0.5 to 20 μg per kilogram per minute seems to be effective. At the lower dosage ranges, pulmonary vasodilatation can often be achieved without concomitant systemic vasodilatation.

Manipulation of Contractility

Contractility, or inotropy, is determined by the level and intensity of activation of the heart muscle. This is the most difficult of the four determinants of cardiac function to measure. Ideally, the other determinants of cardiac function should be optimized prior to the use of inotropic agents. In practice, however, the time for decision making regarding the need for inotropic support is often very limited. Hence, the use of these agents is usually initiated very early in the treatment of a neonate with marked cardiocirculatory embarrassment. The most commonly used intravenous inotropic agents are dopamine and dobutamine; isoproterenol and epinephrine may still be of value, on occasion. Therapy is usually begun with dopamine at a dose of 5 μg per kilogram per minute and is increased, as appears necessary, up to a maximum of 20 μg per kilogram per minute; the usual effective dose, however, is 10 μg per kilogram per minute. It should be emphasized that the doses at which the dopaminergic (renal vasodilatation), beta-adrenergic (inotropy with or without heart rate acceleration), or alpha-adrenergic effects (systemic vasoconstriction) predominate have yet to be established in the neonate. If inadequate inotropic effect is noted, or if excessive tachycardia occurs, the dose of dopamine should be decreased to 5 μg per kilogram per minute to ensure good renal blood flow, and dobutamine should be started at 2.5 μg per kilogram per minute and increased until the desired effect is achieved. Although the maximal recommended dose is 40 μg per kilogram per minute, the usual effective dose is 10 μg per kilogram per minute when used in conjunction with dopamine. If this combination of dopamine and dobutamine (10 μg per kilogram per minute each) is not effective, or if an additional chronotropic response is desired (see below), isoproterenol can be added (0.05 to 0.5 μg per kilogram

per minute). However, vasodilatation, tachycardia, and increased myocardial oxygen consumption (out of proportion to the increase in cardiac output) are associated with the use of isoproterenol; hence, this drug should be reserved for the specific circumstances noted above. If none of the above therapies are effective, epinephrine may be useful (0.05 to 1 μg per kilogram per minute), particularly in neonates who have undergone cardiac surgery.

Digoxin continues to be the drug of choice for subacute or chronic therapy for CHF. The current recommendations for dosages are listed in Table 3. Serum digoxin levels are not of value routinely and are not indicated, unless toxicity is suspected. The level should be drawn 6 to 8 hours after a maintenance dose (never during the digitalization period). A level of greater than 6 ng per milliliter is definitely toxic. A level less than 1.5 ng per milliliter is definitely not toxic and probably not therapeutic. Levels of 1.5 to 3.0 ng per milliliter are considered to be nontoxic and probably therapeutic. However, this obvious uncertainty regarding "therapeutic" and "toxic" levels in neonates underscores the lack of value of "routine" monitoring of digoxin levels. If toxicity is suspected, the therapy should be discontinued, serum potassium concentration checked, and supplemental potassium administered, if necessary. Arrhythmias should be treated specifically. Ventricular tachyarrhythmias due to digoxin toxicity are treated very effectively with phenytoin (1 to 5 mg per kilogram administered intravenously over 5 to 10 minutes). Heart block, or significant bradyarrhythmias, require pacemaker therapy.

Manipulation of Heart Rate

The heart rate affects cardiac function by determining the amount of work performed per unit time. Treatment of specific arrhythmias is discussed below. Occasionally, a neonate may have significant sinus bradycardia (most frequently seen after cardiac surgery) or tachycardia. Symptomatic sinus bradycardia can be treated with atropine (0.01 mg per kilogram per dose intravenously) or isoproterenol. When isoproterenol is used solely for its chronotropic effects, a lower starting dose is indicated (0.01 μg per kilogram per minute intravenously). Pacemaker therapy may eventually be necessary, particularly in the postoperative period. Sinus tachycardia is almost invariably a compensatory mechanism (e.g., as a response to such complications as fever, anemia, volume depletion, hypoxia, and pain). Drugs should not be given to slow the heart rate when sinus tachycardia is present; rather, the *cause* of the tachycardia should be sought and treated.

SPECIAL CIRCUMSTANCES REQUIRING ADDITIONAL THERAPY

When cardiac dysfunction is a result of a specific hematologic, neurologic, endocrinologic, or metabolic disorder, that underlying disorder must be diagnosed and treated appropriately. The cardiocirculatory function may need to be supported in a general manner, as noted above,

TABLE 3 Digoxin Doses

Age and Weight	Dose and Route*	
	Acute Digitalization	Maintenance
Premature newborns		
< 1.5 kg	10–20 μg/kg IV TDD: 1/2, 1/4, 1/4 of dose q8h	4 μg/kg/day IV (may increase to 4 μg/kg q12h at age 1 month)
1.5–2.5 kg	Same as above	4 μg/kg q12h IV
Full-term newborns	30 μg/kg IV, TDD	4–5 μg/kg q12h IV
Infants (1–12 months)	35 μg/kg IV, TDD	5–6 μg/kg q12h IV

* Oral dose approximately 20 percent greater than IV dose.
TDD = total digitalizing dose

until specific therapy for the primary disorder can be instituted. However, there are other cardiorespiratory disorders, including structural abnormalities of the heart, toward which other types of therapies can be directed.

Arrhythmias

The most common arrhythmias in the newborn that result in heart failure are supraventricular tachycardia and complete congenital heart block.

Supraventricular tachycardia (SVT) that is of recent onset, or that occurs without significant cardiovascular compromise, can be treated initially with vagal maneuvers such as gagging the patient, placing the infant in a knee-chest position, or placing an ice pack on the patient's face. While these maneuvers are being performed, intravenous administration of digoxin should be started (dosages as noted in Table 3). The rapidity with which the digitalization is to be achieved should be determined by the severity of the symptoms. After the digoxin is administered, vagal maneuvers can be tried again, if necessary. If digoxin is unsuccessful, propranolol may be added at a dose of 0.01 to 0.1 mg per kilogram per dose intravenously (one-quarter of the dose every 10 minutes). This is followed by 1 to 6 mg per kilogram per day orally in four divided doses every 6 hours. Verapamil should not be used in neonates.

Profound cardiovascular compromise due to SVT may occur if the arrhythmia was present in utero and was not treated effectively; in this situation, synchronous cardioversion using the lowest machine setting (or 1 watt-sec per kilogram), followed by institution of digoxin therapy, may be required.

Most neonates with complete congenital heart block do not require immediate therapy. If signs of heart failure are present, or if the rate is very slow (< 40 beats per minute), acute treatment with isoproterenol may be instituted, beginning at 0.01 μg per kilogram per minute. However, symptomatic patients invariably require a permanent pacemaker.

Structural Heart Disease

Common structural causes of heart failure in the neonatal period are listed in Table 1. Of these, the most common are lesions that result in left ventricular outflow tract obstruction (aortic stenosis, coarctation of the aorta, and hypoplastic left heart syndrome). Heart failure due to left ventricular outflow tract obstruction requires surgical intervention. (The use of cardiac transplantation for the treatment of hypoplastic left heart syndrome is under investigation and is not discussed here.) However, the neonate's condition before surgery can usually be improved by the use of prostaglandin E_1 to maintain patency of the ductus arteriosus. The starting dose is 0.1 μg per kilogram per minute; this should be reduced to 0.05 μg per kilogram per minute whenever possible. Under these circumstances, the patent ductus arteriosus allows blood to shunt right to left (pulmonary artery to aorta), effectively bypassing the obstruction and allowing for adequate systemic flow. Efforts should also be directed toward normalizing metabolic parameters, decreasing metabolic demands, and increasing tissue oxygen supply.

Patent Ductus Arteriosus in a Premature Infant

The premature infant with a symptomatic patent ductus arteriosus who requires mechanical ventilation deserves special attention. Under these circumstances, efforts should be directed toward closing the ductus as rapidly as possible. This usually can be accomplished with *intravenous* indomethacin (Table 4). If there are contraindications to the use of indomethacin, or if it is unsuccessful, surgical closure should be undertaken promptly. Decreasing the amount of fluids administered to no more than 80 ml per kilogram per day, as well as the use of furosemide, may help control the symptoms while medical or surgical closure of the ductus is being accomplished. It should be emphasized that fluid restriction and diuretic therapy represent symptomatic therapy only, not definitive treatment; hence, medical or surgical

TABLE 4 Indomethacin Doses

< 48 hours old:	0.2 mg/kg IV (first dose) followed by 0.1 mg/kg/dose q12h for two additional doses
48 hours–7 days:	0.2 mg/kg IV (first dose) followed by 0.2 mg/kg/dose q12h for two additional doses
> 7 days:	0.2 mg/kg IV (first dose) followed by 0.25 mg/kg/dose q12h for two additional doses

closure of the ductus is still required. Since true myocardial dysfunction is rarely a problem if the patent ductus arteriosus is diagnosed and treated promptly, digoxin is not indicated and, if used, is often associated with toxicity.

Persistent Pulmonary Hypertension of the Newborn

If therapy for persistent pulmonary hypertension of the newborn (PPHN) by mechanical ventilation is unsuccessful, efforts should be directed toward lowering the pulmonary vascular resistance by medical therapy. There has been some recent success with intravenous nitroglycerin. The major advantage of nitroglycerin over other pulmonary vasodilators is that it may have an effect on the pulmonary vascular resistance at doses that do not affect the systemic vascular resistance; this is not true for other vasodilators, such as tolazoline or isoproterenol. In addition to attempts to dilate the pulmonary vessels, inotropic support is often required. Low-dose dobutamine (5 μg per kilogram per minute) or dopamine (5 μg per kilogram per minute) can be used. Pulmonary artery vasoconstriction as a result of dopamine administration has not been documented in neonates.

COPPER DEFICIENCY

ANN M. SUTTON, M.B.B.S., D.C.H., F.R.C.P.

Once copper deficiency has been identified in the neonate, there is no great difficulty in instituting effective replacement therapy. The main problem lies in recognizing the deficiency state. Treatment without an accurate diagnosis is not recommended since, in excess, copper is a metabolic poison and also may interfere with the absorption of other essential elements such as zinc.

IDENTIFYING THE AT-RISK GROUP

True copper deficiency in neonates has been described only in those who (1) are preterm, usually less than 32 weeks of gestation, requiring prolonged, intensive care; (2) are mature but require prolonged, parenteral nutrition; (3) suffer chronic, severe diarrhea; or (4) have had extensive gut resection.

PREVENTION

The vital metabolic functions of copper are well documented in the literature. Those most relevant to the neonate are listed in Table 1 and depend on the activity of cuproenzymes such as superoxide dismutase, cytochrome oxidase, ceruloplasmin, and lysyl oxidase.

It should be possible to prevent clinically important copper deficiency by paying proper attention to the constitution of parenteral and enteral feeds, and by serial monitoring of the copper status of patients at risk.

There are few reliable balance studies in neonates, but it appears that copper deficiency is unlikely to develop in the preterm infant who receives at least 1 μmol per kilogram per day of copper, and in the term infant given at least 0.8 μmol per kilogram per day.

Most low-birth-weight infant formulas now contain reasonable quantities of copper for the preterm infant, provided that adequate volumes can be given into the gut. It must be remembered, however, that (1) the bioavailability of copper from breast milk is higher than that from formula, (2) the concentration of zinc may affect copper absorption by competitive inhibition, and (3) phytates and casein probably precipitate minerals and decrease their bioavailability.

The only sources of copper for infants fed parenterally in the U.K. by current methods are Ped-el added to Vamin Glucose (KabiVitrum, Ltd), which provides 0.9 μmol per 100 ml of fluid when prepared as recommended, and blood and plasma transfusions.

BIOCHEMICAL PARAMETERS

Most laboratories attached to perinatal units are able to measure plasma copper by photon absorption spectrophotometry, and ceruloplasmin by radioimmunoassay. Ceruloplasmin carries the major part of the circulating copper and is therefore useful when taken in conjunction with total plasma copper. Neither is ideal as an indicator

TABLE 1 Metabolic Functions of Copper

Antioxidant mechanisms
Energy production
Iron utilization
Collagen and elastin structure
Nerve myelination and neurotransmission
Melanin synthesis
Synthesis and metabolism of steroid hormones

of body copper, but they are easily available and with careful interpretation they provide important information. Falsely high concentrations of both may occur at times of stress or when biliary excretion of copper is impaired.

Single measurements of plasma copper are difficult to interpret, since there are great variations in the normal population, especially preterm infants (Fig. 1). In mature infants, however, a plasma copper level consistently below 6 μmol per liter with ceruloplasmin less than 0.15 g per liter is abnormal. In preterm infant, serial measurements of both values from birth should show a gradual rise as the infant approaches 38 to 40 weeks, rapidly reaching the concentrations found in term infants. Those who go on to show overt clinical signs of copper deficiency fail to show this increase. Typically their plasma copper level remains below 5 μmol per liter and may even be undetectable by conventional methods. A ceruloplasmin level consistently below 0.1 g per liter in addition to a low copper level supports the diagnosis.

Some physicians have favored the measurement of hair copper, but the results are often unreliable and bear no immediate relationship to body copper. In the future the measurement of superoxide dismutase activity in red blood cells, at present a research tool, should prove a more sensitive indicator of deficiency.

CLINICAL FEATURES

The neonate with copper deficiency can present in a variety of ways. The common clinical findings are listed in Table 2 in descending order of frequency. In the pre-

TABLE 2 Clinical Findings in Copper Deficiency

Bone changes
Neutropenia
Anemia
Poor weight gain
Edema
Apnea
Hypopigmentation
Distended veins

term neonate the signs usually develop between the sixth and tenth weeks of life, although they may take longer to appear in the term neonate who has greater body stores of copper. Copper deficiency should be considered part of the differential diagnosis of any of the listed abnormalities. The characteristic neutropenia and bone changes of severe copper deficiency, namely, subperiosteal new bone formation and bone spurs, are late signs. If we are to recognize early deficiency states, the diagnosis must be borne in mind when less specific features are present, such as poor growth, edema, and osteoporosis.

TREATMENT

After the diagnosis of copper deficiency has been made, a short course of copper supplementation is usually sufficient, provided that the dietary content of copper is improved, since, in my experience, it is usually this that is found to be inadequate. A 7- to 14-day course of oral copper sulfate, giving 4 μmol per kilogram per day of copper (0.2 ml of 0.5 percent solution of copper sulfate as pentahydrate) is safe in the preterm infant. The term neonate may manage with slightly less, but this depends on the clinical and biochemical response. If longer courses are given, other essential elements must be monitored, particularly zinc.

A recognizable response, with weight gain and resolution of edema and apnea, may be expected within 5 to 7 days if the diagnosis is correct. Plasma copper and ceruloplasmin levels begin to rise after 1 to 2 weeks. Anemia and neutropenia gradually resolve over 3 to 4 weeks. Severe bone changes take longer to disappear, but there is usually an improvement in mineralization that is detectable with good quality radiographs within 1 month of treatment. If this improvement is not seen in response to a 7- to 14-day course of treatment, the diagnosis is probably incorrect.

The population we are dealing with is at risk of multiple nutritional deficiencies, in addition to infections, whether routine or opportunistic, and other metabolic derangements. These possibilities should always be rigorously pursued when the diagnosis of copper deficiency is in doubt.

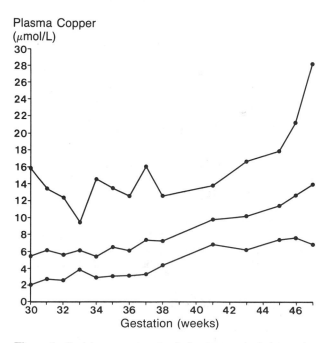

Plasma Copper
(μmol/L)

Gestation (weeks)

Figure 1 Serial measurements of plasma copper (micromoles per liter) in 39 preterm infants (values, geometric mean of 95 percent confidence limit). (From Sutton A, Harvie A, Cockburn F, et al. Copper deficiency in the preterm infant of very low birthweight. Arch Dis Child 1985; 60:644–651.)
Plasma Copper (μmol/L) Gestation (weeks)

SUGGESTED READING

Biological roles of copper. CIBA Foundation Symposium, 1979. Amsterdam, The Netherlands, Excerpta Medica, 1980.
Sutton A, Harvie A, Cockburn F, et al. Copper deficiency in the preterm infant of very low birthweight. Arch Dis Child 1985; 60:644–651.

CRANIOSYNOSTOSIS

AVINOAM SHUPER, M.D.
PAUL MERLOB. M.D.
SALOMON H. REISNER, M.B., Ch.B.

Craniosynostosis is defined as premature closure of one or more sutures of the cranium, resulting in an abnormally shaped skull, described by the term craniostenosis. In most cases the craniosynostosis is primary or idiopathic. However, sutural obliteration may be secondary to some underlying medical disorder or central nervous system malformations. Most primary synostoses have developed before and are detectable at birth, but they are accentuated and more easily observed by cranial growth during the first months of life.

Craniosynostosis represents an etiologically heterogeneous group of craniofacial anomalies that should be classified according to two different perspectives: anatomic and genetic.

ANATOMIC CLASSIFICATION

The anatomic classification describes the ultimate shape of the skull resulting from the premature closure of the relevant suture(s). In *simple* craniosynostosis only one suture is involved. If two or more sutures are prematurely closed, the craniosynostosis is *compound*. Pathologic elongation of the head owing to premature closure of the sagittal suture is called scaphocephaly. Obliteration of the coronal suture results in turricephaly (tower head) and that of the metopic suture causes trigonocephaly (triangular-shaped head). If all the sutures are prematurely closed, oxycephaly results. Plagiocephaly means an asymmetric head resulting from unilateral closure of a coronal or lambdoid suture. In order to avoid confusion with other names describing the same condition, it is recommended that a terminology mentioning the stenosed suture (e.g., premature closure of metopic suture instead of trigonocephaly) be used.

GENETIC CLASSIFICATION

This classification is based on the overall pattern of malformations of the patient and his or her whole family. In this regard, it should be determined whether the craniosynostosis is (1) isolated, complicated (a part of a pattern of morphologic defects not included in a defined syndrome), or syndromic; or (2) sporadic or familial. It is important to emphasize that each case should be classified by both anatomic and genetic perspectives, as the same genetic condition may have different anatomic presentations, involving varying degrees of fusion of different sutures.

INCIDENCE

The estimation of incidence of craniosynostosis should take into account the age at diagnosis, the genetic and anatomic types, and the characteristics of the population. Most of the data in the literature are based on an estimation of the incidence of all genetic types together. These estimations were made by identification of hospitalized patients, and extrapolated percentages were determined from total live births, total admissions, or even based on archeologic skull studies. Thus, estimates have varied in the range of 0.4 to 29 per 1,000 children. The anatomic distribution of craniosynostosis in the general population was determined as sagittal suture 56 to 58 percent, coronal 18 to 29 percent, metopic 3 to 10 percent, and lambdoidal synostosis in 1 to 4 percent.

The incidence of primary isolated (nonsyndromic) craniosynostosis in a newborn population was 0.6 per 1,000 live births. The anatomic distribution in this newborn population was metopic suture 50 percent, sagittal suture 28 percent, coronal suture 16.5 percent, and lambdoidal suture 5.5 percent. The frequency of premature closure of the metopic suture in newborn infants is high in comparison with other populations. It may be assumed that because of the self-correcting characteristic of this type of craniosynostosis, cases of trigonocephaly are easily missed in studies of older children and thus underestimated. Most cases of isolated craniosynostosis are sporadic, the percentage of familial cases being less than 10 percent.

About 60 syndromes were reported that are associated with craniosynostosis. A full list of these syndromes was reported by Cohen. More than ten of these syndromes are due to chromosomal abnormalities, and about half of the rest are monogenic. More new associations and syndromes with craniosynostosis are being reported. Most studies have demonstrated a significant excess of males affected with craniosynostosis: 78 percent for sagittal, 62 percent for coronal, and 75 percent for metopic premature closure.

PATHOGENESIS AND ETIOLOGY

The cause of the premature sutural closure is not fully understood. Theories implicating intrauterine infection, trauma, endocrine dysfunction, radiation during pregnancy, metabolic disorders, and intrauterine constraint have all been mentioned.

The cranial sutures allow the rapid expansion of brain mass during infancy and childhood. Since brain size determines growth and shape of the overlying skull vault, expansion of the cranial vault is uneven when a suture is synostosed. Studies indicate that the dura is the guiding tissue in the morphogenesis of the calvaria and its major sutures. Overlying the central zones between the dural reflections, ossification takes place, whereas none occurs over the reflections of the dura, these being the suture sites. Biomechanical growth-stretch tensile forces that are exerted by the developing brain on the dura mater determine the membranous ossification of the skull. Moss and

Young postulate that intrauterine events affecting the base of the skull modify mechanical conditions along the dural fiber tracts that follow the courses later occupied by the major sutures. These spatially malformed dural attachments cause aberrant tensile forces transmitted through the dura and, as a result, premature fusion of the overlying sutural tissue occurs. On the other hand, craniosynostosis may also result from lack of growth stretch at the sutures due to an underlying developmental brain defect. It is of note that in such cases hair directional patterning may be altered as a clue to the basic pathology.

Recently, fetal head constraint in utero was suggested as a major cause of craniosynostosis. Head constraint may be caused by early fetal head descent, abnormal fetal lie, prolonged breech presentation, multifetal pregnancy, uterine malformation, oligohydramnios, primigravidity, small maternal size, small maternal pelvis, and large fetus. Fetal head constraint in a particular plane could relieve one or more sutural regions of growth stretch, causing synostosis at that region. As there is a more rapid rate of growth and larger head size in the male than in the female fetus during the last trimester of pregnancy, the constraint theory may explain the higher incidence of males with craniosynostosis. It is suggested that in about 60 percent of the cases the premature closure may be related to fetal head constraint, whereas those in whom a genetic etiology is suspected constitute only 23 percent of the cases. In about 15 percent the etiology of the craniosynostosis remains unknown.

DIAGNOSTIC CONSIDERATIONS

The physical examination of every newborn infant should include a careful inspection of the head shape. A fingertip should be run from the glabella to the occiput along the metopic and sagittal sutures, from one temporal region to the other along the coronal sutures, and over the occipitoparietal junction to define the lambdoid suture. The lack of movement across each suture and a palpable ridging, together with abnormal head shape, raise the suspicion of craniosynostosis.

The head shape of an infant with craniosynostosis is distorted according to the closed suture. The growth of adjacent bones is inhibited perpendicular to the course of the obliterated suture. As a result, the diameter of the skull is reduced in this direction, but compensatory and abnormal growth proceed in areas and directions in which open fontanelles or open sutures permit. In premature closure of the sagittal suture (scaphocephaly—boat head) the skull becomes extremely long from front to back and quite narrow from side to side. The typical ridging of the suture is readily detected. The forehead is high and the skull slopes back in the occiput, which is very prominent. If the metopic suture closes prematurely (trigonocephaly), the shape of the head becomes triangular. The eyes are closely set (hypotelorism) with upward slanting. In bilateral coronal synostosis the calvarium is short from front to back and wide from side to side (brachycephaly—short head). Hypertelorism may be present. In unilateral coronal suture synostosis (plagiocephaly), there is flattening of the ipsilateral frontoparietal region. The anterior fontanelle may show unilateral smallness. There may also be a unilateral exophthalmos.

Anthropometric measurements of the skull help to confirm the clinical impression. In each case the occipitofrontal circumference should be measured, as well as the anteroposterior (APD) and biparietal (BPD) diameters. Then the cephalic index (maximum head breadth [BPD]/maximum head length [APD] × 100) may be calculated. The normal range of the cephalic index is 78 to 84. Premature closure of the sagittal suture therefore decreases the cephalic index below 70, whereas in brachycephaly the cephalic index will increase.

A skull roentgenogram is the next step in the confirmation of craniosynostosis. Anteroposterior, lateral, basal, and Towne's projections should be performed. Analysis of skull shape is the best radiologic clue to the diagnosis of craniosynostosis. The suture thought to be involved should be inspected for partial or complete obliteration. A ridge of bone may have been built up along the partially closed suture, and in some cases a sclerotic bone may be found along the margins of the fused suture. Occasionally one will be able to say only that the suture is excessively narrow. In some cases, the convolutional markings adjacent to the closed suture are prominent.

Other imaging modalities should be used if the radiologic findings cannot be interpreted with certainty. Skull scintigraphy may aid in assessing the problem. As the abnormal fusion process extends along the suture, there is a corresponding progression of abnormal accumulation of radioactivity. Uptake is diminished when complete fusion occurs. Computed tomograms of the skull may also be applied in questionable cases or in complex craniofacial anomalies. It has been demonstrated that the overall diagnostic accuracy rate for skull radiology is 89 percent, cranial computed tomography (CT) 94 percent, and skull scintigraphy 66 percent. At present, skull roentgenograms are still the most important and inexpensive aids in the diagnosis. However, CT of the brain is very useful for the exclusion of intracranial malformations.

In every case of craniosynostosis, before deciding on treatment, every effort should be made to determine the following:

1. Is it isolated, complicated, or syndromic?
2. Is it primary or secondary?
3. Is it sporadic or familial?

A thorough search is needed in order to evaluate the presence of all other skeletal and extraskeletal anomalies. In general, associated anomalies are much more common with coronal synostosis than with other sutures. Secondary craniosynostosis may result from disorders such as central nervous system malformations (microcephaly, encephalocele, and shunted hydrocephalus), endocrine disorders (hyperthyroidism), metabolic disorders (rickets or mucopolysaccharidosis), and hematologic disorders (polycythemia vera, thalassemia, erythroblastic anemia, and sickle cell anemia).

FURTHER INVESTIGATIONS

In the follow-up of infants with craniosynostosis, several issues should be taken into consideration:

1. The presence or absence of increased intracranial pressure. (This problem is more severe in cases with the involvement of multiple sutures.)
2. The presence of hydrocephalus. (Hydrocephalus also occurs more frequently in children with complex craniosynostosis syndromes and is very rare in simple craniosynostosis.)
3. Other neurologic abnormalities.
4. Careful ophthalmologic and otologic evaluation.
5. Mental development.

Craniosynostosis may or may not be associated with mental retardation. There is no clear correlation between the degree of synostosis and mental development. However, mental development may be favorably influenced by early surgery. It seems also that multiple associated malformations have no predictive value for mental development.

MANAGEMENT

The treatment of craniosynostosis must be individualized for each patient, depending upon the suture that is closed and the degree of abnormality. Surgery should be considered in order to achieve each of three goals: to allow undisturbed brain growth, to relieve an increased intracranial pressure, and to improve the cosmetic appearance of the child by permitting normal modeling of the skull. If the craniosynostosis is not corrected, the distortion of the skull may be expected to worsen with time as the brain enlarges. Even in the presence of a normal neurologic examination, IQ, and intracranial pressure, the cosmetic deformity of the skull may cause severe emotional stress, and this is an important consideration for surgery.

Some cases of trigonocephaly improve spontaneously with the growth of the child and do not require surgery. In cases of secondary craniosynostosis, surgical intervention is less effective.

The ideal time for operation is between 2 and 3 months of age, when the total blood volume suffices to reduce complications of the operational blood loss. Unless there is involvement of several sutures, causing compression of the developing brain, it is usually safe to defer surgery until 8 months of age at the very latest. If correction is performed before 6 weeks of age, the calvaria may reossify very quickly and the problem remain unsolved.

Many surgical techniques are used. The principle of the surgical operation is to make a craniectomy in the direction of the obliterated suture in order to obtain room for the brain to expand in the previously closed direction. At our center, in cases of sagittal synostosis, two linear craniectomies are performed parallel to the fused suture, which remains in place. Pieces of the removed bone are inserted in the new suture site (Fig. 1). In cases of coronal and metopic synostosis, a wider craniectomy is performed

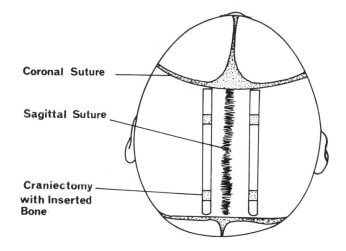

Figure 1 Schematic representation of the craniectomies in sagittal synostosis.

(Fig. 2). The results of this approach are generally very satisfactory, with marked improvement of the shape of the head.

In some centers linear craniectomies are done at the normal site of the missing suture, and the bone edges are lined with an inert (Silastic or polyethylene) film. This film helps to defer the time at which a new bone seals the old bone edges to one another. The new bone regenerates from the dura. The width of the craniectomy is about 1 cm. The craniectomy should be made to extend across the adjacent normal sutures. Then, as the child's head grows, the bone edge that has been filmed becomes longer than the film and allows the sealing of the craniectomy at each end.

In other centers, a wide excision of the bony calvaria is performed from the underlying dura. The excised area

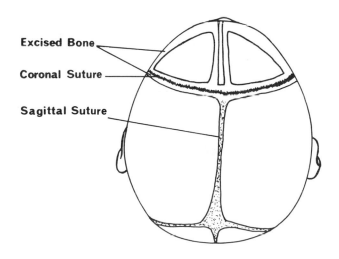

Figure 2 Schematic representation of the craniectomy performed for bilateral coronal synostosis.

generally includes the entire synostotic suture, together with a portion of the deformed bone. After the age of 3 months, small pieces of the bone are replaced into the dura to serve as nidi for new bone growth. Regeneration of the calvaria usually occurs over the next 1 to 2 months.

The rate of potential complications of the surgery is low. The mortality rate was reported to be 0.39 to 1.4 percent. The range of the overall morbidity rate was between 5.5 to 14 percent. The important complications include infection and bleeding. Pressure scars on the forehead may result from a face-down position during the operation, which should be prevented. Wound sepsis and hematoma or cerebrospinal fluid accumulation beneath the scalp require reoperation. The surgical intervention, when performed properly and at the appropriate age, is associated with a low operative risk and marked improvement in the growth and appearance of the child's head.

SUGGESTED READING

Cohen MM Jr. Craniosynostosis and syndromes with craniosynostosis: Incidence, genetics, penetrance, variability and new syndrome updating. Birth Defects: Original Article Series 1979; 15(5B):13.

Cohen MM Jr. Perspectives on craniosynostosis. West J Med 1980; 132:507.

Graham JM Jr. Craniostenosis: A new approach to management. Pediatr Ann 1981; 10:27.

Shillito J Jr. Craniosynostosis. In: Youmans JR, ed. Neurological surgery. Philadelphia: WB Saunders, 1982:1447.

Shuper A, Merlob P, Grunebaum M, Reisner SH. The incidence of isolated craniosynostosis in the newborn infant. Am J Dis Child 1985; 139:85.

CYANOTIC/APNEIC EPISODES

DAVID P. SOUTHALL, M.D., M.R.C.P.
MARTIN P. SAMUELS, M.B., M.R.C.P.

Effective management depends on accurate diagnosis and the availability of adequate therapy. In this chapter, techniques for diagnosing the underlying mechanisms responsible for cyanotic/apneic episodes in the newborn and infant are described, the possible responsible disorders are outlined, and a personal approach to their treatment presented.

FEATURES OF THE CLINICAL HISTORY

The presence of cyanotic episodes during the awake state in response to noxious stimuli or rage associated with an attempt to cry or crying is diagnostic of a condition which includes an intrapulmonary right to left shunt and prolonged expiratory apnea (PEA), or "breath-holding spells". In some patients there is a positive family history with parents, siblings, or more distant relatives having manifested cyanotic breath-holding episodes.

In some infants, generally those born before term or those with respiratory infections, episodes of cyanosis may occur when they are awake, asleep, or feeding. Such episodes also involve an intrapulmonary shunt and PEA.

A history of a recent respiratory tract infection is relevant, since pertussis, respiratory syncytial virus, and other respiratory tract infections may produce cyanotic episodes attributable to this disorder. A repetitive cough that is worse at night and that is not associated with a major systemic illness, in an infant who has not been immunized, is highly suggestive of pertussis.

A history of sudden infant death syndrome in a sibling or, of more concern, in a twin is a feature of the history that must be taken seriously in terms of an increased risk of sudden death in subsequent siblings around four fold higher than in the population as a whole, in surviving twins perhaps as high as 1 in 50.

The onset of cyanotic episodes during sleep in infants younger than 6 months may be due to intrapulmonary shunting and PEA, seizure-induced apnea or, rarely, "imposed" apnea. Additional features that may suggest a seizure disorder include lip smacking or eyelid flickering prior to the apnea.

Features that suggest smothering include the lack of witnesses to the onset of the episodes, inconsistencies in the description of the sequencing of clinical signs, a history of unusual injuries or illnesses in other siblings, and history of abuse of the parent as a child. The very unlikely possibility of such imposed apnea should always be kept in mind when discussing the clinical features of cyanotic episodes with parents.

When episodes are identified by home monitors, inquiries should be made concerning the alarm settings used by the parents.

A history of sleep-related upper airway obstruction should be sought. The following features are relevant to this diagnosis: an intermittent inspiratory stridor, chest wall recession, frequent arousals, and excessive sweating during sleep. In addition, there may be failure to thrive, hypotonia, recurrent upper respiratory tract and middle ear infections, excessive daytime sleepiness, and the adoption of unusual postures during sleep.

The onset of episodes of collapse without initial or early onset cyanosis during fearful or emotionally exciting experiences or during exercise should raise the possibility of either the long Q-T syndrome or a disorder of ventricular repolarization without prolongation of the Q-T interval.

A history of a previous tracheoesophageal fistula or of partial tracheal obstruction from a vascular ring or misplaced innominate artery should also be sought, since these conditions are associated with cyanotic episodes due to intrapulmonary shunting and PEA.

A history of any lesion in the medulla or upper cervical region is also relevant to the occurrence of cyanotic episodes due to intrapulmonary shunting and PEA. This is particularly important in patients with *Arnold-Chiari malformations, meningomyelocele, and achondroplasia*.

INVESTIGATING PATIENTS WITH CYANOTIC/APNEIC EPISODES

The work-up of patients with cyanotic/apneic episodes should follow the balance of probabilities suggested by the history. In all cases, it would be reasonable to perform the following procedures:

1. A standard electrocardiogram (ECG) to exclude the long Q-T syndrome and a 24 hour ECG to exclude ventricular arrhythmias without a prolonged Q-T interval.
2. A full blood count to look for evidence of viral or pertussis infection and to exclude anemia.
3. A multichannel electroencephalogram (EEG) to identify an underlying seizure disorder. However, a normal EEG does *not* exclude the possibility of seizure-induced apnea.
4. An infection screen to exclude pertussis, respiratory syncytial or other viral infection.

In all infants and young children, it is our practice also to perform an overnight 12-hour tape recording of (1) SaO_2 from a beat-to-beat pulse oximeter (Nellcor Respox 2 or N200), (2) the individual pulse waveforms from this latter instrument in order to validate each SaO_2 measurement, (3) abdominal breathing movements (from a Graseby MR10 pressure capsule), and (4) electrocardiogram (ECG). If the history suggests PEA, we also record respiratory air flow from a thermistor or expired CO_2 (sampling from one of the external nares). If the history suggests sleep-related upper airway obstruction, we add respiratory inductance plethysmography (Studley Data Systems), either from an abdominal belt or from a vest covering the rib cage and abdomen (PK Morgan), and transcutaneous Pco_2 (Draeger Electrode and Hewlett Packard). Inductance plethysmography is essential in order to demonstrate any abnormality of the inspiratory waveform engendered by an increased upper airway resistance (Fig. 1). End-tidal CO_2 is useful in detecting and quantifying any alveolar hypoventilation that has resulted from the airway obstruction.

If there is historical evidence to suggest a seizure-induced cyanotic episode, then recordings of SaO_2, two-channel EEG (centrotemporal), and breathing movements should be continued until a cyanotic episode has been captured on tape. Sleep deprivation may help to bring on a seizure that can be documented.

If the history is suggestive of awake-onset intrapulmonary shunting and PEA and the overnight recording is normal, we usually attempt to document SaO_2, breathing movements, ECG, one channel of centrotemporal EEG, and air flow during an episode. However, if episodes are difficult to provoke and there is an adequate history, this diagnosis can usually be made without the need to exclude a seizure-induced apnea.

If the history suggests imposed apnea, attempts must first be made to record physiologic variables during a cyanotic episode. The characteristic features reported during such an episode are the sudden onset of large body movements during patterns of breathing suggesting sleep, associated with sinus tachycardia, absent inspiratory air flow and approximately 60 to 70 sec later, high-voltage slow waves and subsequent flattening of the EEG. Recovery is associated with large-amplitude inspiratory movements linked with a prolonged expiratory phase (gasping). If such features are identified and the history is supportive, it may be appropriate to proceed to *covert* video surveillance (Rosen and Southall have provided further guidance on this problem.) The main differential diagnostic problem is with intrapulmonary shunting and PEA. Clues to the differential diagnosis are first the ability to provoke an episode of PEA in the presence of a third person (which is impossible in imposed apnea), the frequent awake onset of PEA, and the earlier onset of severe hypoxemia and EEG changes (25 to 30 sec) in cyanotic episodes associated with PEA.

In young infants with intrapulmonary shunting and PEA, an overnight tape recording might show combinations of the following three patterns:

1. Hypoxemia associated with prolonged pauses (> 15 sec) in inspiratory efforts.
2. Hypoxemia associated with inspiratory efforts but absent inspiratory air flow.
3. Hypoxemia associated with continued inspiratory efforts and continued inspiratory air flow.

The presence of pattern 3 episodes is confirmatory due to an intrapulmonary shunting and PEA. Pattern 2 may be due to PEA or to sleep-related upper airway obstruction. If there is no evidence of an abnormal inspiratory waveform (see Fig. 1) and no history of stridor or chest wall recession during sleep, then pattern 2 is due to PEA. Pattern 1 may be due to PEA or to seizure-induced apnea. In the additional presence of patterns 2 or 3, pattern 1 is confirmatory of PEA. Without these other patterns it is important to exclude seizure-induced apnea by concurrent EEG recordings (as described above).

If the history suggests sleep-related upper airway obstruction, the following features of the overnight recording provide confirmation of this diagnosis: (1) abnormal dips in SaO_2 accompanied by continued breathing movements showing evidence of increased inspiratory resistance (see Fig. 1). (2) Abnormal inspiratory waveform signals without hypoxemia. An elevation of end-tidal CO_2 levels provides additional information on the degree of alveolar hypoventilation produced by the obstruction. If airway obstruction is identified, upper airway x-ray films, a barium swallow, and fiberoptic endoscopy (2.9 mm Olympus) during free breathing under light general anesthesia should determine the mechanism for the obstruction.

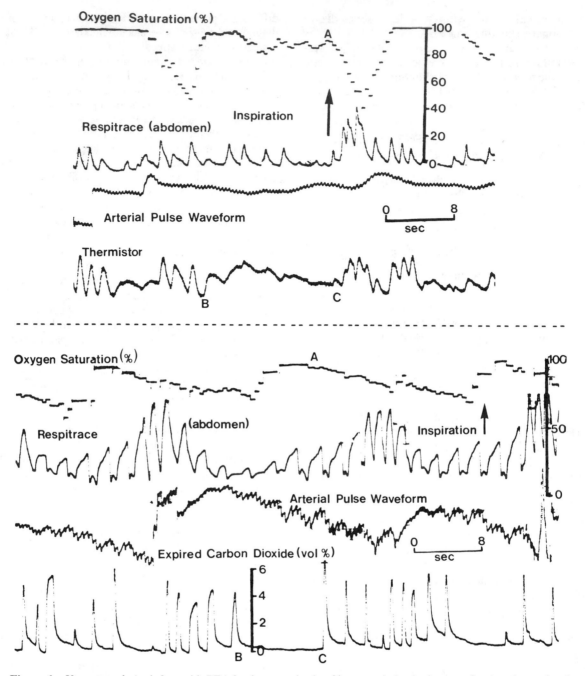

Figure 1 *Upper panel*: An infant with PEA having an episode of hypoxemia beginning at point A and associated with continued breathing movements and absent air flow at the nose, as shown by the thermistor signal (B to C). *Lower panel*: A young child with sleep-related upper airway obstruction having an episode of hypoxemia beginning at point A and associated with continued breathing movements but absent air flow at the nose, as shown by the end-tidal CO_2 signal (B to C). Unlike those in the upper panel, the inspiratory waveforms of the respiratory inductance plethysmograph are abnormal. Inspiration is biphasic, showing an initially rapid and subsequently slower movement, the latter reflecting an increase in airway resistance. (From Southall DP. Role of apnea in the sudden infant death syndrome: a personal view. Pediatrics 1988; 81:73–84.)

TREATMENT

Hypoxemic Episodes Due To Intrapulmonary Shunting and PEA (Cyanotic Breath-Holding) in Response to Noxious Stimuli

No controlled trials have yet been performed but the following outlines our approach to this common problem. Treatment of an acute episode usually involves the parents, since between episodes the infants and children are usually healthy and therefore at home. Mouth-to-mouth resuscitation and/or bag and mask ventilation are usually of little value until the child is extremely hypoxemic and unconscious. Before this time the glottis is closed and it is impossible to inflate the lungs. The child usually recovers by virtue of a large inspiratory effort (a gasp), and it is extremely important that, when it occurs, there is no external obstruction to inspiration, as for example from a face mask. Attempts can be made to stimulate the gasp response as early as possible in the course of the cyanotic episode and might include stimuli used to elicit the first breath of the neonate, for example, cutaneous sensations involving pain or abnormal temperatures. Inspired oxygen is of little value in the initial management of a cyanotic episode, since the child is not inspiring. During the recovery gasp large quantities of air containing oxygen are drawn into the lungs with the rapid recovery of arterial oxygen saturation. If painful cutaneous stimuli are used to induce recovery, it is important that they are not perceived by the child as punishment.

If cyanotic episodes are accompanied by loss of consciousness, we recommend tetrabenazine beginning at a total daily dose of 0.75–1.0 mg per kilogram in three divided doses. The dose is increased gradually until slight drowsiness occurs and is then drawn back to a level which does not produce this side effect but which prevents cyanotic episodes. During times of frequent cyanotic episodes, as may occur during an intercurrent respiratory tract infection or fever, episodes may be reduced in frequency and severity by using a continuous negative extrathoracic pressure tank (Horner and Wells) or by continuous positive airway pressure (CPAP) in addition to the tetrabenazine. Negative pressures of up to −10 cm of H_2O can be given, although −7.5 cm H_2O is usually sufficient to prevent the majority of cyanotic events. There also appears to be a carryover effect from this treatment, in that if it is used overnight, particularly for several successive nights, attacks during the subsequent days may be less frequent and less severe.

The following medications have not been found to be of benefit in preventing these episodes: methylxanthines, steroids (oral and by inhalation), ambroxol, and salbutamol (orally and by inhalation).

One important aspect of these cyanotic episodes is the suffering sustained by the child. Those old enough to provide a description report a feeling of suffocation and an unpleasant nausea and dizziness, the latter presumably associated with the rapid onset of hypoxia. Fortunately, in this particular respect, those episodes occurring with a loss of consciousness are not remembered. Nevertheless, contrary to previous teaching, it is vital that the parent stay with the child for the whole of the episode and be there when he or she recovers.

Hypoxemic Episodes Due To Intrapulmonary Shunting and PEA

Whether or not the infant has an associated respiratory tract infection, the number of hypoxemic episodes can be reduced by increasing the inspired O_2 to around 40 percent using a headbox or special infant nasal cannula at a flow rate of 2 L per minute. If the Hb level is below 12 g per deciliter, we transfuse the infant carefully with partially packed cells to reach an optimal level of greater than 14 g per deciliter. Continuous negative extrathoracic pressure may also be helpful. The latest equipment provides intermittent chest inflations over and above the background subatmospheric pressure. These intermittent inflations can be triggered by the alarm from a blood oxygen or heart rate monitor.

We also have evidence that theophylline or caffeine may be valuable. Theophylline is given at a dose of 2 mg per kilogram every 8 hours, until trough blood levels between 5 and 10 μg per milliliter are obtained. Caffeine citrate is given as a loading dose of 20 mg per kilogram followed by 5 mg per kilogram once daily, the first dose beginning 24 hours after the starting dose. Trough blood levels are kept between 6 and 15 μg per milliliter. To ensure that treatment has been completely effective in abolishing all episodes of abnormal hypoxemia, we restudy infants who have reached adequate blood drug levels using overnight recordings of SaO_2, abdominal breathing movements, and ECG. If abnormal hypoxemia is still present, we give either a further 1-week course of the continuous negative extrathoracic pressure tank or keep the infant under close observation in the hospital and continue the methylxanthine treatment. We send home with a modified $TcPO_2$ monitor (see below) only those infants in whom overnight recordings of SaO_2, breathing movements, and ECG have ceased to show abnormal episodes of hypoxemia. In infants with hypoxemic episodes occurring both in response to crying and during sleep (generally those with brainstem lesions) we use a combination of tetrabenazine and increased inspired oxygen (around 40 percent).

Seizure-Induced Apnea

When the diagnosis of seizure-induced apnea has been confirmed, it is important that the infant or child be referred to a pediatric neurologist for further investigation and treatment. Unfortunately, this form of seizure may be difficult to control with anticonvulsants. We usually begin carbamazepine and if, at adequate blood levels, that alone does not stop apneic episodes we add phenytoin.

Imposed Apnea

With imposed apnea, two objectives should be attained. The first is that the child and his or her siblings must be made safe, and the second is that the parent, usually the mother, should receive adequate psychiatric treatment. We believe that adequate documentation of imposed apnea using covert video surveillance is essential in achieving these objectives.

Sleep-Related Upper Airway Obstruction

The type of treatment given depends on what is found at the time of upper airway endoscopy, the presence of other associated major health problems such as Down syndrome or cerebral palsy, and the degree of severity of the obstruction on the overnight recording. Frequent and severe hypoxemic episodes throughout the recording require more aggressive and urgent treatment than evidence of increased inspiratory airway resistance alone.

Sleep-Related Upper Airway Obstruction in Otherwise Healthy Infants and Children

It is our view that severe sleep-related airway obstruction, by producing hypoxemia and major sleep disturbances, can result in long-term if not permanent developmental impairment. We therefore adopt a fairly aggressive approach to this disorder. If there is any evidence of tonsillar or adenoidal enlargement, these structures are removed. If there is no substantial relief of the obstruction and there is evidence of abnormal hypoxemia, two possible treatments are considered. The first involves continuous positive airway pressure (CPAP) during sleep and the second tracheostomy.

In our hospital, CPAP of +5 to +7.5 cm H_2O has been given using a nasopharyngeal airway inserted every night and removed every morning; other centers have used a close-fitting nasal mask. The technique requires overnight surveillance by a relative or a nurse in conjunction with a transcutaneous (Tc)PO_2 monitor (see below) and is consequently extremely difficult for some families. Nevertheless, since this disorder can improve if not completely disappear with increasing age, this noninvasive form of therapy may be suitable for some patients.

In our unit tracheostomy has been used more frequently than CPAP to date without complications. For 48 hours postoperatively we apply CPAP to the tracheostomy in order to prevent alveolar atelectasis. As soon as possible after the tracheostomy we apply a valve to the tracheostomy opening in order to avoid low lung volumes resulting from the absence of the normal expiratory resistance created by the larynx. This valve freely allows inspiration but provides an expiratory resistance. All our patients with tracheostomies have specially modified $TcPO_2$ monitors in place at home when they are asleep. The monitor ensures that hypoxemia resulting from blockage or displacement of the tracheostomy tube does not go undetected.

Sleep-Related Upper Airway Obstruction in Infants and Children with Down Syndrome

In a continuing prospective study, we have shown that this complication occurs in one-third to one-half of children with Down syndrome. Endoscopy in 15 patients has shown that the main site for obstruction is at the base of the tongue. In some infants there was inward collapse of the hypopharynx and epiglottis during inspiration. In other patients, particularly those over 1 year of age, there may be enlargement of the tonsils and adenoids, which may contribute to the obstruction by adding extra tissue to the tongue base and by increasing negative inspiratory pressure, thus exacerbating the inspiratory airway collapse.

Any degree of tonsillar or adenoidal contribution is therefore first alleviated by tonsillectomy or adenoidectomy. In a proportion of cases this has been completely successful. However, in some, airway obstruction is either not associated with tonsillar or adenoidal enlargement or the removal of these structures produces a relatively small improvement.

Nasopharyngeal intubation, as used in the Pierre Robin syndrome, has also been attempted, but without the additional application of CPAP it has not been successful. Children with Down syndrome appear to have increased upper airway secretions, and these lead to early blockage of the nasopharyngeal tube and an immediate worsening of the obstruction. CPAP is possible but logistically very difficult. Moreover, there is less evidence that the obstruction resolves with time, unlike that in children without Down syndrome.

To date we have become aware of four patients with Down syndrome and sleep-related obstruction who have died from their obstruction during infancy. Death in this disease is not sudden but protracted over many weeks or months and usually results from either a chest infection or the effects of the induced pulmonary hypertension. Prior to death there is intense suffering produced by sleep deprivation, asphyxia, and recurrent upper respiratory tract infections. For these reasons it is our policy to treat upper airway obstruction aggressively in patients with Down syndrome, especially if it is associated with arterial hypoxemia. Attempts are being made in our hospital to develop an appropriate plastic surgical procedure that will create more room in the pharynx and hypopharynx of these infants. In the meantime, with the fully informed support of the parents, we treat patients with hypoxemia by tracheostomy.

Sleep-Related Upper Airway Obstruction in Infants and Children with Cerebral Palsy

In these patients airway obstruction is present in both the awake and the sleep states, and is due to inspiratory collapse of the severely hypotonic or incoordinate oro- and hypopharynx. There is a build-up of secretions in the throat, leading to recurrent upper and lower respiratory tract infections, and the swallowing mechanism may also be seriously impaired, with frequent aspiration into the trachea.

In our experience with such patients, we have been impressed by the serious consequences of this obstruction on the quality of their lives. They have severe sleep disturbances, they fail to thrive, they develop major abnormalities of the chest wall that further embarrass respiratory function, they have extensor spasms that help to open the airway and they suffer from frequent respiratory infections.

As a result of these observations we have performed therapeutic tracheostomies. The response in all cases was dramatic, with loss of obstructive symptoms, recovery from chest wall distortion, lessening of respiratory tract infections and extensor spasms, improvement in affect and in sleep, and weight gain.

Infants with Pierre Robin Syndrome

The standard therapy for this syndrome in the newborn is either use of a nasopharyngeal airway or postural manipulations. Unfortunately, there is little objective data on the efficacy of these methods in preventing abnormal hypoxemia or sudden death.

In some patients who were monitored as described above, nasopharyngeal airways were shown to reduce the incidence of hypoxemia. In others, however, there was only partial relief and in these infants tracheostomies were performed.

We suggest that if procedures less definitive than tracheostomy are used to treat patients with Pierre Robin syndrome, careful monitoring of their effectiveness is required. Under these circumstances, the presence of continuing hypoxemic episodes should perhaps be considered an indication for tracheostomy in view of the reported high risks of sudden death and neurodevelopmental delays in children with this disorder. In all infants with airway obstruction due to Pierre Robin syndrome whether or not they have a tracheostomy, we supply parents with a transcutaneous PO_2 monitor, modified for home use (see below).

HOME MONITORING FOR ABNORMAL HYPOXEMIA

A recent consensus statement from the National Institutes of Health contains a well-balanced review of monitoring for apnea. Our only suggestion concerns the valuable experience we have gained from using $TcPO_2$ monitors at home applied at skin temperatures of 42.5 to 43.0 °C. They do not provide accurate baseline PO_2 values but they do detect sudden falls in $TcPO_2$ and chronic hypoxemia. They can remain in one site up to 8 hours at a time. They are particularly useful in detecting severe hypoxemia associated with continued breathing movements and a lack of bradycardia. We have found them ideal for monitoring infants with tracheostomies. A high PO_2 alarm can be used to detect disconnection of the sensor from the skin. In order to identify the mechanisms for low PO_2 alarms, the monitors also sense breathing movements from a volume expansion capsule taped to the surface of the abdomen (Graseby). The breathing movement signals are not used to provide an alarm but, along with the $TcPO_2$ signals, are constantly sampled by an event recorder based within the monitor. If a low $TcPO_2$ alarm occurs the $TcPO_2$ values and breathing movements are recorded onto a solid state memory card for 20 minutes prior to and 10 minutes after each event.

Acknowledgment. We wish to thank our nursing and medical colleagues at the Brompton Hospital for their invaluable help in managing the patients who provided the experience on which this chapter is based.

SUGGESTED READING

National Institutes of Health, Conference Statement. Infantile apnea and home monitoring. 1986; 6:6.

Rosen CL, Frost JD Jr, Bricker T, et al. Two siblings with recurrent cardiorespiratory arrest: Munchausen syndrome by proxy or child abuse? Pediatrics 1983; 71:715–720.

Rutter N, Southall DP. A family with life-threatening cardiac arrhythmias mistakenly diagnosed as epilepsy. Arch Dis Child 1985; 60:54–56.

Southall DP, Croft CB, Stebbens VA, Ibrahim H, Gurney A, Buchdahl R, Warner JO. Detection of sleep associated dysfunctional pharyngeal obstruction in infants. Eur J Pediatrics 1989; 148:353–359.

Southall DP, Stebbens V, Abraham N, Abraham L. Prolonged apnea with severe arterial hypoxemia resulting from complex partial seizures. Dev Med Child Neurol 1987; 29:784–789.

Southall DP, Stebbens VA, Mirza R, Lang MH, Croft CB, Shinebourne EA. Upper airway obstruction with hypoxemia and sleep disruption in Down's syndrome—clinical implications in children with and without congenital heart disease. Dev Med Child Neurol 1987; 29:734–742.

Southall DP, Stebbens VA, Rees SV, et al. Apnoeic episodes induced by smothering—two cases identified by covert video surveillance. Br Med J, 1987; 294:1637–1641.

Southall DP, Talbert DG, Johnston P, et al. Prolonged expiratory apnea—A disorder resulting in episodes of severe arterial hypoxemia in infants and young children. Lancet 1985; 2:571–577.

DISSEMINATED INTRAVASCULAR COAGULATION

WILLIAM E. HATHAWAY, M.D.

Disseminated intravascular coagulation (DIC) commonly accompanies disorders seen in the critically ill infant. It is an acquired pathologic process characterized by activation of the coagulation system leading to thrombin generation, intravascular fibrin deposition, and platelet consumption. Microthrombi, composed of fibrin and platelets, may produce ischemic tissue damage as well as fragmentation of erythrocytes. The fibrinolytic system is also frequently activated, producing plasmin-mediated destruction of fibrin, fibrinogen, and other clotting factors (factors VIII and V). Degradation or split products of fibrin-fibrinogen (FDP) are formed and function as anticoagulants and inhibitors of platelet function. Clinically, the process may be expressed as diffuse hemorrhage, organ ischemia, and/or hemolytic anemia. Conditions known to trigger DIC include endothelial cell damage (endotoxin, virus), tissue destruction (necrosis, physical injuries), hypoxia (acidosis), ischemic and vascular changes (shock, hemangiomas), and release of tissue procoagulants (malignancies, placental disorders).

ASSESSMENT

Three areas should be considered in planning management of DIC in the sick newborn infant: determination of the cause of the DIC; estimation of the severity of the coagulopathy; and notation of the consequences of the DIC process. The *trigger event* usually is easily determined in the newborn infant, since that episode and evidence of a clinical bleeding tendency are the indications for consideration of DIC. The usual triggers are infection (bacterial or viral sepsis), hypoxia and acidosis, hypotension and shock, placental abnormalities (abruption, previa, dead twin fetus), organ necrosis (thrombosis, necrotizing enterocolitis), and severe erythroblastosis fetalis or hyperviscosity.

The clinical estimation of the severity of the coagulopathy is based on the bleeding manifestations and laboratory measurements. If the infant shows bleeding (persistent oozing from skin wounds, endotracheal or nasogastric oozing, petechiae, ecchymoses, or major hemorrhage), the condition is usually severe. Laboratory tests that are most helpful in assessing the severity are platelet count, fibrinogen level, prothrombin time, estimation of FDP (Thrombo-Wellcotest, d-dimer, or thrombin time), and the activated partial thromboplastin time (APTT). The APTT is less helpful in assessing degree of severity in the small preterm infant because it is often greatly prolonged on a physiologic basis. In the term infant, a markedly prolonged APTT is usually seen in severe DIC. Normal values, minimal hemostatic values, and representative values in severe DIC are shown in Table 1.

The platelet count may be normal or only slightly decreased in severe DIC due to neonatal asphyxia. In early DIC the FDP test may be normal or only slightly elevated. Infants whose screening tests are better than the minimal hemostatic levels rarely display evidence of clinical bleeding in DIC. The exception may be those infants with a brisk fibrinolytic response and with increased FDP (and fibrin monomer-FDP complexes not measured by the Thrombo-Wellcotest), producing significant prolongation of the APTT and, if measured, the bleeding time.

In the severely ill infant, it is frequently difficult to determine whether the clinical manifestations are due to the intravascular coagulation process or are causing the process secondarily. For example, renal ischemia and subsequent necrosis can trigger DIC as well as be caused by microthrombosis. Other organs (heart, liver, brain, and lung) may be similarly affected. Hemorrhage and intravascular hemolysis are more directly attributed to the DIC process. Nevertheless, assessment of the potential consequences of DIC (hemorrhage, hemolysis, organ damage) is important in planning therapy. In particular, the detection of associated large vessel thrombosis is important.

TREATMENT

The major reason for the assessment step in the management of neonatal DIC is to decide whether specific treatment is needed. Table 2 provides guidelines for management. Experience and a few controlled studies have indicated that the most important aspect of therapy of neonatal DIC is removal of the triggering event and stabilization of the infant. Even in severe DIC, if the precipitating cause, infection, placental abnormality, hypoxia, or shock can be quickly controlled, specific therapy, such as replacement of clotting factors and platelets or anticoagulation, is frequently not necessary. However, in the diffusely bleeding patient or the infant with high risk of significant hemorrhage, such as intraventricular hemorrhage or pulmonary hemorrhage, or in the infant who must have a surgical procedure, correction of the coagulopathy and maintenance of minimal hemostatic levels are indicated. An approach to the management of infants with DIC is outlined in Table 2.

Replacement therapy consists of infusions of blood products in an attempt to achieve clinical hemostasis. In general, 10 ml per kilogram of fresh frozen plasma raises the level of coagulation factors by an increment of 15 to 20 percent. A similar dose (10 ml per kilogram) of platelet concentrate will raise the platelet count by about 75,000 to 100,000 per microliter and the clotting factor level by 15 to 20 percent. It is difficult to give enough fresh frozen plasma at one infusion to raise the fibrinogen or antithrombin III level significantly; therefore, in severe depletions of fibrinogen in the bleeding infant, cryoprecipitate (1 bag

TABLE 1 Screening Tests for Disseminated Intravascular Coagulation

Test	Newborn Normal Mean Value (Abnormal Limits)	Minimal Hemostatic Level	Severe DIC
Platelet count	250,000/μl (150,000/μl)	50,000/μl	Normal to <20,000/μl
Fibrinogen	230 mg/dl (150 mg/dl)	100 mg/dl	0–50 mg/dl
Prothrombin time*	13 sec (15 sec)	15 sec	16–30 sec
FDP	<10 μg/ml	—	20 μg/ml

* Currently available reagents have shortened the normal prothrombin time; the values shown are estimates only.

TABLE 2 Management Guidelines in Neonatal Disseminated Intravascular Coagulation

Indications	Treatment
Trigger event relieved	
Mild coagulopathy	None
Severe coagulopathy	Replacement therapy if bleeding or high risk*
Trigger event ongoing	
Mild coagulopathy	Replacement therapy if bleeding or high risk
Severe coagulopathy	Replacement therapy or exchange transfusion
Organ damage (necrosis, thrombosis) with persistent DIC	Replacement therapy plus anticoagulation
Large vessel thrombosis with or without DIC	Anticoagulation

* High risk = preterm (<33 weeks); surgical procedure (any age).

per 3-kg infant,~ 10 ml per kilogram) can raise the fibrinogen level by 50 to 100 mg per deciliter. Antithrombin-III is also found in cryoprecipitate, although most other clotting factors (except factor VIII) are not present. The empiric approach to treatment of the infant with severe DIC is the administration of these products in doses and at intervals to halt bleeding and correct laboratory tests to minimal hemostatic levels (see Table 1). Practically speaking, this may mean giving 10 ml per kilogram of fresh frozen plasma, 10 ml per kilogram of platelet concentrate and, occasionally, 10 ml per kilogram of cryoprecipitate once or twice daily until the desired clinical effect is seen and the trigger for the DIC has been relieved. Severely affected infants, who may not tolerate the infusion volumes and/or who may need rapid and more complete correction of their coagulation status prior to surgery, benefit from an exchange transfusion with fresh (less than 24 hours) whole citrate-phosphate-dextrose blood. Whenever possible, the laboratory effects of replacement therapy should be monitored by repeated platelet counts, fibrinogen levels, and prothrombin times.

Anticoagulation with intravenous heparin is indicated in infants who have large vessel (renal, aorta, or femoral) thromboses with or without evidence for DIC.

Heparinization is achieved by giving 50 U per kilogram of heparin as a bolus followed by the continuous infusion of 20 to 25 U per kilogram per hour (infants weighing less than 1,500 g) or 25 to 30 U per kilogram per hour (infants weighing more than 1,500 g). The effect of heparin can be monitored by a micro whole blood clotting time or APTT in an effort to keep these tests at about one and one-half to two times the pretreatment value. If the pretreatment values for the screening tests are very abnormal, then replacement therapy—fresh frozen plasma, cryoprecipitate, platelet packs—may be needed. A few infants with DIC-associated organ ischemia and necrosis of the skin, kidney, or gut may benefit from heparin in a dose of 10 to 15 U per kilogram continuously plus appropriate replacement therapy. This "low-dose" heparin has been associated with resolution of the ischemic lesions.

Sick newborn infants have low levels of the heparin cofactor antithrombin-III, and heparinization may depend on raising these levels (via fresh frozen plasma, cryoprecipitate). However, in our experience, effective heparinization has been achieved without replacement therapy in nearly all cases of large vessel thrombosis. Bleeding complications of heparin therapy have been seen rarely in the newborn and only in association with major surgery.

COMPLICATIONS

The major complication of neonatal DIC management is liver disease secondary to microthrombosis, ischemia, or viral hepatitis. These infants fail to synthesize clotting factors adequately and to activate intravascular coagulation and fibrinolysis. The result is often a persistent coagulopathy that fails to respond well to replacement therapy. Liver disease is the most common cause of persistent, intractable DIC seen in the newborn in our experience. Treatment is difficult and may consist of repeated exchange transfusions in an effort to support the infant until the damaged liver recovers adequately.

Progressive gangrene associated with DIC, purpura fulminans, is occasionally seen in the newborn infant. Recent reports have demonstrated that neonatal purpura fulminans may be due to hereditary homozygous protein C deficiency. Treatment for this severe coagulopathy involves replacement therapy of protein C using fresh frozen plasma (10 ml per kilogram every 12 hours) as well as anti-coagulation therapy.

DISTURBANCES OF CARDIAC RHYTHM AND CONDUCTION

D. WOODROW BENSON Jr., M.D., Ph.D.

The principal objective in evaluation of a fetus or neonate with suspected disturbance of rhythm or conduction is to obtain echocardiographic (fetus) or electrocardiographic (neonate) documentation of the disturbance, so that a differential diagnosis can be made. This is an important step, since the contemporary approach to cardiac rhythm and conduction disturbances is to individualize the management. Current methods for defining the disturbances and the consequent advances in knowledge about disturbances of rhythm and conduction permit a rational approach to the question of whether or not to treat and if so, then how to choose among available pharmacologic, electrophysiologic, and surgical options. The fundamental differences in treatment strategies between the fetus and the neonate result from the pharmacodynamic and pharmacokinetic barrier to the fetus imposed by the placenta and the relative inaccessibility of the fetus for temporary electrogram recording, cardiac pacing, or electric conversion.

MANAGEMENT OF SPECIFIC DISTURBANCES

Sinus Node Dysfunction

The rhythm disturbances associated with sinus node dysfunction include bradycardia, inappropriately low heart rate response to stress, and tachycardia. The similarity of observed rhythm disturbances to those of the bradycardia-tachycardia syndrome and "sick sinus syndrome" has been apparent, and these terms are used interchangeably. Sinus node function depends on both intrinsic pacemaker automaticity and intra-atrial conduction. Alterations of intra-atrial conduction may interfere with sinus node pacemaker function and thus result in bradycardia, or they may also support re-entry and result in tachycardia. Thus, alterations in intra-atrial conduction rather than dysfunc-tion of the sinus mode per se may be the cause of the rhythm disturbances. Sinus node dysfunction is an uncommon problem in the fetus and neonate, but autonomic nervous system dysfunction is thought to be an important cause of bradycardia. The observation of tachycardia in the patient with a history of bradycardia is important for distinguishing sinus node from autonomic nervous system dysfunction.

The treatment of sinus node dysfunction with antiarrhythmic drugs (tachycardia) or pacemaker (bradycardia, tachycardia) is symptomatic. This approach to therapy, i.e., alleviation of symptoms rather than correction of the underlying disorder, emphasizes the importance of documentation of the rhythm disturbance.

Atrioventricular Conduction Abnormalities

Disorders of atrioventricular (AV) conduction are recognized in the fetus and neonate. Impaired conduction (first-, second-, and third-degree heart block) and apparently abbreviated conduction generally in association with metabolic disease are usually noted.

Heart Block

The conventional classification of heart block is based on selected electrocardiographic findings. First-degree heart block is said to be present when the P-R interval is prolonged for age and heart rate. Second-degree heart block is characterized by intermittent AV conduction. Third-degree heart block is present when there is no evidence of AV conduction (atrial rate exceeds ventricular rate and there is no relationship between atrial and ventricular depolarization). In the fetus and neonate, third-degree heart block is more common than second- or first-degree heart block. Congenital third-degree heart block can be divided into cases that occur in congenitally malformed hearts and those that occur in otherwise anatomically normal hearts. In cases with severe malformation, it is thought that the cardiac anomaly disrupts the cardiac conduction system. In contrast, in hearts that appear normal otherwise it is thought that a primary malformation of the conduction system has occurred at one of several sites. Recently, the association of maternal connective tissue disease with heart block due to discontinuity between the atrial myocardium and the distal portion of the AV node has been well established. Thus, much has been learned on the etiology of third-degree heart block in the fetus and neonate, but it is not known to what extent the etiology of first- and second-degree block relates to the etiology of third-degree block.

The major emphasis in the treatment of symptoms associated with heart block has focused on the use of cardiac pacemakers. In the fetus and neonate, symptoms are usually the result of low cardiac output associated with bradycardia, rather than syncope due to *torsade de pointes*, as seen in older children. At this time, there appears to be no indication to pace asymptomatic fetuses or neonates with first-, second-, or third-degree heart block, whereas symptoms of heart failure associated with second- or third-degree block are a clear indication for pacing. Recently it has become feasible to temporarily pace bradycardic fetuses with hydrops fetalis, but pacing has not been shown to alter morbidity or mortality. Neonates with surgically acquired third-degree block should be seriously considered for pacing, regardless of symptom status.

Abbreviated AV Conduction

Conditions resulting in a shortened P-R interval are rarely recognized in the fetus and neonate. The causes of shortened P-R interval are heterogenous. Lown-Ganong-Levine syndrome (shortened P-R interval and palpitations) has not been studied in young patients, but the characteristic electrocardiographic features of short P-R interval and normal QRS complex duration has been found, in older patients, to be a variant of Wolff-Parkinson-White syndrome. Type II glycogenosis (Pompe's disease) and Fabry's disease are also associated with a short P-R interval. The electrophysiologic basis of the short P-R interval is not known. In asymptomatic patients, this finding has little implication for treatment.

Abnormalities of Ventricular Depolarization and Repolarization

Alterations of QRS waveform configuration result from aberrancy, pre-excitation, or ectopic ventricular depolarization. Alterations in ventricular depolarization have a major impact on the ST-T wave. On the other hand, the disorders associated with prolongation of the Q-T interval are thought to be due to a neurogenically induced abnormality of repolarization in the presence of normal depolarization.

Aberrancy

Altered QRS configuration associated with depolarization initiated via the normal conduction system is termed aberrancy. Little management of aberrancy is required, but its recognition is important relative to associated underlying disorders. Right bundle branch block (RBBB) results from delay in right ventricular depolarization. Consequently, ventricular depolarization is sequential (left, then right) rather than simultaneous, as is characteristic of normal ventricular depolarization. In neonates, the electrocardiographic patterns of RBBB include a QRS complex of prolonged duration (exceeding 80 msec, 0.08 sec), a dominant R wave in lead V_1, and a dominant S wave in lead V_6. RBBB may be observed following cardiac surgery, during atrial extrasystoles, during tachycardia, or in association with Ebstein's anomaly of the tricuspid valve. Left bundle branch block (LBBB) results from delay in left ventricular depolarization. In neonates, LBBB is most often observed as rate-dependent block at the onset of tachycardia, but it may be observed following cardiac surgery. LBBB is characterized by prolonged QRS duration, a dominant S wave in lead V_1 and a dominant R wave in V_6. The QRS axis may be normal or shifted to the left. When the QRS duration is prolonged but not in a pattern typical of RBBB or LBBB, intraventricular conduction delay is said to be present.

Axis deviation may be interpreted in terms of fascicular block (hemiblock), but other considerations apply to neonates. For example, left axis deviation seen in endocardial cushion defects is due to early depolarization of the diaphragmatic surface of the left ventricle, which is the result of the well-known posterior and inferior displacement of the specialized conduction system in this defect. Left axis deviation, commonly observed in tricuspid atresia, is due to early right ventricular depolarization with relative delay, primarily in the base, of left ventricular depolarization.

Pre-Excitation

Pre-excitation of the ventricles is said to be present if ventricular depolarization is initiated, by an impulse originating in the atrium, earlier than would be expected if ventricular depolarization proceeded entirely via the normal conduction system. Wolff-Parkinson-White syndrome is a common variety of pre-excitation syndromes. There are two principal electrocardiographic features of the pre-excitation syndromes: short P-R interval and/or prolonged QRS complex for age. Ventricular pre-excitation in the Wolff-Parkinson-White syndrome is the result of fusion of ventricular depolarization via the normal conduction system and an accessory AV connection. Thus the short P-R interval is the result of early ventricular activation, inscribed by the delta wave, via the accessory connection. In the neonate, no specific management is required, but an association with paroxysms of tachycardia should be appreciated.

Ectopic Ventricular Depolarization

The prolonged QRS duration that results from endocardial or epicardial ectopic ventricular depolarization is the result of protracted ventricular depolarization. This situation may be encountered during premature ventricular contractions, ventricular tachycardia, or cardiac pacing. It is usually possible to estimate crudely the pacing initiated site at which ventricular depolarization begins by noting the electrocardiographic similarity of the paced complexes to RBBB (early left ventricular depolarization) or LBBB (early right ventricular depolarization). From an electrophysiologic standpoint there is little similarity between intraventricular conduction disorder (bundle branch block) and initiation of ventricular activation from an ectopic site on the contralateral ventricle (pacing), but the electrocardiographic similarity is well-recognized.

Prolonged Q-T Interval

The significance of a prolonged Q-T interval on the electrocardiogram of an asymptomatic neonate is not precisely known. Q-T interval prolongation may indicate an antiarrhythmic drug effect (e.g., of procainamide) or metabolic derangement (e.g., hypocalcemia). On the other hand, it may indicate a propensity to syncope and to sudden death due to ventricular tachycardia (*torsade de pointes*). The latter situation is a heritable disorder that may be associated with deafness or normal hearing. In infants with hereditary prolonged Q-T interval, symptoms rarely occur during the first year of life, but cases in fetuses and neonates have been reported. Current evidence suggests that life-threatening rhythm disturbances may be the result of a centrally mediated discharge of left-sided sympathetic nerves. Therapy for symptomatic patients with prolonged Q-T interval includes beta-adrenergic blocking drugs, cardiac pacing, and a left stellectomy.

Irregularities of Cardiac Rhythm: Extrasystoles and Escape Beats

Irregularities of heart beat occur commonly in the fetus and neonate. Atrial extrasystoles are most commonly documented during electrocardiographic and echocardiographic studies. Ventricular extrasystoles and sinus pause with junctional escape beats occur less commonly. These conditions rarely require treatment; they do not imply other heart disease. Although they are usually benign in their own right, they may serve as initiating events for tachycardia in susceptible patients (Fig. 1).

Tachycardia with Normal QRS Complex

General Comment and Nomenclature

In the fetus and newborn, tachycardia is a relatively common rhythm disturbance. A strict, numerical definition of tachycardia poses some difficulty because the normal heart rate range for neonates includes rapid rates during normal sinus rhythm. However, heart rates in excess of 200 beats per minute should be evaluated for their potential as pathologic conditions. Other factors such as loss of heart rate variation of excessive variation (irregularity) should also stimulate evaluation of possible rhythm disturbance.

With the advent of modern investigative electrophysiologic techniques, it has become apparent that *different electrophysiologic mechanisms can result in tachycardias with similar electrocardiographic features*. For example, now we can think of three types of paroxysmal atrial (supraventricular) tachycardia. In primary atrial tachycardia, the

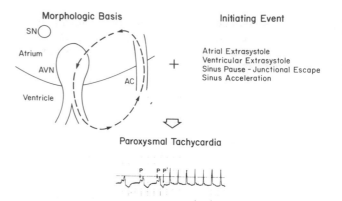

Figure 1 Paroxysmal tachycardia results from two ingredients: a morphologic/functional basis and an initiating event. The morphologic basis can be considered as two limbs: the antegrade limb (atrioventricular node, AVN) and the retrograde limb (accessory atrioventricular connection, AC). In this example, orthodromic tachycardia (dashed line) is initiated by atrial extrasystole in an infant with Wolff-Parkinson-White syndrome. The sinus node (SN) does not actively participate in the tachycardia.

rhythm disturbance is confined to the atrium and consequently describes a true atrial tachycardia. On the other hand, when tachycardia is due to re-entry within the AV node, the precise contribution of the atria is unclear. Furthermore, when re-entry utilizes an accessory AV connection, both the atria and ventricles are equally critical to maintenance of re-entrant tachycardia. The two tachycardias with a normal QRS complex that occur most commonly in the fetus and neonate will be discussed.

Orthodromic Reciprocating Tachycardia

Recent investigation has shown that common paroxysmal atrial tachycardia in the fetus and neonate is a re-entrant rhythm, termed orthodromic reciprocating tachycardia. In this setting there are two limbs of the tachycardia circuit: the normal conduction system (antegrade) and the accessory AV connection (retrograde) (see Fig. 1). The tachycardia circuit is composed of these two limbs and the atrium and ventricle. During tachycardia, depolarization advances from atrium to ventricle via the normal conduction system and from the ventricle back to the atrium via the accessory connection.

In the fetus, echocardiographic features include a regular rhythm with a 1:1 AV relationship. Electrocardiographic features in the neonate include a rapid, regular heart rate with a normal QRS morphology and no evidence of AV dissociation. At tachycardia onset, the QRS complex may be transiently prolonged because of rate-related bundle branch block. Usually, P waves are not seen during tachycardia, because of the superposition of the P wave on the ST-T wave during the short tachycardia cycle length.

In the fetus and newborn, the heart rate is usually 200 to 320 beats per minute. Abrupt or paroxysmal onset of termination of tachycardia are characteristic features.

Orthodromic reciprocating tachycardia has not been reported prior to 20 weeks' gestation. It is a common problem, but its exact incidence is not known. In some infants, ventricular pre-excitation is noted during sinus rhythm. Thus, these infants have Wolff-Parkinson-White syndrome. Patients with orthodromic tachycardia who do not have pre-excitation during sinus rhythm are said to have concealed accessory connections.

The consequences of tachycardia may be life-threatening, but overall tachycardia is thought to have a good prognosis, since clinically apparent episodes cease during the first year of life. The presence of the accessory AV connection allows the potential for tachycardia, but it is the occurrence of the initiating event that determines the precise moment of tachycardia onset (see Fig. 1). Changes in the occurrence of initiating events—e.g., disappearance of atrial extrasystole during the first postnatal year—or changes in the morphologic or functional characteristics of the tachycardia circuit are important elements in the natural history of tachycardia recurrence or cessation.

Orthodromic reciprocating tachycardia provides a useful model for evaluating the relationship between morphologic and functional determinants of tachycardia, and consideration of these elements can be useful in planning treatment strategy. For example, termination of an established tachycardia episode may be accomplished by impairing conduction in the antegrade (e.g., with verapamil, adenosine phosphate or adenosine triphosphate) or retrograde (e.g., with procainamide) limbs or by interrupting the re-entry circuit with electrical stimulation (e.g., transesophageal pacing or direct current cardioversion) (Fig. 2). When necessary, treatment to prevent recurrences of tachycardia may be accomplished by prophylactic therapy to impair conduction in the antegrade (with propranolol or verapamil), retrograde (with quinidine-like

drugs), or both (with amiodarone) limbs. Alternatively, suppression of the initiating event (e.g., atrial extrasystoles) would prevent tachycardia recurrence.

Primary Atrial Tachycardia

Here the rhythm disturbance is confined to the atria, as opposed to the previous example in which nonatrial tissue was important in tachycardia maintenance. Examples of primary atrial tachycardia include atrial fibrillation, atrial flutter, and other intra-atrial re-entry and chaotic atrial rhythms (Table 1). The common features are that the rhythm disturbances are confined to the atria and they are often associated with underlying heart disease. One of the distinguishing electrocardiographic features of primary atrial tachycardias is that the P waves are usually visible, whereas for other tachycardias with normal QRS complexes they usually are not.

Atrial fibrillation occurs rarely in very young patients, whereas atrial flutter occurs more frequently. Both atrial fibrillation and atrial flutter have been reported in association with Wolff-Parkinson-White syndrome in a fetus. Atrial flutter has also been noted as a complication of prolonged umbilical venous catheterization. Electrical cardioversion may be sufficient treatment and should be employed prior to drug administration.

In ectopic atrial tachycardia, it is believed that a non-sinus atrial pacemaker controls the heart rate. These ectopic pacemakers are often responsive to changes in autonomic tone, and tachycardia rate may vary. Chaotic (multifocal) atrial tachycardia has been recognized as a distinct electrocardiographic entity characterized by atrial tachycardia (rate exceeding 100 beats per minute) with at least three different P-wave morphologies, variation in the P-R and P-P intervals, and an isoelectric baseline. In older patients it is often associated with severe cardiopulmonary disease, but in neonates the severity of the underlying disease and the clinical significance of the rhythm disturbance are more variable. Treatment strategy in ectopic and chaotic atrial tachycardia may be aimed at controlling ventricular rate with drugs that impair AV conduction (e.g., digoxin, propranolol, or verapamil). Alternatively, tachycardia may be abolished with calcium-channel blockers, type I antiarrhythmic drugs, or amiodarone (Fig. 3).

Tachycardia with Prolonged QRS Complex

Tachycardias with a prolonged QRS complex have been infrequently described in the fetus and newborn, but this is partly the result of under-recognition. From the standpoint of electrocardiographic features, these tachycardias can be categorized depending on whether QRS morphology is uniform and whether the rate is regular or irregular. Since tachycardia with a prolonged QRS complex may be due to a variety of mechanisms, it is important to think in terms of a differential diagnosis when evaluating an individual patient. The differential diagnosis includes ventricular tachycardia as well as unusual tachycardias associated with pre-excitation syndromes.

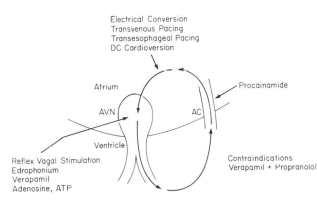

Figure 2 Treatment strategy for established orthodromic reciprocating tachycardia. In a simple way, therapy can be considered in terms of an effect on a portion of the re-entry circuit. AC = accessory atrioventricular connection; ATP = Adenosine triphosphate; AVN = atrioventricular node.

TABLE 1 Terminology for Tachycardia with Normal QRS Complex Duration

Previous	Preferred
Supraventricular tachycardia or Paroxysmal atrial tachycardia	Orthodromic reciprocating tachycardia or Re-entry within the atrioventricular node or Primary atrial tachycardia
Atrial flutter Atrial fibrillation Ectopic atrial tachycardia Intra-atrial re-entry tachycardia	Primary atrial tachycardia (with description of rate and rhythm)
Ectopic junctional tachycardia	Same

Regular Rate, Uniform QRS Morphology

The differential diagnosis of regular tachycardia with a prolonged QRS complex duration includes ventricular tachycardia, orthodromic reciprocating tachycardia with bundle branch block, and tachycardia associated with pre-excitation syndromes. At present it is usually not possible to make the distinctions from analysis of the QRS complex on standard electrocardiographic recordings. Analysis of heart rate is not useful either. In young patients, ventriculoatrial conduction may be present during ventricular tachycardia, so that this feature may not be useful in making a distinction among types of tachycardia with prolonged QRS complex duration.

Irregular Rate, Varying QRS Morphology

In patients of any age, the paradigm of irregular tachycardia is atrial fibrillation whether QRS complex duration and morphology are normal, prolonged, or vari-

able. Atrial fibrillation is infrequently reported in the fetus and neonate. When atrial fibrillation occurs in association with ventricular pre-excitation (Wolff-Parkinson-White syndrome), a prolonged QRS complex duration results. There may also be intermittent bundle branch block during atrial fibrillation, so that, in addition to irregularity of heart rate, QRS morphology may vary. In some young patients with nonsustained ventricular tachycardia, irregularity and variation in QRS morphology have been noted. *Torsade de pointes* may also be associated with variation in heart rate and QRS morphology, and this has been observed in the fetus and neonate.

The variety of mechanistic possibilities associated with tachycardia with a prolonged QRS complex makes a simple, comprehensive treatment regimen difficult. Digitalis derivatives and verapamil should not be used. For critically ill neonates with tachycardia, direct current cardioversion is the treatment of choice for established tachycardia. If direct current cardioversion is ineffective, it may be repeated following administration of lidocaine or procainamide. Cardiac pacing with a temporary transvenous pacing catheter may be useful for tachycardia conversion or prevention of tachycardia recurrence by pacing. Prior to commencing prophylactic antiarrhythmic drug therapy, a precise electrophysiologic diagnosis should be established.

SUGGESTED READING

Benson DW Jr, Dunnigan A. Treatment of pediatric patients with preexcitation syndromes. In: Benditt DG, Benson DW Jr, eds. Cardiac preexcitation syndromes: Origins, evaluation and treatment. Hingham, MA: Martinus Nijhoff, 1986:465.

Benson DW Jr, Dunnigan A, Benditt DG. Follow-up evaluation of infant paroxysmal atrial tachycardia: Transesophageal study. Circulation 1987; 76:542–549.

Kugler JD. Evaluation of pediatric patients with preexcitation syndromes. In: Benditt DG, Benson DW Jr, eds. Cardiac preexcitation syndromes: Origins, evaluation and treatment. Hingham, MA: Martinus Nijhoff, 1986:361.

Strasburger JF, Huhta JC, Carpenter RJ, et al. Doppler echocardiography in the diagnosis and management of persistent fetal arrhythmias. J Am Coll Cardiol 1986; 7:1386–1391.

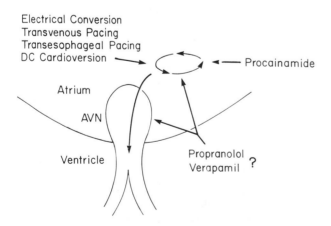

Figure 3 Treatment strategy for established primary atrial tachycardia. The aim of therapy is either to disrupt the electrophysiologic disturbance in the atrium or limit the ventricular response by impairing conduction in the atrioventricular node (AVN).

EARLY CONGENITAL SYPHILIS

CAROL I. EWING, M.B., Ch.B., B.Sc., M.R.C.P.(UK), D.C.H., D.R.C.O.G.
OM P. ARYA, M.B.B.S., D.T.M.&H., D.P.H., D.I.H., Dip. Ven.

Congenital syphilis is a totally preventable disease that still occurs today. We will outline the prevention and management of early congenital syphilis, defined as syphilis diagnosed in a patient under the age of 2 years.

PREVENTION

The Problem

In countries with established screening programs, the incidence of early congenital syphilis (ECS) has been reduced to very low levels. Only three cases were recorded in England and Wales in 1985. Screening for syphilis is not a legal requirement in all states in the United States, where 268 cases were recorded in 1985.

Early syphilis is very common in many developing countries. In Zambia, for example, where there is a high incidence of venereal syphilis in pregnant women and where a screening program is not socioeconomically possible at present, serologic tests were positive in 18.7 percent of women who aborted and 42 percent of those whose pregnancies ended in stillbirths. Fifteen cases of ECS were seen over a period of 4 weeks in the university teaching hospital in Lusaka.

A significantly high incidence of ECS contributes greatly to perinatal and infant morbidity and mortality.

Case Finding

The introduction of serologic testing for syphilis at an expectant mother's first antenatal visit is the first step toward reduction of the incidence of ECS. If a woman is thought to be at high risk of harboring venereal syphilis, serologic testing should be repeated in the third trimester to discover if the infection was being incubated at the time of the first test or if it was acquired subsequently. In the United States, high risk factors identified for the emergence of ECS were inadequate antenatal care and ethnic origin of the mother. In the United Kingdom, factors such as multiple consorts, occupation of consort, or history of a sexually transmitted disease in the expectant mother (who is often single) should alert the obstetrician to the possibility of syphilitic infection.

Contrary to prior opinion, it has been shown in recent years that transplacental infection by *Treponema pallidum* can occur at much earlier stages of pregnancy. Also, the stage of maternal syphilis is important in determining the outcome of pregnancy. If the mother has untreated primary or secondary disease, infectivity is usually 100 percent whereas in late maternal syphilis (of more than 2 years' duration), fetal infection is uncommon.

To test the efficacy of a screening program, one can look at the Vertical Transmission Index. This is the number of cases of congenital syphilis diagnosed in those under 1 year of age per 1,000 cases of primary and secondary syphilis confirmed in mothers in the preceding year. Indices above 20 to 25 should prompt evaluation of maternal health care in that population.

Serologic Testing of the Expectant Mother

This usually consists of a nontreponemal test such as the rapid plasma reagin (RPR) or the Venereal Disease Research Laboratory (VDRL) test. If the RPR or the VDRL test is positive, the expectant mother should be asked for a detailed history and given a thorough clinical examination. Serologic confirmation should be obtained by use of the specific tests, such as the *Treponema pallidum* hemagglutination assay or the fluorescent treponemal antibody absorption test.

Treatment of the Expectant Mother

If the diagnosis is confirmed or if the disease cannot be excluded, the woman should be given appropriate treatment with the aim of completing the course of antibiotic at least 2 weeks before delivery. However, to ensure the prevention of the stigmata of congenital syphilis, one should aim to complete treatment of the mother during the first trimester.

In all trimesters of pregnancy, dosage regimens are the same as for the treatment of nonpregnant patients. Table 1 shows the minimum treatment regimens defined by the World Health Organization (1982), and the physician should not use less than the recommended dosages. Indeed, many specialists use higher dosage regimens, particularly if the nervous system is involved.

A problem arises if the mother has a history of penicillin allergy. The recommended alternative antibiotic is erythromycin (not estolate), although there is uncertainty about its efficacy during pregnancy and in the prevention of congenital syphilis.

Following treatment of the mother, serologic testing should be repeated at monthly intervals until delivery; a second course of treatment is given if there is any evidence of reinfection, serologic relapse (e.g., a fourfold rise in titer), or serologic resistance; thereafter the follow-up is as for nonpregnant patients. Blood tests should be repeated during subsequent pregnancies. If the nontreponemal tests have become negative and the patient is known to have received adequate treatment, there is no need for further therapy. The infant should, however, be followed up as described below.

Failure of Treatment as Regards the Outcome of Pregnancy

Such failure of treatment may be due to (1) an already severely diseased fetus that may abort shortly after antibiotic treatment; (2) reinfection or possible relapse in the mother prior to delivery of the infant; (3) treatment not

TABLE 1 Treatment of Syphilis in the Expectant Mother

Type of Syphilis	Aqueous Procaine Penicillin G	Benzathine Penicillin G*
Early (primary, secondary, early latent, i.e., less than 2 yr duration)	0.6 Megaunit IM daily for at least 10 days	OR 2.4 Megaunits at one session (1.2 megaunits IM into each buttock)
Late latent syphilis and late benign syphilis	0.6 Megaunit IM daily for at least 15 days	OR 2.4 Megaunits IM once weekly for 3 weeks
Cardiovascular syphilis and neurosyphilis	0.6 Megaunit IM daily for at least 20 days	–

* Benzathine penicillin does not penetrate into the CSF and therefore should be used only if the CSF is normal. It is no longer available in the United Kingdom.

completed at least 2 weeks before delivery; (4) inadequate or ineffective treatment, such as with erythromycin; and (5) precipitation of a Jarisch-Herxheimer reaction.

MANAGEMENT OF THE INFANT

Babies in Whom Follow-Up Is Adequate

All babies of seropositive mothers who have been adequately treated before or during pregnancy should be examined at birth and at monthly intervals until RPR or VDRL tests are confirmed as negative. The nontreponemal antibodies that are carried over from the mother to the infant usually fall fourfold within 2 months and disappear by 6 months after birth. Treatment is necessary only if there is a rise or persistence of serologic titer, clinical or radiologic evidence of the disease.

Other Criteria for Treatment

Infants should be treated at birth if (1) treatment of the mother was inadequate, late, or unknown, including treatment of the mother with erythromycin; or if (2) clinical and serologic follow-up of the child cannot be ensured.

Awareness of the Condition

The pediatrician must maintain a high index of suspicion of ECS, particularly in countries where syphilis is prevalent. There is a wide variation in the clinical presentation of ECS when there has been failure to diagnose and treat venereal syphilis in the expectant mother. Moreover, infants of untreated mothers may be asymptomatic at birth. Table 2 shows the physical symptoms and signs that should alert the pediatrician to consider ECS in the differential diagnosis.

To confirm the diagnosis of ECS, demonstration of *Treponema pallidum* by dark-field microscopic examination (for example, of the fluid from bullous lesions that may occur on the palms or soles and are full of spirochetes) provides a definite criterion for treatment. When treponemes cannot be demonstrated, confirmation of the diagnosis relies on serologic tests. A sample of cord blood is routinely obtained whenever congenital syphilis is a pos-

sibility. However, because cord blood can be easily contaminated by maternal blood or mucoid material from the outer surface of the cord, it is preferable to take blood directly from the infant. In view of the possibility of maternal-fetal transfer of antibodies (excluding IgM) and in the absence of positive lesions on dark-field microscopy, rising titers of RPR or VDRL tests should be sought to confirm active disease. A titer of the RPR or VDRL test that is higher in the infant than in the mother also indicates congenital syphilis. There is much debate as to the diagnostic value of the fluorescent treponemal antibody absorption IgM test. In most cases and in the absence of placental leakage, a positive fluorescent treponemal antibody absorption IgM test confirms congenital syphilis. The test is very sensitive in infants who have symptomatic syphilis at birth but may give false-negative results in those with delayed onset of the disease. Also, any congenital infection associated with an elevated anti-IgG IgM from the fetus may result in a false-positive fluorescent treponemal antibody absorption IgM test. In these cases the specific treponemal fraction may be detected by the 19S IgM fluorescent treponemal antibody test.

The infant may have a normochromic normocytic anemia; sometimes a reticulocytosis is present. Autoimmune hemolysis can be associated with cryoglobulinemia, macroglobulinemia, or the presence of circulating immune complexes. Thrombocytopenia may lead to life-threatening bleeding episodes. Liver function tests may

TABLE 2 Symptoms and Signs of Early Congenital Syphilis

Failure to thrive
Hematologic abnormalities
Condylomata lata
Snuffles (may be blood-stained)
Maculopapular/exfoliative/vesicobullous rash
Osteochondritis/periostitis
Hepatosplenomegaly
Generalized lymphadenopathy
Perioral and perianal fissures
Mucous patches
Central nervous system signs
Cerebrospinal fluid abnormalities
Nephrotic syndrome or glomerulonephritis

show a conjugated hyperbilirubinemia as well as raised serum glutamic-oxaloacetic and serum glutamic-pyruvic transaminase values.

Radiologic changes are reasonably specific for ECS and may be associated with clinical signs of epiphyseal swelling and tenderness of long bones. Radiologic changes occur in areas of rapid bone growth, such as the periosteum and at the metaphyseal-epiphyseal junctions. Cortical destruction may occur bilaterally on the medial aspect of the upper ends of the tibia, giving the characteristic rat-bite or Wimberger's sign. Later, parallel lines or rarefaction may appear in the diaphysis, giving a "celery-stick" appearance. When there is new bone formation, the "onion-peel" periosteal changes are seen. If ECS is a diagnostic possibility, a skeletal survey should be included as part of an investigative screening.

Examination of the cerebrospinal fluid, including the VDRL test, must be undertaken in all children, especially in the presence of neurologic features when ECS is suspected or confirmed, since this will determine the nature and duration of treatment. Apart from the VDRL reactivity, the changes include a lymphocytosis and a raised protein level. Untreated neurosyphilis can lead to a chronic meningovascular process that results in hydrocephalus, cranial nerve palsies, and cerebral infarction, even in the first year of life.

Human Immunodeficiency Virus (HIV) Infection and Congenital Syphilis

The immunosuppression associated with concurrent HIV infection may alter the natural history of syphilitic infection, which may pursue a more aggressive course. At the present time there is not enough information on the interaction between these two infections, including diagnostic and therapeutic implications, in the infant.

Treatment

The child should be admitted to the hospital. In ECS, procaine or crystalline penicillin G, 50,000 U per kilogram of body weight (the latter in two divided doses), should be given intramuscularly daily for 10 days; (crystalline penicillin G can be given intravenously). Crystalline penicillin G, given in two divided doses intravenously daily for at least 10 days, is the preferred treatment if the cerebrospinal fluid is abnormal or if there is a possibility of concurrent HIV infection.

Alternatively, benzathine penicillin, 50,000 U per kilogram of body weight, given intramuscularly in a single

dose, can be used provided the cerebrospinal fluid is normal; the drug does not penetrate into the cerebrospinal fluid. (Benzathine penicillin is no longer available in the United Kingdom.)

Prognosis

Most children respond well to the above treatment. Full recovery may be slow in those who are severely affected. The prognosis is worse in infants born with actual physical signs of the disease. Some of the seriously ill infants may succumb to intercurrent infection, such as pneumonia or gastroenteritis.

Follow-Up of Infants

Infants should be followed up for at least 2 years at 3-month intervals. RPR and VDRL titers will fall, with eventual reversion to negative serologic results.

Resolution of bone lesions and hepatosplenomegaly is usually achieved by about 3 months after treatment. Lumbar puncture should be repeated if the cerebrospinal fluid was abnormal before treatment. If all tests, including cerebrospinal fluid, are normal at the end of 2 years, the child can be discharged.

SUGGESTED READING

Adler MW. Pregnancy and the neonate. Br Med J 1984; 288:624–627.

Arya OP, Osoba AO, Bennett FJ. Syphilis. Tropical venereology. 2nd ed. Edinburgh: Churchill Livingstone, 1988: 39–132.

Ewing CI, Roberts C, Davidson DC, Arya OP. Early congenital syphilis still occurs. Arch Dis Child 1985; 60:1128–1133.

Harter CA, Benirschke K. Fetal syphilis in the first trimester. Am J Obstet Gynecol 1976; 124:705–711.

Hashisaki P, Wertzberger GG, Conrad GL, Nichols CR. Erythromycin failure in the treatment of syphilis in a pregnant woman. Sex Transm Dis 1983; 10:36–38.

Hira SK, Hira RS. Congenital syphilis. In: Osoba AO, ed. Clinical tropical medicine and communicable diseases 2:1. London: WB Saunders, 1987: 113–127.

Mascola L, Pelosi R, Blount JH, et al. Congenital syphilis. Why is it still occurring? JAMA 1984; 252:1719–1722.

Murphy KF, Patamasucon P. Congenital syphilis. In: Holmes KK, Mardh PA, Sparking PF, Weisner PJ, eds. Sexually transmitted diseases. New York: McGraw-Hill, 1984:352–371.

Rosen EU, Richardson NJ. A reappraisal of the value of the IgM fluorescent treponemal antibody absorption test in a diagnosis of congenital syphilis. J Pediatr 1975; 87:38–42.

Thompson SE. Treatment of syphilis in pregnancy. J Am Vener Dis Assoc 1976; 3:159–167.

World Health Organization. Treponemal infections. Repeat of a WHO scientific group. Tech Rep Ser 674, Geneva, 1982.

EARLY METABOLIC ACIDOSIS

HENRIK EKBLAD, M.D., Ph.D.
PENTTI KERO, M.D., Ph.D.
JUKKA TAKALA, M.D., Ph.D.

In 1916 Ylppö showed that premature infants readily develop acidosis, and in 1964 Kildeberg (1964a) introduced the term "late metabolic acidosis" to describe apparently healthy premature infants with metabolic acidosis and growth failure at 1 to 3 weeks of age. Metabolic acidosis in premature infants has subsequently been described by several groups (Kerpel-Fronius et al, 1970; Sulyok et al, 1972). *Acidosis in premature infants during the first week of life is primarily related to perinatal events and respiratory function, while "late metabolic acidosis" seems to be due to immature renal function* (Kildeberg, 1964b; Kerpel-Fronius et al, 1970; Sulyok et al, 1972; Svenningsen, 1974; Zilleruelo et al, 1986).

The treatment of metabolic acidosis is a relatively common clinical problem in critically ill premature infants during the first days of life. The use of "push" doses of hypertonic sodium bicarbonate to correct acidosis has been criticized. It brings about abrupt rises in osmolality, which may adversely affect the developing central nervous system (Finberg, 1977). Sodium acetate is a potential alternative to bicarbonate, since it is rapidly converted to bicarbonate in the body. A slow and continuous infusion of base, without the problems of incompatibility associated with sodium bicarbonate, is the practical advantage of acetate in fluid therapy for the neonate.

RENAL FUNCTION AND ACID-BASE BALANCE

The kidney regulates acid-base balance by reabsorption of filtered bicarbonate and excretion of hydrogen ion as titratable acid and ammonia. The urine is mainly acidified in the proximal tubule by active hydrogen ion secretion via Na^+-H^+ exchange. Several mechanisms influence the acidification process: extracellular water compartment, plasma potassium level, arterial PCO_2, luminal bicarbonate concentration, peritubular pH, luminal flow rate, serum calcium concentration, acid load, and mineralocorticoid and parathyroid hormone activity (Toto, 1986).

The mechanism for the limited renal response to metabolic acidosis in premature infants is unknown. The "physiologic acidosis" in these infants is probably due to a low renal threshold level for plasma bicarbonate. The capacity to excrete hydrogen ions is reduced, whereas the tubular reabsorption of bicarbonate is presumably adequate (Kerpel-Fronius et al, 1970; Sulyok et al, 1972; Svenningsen, 1974; Schwartz et al, 1979; Zilleruelo et al, 1986). Sulyok and Varga (1978) investigated the relationship between renal bicarbonate threshold and urinary sodium loss in 1- to 6-week-old premature infants. They proposed that the high urinary sodium excretion during the first 2 weeks of life may, at least in part, account for the low renal threshold bicarbonate reabsorption. This finding suggests that renal sodium handling is important in the maintenance of acid-base balance.

HEMODYNAMICS, FLUID BALANCE, AND ACID-BASE BALANCE

Renal function is one determinant of acid-base balance; others include pulmonary gas exchange, tissue perfusion, and nutrition. Acid-base balance during the first week of life is more dependent on other factors than on renal function. Disturbances of hydrogen ion homeostasis occur frequently in premature infants during the first week of life, most typically taking the form of a combined respiratory and metabolic acidosis (Kildeberg, 1964b). Acidosis due to hypercapnia can be treated by appropriate ventilatory support. The maintenance of adequate cardiac output, peripheral perfusion, and nutrition, as well as control of infection, all reduce the risk of metabolic acidosis in the critically ill premature infant.

One of the premises in seeking an appropriate internal milieu for the premature infant is stable osmolality, which means that wide variations in blood concentrations of Na^+, K^+, PCO_2, HCO_3^-, and glucose are undesirable (Avery and Hodson, 1966; Finberg, 1977). Osmoregulation in the neonate is complex since the urine concentrating mechanism is limited, insensible water loss is high, and water turnover is high. Consequently, the neonate is prone to wide swings in plasma osmolality (Bevan, 1978).

Changes in osmolar concentration are especially hazardous to the central nervous system (Finberg, 1977). Osmolar concentration gradients between plasma and the central nervous system can be deleterious: high plasma osmolality may cause cerebral hemorrhage, and a gradient in the opposite direction will result in cerebral edema.

Usher (1963) introduced the early administration of sodium bicarbonate for the correction of acidosis in premature infants suffering from the respiratory distress syndrome. Subsequently the liberal use of rapid infusions of bicarbonate became a custom (Hobel et al, 1972).

Laboratory and experimental studies indicate that rapid infusion of hypertonic sodium bicarbonate may actually worsen the acidosis temporarily, owing to a rapid increase in PCO_2 level and a consequent fall in pH, and that it also causes sharp fluctuations in cerebrospinal fluid pressure (Kravath et al, 1970; Steichen and Kleinman, 1977). Other studies show no beneficial effects from rapid infusion of sodium bicarbonate (Bland et al, 1975; Corbet et al, 1977). Studies in neonates indicate that the use of rapid infusion of sodium bicarbonate may be related to the development of intraventricular hemorrhage (Papile et al, 1978; Dykes et al, 1980).

SODIUM ACETATE AND METABOLIC ACIDOSIS

Sodium bicarbonate has practical disadvantages, such as incompatibility with calcium and magnesium, that make a slow and continuous infusion difficult (Kirkendol et al, 1980). Acetate is rapidly converted to bicarbonate in man

(Mudge et al, 1949). It has widely replaced bicarbonate in dialysis. The amounts used in dialysis may elevate the blood acetate concentration and lower the blood pressure, probably by vasodilatation (Kirkendol et al, 1977). When given as a slow and continuous infusion, the blood concentrations are low and reduction of the blood pressure has not been observed (Kirkendol et al, 1978; Ekblad et al, 1987a). In acute hypoxia the use of sodium acetate can be criticized because of its aerobic metabolism (Randle et al, 1970).

In premature infants with gestational ages between 27 and 34 weeks treated in incubators with high air humidity, hemodynamics, fluid balance, and sodium balance remained stable with low fluid intake and a sodium supply of 3 to 4 mmol per kilogram daily from the first day of life (Ekblad et al, 1987a). Fluid restriction and early enteral feeding decreased the total amount of glucose given parenterally, and thereby the risk of hyperglycemia. Under these conditions, glucose homeostasis was efficiently maintained, and hydration by intravenous infusion of 5 and 10 percent glucose appeared equally well tolerated (Ekblad et al, 1987b).

We have investigated whether a slow infusion of sodium acetate is suitable for the prevention and correction of metabolic acidosis and the supply of sodium in the premature infant (Ekblad et al, 1985). The study population consisted of appropriate-for-gestational age infants with gestational ages between 27 and 34 weeks, and birth weights between 925 and 2,420 g. Seven infants of 11 developed the respiratory distress syndrome; all were treated in incubators with high air humidity to minimize insensible water loss. Fluid intake was low (Table 1), consisting of intravenous infusion of 5 percent glucose from the first day of life. Small amounts of 5 percent glucose and human milk were added enterally beginning on the second to third day of life. The daily intravenous supply of sodium was set at 3 mmol per kilogram, and consisted of sodium acetate during the first day of life and both sodium acetate and sodium chloride thereafter (Table 1).

The use of sodium acetate as a slow and continuous infusion of base was both efficient and practical in preventing metabolic acidosis (Table 2). The effect on acidosis was demonstrated by the number of infants with a pH of less than 7.30 at different periods, with values as follows: at 1 to 3 hours, four of 11; at 24 hours, two of 11; at 48 hours, one of 11; and at 72 hours, one of 11. The metabolic component was characterized by the base deficit: the number of infants with a base deficit of more than five was four of 11 at 1 to 3 hours, one of 11 at 24 hours, one of 11 at 48 hours, and zero of 11 at 72 hours. Hypercapnia was never the cause of acidosis. The serum sodium concentrations were normal, with no values below 130 or above 150 mmol per liter (Table 2). Weight loss was appropriate and fell to a mean of 94 percent of birth weight by 72 hours of age.

We propose that the protocol of (1) low fluid intake (first day, 50 ml per kilogram; second day, 70 ml per kilogram; third day, 90 ml per kilogram; fourth day, 110 ml per kilogram;(2) high air humidity minimizing insensible water loss; (3) a sodium supply of 3 mmol per kilo-

TABLE 1 Fluid and Sodium Intake

Day	Planned Intake mL/kg	Actual Intake* mL/kg	(range)	Sodium Acetate mmol/kg	Sodium Chloride mmol/kg
1	50	49 ± 2.8	(43–55)	3.0	—
2	70	71 ± 8.7	(61–90)	1.5	1.5
3	90	97 ± 16.0	(65–131)	—	3.0
4	110	122 ± 17.8	(88–149)	—	3.0

* Values are mean ± SD.

TABLE 2 Acid-Base Balance, Serum Lactate Concentrations, and Serum Sodium Concentrations*

	Age (Hours)			
	1 – 3	24	48	72
pH range	7.34 ± 0.07 7.26 – 7.45	7.37 ± 0.07 7.24 – 7.47	7.38 ± 0.06 7.28 – 7.45	7.37 ± 0.05 7.29 – 7.43
P_{CO_2} (kPa) range	5.24 ± 1.14 3.4 – 6.7	5.13 ± 0.69 4.0 – 6.7	5.25 ± 0.97 3.9 – 7.4	5.63 ± 1.21 4.2 – 7.3
Base excess, mmol/L range	-4.47 ± 2.21 -8.8 – 1.6	-1.93 ± 3.04 -9.9 – 1.1	-1.48 ± 3.36 -5.7 – 5.1	-1.08 ± 2.73 -3.4 – 3.1
Lactate, mmol/L range	2.9 ± 2.85 1.3 – 10.3	2.9 ± 3.02 1.2 – 11.2	2.0 ± 0.51 1.2 – 2.8	1.6 ± 0.81 0.8 – 2.9
Sodium, mmol/L range	133 – 141	131 – 141	137 – 145	139 – 144

* Values are mean ± SD.

gram per day from the first day of life, and (4) slow infusion of sodium acetate to prevent metabolic acidosis yields suitable guidelines for planning fluid and electrolyte therapy for the premature infant with a gestational age between 27 and 34 weeks.

SUGGESTED READING

Avery ME, Hodson WA. The first drink reconsidered. J Pediatr 1966; 68:1008–1010.

Bevan DR. Osmometry. 2. Osmoregulation. Anaesthesia 1978; 33:801–808.

Bland RD, Clarke TL, Harden LB. Rapid infusion of sodium bicarbonate and albumin into high-risk premature infants soon after birth: A controlled, prospective trial. Am J Obstet Gynecol 1975; 124:263–267.

Corbet AJ, Adams JM, Kenny JD, et al. Controlled trial of bicarbonate therapy in high-risk premature newborn infants. J Pediatr 1977; 91:771–776.

Dykes FD, Lazzara A, Ahmann P, et al. Intraventricular hemorrhage: A prospective evaluation of etiopathogenesis. Pediatrics 1980; 66:42–49.

Ekblad H, Kero P, Takala J, et al. Water, sodium and acid-base balance in premature infants: Therapeutical aspects. Acta Paediatr Scand 1987a; 76:47–53.

Ekblad H, Kero P, Takala J. Stable glucose balance in premature infants with fluid restriction and early enteral feeding. Acta Paediatr Scand 1987b; 76:438–443.

Ekblad H, Kero P, Takala J. Stable glucose balance in premature infants with fluid restriction and early enteral feeding. Acta Paediatr Scand, in press.

Finberg L. The relationship of intravenous infusions and intracranial hemorrhage—a commentary. J Pediatr 1977; 91:777–778.

Hobel CJ, Oh W, Hyvarinen MA, et al. Early versus late treatment of neonatal acidosis in low-birth-weight infants: Relation to respiratory distress syndrome. J Pediatr 1972; 81:1178–1187.

Kerpel-Fronius E, Heim T, Sulyok E. The development of the renal acidifying processes and their relation to acidosis in low-birth-weight infants. Biol Neonate 1970; 15:156–168.

Kildeberg P. Disturbances of hydrogen ion balance occurring in premature infants. II. Late metabolic acidosis. Acta Paediatr 1964a; 53:517–526.

Kildeberg P. Disturbances of hydrogen ion balance occurring in premature infants. I. Early types of acidosis. Acta Paediatr 1964b;53:505–516.

Kirkendol PL, Devia CJ, Bower JD, Holbert RD. A comparison of the cardiovascular effects of sodium acetate, sodium bicarbonate and other potential sources of fixed base in hemodialysate solutions. Trans Am Soc Artif Intern Organs 1977; 23:399–405.

Kirkendol PL, Robie NW, Gonzalez FM, Devia CJ. Cardiac and vascular effects of infused sodium acetate in dogs. Trans Am Soc Artif Intern Organs 1978; 24:714–718.

Kirkendol PL, Starrs J, Gonzalez FM. The effects of acetate, lactate, succinate and gluconate on plasma pH and electrolytes in dogs. Trans Am Soc Artif Intern Organs 1980; 26:323–327.

Kravath RE, Aharon AS, Abal G, Finberg L. Clinically significant physiologic changes from rapidly administered hypertonic solutions: Acute osmol poisoning. Pediatrics 1970; 46:267–275.

Mudge GH, Manning JA, Gilman A. Sodium acetate as a source of fixed base. Proc Soc Exp Biol Med 1949; 71:136–138.

Papile L, Burstein J, Burstein R, et al. Relationship of intravenous sodium bicarbonate infusions and cerebral intraventricular hemorrhage. J Pediatr 1978; 93:834–836.

Randle PJ, England PJ, Denton RM. Control of the tricarboxylate cycle and its interactions with glycolysis during acetate utilization in rat heart. Biochem J 1970; 117:677–695.

Schwartz GJ, Haycock GB, Edelmann CM Jr, Spitzer A. Late metabolic acidosis: A reassessment of the definition. J Pediatr 1979; 95:102–107.

Steichen JJ, Kleinman LI. Studies in acid-base balance. I. Effect of alkali therapy in newborn dogs with mechanically fixed ventilation. J Pediatr 1977; 91:287–291.

Sulyok E, Heim T, Soltész G, Jászai V. The influence of maturity on renal control of acidosis in newborn infants. Biol Neonate 1972; 21:418–435.

Sulyok E, Varga F. Relationship of renal threshold for bicarbonate reabsorption to urinary sodium excretion in premature infants. Acta Paediatr Acad Sci Hung 1978; 19:281–284.

Svenningsen NW. Renal acid-base titration studies in infants with and without metabolic acidosis in the postneonatal period. Pediatr Res 1974; 8:659–672.

Toto RD. Metabolic acid-base disorders. In: Kokko JP, Tannen RL, eds. Fluids and electrolytes. Philadelphia: WB Saunders, 1986:229.

Usher R. Reduction of mortality from respiratory distress syndrome of prematurity with early administration of intravenous glucose and sodium bicarbonate. Pediatrics 1963; 32:966–975.

Ylppö A. Neugeborenen-, Hunger- und Intoxikationsacidosis in ihren Beziehungen zueinander. Studien uber Acidosis bei Säuglingen, insbesondere im Lichte des Wasserstoffionen-"Stoffwechsels." Zeitschr Kinderheilk 1916; 14:1–184.

Zilleruelo G, Sultan S, Bancalari E, et al. Renal bicarbonate handling in low birth weight infants during metabolic acidosis. Biol Neonate 1986; 49:132–139.

GASTROESOPHAGEAL REFLUX

JOHN J. HERBST, M.D.
LOUIS L. MIZELL, M.D.

Most infants spit up occasionally, but in some, regurgitation can be so severe that they are unable to retain adequate calories and fail to grow. They may develop aspiration pneumonia, esophagitis, blood loss, stricture, or dysphagia.

Newborn intensive care nurseries have a high proportion of very ill infants who are likely to have apnea, worsening pulmonary disease, gagging, and choking as common presenting symptoms of reflux. In such a setting it is often difficult to determine whether gastroesophageal reflux is causing apnea and other pulmonary symptoms or whether these problems are primarily due to prematurity, respiratory distress syndrome, or sepsis, with reflux and vomiting occurring as late secondary or even agonal events.

FACTORS FAVORING REFLUX

Factors that may enhance the severity of reflux in these infants include problems inherent in the physiology of the premature or sick newborn (Table 1). Pressures in the lower esophageal sphincter are lower in infants and prematures, and the sphincter is shorter and predominantly intrathoracic. These factors all decrease the efficiency of the sphincter. Swallowing saliva initiates esophageal peristalsis that clears the esophagus, and the saliva washes any remaining gastric acid into the stomach. Esophageal clearance is impaired in neonates because salivation is less copious in neonates and prematures. Clearance of refluxed material from the esophagus is also inhibited because esophageal peristalsis is uncoordinated in premature infants. Very small infants have poor gastric emptying and intestinal peristalsis, usually described as obstipation of the premature. The associated distention and increased abdominal pressure predispose to reflux. Pharyngeal clearance and swallowing mechanisms are not well coordinated in premature infants, and aspiration of refluxed material during inspiration occurs more frequently in neonates. The resultant aspiration pneumonia may produce radiologic changes that mimic bronchopulmonary dysplasia. Infants have sensitive chemoreceptors in the esophagus and larynx which, when stimulated by mechanical means, weak acid solutions, or milk from other species (including formula), may cause apnea and bradycardia.

Factors associated with illnesses common to the neonatal intensive care unit also encourage reflux: wide swings in thoracic and abdominal pressures among infants with respiratory distress, and abdominal distention and poor gastric emptying related to sepsis or necrotizing enterocolitis. These infants have a high incidence of cerebral anoxia and intracranial bleeding associated with intracranial hypertension that may lower esophageal sphincter pressure and encourage reflux. Theophylline, a drug used to prevent central apnea, also decreases lower esophageal sphincter pressure and encourages reflux.

Despite all this, our own experience indicates that premature and full-term infants under 6 weeks of age do not usually have a higher incidence of reflux than normal older children. However, once reflux occurs, the extent and severity of symptoms are often exacerbated by the factors noted.

CLINICAL FEATURES

Rarely, regurgitating infants may have blood-tinged vomitus or even coffee-ground–appearing emesis. This indicates severe esophagitis and is usually associated with multiple continuing symptoms of reflux.

Signs of recurrent aspiration pneumonia should be actively sought, since vomiting is often not a prominent symptom and it is difficult to separate the findings of bronchopulmonary dysplasia from those of aspiration on x-ray examination. Rapid changes in radiologic findings are often noted if formula is aspirated from the pharynx or trachea.

In full-term infants, reflux to the pharynx may be associated with gagging, opisthotonos or arm movements that may resemble seizures. These actions are usually not associated with massive aspiration and may be part of an exaggerated response to minor or aborted aspiration. In sick or premature infants these findings are often absent,

TABLE 1 Factors Encouraging Reflux

Related to early development:
  Decreased esophageal sphincter pressure
  Shorter esophageal sphincter
  Thoracic position of sphincter
  Increased abdominal pressure
  Poor esophageal clearance

Related to illness in neonates:
  Increased abdominal pressure with dyspnea
  Abdominal distention
  Poor gastric emptying
  Central nervous system disease

so that bradycardia and apnea may be the only signs, possibly mediated by stimulation of receptors in the larynx and esophagus by refluxed gastric contents.

DIAGNOSTIC TESTS

If symptoms are not immediately life-threatening, it is reasonable to stop oral feedings and maintain nutrition by shifting to continuous nasojejunal or total parenteral nutrition for a short period to see if symptoms improve.

An upper gastrointestinal series with fluoroscopy is not often feasible in neonatal intensive care units, especially if the patient is on a respirator, but a small amount of barium can be instilled into the stomach and portable x-ray films obtained to document the absence of mechanical obstruction.

Reflux can be documented by monitoring esophageal pH. Milk feeding will neutralize gastric acidity for about an hour, but detection of postprandial reflux in the rare achlorhydric premature can be facilitated by a small feeding of apple juice, which is weakly acidic.

Since the esophageal pH probe is only 1.4 mm in diameter, it is well tolerated by even the smallest infant. The temporal occurrence of unusual events, such as apnea or bradycardia, should be noted on the pH record. In some patients, refluxed material may induce laryngospasm and obstructive apnea. Stimulation of the pharyngeal area with a nasogastric tube can cause the same effect in many small premature infants. *If episodes of apnea or bradycardia are not simultaneous with documented reflux, it is highly unlikely that the apnea is related to reflux.*

In patients with a history of hematemesis or chronic blood loss, esophagoscopy may be necessary to document gross esophagitis. Compression of the airway by the endoscope can be a major problem in smaller neonates, but we have found it possible to view the esophagus by using a pediatric flexible endoscope in infants as small as 1,800 g. In smaller patients, use of the small-diameter flexible bronchoscope, with manual insufflation of air through the suction port, has allowed visualization of the esophagus.

Esophageal biopsies (usually using a Rubin tube) obtained 2 cm above the lower esophageal sphincter can be taken to evaluate the severity of esophagitis. Among prematures, the dermal papillae are often widely spaced, even with esophagitis, and the most obvious early sign is a marked increase of the germinative layer of the epithelium from a normal 10 percent to more than 50 percent of the thickness of the mucosa. In more severe cases, polymorphonuclear leukocytes and eosinophils are present in the mucosa.

Diagnostic tests less useful in the newborn period in our experience include the gastric scintiscan and esophageal manometry.

Detection of formula in pharyngeal or endotracheal aspirates should heighten suspicions of reflux. *Detection of lipid-laden macrophages in tracheal aspirates is a more sensitive sign of aspiration of milk.* It has recently been suggested that assaying endotracheal aspirations for lactose can also be a very sensitive and specific test of aspiration.

MEDICAL TREATMENT

Treatment of gastroesophageal reflux in neonates is based upon the same principles used in older patients but adapted to their special situation (Table 2). Placing the patient prone with the head elevated is an effective maneuver. We find that this is easily accomplished in an Isolette or radiant warmer by placing the child prone on a small padded board with the cephalic end raised 30 degrees. The infant's position can be maintained by use of a cloth harness anchored to the board that passes between the legs and about the chest and is secured with Velcro. Alternatively, the infant can be placed so as to straddle a padded peg. Such a position does not interfere with the use of a respirator or other care. If the patient is being fed, it is often *useful to switch to constant gastric or transpyloric gavage feeding.* In rare cases parenteral nutrition might be used to minimize gastric contents. It is wise to check for significant gastric residual with nasogastric feedings or for reflux of formula into the stomach in the case of nasojejunal feedings. In a few rare instances, we have even employed constant or intermittent gastric aspiration to prevent reflux of basal gastric secretions.

When considering the use of drugs to treat gastroesophageal reflux in very small infants, one is faced with the common problem that most drugs are not specifically recommended or even approved for this age group. Considering the seriousness of complications of reflux and that the surgical approach involves major abdominal surgery, we feel that the cautious use of drugs to augment therapy is reasonable.

If there is evidence suggestive of esophagitis, antacids or cimetidine can be used. One or 2 ml of antacids are administered every 2 to 3 hours or midway between feedings. Alternatively, 20 mg per kilogram per day of cimetidine given in three doses may be used. Although we have not observed adverse side effects of cimetidine in prematures, we do watch closely for signs of sedation or leukopenia, known but rare complications. Antacids, on the other hand, may in some instances be associated with bezoars or diarrhea. Because of the amounts of antacids used, it is wise to monitor serum calcium, phosphorus, and magnesium levels.

Drugs that stimulate motor function (e.g., bethanechol, metoclopramide) have been widely used in older infants and children. The rationale is that they stimulate gastric emptying, which is clearly delayed in approximately two-thirds of children and adults with reflux. These drugs also stimulate esophageal motor activity to increase esophageal sphincter pressure and thus may stimulate esophageal peristaltic waves to clear the esophagus of gastric contents. Metoclopramide is used most often, partially because it is available as a syrup. We use a dose of 0.1 mg per kilogram every 8 hours, which may be increased to every 6 hours. Doses of 2 mg per kilogram have been used to suppress vomiting after chemotherapy, suggesting a high toxic-therapeutic ratio. Since the drug is partially metabolized in the liver and there are few pharmacokinetic studies in the newborn, we routinely observe the infant carefully for toxic side effects such as irritability, lethargy, or extrapyramidal signs. A rare case of irritability is the only toxic effect we have observed. The recommended dose of bethanechol is 8.7 mg per square meter of body surface area per day, divided into three doses given one-half hour before feedings. There are no oral liquid preparations, and so it is usually easiest to dilute the intramuscular preparation to 1 mg per milliliter.

SURGICAL THERAPY

Most patients improve if treated with one or more of the aforementioned therapies, but a small number continue to have symptoms even after a prolonged trial of intensive medical therapy (usually 6 weeks). In these patients, surgical correction of reflux must be considered. If the patient continues to have major life-threatening complications, such as repeated bouts of choking, apnea, laryngospasm, or deteriorating lung function and failure to thrive due to continuous aspiration of refluxed material, we consider an early surgical approach.

The Nissen fundoplication or a modification employing a partial wrap is the usual surgical procedure. Infants of 1 to 1.5 kg have tolerated the procedure well, even when they require the constant use of mechanical respirators. In several cases, not until severe reflux was surgically con-

TABLE 2   Therapy of Gastroesophageal Reflux

Medical
  Positioning
  Feeding technique
    Small frequent bolus
    Continuous nasogastric feeding
    Continuous nasojejunal feeding
    Parenteral nutrition

  Drugs
    Antacids
    Cimetidine
    Bethanechol
    Metoclopramide

Surgical
  Nissen fundoplication

trolled did the pulmonary status improve so that FiO_2 could be reduced and the patient weaned from the respirator. In other patients the pulmonary disorder has proved to be a combination of bronchopulmonary dysplasia and chronic aspiration. The improvement in the immediate postoperative period in these cases, while marked, was less dramatic but consisted of a cessation of sudden deterioration in pulmonary function associated with increased infiltrates on the chest x-ray film.

The early results of surgery indicate that we are able to control vomiting and reflux in approximately 95 percent of cases. Several other centers have had similar results with a surgical mortality rate of less than 1 percent. Several centers, including ours, have performed over 100 operations each without a death, despite the inclusion of extremely sick infants on supplemental oxygen or respirators.

One concern has been the long-term control of reflux. Evidence from the adult literature indicates that approximately one-half of the patients experience return of some reflux symptoms within 5 years. In surgical follow-up of our patients who underwent antireflux surgery a mean of 5.7 years previously, reflux was still controlled in all but one. As a group, they have actually experienced less reflux on prolonged pH testing than do normal infants. Parents have been universally satisfied, but approximately one-third of the children have had some minor problems, such as minor gas bloat, inability to burp or vomit, a tendency to gag occasionally on eating fresh vegetables or nuts, or requiring more time to eat than their siblings.

Thus, most small infants with reflux can be successfully managed by medical therapy alone. Those who do not respond and have serious or life-threatening complications of their gastroesophageal reflux should be considered for a surgical antireflux procedure. The surgical control of reflux is excellent, even after prolonged follow-up, but problems of major abdominal surgery encountered in a third of our patients emphasize the wisdom of reserving surgery for the most severe cases.

GROUP B STREPTOCOCCAL INFECTIONS

KATHLEEN A. VENESS-MEEHAN, M.D.
DONALD L. SHAPIRO, M.D.

The group B streptococcus is a major pathogen in neonates. The organism is part of the genital tract flora of many women, and it is a common organism among hospital personnel. Because of the ubiquitous nature of the organism, many newborns become colonized with group B streptococci. Few, however, develop sepsis. The variables that distinguish these cases probably involve the size of the inoculum, the establishment of the organism in a compromised tissue, and the immunologic status of the mother vis à vis the group B streptococcus.

PREVENTION OF INFECTION

Attempts have been made to diminish the risk of colonization by this organism by treating the mother or the infant with prophylactic antibiotics. If the mother is colonized with group B streptococci, antibiotic therapy (usually penicillin) does eliminate the colonization. However, because recolonization occurs readily, prophylaxis, even when applied on a broad scale to all colonized women at an early stage of pregnancy, has not significantly diminished the incidence of neonatal infection. More recently, selective approaches to prophylactic treatment have had more success. If mothers are known to be colonized with group B streptococci and if they develop risk factors for neonatal sepsis during labor (such as prematurity or premature rupture of membranes), treatment of mothers before delivery (with ampicillin, 2 g intravenously followed by 1 g intravenously every 4 hours) in conjunction with treatment of the newborn until cultures are negative reduces neonatal colonization and sepsis. Of course, this approach is effective in only a percentage of all infants who are destined to be infected by the group B streptococcus.

Prophylactic treatment of all newborn infants with penicillin has been investigated as a means of eliminating the disease. Although this approach does seem to diminish somewhat the incidence of neonatal infection, the incidence of later infections with resistant organisms is higher in infants who have undergone treatment, and as a result, this approach is not recommended.

A very promising therapy is the immunization of mothers with a polysaccharide vaccine of group B streptococcus used to raise maternal serum antibody levels. It has been shown that *invasive group B streptococcal disease is associated with low levels of the maternal antibody*. Immunization with group B streptococcal capsular polysaccharide has been shown to increase IgG levels significantly in 57 percent of women immunized at 31 weeks' gestation. In this study, increased maternal serum IgG correlated strongly with higher newborn serum antibody levels and enhanced opsonization, phagocytosis, and bacterial killing of group B streptococci. Although transplacental passage of maternal IgG is low during the first and second trimesters, transfer increases markedly during the third trimester, affording some protection to even the premature infant. A still more effective vaccine may soon be made possible through the use of capsular polysaccharide covalent linkage to a protein carrier to improve immunogenicity, thereby increasing maternal and fetal antibody titers. However, maternal and fetal safety issues must first be addressed before immunization can be considered an effective approach toward preventing group B streptococcal disease in the newborn.

At present there is no way to eliminate infection from the organism, but postnatal colonization can be minimized by certain traditional procedures that apply specifically to hospital personnel. For example, careful attention to aseptic technique, particularly thorough hand-washing, may prevent a number of nosocomially acquired cases of group B streptococcal infection.

DIAGNOSIS

The group B streptococcus has become the most common organism causing sepsis in neonates. In any setting in which sepsis is a possibility based on known risk factors, such as the presence of chorioamnionitis or prematurity, infection with group B streptococcus should be suspected. This is particularly true when there is unexplained tachypnea or the infant's behavior is altered. Because of the fulminating nature of some group B streptococcal infections, a highly aggressive approach to diagnosis of infection, even when there are minimal symptoms, has become current practice. In cases in which clinical signs are equivocal, laboratory studies can be helpful. Significant elevation or depression of the white blood cell count or an abnormally high ratio of band forms to mature neutrophils can be an early sign.

The blood culture remains the mainstay of diagnosis for neonatal sepsis. At least 1 ml of blood should be obtained from a peripheral venous site after careful skin preparation. In addition to blood cultures, countercurrent immunoelectrophoresis or a latex particle agglutination test for group B streptococcal antigens should be performed on a concentrated urine specimen; either may provide an early diagnosis.

The extent of the infection should be determined by additional diagnostic studies, since this information has a bearing on the dose of antibiotic to be used and the duration of therapy. Because the initial site of infection is almost always the lungs, a chest roentgenogram helps determine the presence of pneumonia. A spinal tap should be performed to determine whether meningitis is present.

THERAPY

Antibiotic therapy is the mainstay of treatment for group B streptococcal infections. Some clinical problems associated with the infection will require additional therapy. For example, infection is sometimes fulminating and associated with circulatory collapse, in which case therapy with volume expanders and cardiac supportive agents would be indicated. A particular problem associated with the group B streptococcus is pulmonary hypertension, because the organism elaborates a toxin that can produce pulmonary vascular constriction. (Therapeutic strategies for pulmonary hypertension are discussed elsewhere in this book.) In general, the group B streptococcus is highly sensitive to penicillin. Penicillin can be administered readily to the neonate, and high drug levels can be achieved in virtually all organs. The major questions regarding antibiotic therapy for group B streptococcal infections are as follows:

1. Is the organism typical, i.e., highly sensitive to penicillin, or is it relatively resistant or "tolerant"?
2. Would the addition of other antibiotics offer a synergistic effect against the organism?
3. What duration of therapy is needed to eliminate the organism completely?

When group B streptococcal infections were first described, all the organisms isolated were highly sensitive to penicillin. With more experience, a small number of strains (4 to 5 percent) have been found to be more resistant. These "tolerant" strains are inhibited but not always killed by the usual penicillin dosages. In addition, some strains of group B streptococcus also show an "inoculum effect;" they may appear sensitive at the bacterial densities usually seen (approximately 10^6 organisms per milliliter), but at the higher bacterial densities sometimes seen in blood or cerebrospinal fluid (10^7 to 10^8 organisms per milliliter), they may be more resistant. Consequently, the dose of penicillin recommended has been raised from that originally used. Moreover, routine determination of minimum inhibitory and bactericidal concentrations should be performed on all group B streptococci isolated from newborn infants.

The initial broad-spectrum treatment of neonatal infections for which an organism has not been identified is a combination of a penicillin (usually penicillin G or ampicillin) and an aminoglycoside (usually gentamicin, kanamycin, or amikacin sulfate). This therapy is a good choice for group B streptococcal infections. The combination of a penicillin and an aminoglycoside works so well against the group B streptococcus that a possible synergistic effect has been suggested. Some laboratory studies have supported this concept. It seems prudent, in light of the foregoing information, to continue this combination of antibiotics until the sensitivity of the organism has been determined. Most infections with group B streptococcus can be treated with penicillin G alone once the diagnosis has been made. However, if the organism is tolerant or if the minimal inhibitory concentration–minimal bactericidal concentration (MIC/MBC) values cannot be obtained and meningitis is present, the penicillin-aminoglycoside combination should be continued for the duration of therapy. Ampicillin and cefotaxime are good second and third choices for single-antibiotic therapy of sensitive organisms.

Because the renal clearance is affected by the infant's maturity, the dosage for penicillin depends on whether meningitis is present and on the age of the infant. Table 1 summarizes the recommended dose.

In treating the neonate, a 10-day course of therapy for sepsis has been traditional and seems to be effective for infections in which no other organs are seeded. However, an occasional neonate continues to have organisms in the blood after this course of therapy. For this reason, some

TABLE 1 Recommended Dose of Penicillin for Sepsis and Meningitis

	Age 0–7 Days	Age >7 Days
Sepsis	100,000 U/kg/day (50,000 U/kg q12h IV)	150,000 U/kg/day (50,000 U/kg q8h IV)
Meningitis	200,000 U/kg/day (50,000 U/kg q6h IV)	300,000 U/kg/day (75,000 U/kg q6h IV)

have suggested that a longer initial course of therapy be used. Nevertheless, it seems just as reasonable to perform a blood culture 24 to 48 hours after discontinuation of the 10-day course of antibiotics to ensure that there are no remaining organisms.

When the central nervous system or bone has been seeded with organisms, a longer course of therapy is recommended. For meningitis, a 14- to 21-day course of therapy is recommended, depending on the severity of the initial infection and the response to antibiotic therapy. A lumbar puncture performed 24 to 48 hours after discontinuation of therapy should be sterile. The presence of osteomyelitis requires even more prolonged therapy, depending on the status of the lesion and its response to treatment.

Adjunctive therapies should be considered, particularly for the patient with severe infection. When true neutropenia (defined by diminished neutrophil precursors in the bone marrow) is present, white blood cell transfusion may alter the course of the disease. The use of hyperimmune anti–group B streptococcus intravenous immunoglobulin has been shown to provide protective immunity in experimental models, and immunoglobulin infusion may improve survival in some neonates with bacterial infections. Other therapies that have been suggested but for which there is less evidence of efficacy include exchange transfusion and the use of fresh frozen plasma.

HEMORRHAGIC DISEASE (VITAMIN K DEFICIENCY)

MARY E. O'CONNOR, M.D., M.P.H.

An infant less than 2 months of age who presents with severe bleeding is cause for immediate concern. The differential diagnosis can be divided into congenital causes, such as hemophilia, and acquired causes, including disseminated intravascular coagulation and hemorrhagic disease of the newborn. Because of the gravity of some situations, therapy is often immediate and broad in spectrum, including antibiotics, fresh frozen plasma, blood, and vitamin K, even before an exact diagnosis is made. The physician is then left 24 hours later with a clinically improved infant and turns to trying to reconstruct the cause of the bleeding.

Hemorrhagic disease of the newborn was first described in 1894 by Townsend, who noted babies that bled in the first 2 weeks of life. The hemorrhage usually began on the second or third day of life and, if it was not severe, soon stopped; these infants had no bleeding problems in later life. The transient nature of the bleeding tendency differentiated this entity from hemophilia. The etiology of hemorrhagic disease of the newborn was unknown until the 1930s and 1940s, when vitamin K was discovered. Vitamin K corrected the prolonged prothrombin time (PT) in some individuals who had bleeding. Among these patients were newborns, many of whom had cessation of bleeding and no further problems. In the 1950s and the early 1960s, prevention of neonatal hemorrhage was attempted with vitamin K. By 1961 the recommendation of the American Academy of Pediatrics that all newborns receive 1.0 mg of intramuscular vitamin K_1 soon after birth became standard practice in the United States.

By the late 1960s and early 1970s, mention of hemorrhagic disease of the newborn disappeared from the medical literature. However, in the early 1980s reports appeared from England, Japan, Germany, New Zealand, and the United States of 1- to 2-month-old infants who had been solely breast-fed, had not received vitamin K, and who had experienced significant bleeding. Many of these infants had an intracranial hemorrhage and died as a result of the consequences of increased intracranial pressure, although the acute coagulopathy was brought under control rapidly. These reports played a role in the development of recent research on hemorrhagic disease of the newborn.

This research has been supported by the development of specialized tests of the coagulation system. The coagulopathy in hemorrhagic disease of the newborn is due to a deficiency of the vitamin K–dependent procoagulants, factors II, VII, IX, and X. The last step in the formation of these functional (carboxylated) procoagulants is a carboxylation step using vitamin K. Nonfunctional (noncarboxylated) prothrombin reacts with vitamin K in the liver and yields functional prothrombin and an inactive vitamin K_1 molecule, which can then be enzymatically regenerated. The ability to differentiate between functional and nonfunctional prothrombin is the basis of new assays for the detection of vitamin K deficiency.

Traditionally, the diagnosis of vitamin K deficiency was made in a person with bleeding and a prolonged PT who received vitamin K with correction of the PT and cessation of the bleeding. One new method compares the level of prothrombin measured functionally with that measured antigenically. Both nonfunctional and functional prothrombin are alike antigenically. A ratio of functional to antigenic prothrombin that approaches 1 indicates vitamin K sufficiency, as all nonfunctional prothrombin has been converted to functional prothrombin. A low functional-antigen ratio indicates the presence of nonfunctional prothrombin, as is seen in vitamin K deficiency. This assay is usually performed using *Echis carinitus* (snake) venom to activate the nonfunctional prothrombin and is referred to as functional factor II/total factor II, factor II/*Echis* II, or coagulant/antigen ratio. The second method, PIVKA II (protein induced in vitamin K absence) measures inactive prothrombin in a more direct manner either immunologically or using electrophoresis. Any amount of PIVKA present is abnormal and indicative of vitamin K deficiency. Assays to measure vitamin K itself using high-performance liquid chromatography have been developed in several research laboratories around the world. Vitamin K_1 is present in serum in only nanogram per milliliter amounts in adults. Measuring these minute amounts of vitamin K_1 necessitates using large amounts of blood and makes studies in neonates difficult.

Ideally, the diagnosis of vitamin K deficiency should be documented by measurement of a low functional factor II/total factor II or a positive PIVKA. Supporting evidence includes an increased PT and partial thromboplastin time, decreased levels of factors II, VII, IX, and X, normal platelet count, normal fibrinogen and thrombin time, and normal factors V, VIII, XI, and XII. The confirmatory evidence is a response of the PT as well as other coagulation parameters to vitamin K administration, along with cessation of bleeding. The diagnostic picture is not always clear, because in those infants presenting with severe bleeding, cardiovascular collapse may have occurred with resulting disseminated intravascular coagulation. When PIVKA is present in plasma, the 50 percent disappearance time after the administration of vitamin K_1 ranges from 40 to 70 hours. Consequently, measurement of PIVKA even after treatment of the acute bleeding episode should be helpful in making a diagnosis of vitamin K deficiency.

In a recent review article, Lane and Hathaway characterized infantile vitamin K deficiency as falling into three patterns: early hemorrhagic disease in the newborn, classic hemorrhagic disease in the newborn, and late hemorrhagic disease. The manifestations and characteristics of each of these are listed in Table 1.

The early hemorrhagic disease of the newborn occurs in the first 24 hours of life, most commonly following maternal ingestion of drugs that affect vitamin K metabolism. These drugs include warfarin, anticonvulsants (most commonly phenytoin and phenobarbital), and antituberculous chemotherapeutic agents (especially rifampin). Bleeding in these infants may not be prevented by administration of vitamin K at birth because the bleeding may have begun during labor. Giving vitamin K_1 to an at-risk mother prior to delivery may prevent neonatal hemorrhage, but there is no standardized treatment regimen.

The classic hemorrhagic disease of the newborn remains as described by Townsend, and this concept is supported by work of O'Connor and Addiego. They studied a group of 37 women who gave birth at home. Half the babies received oral vitamin K_1, and half received no vitamin K. A third group of babies born in the hospital received intramuscular vitamin K_1. There was no difference among the three groups in the ratio of factor II to *Echis II* in the cord blood. At 2 to 3 days of age, the average of the ratio of the factor II to *Echis II* was significantly lower in the infants who had not received vitamin K than in those who received vitamin K. There was no difference between the groups receiving oral or intramuscular vitamin K_1. This supports the hypothesis that some breast-fed infants who do not receive vitamin K_1 have adequate

TABLE 1 Vitamin K Deficiency in Infancy

	Age	Sites of Bleeding	Cause

Early hemorrhagic disease	0–24 hr	Cephalohematoma
		Scalp monitor
		Intracranial
		Intrathoracic
		Intra-abdominal
			Maternal drugs
			  Warfarin
			  Anticonvulsants
			  Antituberculosis therapy
			Idiopathic

Classic Hemorrhagic disease	1–7 days	Gastrointestinal Skin Nasal Circumcision	Idiopathic Maternal drugs Increased with breast feeding or delayed feeding

Late hemorrhagic disease	1–6 mo	Intracranial
		Skin
		Gastrointestinal
			Idiopathic
			Oral antibiotics
			Malabsorption
			  Diarrhea
			  Cystic fibrosis
			  Biliary atresia
			  Alpha$_1$-antitrypsin
			    deficiency
			  Abetalipoproteinemia
			Associated with breast-feeding

vitamin K–dependent clotting factors at birth but by 3 days of age develop a mild form of vitamin K deficiency. In most infants this deficiency improves without treatment by 7 to 10 days of age. It has been postulated that circumcision of Jewish males was set for 7 days of age because bleeding was increased when it was performed at an earlier age.

The incidence of detectable vitamin K deficiency at birth has been studied by Shapiro and coworkers. They assayed 934 cord blood samples for vitamin K deficiency using the PIVKA-II assay. Of these infants, 2.9 percent were positive for PIVKA, suggesting vitamin K deficiency at the time of birth. This result was greater in the group that was small for gestational age than in the groups that were appropriate or large for gestational age. However, other perinatal risk factors could not be associated with positive PIVKA, and the majority of infants who were PIVKA-positive were products of a normal pregnancy, labor, and delivery. All of these infants received prophylactic vitamin K_1 in the newborn period and no infant subsequently had bleeding.

Two studies have attempted to measure vitamin K_1 levels in cord blood. Shearer found nondetectable or very low levels, and Sann found levels comparable to maternal levels. This discrepancy needs to be resolved by further studies.

Late hemorrhagic disease has occurred in healthy breast-fed infants and in infants with underlying malabsorption. The absorption of vitamin K requires the presence of bile acids. Decreased bile acid production leads to decreased vitamin K absorption. This fact and generalized fat malabsorption are the predisposing factors for vitamin K deficiency in infants with cystic fibrosis, biliary atresia, alpha$_1$-antitrypsin deficiency, and abetalipoproteinemia. Any infant with late hemorrhagic disease needs to be screened for these predisposing factors.

The late hemorrhagic disease in healthy infants has been attributed largely to the increased incidence of breast-feeding in the last 15 years. The vitamin K_1 content of cow's milk is much higher than that of human milk, and all of the infant formulas in the United States have vitamin K_1 added to them. The concentration of vitamin K_1 in formula is at least 50 μg per liter. The concentration of vitamin K_1 in breast milk is generally less than 20 μg per liter and often less than 5 μg per liter. These values vary markedly from woman to woman and from breast-feeding to breast-feeding. The newborn fed breast milk exclusively receives much less vitamin K_1 than does the infant who is fed cow's milk or formula. The volume of colostrum in the first 2 to 3 days of life is much less than the volume of formula taken by a formula-fed infant. This small volume of low vitamin K–concentration breast milk contributes to the transient vitamin K deficiency at 3 to 4 days of age. Vitamin K_2 is synthesized by certain bacteria in the intestine. However, the relative importance of vitamin K_2 in providing vitamin K to the infant is unknown.

Studies of Shapiro and O'Connor support the hypothesis that the vast majority of normal infants are not vitamin K–deficient at birth, but without adequate supplementation, mild deficiency may develop by 3 days of age or later. Infants with a positive cord blood PIVKA value may be at greater risk for developing vitamin K deficiency if supplementation is not given. If one of these infants is breast-fed by a mother with very low vitamin K_1 content in her milk, this scenario could set the stage for the development of clinically significant vitamin K deficiency. The vitamin K deficiency could manifest with bleeding in the infant as early as 3 days of age. However, the deficiency might remain present for as long as the first several months of life, leaving the infant at risk for late-onset hemorrhage. At present, we have no way of knowing which few of these healthy infants are at high risk for development of vitamin K deficiency. The only accepted risk factor is breast-feeding. Since 50 to 70 percent of infants in the United States are now breast-fed, the vast majority would be at risk for vitamin K deficiency.

The recommendation remains that all infants need supplemental vitamin K. In the United States the standing recommendation is the administration of 1.0 mg of vitamin K_1 intramuscularly soon after birth. The universality of this treatment has eliminated classic hemorrhagic disease of the newborn from the United States and also probably caused the markedly lower numbers of infants with late hemorrhagic disease in the United States compared with countries like Japan where vitamin K prophylaxis is not universally given.

What should the physician do when presented with parents who refuse vitamin K administration for their infant? Many of these parents want a "totally natural delivery," and the mother plans unsupplemented breast-feeding. O'Connor and Addiego showed in a small number of infants that giving 2.0 mg of oral vitamin K_1 within 2 hours of delivery produced normal levels of vitamin K–dependent clotting factors at 3 days of age. Whether this protection lasts as long as the 1 to 3 months of age that the infant may be at risk for late hemorrhage is unknown. This treatment method was supported by the use of oral vitamin K_1 in many of the European countries in the 1950s. For parents who refuse any administration of vitamin K to their baby, consideration should be given to administering vitamin K to the mother prior to delivery. Shearer gave high doses of intravenous vitamin K to a small number of mothers in labor and found increased vitamin K levels in the infants' cord blood. Whether this prevents development of vitamin K deficiency in the infant is unknown. Giving vitamin K_1 to breast-feeding women does increase the vitamin K_1 content of their milk. Whether this increased concentration is enough to prevent vitamin K deficiency in the nursing infant is unknown. The vitamin K content of most foods is not known. High values are found in green leafy vegetables such as spinach, broccoli, and kale. Whether the vitamin K intake of a pregnant woman can be increased enough to prevent neonatal vitamin K deficiency by using dietary manipulation prenatally or during nursing is unknown.

In Africa, Asia, and Central and South America, the majority of births occur at home or in small health centers with midwife supervision and minimal supplies. The incidence of hemorrhagic disease of the newborn in these areas is unknown. Intramuscular administration of vitamin K is impractical and oral vitamin K is not available; therefore, dietary manipulation may be the only method available for prophylaxis.

For an infant who has bleeding due to vitamin K deficiency, 1 to 2 mg of vitamin K_1 given intramuscularly or intravenously over 15 to 20 minutes is the treatment of choice. Infants with serious bleeding may also need fresh frozen plasma, 10 to 15 ml per kilogram, or heat-treated lyophilized factor IX preparations. Fresh frozen plasma or factor IX preparations supply functional factor II immediately. Vitamin K administration corrects the vitamin K deficiency within several hours. Other therapies appropriate to the child's condition can be pursued concomitantly.

Recent studies on the mechanism of vitamin K action and the incidence of neonatal vitamin K deficiency have helped define hemorrhagic disease of the newborn more precisely. Much research remains to be done, especially in areas of risk factors for vitamin K deficiency and methods of prophylaxis.

SUGGESTED READING

Lane PA, Hathaway WE. Vitamin K in infancy. J Pediatr 1985; 106:351–359.

O'Connor ME, Addiego JE. Use of oral vitamin K_1 to prevent hemorrhagic disease of the newborn infant. J Pediatr 1986; 108:616–619.

Sann L, Leclercq M, Troncy J, et al. Serum vitamin K_1 concentration and vitamin K dependent clotting factor activity in maternal and fetal cord blood. Am J Obstet Gynecol 1985; 153:771–774.

Shapiro AD, Jacobson LJ, Armon ME, et al. Vitamin K deficiency in the newborn infant: Prevalence and perinatal risk factors. J Pediatr 1986; 109:675–679.

Shearer MJ, Barkhan P, Rahim S, Stimmler L. Plasma vitamin K_1 in mothers and their newborn babies. Lancet 1982; 2:460–463.

HIRSCHSPRUNG'S DISEASE

THOMAS V.N. BALLANTINE, M.D., F.A.C.S.

The first sign of Hirschsprung's disease in the neonatal unit is failure to pass stool, with or without bilious vomiting. Failure to pass stool may also occur as a result of a number of other perinatal events: prematurity, maternal drug addiction, "lazy left colon syndrome," or diabetes in the mother, among others.

Barium enema is *not* an appropriate way to establish the diagnosis of Hirschsprung's disease in the newborn. Because the colon has been inactive throughout gestation, no transition zone will have developed. Thus, the typical radiologic appearance of a dilated proximal segment, separated from the distal aganglionic portion by the transition zone, is *not* seen. However, if a barium enema is performed, the single most important radiologic finding is the retention of barium 24 and 48 hours after the procedure. Accordingly, it is the responsibility of the pediatrician, not of the radiologist, to assure that two follow-up films, 1 and 2 days after the procedure, are obtained. If barium is retained, rectal biopsy is indicated.

In previous years, rectal biopsy necessitated relaxation of the infant and an open technique with the associated complications of general anesthesia and the possibility of hemorrhage. Today, adequate tissue may be obtained for pathologic examination using the suction rectal biopsy techniques. Biopsy samples should be taken at 2, 4, and 6 cm above the anal verge to assure adequate sampling. One biopsy specimen at each level is sufficient. When the procedure is performed by a well-trained operator, three adequate specimens can easily be obtained in 10 or 15 minutes. The specimens are immediately placed in 10 percent formalin solution. Frozen-section diagnosis is less reliable than when the tissue has been properly fixed and processed for permanent sections. In addition, more levels may be obtained from the biopsy specimen, as needed.

We usually see three different types of Hirschsprung's disease, based on the length of the aganglionic segment: short, usual, and total colonic. If the aganglionic segment is less than 6 to 8 cm above the anal verge, the persistent rectal tone (a consequence of the lack of ganglionic cells in Meissner's and Auerbach's plexus) may be remedied by the transanal approach and excision of a 1-cm wide strip of rectal mucosa. The child with short segment disease is seldom seen in the newborn period. Infants with standard or ultra-long segment disease are managed similarly in the newborn unit. *The goal of management is to assure that the fecal stream terminates in ganglionated bowel.* Accordingly, a diverting stoma must be created.

When the diagnosis is established, the infant must be prepared for surgery, first ensuring that no infection or dehydration is present. The infant is "covered" with perioperative antibiotics selected for treatment of gut flora.

There are at least two appropriate procedures for Hirschsprung's disease: a simple diverting colostomy and a leveling colostomy. The decision as to which operation is appropriate is predicated on the surgeon's choice of definitive pull-through. Many surgeons prefer to protect the pull-through operation with a colostomy. Accordingly, the surgeon usually elects a right transverse colostomy because, more than 80 percent of the time, the right transverse colon contains ganglion cells.

If the operating surgeon does not elect to protect the pull-through with a colostomy, thus performing corrective surgery in two rather than three stages, a leveling colostomy is carried out. In this instance a formal laparotomy is often required, and multiple biopsies are performed until the transition zone is identified. The colostomy is brought out immediately proximal to the transition zone. At the time of definitive repair, the transition zone is used to form the neo-anus. Irrespective of the level of colostomy, postoperatively the patient is maintained on nasogastric suction until the ileus has resolved. Clear liquids are initiated, followed by an appropriate diet, including breast milk as indicated.

Physicians should be sure that both parents understand the principles of colostomy care before the child is discharged from the hospital.

HYDROCEPHALUS

BENJAMIN S. CARSON, M.D.
JOHN M. FREEMAN, M.D.

Hydrocephalus results from the abnormal accumulation of cerebrospinal fluid (CSF) within the intracranial ventricular system. Although on rare occasions this excess accumulation results from overproduction of CSF, in most cases it is the result of the blockage of flow of this fluid at the level of the cerebral aqueduct, at the fourth ventricle, and over the surface of the brain at the arachnoid granulations where the spinal fluid is absorbed. Blockage of the flow of fluid can occur at any location, but when it occurs within the ventricular system this results in what is called noncommunicating hydrocephalus. When the blockage is over the surface of the brain or is due to inadequate absorption through the arachnoid villi, it is called communicating hydrocephalus. Noncommunicating hydrocephalus may occur as a result of tumors, maldevelopment or scarring of the aqueduct (aqueductal stenosis), congenital defect of the fourth ventricle (Dandy-Walker syndrome), or any other discontinuity in the pathway. Communicating hydrocephalus may be due to scarring of CSF pathways at the base, over the surface, or at the arachnoid granulations. Transient clogging of these granulations may also occur from blood (secondary to intraventricular hemorrhage or subarachnoid hemorrhage), infection (meningitis), or proteinaceous fluid (e.g., tumors, Guillain-Barré syndrome).

SIGNS AND SYMPTOMS

Signs and symptoms vary with age and with the severity and rate of progression of the hydrocephalus.

In the newborn and young infant whose sutures have not yet closed, hydrocephalus may be asymptomatic and manifest only by progressive enlargement of the head. The rate of enlargement varies with the severity of the hydrocephalus. With rapidly progressive hydrocephalus, the young infant may show a poor suck, irritability, vomiting, and, occasionally, depressed levels of consciousness. The common signs, however, include a bulging fontanelle, sometimes accompanied by a "sunset" sign with downward deviation of the eyes.

In the older child, after the age of 18 months to 2 years, when the sutures have begun to close and the fontanelle is fibrotic, hydrocephalus may be manifested by the usual signs of increased intracranial pressure. These classic signs include sixth nerve palsy, papilledema, vomiting, headache, spasticity in the lower extremities, and decrease in mental performance. When increased pressure is severe, it may be accompanied by decrease in level of consciousness and alteration of vital signs. However, even at this age, slowly progressive hydrocephalus may be asymptomatic for prolonged periods.

EVALUATION OF AN ENLARGING HEAD

Serial measurements of head circumference are a part of the standard well baby examination. These measurements should be plotted serially on a standard head growth chart. *When the rate of head growth crosses percentiles on this chart, hydrocephalus should be suspected.* Low-birth-weight infants have a more rapid rate of head growth than infants at term and should be plotted on an appropriate growth chart. Children who have been starved, are small for dates, or have been severely ill will, when re-fed and beginning to grow, have an excessive rate of head growth. *Charting on an appropriate scale for gestational age and sickness or health helps to determine which head growth patterns should be of concern.*

A child whose head is growing more rapidly than appropriate should be evaluated with a computed tomography (CT) scan; ultrasonography can be performed in children and infants with an open fontanelle. This provides an excellent measurement of ventricular size, but may be less reliable in detecting subdural collections or other abnormalities causing enlargement of the head. However, *once a CT scan has been taken and other abnormalities have been ruled out, ultrasonography provides an excellent, risk-free approach to the monitoring of ventricular size.* The CT scan not only documents ventricular size, but may differentiate communicating from noncommunicating hydrocephalus and rule out other substantial abnormalities that could cause enlargement of the head.

The most common abnormality confused with hydrocephalus on CT scan is cortical atrophy. Infants who have an excessive rate of head growth, and who on CT scan show excessive fluid over the surface of the brain but without substantial ventricular enlargement, do *not* have cortical atrophy. Cortical atrophy of itself is incompatible with an excessive rate of head growth. Some such children have familial megaloencephaly. They do not require therapeutic intervention and are usually normal, albeit with large heads. However, a CT scan is still important to ensure that a treatable cause of progressive head enlargement is not present.

WHY DO YOU TREAT HYDROCEPHALUS?

Hydrocephalus is treated *only* when it is clearly progressive. In many patients with slowly progressive hydrocephalus, head growth may arrest spontaneously; they remain with slightly large ventricles but perfectly normal intellectual and motor performance. Hydrocephalus, of itself, does not necessarily cause permanent damage to the brain unless it is severe and prolonged. *Hydrocephalus is not usually associated with poor neurologic function unless the cortical mantle is less than 0.5 cm.* Even in these situations, shunting may allow the cortical mantle to re-expand and the child to improve. Therefore, slight dilatation of the ventricles is not an ominous sign unless it is clearly progressive.

The second reason for treatment of hydrocephalus is to facilitate better head control and nursing care. Even in the child with profound brain damage or with hydranencephaly and hydrocephalus, we usually treat to allow better caretaking. Most children with hydrocephalus alone are of normal intelligence. Retardation associated with hydrocephalus is usually due to other developmental abnormalities, or damage to the cortex by the process that also led to the hydrocephalus.

WHEN DO YOU TREAT HYDROCEPHALUS?

It is difficult to state a specific time, thickness of cortical mantle, or rate of progression when treatment should be initiated. A child whose rate of head growth is rapidly crossing percentiles should be treated sooner. An asymptomatic child whose rate of head growth is slowly crossing percentiles can be carefully observed until the situation stabilizes or the need for shunting becomes apparent. It must be remembered that treatment of hydrocephalus by either medical or surgical management carries potential complications.

TREATMENT

The standard treatment of hydrocephalus is with a shunt from the lateral ventricle to the peritoneal cavity, or into the right atrium of the heart. Shunting of hydrocephalus is discussed below. Occasionally and for slowly progressive hydrocephalus, or for the temporary treatment of hydrocephalus after intraventricular hemorrhage or infection, medical management of hydrocephalus is now possible.

Medical

The production of CSF both by the choroid plexus and across the ventricular wall is an active process.

Acetazolamide, a carbonic anhydrase inhibitor, and furosemide (a loop diuretic) have been shown to inhibit the formation of CSF to 20 percent or less of its normal rate. Recent studies have shown that treatment with these two diuretics for 3 to 6 months can allow the rate of head growth to become normal and the cranial sutures to become partially fused, allowing slight increase in intracranial pressure and arrest of the hydrocephalus. Acetazolamide is begun at 25 mg per kilogram and increased every 1 to 2 days by 25 mg to a total of 100 mg per kilogram, in four divided doses. Furosemide, 1 to 2 mg per kilogram per day in four divided doses, may be used in addition. The most common side effect of medical therapy is acidosis, which should be treated prophylactically with Polycitra, 3 to 4 ml per kilogram per day in four divided doses, gradually increased until the acidosis is compensated.

The patient is followed with frequent assessment of serum electrolyte levels, weekly monitoring of head circumferences, and monthly measurements of ventricular size by ultrasonography. If the hydrocephalus is progressive, a shunt should be implanted. If the head size stabilizes despite moderately enlarged ventricles, the child is continued on medications until 6 months of age. The medication is then gradually tapered with close observation for recurrence of hydrocephalus. This form of therapy appears effective in 50 percent of children with hydrocephalus. It does not appear to be effective in children with spina bifida. Children with arrested hydrocephalus after this treatment appear normal, but long-term comparative studies have not been undertaken.

Medical treatment can also be effective when children have hydrocephalus and spinal fluid that is too bloody or too proteinaceous to permit shunting, or when infection prohibits reinsertion of a shunt. In these cases it is useful as a temporizing procedure.

Surgical

On rare occasions, hydrocephalus may be due to a choroid plexus papilloma, a tumor that causes excessive secretion of CSF. Such a tumor should be ruled out by CT scan. Choroid plexus papilloma is one of the few curable causes of hydrocephalus.

Except in the rare instance when hydrocephalus is produced by a mass lesion causing obstruction to flow, and which can be directly removed, allowing normal CSF flow patterns, all other forms of hydrocephalus (communicating and noncommunicating) are treated by diverting the CSF with an implantable shunting device.

Although CSF has been diverted into virtually every known body orifice, most neurosurgeons divert it to the peritoneal cavity (ventriculoperitoneal shunt), less commonly to the right atrium (ventriculoatrial shunt), and, occasionally in older children and adults, to the pleural space.

A ventriculoperitoneal shunt is easily inserted. One can place enough tubing to allow for body growth. Such shunts usually are easily revised. A ventriculoatrial shunt is less desirable in young infants because of the difficulties in allowing for growth, and because placement of the distal tip in the right atrium can produce arrhythmias. Other known complications include distal tip embolization to the lung and glomerulonephritis. Ventriculopleural shunts cannot be used in young infants because of their inability to tolerate the continued pleural infusion. However, in older children or adults when the peritoneal cavity cannot be used or when ventriculoatrial shunts are inadvisable, a pleural shunt may be inserted and well tolerated.

COMPLICATIONS OF SHUNTS

The major complications of shunts are obstruction and infection. It would appear that these are far more common in young infants and less common as they grow older. In one study, approximately half of the children experienced no complications, while in the other half there were repeated complications. There was no ability to predict which child would fall into which group, or for what reason.

Shunt Infections

Shunt infections occur in 1.5 to 5 percent of shunt insertions. This is true each time a shunt is revised. We have been able to keep our incidence of infection below 2 percent by meticulous aseptic technique. *The incidence of shunt infection appears related partly to the surgeon who inserts the shunt, partly to the rapidity with which the shunt procedure is performed, and partly to the frequency with which the surgeon does the procedure.* We advocate a meticulous surgical preparation, which includes close shaving immediately before surgery using antiseptic solutions with both a prescrub and a final scrub. This is followed by placement of an antiseptic-impregnated adhesive plastic drape on the operative field to prevent contamination of shunt components with skin flora. A broad-spectrum antistaphylococcal antibiotic is administered intravenously before surgery and for 72 hours postoperatively. Additionally, we instill 40 mg of cephalothin intraventricularly through the shunt reservoir at the time of surgery, as well as on a daily basis for the first two postoperative days by way of a shunt tap. CSF is analyzed at the time of these shunt taps for evidence of infection.

Diagnosis of Shunt Infection

Diagnosis of shunt infection requires a high degree of suspicion. *Infections are most common in the first several weeks after insertion of a new shunt, and decrease in frequency over the following 6 months.* They may be subtle and present as shunt obstruction. A child with a ventriculoperitoneal shunt who has fever or is doing poorly should have a shunt tap performed by someone familiar with the anatomy of the shunt itself. Such a tap should measure pressure, and CSF should be inspected for white cells and cultured.

When shunt infection is documented, the child is treated with appropriate antibiotics intravenously for 2 to 5 days and recultured. The shunt is then removed and a new shunt placed with continued antibiotic coverage for 7 to 10 days. If CSF is not sterile at the time a new shunt is to be inserted, the shunt should be removed and the child maintained on antibiotic therapy under close observation until the CSF is sterile. If the child is shunt dependent, he or she should be placed on external ventricular drainage until sterility can be achieved, after which a new shunting system is placed.

Shunt Obstruction

ANYTHING that goes wrong in a child with a shunt must be presumed to be due to the shunt until proven otherwise. Many children with shunt obstruction present with the classic signs and symptoms of increased pressure; bulging fontanelle, poor feeding, and (in the older child) headache, vomiting, and lethargy or increasing spasticity or sixth nerve palsy. In some children and adults, symptoms of shunt obstruction may be subtle, including poor school work, decreased attention span, and increased irritability. While the ventricles commonly increase when the shunt is obstructed, some children develop the "slit ventricle" syndrome in which the ventricular wall becomes fibrosed and cannot expand. In these children, shunt obstruction may be acute and fatal. Parents should be educated regarding the signs of shunt obstruction and a child with this complication should be seen *day or night* by a physician familiar with the signs and symptoms of shunt obstruction. The shunt should be evaluated by pumping, CT scan, and, if necessary, shunt tapping to measure pressure and obtain CSF for laboratory studies. If there is doubt, the child should be admitted to the hospital for observation. The signs and symptoms may mimic viral infections, but it is better to admit the child for observation than to ascribe symptoms to a viral infection that may prove fatal.

OUTCOME

Hydrocephalus, appropriately treated, usually results in a child who is normal and of average intellect with no motor deficits. The outcome of hydrocephalus is directly related to its etiology and the coexistence of other congenital or developmental abnormalities. CNS infection has been documented to decrease IQ. In general, however, close attention to CSF infection, and careful evaluation and treatment of signs and symptoms of shunt obstruction, should allow most children with hydrocephalus to function normally.

SUGGESTED READING

Alvarez LA, Maytal J, Shinnar S. Idiopathic external hydrocephalus: natural history and relationship to benign familial macrocephaly. Pediatrics 1986; 77:901–907.

Freeman JM, D'Souza B. Obstruction of CSF shunts. Pediatrics 1979; 64:111–112.

Shinnar S, Gammon K, Bergman EW, et al. The medical management of hydrocephalus in infancy: use of acetazolamide and furosemide. J Pediatr 1985; 107:31–37.

HYDRONEPHROSIS

MARK F. BELLINGER, M.D.

Hydronephrosis is a generic term, signifying dilatation of the upper urinary tract without regard to pathogenesis or degree. Many factors may lead to the development of hydronephrosis, and because of the extreme distensibility of the urinary tract in the fetus and infant, a consideration of therapy requires delineation not only of anatomic but also of functional parameters. It is important to keep in mind that *dilatation does not equate to poor function*.

In considering both the nature of and appropriate intervention for perinatal hydronephrosis, a coordinated evaluation may include radiologic, radionuclide, and sonographic studies designed to investigate obstruction, reflux, and bladder emptying. These examinations, when ordered appropriately and monitored closely, can minimize radiation exposure and be tailored to providing the information required in spite of the diminished glomerular filtration rate (GFR) of the perinatal period. It is appropriate to consider perinatal diagnostic imaging briefly.

IMAGING

The *plain abdominal radiograph* should be examined for evidence of vertebral or sacral anomalies that may be associated with either renal agenesis or neuropathic bladder dysfunction.

Diagnostic ultrasound, the initial screening of choice for infants with abdominal or renal anomalies, should offer more than just structural evidence of hydronephrosis or cystic dilatation. Real-time and serial examinations may assess renal size, cortical thickness and consistency, bladder emptying, and ureteral peristalsis.

Intravenous urography offers limited information in the newborn period. Diminished GFR and overlying bowel gas contribute to poor detail and limited functional data. *Radionuclide imaging* offers increasingly sophisticated diagnostic ability. DTPA (^{99m}-Tc diethylenetriaminepentaacetic acid) scanning requires no bowel preparation or fasting, is not influenced by bowel gas, and, with computerized interpretation, allows both evaluation of differential function and diuretic renography to distinguish dilated from obstructed renal units.

Voiding cystourethrography is extremely important in the evaluation of hydronephrosis. Urethral obstruction in the male may be a cause of vesical as well as upper tract dilatation, and vesicoureteric reflux (VUR) may result in upper tract fullness. VUR is diagnosed only by cystography.

FETAL HYDRONEPHROSIS

Prenatal detection of fetal urinary tract dilatation is a well-documented capability of ultrasound examination. Real-time studies and serial examinations are important to evaluate transient hydronephrosis and to assess bladder emptying but offer little in the way of functional data. Sonographic assessment of diminished amniotic fluid volume is important but is not diagnostic of a tendency toward pulmonary hypoplasia. A growing body of experience supports a conservative approach to late gestational fetal hydronephrosis and to unilateral lesions at any gestational age. The role of intervention in bilateral hydronephrosis detected in early gestation remains controversial and will require well-controlled trials in the handful of centers with clinical experience and ongoing research. The current aim of prenatal detection is to offer parental counseling and close prenatal monitoring and to allow for prompt perinatal evaluation and treatment.

POSTNATAL HYDRONEPHROSIS

Ureteropelvic Junction Obstruction

The most common cause of hydronephrosis in the infant is ureteropelvic junction (UPJ) obstruction. In our recent experience with prenatal ultrasound detection, we have found that many infants have a very soft hydronephrosis at birth, which becomes gradually more tense (palpable) over 12 to 36 hours. Ultrasound findings may be diagnostic, but radionuclide studies should be performed to rule out multicystic dysplasia and to evaluate the contralateral kidney. The voiding cystourethrogram is necessary to rule out VUR with a UPJ obstruction secondary to kinking of a tortuous ureter.

Traditionally, perinatal repair has been preferred in the otherwise healthy neonate. However, recent experience with larger numbers of infants studied in the postnatal period with radionuclide scanning and followed nonoperatively has shown that, in selected cases, function and drainage may improve spontaneously or at least remain stable for several months. This experience has led to a reconsideration of the timing of surgical intervention in neonatal and infant hydronephrosis, a debate that is currently in progress. These renal units, although tremendously dilated, usually have good function and little or no evidence of dysplasia. The standard of repair is the dismembered pyeloplasty—excising the stenotic segment and performing a dependent, spatulated anastomosis. Optical magnification has allowed successful repair in 95 percent of cases. Such repairs, when uncomplicated and in the face of sterile urine, may be left unstented and without nephrostomy tubes, using only a small perirenal drain. Complicated or bilateral procedures or repairs in solitary kidneys require stent and nephrostomy drainage for 5 to 7 days in the event of temporary postoperative edema. An alternative to immediate pyeloplasty is (1) surgical or percutaneous nephrostomy placement with delayed repair, or (2) cutaneous pyelostomy. Intubated diversions are rarely indicated in the perinatal age group, but temporary percutaneous drainage may be necessary in the face of sepsis or serious impediments to repair. Cutaneous pyelostomy is an important alternative in the small infant when repair may be technically difficult. The dilated renal pelvis is merely opened to the skin and covered with the child's diaper.

When conditions are optimal and the child is several months of age, closure and pyeloplasty are performed. Prolapse of the dilated renal pelvis may occur, but the tubeless pyelostomy in general is an excellent temporary diversion.

Pyeloplasty is a highly satisfactory procedure. Anastomotic stricture may occur, but results of repair and long-term renal function are excellent. The furosemide (Lasix) washout renal scan (diuretic renogram) may be important in postoperative evaluation, since chronic caliectasis and renal pelvic dilatation may persist in spite of an adequate repair.

Ureteral Valves or Ureteral Stenoses

These are uncommon entities, but they do occur. Evaluation and treatment are the same as for UPJ obstruction.

Primary (Obstructive) Megaureter

This condition is less common than UPJ obstruction. Megaureter simply means a large ureter, classically larger than 1 cm in diameter. Many classification systems exist. Because primary megaureter usually results in less renal pelvic dilatation and a less tense hydronephrosis, a mass may not be palpable and the usual presentation occurs later, with infection, hematuria, or sepsis. The intravenous pyelogram classically shows a large, rather straight ureter with variable degrees of caliectasis. The distal ureter is usually widest, narrowing to a thin spindle. The voiding cystourethrogram is important to rule out reflux.

Therapy is based on a clinical impression of the degree of hydronephrosis and functional impairment. An acutely infected system with diminished peristalsis may improve dramatically with antibiotic therapy, and so in moderate cases imaging should be repeated after treatment and 1 to 2 months of urinary suppression. The diuretic renogram is extremely helpful in evaluation and may be a significant factor in determining the need for surgical intervention. Recurrent infections, high-grade obstruction, or increased hydronephrosis may necessitate early repair.

Surgical treatment of primary obstructive megaureter involves resection of the distal ureter and creation of a nonrefluxing submucosal tunnel. This commonly necessitates tapering of the distal ureteral segment. Here, ureteral splinting is necessary for 5 to 7 days. Repair is generally successful, although continued obstruction or reflux may result more commonly (15 percent) than in reimplantation of nondilated ureters (5 percent).

Vesicoureteral Reflux

In all cases of hydronephrosis, VUR must be excluded. It is generally agreed that sterile reflux is not a cause of renal scarring, but the role of pressure atrophy in higher grades of reflux is poorly understood. Infants are known to void with high intravesical pressure, thus accentuating the problem.

The presentation of reflux in the perinatal period is usually that of urinary tract infection. Renal failure associated with massive reflux into dysplastic kidneys is uncommon but may manifest as failure to thrive or uremia.

The role of infection in causing renal scarring is well documented, and the role of nonsurgical management of reflux is well established. Daily suppressive antibacterial therapy, frequent urine monitoring for infection, and close surveillance with documentation of good renal growth may allow for long-term follow-up and spontaneous cessation of reflux. Reflux of enough volume to cause hydronephrosis, particularly in the infant, may demand surgical intervention. Such massively dilated ureters are commonly related to grossly incompetent orifices and degrees of renal dysplasia. Reimplantation in such situations may be technically difficult and fraught with a significant complication rate. Temporary cutaneous vesicostomy offers a rapid, easily reversible alternative to primary reimplantation. By lowering intravesical pressure and decompressing the bladder, VUR is effectively minimized. The infant must remain on urinary suppression and merely wears a diaper over the stoma. When the child is older, vesicostomy closure is combined with ureteral reimplantation if reflux is persistent.

In moderate grades of reflux with minimal hydronephrosis, nonsurgical management may be sufficient. If indications for surgery arise, reimplantation may be performed successfully even in small bladders by the Cohen cross-trigonal technique with a higher than 95 percent success rate. Reflux may persist or obstruction occur in 5 percent of cases, but a second procedure usually is successful.

Ureteroceles

These are cystic dilatations of the terminal ureter. In children, ureteroceles commonly subtend the upper segment of a completely duplicated ureter, causing obstruction and frequently nonfunction of the upper renal unit (which may demonstrate severe renal dysplasia). The cystic intravesical ureterocele may cause contralateral hydronephrosis or bladder outlet obstruction, or it may prolapse through the urethral orifice. Large ureteroceles may distort the bladder neck or extend into the urethra (cecoureterocele), affecting continence. Sepsis related to the obstructed unit is the most common presentation in infants, and reflux to the lower renal segment is common. Ultrasonography, voiding cystourethrography, and urography may delineate the pathology. A distorted or anomalous radiologic appearance should always bring to mind a duplication anomaly, since the configuration may be extremely variable.

Treatment of ectopic ureteroceles may be complicated. Appropriate therapy is individualized according to the pathology involved, the degree of function of the upper segment, and bladder anatomy. If the lower kidney is functioning well, the nonfunctioning upper segment is best treated by heminephrectomy and subtotal ureterectomy, decompressing the distal ureter and leaving the ureterocele in situ. In 75 percent of cases, this treatment suffices, leaving a functioning lower segment. If infections, persistent reflux, or bladder outlet obstruction due to the ureterocele remnant occur, reconstruction necessitates ureterocele excision, strengthening of the bladder floor, and reimplantation of the lower pole ureter. This is a technically tedious procedure, but results are good in almost all cases of secondary lower tract reconstruction as opposed to the 50 percent success rate with simultaneously upper and lower procedures. A well-functioning upper pole unit is less common, but if hydronephrosis is only moderate and reflux to the lower segment is present, ureterocele excision with reimplantation of both ureters is highly successful. Rarely, ureteropyelostomy, or connection of the obstructed but functioning upper pole ureter to a nonrefluxing lower pole ureter, may be a viable alternative. Transurethral incision of the ureterocele, one of the earliest treatments, has virtually gone out of favor since it trades obstruction for reflux. However, in the septic neonate who is a poor operative risk, this may be a lifesaving temporary measure. The evaluation and treatment of the infant with ureterocele thus is highly individualized and must take into consideration both functional parameters and long-term goals.

Failure of Bladder Emptying

Abnormal bladder emptying may be a cause of reflux or hydronephrosis. Mechanical obstruction (posterior urethral valves, anterior urethral pathology) and neurogenic bladder dysfunction (spina bifida, sacral agenesis) are the most common etiologies.

Posterior and anterior urethral pathology in the male is common and is diagnosed by voiding cystourethrography. Treatment is individualized and must initially be aimed at improvement in bladder drainage by primary treatment of obstruction or temporary vesicostomy.

Neuropathic bladder function similarly may be associated with hydronephrosis from reflux or simply from a full bladder not permitting free upper tract drainage. Voiding studies must rule out reflux.

No study (urogram or scan) with upper tract dilatation should end with a full bladder, especially in cases of neurogenic dysfunction. It is imperative to document whether bladder drainage by voiding or catheterization diminishes upper tract fullness. If it does, intermittent catheterization or cutaneous vesicostomy is effective treatment for the hydronephrosis; if not, temporary upper tract diversion or primary repair may be indicated. Intermittent catheterization is feasible even in the small infant (male or female). During hospitalization, sterile technique must be used, but the parents should be instructed in a clean technique, reusing small (No. 5 or 8 French) catheters for 1 week. The infant should remain on antibiotic prophylaxis (preferably a penicillin in the first month of life). In the face of massive reflux, parental reluctance to catheterize, parental noncompliance, or parental inability to perform intermittent catheterization on a regular (every 4 hours) schedule, cutaneous vesicostomy offers a simple, quick, and easily managed temporary urinary diversion. A small subumbilical stoma is formed, and the infant is simply managed in diapers. The vesicostomy is closed at a later date, in conjunction with ureteral reimplantation and the institution of intermittent catheterization. Reversal of the diversion may thus be postponed until the age when the child is motivated to learn self-catheterization. Vesicostomy in the spina bifida group has a greater than 95 percent success rate in improving and stabilizing upper tract dilatation, has a high rate of parent satisfaction, and has few complications. Stomal stenosis and prolapse may occur, requiring revision, but in general results are excellent and undiversion is simple.

Many other, less common causes of hydronephrosis include horseshoe kidneys or renal ectopias, ectopic ureters, prune belly syndrome, megalourethra with upper tract anomalies, retrocaval ureter, and countless other lesions. The most important aspect of considering therapy for these lesions is accurate anatomic and functional evaluation, which, as with hydronephrosis from other causes, contributes significantly to a rational therapeutic plan.

HYDROPS FETALIS

MICHAEL F. EPSTEIN, M.D.

Hydrops fetalis refers to a condition in the fetus characterized by generalized edema, collections of fluid in the pleural, pericardial, and peritoneal spaces, and usually enlargement of the liver, spleen, and heart. Although considerable confusion surrounds the pathophysiology of this condition, most instances of hydrops fetalis involve congestive heart failure, anemia, hypoproteinemia, or a combination of those factors. Since

the treatment of hydrops depends largely on the specific etiology, I will briefly describe the differential diagnosis and the antenatal evaluation of the fetus with hydrops fetalis, as well as the perinatal management of these infants.

DIFFERENTIAL DIAGNOSIS AND ANTENATAL EVALUATION

The two broad diagnostic categories of hydrops fetalis are comprised of entities leading to fetal anemia and of those not associated with anemia.

I. Anemia-related hydrops
  A. Hemolysis

1. Isoimmune disease—Rh, Kell, rarely ABO "private antigens"
2. Hemoglobinopathies—most commonly homozygous alpha-thalassemia seen in Oriental or Mediterranean ethnic groups
3. Macroangiopathic—secondary to red blood cell destruction in an arteriovenous malformation
   B. Fetal-maternal hemorrhage
II. Nonanemia–related hydrops
   A. Congenital heart disease
   1. Structural—endocardial fibroelastosis, ventricular septal defect, tetralogy of Fallot, transposition of the great vessels, and others
   2. Rhythm disturbances, both tachyarrhythmias (paroxysmal atrial tachycardia or atrial flutter) and heart block
   B. Chromosomal aberration
   C. Congenital viral infection—cytomegalovirus
   D. Arteriovenous malformations in fetus or placenta
   E. Associated anomalies
   F. Idiopathic

A vigorous attempt should be made to identify the etiology of fetal hydrops when the diagnosis is made in the last trimester of pregnancy. Women usually present with polyhydramnios, or undergo an ultrasound examination for discrepancy of gestational size and date. A careful ultrasonographic evaluation of the fetus, with particular attention to the placenta and to cardiac structure and rate, is indicated to detect abnormalities. Maternal serum analysis for blood type and antibody screen and a Kleihauer-Betke test for fetal red cells are important to detect isoimmune disease or fetal-maternal hemorrhage. Maternal red cell morphology, mean corpuscular volume, and mean corpuscular hemoglobin concentration should indicate whether hemoglobin electrophoresis is necessary. Titers for cytomegalovirus, *Toxoplasma*, and rubella virus, as well as a serologic test for syphilis, should be obtained.

Amniocentesis should be performed. If the maternal antibody screen is positive, amniotic fluid should be sent for OD_{450} measurements as an indicator of fetal hemolysis. Amniotic fluid fibroblasts can be sent for karyotyping and lecithin/sphingomyelin ratio and saturated phosphatidylcholine measured to indicate the status of fetal lung maturity in the event that early delivery is necessary. The presence of *isoimmunization appears to increase the risk of respiratory distress syndrome* in the presence of a (usually mature) lecithin/sphingomyelin ratio of higher than 2.0 and a saturated phosphatidylcholine of higher than 500. In affected pregnancies, we use a lecithin/sphingomyelin ratio of above 3.0 and a saturated phosphatidylcholine measure of over or equal to 1,000 μg per milliliter to define biochemical maturity of the lungs.

If the etiology of the hydrops fetalis remains unclear, obtaining a percutaneous blood sample from the fetal umbilical cord should be seriously considered. When safety is assured in the hands of an experienced operator working under direct ultrasound guidance, a fetal blood sample allows direct determination of fetal hematocrit, reticulocyte count, red blood cell morphology, blood type, Coombs' test, and hemoglobin electrophoresis. Moreover, fetal lymphocytes can be obtained to yield an accurate karyotype in several days compared with the 2-week wait for results from amniotic fluid fibroblasts.

Once a diagnosis is made (or the hydrops fetalis remains idiopathic), a coordinated plan for fetal therapy, delivery, delivery room, and neonatal intensive care unit management should be established by the perinatologist, the neonatologist, and the parents. Consideration should be given to fetal transfusion or exchange transfusion via the umbilical cord for severe isoimmune disease or fetal-maternal hemorrhage, to maternal drug therapy with digoxin or propranolol for fetal tachyarrhythmias, or to drainage of the pleural effusions and ascites immediately prior to delivery to achieve optimal lung inflation in the delivery room. The diagnosis of a fatal trisomy (13 or 18) would also have importance for the timing and route of delivery as well as for immediate and ongoing neonatal management.

DELIVERY ROOM MANAGEMENT

Delivery room measures are similar for all babies with hydrops fetalis, but after establishment of adequate gas exchange and heart rate, management must be individualized according to underlying diagnosis. As for all infants, initial attention should focus on establishing a clear airway and adequate gas exchange. Since these infants are often critically ill immediately after delivery, a team of physicians and nurses should be prepared for the multiple roles that may be necessary in the first few minutes after delivery. Most neonates with hydrops have abundant lung fluid, pleural effusions and ascites, and thick body wall edema. All these factors limit initial lung expansion, and one should be prepared to rapidly intubate the baby if respiratory efforts appear to be ineffective. In those babies with large collections of pleural and peritoneal fluid, one must be prepared to perform thoracentesis and paracentesis to drain the fluid and allow lung expansion.

Pleural and peritoneal drainage in the delivery room is best accomplished with 20-gauge intravascular catheters and 20-ml syringes attached via a stopcock. The placement of chest tubes for continuous drainage should generally be reserved for the sterile conditions and monitored setting of the neonatal intensive care unit.

Once a secure airway is achieved, mechanical ventilation should proceed as in routine resuscitation. Inspiratory pressures greater than those usually used may be necessary to achieve lung expansion. The usual guides of upper chest movement and breath sounds in the axillae should serve to direct optimal inspiratory pressure. A positive end-expiratory pressure of 4 to 6 cm H_2O should be maintained with an inspiratory time of 0.6 to 1.0 sec.

Even in the presence of severe anemia, it is generally best to move the patient to the neonatal intensive care unit at this point if the heart rate is higher than 100 beats per minute and the infant's gas exchange is adequate.

Before leaving the delivery room, a cord blood specimen should be obtained for cord pH, hematocrit, erythrocyte morphology, reticulocyte count, blood type, Coombs' test, hemoglobin electrophoresis, and bilirubin level. Another cord blood specimen should be sent to the blood bank for typing and cross-matching.

Neonatal intensive care unit management depends on the specific etiology of the hydrops fetalis. In all hydropic infants who present with severe respiratory failure at birth, however, placement of an umbilical artery catheter and umbilical venous catheter (in the inferior vena cava or right atrium) provides important access for physiologic monitoring and for administration of fluid and medications. Direct and continuous arterial blood pressure and central venous pressure measurements are important to guide volume, pressor, and diuretic therapy. The placement of these catheters, the location of the endotracheal tube, and the presence of pleural effusions should be checked with chest and abdominal x-ray films before additional procedures begin. The presence of large pleural effusions and persistent hypoxia and hypercarbia indicates the need for the placement of chest tubes for continuous pleural drainage. The presence of a large amount of ascites or the remnants of a recent intraperitoneal fetal transfusion may require aspiration of the peritoneal space. In addition, although transcutaneous monitoring of Po_2 and Pco_2 may be affected by the peripheral edema, oximetry should be accurate and is useful in this situation.

HYDROPS SECONDARY TO FETAL ANEMIA

The major therapeutic intervention in this group of infants is correction of the anemia. Since it is unusual for fetal anemia to lead to hydrops fetalis unless the hematocrit is lower than 20 to 25 percent, elevation of the hematocrit by simple transfusion would result in volume expansion and the risk of worsened congestive heart failure. To avoid this risk, an exchange transfusion should be carried out as soon as adequate mechanical ventilation is achieved and umbilical catheters are in place. Delay until the infant's blood can be cross-matched is not desirable; rather, freshly drawn (less than 6 to 12 hours) O-negative red blood cells suspended in AB-negative plasma and cross-matched before delivery with the mother's blood should be ready for use immediately after delivery. The blood should be packed to achieve a hematocrit of 55 to 70 percent, depending on the severity of the anemia. A single-volume exchange transfusion should suffice for nonhemolytic anemia; double-volume exchange is more effective in replacing sensitized fetal cells in cases of isoimmune disease.

The optimal technique for exchange transfusion continues to be debated. We withdraw blood from the umbilical artery and infuse it into the umbilical vein cannula at a continuous, matched rate of 2 to 4 ml per kilogram per minute. This should allow establishment of an acceptable hematocrit value within 30 to 60 minutes of delivery. Careful monitoring of the heart rate, blood pressure (via Dynamap oscillometry once the umbilical artery catheter is in use), arterial blood gases, and hematocrit is performed during the exchange transfusion. The need for subsequent exchange transfusions can be determined by following the hematocrit in cases of fetal-maternal hemorrhage or the hematocrit and bilirubin levels in cases of isoimmune disease.

The first exchange transfusion usually is adequate to treat the anemia, hypoproteinemia, and volume problems seen in hydrops fetalis secondary to isoimmune disease. Albumin or fresh frozen plasma infusions are usually not needed and may prove detrimental because increasing oncotic pressure may lead to rapid mobilization of the peripheral edema and worsened congestive heart failure. Once the hematocrit has been corrected, support of ventilation with positive end-expiratory pressure is usually sufficient to allow gradual mobilization of the 25 to 30 percent of birth weight that is excess fluid. If cardiomegaly, hepatomegaly, and persistent pulmonary fluid persist, judicious use of cardiotonic drugs and diuretics may be useful. Dopamine in a dose of 2.5 to 5.0 μg per kilogram per minute intravenously and furosemide in a dose of 0.5 to 1.0 mg per kilogram given intravenously will assist in the diuresis in those cases.

Fluid administration should be kept to a minimum, since there is usually 30 percent excess extravascular water mobilized postnatally. The provision of 40 to 60 ml per kilogram per day as dextrose-containing fluid is usually sufficient until diuresis is accomplished. Care must be taken to provide a high enough glucose concentration to meet the usual 4 to 8 mg per kilogram per minute glucose requirement. Provision of 12.5 to 20 percent dextrose via the umbilical venous catheter located in the inferior vena cava or right atrium may be needed. Maintenance electrolytes should be added after 24 to 48 hours. Total output, including urine and chest tube drainage, should be carefully measured to guide fluid administration.

HYDROPS SECONDARY TO CONGENITAL HEART DISEASE

A chest x-ray film, ultrasonographic examination, and an electrocardiogram should be done on all nonanemic hydropic infants. Even in the presence of normal sinus rhythm and a structurally normal heart, intermittent tachyarrhythmia as the cause of hydrops cannot be completely ruled out.

If the infant has a tachyarrhythmia at birth and is hydropic, immediate measures to correct the arrhythmia should be taken. Vagal stimulation by rectal examination, ice applied to the face, and even intubation are frequently unsuccessful. Digoxin administration using a total intravenous loading dose of 20 to 30 μg per kilogram can be administered as half followed by one-quarter at 8 to 12 hour intervals. This may not be effective in establishing normal sinus rhythm for several hours, and the severely compromised infant should be treated with cardioversion. A synchronized direct current defibrillator beginning at 1 to 2 ws per kilogram should be applied to achieve normal sinus rhythm. Our limited experience with the calcium-channel blocker, verapamil, has been unsatisfactory, with electromechanical dissociation and circulatory collapse having occurred in the one infant in whom we used this medication.

The presence of congenital heart block should alert the obstetrician to the possibility of lupus erythematosus in the mother. Also, nearly half of these infants have an associated structural heart defect. The hydropic baby with a very slow heart rate should received intravenous isoproterenol (Isuprel, 0.1 μg per kilogram per minute) until a transvenous pacemaker can be inserted.

The supportive care for infants with the unusual case of hydrops secondary to congenital infection, aneuploidy, or idiopathic cause is similar to that discussed under anemia-related hydrops. Careful attention to adequate ventilation, maintenance of a normal hematocrit, fluid restriction, use of diuretics and cardiotonic drugs as indicated by blood pressure, central venous pressure monitoring, and striving for a gradual consistent diuresis over 5 to 7 days should result in recovery. Infants with trisomy 13 or 18 or complex congenital heart disease and those who are premature and have hyaline membrane disease in addition to hydrops fetalis contribute to an overall mortality of 40 to 50 percent in this condition.

HYPERAMMONEMIA

DENNIS W. BARTHOLOMEW, M.D.
MARK L. BATSHAW, M.D.

Neonatal hyperammonemia may result from various inborn errors of metabolism, including urea cycle defects, organic acidemias, and congenital lactic acidosis as well as from nongenetic causes such as transient hyperammonemia of the neonate, hepatic failure, and herpesvirus infection. Hyperammonemia is a potentially lethal condition requiring prompt and aggressive intervention if the infant is to have a chance of surviving intact. However, most affected infants are born into families in which the disorder has not previously been identified and therefore is not suspected. Delays in detection of a markedly elevated plasma ammonium level (500 to 2,000 μM, normal <50 μM) are likely to be catastrophic. Even with optimal therapy, almost half of affected newborns do not survive. On the other hand, prospective therapy from birth for infants detected as having a urea cycle defect (because of a previously affected sibling) has been shown to be effective in preventing neonatal hyperammonemic coma, although it does not necessarily ensure normal intellectual development.

Severe neonatal hyperammonemia is most commonly the result of a urea cycle defect (Fig. 1). Of the six inborn errors of urea synthesis, the X-linked condition ornithine transcarbamylase deficiency is the most frequent, with an estimated incidence of 1:50,000 live births. A maternal family history of male infant deaths or of recurrent Reye's syndrome and protein intolerance in females is helpful. In the other defects, a history of consanguinity increases the likelihood of these disorders, since they are inherited as autosomal recessive traits.

Hyperammonemia may also occur secondary to other disorders, both genetic and nongenetic. Organic acidemias, including propionic acidemia, methylmalonic acidemia, glutaric aciduria type II, multiple carboxylase deficiency, isovaleric acidemia, and 3-hydroxymethylglutaryl-CoA lyase deficiency, may be manifested by moderate to severe hyperammonemia (range 150 to 1,000 μM) associated with profound metabolic acidosis. The congenital lactic acidoses, caused by deficient activity of pyruvate carboxylase, pyruvate dehydrogenase or the electron transport chain, may also manifest in this manner. Presumably the hyperammonemia in these disorders is secondary to an inhibition of the urea cycle by accumulating metabolic intermediates.

Nongenetic causes of neonatal hyperammonemia include hepatic failure, systemic herpesvirus infections, and transient hyperammonemia of the newborn. The last is a poorly understood entity affecting mostly premature infants who have respiratory distress in the first 24 hours of life. Resolution of the hyperammonemia following treatment of the underlying pulmonary disease is the rule, and episodes do not recur. However, the mortality rate is high, and severe brain damage may occur.

Regardless of cause, the consequences of prolonged hyperammonemia in newborn infants are devastating, and early aggressive treatment is mandatory. The onset of hyperammonemia is usually heralded by respiratory distress, irritability, poor feeding, and emesis. Except for transient hyperammonemia of the newborn, symptoms usually become manifest on the second or third day of life. They are sufficiently nonspecific to prompt an evaluation for other causes of clinical deterioration, including sepsis, gastrointestinal obstruction, cardiac abnormalities, and intraventricular hemorrhage. A good rule of thumb is that unless the cause of sepsis is evident, *any infant who is doing poorly enough to warrant a work-up for sepsis deserves a plasma ammonium determination.*

In the absence of proper treatment, hyperammonemia is inexorably progressive, and deep coma and death result. Tachypnea is a frequent early sign and is a direct result of the stimulation of the respiratory center in the brain stem by ammonium ions. Respiratory alkalosis may be useful in distinguishing a urea cycle defect from an organic acidemia or lactic acidemia, both of which generally manifest as metabolic acidosis. Other signs may include seizures, apnea, and ultimately cardiovascular collapse.

A knowledge of the precise underlying metabolic defect causing the hyperammonemic coma is not a prerequisite for initial therapy. Ideally, plasma amino acids and lactate levels should be obtained and urine collected for

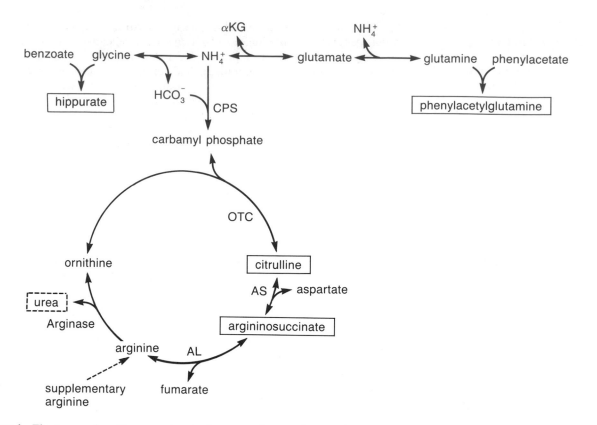

Figure 1 The urea cycle with approaches to alternate pathways of waste nitrogen excretion using arginine, sodium benzoate, and sodium phenylacetate. Boxed compounds are alternate waste nitrogen products; CPS, carbamyl phosphate synthetase; OTC, ornithine transcarbamylase; AS, argininosuccinate synthetase (deficiency is citrullinemia); AL, argininosuccinate lyase (deficiency is argininosuccinic aciduria); αkG, α-ketoglutarate.

orotic acid and organic acid analysis, although results of these tests are seldom immediately available. Serial plasma ammonium levels are necessary to monitor therapy.

Several therapeutic steps should be undertaken while diagnostic testing is under way (Fig. 2). Protein-containing feedings should be withdrawn, although this is insufficient in itself to improve hyperammonemia due to the large endogenous protein turnover during the first few days of life. The infant is given 60 to 100 kcal per kilogram per day by peripheral hyperalimentation with a hyperosmolar dextrose solution and supplemental lipids. Removal of protein from the diet for several days does no harm, and the provision of adequate calories from carbohydrate and fat sources reduces protein turnover for gluconeogenesis.

A rapidly rising plasma ammonium level results in profound clinical deterioration and requires immediate intervention with hemodialysis or peritoneal dialysis. Hemodialysis is the preferable treatment. Access to the circulatory system for hemodialysis may be gained by the use of the femoral or umbilical vessels. Umbilical artery catheters should be at least No. 5 French, preferably No. 8 French, to ensure adequate blood flow to the dialyzer. The dialysis unit itself should be well heparinized and of the smallest possible volume (30 ml). Wide swings in pulse rate and blood pressure during dialysis are frequent and may necessitate transfusion. Only fresh whole blood

should be administered, since ammonium concentration in stored blood may reach high levels.

If hemodialysis is not available, peritoneal dialysis should be instituted. There are only a few absolute contraindications to peritoneal dialysis in an infant: diaphragmatic hernia and open abdominal defects. Standard dialysis fluid containing 1.5 percent added glucose may be used in a volume of 50 to 100 ml per kilogram per pass with a dwell time of 20 to 30 minutes. To assist effluent flow, a second peritoneal opening may be established. The potential for immediate hemodynamic disturbances is considerably less than for hemodialysis, and close monitoring of weight, electrolyte, and acid-base status reduces the risk of secondary metabolic complications. However, the rate of fall in plasma ammonium in response to peritoneal dialysis is seldom as vigorous as that seen with hemodialysis.

In contrast to hemodialysis and peritoneal dialysis, exchange transfusions have been shown to be of little value in lowering plasma ammonium levels, probably because unlike bilirubin, ammonium is fairly uniformly distributed throughout the body water. Charcoal hemoperfusion has been used but is of unproven benefit.

Cerebral edema is commonly associated with hyperammonemic coma. However, elevations in intracranial pressure are not always evident in the newborn because

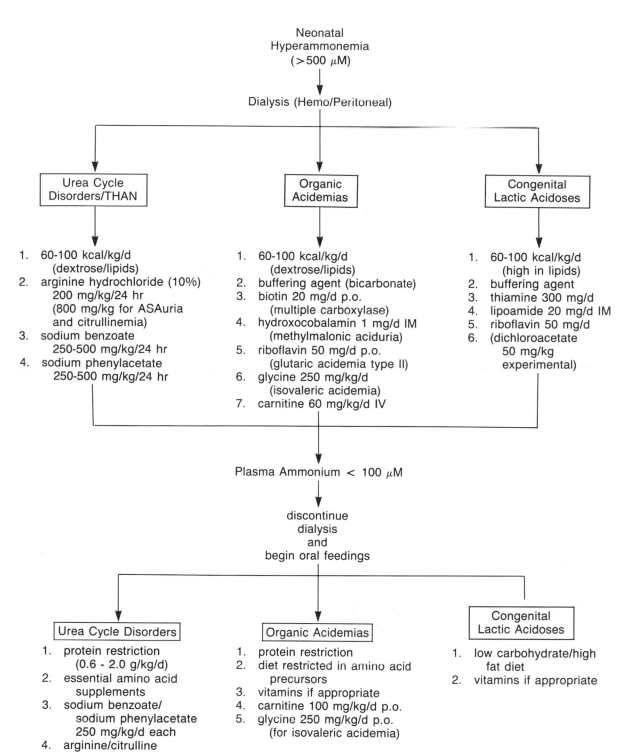

Figure 2 Flow diagram for treatment of neonatal hyperammonemic coma. ASAuria = argininosuccinic aciduria; THAN = transient hyperammonemia of the neonate.

of patent cranial sutures. If therapy is deemed necessary, intravenous osmotic agents such as mannitol may be of benefit. Mechanically assisted hyperventilation as a means of decreasing intracranial pressure should be avoided because of the risk of increasing the intracellular shift of ammonium ions. Steroids are contraindicated because they promote catabolism.

Although dialysis is the most efficient means of removing ammonium ions and other small organic molecules, several ancillary treatments may help to decrease ammonium levels. These approaches vary, depending on the suspected underlying disorder, and should be used in combination with dialysis.

UREA CYCLE DISORDERS

In urea cycle defects ancillary therapy involves the use of arginine, sodium benzoate, and sodium phenylacetate (see Fig. 1). With the sole exception of the presence of arginase deficiency, any interruption of the urea cycle will curtail synthesis of arginine. As a result, patients with urea cycle disorders invariably become arginine-deficient in the absence of supplementation. This results in an inhibition of residual urea cycle activity. This is particularly true of argininosuccinic aciduria and, to a lesser extent citrullinemia, in which vast quantities of the arginine precursors, argininosuccinic acid and citrulline, respectively, are lost in the urine. For this reason, a solution of 10 percent arginine hydrochloride (R-Gene, KabiVitrum) should be administered intravenously as a bolus of 800 mg per kilogram at the initiation of therapy. This is followed by a continuous infusion of 800 mg per kilogram per day until the diagnosis of argininosuccinic aciduria or citrullinemia has been excluded. At this point, the dosage may be decreased to 200 mg per kilogram per day. Hyperchloremic acidosis often occurs with prolonged infusion of the arginine hydrochloride salt and may require buffering with bicarbonate. Arginine is obviously contraindicated in the treatment of arginase deficiency, but this disorder does not result in clinical symptoms in the newborn period.

The medications sodium benzoate and sodiumphenyl acetate (Ucephan, Kendall-McGaw) provide alternate pathways of waste nitrogen disposal that bypass the urea cycle. Their efficacy in the prevention and treatment of hyperammonemia is now well established. The rationale for their use lies in the observation that following activation with coenzyme A, they bind to specific amino acids and are then rapidly excreted in the urine. Sodium benzoate combines with glycine to form hippurate, whereas sodium phenylacetate reacts with glutamine to form phenylacetylglutamine. Both amino acids are nonessential and are rapidly resynthesized from available nitrogen-containing precursors. Whereas glycine contains only a single nitrogen atom, glutamine contains two; hence, on a molar basis, phenylacetate should remove about twice as much nitrogen as benzoate. These drugs appear to work synergistically, and therefore combined therapy is suggested.

It should be emphasized that these drugs are of limited benefit in the face of marked hyperammonemia (higher than 500 μM), and the institution of dialysis should not be delayed by attempts at drug therapy alone. Since neurologic outcome appears to be directly related to the duration of hyperammonemic coma, the simultaneous use of dialysis and alternate pathway drug therapy would appear to offer the best hope for the rapid resolution of hyperammonemic coma. Sodium benzoate and sodium phenylacetate are given in a bolus of 250 mg per kilogram, each mixed in 25 ml per kilogram of 10 percent dextrose over 90 minutes. This is followed by a continuous infusion of each at 250 to 500 mg per kilogram per day. Both drugs

may be mixed in the same intravenous bottle. Remember that this infusion represents a sodium load of 3.5 to 7.0 mEq per kilogram per 24 hours, so that additional sodium should not be given. Emesis is common following a bolus injection of benzoate or phenylacetate. Plasma drug levels should be monitored if possible. Overdose is characterized by a metabolic acidosis with a large anion gap. An accidental administration of tenfold the prescribed intravenous dose of benzoate and phenylacetate to a 1-year-old child resulted in death. The use of lactulose or bowel sterilization with neomycin is of unclear benefit in neonatal hyperammonemia, since ammonium production from urea-splitting organisms is negligible in newborns.

When the plasma ammonium level has fallen below 100 μM (twice that of normal), nitrogen may be cautiously reintroduced in the form of a combination of natural protein and essential amino acids to a total of 1.5 g per kilogram per day (Table 1). Alternatively, essential amino acid formulas such as UCD-1 (Mead-Johnson) may be used. Infants with deficiencies of ornithine transcarbamylase or carbamyl phosphate synthetase may be less tolerant of excess nitrogen and require an essential amino acid mixture as one-half of their daily nitrogen intake. Those with citrullinemia or argininosuccinic aciduria may tolerate up to 2 g of protein per kilogram per day from natural sources such as infant formulas. Non-nitrogen calories up to 120 kcal per kilogram per day may be provided with a protein-free formula such as Mead Johnson Product 80056. Children with urea cycle defects continue to need sodium benzoate 250 mg per kilogram per day and/or sodium phenyl acetate 250 mg per kilogram per day, both of which can be added to the child's formula. L-Arginine free base 600 to 700 mg per kilogram per day is continued in patients with citrullinemia and argininosuccinic aciduria. We routinely substitute oral citrulline 175 mg per kilogram per day for arginine in children with ornithine transcarbamylase or carbamyl phosphate synthetase deficiencies.

ORGANIC ACIDEMIAS

Besides dialysis, therapy in organic acidemias involves nitrogen restriction, vitamin supplementation, and carnitine administration. Precursor formation is reduced by protein withdrawal and adequate caloric supplementation. The correction of metabolic acidosis is enhanced by the use of intravenous buffering solutions. Vitamin cofactors activate some of the deficient enzymatic pathways, and the toxic metabolites that accumulate in organic acidemias, such as propionate and methylmalonate, are amenable to removal as carnitine or glycine conjugates.

Biotin, 20 mg per day, hydroxocobalamin, 1 mg per day intramuscularly, and riboflavin (50 mg per day) have been used in treating methylmalonic acidemia, multiple carboxylase deficiency, and glutaric acidemia type II, respectively. These three vitamins may be given together if the specific defect is unknown. Continued treatment with vitamin supplements depends on establishing a specific diagnosis and demonstrating whether the defect is vitamin-responsive. Carnitine is given at a dosage of 60 mg per kilogram per day intravenously or 100 mg per kilogram

TABLE 1 Long-Term Therapy of Urea Cycle Disorders (g/kg/day)

Disorders	Natural Protein	Essential Amino Acids	Citrulline	Arginine	Sodium Benzoate	Sodium Phenyl Acetate
Carbamyl phosphate synthetase deficiency	0.6	0.6	0.18	—	0.25	0.25
Ornithine trans-carbamylase deficiency	0.6	0.6	0.18	—	0.25	0.25
Citrullinemia	1.2–1.5	—	—	0.4–0.7	0.25	0.25
Argininosuccinic aciduria	1.2–1.5	—	—	0.4–0.7	—	—

Calories supplemented with Mead Johnson Product 80056.
Essential amino acids provided as UCD-1 (Mead-Johnson).

per day by mouth. In isovaleric acidemia, glycine is administered at a dose of 250 mg per kilogram per day.

Long-term therapy requires the restriction of intake of precursor amino acids only to that required to sustain growth. Formulas low in branched chain amino acids such as OS-1 and S-14 have been useful. Caloric supplementation with low-protein solids and protein-free formulas such as Product 80056 keeps endogenous protein catabolism to a minimum. L-Carnitine 100 mg per kilogram per day by mouth replaces depleted tissue carnitine stores and enhances the urinary excretion of toxic organic acid intermediates in the form of acylcarnitine derivatives such as propionylcarnitine in propionic acidemia.

CONGENITAL LACTIC ACIDOSES

Ancillary therapy for lactic acidosis has involved a ketogenic diet, vitamins, and dichloroacetate. These rare disorders of pyruvate metabolism or of the electron transport chain often manifest on the first days of life with respiratory distress and coma associated with profound lactic acidosis and secondary hyperammonemia (range 100 to 2,000 μM). Since an enzyme diagnosis is made in less than half the cases of congenital lactic acidosis, firm conclusions regarding therapy are lacking. Isolated reports have suggested some improvements in patients with pyruvate dehydrogenase deficiency who received the cofactors thiamine hydrochloride, 300 mg per day by mouth, and lipoamide, 20 mg per day intramuscularly. Riboflavin, 100 mg per day by mouth, has been used to treat certain defects in the mitochondrial respiratory chain causing lactic acidosis. Intravenous dichloroacetate (50 to 100 mg per kilogram per day), is known to activate residual pyruvate dehydrogenase activity by inhibiting pyruvate dehydrogenase kinase. Dichloroacetate is considered an experimental medication.

TRANSIENT HYPERAMMONEMIA OF THE NEWBORN

Despite the self-limited nature of this nongenetic disorder, the consequences of untreated neonatal hyperammonemia may be devastating. Plasma ammonium levels generally exceed 1,000 μM and necessitate dialysis. However, transient hyperammonemia of the newborn should be distinguishable from urea cycle disorders and organic acidemias by its early onset, lack of family history, and generally normal pattern of plasma amino acids and urinary organic acids. Episodes do not recur after the newborn period, and long-term drug therapy and protein-restricted diets are not required. Thus, therapy is directed at the rapid removal of ammonia by dialysis.

RESULTS OF TREATMENT

Early intervention with protein withdrawal, adequate calories by means of hyperalimentation, dialysis, and ancillary therapy hopefully result in a significant fall in plasma ammonium levels within 24 to 48 hours. Neurologic improvement in all these disorders generally lags behind the biochemical correction of hyperammonemia by 12 to 24 hours. By this time, a tentative diagnosis has been established in most cases, and long-term management may begin. In urea cycle defects, eventual neurologic outcome depends on the duration of hyperammonemic coma. Over half of surviving children have been developmentally disabled, and all who have been in hyperammonemic coma more than 72 hours have been mentally retarded.

Since approximately half of the infants with neonatal hyperammonemia expire during the first week of life, definitive diagnostic procedures such as liver biopsy or skin fibroblast cultures should be obtained at the time of death in order to provide accurate genetic counseling to parents regarding future pregnancies.

Supported by RO1-NS 28033. Neurotransmitters, appetite and inborn metabolism errors.

SUGGESTED READING

Batshaw ML. Hyperammonemia. Curr Prob Pediatr 1984; 14:1–69.

Batshaw ML, Brusilow SW. Treatment of hyperammonemic coma caused by inborn errors of urea synthesis. J Pediatr 1980; 97:893–900.

Brusilow SW, Batshaw ML Waber L. Neonatal hyperammonemic coma. Adv Pediatr 1982; 29.69–103.

Hudak ML, Jones MD, Brusilow SW. Differentiation of transient hyperammonemia of the newborn and urea cycle enzyme defects by clinical presentation. J Pediatr 1985; 107:712–719.

Msall M, Batshaw ML, Suss R, et al. Neurologic outcome of children with inborn errors of urea synthesis. N Engl J Med 1984; 310:1500.

Robinson BH, Sherwood WG. Lactic acidemia. J Inherited Metab Dis 1984 (Suppl 1); 7:69–73.

Tuchman M, Ulstrom RA. Organic acids in health and disease. Adv-Pediatr 1985; 32:469–506.

HYPERBILIRUBINEMIA

M. JEFFREY MAISELS, M.B., B.Ch.

We know how to treat hyperbilirubinemia; we are less sure about *when* to treat it. What follows reflects my personal practice. For "practice," do *not* read "recommendations." *We should make recommendations only when there are sufficient experimental or epidemiologic data to support them.* With the exception of the infant with erythroblastosis fetalis, such evidence is lacking.

By 1952, two studies had established a strong association between severe hyperbilirubinemia and the clinical syndrome of kernicterus in newborn infants with Rh erythroblastosis fetalis. However, if the serum bilirubin concentration was maintained below 20 mg per deciliter, clinical kernicterus was not seen. These studies were not randomized clinical trials, but they satisfied the criteria for contributory cause: (1) there was a strong association between hyperbilirubinemia and kernicterus (and a strong "dose-response" gradient); (2) the putative cause (hyperbilirubinemia) preceded the effect (kernicterus); and (3) altering the cause (lowering serum bilirubin level by exchange transfusion) dramatically altered the effect (decreased kernicterus). The level of 20 mg per deciliter is still considered an appropriate maximum for infants with erythroblastosis fetalis.

The clinical syndrome of kernicterus is rarely seen today, but some studies have identified an association between increasing bilirubin levels during the neonatal period and subsequent poor developmental outcome. Others have not found this association, but the possibility of subtle brain damage remains the major rationale for attempting to lower the serum bilirubin.

In small premature infants, bilirubin staining of the brain is still found occasionally at autopsy, even when these infants were exposed to low serum bilirubin levels (as low as 3.3 mg per deciliter in one reported case). Presumably, these infants did not die *from* kernicterus, and whether they died *with* kernicterus is a matter of some debate. It has been argued by some pathologists that, in many such cases, the bilirubin staining is secondary to prior nonspecific cell damage rather than an indication of bilirubin toxicity itself. Other pathologists contest this viewpoint.

The association between increasing serum bilirubin concentration and developmental outcome, in both full-term and preterm infants, has been examined many times. Most of these studies are flawed and the results are conflicting, permitting neither a consistent nor a rational approach to therapy. It is not difficult to understand, therefore, why we approach the management of jaundiced newborn infants with little confidence.

PREMATURE INFANTS

Most current autopsy diagnoses of kernicterus are made in infants with birth weights of less than 1,500 g. Since such infants are the sickest occupants of our Neonatal Intensive Care Units and most likely to die, this is not surprising. In preterm infants, however, it is important to note that the association between increasing serum bilirubin levels and clinical or pathologic kernicterus is poor, provided the bilirubin level remains below 18 mg per deciliter. Thus, it is difficult to offer a *scientific* rationale for treating (on the basis of birth weight alone) a 900-g baby more vigorously (i.e., at a lower bilirubin level) than a 1,400-g baby, or, indeed, an 1,800-g baby.

In the recent prospective randomized trial of phototherapy, conducted in six centers by the National Institutes of Child Health and Human Development (NICHD), there were four cases of kernicterus documented at autopsy. None of these infants received phototherapy, and their birth weights ranged from 760 to 1,270 g. A 6-year follow-up of the surviving infants with birth weights of 2,000 g or less has been completed. Although phototherapy reduced peak serum bilirubin levels significantly (by about 4 mg per deciliter), there were no differences in the incidence of motor deficits or cerebral palsy between the phototherapy and control groups, and there was no effect on IQ scores. A recent study from Holland evaluated the neurodevelopmental outcome in 831 surviving infants of less than or equal to 32 weeks' gestation or birth weights of 1,500 g or less. At a corrected age of 2 years, a significant association was found between increasing maximal neonatal bilirubin concentrations and neurodevelopmental handicaps (mainly cerebral palsy). The risk of handicaps increased by 30 percent for each 3 mg per deciliter increase in the maximal bilirubin level.

These two studies are the first evaluations of the relationship between hyperbilirubinemia and developmental outcome in surviving low birth weight infants in the modern era of intensive care, and the results are conflicting. Although the Dutch study suggests a cause-and-effect relationship between hyperbilirubinemia and neurodevelopmental outcome in infants weighing 1,500 g or less, it provides *no evidence that treatment to reduce the maximal serum bilirubin concentration would also reduce the incidence of neurologic handicap.* Such evidence can only be obtained by randomized clinical trials, which are necessary before we can make therapeutic recommendations.

Data from the NICHD study and from numerous other studies suggest that phototherapy is a safe procedure. No overt, short-term toxicity has been identified in the human neonate. The ease with which it is used and its apparent safety have, in fact, removed much of the clinical decision-making from the treatment of hyperbilirubinemia in the low birth weight infant. This may not be a rational approach, and it is certainly not a scientific one, but it is a fact. For infants with a birth weight of less than 1,500 g, I generally initiate phototherapy when the serum bilirubin level approaches 5 mg per deciliter. For those weighing between 1,500 and 2,000 g, phototherapy is started at a bilirubin level of 8 to 12 mg per deciliter. (In view of what has been stated above, the inconsistency of this approach is obvious! I can offer no defense.) Lower levels are selected for infants who are septic, acidotic, hypoxic, or hypercarbic, and those who have an obvious cause for hyperbilirubinemia, such as severe bruising. In such cases, hyperbilirubinemia can be anticipated, and "prophylactic" phototherapy seems reasonable.

Over the last 12 years, I have not seen a single case of autopsy-proven kernicterus. I do not know whether this has anything to do with our liberal use of phototherapy, nor do I know whether treating mild jaundice in these infants has had any effect on the incidence of neurodevelopmental handicap. However, the experience of most neonatal units in this country is similar to ours. Most report a decreasing incidence of kernicterus in their low birth weight population over the last 5 years.

It is tempting to conclude that this is related to the more liberal use of phototherapy, as suggested by data from the NICHD project. In that study, infants weighing less than 2,000 g were treated with phototherapy (irrespective of serum bilirubin levels) at age 24±12 hours and received treatment for a total of 96 hours. Infants in the control group did not receive phototherapy. Phototherapy was effective. In the phototherapy group, serum bilirubin was greater than or equal to 10 mg per deciliter in only 17.7 percent of infants weighing less than 2,000 g versus 62.8 percent of those in the control group. In both groups, exchange transfusion was performed at serum bilirubin levels of 13 mg per deciliter (less than 1,250 g) or 15 mg per deciliter (1,250 to 1,499 g), unless the infant's course was complicated by perinatal asphyxia, respiratory distress, acidosis, hypothermia, low serum protein level, or evidence of central nervous system deterioration. In such cases, exchange transfusions were performed at bilirubin levels of 10 mg per deciliter (less than 1,250 g) and 13 mg per deciliter (1,250 to 1,499 g), respectively. Of infants weighing less than 1,500 g, 40 in the phototherapy group and 29 in the control group came to autopsy. No kernicterus was found in the phototherapy group, but three cases (10.3 percent) occurred in infants who did not receive phototherapy. A fourth case occurred in an infant who was assigned to the phototherapy group but, due to an error, did not receive phototherapy until age 48 hours, 1 hour before an exchange transfusion was performed. The serum bilirubin levels in the four infants who had kernicterus were 6.5, 8.6, 14.0, and 14.2 mg per deciliter. Although these findings suggest that the liberal use of phototherapy reduced the risk of bilirubin staining of the brain in infants weighing less than 1,500 g, it should be noted that 25 percent of the infants who died did not have autopsies. No kernicterus was seen in infants with birth weights higher than 1,500 g. Only eight such infants were examined by autopsy, however. *Given the absence of toxicity related to phototherapy, I consider its liberal use in this group of infants appropriate.*

Based on the available data, selecting a higher bilirubin level at which to institute phototherapy for infants weighing between 1,500 and 2,000 g (versus those weighing less than 1,500 g) makes little sense but has achieved widespread acceptance. One explanation is that infants weighing less than 1,500 g are more likely to be sick, acidotic, hypoxic, hypercarbic, or septic. Interestingly, in one study, kernicterus was found in 1.6 percent of autopsies on patients between 1,500 and 2,000 g, whereas the incidence in those weighing 2,000 to 2,500 g was 13.8 percent.

For infants weighing between 2 and 2.5 kg (approximately 34 to 36 weeks' gestation), I use phototherapy when the total serum bilirubin level reaches 13 to 15 mg per deciliter. Some experts recommend that the presence of the risk factors listed for NICHD study requires treatment at a lower serum bilirubin level. In two recent studies of low birth weight infants, however, many of these frequently mentioned risk factors, when present, did *not* increase the risk of kernicterus at any given level of serum bilirubin. It is possible that the presence of various risk factors might alter the permeability of the blood-brain barrier to bilirubin or render brain cells more susceptible to damage by bilirubin. If so, a strong association between total bilirubin or free (unbound) bilirubin levels and kernicterus is unlikely.

During the last 10 years, I have not performed a single exchange transfusion for hyperbilirubinemia in a low birth weight infant, unless it was associated with severe bruising or hemolytic disease. Rising bilirubin levels in these infants are controlled by the use of phototherapy. If one phototherapy light is not effective, I use two or three lights, placing the light source as close as possible to the incubator surface to increase the radiant intensity. If serum bilirubin levels cannot be controlled by phototherapy, I consider performing an exchange transfusion at a level of approximately 13 mg per deciliter in infants weighing less than 1,500 g and 15 mg per deciliter for infants weighing between 1,500 and 2,000 g.

FULL-TERM INFANTS

Most premature infants must remain in the hospital for some time. Thus the decision to use or not to use phototherapy has no effect on the length of stay and minimal impact on considerations such as cost and parent-infant bonding. Under these circumstances, and because phototherapy is so easy to use, the decision to use it rather liberally is easily understood and, on balance, defensible. The presence of jaundice in a healthy full-term infant, however, engenders substantial anxiety in the parents and perhaps even more in the physician. Here, decisions regarding continued hospitalization, the need for repeated serum bilirubin determinations, and the use of phototherapy raise issues that need not be confronted in the treatment of the low birth weight infant.

Because the syndrome of clinical kernicterus in full-term infants is essentially unknown today, we treat them to avoid the (presumed) risk of subtle neurologic damage. But the management of hyperbilirubinemia in the full-term infant also depends on the etiology of the jaundice.

Breast-Feeding and Jaundice

The association between breast-feeding and jaundice in the healthy term infant has been divided into two categories: (1) the jaundice that is "associated with breast-feeding, and (2) "true breast-milk jaundice." The difference between these two entities may be more apparent than real. True breast-milk jaundice is a well-described syndrome said to occur in 1 to 2 percent of breast-fed babies. In these infants, the bilirubin concentration rises progressively from the fourth day of life, reaching a maximum of 10 to 30 mg per deciliter by 10 to 15 days. If breast-feeding continues, elevated levels may persist for 4 to 10 days and then decline slowly, reaching normal values by 3 to 12 weeks. If breast-feeding is interrupted, there is usually a prompt decline in serum bilirubin levels within 48 hours. With the resumption of nursing, bilirubin concentrations may rise by 1 to 3 mg per deciliter but do not reach the previous level. Several recent studies, however, suggest that the syndrome of prolonged hyperbilirubinemia, in association with breast-feeding, occurs in as many as 30 percent of breast-fed babies. In one study, 11 of 27 breast-fed infants had bilirubin levels higher than 12 mg per deciliter at 1 week (five had levels higher than 15 mg per deciliter). The mean serum bilirubin level for 27 breast-fed babies at age 21 days was 5.0 mg per deciliter. There is little doubt, therefore, that the syndrome of breast-milk jaundice is more common than previously realized. There is probably a wide spectrum of such infants, some of whom have mild and others pronounced hyperbilirubinemia but in whom the pathogenesis is likely to be similar.

Heretofore, there has been little evidence to support the contention that breast-fed infants, in the first 3 days of life, have serum bilirubin levels that are higher than those of their formula-fed peers. However, more recent evidence from our own institution and others clearly demonstrates that this contention was correct. There is now overwhelming evidence that there *is* a significant association between breast-feeding and the incidence of non-physiologic jaundice in a normal newborn population as early as the third day of life. Of infants with no identifiable cause for hyperbilirubinemia (55 percent in our full-term population), 81 percent are breast-fed. This suggests that the approach to the management of jaundice in the breast-fed and bottle-fed populations should be different.

I treat full-term formula-fed infants without hemolytic disease by using phototherapy when the serum bilirubin concentration exceeds 15 mg per deciliter. *In breast-fed infants, in the absence of other obvious causes, I assume that breast-feeding is contributing to hyperbilirubinemia.* Initially, I encourage breast-feeding mothers to nurse as frequently as possible, as there appears to be an association between a decreased frequency of nursing and higher bilirubin levels. This conclusion is reinforced by the data from the NICHD study, which showed an inverse relationship between caloric intake and serum bilirubin levels. Higher fluid and caloric intakes were associated with lower daily mean serum bilirubin levels, in both infants receiving and those not receiving phototherapy. Thus, it seems appropriate to encourage breast-feeding mothers to nurse their infants as frequently as possible, particularly if the serum bilirubin level is rising. *If it appears that the bilirubin concentration will reach 20 mg per deciliter, I recommend that nursing be interrupted for 48 hours* and almost invariably observe a prompt decline in bilirubin levels. Nursing can then be resumed. If positive and enthusiastic support is provided for these mothers and they are encouraged to maintain lactation by using a breast pump during the period of interrupted nursing, they will invariably return to nursing their infants. A decline in serum bilirubin levels removes the necessity for concern about bilirubin or further blood tests which, in my experience, is more than sufficient to make up for the inconvenience of interrupting nursing. This approach obviates the use of phototherapy in the vast majority of breast-fed infants with hyperbilirubinemia.

What is the risk of hyperbilirubinemia in an infant without hemolytic disease? The answer is unknown and the data are conflicting, but some studies have found no evidence for a relationship between serum bilirubin levels below 20 to 25 mg per deciliter and developmental outcome. More recently, however, measurements of brain stem auditory-evoked responses showed abnormalities in approximately one-third of infants with serum bilirubin concentrations between 15 and 25 mg per deciliter and changes in infant behavior and crying have also been observed at similar bilirubin levels. Although the changes reversed rapidly when serum bilirubin levels decreased to within normal range, these observations again raise questions regarding the possibility of subtle bilirubin damage in an otherwise healthy population.

Hemolytic Disease

In my practice, management of hemolytic disease, whether due to Rh or ABO incompatibility, is based on the rate of rise of serum bilirubin. In infants with documented hemolysis and a rapidly rising serum bilirubin level, the early use of phototherapy is appropriate. Hemolysis associated with Rh hemolytic disease is usually but not always more severe than that with ABO hemolytic disease, and the majority of such infants require early phototherapy. A rapid rise of serum bilirubin is defined as an increase of 1 mg per deciliter per hour or more. Experts continue to argue about the necessity for early versus late exchange transfusions. "Early" exchange transfusions are performed based on the prediction that the serum bilirubin concentration will reach 20 mg per deciliter. The rationale for early intervention is the removal of sensitized red cells from the blood, thus aborting the hemolytic process. An early exchange transfusion also corrects anemia and removes some bilirubin before large amounts are distributed into the extravascular space. In Rh hemolytic disease, in particular, I perform an exchange transfusion if the shape of the bilirubin curve indicates that it will exceed 20 mg per deciliter.

Recent studies suggest that the approach to infants with ABO incompatibility can be modified. Although these infants may have a fairly rapid increase of serum bilirubin in the first 12 hours of life, many do not develop significant hyperbilirubinemia subsequently. In a study of full-term infants at the University of California, Los Angeles, infants received phototherapy only if their serum bilirubin levels exceeded 10 mg per deciliter by 12 hours of life, 12 mg per deciliter by 18 hours, 14 mg per deciliter by 24 hours, or 15 mg per deciliter thereafter. Using these criteria for the initiation of phototherapy, the investigators found that only 9 percent of infants with evidence of ABO incompatibility subsequently required phototherapy, and none required an exchange transfusion. Occasionally, infants with severe AO hemolytic disease do require exchange transfusion. The use of intensive phototherapy, however, has made this an infrequent occurrence.

It is important to note that *the majority of infants who are ABO incompatible and have positive indirect Coombs' tests (presence of anti-A or anti-B antibodies in the plasma) do not, in fact, have hemolytic disease and have serum bilirubin levels that are no different from those of the normal nursery population.*

Severe Hemolytic Disease and Hydrops Fetalis

Current obstetric management allows us to anticipate the delivery of these infants. They suffer significant hypoxia in utero, and women who are likely to deliver such infants should be handled exclusively in perinatal centers capable of the full range of obstetric and neonatal intensive care. The management of these infants demands a comprehensive approach that includes intensive monitoring and vigorous treatment of asphyxia, acidosis, hypoglycemia, and hypothermia. *I do not perform routine phlebotomy on these infants because they are usually normovolemic and may be hypovolemic.* In fact, no manipulation of the blood volume should be performed without appropriate measurements of central venous and aortic blood pressure. In order to monitor the central venous pressure accurately, the umbilical venous catheter must enter the inferior vena cava (by way of the ductus venosus). If the catheter is in a portal vein or the umbilical vein, the pressures so measured are meaningless and preclude interpretation of the infant's circulatory status. The practice of measuring "central venous" pressure by means of an umbilical vein catheter may lead to serious therapeutic error unless the position of the catheter is confirmed radiologically or by pressure tracing. Before making therapeutic decisions based on measurements of central venous pressure, it is also necessary to correct acidosis, hypercarbia, hypoxia, and anemia. Serum glucose levels are monitored carefully because hypoglycemia is common. Exchange transfusion with citrate-phosphate-dextrose blood provides a significant glucose load and may lead to rebound hypoglycemia following the procedure.

Hydropic infants or those who are severely anemic (hematocrit of less than 35 percent) and asphyxiated demand immediate treatment. In these infants, *I perform an exchange transfusion of about 40 ml per kilogram of packed cells soon after birth to raise the hematocrit to about 40 percent.* Otherwise, therapy is based on serial hemoglobin and bilirubin determinations. The technique for exchange transfusion is described in detail elsewhere in this volume.

PHOTOTHERAPY

Phototherapy has been accepted as an effective method for reducing serum bilirubin concentrations. It appears to be *more effective than exchange transfusion in achieving prolonged reduction of bilirubin levels in infants with nonhemolytic jaundice* and, if used early, will modify the course of hyperbilirubinemia in ABO and Rh hemolytic disease and may reduce but not eliminate the need for exchange transfusion.

Various types of fluorescent light have been used for phototherapy, and any light that has a significant output in the blue spectrum (425 to 475 nm) is effective in reducing serum bilirubin levels. I use a combination of four special blue lamps (Westinghouse 20-watt F20T12BB) placed in the center of the phototherapy unit with two daylight lamps on either side. This provides effective irradiance without producing discomfort among the nursery staff. There is a clear dose-response relationship, the response increasing with increased dose until a saturation point is reached at an irradiance of approximately 25 to 30 μw per square centimeter per nanometer in the blue spectrum. This produces a 40 to 50 percent decline in the serum bilirubin level over the first 24 hours. Subsequently, the bilirubin concentration continues to fall, but at a decreased rate.

It is important to recognize that this level of irradiance cannot be achieved by a standard phototherapy lamp placed 18 inches above the baby. If necessary, the lamp should be positioned as close as possible to the infant (taking care not to overheat the baby) and, if this is not effective, two or three lamps (on either side) should be used. Note that phototherapy lamps deliver considerable amounts of heat, and the infant's temperature must be monitored to prevent overheating. Because phototherapy lamps deliver a horizontal band of light to the baby, the irradiance is maximal at the surface of the infant closest to the lamp but there is a rapid decline in the radiant energy reaching the lateral surfaces of the body. Additional lamps placed on either side deliver a higher dose of phototherapy to a greater surface area and are therefore more effective than a single lamp. Lining the incubator walls with a white reflecting material (such as a sheet) also increases the efficacy of phototherapy. It has recently been shown that green light ($\approx$ 525 nm) is as effective (or more effective) as blue light in reducing serum bilirubin levels. It seems unlikely, however, that "green" infants will be readily accepted by nursing staff or parents.

Side Effects of Toxicity of Phototherapy

Infants receiving phototherapy pass more frequent and loose stools. They may also develop a transient rash and, on occasion, lethargy and abdominal distention. Some infants develop a dark gray-brown discoloration of their skin, serum, and urine known as the "bronze baby syndrome." Because this occurs almost exclusively in infants with some degree of cholestasis, it seems reasonable to assume that the retention of some product of phototherapy produces the color change. Most infants with the syndrome do not appear to have suffered deleterious consequences, and discontinuance of phototherapy generally results in the disappearance of the bronze pigment.

No significant acute toxicity of phototherapy has been reported. Nevertheless, phototherapy has many biologic effects, and long-term follow-up studies of such infants are still needed. *Because animal experiments have documented retinal damage from phototherapy, I cover the infants' eyes* with opaque patches. These patches can be displaced, obstruct the nares and cause apnea, and constant supervision is necessary to avoid this potential hazard. *Stool water and insensible water losses are increased in infants undergoing phototherapy.* Some experts recommend that additional fluid (25 ml per kilogram per 24 hours) should be given to compensate these infants for their anticipated losses. We do not follow this rule of thumb, preferring to assess the state of the infants' hydration on a daily basis (e.g., based on weight loss, urine output, urine specific gravity) and to adjust fluid balance accordingly. In infants with respiratory disorders, this increased water loss may actually have a salutary effect on interstitial lung fluid and therefore may be a desirable side effect.

TESTS OF THE BINDING OF BILIRUBIN TO ALBUMIN

Some experts believe that measurements of "free" or "loosely bound" bilirubin, or the reserve binding capacity of albumin, predict more accurately the need for exchange transfusion. *To date, no studies have satisfactorily documented the usefulness of these tests.* In the infants in the NICHD cooperative phototherapy study, the hydroxybenzene azobenzoic acid (HABA) binding test was low or "inappropriate" in all four infants who had kernicterus but in only five of 43 infants without kernicterus in whom these studies were done (p = 0.001). The Sephadex binding test and the salicylate saturation index, on the other hand, were less predictive and did not agree with the HABA binding test. Three of the four infants who developed kernicterus had negative Sephadex (Kernlute) tests and normal salicylate indices. One infant had a positive Sephadex test and a normal salicylate saturation index (5.2), and another had a high salicylate index (8.1) and a negative Sephadex test. It is not known whether exchange transfusion in the infants with low HABA values would have prevented kernicterus. The authors of a recent study evaluating the peroxidase technique for the measurement of free bilirubin concluded that this method was "not yet suitable for clinical use." No studies have been done to show that treatment based on the results of binding tests will lead to a different outcome. Indeed, which treatment is appropriate for a serum bilirubin of 6.5 mg per deciliter is open to debate. Currently, we do not use these tests, although some neonatal units do.

COMPLICATIONS OF EXCHANGE TRANSFUSION

Previous data suggested a mortality rate associated with exchange transfusion that approached 1 percent. In the NICHD cooperative phototherapy study, no infant who was not critically ill died following exchange transfusion. The overall death rate from exchange was 0.53 percent of patients or 0.3 percent of exchange transfusions. Only one death occurred, and that was in a critically ill child who died within 6 hours of the procedure. Severe complications (cyanosis, severe bradycardia, or respiratory arrest) occurred in 3.6 percent of those who received exchange transfusions. In expert hands, the mortality from exchange transfusions is low, although significant morbidity may still occur.

PHARMACOLOGIC TREATMENT

Phenobarbital is a potent inducer of microsomal enzymes. In fact, phenobarbital acts on the whole hepatic transport system for organic anions, enhancing uptake and excretion of bilirubin and stimulating bile flow. *I do not administer phenobarbital, except when severe hemolytic disease is predicted.* Given to the Rh-sensitized mother in a dose of 50 to 125 mg per day for 2 weeks prior to delivery, phenobarbital leads to a slower postnatal rise of bilirubin than in nontreated controls and reduces the need for exchange transfusions. If the mother has not received phenobarbital, I usually give a loading dose of 15 to 20 mg per kilogram intravenously or intramuscularly soon after birth to infants with significant Rh hemolytic disease.

An exciting new development in pharmacologic treatment is the use of tin protoporphyrin. This is one of several synthetic metalloporphyrins that competitively inhibit heme oxygenase. By so doing, tin protoporphyrin inhibits the conversion of heme to bilirubin and, potentially, can prevent hyperbilirubinemia. In a study of Coombs' test positive, ABO incompatible full-term infants, the administration of tin protoporphyrin soon after birth significantly decreased plasma bilirubin levels. Further studies are necessary, however, to document both the efficacy and lack of toxicity before this drug can be recommended for widespread use.

HYPOGLYCEMIA

MARVIN CORNBLATH, M.D.

Hypoglycemia refers to an abnormally low value of blood glucose for a well-defined population at a given age and nutritional status. The values are based on data utilizing specific, reliable laboratory analyses and blood sampling techniques that protect against the increased glycolysis in newborn red cells and the increased nonspecific nonglucose-reducing substances also present. Thus, blood samples must be kept iced and/or contain a glycolytic inhibitor, e.g., sodium fluoride, to provide reliable results. With these precautions, hypoglycemia in the neonate has been defined according to values given in Table 1.

TABLE 1 Hypoglycemic Glucose Levels

Neonate	Glucose (mg/dl)	
	Whole Blood	Serum/Plasma
Preterm or low birth weight	<20 (1.1 mM)	<25 (1.4 mM)
Term or full-sized		
Birth to 72 hr of age	<30 (1.7 mM)	<35 (1.9 mM)
>72 hr of age	<40 (2.2 mM)	<45 (2.5 mM)

To establish the validity of these values, either two blood samples or one blood sample and one cerebrospinal fluid sample must confirm that hypoglycemia is indeed present. Chemstrip Bg or Visidex or Dextrostix may be used for screening (to be discussed) but cannot be regarded as a blood glucose determination to establish that hypoglycemia is or is not present. Even when read in their appropriate reflectometers, these glucose oxidase sticks represent screening techniques only and not a laboratory glucose determination.

Clinical manifestations of hypoglycemia are never specific, especially in the neonate, and may include a wide range of local or generalized manifestations that are common in the sick neonate. Seizures, episodes of cyanosis, apnea, limpness, irregular respirations, apathy, difficulty in feeding, and an abnormal cry have all been attributed to or have resulted from significant hypoglycemia. All have occurred with sepsis, asphyxia, intracranial hemorrhage, and multiple other illnesses that are prevalent in the newborn period. Therefore, to establish the diagnosis of symptomatic neonatal hypoglycemia it is critical, after two reliable glucose determinations have been obtained, to demonstrate that the clinical manifestations disappear promptly following the parenteral administration of adequate amounts of glucose. Only then can the infant's problems be attributed to symptomatic neonatal hypoglycemia.

Some infants may have significantly low blood glucose levels without any overt signs or symptoms. Thus, while any infant with clinical manifestations suggestive of hypoglycemia should be screened for a low blood glucose level, it is prudent to establish a routine for testing all infants who might have significantly low blood glucose levels.

Our management of neonatal hypoglycemia is based on three basic principles: (1) screening infants at highest risk, (2) verifying that the blood glucose is low and responsible for the clinical manifestations, and (3) noting that symptoms clear with glucose therapy.

Routine screening for infants at highest risk, regardless of their symptoms, would include the following:

1. Small for gestational age (SGA) (<3rd percentile)
2. Smaller of discordant twins
3. Large for gestational age (LGA) (>95th percentile)
4. Infants of diabetic mothers (IDM)
5. Infants of gestational diabetic mothers (IGDM)
6. Isolated hepatomegaly
7. Significant anoxia
8. Perinatal distress
9. Apgar scores lower than 5 at 5 or 10 minutes
10. Severe erythroblastosis
11. Appropriate for gestational age (AGA) or LGA infants with microphallus or anterior midline defect
12. Family history of neonate with hypoglycemia or unexplained death
13. AGA or LGA infant with exomphalos, macroglossia, and gigantism

Routine screening can be done conservatively at 2, 4, 6, 12, 24, and 48 hours of age or whenever any of the aforementioned symptoms occurs. Obviously, it is necessary to repeat any low blood glucose value to be sure that it has returned to normal. If symptoms then occur after the first hours of life, another blood sample for glucose is indicated.

With these principles in mind, refer to Figure 1, which is a graphic flow sheet to be used in screening, confirming, and treating the most common types of hypoglycemia encountered in level 1, 2, and 3 nurseries in 1988.

ASYMPTOMATIC, TRANSITIONAL HYPOGLYCEMIA (>50 Percent)

Low blood glucose values are often seen within 4 to 6 hours of life or within the first 12 hours after birth and may be associated with perinatal distress (low Apgar scores), delayed feeds, or diabetes in the mother. Initial therapy consists of initiating oral feedings, first glucose water and then breast or formula. If the blood glucose remains significantly low, an intravenous infusion of glucose at a rate of 4 to 8 mg per kilogram per minute should be started, using 5 percent or 10 percent concentrations of glucose. In IDM or IGDM, glucagon at a dose of 0.3 mg per kilogram body weight, but not to exceed 1.0 mg total dose, given intramuscularly or intravenously, may restore the blood glucose to within normal values for up to 2 hours. This is indicated especially if an intravenous line is difficult or impossible to start in some LGA infants who may weigh in excess of 4.0 to 4.5 kg and essentially have no available veins or sites for a parenteral glucose infusion other than the umbilical vessels.

In this type of asymptomatic hypoglycemia of a transitional nature, the prognosis is so good that the risk of using hypertonic fluids, especially in the umbilical veins, is greater than that of neuroglucopenia. If hypoglycemic clinical manifestations occur or according to a reliable laboratory determination the blood glucose remains persistently low after these simple measures, only then is one justified in giving larger amounts of hypertonic glucose by whatever parenteral route is required.

HYPOGLYCEMIA SECONDARY TO OR ASSOCIATED WITH OTHER DISEASES (35 to 40 Percent)

The persistence of symptoms or failure to respond completely after correction of the hypoglycemia indicates that the low blood glucose level was secondary to or associated with a primary abnormality that was responsible

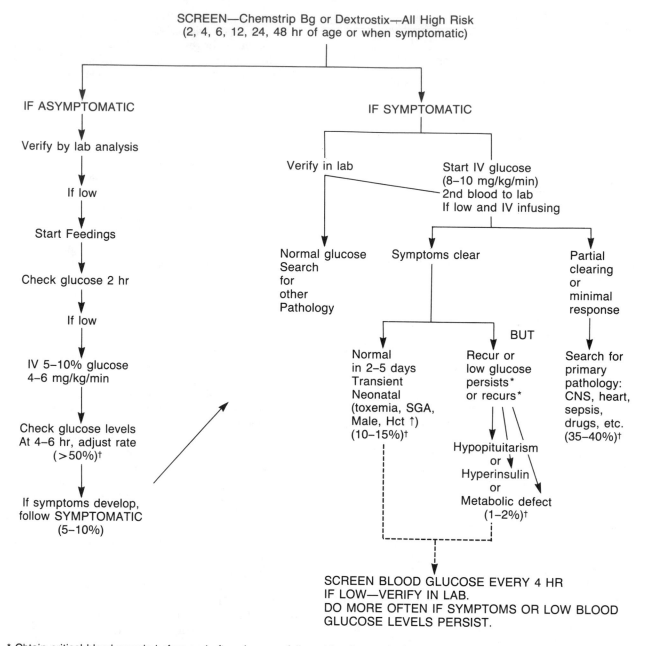

Figure 1 Flow sheet for screening, confirming, and treating hypoglycemia in the neonate. (Modified from Cornblath M, Poth M. In: Kaplan S, ed. Clinical pediatric and adolescent endocrinology. Philadelphia: WB Saunders, 1982: Chapter 5.)

* Obtain critical blood sample before and after glucagon followed by diagnostic-therapeutic trial.
† % Frequency among cases of neonatal hypoglycemia.

for the clinical manifestations noted. A search for the primary disease is critical, since hypoglycemia may be secondary to a number of neonatal conditions that in themselves may be life-threatening or debilitating. These include:

1. Central nervous system pathology (intrauterine or perinatal infections, congenital defects, or hemorrhage),
2. Sepsis,
3. Congenital heart disease,
4. Anoxia and/or asphyxia,
5. Adrenal hemorrhage,
6. Hypothyroidism,
7. Multiple congenital anomalies,
8. Neonatal tetany,
9. Postexchange transfusion,
10. Drugs given to or taken by the mother.

A large number of other abnormal conditions also occur frequently among very low and low birth weight neonates. Perhaps the most common association is with the abrupt cessation, often due to infiltration, of a hypertonic parenteral glucose solution being given to these high-risk infants for purposes other than blood glucose support. Although support of the glucose level is indicated in the conditions just listed, the primary disease is often the cause of any morbidity or mortality in these infants and the secondary hypoglycemia is not involved.

SYMPTOMATIC, TRANSIENT HYPOGLYCEMIA (10 to 15 Percent)

In the presence of symptoms already noted, our current approach to the management of the high-risk infant who has been documented to have significant hypoglycemia as defined here includes the following:

1. Give an intravenous bolus of glucose, 0.2 to 0.5 g per kilogram body weight as a 10 or 25 percent solution at the rate of 1.0 ml per minute.
2. Continue the intravenous glucose in water at a rate of 8 to 10 mg per kilogram per minute for the first 12 hours, then add sodium chloride (2 to 3 mEq per kilogram per day), and after 24 hours add potassium chloride (1 to 2 mEq per kilogram per day).
3. Oral feedings should be introduced as quickly as tolerated.
4. Blood glucose values should be monitored at 4- to 6-hour intervals until normal values persist for a period of 24 hours.
5. Then, the hypertonic parenteral glucose infusion is slowly discontinued by reducing the rate of administration from 10 to 8 to 6 to 4 mg per kilogram per minute as a 5 percent glucose solution.

Parenteral glucose therapy can usually be discontinued after 48 to 72 hours, but normoglycemia must be demonstrated for at least 24 hours prior to stopping therapy.

RECURRENT OR PERSISTENT SEVERE HYPOGLYCEMIA (1 to 2 Percent)

In rare instances, an infant continues to show clinical manifestations or persistently low blood glucose concentrations even with rates of glucose infusions as high as 12 to 16 mg per kilogram per minute. In these neonates, it is critical to establish the specific primary cause of the low blood glucose in order to institute appropriate therapy. Thus, the management of these rare conditions begins with obtaining the critical blood sample prior to and 15 minutes following the parenteral administration of glucagon (0.1 to 0.3 mg per kilogram body weight) in order to ultimately establish the diagnosis (Table 2). Until the results are available, management consists of the diagnostic-therapeutic trial as follows (it is not necessary to discontinue any ongoing therapies while adding the next one):

1. Increase intravenous glucose to 12 to 16 mg per kilogram per minute.

2. Monitor blood glucose values at 4- to 6-hour intervals.
3. Add in sequence for trial periods of 3 to 5 days: Solu-Cortef, 5 mg per kilogram per day intravenously, or prednisone, 2 mg per kilogram per day orally; Human growth hormone, 1 unit per day intramuscularly or subcutaneously; Diazoxide, 10 to 25 mg per kilogram per day orally in three divided doses.
Surgery to remove islet-cell tumor or 95 percent pancreatotomy for beta-cell hyperplasia or nesidioblastosis. Do not remove the spleen!

TABLE 2 The Critical Blood Sample in Hypoglycemia

Substrates	5–10 ml Hormones
Glucose*†‡	Insulin*†‡
Ketones*‡	Human growth hormone*
Free fatty acids*	Cortisol*
Lactate‡	Glucagon
Alanine‡	(Trasylol)
Uric acid‡	Thyroid stimulating hormone, thyroxine, triiodothyronine*

Before and after glucagon
* Helpful in neonatal hyperinsulinism.
† Helpful in congenital hypopituitarism.
‡ Helpful in hereditary defects in carbohydrate and amino acid metabolism.
From Cornblath M. Hypoglycemia in infants and children. Pediatr Ann 1981; 10:356–363.

If *congenital hypopituitarism* is the diagnosis, the hypoglycemia usually responds to cortisone and intravenous glucose therapy and human growth hormone may be necessary as well. The microphallus usually responds to the human growth hormone therapy; thyroid extract may be necessary later, if indicated.

If *hyperinsulinism* (i.e., insulin elevated relative to glucose value) is the diagnosis, in my experience all of these infants have required pancreatotomy. If hypoglycemia still persists, as may be the case with nesidioblastosis, both long-acting protamine zinc-glucagon (2 to 5 mg per day) and in an older child tapioca starch (1.5 to 2.0 g per kilogram per day every 6 hours) have been effective in controlling the hypoglycemia.

If a *metabolic defect* is the diagnosis, specific therapy is necessary, for example:

1. For glycogen storage disease type I: frequent low fructose-galactose feedings until 8 to 10 months of age and then supplement with raw cornstarch (1.5 to 2.0 g per kilogram every 6 hours day and night).
2. For hereditary fructose intolerance: a fructose-free diet.
3. For galactosemia: a galactose-free diet.

Thus, the specific diagnosis determines the management of the neonate who has hypoglycemia that is severe, persistent, or recurrent. Parenteral glucose and steroids are used initially until a definitive diagnosis is made.

HYPOKALEMIA

HANNSJÖRG W. SEYBERTH, M.D.
P. GONNE KÜHL, M.D.

Potassium is the major intracellular cation. Thus, its serum concentration only roughly reflects total body potassium. Hypokalemia is defined as a serum level of less than 3.5 mEq per liter. Imbalances in potassium homeostasis develop when there is a low intake, increased output, or both. Provided there is an adequate intake (2 mEq per kilogram per day), potassium depletion with resultant hypokalemia may occur as a consequence of a variety of conditions, including increased renal and extrarenal, principally gastrointestinal, losses. However, one should keep in mind that a shift of potassium into cells (e.g., in acid-base imbalances) may rapidly cause hypokalemia without any potassium loss from the body.

This article focuses especially on the role of prostaglandins in renal and gastrointestinal losses of potassium. The pathophysiology of prostaglandin-mediated hypokalemia is best demonstrated in a congenital renal tubular disorder. In such a syndrome, marked renal and gastrointestinal electrolyte and water losses are associated with increased prostaglandin (PG) E_2 activity. Since PGE_2 plays a key role in the manifestation of this complex disease, the term "hyperprostaglandin E_2 syndrome" has been introduced. The physiology and pathophysiology of renal prostaglandins provide the basis for understanding the treatment of prostaglandin-mediated hypokalemia and of hypokalemia iatrogenically induced by furosemide. Moreover, the tendency toward hyperkalemia, frequently observed in preterm infants with patent ductus arteriosus during treatment with indomethacin (a potent inhibitor of renal prostaglandin synthesis), can be explained on the same basis.

PHYSIOLOGY OF RENAL PROSTANOIDS

In the last decade the important role of renal prostaglandins in kidney function has become more and more apparent (Table 1). The vasodilators PGI_2 and PGE_2 attenuate vasoconstriction in stress situations with an insufficient circulatory volume and secondary hyperaldosteronism (e.g., in heart failure, sodium depletion, and patent ductus arteriosus). On the other hand, these prostanoids, like adrenergic stimuli, are important mediators of renin release. At the tubule, PGE_2 is a potent inhibitor of sodium, potassium, and probably calcium reabsorption. This direct effect and the activation of the renin-angiotensin-aldosterone system augments reabsorption of the increased sodium load by the distal tubule in exchange for potassium, and leads to an aggravation of potassium and proton losses. Free-water diuresis is increased by a PGE_2-mediated antagonism to antidiuretic hormone (ADH). This effect is enhanced by vasodilatation in the medulla through locally released PGE_2, which leads to hyperperfusion and a wash-out of the transtubular osmotic gradient.

HYPERPROSTAGLANDIN E SYNDROME

This congenital tubular disorder may often have been misdiagnosed, undiagnosed, or even not observed at all, before the advent of neonatal intensive care. Although described 30 years ago by the pediatricians Rosenbaum and Hughes, it was the internist Bartter and his colleagues who studied the pathophysiology of renal potassium wasting in more detail in a similar entity, designated Bartter's syndrome. Today it can be stated that *excessive activity of PGE_2 is one of the most common humoral causes of hypokalemia in pediatric patients*. Clinically, this apparently hereditary disease, which occurs almost exclusively in preterm infants, overlaps with Bartter's syndrome, nephrogenic diabetes insipidus, chloride diarrhea, idiopathic hypercalciuria, primary hyperparathyroidism, and Fanconi's syndrome. Most clinical features and the possible underlying mechanism can be deduced from the complex renal (Table 1) and extrarenal profile of the biologic activities of PGE_2, such as mediation of fever, secretory diarrhea, osteolysis, immune suppression, and uterine contraction. The disease entity is described as follows: pregnancies complicated by polyhydramnios and premature birth, hypokalemic alkalosis, isosthenuria, and hypercalciuria with nephrocalcinosis. Beside these renal manifestations, systemic features of increased PGE_2 activity include noninfectious fever, episodic diarrhea, osteopenia with transitory hypercalcemia, susceptibility to infections, and failure to thrive.

This complex clinical presentation and the varying postnatal time of onset may result in several misleading preliminary diagnoses. Hypercalcemia and nephrocalcinosis frequently are the first detectable features of the disorder; hence, primary hyperparathyroidism may be diagnosed. Subsequently, the disturbed tubular sodium reabsorption causes hyponatremia with volume contraction. At the same time, the serum potassium level still is normal or even slightly elevated, probably because of a physiologically low glomerular filtration rate and/or a relative tubular unresponsiveness to aldosterone. This situation resembles pseudohypoaldosteronism. If diarrhea with hypochloremia is the predominant feature, the diagnosis

TABLE 1 Renal Activities of Prostaglandins

Cortex (PGI_2, PGE_2):
  Direct vasodilatation (perfusion ↑)
  Indirect vasoconstriction (renin ↑)

Medulla (PGE_2):
  Tubule: direct saluresis (Na^+, K^+, Ca^{++}
      indirect sodium reabsorption (aldosterone ↑)
      indirect free-water diuresis ↑ (ADH
      antagonism)

  Vasculature: direct vasodilatation (perfusion and
      diuresis ↑)

of congenital chloride diarrhea may be justified. Finally, if the infant has hypokalemic alkalosis, fever, excessive free-water loss, isosthenuria (less than 100 mOsm per kilogram), and high vasopressin plasma levels, Bartter's syndrome or nephrogenic diabetes insipidus, respectively, appear to be the most likely diagnoses. However, at the age of 4 to 8 weeks all features, including massive hypercalciuria (greater than 10 mg per kilogram per day), are present and the definitive diagnosis can be made. If the gestational history reveals polyhydramnios, which has led to premature birth, the diagnosis of the hyperprostaglandin E_2 syndrome is unequivocal. Polyhydramnios is typical neither for Bartter's syndrome nor for nephrogenic diabetes insipidus. In all these tubular syndromes, similarly affected siblings are quite common.

What is the evidence that most of the complex features of this entity are the result of increased PGE_2 activity?

1. Increased excretion of PGE_2 and PGE-M, the major urinary metabolite of the E prostaglandins, indicates activated renal and systemic PGE_2 production.
2. Indomethacin, a prostaglandin synthesis inhibitor, is the most effective treatment for these infants, who otherwise require prolonged hospitalization for electrolyte and water substitution.
3. Intravenous infusion of PGE_1 or PGE_2 induces some of the systemic symptoms such as fever, diarrhea, and high susceptibility to infections.
4. Furosemide, a potent stimulator of renal PGE_2 synthesis, causes hypokalemic alkalosis, hypercalciuria, and nephrocalcinosis when used chronically.

This last observation helps to explain the prostaglandin-mediated hypokalemia in the hyperprostaglandin E_2 syndrome. The primary target of furosemide is the proximal tubule, leading to increased salt loading of the distal tubule, with increased sodium exchange against potassium and hydrogen. In analogy, this appears in part to be the mechanism of hypokalemia in the hyperprostaglandin E_2 syndrome. Further evidence for this hypothesis is provided by reports of a disease entity with hyperkalemia, acidosis, and hypertension, associated with an endogenous defect of renal prostaglandin release. This disorder is most effectively treated with furosemide. Moreover, preterm infants with patent ductus arteriosus, who are treated with indomethacin, present features contrasting with those of infants with the hyperprostaglandin E_2 syndrome. These features are, in particular, hyperkalemia, oliguria, and hypocalciuria.

TREATMENT

Since the primary cause of stimulated renal and systemic PGE_2 synthesis is not yet known, only symptomatic treatment regimens can be offered (Table 2). As the first step, adequate potassium intake (2 mEq per kilogram per day) should be guaranteed. If urinary excretion of potassium exceeds the dietary supply, intake should be increased until the serum concentration of potassium is in the normal range. In case of excessive renal sodium loss, sodium has to be substituted as well. Frequently this supplementation can be adequately provided only by parenteral infusion in infants with a severe course of renal and gastrointestinal electrolyte and water losses. At that stage, additional pharmacotherapeutic interventions need to be considered. Previously, the aldosterone antagonist spironolactone was recommended. However, as hyperaldosteronism is only a consequence of the excessive electrolyte and water losses, this treatment is without any significant effect. The somewhat more proximal intervention with beta-adrenergic blocking agents such as propranolol appears to be not very efficacious in prostaglandin-mediated hyperreninemia. Thus, the current treatment of choice is the administration of a nonsteroidal antiinflammatory drug, preferably indomethacin. Aspirin is by far the less potent inhibitor of renal and systemic prostaglandin synthesis, and in addition infants frequently exhibit an unacceptable gastrointestinal intolerance for this agent.

It must be mentioned that chronic indomethacin treatment in infants has to be considered as an experimental therapy. Although we and others have collected a significant amount of experience in the short-term treatment of preterm infants with indomethacin, much less experience is available in the treatment of older infants and children over a period of years. Therefore, several requirements must be fulfilled by the institution in which these patients are to be closely followed. These are (1) a reliable assay of serum indomethacin levels; (2) a reliable assay of urinary PGE_2 levels, preferably gas chromatography–mass spectrometric assays or a carefully validated radioimmunoassay (most commercially available kits do not fulfill essential validation criteria—e.g., tests with several antisera, preassay chromatography, mass spectrometric validation); and (3) a microassay for plasma renin activity. The last-named parameter provides an additional index of effective inhibition of renal PGE_2 synthesis and is more readily available in academic pediatric centers.

Indomethacin treatment is started when (1) electrolyte and water balances cannot be maintained by plain supplementation (see above); (2) urinary PGE_2 levels are

TABLE 2   Treatment of Prostaglandin-Mediated Hypokalemia

Interventions	Efficacy
Potassium and sodium (if necessary) supplementation	Moderate
Aldosterone antagonism, e.g., spironolactone	Hardly any
Inhibition of renin release, e.g., beta-blocker (propranolol)	Hardly any
Cyclo-oxygenase inhibition Indomethacin* (2–8 mg/kg/day) Aspirin* (50–100 mg/kg/day)	Effective Moderate

* Drug level monitoring is essential.

found to be definitely above the normal range of 16 ng per kilogram per 1.73 m² for all ages (at least two determinations are desirable); and (3) the infant is not thriving. Indomethacin treatment should not be started later than the second to third month of life, since rapid fluctuation in water balance may cause cerebral damage, and several patients transferred to our institution from other hospitals as early as 2 to 3 months of age have already displayed signs of cerebral atrophy on CT scan and were already receiving anticonvulsive therapy.

The usual starting dose for indomethacin is 2 mg per kilogram per day, preferably as syrup, which is commercially available in some countries (e.g., West Germany). After only 2 to 3 days, the serum level of potassium starts to rise, metabolic alkalosis disappears, there is significant weight gain, and fever and episodic diarrhea stop. Usually the indomethacin dosage has to be tailored individually according to the drug level, the urinary PGE_2 excretion, and the activity of plasma renin. The therapeutic window of indomethacin serum concentration, 4 hours after the last oral dose, ranges from 1 to 3 μg per milliliter, and should suppress urinary PGE_2 excretion and plasma renin activity well below the upper-normal range. To maintain these levels, the indomethacin dose sometimes has to be increased up to 8 mg per kilogram per day. Beside marked interindividual differences in indomethacin disposition, coadministration of phenobarbital may stimulate hepatic biotransformation of indomethacin, with the need to choose a higher maintenance dose. If sufficient suppression of PGE_2 biosynthesis has been achieved, no additional potassium supplementation is needed to maintain the serum concentration in the normal range (3.5 to 5.0 mEq per liter). Urinary excretion of calcium, however, decreases only over several weeks of indomethacin treatment. Unfortunately, it rarely reaches normal excretion rates (less than 5 mg per kilogram per day). Additional treatment with hydrochlorothiazide (1 mg per kilogram per day) is effective in achieving normocalciuria, but this has to be paid for by a significant drop in glomerular filtration rate, by hyperuricemia, and by the reappearance of hypokalemia. At present, no effective and acceptable treatment can be offered that completely corrects urinary calcium excretion. Fortunately, no apparent progression of nephrocalcinosis or deterioration of glomerular filtration rate has been observed in eight patients of ours during chronic indomethacin treatment over a period of 3 to 4 years.

Follow-up at least every 6 months is recommended. In addition to adjusting the dose of indomethacin, adverse reactions to indomethacin have to be sought. Most critical are kidney function, gastrointestinal tolerance (ulcers), hemostasis, and bone marrow suppression. For this reason, we frequently determine endogenous creatinine clearances, which are validated by ⁵¹Cr-EDTA or inulin clearance. Stool is regularly tested for blood contamination. The blood count, hepatic function, and coagulation status are frequently monitored. Certainly, relevant defects or dysfunctions in these organs or systems have to be considered as contraindications to indomethacin treatment.

This mode of treatment is also effective for other prostaglandin-mediated nephropathies, such as Bartter's syndrome and nephrogenic diabetes insipidus. There is no evidence of incomplete efficacy or tachyphylaxis in hyperprostaglandin E_2 (and related) tubulopathies, as suggested by other authorities, provided that indomethacin treatment is frequently adjusted according to the procedure described above.

FUTURE ASPECTS

Two major objectives for future research efforts should be (1) to prevent this disorder by family counseling and (2) to elucidate the most proximal event in the pathophysiology, which might suggest a more specific pharmacotherapeutic intervention with less potential side effects. At present we know only that there is an approximately 50 percent chance that the next child of an affected family will have the same disorder, and that the development of polyhydramnios is the earliest manifestation of the disease. It is still a matter of debate whether this is a consequence of increased fetal PGE_2 activity or of the primary disorder, which stimulates renal and systemic PGE_2 production after birth. Nevertheless, the possibility of a prenatal presentation of a hyperprostaglandin E_2 syndrome appears to be important enough to be included in the differential diagnosis of polyhydramnios with no other apparent explanation.

SUGGESTED READING

Bartter FC, Pronove P, Gill JR Jr, Mac Cardie RC, Diller E. Hyperplasia of the juxtaglomerular complex with hyperaldosteronism and hypokalemic alkalosis: A new syndrome. Am J Med 1962; 33:811.

Rosenbaum P, Hughes M. Persistent, probably congenital, hypokalemic metabolic alkalosis with hyaline degeneration of renal tubules and normal urinary aldosterone. Am J Dis Child 1957; 94:560.

Seyberth HW, Rascher W, Schweer H, Kühl GP, Mehls O, Schärer K. Congenital hypokalemia with hypercalciuria in preterm infants: A hyperprostaglanduric tubular syndrome different from Bartter syndrome. J Pediatr 1985; 107:694.

HYPOPLASTIC LEFT HEART SYNDROME

WILLIAM I. NORWOOD, M.D., Ph.D.
JOHN D. PIGOTT, M.D.

Hypoplastic left heart syndrome is the fourth most common congenital cardiac anomaly presenting in the first year of life. The central anatomic features are aortic valve atresia or severe stenosis, with associated marked hypoplasia or absence of the left ventricle. The aortic arch and ascending aorta are functionally a branch of the thoracic aorta, with retrograde flow through the aortic arch and diminutive ascending aorta. Most commonly the aortic valve is atretic, and the ascending aorta carries only coronary flow retrograde from the ductus arteriosus. It is therefore correspondingly small, measuring 1 to 3 mm in diameter. In our series of 166 patients with hypoplastic left heart syndrome from January 1984 to August 1987, 78 percent had normally related great arteries, 10 percent had double-outlet right ventricle and severe hypoplasia of the left ventricle, and 12 percent had malalignment of the atrioventricular canal with right ventricular dominance and hypoplasia of the left ventricle.

A physiologic consequence of this anatomy is that the systemic circulation is supported virtually in its entirety by flow through the ductus arteriosus. Pulmonary venous return passes through a patent foramen ovale or, occasionally, a true atrial septal defect to the right atrium and right ventricle. This physiology allows normal growth and development in utero. Newborns with hypoplastic left heart syndrome generally are only mildly cyanotic, with a PaO_2 of 50 to 60 mm Hg, and their cardiac disease may go unrecognized until pallor, limpness, and metabolic acidosis develop when the ductus arteriosus begins to close. When the disorder is unrecognized and untreated, most infants with aortic atresia die in the first days after birth. Occasionally, the ductus arteriosus remains patent, and intractable congestive heart failure ensues as the pulmonary vascular resistance naturally decreases in the first month or two of life. *The distressed newborn may be readily resuscitated by continuous infusion of prostaglandin E_1 to maintain patency of the ductus arteriosus and a bolus of sodium bicarbonate to reverse metabolic acidosis.* If apnea occurs secondary to PGE_1 infusion, ventilatory support may be necessary as well. Catecholamine infusion is rarely necessary and actually may increase pulmonary blood flow at the expense of systemic circulation by increasing systemic resistance.

Since the lungs, coronary anatomy, and myocardial biochemistry are otherwise inherently normal in this condition, hypoplastic left heart syndrome may be considered one of several cardiac malformations with only one effective ventricle, which in principle is treatable by a modification of Fontan's procedure (connection of the right atrium to the main pulmonary artery). It has been demonstrated that a good functional result following a Fontan procedure can be expected when the pulmonary artery architecture is near normal, the pulmonary vascular resistance is that of the normal mature lung, and ventricular function has been preserved (low end-diastolic pressure). Since the systemic circulation in neonates with hypoplastic left heart syndrome is dependent on the patency of the ductus arteriosus, which characteristically closes in the first days of life, urgent surgery is necessary. However, *the pulmonary vascular resistance of the newborn is prohibitively high for a Fontan procedure, and staged surgical therapy is therefore necessary.* The general goals of the initial palliation are to establish unobstructed systemic output from the right ventricle, to ensure normal maturation of the pulmonary vasculature by regulating pulmonary arterial blood flow and pressure, and to ensure a widely patent interatrial communication, thereby avoiding pulmonary venous hypertension. Although several approaches to these goals have been conceived, the surgical techniques outlined here are designed additionally to incorporate, as much as possible, the patient's own tissues and to avoid conduits or circumferential suture lines, thus minimizing the number of surgical interventions.

PALLIATION (STAGE I)

Since circulatory arrest is necessary for the aortic reconstruction, the operating room is maintained at 20°C to promote surface cooling of the patient. Induction of general anesthesia with pancuronium bromide (Pavulon) (0.1 mg per kilogram) and Fentanyl (25 μg per kilogram in 10 μg per kilogram increments) is achieved. The left radial artery is cannulated with a 22-gauge indwelling catheter, and a urinary bladder drainage tube, a nasogastric tube, and nasopharyngeal, esophageal, and rectal temperature probes are placed. During this preparatory time the rectal temperature typically decreases to about 33°C.

Through a conventional midline sternotomy incision, the thymus gland is excised, exposing the diminutive aortic arch and its branch vessels (Fig. 1). Cannulation for arterial infusion is conveniently achieved in the proximal main pulmonary artery just above the sinuses of Valsalva. The tip of a 10-French aortic cannula is introduced 3 to 4 mm into the artery. Threading of the cannula through the ductus arteriosus is to be avoided; it is unnecessary and requires excessive manipulation of the cardiovascular structures. A minimal amount of distortion, manipulation, and trauma to the delicate neonatal cardiovascular structures is essential to preserve anatomy and function. A single venous cannula is placed through the right atrial appendage, and cardiopulmonary bypass is instituted. The right and left pulmonary artery branches are rapidly occluded (Fig. 2) to ensure systemic perfusion through the ductus arteriosus. The baby is cooled on bypass while esophageal, nasopharyngeal, and rectal temperatures are monitored. The rectal temperature reaches 20°C after approximately 15 minutes of cardiopulmonary bypass. During this time, the branch vessels of the aortic arch are exposed and looped with suture tourniquets in preparation for circulatory arrest. Dissection is carried around

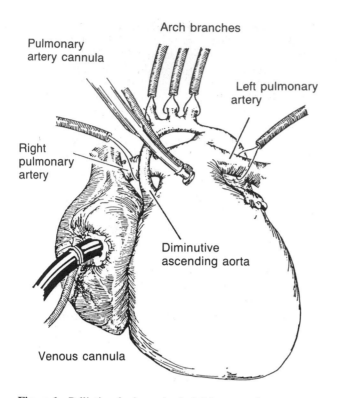

Figure 1 Palliation for hypoplastic left heart syndrome: external anatomy.

After removal of the arterial and venous cannulas, the atrial septum is excised to allow unimpeded pulmonary venous return to the right atrium. The main pulmonary artery, which has been separated from the diminutive ascending aorta during the cooling phase of cardiopulmonary bypass, is transected adjacent to the takeoff of the right pulmonary artery, and the distal stump of the main pulmonary artery is closed with a patch (Fig. 3). Patch closure is recommended in order to ensure continuity between the right and left pulmonary artery branches. The ductus arteriosus is then exposed, ligated, and transected at its entrance into the thoracic aorta. An incision in the aorta is carried distally 1 to 2 cm into the thoracic aorta (Fig. 4) and also proximally into the aortic arch and ascending aorta to the level of the rim of the transected proximal main pulmonary artery. Because the isthmus of the aorta and the aortic arch actually function as a branch of the main pulmonary artery–ductus–thoracic aorta continuum, the junction of the isthmus and thoracic aorta is gusseted with a patch in order to avoid subsequent development of distal aortic arch obstruction (Fig. 5). A piece of pulmonary homograft is used for this patch because it is thin, pliable, and hemostatic.

At this point, we favor the construction of a short central shunt of 4-mm tube graft between the inferior aspect of the augmented aortic arch and the confluence of branch

the aortic arch onto the thoracic aorta in the posterior mediastinum. At this point the branch vessels of the aortic arch are occluded, the circulation is discontinued, and the blood is drained into the venous reservoir.

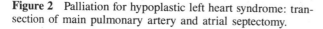

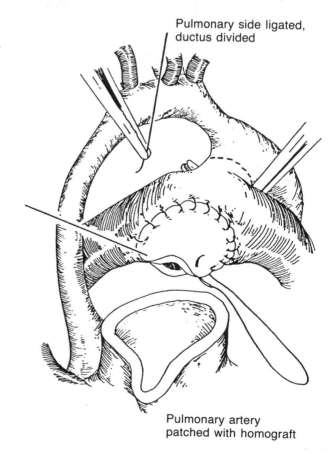

Figure 2 Palliation for hypoplastic left heart syndrome: transection of main pulmonary artery and atrial septectomy.

Figure 3 Palliation for hypoplastic left heart syndrome: creation of pulmonary atresia and ligation of ductus arteriosus.

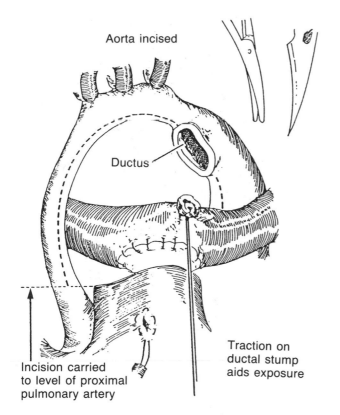

Figure 4 Palliation for hypoplastic left heart syndrome: aortic incision.

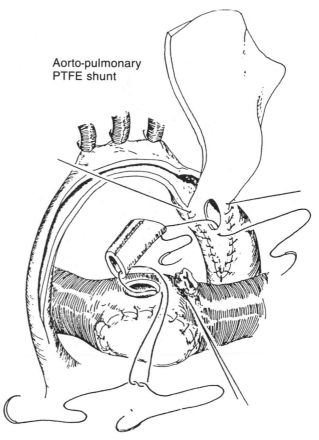

Figure 6 Palliation for hypoplastic left heart syndrome: central 4 mm PTFE shunt.

pulmonary arteries (Fig. 6). The rationale for a central shunt is to obtain more even distribution of flow and thus uniform growth of the right and left pulmonary arteries. The remaining pulmonary homograft gusset is then car-

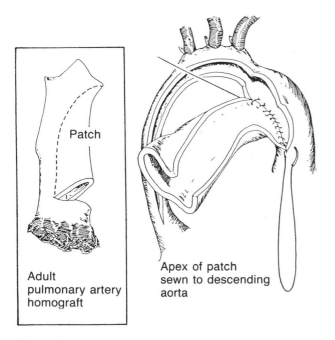

Figure 5 Palliation for hypoplastic left heart syndrome: augmentation of aorta using pulmonary artery homograft.

ried to 5 mm above the end of the most proximal incision in the ascending aorta (Fig. 7). The proximal transected main pulmonary artery is then anastomosed to the ascending aorta and homograft gusset, thus creating outflow from the right ventricle to the augmented aorta through the pulmonary valve (Figs. 8, 9).

Cardiopulmonary bypass is reinstituted and the patient is rewarmed to 37 °C. The tourniquets on the branch vessels of the aortic arch are removed, but those on the branch pulmonary arteries remain until the time of weaning from cardiopulmonary bypass. After weaning, the cannulas are removed and a pressure monitoring line is placed through the right atrial appendage cannulation site.

Using the lowest possible mean airway pressure, ventilation is adjusted to maintain the Pco_2 between 20 and 30 mm Hg in order to minimize pulmonary vascular resistance. Generally the Po_2 ranges from 40 to 45 mm Hg. However, a PaO_2 of 50 mm Hg or greater suggests a large pulmonary-to-systemic flow ratio, which may result in inadequate systemic perfusion. When this occurs, the ventilator may be used to adjust the pulmonary-to-systemic flow ratio by rapidly decreasing FIO_2 to 30 mm Hg and allowing Pco_2 to increase to 40 mm Hg, with a concomitant increase in pulmonary vascular resistance. Pharmacologic support is rarely necessary in the postoperative period.

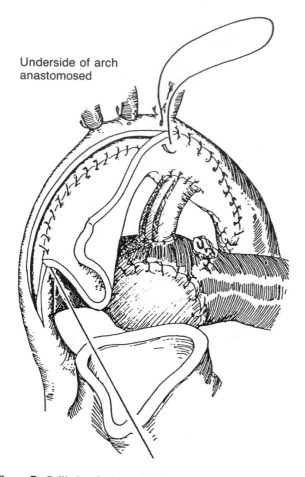

Underside of arch anastomosed

Figure 7 Palliation for hypoplastic left heart syndrome: completion of aortic augmentation.

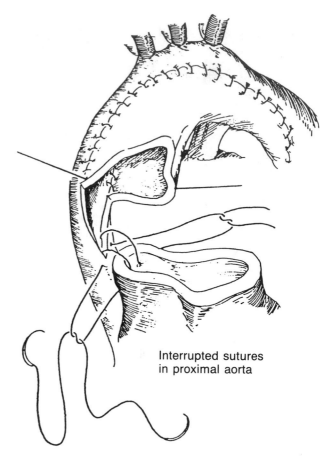

Interrupted sutures in proximal aorta

Figure 8 Palliation for hypoplastic left heart syndrome: pulmonary artery to aortic anastomosis.

FONTAN'S PROCEDURE (STAGE II)

After the previously described palliative surgery, the right ventricle is subjected to both volume and pressure load greater than normal for a right ventricle. With a view to long-term preservation of ventricular function, early assessment for suitability for Fontan's procedure is undertaken when the infant is 12 to 18 months of age. At this age, the pulmonary resistance generally has decreased to less than 2.5 Woods units and the ventricular end-diastolic pressure has remained normal (less than 7 to 8 mm Hg). The following surgery may then be planned.

Again the heart is exposed through a midline sternotomy, and cannulation for cardiopulmonary bypass is achieved by placement of an arterial cannula in the ascending aorta and a single venous cannula through the right atrial appendage. The systemic-to-pulmonary artery shunt is exposed and occluded as cardiopulmonary bypass is begun, and the patient's core temperature is reduced to 20 °C.

During this cooling phase on cardiopulmonary bypass, the right and left pulmonary artery branches are exposed from pericardial reflection to pericardial reflection. This exposure is in preparation for widely augmenting the pulmonary arteries, in order to avoid proximal pulmonary arterial obstruction from unrecognized irregularities in size.

During a period of circulatory arrest, the pulmonary arteries are opened and an incision in the right atrium is made from the sulcus terminalus superiorly to the right lateral insertion of the eustachian valve inferiorly. The interatrial communication is inspected and enlarged if pos-

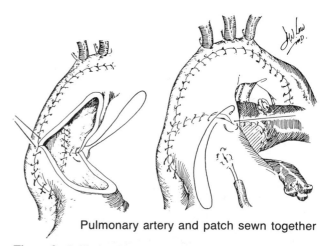

Pulmonary artery and patch sewn together

Figure 9 Palliation for hypoplastic left heart syndrome: completion of aortic reconstruction.

sible. A final incision is then made in the superior right atrium adjacent to the right pulmonary artery, and carried into the posterior aspect of the right superior vena cava immediately adjacent to the most rightward aspect of the incision in the right pulmonary artery. A suture line is begun between the inferior lip of the incised right pulmonary artery and the posterior lip of the right superior vena caval–right atrial incision. This will provide the floor for the anastomosis of the systemic venous return to the pulmonary arterial tree.

A piece of tube graft 10 mm in diameter, of sufficient length to extend from the inferior vena caval–right atrial junction to the right superior vena caval–right atrial junction, is cut in half lengthwise. This is for use as a baffle to channel inferior vena caval flow along the right lateral aspect of the right atrium to the anastomosis between the right atrium and the pulmonary arterial tree superiorly. The baffle is sutured around the orifice of the inferior vena cava along the right lateral floor and freewall of the right atrium, and around the patulous orifice in the superior dome of the right atrium. This particular baffling technique was introduced to minimize problems associated with tricuspid prolapse or regurgitation, or obstruction of pulmonary venous return to the right ventricle, which was experienced early in this series with an alternative baffling technique.

The construction of the systemic venous pulmonary arterial system is completed by gusseting the pulmonary arterial incision with an elongated triangular patch, beginning on the left pulmonary artery. As one approaches the right pulmonary artery and adjacent right superior vena cava, the base of the triangular patch is sutured onto the anterior lip of the right superior vena caval–right atrial incision, providing a roof for the anastomosis. The patient is placed back on cardiopulmonary bypass after closure of the initial right atriotomy, and rewarmed to 37 °C.

RESULTS

From August 1985 to September 1987, 104 newborns underwent palliative surgery as described above for hypoplastic left heart syndrome at The Children's Hospital of Philadelphia. The hospital mortality among these patients was 30 percent, and to date 33 patients have undergone application of Fontan's procedure for the treatment of hypoplastic left heart syndrome. Among these 33 patients, there were 11 early deaths and one late death. The results continue to improve, both for initial palliation and later reconstructive surgery, as we gain ever-increasing knowledge of the anatomy and physiology of this complex group of patients, and of the surgical procedures required for them.

SUGGESTED READING

Noonan JA, Nadas AS. The hypoplastic left heart syndrome: An analysis of 101 cases. Pediatr Clin North Am 1958; 5:1029–1056.

Doty DB, Marvin WJ Jr, Schieken RM, Lauer RM. Hypoplastic left heart syndrome: Successful palliation with a new operation. J Thorac Cardiovasc Surg 1980; 80:148–152.

Norwood WI, Lang P, Castaneda AR, Campbell DN. Experience with operations for hypoplastic left heart syndrome. J Thorac Cardiovasc Surg 1980; 82:511–519.

Norwood WI, Lang P, Hansen DD. Physiologic repair of aortic atresia-hypoplastic left heart syndrome. N Engl J Med 1983; 308:23–26.

Helton JG, Aglira BA, Chin AJ, et al. Analysis of potential anatomical or physiological determinants of outcome of palliative surgery for hypoplastic left heart syndrome. Circulation 1986; 74 (Suppl I):70–76.

HYPOTHYROIDISM

OSAMU NOSE, M.D., Ph.D.

Neonatal hypothyroidism is a congenital disease caused by a deficiency in circulating thyroid hormone. The major effects of thyroid hormones include the stimulation of cellular metabolism and of growth and maturation of all the organs. Thus, insufficient circulating thyroid hormone leads to depression of oxygen consumption and all metabolism of proteins, carbohydrate, and fats and results in developmental disturbances. In this respect thyroid hormone is of critical importance for normal brain growth and development during the first 2 to 3 years of life and is especially important in the neonatal period. The degree of mental disturbance in neonatal hypothyroidism depends mainly on the degree and duration of the lack of thyroid hormones during the fetal to infant period. Therefore, early diagnosis and treatment are of major importance to prevent mental retardation in neonatal hypothyroidism. In light of these facts, a mass screening program for detecting neonatal hypothyroidism is necessary, and since around 1975, mass screening programs for neonatal hypothyroidism have been established in North America, Europe, and Japan.

In recent decades, hypothyroidism in neonates has been detected exclusively by such mass screening. But some cases with especially severe manifestations of characteristic neonatal cretinism (e.g., moderate and/or prolonged jaundice, poor feeding, vomiting, lethargy, poor peripheral circulation with cool, mottled skin, and facial edema) can be diagnosed prior to learning the results of filter paper blood studies. The incidence of neonatal hypothyroidism is approximately 1 in 3,000 to 1 in 4,000 births in North America and 1 in 5,000 to 1 in 7,000 births in Japan.

Since the introduction of mass screening programs, various types of abnormal pituitary thyroid functions have been found, in addition to congenital hypothyroidism. Infantile transient hyperthyrotropinemia (normal free thyroxine, thyroxine, and triiodothyroxine with slight elevation [17 to 50 μU per milliliter] of thyroid-stimulating hormone; normal size, shape, and location of thyroid gland in I^{123} scintigram; thyroid-stimulating hormone level spontaneously returning to normal within 1 year), and transient hypothyroxinemia (low serum thyroxine levels without an increase in serum thyroid-stimulating hormone and low serum free thyroxine values by term infant standards but in the normal adult range; usually found in premature babies) are examples. Available evidence indicates that treatment of such infants is not necessary. In addition, congenital thyroxine-binding globulin deficiency is also found in mass screening, but this condition can easily be differentiated by measurement of serum triiodothyroxine resin uptake or direct measurement of thyroxine-binding globulin. These syndromes do not produce any hypothyroid state and do not need to be treated with thyroid hormone.

The hypothyroid state in congenital hypothyroidism may be permanent or transient. Permanent congenital hypothyroidism usually (in 85 to 90 percent of cases) is due to an abnormality in the thyroid gland embryogenesis (thyroid dysgenesis), but it may be due (in 8 to 12 percent of cases in North America) to a hereditary defect in thyroid hormone biosynthesis (thyroid dyshormonogenesis) or rarely (in 0.2 to 0.3 percent of cases) to a deficiency of thyroid-releasing hormone and/or thyroid-stimulating hormone secretion (hypothalamic-pituitary hypothyroidism). Transient hypothyroidism (2 to 5 percent in North America, 5 to 10 percent in Japan of all cases of hypothyroidism) is most often secondary to intrauterine exposure to pharmacologic doses of iodide or antithyroid drugs or to maternal thyroid-stimulating hormone binding inhibitor immunoglobulins (TBII), which block the effects of thyroidal thyroid-stimulating hormone. Such infants with TBII have mothers with Hashimoto's thyroiditis or Graves disease. More recently, neonatal immaturity of thyroidal iodine organification has also been attributed to a transient cause.

The diagnosis of congenital hypothyroidism is established on the basis of low serum concentrations of thyroxine and/or free thyroxine (FT_4, or free T_4 index) in association with elevated serum levels of thyroid-stimulating hormone. When there is significant residual thyroid function (an ectopic gland of moderate size), excessive thyroid-stimulating hormone increases the thyroid triiodothyroxine-thyroxine secretion ratio. In these instances, the serum triiodothyroxine concentration may be normal. In infants with a low serum thyroxine level and a normal thyroid-stimulating hormone level, hypothalamopituitary hypothyroidism is suspected. Measurement of low free thyroxine level for gestational age is helpful. Most cases with this type of hypothyroidism have associated deficiency of growth hormone, gonadotropin, and/or adrenocorticotropic hormone. Therefore, hypoglycemia due to lack of growth hormone and/or adrenocorticotropic hormone is manifest in the early weeks of life. Absent or prolonged thyroid-stimulating hormone response to thyrotropin-releasing hormone confirms the diagnosis of hypothalamopituitary origin. The differential diagnosis of these types of hypothyroidism, in relation to the serum level of thyroid-stimulating hormone (TSH) and thyroxine, is listed in Table 1.

AVAILABLE PREPARATIONS FOR REPLACEMENT THERAPY

Several thyroid hormone preparations are available. These include synthetic USP (desiccated thyroid thyroglobulin), synthetic Na-l-thyroxine (levo-thyroxine) (NaT_4), and synthetic Na-l-triiodothyronine (NaT_3). But the recent trend toward replacement therapy for neonatal hypothyroidism reflects exclusive use of levo-thyroxine because of the indefinite potency of USP. Moreover, L-triiodothyronine is not recommended because of rapid fluctuations of circulating triiodothyronine with levels in the hyperthyroid range after ingestion of this hormone.

On the other hand, NaT_4 binds to carrier serum proteins with high affinity, and therefore the serum concentrations and tissue availability are less variable. Moreover, thyroxine is deiodinated to triiodothyronine by a tissue $5'$-iodothyronine deiodinase, greatly augmenting the metabolic potency, and there are endogenous control systems regulating the activity of the thyroxine to triiodothyronine conversion step. This provides additional control or buffering of the tissue levels of active thyroid hormone and is of advantage in long-term replacement therapy. Thus, NaT_4 is the medication of choice in most instances; NaT_3 is reserved for short-term treatment and for situations in which it is desirable to measure endogenous thyroxine secretion (serum concentration) during replacement.

THYROID HORMONE REPLACEMENT THERAPY

Replacement therapy in neonatal hypothyroidism is divided into two steps: (1) initial treatment in the early neonatal period (before 2 months of age), and (2) maintenance therapy (after 2 months of age, i.e., after the thyroid-stimulating hormone level returns almost to normal [<50 μU per milliliter]). Both treatments consist exclusively of oral L-thyroxine replacement.

Initial Therapy

In the past, initial treatment for cretinism started with a low dose of a thyroid hormone preparation, followed by increasing the dose gradually up to the maintenance level within 1 month. In treating neonatal hypothyroidism,

TABLE 1 Type and Biochemical Indices of Hypothyroidism

| Type | Prevalence | Serum Thyroid Hormone | | | |
		T_4	T_3	rT_3	TSH
Hypothalamic pituitary	<0.3%	↓	↘	↘	↓
Primary	>90%	↓↓	↘	↘	↑↑↑

however, a sufficient dose should be given from the beginning to prevent early brain damage immediately after biochemical confirmation of the diagnosis of hypothyroidism has been obtained. Most treatment regimens for full-term infants around the world are similar at present. In severe cases, an initial dose of 10 μg per kilogram per day of L-thyroxine is recommended. However, in our experience, if we start the therapy of mild cases (high serum thyroid-stimulating hormone but low normal serum thyroxine and no symptoms) with a dose of 10 μg per kilogram per day, some infants develop a hyperthyroid state, so we usually start treating full-term infants with a dose of 5 μg per kilogram per day of L-thyroxine for the first week and then increase the dose up to 10 μg per kilogram per day in the second week, monitoring the serum thyroxine level. The suggested absolute prescribed doses were 25, 37.5, and/or 50 μg per day, rounded off to the nearest one-half 25-μg tablet according to the body weight. Premature infants can be started on 25μg per day. Infants with congenital hypothyroidism usually have a high threshold of the negative feedback control loop for regulation of thyroid-stimulating hormone secretion at the level of the pituitary gland. As a result, they may have relatively elevated serum thyroid-stimulating hormone concentrations when the serum thyroxine level is in the normal or high normal range, e.g., higher than 8 μU per milliliter with a serum thyroxine concentration higher than 10 μg per deciliter. Thus, the serum thyroid-stimulating hormone measurement value must be interpreted with caution in adjusting the thyroxine dosage. Short-term dosage adjustments are based primarily on the measured serum thyroxine value and clinical response. The serum thyroxine level usually equilibrates to a prescribed dosage within 1 to 2 weeks. Thus, the dosage can be easily varied in 5-μg increments at 1-week intervals monitoring the serum thyroxine level. Then we can adjust the patients' circulating thyroxine concentration in the upper half of the normal range for their age. In the first 2 months of life, this is 10 to 15 μg per deciliter. Usually the clinical symptoms of hypothyroidism gradually disappear when the patient is on this replacement therapy. But in-hospitalized treatment is desirable for the first 3 to 4 weeks of initial treatment because of the complications associated with overtreatment, such as irritability and/or vomiting. After 2 months of age, patients can attain the maintenance dose and the thyroid-stimulating hormone level comes down to near normal (<50 μU per milliliter).

Maintenance Therapy

After 2 months of age, because of the rapid weight gain during infancy, serum thyroxine and thyroid-stimulating hormone should be measured, and if necessary, the dose of L-thyroxine should be adjusted once a month during the first 6 months; then, testing should be carried out twice monthly over the next 6 months, every 6 months through 3 years, and yearly thereafter. Minute dosage adjustment is recommended, to be performed by measuring the serum thyroid-stimulating as an index of the optimal replacement therapy dose. Adequate treatment should normalize the growth rate and bone maturation,

and longer-term dosage adjustments are also based on serial measurements of the length and bone age. Careful periodic assessments of maturational events and the developmental quotient, including Denver development (or similar) scoring, should also be conducted. If patients have histories of exposure to excessive iodine, antithyroid drugs, or antithyroid antibody, they can be weaned off thyroid hormone within 12 weeks after initiation of therapy. Serum thyroxine and thyroid-stimulating hormone remain normal as the thyroxine replacement dose is reduced. After 1 year of age, permanent diseases require increasing the maintenance dose of L-thyroxine to around 50 to 80 μg per day (group A in Fig. 1); conversely, transient hypothyroidism cases (group B in Fig. 1) without any specific history of exposure during fetal life (probably due to immaturity of thyroidal iodine organification) do not require an increase in the maintenance dose above the initial dose, even after 1 year of age. Thus, hypothyroid infants suspected of having this type of transient disease can also be weaned off thyroid hormone at around 1½ years of age with normal thyroxine and thyroid-stimulating hormone, even though the thyroxine replacement dose is reduced. In hypothyroid infants without an etiologic diagnosis, treatment is discontinued after 2 years (when central nervous system development is not thyroid-dependent) for differential diagnostic work-up.

Side Effects and Complications

Side effects of thyroid hormone replacement itself are uncommon. Thyroid hormone toxicity may occur at excessive dosages. This is associated with irritability, hyperactivity, loose stools, or diarrhea in mild toxicity. In prolonged, severe toxicity, accelerated linear growth and premature synostosis of cranial sutures are produced.

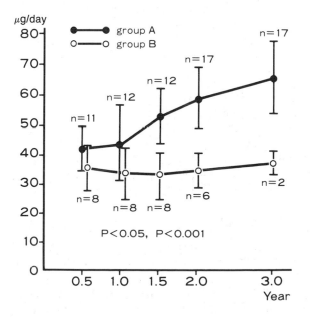

Figure 1 Relationship between age and dose of L-thyroxine.

HYPOXIC-ISCHEMIC ENCEPHALOPATHY

MICHAEL V. JOHNSTON, M.D.
STEVEN DONN, M.D.

Therapy for infants with hypoxic-ischemic encephalopathy (HIE) is aimed at correcting physiologic changes in peripheral organs that could worsen brain injury and at reversing events that may cause progressive cell death within the brain. *Aside from effective cardiopulmonary resuscitation when indicated, no specific therapies have been shown unequivocally to improve the neurologic outcome from perinatal hypoxic-ischemic encephalopathy and no consensus of practice exists.* Nevertheless, more is being learned about the pathophysiology of brain injury from this insult. This new information provides a framework for assessing current protocols and suggests directions for therapeutic innovation in the future. Some infants are seen in the nursery after a major hypoxic-ischemic insult but before the onset of HIE. Others have an evolving injury in which certain cell populations might be salvageable with appropriate interventions. This chapter describes a schematic and conceptual framework for thinking about this topic as well as some specific guidelines for management.

PATHOPHYSIOLOGY OF HYPOXIC-ISCHEMIC ENCEPHALOPATHY

Multi-Organ Involvement

Significant HIE is usually accompanied by one or more complications in the cardiovascular, respiratory, hematopoietic, genitourinary, endocrine, or integumentary system. For example, hypoxia-ischemia severe enough to cause encephalopathy may also cause arrhythmias, myocardial insufficiency, and shock lung, which may further compromise blood flow to the brain. Renal failure and the syndrome of inappropriate antidiuretic hormone secretion may also complicate management, especially for therapy of complications of encephalopathy, such as cerebral edema. Hypoglycemia may increase the evolution of brain injury under certain circumstances. As described below, the brain with HIE may be especially vulnerable to metabolic and circulatory disorders. Recognition and appropriate therapy of these complications are important supportive measures that could influence the outcome of HIE.

Behavioral Syndrome of Encephalopathy

Behavioral abnormalities may progress from an early period of relative hyperalertness and tachycardia with apparent sympathetic overdrive to a later state of lethargy, hypotonicity, and obtundation with more evidence of parasympathetic activity. These stages undoubtedly have their foundation in progressive changes in neuronal and glial function as outlined below, but the direct relationship between the physiology of encephalopathy and these manifestations is incompletely understood.

Evolution of Cell Death in Encephalopathy

The diagram in Figure 1 is useful for visualizing and organizing the interrelated events causing cell death in the brain from hypoxia-ischemia. The syndrome of HIE is usually caused by a combination of an extended period of moderate to severe hypoxemia and systemic hypotension, leading to decreased regional cerebral blood flow. The cerebral circulation during HIE may be less capable of maintaining cerebral blood flow in the face of a fluctuating cardiac output and blood pressure. At present, the methods for studying regional cerebral blood flow in asphyxiated infants are available only at a few centers, but preliminary information suggests that *significant hypoperfusion may occur in the postasphyxial period.* Nevertheless, it is difficult to assess the status of the infant's brain circulation from the history and physical examination alone. Availability of a practical method for assessing blood flow in the nursery might help to classify infants who could benefit from specific therapies. This indicates the need for careful attention to peripheral factors that could further reduce cerebral blood flow.

Reduction in oxygen and substrate delivery to the brain triggers a cascade of biochemical events responsible for

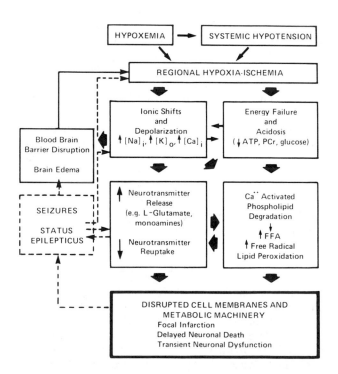

Figure 1 Pathogenesis of events that may mediate hypoxic-ischemic injury to neurons and other tissues in the brain in the hours after asphyxia.

the behavioral manifestations and progressive pathologic evolution seen in HIE.

The most immediate effects on level of consciousness are probably produced by rapid depolarization of cell membranes and ionic shifts during profound asphyxia. Depletion of high-energy phosphate compounds and instability of injured neuronal membranes contribute to the delayed abnormalities in cerebral function. During the hours after a hypoxic-ischemic insult, the oxygen delivered to ischemic areas probably leads to increased lipid peroxidation and free radical generation, as well as to an increase in free fatty acids liberated from membranes triggering the arachidonic acid cascade. Excessive entry of calcium into cells and diminished ability of buffers within the cell to sequester calcium lead to destruction of membranes through calcium-activated phospholipid degradation and other lethal events.

Enhanced release of certain neurotransmitters, such as the excitatory amino acid glutamate and of catecholamines, may also participate in cellular necrosis. Neurotransmitter release could potentially have an impact on local control of cerebral blood flow and may augment the entry of potentially lethal cations such as calcium into cells. Local release of neurotransmitters such as glutamate may account for patterns of selective regional vulnerability. Sensitive regions such as the hippocampus and the basal ganglia are relatively rich in nerve endings and receptors for excitatory amino acids.

The four major groups of biochemical events outlined in the diagram in the boxes in Figure 1 probably lead to relatively rapid destruction of many cells in the hours after asphyxia. However, it is likely that another significant population of brain structures exists that remains alive but with disordered metabolism and physiologic dysfunction. This tissue is the target for strategies to improve neurologic outcome.

Seizures and brain edema are major manifestations of disrupted metabolism and function in this group of brain structures. Seizures result from abnormalities in synaptic function, a disruption of the normal balance between excitatory and inhibitory neuronal systems. The clinical delay between a hypoxic-ischemic insult and seizures suggests that seizures result from evolving biochemical events in HIE. Brain edema is another manifestation of transient disruption of ion and water balance in neurons, glia, and the endothelial blood-brain barrier. Seizures and to a lesser extent edema may participate in a positive feedback loop that acts to enhance brain injury. Seizures increase the energy requirements of dysfunctional cells with limited metabolic reserves. Excessive release of excitatory neurotransmitters may add additional injury directly and stimulate the energy requirements of neurons and glia. Also, seizures may produce disruptive physiologic effects that diminish blood and substrate delivery to the brain. Severe brain edema may reduce local cerebral blood flow by reducing capillary diameter. Brain edema itself probably does little to impede cerebral blood flow in the early stages of HIE but when severe is a sign of potentially lethal injury.

MANAGEMENT

Assessment and Supportive Care

Clinical signs of encephalopathy call for a thorough assessment for infection and metabolic disturbances (e.g., calcium, glucose, electrolytes) as well as appropriate supportive care for other complications.

Optimizing Cerebral Blood Flow

Optimal matching of regional cerebral blood flow with the metabolic needs of the injured brain is a major goal of therapy. Despite our inability to quantitate cerebral blood flow accurately, it is worthwhile to consider this variable as a total plan of care is devised. Maintenance of optimal cardiac output and blood pressure is likely to influence cerebral blood flow in the postasphyxial period. The value of severe fluid restriction to treat edema must be weighted against the dangers of hypovolemia. Hyperventilation using assisted respiration may be helpful to reduce intracranial pressure from cerebral edema, but it may also reduce cerebral blood flow. In situations in which there is significant edema, marked hyperventilation could be potentially harmful if it reduces cerebral blood flow below the threshold for neuronal survival. Mild hypercarbia might be expected to increase cerebral blood flow, although it is possible that this would occur in areas of the brain with normal autoregulation at the expense of compromised areas. Marked hypercarbia may lead to dangerous increases in cerebral blood flow and tissue acidosis.

The rational basis for modifying cerebral blood flow by manipulating arterial blood gases or drugs is an area in which some progress can be expected over the next several years. At present, it seems prudent to monitor respiratory function carefully and to maintain normal arterial blood gases with perhaps mild hypocarbia when signs of increased intracranial pressure are present. Maintenance of normoxia is also imperative.

Blood Glucose

The appropriate blood glucose concentration for management of HIE has been controversial. Hypoxia-ischemia and hypoglycemia may damage the brain by common mechanisms, and hypoglycemia may extend hypoxic-ischemic injury. The brain content of glucose is reduced during hypoxia. This appears to result from reduced delivery, increased consumption during glycolysis, and a defect in transport of glucose across the blood-brain barrier. However, *the neonatal brain may also use alternate fuels such as ketone bodies, partially compensating for the glucose deficiency.* Raising blood glucose levels may seem desirable to overcome the tissue deficiency, but excessive glucose has been reported to lead to high lactic acid levels, acidosis, and enhanced injury in adult ischemia models. This may be less important in the immature brain. A reasonable approach at present is to correct hypoglycemia promptly but to avoid excessive infusion of glucose and consequent high glucose levels.

Monitoring Brain Structure and Function

Monitoring of brain structure has been shown to be a useful prognostic technique in infants with HIE. Bedside real-time cranial sonography is noninvasive and provides detailed anatomic images of structures likely to be affected, including the basal ganglia, the thalamus, and the cortex. Vascular pulsatility may also be estimated. Computed tomographic brain scanning may give a better overall representation of the brain, especially the posterior fossa and superior aspects of the cerebral cortex, but it involves radiation and is not portable. Newer quantitative imaging techniques such as magnetic resonance imaging, positron emission tomography, and single photon emission tomography show great promise as tools that will further our understanding of the mechanisms of HIE, but at present they remain research instruments. Nuclear magnetic resonance spectroscopy for energy-containing phosphorus compounds and pH may also be useful for monitoring brain dysfuction in HIE. Brain stem auditory evoked potentials have been demonstrated to correlate with asphyxial injury and may be a useful screening device. The electroencephalogram is useful for staging the severity of HIE and assessing epileptic activity (see further on).

Seizures and Anticonvulsant Drugs

As noted above, seizures are a sign of dysfunction in neuronal circuits following significant HIE and may also play a role in further extending injury. HIE is the most common cause of neonatal seizures, and seizures following HIE are often a marker for significant neurologic injury. Along with understanding and managing cerebral blood flow, the detection and treatment of epileptic electrical activity are areas of routine care that may be expected to change over the next several years. *There is an imperfect correlation between electrical seizure activity (as seen on the electroencephalogram) and clinical manifestations.* If the relationship between seizure activity and poor outcome is demonstrated in future studies, continuous electroencephalographic monitoring may become advisable for determining appropriate treatment, especially in infants who require elective paralysis for effective ventilation.

Seizures should be anticipated in the HIE infant and treated vigorously with anticonvulsants. Reassessment for metabolic disturbances (e.g., hypoglycemia) may also be appropriate when seizures occur. Loading doses of phenobarbital of up to 30 mg per kilogram are safely tolerated when given slowly. Blood concentrations as high as 50 μg per milliliter are usually well tolerated and may be necessary to control seizures. Higher levels may compromise cardiac output. Maintenance is continued with 3 to 5 mg per kilogram per day with anticonvulsant monitoring. The usefulness of phenobarbital given before the onset of seizures is under investigation. *If clinical seizures continue despite phenobarbital, phenytoin in a loading dose of 10 to 20 mg per kilogram can be administered* to produce blood levels of up to 20 μg per milliliter. Phenytoin is difficult to use as an oral maintenance drug in the newborn because of poor absorption, but it may be con-

tinued in a dose of approximately 5 mg per kilogram per day given intravenously in divided doses with therapeutic monitoring. Primidone (15 to 25 mg per kilogram oral loading dose, 12 to 20 mg per kilogram per day maintenance) may also be useful as a third drug in some infants, especially if intermittent seizures continue beyond several days. Although it is not recommended as a first-line drug, diazepam 0.1 mg per kilogram intravenously may be used for treatment of electrical status epilepticus. In rare instances, a continuous infusion of diazepam has been used to treat status epilepticus in ventilated infants. Paraldehyde may also be used to stop refractory seizures. Use of oral carbamazapine to treat seizures in neonates is being explored.

Despite the fact that many seizures in HIE are relatively refractory to treatment, a vigorous attempt to control them seems warranted because of their potential for extending injury. Other metabolic causes (e.g., hyperammonemia, organic aciduria) should be considered as causes for refractory seizures, and a pyridoxine trial (50 to 100 mg per day) may be warranted.

Assessment of the brain's electrical activity using an electroencephalogram is important to monitor the response to therapy. At present, continuous on-line monitoring is not available in most nurseries. However, it is useful to obtain an electroencephalogram in infants with HIE within the first 24 hours, even if clinical seizures are not apparent. This provides a semiquantitative rating of encephalopathy and serves as a screen for a occult seizure activity. The expertise of an electroencephalographer skilled in neonatal electroencephalograms is helpful for interpretation of these studies. An electroencephalogram should be obtained as soon as feasible after overt seizures have been treated to determine that subclinical seizure activity is not present. If clear-cut seizure activity is detected on the electroencephalogram but there are not clinical signs, anticonvulsant medication should be increased in an attempt to reduce seizure activity, and the electroencephalogram should be assessed in 6 to 24 hours. Given the present uncertain significance of seizure activity in extending injury, a cautious but deliberate approach seems warranted. Definite guidelines are not available at this time.

Cerebral Edema

Mild fluid restriction is used in many nurseries to help prevent cerebral edema, especially in the face of congestive heart failure, renal insufficiency, syndrome of inappropriate antidiuretic hormone. However, management of fluid balance should be assessed carefully to avoid degrees of restriction that would negatively impact on cardiac output and perhaps cerebral blood flow. Similarly, vigorous prophylactic hyperventilation does not seem warranted because of its potential to reduce cerebral blood flow. Corticosteroids have not been shown to be helpful in cerebral edema from HIE. Furthermore, some evidence from animal studies suggests that steroids may enhance neuronal injury from ischemia. Therefore, steroids are not recommended for this indication. Also, mannitol is not likely to be useful for edema in this context. At present, the use of pentobarbital coma for status epilepticus and cerebral edema does not seem warranted considering the possible side effects of reduction in cardiac output. Similarly, the use of hypothermia does not seem warranted considering the possible complications.

SUGGESTED READING

Donn SM, Goldstein GW. Application of newer brain imaging techniques to neonatal cerebrovascular disease. In: Swaiman K, ed. Pediatrics update 1986. New York: Elsevier Science Publishing Co, 1986:111-129.

Donn SM, Goldstein GW, Schork MA. Neonatal hypoxic-ischemic encephalopathy: Current management practices. J Perinatol, in press.

Johnston MV, Silverstein FS. New insights into mechanisms of neuronal damage in the developing brain. Pediatr Neurosci 1986; 12:87-89.

Lockman LA, Kriel R, Zoske D, et al. Phenobarbital dosage for control of neonatal seizures. Neurology 1979; 29:1445.

MacKintosh SA, Baird-Lampert J, Buchanan M. Is carbamazapine an alternative maintenance therapy for neonatal seizures? Dev Pharmacol 1987, 10.100-106.

Painter MJ, Pippenger C, MacDonald H, Pitlick W. Phenobarbital and diphenylhydantoin levels in neonates with seizures, J Pediatr 1978; 92:315.

Powell C, Painter MJ, Pippenger CE. Primidone therapy in refractory neonatal seizures. J Pediatr 1984; 105:651.

INFANT OF A DIABETIC MOTHER

WILLIAM OH, M.D.

It is now well-established that control of maternal diabetes is an important factor in the outcome of the fetus. If diabetes is not controlled by dietary management and insulin therapy, perinatal morbidity and mortality will be high, whereas the incidence of fetal and neonatal complications of well-managed diabetic pregnancies is very low; indeed, the infants are often indistinguishable from normal neonates.

Unfortunately, good control of pregnant diabetic mothers is often not achieved for a variety of reasons. Hence, the pediatrician must often deal with complications among infants of diabetic mothers. With increased understanding of the pertinent pathophysiologic processes, we can now predictably identify and manage successfully such problems as congenital malformations, neonatal asphyxia, birth injury, hypoglycemia, hyaline membrane disease, and respiratory distress resulting from causes other than surfactant deficiency, polycythemia and hyperviscosity, hyperbilirubinemia, hypocalcemia, and renal vein thrombosis. We will discuss these problems in their usual order of appearance from the time of birth.

CONGENITAL MALFORMATIONS

The infant of the diabetic mother (IDM) is known to experience a higher incidence of congenital malformations than does the general newborn population, although the precise etiology and mechanism of this are still unclear. Caudal regression syndrome is often associated with IDM, and other congenital malformations have also been observed. The most common organs involved are the heart and gastrointestinal tract. Careful physical examination of the newborn at birth is mandatory to detect these abnormalities as early as possible.

NEONATAL ASPHYXIA

Asphyxia at birth is commonly observed in the IDM as a continuum of fetal distress. When fetal distress is recognized, the pediatrician should immediately be notified to prepare for resuscitation of the infant at birth by assembling the requisite equipment, drugs, and expert personnel. If the infant is asphyxiated at birth, immediate resuscitation should be undertaken by establishment and maintenance of the airway, administration of oxygen as needed, keeping the infant warm, and administration of a volume expander in the event of hypotension. Since polycythemia and hyperviscosity are common complications in the IDM, we clamp the umbilical cord within 15 to 30 seconds of birth to prevent an excessive placental transfusion. This is particularly true for those infants delivered by the vaginal route.

BIRTH INJURY

Since the IDM is often macrosomic (birth weight exceeding two standard deviations of the mean for gestation), birth injury is a significant risk if vigorous attempts are made to deliver a large infant vaginally and, occasionally, even by cesarean section. The most common type of birth injury is a fracture of the clavicle or humerus. Although it is rare, injury to the central nervous system can also occur. Hence, in the initial evaluation of the IDM, particularly those with macrosomia, it is essential that the possibility of a fractured clavicle or humerus be considered by (1) observation of the infant's upper extremity movements during a Moro reflex maneuver, (2) palpation of the clavicular area for crepitation at the fracture site, and (3) radiologic examination of the clavicle and upper extremities. If injury to the central nervous system is suspected, roentgenologic examination of the skull for fracture should be performed as should ultrasonography or computed tomography to detect intracranial hemorrhage.

Management of this sort of birth injury is generally supportive in nature. Injury to the central nervous system can be associated with a seizure disorder, which is best treated by the use of phenobarbital. Fracture of the clavicle and upper extremity can be treated conservatively by immobilizing the affected upper extremity with an elastic binder. An orthopaedic consultation should be obtained.

HYPOGLYCEMIA

This is directly related to the fetal hyperinsulinemia that results from maternal hyperglycemia and usually occurs between 1 and 3 hours of age. The diagnosis is based on blood or plasma glucose determination. A *blood* glucose level below 30 mg per deciliter in term infants or 20 mg per deciliter in preterm infants establishes the diagnosis. If *plasma* glucose is used, the lower limit of normal is 35 and 25 mg per deciliter for term and preterm infants, respectively. Hypoglycemia in these first hours of life can often be asymptomatic, possibly because newborn infants (including infants of diabetic mothers) have the capability to utilize alternative substrates, such as ketone bodies, in the event of hypoglycemia.

Glucose infusion should be given as early as possible, despite the lack of symptoms, to correct the biochemical deficiencies and avoid frank clinical manifestations and possible injury to the central nervous system. Glucose should be infused intravenously at a dose of 6 mg per kilogram per minute by a constant infusion pump. A peripheral vein is the preferred site of infusion, but in many infants, particularly those who are macrosomic, venipuncture is often difficult. In these circumstances, we use an umbilical venous catheter, provided it can be placed either in the ductus venosus or, even better, in the inferior vena cava; a radiologic confirmation of location is recommended. An umbilical arterial catheter can be used as another alternative, provided the glucose concentration does not exceed 12 percent and the catheter tip is placed below the diaphragm to avoid the direct infusion of glucose into the celiac artery (which can produce persistent hypoglycemia because of the direct pancreatic infusion of glucose and resultant marked increase in insulin secretion).

If the infant's cardiorespiratory condition remains stable, we consider feeding by mouth as early as 4 to 6 hours of age. The first feeding is in the form of 5 to 10 percent glucose in water, followed by formula feeding. This early small glucose feeding, particularly when followed by a milk formula, has the beneficial effect of releasing pancreatic and gut glucagon to produce sustained gluconeogenesis, which helps to stabilize glucose homeostasis.

Glucagon and epinephrine have been used as alternative pharmacologic agents for the treatment of hypoglycemia in the IDM, the rationale being that in the IDM there is an abundance of liver glycogen to generate glucose from the glycogenolysis produced by these hormones. Our own clinical experience indicates, however, that simple glucose infusion and feeding are still the methods of choice for treatment of hypoglycemia in the IDM.

It is important to avoid hyperglycemia during treatment, because the IDM has active beta-cell function that responds very effectively to a rapid increase in blood glucose by producing a marked increase in insulin concentration, which may produce "rebound" hypoglycemia. Moreover, since hypoglycemia is often asymptomatic, there is no real reason for too rapid a restoration of blood glucose concentration. Furthermore, hypertonic glucose infusion can produce intraventricular hemorrhage; although this observation has not been documented in human infants, it raises significant concern over the use of any hypertonic glucose infusion in the treatment of hypoglycemia.

With early oral feeding and the institution of the continuous glucose infusion described, the large majority of hypoglycemic IDMs respond very nicely. A normal blood glucose level is generally achieved by the second or third day of life and should be documented by monitoring blood or plasma glucose during the course of treatment. The Dextrostix method may be used to minimize blood removal, but it is only semiquantitative, so that periodic actual biochemical confirmation should be done.

Persistent hypoglycemia may occur on rare occasions and is generally the result of (1) inappropriate treatment with hypertonic glucose infusion, (2) hyperplasia of pancreatic beta cells with resultant hyperinsulinemia, and (3) placement of an umbilical arterial catheter tip above the diaphragm for glucose infusion.

RESPIRATORY DISTRESS SYNDROME

Respiratory distress syndrome is commonly seen in the IDM, possibly because fetal hyperinsulinemia inhibits surfactant production and thus delays fetal lung maturation. This abnormality affects both the synthesis of phosphatidyl choline (lecithin) and phosphatidyl glycerol (PG). Therefore, in monitoring fetal lung maturity during a diabetic pregnancy, amniocentesis for the assessment of both the amniotic fluid lecithin-sphingomyelin ratio and, if possible, PG should be done. As in a nondiabetic pregnancy, a lecithin-sphingomyelin ratio of less than 2:1 indicates a high potential risk for respiratory distress syndrome. In addition, because of the delay in the appearance of PG among IDM, the usually adequate lecithin/sphingomyelin ratio of 2:1 may not ensure a low risk for respiratory distress syndrome, since low PG may also produce respiratory distress syndrome despite a normal lecithin/sphingomyelin ratio. Hence, amniotic PG measurements should also be done. In the absence of an available biochemical assay for PG, a lecithin/sphingomyelin ratio greater than 3:1 generally suggests a good level of PG as well.

With such careful attention to prenatal assessment of fetal maturity before terminating pregnancy, the risk of respiratory distress syndrome in all infants, including IDMs, should be low.

RESPIRATORY DISTRESS RESULTING FROM CAUSES OTHER THAN RESPIRATORY DISTRESS SYNDROME

Not all infants with respiratory distress at birth have respiratory distress syndrome due to surfactant deficiency (hyaline membrane disease). This is particularly true in IDMs who are also prone to conditions such as asphyxia, hypoglycemia, retained lung fluid (particularly those delivered by cesarean section), polycythemia, and congestive heart failure—all potential causes of respiratory distress in the first few hours of life. Therefore, in the IDM with respiratory distress in the first hours of life with documented adequate fetal lung maturity and no evidence of respiratory distress syndrome on chest roentgenogram, these various causes must be entertained and diagnosed and appropriate specific therapy instituted. Beyond any such specific treatment, the management of respiratory distress is supportive and includes oxygen therapy, maintenance of systemic perfusion and acid-base balance, as careful monitoring of blood gases as a guide to respiratory management.

HYPERBILIRUBINEMIA

The incidence of hyperbilirubinemia in IDMs is significantly higher than in other newborns, but the reasons are not entirely clear. Recent investigations have shown that the incidence of hyperbilirubinemia is still high even when corrected for gestational age and that it may be related to polycythemia with increased bilirubin production by a physiologic hemolysis during the first few days of life.

In spite of the high incidence of jaundice, the occurrence of kernicterus in IDMs is relatively rare, but the clinician should not be complacent about the potential risk of bilirubin encephalopathy. The accepted methods of management of hyperbilirubinemia are phototherapy and, if necessary, exchange transfusions in both IDMs and non-IDMs.

POLYCYTHEMIA AND HYPERVISCOSITY

We define polycythemia as a condition in which the infant's *venous* hematocrit exceeds 65 percent and the blood viscosity exceeds two standard deviations of the mean. Hyperviscosity is most often secondary to polycythemia. The IDM is at higher risk for polycythemia and hyperviscosity because chronic fetal hypoxia results from insufficient control of diabetes during pregnancy. Furthermore, acute hypoxia may also occur during labor and result in an intrauterine placental transfusion. Hence, we believe it advisable to clamp the umbilical cord of these infants within 15 to 30 seconds following the delivery of the body to minimize further placental transfusion postnatally. If the infant receives a sizeable amount of placental blood transfusion acutely, either during labor or within the first 3 minutes after birth, hemoconcentration occurs during adjustment of the circulating blood volume in the first few hours of life. This process of hemoconcentration entails transudation of fluid into the interstitial tissues and may partly account for some of the symptoms observed in the IDM with polycythemia. These symptoms of polycythemia and hyperviscosity are not specific and are generally secondary to one or more of the following: (1) perinatal asphyxia, (2) fluid transudation into the interstitial tissue of various organs, (3) hyperviscosity per se, and (4) increased red cell mass.

The treatment for polycythemia and hyperviscosity is a partial exchange transfusion (removal of blood with isovolemic replacement by a volume expander, usually Plasmanate).

The formula used for calculation of volume to be removed and replaced is as follows:

Volume of partial exchange transfusion (ml) =

$$\frac{\text{Hematocrit} - 55}{\text{Hematocrit}} \times \begin{array}{c}\text{Body}\\\text{Weight}\\\text{(kg)}\end{array} \times \begin{array}{c}\text{Blood}\\\text{Volume}\\\text{(80 ml/kg)}\end{array}$$

Although most agree on the need for treatment in symptomatic cases of polycythemia and hyperviscosity, there are instances when an infant may be completely asymptomatic despite the presence of polycythemia and hyperviscosity, and there is controversy regarding the indications for treatment of these asymptomatic cases. There is a current lack of good long-term follow-up data to support the indications for therapy. Therefore the choice for treatment should be individualized, depending on the level of the hematocrit, the age of the infant, and the certainty of clinical observations. In infants with a hematocrit of 65 to 70 percent at 24 to 48 hours of age and no symptoms, the indication for treatment is not pressing, we believe. But when the hematocrit is between 70 and 75 percent at less than 12 hours of age and with equivocal clinical manifestations, it would be best to treat with partial exchange transfusion.

RENAL VEIN THROMBOSIS

This condition is traditionally associated with the IDM, but it is actually a relatively rare complication and, as a matter of fact, the reason for its occurrence in IDMs is not clear. It is likely that it is secondary to hyperviscosity, hypotension, or disseminated intravascular coagulation. The symptom complex consists of hematuria, palpable renal mass, and signs of acute renal failure. Treatment consists of restriction of fluid and electrolyte intake in the presence of acute renal failure and supportive treatment to provide for adequate circulation. Heparin therapy may also be a consideration to prevent further coagulation, but if the thrombosis is unilateral and if the infant is acutely ill with no response to medical treatment, nephrectomy may be indicated.

NEONATAL MACROSOMIA AND ADOLESCENT OBESITY

It has been shown that infants who are macrosomic are more likely to become obese during the adolescent period, probably because of the increased number of fat cells resulting from increased fat deposition during the fetal period. Although the data documenting the association between neonatal and adolescent obesity are based on a retrospective analysis (which demands further prospective confirmation), the pediatrician should be aware of this correlation. If obesity is detected early in the childhood of offspring who were macrosomic at birth to diabetic mothers, appropriate dietary advice should be instituted to reduce caloric intake.

INGUINAL HERNIA IN THE PERINATAL PERIOD

JAY L. GROSFELD, M.D.

Inguinal hernia is a common condition in the neonate and is often a cause of considerable parental and physician concern. Congenital indirect inguinal hernia is related to the descent of the testes from its origin at a retroperitoneal site near the developing renal tissues. Following the gubernaculum testis, the gonad descends through the internal inguinal ring traversing the inguinal canal, passing through the external inguinal ring to its ultimate position within the scrotal sac. As the testis descends through the internal inguinal ring, it takes with it a portion or diverticulum of the peritoneal lining, referred to as the processus vaginalis. In the majority of full-term infants, the processus vaginalis undergoes spontaneous involution or obliteration, leaving a remnant on the anteromedial surface of the testis, which becomes the anatomic tunica vaginalis. In 5 to 10 percent of newborns, portions of the processus vaginalis persist, resulting in a variety of inguinal anomalies, including scrotal hernia, proximal inguinal hernia, communicating hydrocele, hydrocele of the spermatic cord in boys or the canal of Nuck in girls, and finally an isolated hydrocele of the tunica vaginalis. Except for the latter defect, all the other anomalies of the inguinal canal communicate with the free peritoneal cavity and therefore have the potential risk of bowel incarceration. Inguinal hernias are considerably more common in boys than in girls (9:1) and have a strong tendency to occur in multiple family members. Hernias are more frequently observed in infants with ascites, meconium peritonitis, hydrops, and abdominal wall defects (e.g., omphalocele and gastroschisis), in which an increase in intra-abdominal pressure may play a role. An increased incidence of inguinal hernia is also seen among infants with ambiguous genitalia and genitourinary anomalies, including hypospadias, epispadias, and cryptorchidism. The highest incidence of inguinal hernia is seen in the premature infant, as those factors that result in obliteration of the processus vaginalis do not have a chance to effect this change (Table 1).

TABLE 1 Increased Incidence of Inguinal Hernia

Prematurity
Positive family history
Hydrops
Meconium peritonitis
Chylous ascites
Abdominal wall defects
Ambiguous genitalia
Hypospadias, epispadias
Exstrophy of bladder, cloaca
Cryptorchid testis
Ventriculoperitoneal shunt
Liver disease with ascites

With the development of contemporary neonatal intensive care facilities in most urban areas, many premature infants who previously succumbed from a variety of causes (especially birth asphyxia) now survive and frequently present with clinically symptomatic inguinal hernia.

Body temperature should be closely monitored in these infants to avoid hypothermia. When the infant is relaxed and quiet, gentle taxis is employed in an attempt to reduce the incarceration and avoid the need for an emergency operation. This was successful in 22 of 31 cases of incarceration that subsequently underwent elective hernia repair 24 to 48 hours following reduction. Toxicity is defined as severe tachycardia (>180 beats per minute), leukocytosis (>15,000 white blood cells per mm³), a shift to the left on differential smear, abdominal distention, bilious vomiting, an obstructive small bowel pattern on abdominal x-ray films in the erect and recumbent positions, and black or dusky-blue discoloration of the trapped viscera. Infants with these clinical findings require an emergency operation, since manual reduction should not be attempted under these circumstances because of the risk of reducing necrotic bowel. In nontoxic patients, a waiting period of 4 to 6 hours for the bowel to reduce may be reasonable as long as the infant is comfortable.

Parenteral antibiotics are given in instances of irreducible incarceration requiring an emergency operative procedure. Prophylactic antibiotics are also utilized in elective procedures in infants with preexisting ventriculoperitoneal shunt catheters placed for hydrocephalus and those with congenital heart defects. Ampicillin (100 mg per kilogram per day) and gentamicin (5 mg per kilogram per day) or tobramycin (5 mg per kilogram per day) is the drug combination usually employed. Intravenous antibiotics are started preoperatively to effect an adequate blood level during the procedure and are continued for 48 hours.

Preterm infants who are evaluated for the first time after previous discharge from the nursery or hospital neonatal unit are usually admitted to the hospital and managed as inpatients. Full-term infants who had no prior neonatal difficulties and are otherwise thriving except for their hernias are managed as outpatients and are discharged shortly following their operation.

PREOPERATIVE PREPARATION

Preoperative preparation varies with the type of patient encountered. Full-term outpatients are kept without oral intake for 4 hours prior to the procedure. Atropine, 0.1 mg, is usually given intravenously just prior to induction. This reduces excessive airway secretions and maintains the pulse rate and may prevent cardiovascular depression associated with anesthesia. Babies with irreducible hernias and bowel obstruction require insertion of an orogastric tube to prevent distention from swallowed air and to empty and decompress the stomach in order to reduce the risk of aspiration. Fluid resuscitation may be necessary to correct hypovolemia related to sequestration of fluids into the obstructed bowel lumen and edematous inguinal tissues. Intravenous fluid should contain 5 to 10 percent glucose in lactated Ringer's solution to prevent hypoglycemia and deliver adequate crystalloid to restore circulating volume.

282

Although inguinal hernia repair is one of the most commonly performed operations in childhood, controversy exists concerning the most appropriate timing and actual safety of hernia repair in the perinatal period. These concerns are of special importance in the premature or seriously ill neonate who is hospitalized with a concurrent illness. To evaluate this problem we recently reviewed 100 consecutive herniorrhaphies performed in infants under 8 weeks of age at the James Whitcomb Riley Hospital for Children, Indiana University Medical Center, Indianapolis.

Eighty-five of the infants were boys and 15 were girls. Thirty of the babies were premature (< 36 weeks' gestation). Forty-two infants had been hospitalized: 16 for respiratory distress syndrome requiring assisted ventilation, 7 for hydrocephalus requiring a ventriculoperitoneal shunt procedure, and 19 for congenital heart disease with cyanosis, congestive heart failure, or both. Clinically, hernia was present on the right side in 44 cases, was bilateral in 42 patients, and on the left side in 14 infants. Thirty-one infants had an incarcerated hernia; 9 had overt intestinal obstruction. Eleven of the 85 boys (12.9 percent) had cryptorchid testis, while three of the 15 girls presented with a palpable ovary in the upper labia. This rate of incarceration (31 percent) is 2 to 2.5 times greater than the incidence of incarceration (12 to 15 percent) reported throughout childhood (0 to 16 years). The incidence of cryptorchidism is more than twice that usually reported for the newborn (5 percent) and more than 24 times that reported for males during the childhood years (0.5 percent).

MANAGEMENT

In infants already hospitalized with clinically apparent but asymptomatic inguinal hernia, the timing for operative repair depends on the overall condition of the patient. It is reasonable to await improvement in the general status of the condition that initially required hospitalization, such as respiratory distress syndrome on ventilator support, hydrocephalus, heart failure due to congenital cardiac defects, meconium peritonitis, or peritonitis due to necrotizing enterocolitis. In addition, some delay in operative repair would seem indicated for the infant with a very low birth weight who has an asymptomatic hernia. When the underlying condition improves and the infant weighs more than 2,200 g, elective inguinal hernia repair is carried out, usually just prior to discharge from the hospital.

For hospitalized infants who have an incarcerated hernia, manual reduction of the hernia is attempted in nontoxic cases. The baby may be sedated with a short-acting barbiturate such as secobarbital (Seconal 1.0 mg per kilogram) or sodium pentobarbital (Nembutal, 1.0 mg per kilogram) intramuscularly to diminish straining. Morphine sulfate should be avoided because of its exaggerated depressive effect on the respiratory center in the medulla oblongata in infants. The only exception to this rule concerning morphine is in the infant who is already receiving respiratory support with mechanical ventilation. A suggested sedative dose for this specific situation would be 0.2 mg per kilogram of morphine sulfate intramuscularly. The infant is placed in the Trendelenburg position in an effort to reduce edema by the effect of gravity, and a "cool pack" over a sheet of petrolatum-impregnated gauze is placed over the inguinal-scrotal region.

Anesthesia

In all infants with incarcerated hernias, endotracheal anesthesia is administered following an awake intubation technique. In full-term babies who are undergoing elective herniorrhaphies, anesthesia is often induced with thiopental prior to intubation. Warm humidified gases are employed, with halothane being the usual agent. The infant is carefully monitored with electrocardiogram leads, Doppler for pulse and blood pressure, cutaneous Po_2 probe, and an axillary skin temperature probe. Body temperature is maintained at 96.5°F with the aid of overhead radiant warmers, heat lamps, warming aqua-blankets, and swaddling cloth for the extremities. A hat is also useful to cover the small infant's head, with its 19 to 20 percent of total body surface area, in order to prevent radiant heat loss.

Operation

The operative field is prepared with a warm iodophor preparation solution applied to the abdomen, groin, scrotal, and perineal areas. After appropriate linen draping, operation is carried out initially on the most symptomatic side. The operation is accomplished through a short transverse incision in the lowest inguinal crease. Hemostasis is achieved using a fine-tipped infant electrocoagulator to minimize blood loss. The subcutaneous (Scarpa's) fascia is opened, and the external oblique fascia is identified and traced laterally to the inguinal ligament and then inferiorly to demonstrate the external inguinal ring. The external oblique fascia is opened perpendicular to the ring in the long axis of its fibers, with care being taken to identify and preserve the ilioinguinal and iliohypogastric nerves. The cremasteric muscle fibers are teased open, and the hernial sac is encountered on the anteromedial surface of the spermatic cord. The sac is carefully separated from the spermatic vessels and vas deferens by sharp and blunt dissection. The proximal limit of dissection is at the internal inguinal ring, where the base of the sac is suture ligated with two separate 4-0 silk sutures. A free tie at the neck of the sac is to be avoided, as it may be dislodged if postoperative abdominal distention occurs. If the distal sac freely communicates with the scrotal component of the hernia, the anterior wall of the distal sac is simply incised but left in place to reduce the risk of bleeding. However, if a separate, noncommunicating hydrocele is present distally, this is excised by means of the electrocoagulator, leaving that portion of the peritoneum adherent to the epididymis and testis in place.

If an undescended testis is present, freeing of the hernial sac from the cord vessels and vas deferens frequently increases the spermatic cord length significantly. Further length of the spermatic cord is obtained by division of bands of lateral spermatic fascia along the testicular vessels as they pass cephalad through the internal ring up into the retroperitoneal space. The previously empty scrotal sac is prepared for orchiopexy by digital (fingertip) stretching. The testis is fixed in a dartos muscle pouch with 4-0 chromic catgut sutures to complete the orchiopexy and prevent retraction. This is best accomplished by a small, low, transverse scrotal incision near the midline raphe.

Should the internal ring be excessively large or the floor of the inguinal canal (e.g., the transversalis fascia) seem weak, this is repaired with one or two interrupted 4–0 sutures. In little girls, the internal ring is usually sutured closed with a 4–0 silk suture. Wound closure is accomplished by means of interrupted 5–0 silk sutures (inverting the knots) on the external oblique and subcutaneous fasciae and interrupted 4–0 plain catgut subcuticular sutures to oppose the skin edges. A collodion dressing is applied to seal the wound and protect it from urinary and fecal contamination. An alternative closure involves the use of Steri-strips to oppose the skin and an Op-site dressing to prevent contamination.

In emergency cases of incarceration and bowel obstruction, only the symptomatic side is repaired. In elective cases, bilateral inguinal exploration is routinely carried out in this group of very young patients. Forty-two percent of the infants in the present review had bilateral hernias. In addition, the high incidence of prematurity and the fact that a contralateral patent processus vaginalis is so common in this age group would suggest that bilateral exploration is a reasonable approach. More than 90 percent of the cases had either a second hernia or a patent processus vaginalis. In elective cases, circumcision can also be done as a complementary procedure if the parents of the baby so desire. Such adjunctive procedures have not affected morbidity.

POSTOPERATIVE CARE

At the end of the procedure, following extubation, infants are either placed in heated Isolettes or wrapped in warm blankets and, when active, are transferred to the recovery room. Infants managed as outpatients are kept in a separate alcove area away from the inpatients to reduce the number of contacts for potential nosocomial infection. Appropriate monitoring is continued during the sojourn to the recovery room suite. When the baby is active and vital signs are stable, preterm infants are transferred to the neonatal or infant units for overnight observation.

RESULTS

There was no operative mortality in this group of 100 patients. One infant with incarceration and undescended testis had acute gonadal infarction. Although the bowel was dusky in three other infants with incarceration and obstruction, none required bowel resection as normal color, peristalsis, and sheen were restored following reduction. In one instance, the obstructed viscera reduced during operative manipulation of the sac without adequate examination of the bowel. As cloudy peritoneal fluid was noted, a laparotomy was done through a separate incision to explore the peritoneum and inspect the bowel. Fortunately, the dusky antimesenteric bowel wall became pink and had good Doppler pulses. One infant girl with incarceration of an ovary had torsion and gonadal gangrene, requiring oophorectomy at the time of hernia repair.

Postoperative complications occurred in eight cases (Table 2). Four premature infants required postoperative mechanical ventilation for 24 hours in three instances and 48 hours in one. This was related to apnea and bradycardia in two, digoxin toxicity due to hypokalemia in one, and *Klebsiella* sepsis in one infant who had an incarcerated hernia. Two infants developed scrotal hematomas, which spontaneously resolved. One baby developed a late wound infection at 6 weeks, and there was one recurrent hernia at 6 months in a baby with cerebrospinal fluid ascites related to a ventriculoperitoneal shunt. All full-term infants treated as outpatients had uncomplicated postoperative courses.

These observations indicate that inguinal hernia is extremely common in prematures and neonates and is associated with a high incidence of incarceration (31 percent), intestinal obstruction (9 percent), and cryptorchidism (12.9 percent) in this age group. The high risk of complications in the perinatal period further suggests that early elective hernia repair should be accomplished when the infant's general condition is stable. Inguinal hernia repair can be done safely in the neonatal period with a relatively low morbidity and zero mortality. Preterm infants and other neonates with associated illnesses should be managed as inpatients. Preterm infants are more susceptible to episodes of apnea and bradycardia following general anesthesia. The actual cause of apnea in these infants is not entirely clear. Halogenated anesthetic agents may be implicated in the immediate postoperative phase, as even low blood levels of these agents may cause depression of chemoreceptor response to hypoxemia. Preterm infants demonstrate easy fatigability of ventilatory muscles. Muscle fatigue may be related to the relatively few high oxidative fatigue-resistant fibers present in the diaphragm of small infants. Whatever the reason, premature and previously seriously ill babies should be carefully monitored and observed postoperatively for a 24-hour period within the hospital confines. Full-term infants who are otherwise well can safely undergo hernia repair on an outpatient basis. Careful parental instruction is necessary for proper home care following outpatient cases regarding fever, diet, breathing problems, adequate urination, activity, bathing, and pain. Acetaminophen is usually prescribed as an analgesic. Baby aspirin should be avoided owing to the inhibitory effect of platelet aggregation by the acetylsalicylic acid molecule and the risk of postoperative hematoma.

TABLE 2 Postoperative Complications: 8/100 Cases (8%)

Apnea and bradycardia	2
Digoxin toxicity	1
Klebsiella sepsis	1
Scrotal hematoma	2
Wound infection	1
Recurrent hernia	1

INTRAUTERINE GROWTH RETARDATION: PEDIATRIC ASPECTS

STEWART LAWRENCE, M.D.
EDWARD R. YEOMANS, M.D.
CHARLES R. ROSENFELD, M.D.

Management of the infant with intrauterine growth retardation should be a joint effort of the obstetrician and neonatologist; thus, it is assumed that the diagnosis and management should begin in utero. Since this approach is used in our institution, a description of our management begins in utero.

PRENATAL DETECTION

Intrauterine growth retardation (IUGR) is defined by the obstetrician as a fetal weight below the tenth percentile for gestational age and is associated with a perinatal mortality rate four to eight times greater than that for the general population. Early detection of IUGR in pregnancy remains a difficult task, despite significant improvements in the obstetrician's ability to monitor fetal growth and "well-being." Therefore, the first prerequisite for making the diagnosis of IUGR is a high degree of clinical suspicion.

There are numerous causes of abnormal fetal growth. This is illustrated in a 1986 review of the subject in which more than 50 entities were cited that predispose to IUGR. Nevertheless, the most common causes of IUGR can be conveniently grouped as maternal, placental, and fetal; these are listed in Table 1. Knowledge of the various causes of IUGR enables the practicing physician to identify the pregnancy that is at greatest risk for this complication. It has been estimated that, although one-third of all pregnancies are associated with at least one identifiable risk factor for IUGR, two-thirds of all identified growth-retarded infants are the product of pregnancies complicated by one of these factors.

Early detection of abnormal fetal growth depends on careful serial physical examinations. Measuring the distance in centimeters from the top of the symphysis pubis to the top of the uterine fundus palpated through the abdominal wall (McDonald measurement) is a simple technique that should be used routinely in prenatal care. Its utility in screening for IUGR varies widely, highlighting both the importance of early prenatal care and the need for precise measurement, preferably by the same examiner. Obviously, a number of factors, including maternal body habitus, degree of bladder distention, and position on the examining table, can affect this measurement; however, there is general agreement that a fundal height 4 cm or more less than the estimated gestational age in weeks is a suspicious indication of possible IUGR and warrants further investigation. In current obstetric practice this usually entails some application of diagnostic ultrasonography.

An understanding of the patterns of abnormal fetal growth is a prerequisite to interpreting any sonographic data. Campbell and Dewhurst first distinguished "low profile" or symmetric IUGR from "late flattening" or asymmetric (head-sparing) IUGR. There is, however, a spectrum of abnormally decreased fetal growth, rather than two distinct categories, with the onset varying from early gestation (predominantly due to viral infections or genetically determined decreased growth potential) to late gestation (predominantly secondary to inadequate delivery of substrate and/or oxygen). The existence of at least two patterns of abnormal fetal growth helps to explain why multiple sonographic measurements are more reliable than are single measurements of individual variables.

Clearly, a single measurement of the biparietal diameter (BPD) is an unreliable indicator of abnormal growth. Even serial BPD measurements can fail to detect asymmetric IUGR, since, by definition, the head is relatively spared until quite late in gestation. We therefore use the head-abdomen ratio (head circumference divided by abdominal circumference) to improve our detection of the late-flattening or asymmetric variety of IUGR. The normal head-abdomen ratio is greater than 1 until 32 weeks, approximately 1 from 32 to 36 weeks, and less than 1 from 36 weeks to term, reflecting the deposition of subcutaneous fat and hepatic glycogen in the latter part of pregnancy. An estimate of fetal weight is obtained from tables that

TABLE 1 Etiology of Intrauterine Growth Retardation

Maternal	*Placental*	*Fetal*
1. Prepregnancy weight < 50 kg	1. Circumvallate placenta	1. Infections, especially viral
2. Poor weight gain during pregnancy	2. Multiple fetuses	2. Malformations
3. Chronic maternal disease	3. Chronic abruption	3. Genetic abnormalities
Hypertensive vascular disease	4. Infarct or hemangioma	
Cyanotic heart disease		
Sickle cell anemia		
Diabetes mellitus		
(class D–F)		
4. Drug ingestion		
5. Smoking (excessive)		
6. History of previous growth-retarded infant		

require as input parameters a BPD and abdominal circumference. If this estimate falls below the tenth percentile for gestational age, the diagnosis of IUGR is considered.

Measurement of fetal femur length also has been recommended as an aid to the diagnosis of abnormal fetal growth. It has been incorporated into formulas for calculating a sonographic fetal ponderal index, which, analogous to the neonatal ponderal index, could potentially identify fetuses with abnormal weight for length relationships. However, femur length in the latter half of gestation is a relatively inaccurate measurement, and it appears in the formula for ponderal index as a factor in the denominator raised to the third power, thereby compounding any inaccuracy of this measurement. In our institution, femur length is used only to help corroborate the estimation of gestational age before 22 weeks or the early diagnosis of a fetal dwarf.

In addition to fetal mensuration, estimation of amniotic fluid volume has been used as a means of diagnosing IUGR. It has been suggested that in IUGR the distribution of fetal cardiac output is directed away from the kidneys with sparing of the brain, heart, placenta, and adrenals, thereby reducing fetal urine output and, as a direct consequence, amniotic fluid volume. Oligohydramnios has been defined sonographically as the absence of at least one pocket of amniotic fluid measuring 1 cm in its broadest diameter. However, others have concluded that, although severe oligohydramnios was indeed present when pocket size was less than 1 cm, many cases of IUGR would be missed by adoption of such a stringent criterion. At the present time we prefer to estimate the volume of amniotic fluid subjectively as increased, normal, or decreased for gestational age.

The latest modality to be employed in the detection of fetal growth retardation is Doppler velocimetry. Developments in this area have been rapid. It is possible to assess blood flow "indirectly" through both the uterine and umbilical arteries, and even to measure "flow" selectively through the fetal carotid arteries. As might be expected, blood flow through the carotid arteries appears to be relatively maintained in the brain-sparing or asymmetric type of IUGR. Although Doppler studies may have a potential for clinical use, they should be regarded at this time only as investigational. We are currently investigating Doppler velocimetry at our institution in several settings: hypertensive disease, suspected fetal growth retardation, discordant twins, and post-term pregnancy. Results are not as yet used for determining clinical management.

In summary, IUGR is a condition with a relatively low prevalence for which methods of detection remain imperfect. It is, therefore, a condition that is exceedingly difficult to predict; i.e., the positive predictive value of any of the several tests discussed, alone or in combination, is low. This is a critical factor to consider in the management of the pregnancy in which retarded fetal growth is suspected. Hence, decisions in our center concerning early intervention to terminate an increasingly high-risk pregnancy, the relative safety of allowing a trial

of labor, and the most appropriate route of delivery are discussed jointly among perinatologists and neonatologists.

PRENATAL MANAGEMENT

Once IUGR is clinically suspected, careful antepartum and intrapartum management is required to obtain a good perinatal outcome. The most important factor for the successful management of a pregnancy complicated by IUGR is precise knowledge of the gestational age of the fetus. If the length of gestation is known and the pregnancy is thought to be at or near term, delivery is indicated soon after IUGR is diagnosed. However, before term, the risks of preterm birth must be weighed against the risks of IUGR. If maternal disease, especially hypertensive disease, is associated with IUGR, delivery not only removes the fetus from a hostile environment, but also may arrest the progression of maternal disease in many cases. If the mother's condition is stable, we employ amniocentesis to assess pulmonary maturity before delivery. Occasionally, expectant management allows for the modification of certain risk factors for decreased fetal growth, such as provision of better nutrition, cessation of substance abuse, and bed rest.

The role of antepartum testing by either biophysical or biochemical methods is highly variable from one institution to another. We presently do not employ serum or urine estriol measurements or human placental lactogen (HPL) measurements in the management of IUGR or any other complications of pregnancy, since they appear to have low predictive value and reproducibility, can be interfered with by a variety of agents, and are quite expensive. The biophysical profile (which combines a number of sonographic observations with a nonstress test) is probably of greater value in the antepartum management of preterm IUGR; we use a simplified "profile," consisting of the mother's perception of fetal movements and the examiner's assessment of amniotic fluid volume. Amniocentesis is employed to assess fetal lung maturity in pregnancies in which the estimate of gestational age is uncertain or those with a borderline gestational age for lung maturity (33 to 36 weeks).

DELIVERY ROOM MANAGEMENT

The birth process itself represents a potential asphyxial stress, even for an appropriately grown, previously uncompromised fetus. The fetus with IUGR is, therefore, at an even greater risk of suffering the consequences of birth anoxia; this is evidenced by the high frequency of low Apgar scores, meconium expulsion into the amniotic fluid, and intrapartum death reported to occur in these infants. Therefore, fetal monitoring during the intrapartum period is essential. If fetal distress is detected and vaginal delivery is not imminent, immediate cesarean section is performed. A member of the neonatal staff is present at all deliveries of prenatally identified infants with IUGR in order to provide skilled resuscitation, and to prevent or minimize further anoxia secondary to cardiopulmonary depression or meconium aspiration. When meconium-stained amniotic fluid has been observed, the infant's posterior oropharynx and nasopharynx *must be cleared* of meconium by bulb (preferred) or DeLee suction *on the perineum,* immediately upon delivery of the head. Following delivery, the infant's trachea is visualized and cleared of meconium if the meconium was thick or if there was previous evidence of fetal distress. Supplemental oxygen and positive-pressure ventilation is provided as necessary to stabilize the infant before transport to the Special Care Nursery.

NEONATAL DETECTION

IUGR not identified during pregnancy can be detected shortly after birth. All low-birth-weight infants (2,400 g or less) are initially evaluated in the triage area of the Special Care Nursery, where their growth parameters, i.e., height, weight, head circumference, and ponderal index, are measured and recorded against the estimated gestational age. The latter is determined primarily by obstetric criteria: last menstrual period, onset of fetal heart tones, serial measurements of uterine fundal height, and early sonographic (12 to 24 weeks gestation) measurements of fetal crown-rump length and biparietal diameter. When obstetric criteria are poor, pediatric assessments of gestational age are used; these include a Finnstrom examination by a research nurse on all infants with birth weight less than 1,500 g (for the purpose of data collection) and a Ballard assessment by the infant's primary physician. The growth grids compiled by Lubchenko at the University of Colorado Medical Center are presently used for the purpose of widespread comparison with fetal growth data from other centers. Data are presently being compiled in order to correlate newborn growth parameters with neonatal morbidity and mortality rates in our predominantly inborn population.

In addition to having their growth and gestational age assessed, infants are examined carefully for features suggestive of chronic intrauterine hypoxemia or placental insufficiency: e.g., decreased subcutaneous tissue and fat; meconium staining of the nails, skin, or umbilical cord; and rough, parchment-like skin that desquamates easily. Late-term (40 to 42 weeks' gestation) or post-term (more than 42 weeks' gestation) infants possessing these characteristics may not fulfill the definition currently used for small for gestational age (SGA), i.e., less than the tenth percentile for weight, but may demonstrate an abnormality of the ponderal index (less than 10 percent). These infants, who are at risk for many of the neonatal problems of the SGA infant, are identified as having IUGR.

MANAGEMENT OF NEONATAL PROBLEMS

Temperature Regulation

Thermoregulation may be impaired in the SGA infant secondary to diminished subcutaneous fat, with resultant increased convective heat losses. The SGA infant also may have decreased brown fat stores, resulting in a limited capacity to produce heat to counteract cold stress. Immediately after the umbilical cord is clamped in the delivery room, the infant is placed on sterile drapes and dried thoroughly on a radiantly heated resuscitation table. Once the cardiopulmonary status has stabilized, the infant is placed in an incubator in a thermoneutral environment provided by servocontrolled heating. We use an additional heat shield or bordered plastic blanket in all our low-birth-weight infants to minimize radiant heat loss, as well as evaporant water loss.

Metabolic Problems

The SGA infant is at substantial risk for the occurrence of hypoglycemia, secondary to diminished glycogen stores and defective gluconeogenesis. Careful monitoring of blood glucose following birth (hourly for 4 hours and every 4 hours until at least 24 hours of age) allows for early detection and expectant management of hypoglycemia before the onset of symptoms. In most cases we either initiate early feeds at 1 to 3 hours of life or start an intravenous infusion of 10 percent dextrose in water at 60 to 80 ml per kilogram per day. When hypoglycemia occurs (i.e., a Dextrostix test result of less than 25 mg per deciliter), therapy is initiated. Blood glucose level is determined to confirm the diagnosis of hypoglycemia, and an intravenous dextrose infusion (200 mg per kilogram "minibolus" over 15 to 20 minutes, followed by a continuous dextrose infusion of 5 to 8 mg per kilogram per minute) is started. The use of early enteral feeding alone is sometimes successful in achieving glucose homeostasis among SGA infants in whom there has been little or no evidence of perinatal anoxia and in whom the likelihood of gastrointestinal ischemia is minimal (Table 2).

Hypocalcemia has been observed in SGA infants who also appeared to have suffered perinatal anoxia. All infants admitted to our nursery with evidence of anoxia are screened for hypocalcemia at 12 to 24 hours of life. Calcium gluconate therapy (200 to 400 mg per kilogram per

TABLE 2   Clinical Manifestations of Perinatal Anoxia

Fetal heart rate abnormalities: Tachycardia, decreased beat-to-beat variability, decelerations

Meconium staining of amniotic fluid, skin, nails, or umbilical cord

Cord blood acidosis: pH < 7.20

Low Apgar scores: less than 6 at 5 and 10 minutes of life

Neurologic abnormality: muscle flaccidity, poor responsiveness to stimulation, apnea, seizures

Renal abnormality: oliguria, anuria, hematuria

Cardiovascular abnormality: persistent bradycardia, cardiogenic shock secondary to myocardial dysfunction, tricuspid insufficiency day divided into four doses and administered intravenously over 5 to 10 minutes with careful heart rate monitoring) is initiated in asymptomatic infants with a serum calcium level less than 6.0 mg per deciliter and in infants with symptoms attributable to hypocalcemia, e.g., jitteriness, apnea, or seizures and serum calcium levels below 7.0 to 7.5 mg per deciliter. Obviously, it may be difficult to distinguish neurologic symptoms secondary to asphyxia from those of hypocalcemia.

Polycythemia-Hyperviscosity Syndrome

The polycythemia-hyperviscosity syndrome occurs more frequently in SGA infants than in other groups of neonates, probably as a consequence either of elevated erythropoietin levels after chronic hypoxemia or of placental-fetal transfusions during acute episodes of fetal hypoxia. Polycythemia is generally defined as a peripheral venous hematocrit > 65 percent. Because of concerns about measurement reliability, we do not perform blood viscosity measurements, which have been demonstrated to increase exponentially as the hematocrit rises over 65 percent and would be expected to correlate closely with adverse sequelae. Infants are therefore managed conservatively; those with a venous hematocrit between 65 and 70 percent and any symptoms associated with the polycythemia-hyperviscosity syndrome (e.g., tachypnea, poor feeding, hypoglycemia, lethargy, jitteriness, irritability, or seizures) receive a partial exchange transfusion. Either 5 percent albumin, plasmanate, or fresh-frozen plasma is used to replace the infant's whole blood to produce a subsequent venous hematocrit of 50 to 55 percent. An exchange transfusion is generally performed when the venous hematocrit is 70 percent or greater, even in the absence of symptoms.

Diagnostic Evaluation and Developmental Follow-Up

Once infants are defined as being SGA or having IUGR, they are carefully evaluated to determine the etiology of the aberrant fetal growth. A prenatal history is obtained to identify maternal factors that could have resulted in limited fetal growth (see Table 1). The placenta is examined for abnormalities that might have caused impaired support for fetal growth, such as infarcts, hemangiomas, aberrant cord insertions, occult abruption, and abnormal implantation. The infant is examined thoroughly for dysmorphic features and gross anomalies suggestive of conditions with an altered growth potential, such as congenital malformation syndromes, chromosomal defects, and exposure to teratogens. Intrauterine viral infection (TORCH) is suspected and screened for in all SGA infants when another cause has not been clearly identified. Many of these infections are clinically silent in the neonatal period, but are likely to compromise infant growth and development, and also are transmissible to health care personnel.

Previous follow-up studies have demonstrated an increased risk of developmental disabilities among SGA infants, particularly those with microcephaly, intrauterine viral infection, perinatal asphyxia, symptomatic hypoglycemia, the polycythemia-hyperviscosity syndrome, chromosomal abnormality, or teratogenic exposure. These developmental abnormalities encompass a wide spectrum of severity, from mild learning disorders and slight vision or hearing deficits to severe mental retardation and spastic diplegia. Follow-up evaluation and surveillance is arranged in accordance with the likelihood of developmental disability in each individual infant, as predicted by the coexistence of other neonatal problems. Comprehensive developmental follow-up evaluation and care of the high-risk SGA infant is currently provided in our Low-Birth-Weight Clinic at Children's Medical Center of Dallas.

SUGGESTED READING

Campbell S, Dewhurst CJ. Diagnosis of small-for-dates fetus by serial ultrasonic cephalometry. Lancet 1971; 2:1002.

Crane JP, Kopta MM. Prediction of intrauterine growth retardation via ultrasonically measured head/abdominal circumference ratio. Obstet Gynecol 1979; 54:597.

Fitzhardinge P, Steven E. The small-for-date infant. II. Neurological and intellectual sequellae. Pediatrics 1972; 50:50.

Fleischer A, et al. Umbilical arterial velocity waveforms and intrauterine growth retardation. Am J Obstet Gynecol 1985; 151:502.

Lilieu LD, et al. Treatment of neonatal hypoglycemia with minibolus and intravenous glucose infusion. J Pediatr 1980; 97:295.

Lockwood CJ, Weiner S. Assessment of fetal growth. Clin Perinatol 1986; 13:3.

Vintzileos AM, et al. Value of fetal ponderal index in predicting growth retardation. Obstet Gynecol 1986; 67:584.

Wladimiroff J, et al. Cerebral and umbilical arterial blood flow velocity waveforms in normal and growth retarded pregnancies. Obstet Gynecol 1987; 69:705.

INTRAVENTRICULAR HEMORRHAGE

THOMAS HEGYI, M.D.

Modern perinatal care has greatly improved the outcome for small preterm infants and led to a 75 to 85 percent survival rate in infants with birth weights less than 1,500 g. However, 40 to 50 percent of preterm newborns born before 35 weeks of gestation suffer from germinal matrix hemorrhage (GMH) and/or intraventricular hemorrhage (IVH), recognized by computer tomographic (CT) scanning or neurosonography. The clinical manifestations can vary from a dramatic neurologic deterioration to an extremely subtle, perhaps even silent presentation. Moderate to large IVH has been associated with increased mortality, in addition to the development of posthemorrhagic hydrocephalus (PHH) among the survivors.

DIAGNOSIS AND MONITORING

Before the advent of routine screening with CT scans or ultrasonography, the clinical diagnosis of IVH was based on symptoms. These manifestations include hypotension, acute anemia, metabolic acidosis, full fontanelle, and altered sensorium, as well as apnea and bradycardia, all of which together demonstrate high sensitivity in the diagnosis of a large hemorrhage. Seizure activity during the first days of life is often an accompanying event. The careful observer can successfully identify subtle neurologic abnormalities, such as impaired visual tracking, abnormal popliteal angle, and roving eye movements. However, as demonstrated by the routine scanning of the past 10 years, most cases of IVH are asymptomatic, so that the diagnosis can no longer be based on clinical manifestations. The prevalence of IVH in different populations of very-low-birth-weight infants has been consistently documented to range between 30 and 60 percent by CT, and between 36 and 90 percent by ultrasound examination.

The widespread use of routine ultrasound scanning in intensive care nurseries has yielded various grading systems, causing some confusion in the comparison of experiences among different clinical services. More important, the interobserver variability and the validation of the ultrasonographic reading with a postmortem evaluation have not received the necessary emphasis. False-negative findings can be caused by small germinal matrix hemorrhages and occipital and frontal parenchymal hemorrhages, and false-positive evaluations can be derived from a large choroid plexus or from parenchymal echoes without infarction or hemorrhage that are interpreted as IVH.

In a recent preliminary trial we tested the interobserver reliability of ultrasound readings and concluded that both observation of abnormalities and interpretation of hemorrhage vary, the diagnosis of germinal matrix hemorrhage being particularly difficult. Agreement on specific abnormalities on individual films was lower than that for the final diagnosis, usually based on the review of a series of films. Autopsy validation revealed that the ultrasonographic diagnosis of hemorrhage was usually correct; however, early ultrasound scans tended to miss lesions found at the postmortem examination. Intraparenchymal echodensities (IPE) did not yield such consistent results and represented a variety of findings. During the first day, they rarely represented a focal infarctive or hemorrhagic lesion; by 1 week they usually represented parenchymal infarction, sometimes associated with extension of the ventricular hemorrhage. At no time were these lesions specific for hemorrhage or infarction.

In spite of the limitations of the CT and ultrasound scans, routine evaluation of intracranial state is warranted in all infants weighing less than 1,500 g and in selected infants over this weight. Early CT studies yielded a grading system, first proposed by Papile and coworkers: Grade 0, no GMH or IVH; Grade I, blood in the periventricular germinal matrix regions, or GMH; Grade II, blood within the lateral ventricular system without ventricular dilatation; Grade III, blood within and distending the lateral ventricles; and Grade IV, blood within the ventricular system accompanied by parenchymal extension. Although this system has not been adopted by all, it has served a useful clinical role in the classification of hemorrhages. Our recent autopsy validation studies, however, have identified a flaw in this grading system: clear differences between Grades III and IV hemorrhages are often not present.

Expense, radiation exposure, availability, and distance from the intensive care nursery has limited the usefulness of CT scanning as a general screening procedure. Newer ultrasound technology, providing clearer visualization of intracranial anatomy, has replaced CT for routine scanning. With a transfontanelle approach, coronal and sagittal views, defined by anatomic landmarks, are obtained at specific periods during the first week of life. In our center the scans are taken at postnatal ages of 1, 3, and 7 days; they are repeated at weekly intervals in infants diagnosed to have IVH, until the ventricular size remains unchanged for 2 consecutive weeks. Scans are repeated less often thereafter, until the ventricular size becomes normal or remains unchanged. The hemorrhages are graded according to a modification of the classification of Papile, and any Grade IV ultrasonographic diagnosis is usually confirmed by CT scanning. Among infants without IVH, routine scans are repeated less frequently, but are readily obtained for specific clinical indications.

RISK FACTORS AND PATHOGENESIS

Hypotheses regarding the pathogenesis of intraventricular hemorrhage have been obtained from pathologic data and clinical studies focusing on the identification of risk factors associated with hemorrhage. The two most important factors associated with this disorder are prematurity and the respiratory distress syndrome. Table 1 lists established risk factors for IVH. The importance of maturation in the development of hemorrhages is documented by the inverse relationship between incidence and gesta-

TABLE 1 Established Risk Factors for Intraventricular Hemorrhage

Birth weight
Gestational age
Birth asphyxia
   Low Apgar scores
   Resuscitation
Respiratory problems
   Respiratory distress syndrome
   Pneumothorax
   Apnea
   Patent ductus arteriosus
Therapy
   Mechanical ventilation
   Continuous positive airway pressure
   Bicarbonate infusion
   Volume expansion
Miscellaneous
   Hypotension
   Hypothermia
   Outborn state

tional age. Possible diagnoses derived from this observation include poor vascular support of the germinal matrix, tenuous integrity of the periventricular capillary network, altered coagulation status, and the presence of a pressure-passive cerebral circulation existing at the mercy of the fluctuations of systemic arterial pressure.

Respiratory distress accompanied by perturbations in oxygenation and metabolic state, and by the stresses of modern therapeutic interventions, is the other consistent factor associated with IVH. Hypoxia, hypercarbia, acidosis, increased intrathoracic pressure, and blood pressure changes can influence cerebral blood flow and result in ischemia, hemorrhage, or both. The use of hypertonic infusions, hypertensive agents, and antiprostaglandin medication can further compromise cerebral perfusion.

Preterm infants suffering from the respiratory distress syndrome often reveal other factors that predispose to hemorrhage. Perinatal asphyxia can result in hypertension, hypercarbia, hypoxia, and acidosis, with the resultant changes in systemic pressure transmitted to the cerebral blood flow, where a tenuous capillary system is easily overwhelmed. Increased fibrinolytic activity in the periventricular area can transform a collection of ruptured capillaries into a major hemorrhage. Other conditions contributing to risk status include patent ductus arteriosus, apnea, pneumothorax, hyperosmolality, and dehydration.

PREVENTION

Elimination of the two most important predisposing factors is the best way to prevent intraventricular hemorrhage. Although early eradication of prematurity is not to be expected, efforts at eliminating or, more likely, reducing the incidence of the respiratory distress syndrome may be successful. The use of tocolytic agents, combined with prenatal steroid therapy, has already resulted in a reduced incidence of this syndrome in select populations. The postnatal instillation of exogenous surfactant holds promise for further reducing the prevalence of this disorder.

Management of labor and delivery constitutes an area of controversy in the prevention of hemorrhage. The ad-

vantages of cesarean section over vaginal delivery have been suggested, but the lack of conclusive data precludes the adoption of rigid policies for the delivery of preterm infants. Obstetric management should be aimed at delivering the high-risk infant in an optimal condition by the best possible route, preventing trauma and asphyxia. After delivery, nursery routines must emphasize limited handling and limited interventions that are associated with abrupt changes in blood pressure and oxygenation status. Pharmacologic agents influencing blood pressure and serum osmolality should be carefully used and noxious procedures limited. Maintenance of normal oxygen and stable carbon dioxide and pH status, and ventilatory procedures emphasizing low airway pressure, can contribute to the protection of the infant. Complications of intensive care, such as hypotension, pneumothorax, or overhydration, should be rapidly recognized and treated.

In spite of well-defined guidelines for optimal care, the management alternatives available to clinicians are often limited. Other preventive efforts have focused on the use of pharmacologic agents and their ability to prevent cerebral hemodynamic perturbations. Monitoring cerebral blood flow with Doppler ultrasonography, and quantitating observations of cerebral blood flow velocity by the pulsatility index, led Perlman and coworkers to identify a specific, fluctuating pattern in Doppler tracings that they associated with the development of hemorrhage. Paralysis induced by pancuronium administration eliminated the fluctuating pattern and may have afforded some protection against IVH among treated infants. Although this was useful in demonstrating that manipulations of cerebral blood flow may affect the clinical status, further studies of this mode of therapy are required before it can be recommended.

Among other pharmacologic agents, the drug that has been most closely scrutinized is phenobarbital. This agent has been shown in several investigations to have protective effects, its potential benefit supported by data that acute elevations in systemic blood pressure were controlled by phenobarbital's sedative effects (Table 2). These results, however, are not yet confirmed. Recent studies of the capillary stabilizing drug ethamsylate report a reduction in incidence of IVH by approximately 50 percent, the effect being limited to the less severe hemorrhages, with little effect on intraventricular hemorrhage with ventricular dilatation or with parenchymal involvement. Correction of hemostatic disturbances may also have a role in prophylaxis, and supplemental vitamin E administration studied in several centers has demonstrated some beneficial effects.

TABLE 2 Neuroprotective Effects of Phenobarbital: Proposed Mechanisms

Decreased cerebral metabolic rate
Decreased catecholamine release
Free radical inactivation
Decreased intracellular and extracellular edema
Decreased intracranial pressure
Anticonvulsant effect
Sedative effect

However, in spite of the apparent success of these various drugs in reducing the incidence and severity of IVH, no agent has been clearly shown to be effective in preventing hemorrhage, and the use of drug therapy must still be controlled by strict criteria.

MANAGEMENT

After the diagnosis of IVH, the management protocol must focus on three important areas: (1) maintenance of cerebral perfusion, (2) treatment of associated clinical symptoms that can potentially exacerbate the primary condition, and (3) surveillance for the development of posthemorrhagic hydrocephalus.

Cerebral perfusion is at risk of compromise in the unstable, sick, preterm infant. Utilizing the positron emission tomography scanner, Volpe demonstrated areas of ischemic involvement far more extensive than that of the hemorrhage itself. The pressure-passive cerebral circulation must therefore be protected against abrupt changes in blood pressure.

Associated clinical symptoms reflecting disturbed homeostasis must be recognized early and rectified in order to prevent the additional risk to the infant created by conditions that further compromise cerebral perfusion, or damage the integrity of the cerebral capillary network. Systemic hypotension due to anemia, acidosis, or hypovolemia exacerbate the ischemic insult, and hypertension caused by aggressive bicarbonate and pressor therapy, or overhydration, can increase cerebral blood flow and cause additional bleeding. Hyperkalemia, hyperglycemia, and hyperbilirubinemia often follow the hemorrhagic event and have the capacity to further endanger the infant. Apnea is a common clinical problem in infants with IVH, and although a cause-and-effect relationship has not yet been demonstrated, apnea may be a manifestation of the hemorrhage itself. Respiratory neurons are influenced by the maturity and functional state of the rest of the central nervous system, an equilibrium potentially disturbed by an untoward intracranial event. Although this latter hypothesis is as yet unproved, a common clinical observation is prolonged respiratory dependence.

Monitoring for the development of posthemorrhagic hydrocephalus is mandatory in all infants with IVH. We perform bedside cranial ultrasonography approximately twice a week after the diagnosis. The subsequent frequency of examinations is determined by the rate of change of ventricular size, with routine examinations once a week until it remains unchanged for 2 weeks. Ultrasonographic findings are accompanied by daily clinical evaluation for signs of increased intracranial pressure. Intracranial pressure can also be checked by a noninvasive monitor, which can provide further information on the evolution of pressure-related phenomena, but is not useful in the presence of low-pressure hydrocephalus.

POSTHEMORRHAGIC HYDROCEPHALUS

Posthemorrhagic hydrocephalus is a common sequel to moderate or severe intraventricular hemorrhage. One center reported an incidence of 15 to 25 percent after moderate, and 65 to 100 percent after severe, hemorrhage. The cause of hydrocephalus in these infants is usually an obliterative arachnoiditis, due to collection of blood products in the posterior fossa. This process obstructs the flow of cerebrospinal fluid (CSF) either out of the fourth ventricle or through the tentorial notch. Experimental and clinical observations indicate that progressive ventricular dilatation can cause brain injury (Table 3). Ventricular dilatation and increased intracranial pressure usually occur between 2 and 3 weeks of age, with early changes beginning slowly and usually under low pressure. The change in ventricular size is not always progressive, a phenomenon that has confounded early studies dealing with prevention or treatment. In approximately one-half of the infants, ventricular dilatation arrests without intervention.

Several methods have been attempted to prevent hydrocephalus following hemorrhage. These have included methods to decrease CSF production, and intermittent drainage procedures such as serial lumbar punctures, to decrease intracranial pressure and remove blood products. Several investigators have attempted to prevent hydrocephalus or delay the insertion of a shunt with medications. Bergman and associates used high doses of acetazolamide and furosemide with success. Carbonic anhydrase is important in the development of myelin, and high doses of acetazolamide, a carbonic anhydrase inhibitor, may have long-term toxic effects. Volpe used glycerol and Lorber and associates used isosorbide, with positive results. Glycerol and sorbitol are both osmotic agents with side effects that include vomiting, diarrhea, weight loss, dehydration, azotemia, hypernatremia, and acidosis. These drugs have not yet been studied in prospective, controlled trials. Select studies have demonstrated that intermittent lumbar punctures can be effective in eliminating the need for shunting. However, these findings have not been easily replicated, so that this approach remains controversial.

Progressive hydrocephalus mandates close monitoring with frequent ultrasound examinations and medical-surgical intervention. It is unclear why hydrocephalus progresses in some infants yet regresses in others. Perhaps if the process is slowly evolving, alternative pathways for CSF absorption can compensate and the hydrocephalus may be arrested. Mechanical removal of CSF by repeated spinal taps may give these infants more time to compensate and can alter the pressure-volume curve of the ventricles, so that CSF absorption may be improved. These processes seem to differ in individual infants, and some patients may benefit from the use of spinal taps. Daily lumbar punctures provide a simple mechanism for relief of increasing intracranial pressure and may prevent further

TABLE 3 Mechanism of Brain Injury in Intraventricular Hemorrhage

Preceding hypoxic-ischemic insult
Intracranial hypertension and impaired cerebral perfusion
Destruction of periventricular white matter
Destruction of germinal matrix (and glial precursors)
Focal brain ischemia secondary to vasospasm
Posthemorrhagic hydrocephalus

surgical therapy. CSF is drained in amounts ranging from 5 to 20 ml, or until flow stops. Lumbar punctures are performed every other day, or less often if the amount of CSF removed at each tap is less than 3 ml. If successful, lumbar punctures are continued until the ventricular size decreases or remains unchanged for 2 consecutive weeks. Failure is defined as a progressive increase in ventricular size, as measured by neurosonography, in association either with signs of increased intracranial pressure or with an increase in head circumference of more than 2 cm per week for at least 2 weeks. The following signs indicate increased intracranial pressure if no other abnormalities are present: episodes of apnea and bradycardia, feeding difficulties with regurgitation and vomiting, change in sensorium with lethargy, change in muscle tone, seizures and a bulging, and a tense fontanelle associated with split sutures.

Among infants not responding to therapy with serial spinal puncture, or when technical failures preclude obtaining fluid, the administration of medications to reduce CSF production may be helpful (Table 4). The timing, dosage, and efficacy of these drugs still need to be further clarified; therefore, routine use should be limited to experimental protocols. Moreover, in the face of rapidly progressive hydrocephalus, these drugs often do not have time to work.

Progressive hydrocephalus is treated with a ventriculoperitoneal (VP) shunt, if the ventricular fluid is clear and the infant weighs close to 2,000 g. In infants who are unfit for a VP shunt, a subcutaneous ventricular catheter reservoir can be inserted for intermittent drainage of ventricular fluid until they are ready for a shunt. Alternative therapies have consisted of repeated ventricular punctures

TABLE 4 Management of Progressive Posthemorrhagic Hydrocephalus

Serial lumbar punctures
Medications to reduce production of CSF
  ATP-ase inhibitors—digoxin
  Carbonic anhydrase inhibitors—acetazolamide, furosemide
  Osmotic agents—glycerol, isosorbide
External ventriculostomy
Internal ventricular drainage
  Subcutaneous ventricular reservoir
  Ventriculoperitoneal shunt

and external ventricular drainage. Repeated ventricular taps may further damage brain parenchyma, and cerebral cavitation has been described following needle puncture of the lateral ventricles. Although favorable results have been reported from an external ventricular drain, infection can be a common complication.

Subcutaneous ventricular catheter reservoir placement is a relatively safe procedure that is very effective in controlling the hydrocephalic process. The reservoir is punctured daily and cerebrospinal fluid removed. The frequency of the taps is controlled by clinical signs of increased intracranial pressure and by ventricular size, as monitored by frequent ultrasound examinations. Dependence on daily taps to control ventricular size warrants the insertion of a shunt; if the size of the ventricle remains stable without any tapping for 1 to 2 weeks, the infant can be discharged with the reservoir in place and followed with serial neurosonograms, in the attempt to obviate permanent shunting.

LARYNGOTRACHEAL STENOSIS

JAMES A. STANKIEWICZ, M.D.

Laryngotracheal stenosis can pose a very difficult treatment problem. It is the purpose of this presentation to inform the practitioner about the various aspects of this disorder, moving step by step from the initial evaluation through treatment.

DEFINITION

Laryngotracheal stenosis can be divided into two distinct areas: (1) congenital and (2) acquired. The components of stenosis are fibrous scar, cartilaginous scar, or a combination of both. Usually, stenosis occurs in the smallest areas of the airway: the cricoid cartilage ring and the laryngeal inlet; these are especially susceptible to acquired injury.

Congenital Laryngotracheal Stenosis

Congenital laryngeal stenosis is very rare. A congenital web, however, can act as a stenosis and obstruct the airway. Congenital subglottic webs and stenosis have been reported along with tracheal webs, stenosis, and rarely stenosis with a tracheoesophageal fistula.

At birth the normal infant larynx is about one-third the size of the adult larynx. The glottis measures 7 mm in the sagittal (anteroposterior) plane and 4 mm in the coronal (width) plane, with the vocal cords 6 to 8 mm in length. The premature child has an even smaller larynx. The normal subglottic diameter is 3.5 mm from birth to 3 months of age, and 4.0 mm at 3 to 9 months (Fig. 1). However, the premature subglottis can be as small as 2.5 to 3.0 mm. These diameters are borderline for airway patency, and it can be readily appreciated how the slightest edema may precipitate respiratory distress: 1 mm edema causes a 60 percent or greater decrease in the airway. Newborn airway sizes less than 3.0 to 3.5 mm (cricoid-subglottic) have some degree of associated subglottic stenosis.

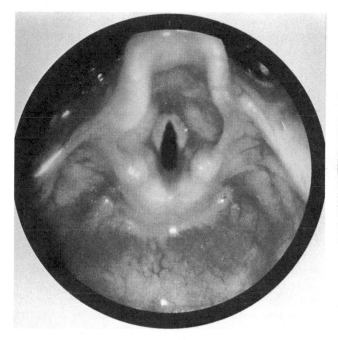

Figure 1 A normal 6-month-old glottis. (Courtesy of Oxford Medical Publications.)

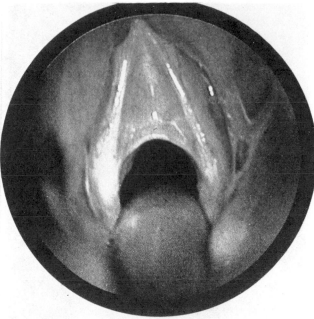

Figure 2 Laryngeal web with the endotracheal tube in place. (Courtesy of Oxford Medical Publications.)

The clinical symptoms associated with congenital stenosis include (1) respiratory obstruction, (2) stridor, (3) weakened or absent cry, (4) dyspnea, (5) tachypnea, (6) aspiration, and (7) sudden death. Stridor is usually inspiratory. As the obstruction moves toward the carina, an expiratory component may be noted as well.

A laryngeal web is a membrane of varying thickness that partially occludes the lumen. While a small web may cause only slight voice change, the degree of respiratory distress depends on the lumen. A small web in a premature child may cause respiratory distress, whereas in a newborn it may cause voice change alone. Seventy-five percent of webs are glottic at the level of the vocal cords. Most webs are anterior in position and are thick and fibrous, with some element of subglottic extension (Fig. 2). The birth of a child with an obstructing web is a true emergency, and emergency intubation is required. Thin webs may be penetrated easily with an endotracheal tube or a bronchoscope. Thick webs may present a situation in which tracheotomy is necessary because of inability to pass an endotracheal tube; fortunately, these are very rare. After an airway is established, the remainder of the web can be removed endoscopically with microsurgery involving microinstruments, the CO_2 laser, or both. Follow-up laryngoscopy-bronchoscopy with dilatation of the larynx may be required. A thick web may not be amenable to microsurgery and may require tracheotomy and an external laryngeal approach through the thyroid cartilage (thyrotomy), lysis of the web, and implantation with a stent (keel) to keep the web from regrowing. The stent is removed in 4 to 6 weeks.

Laryngeal atresia represents a complete failure during embryogenesis to form a laryngeal lumen. Fortunately, only a handful of cases have been reported. If this can be recognized at birth (no respiratory effort is seen), tracheotomy is the treatment. A concomitant tracheoesophageal fistula is noted on occasion, which will maintain an airway until a tracheotomy can be performed.

A web can also form in the subglottis and may be appreciated as a subglottic stenosis or a cricoid cartilage deformity. The webs are usually positioned anteriorly and may have a pinpoint opening posteriorly. If respiratory distress is present, the web requires surgical division. Endoscopic division with a bronchoscope and CO_2 laser may work well. If this is unsuccessful, an open procedure with a stent or keel is required with tracheotomy; this is very rarely necessary.

Congenital subglottic stenosis has been defined as a lumen in the normal neonate less than 3.5 mm in diameter without a history of trauma or intubation. Histologically, the stenosis reveals a soft tissue thickening of the subglottis with thickening of the true vocal cords (Figs. 3 and 4).

Patients with a marginal airway sometimes present in the first 6 months of life with a history of recurrent upper respiratory infections and increasing respiratory distress. The cricoid cartilage as a complete ring prevents outward expansion, allowing edema to occur internally, usually about 2 to 3 mm below the true vocal cords. Radiographic evaluation using lateral neck and anteroposterior chest views often shows the narrowing in a child without distress. Diagnosis is confirmed by direct laryngoscopy and bronchoscopy.

Treatment in 40 percent of cases involves tracheotomy and observation; the latter alone is necessary for the other 60 percent. The larynx and trachea will grow, and most children can have the tracheotomy tube removed within 24 to 36 months. It must be kept in mind that 15 to 20 percent of these children will have other associated con-

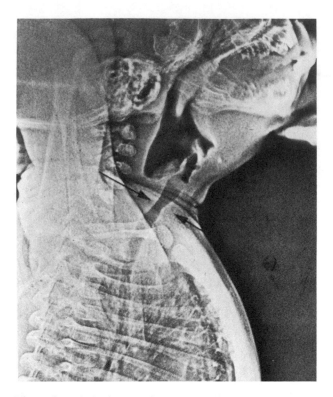

Figure 3 Subglottic stenosis (*arrows*): 8-week-old xerogram. (Courtesy of Oxford Medical Publications.)

genital lesions and syndromes. Upper respiratory infections and recurrent croup need to be treated aggressively in a patient without tracheotomy in order to avoid intubation.

Tracheal constrictions are divided into fibrous strictures and absence or deformity of tracheal cartilages; all of these are very rarely encountered in clinical practice.

Tracheal webs can occur and are usually thin and fibrous. The underlying cartilage is usually normal. The thickness and aperture of the web can vary. Usually, simple dilatation or web rupture is sufficient. Repeated dilatations or CO_2 laser bronchoscopy (in older children) may be necessary.

Tracheal stenosis can occur anywhere in the trachea. These stenoses are usually thicker, with greater depth than a simple web. Diagnosis is made with bronchoscopy, but radiography can help identify the problem and locate the narrowing. Treatment usually involves multiple careful dilatations by means of bronchoscopy. If dilatation is unsuccessful, an endotracheal tube or tracheotomy may be necessary. A short segment stenosis may be primarily resected and an end-to-end reanastomosis performed.

Stenosis associated with a tracheoesophageal fistula has been noted. This is usually found postoperatively and may be related to surgical correction.

Two cases of congenitally narrowed trachea have been seen. The whole of the trachea is involved. The children presented with recurrent pneumonia and crouplike illness. The pneumonias were secondary to an inability to cough out secretions owing to the narrowed trachea. Diagnosis was made by chest x-ray study and bronchoscopy. Treatment is expectant. One child died because of multiple congenital complications. The other, who has trisomy 21, has done well with growth and his infections have disappeared.

Tracheomalacia can occur independent of laryngomalacia or may be associated with it. This can create an apparent stenosis. The problem occurs because weakened tracheal cartilages do not properly support the airway. With respiration, a markedly exaggerated mobility or flaccidity of the posterior membranous tracheal wall occurs, which can occlude the lumen. The child presents with cough and inspiratory-expiratory stridor, which is high-pitched and almost reminiscent of asthmatic wheezing. Although this may be noted at birth, it may also be seen in the older child. Rarely, a tracheotomy is necessary and the problem usually disappears with growth by 12 to 18 months. Aggressive treatment of respiratory infections is necessary, and the environment (e.g., the humidity) has to be controlled, particularly in colder winter climates.

Although vascular anomalies will not be discussed at length, a few comments are appropriate. Vascular rings or innominate artery compression create a segment of weakened cartilage (tracheomalacia) that remains after correction and can account for persistent symptoms such as barking coughs, mild respiratory distress, and stridor. With growth, this segment strengthens and problems eventually disappear.

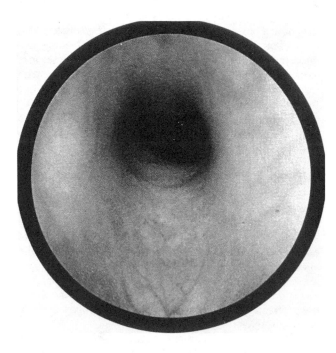

Figure 4 Subglottic stenosis, 2.5-mm opening. (Courtesy of Oxford Medical Publications.)

Acquired Laryngotracheal Stenosis

Acquired laryngotracheal stenosis in neonates is most commonly related to the trauma of prolonged endotracheal intubation (Fig. 5). Rigorous guidelines have been developed regarding the size of endotracheal tubes in premature infants, and it is known that these children tolerate prolonged intubation for 3 to 4 months very well. This is because the larynges are very compliant and the amount of movement the child makes is minimal. When the child is old enough (4 to 5 months after birth in the premature child, 2 to 3 months in the normal neonate) to use his hands, turn his head, and chew or suck on the endotracheal tube, trauma occurs in the airway and acquired stenosis can result. Thus, appropriate tube size for the premature and newborn child, and timing of extubation or tracheotomy, are necessary to avoid subglottic stenosis. Children who are intubated because of infectious disease such as croup are also likely to develop stenosis. Once a child is intubated for croup, the endotracheal tube is usually required for 7 to 8 days. With the subglottic area already compromised because of infection, further irritation from the tube can lead to stenosis (Fig. 6). For infants with croup who require intubation (5 to 10 percent of all cases of croup), it is paramount that an endotracheal tube one to two sizes smaller than normal be used, and extubation attempted as soon as possible. Appropriate sedation to minimize activity is extremely important.

In bronchopulmonary dysplasia (BPD), if a child is intubated for 2 to 3 months and further ventilator support is necessary, a tracheotomy should be placed sooner rather

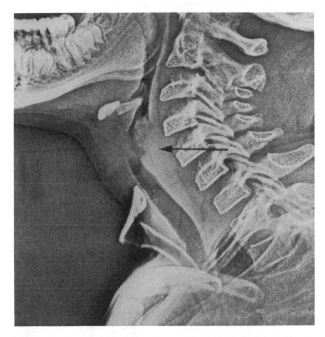

Figure 6 Acquired subglottic stenosis following intubation in croup seen on the xerogram. Posterior glottic stenosis (*arrow*) is apparent. (Courtesy of Oxford Medical Publications.)

than later. Recently a premature child who was intubated for 5 months with BPD underwent tracheotomy; this had been requested 6 weeks earlier, but the parents refused. At the time of surgery, bronchoscopy revealed a marked ulceration with granulation at the level of the cricoid cartilage. Follow-up bronchoscopy showed marked subglottic stenosis. More than 50 tracheotomies have been performed for BPD over the past 7 years, and this was the first child to demonstrate such a finding. Because of the child's activity and age, it was predicted before surgery that there would be complications.

Two types of stenosis are apparent: hard and soft. Hard stenosis is made up of firm cicatricial scar or distorted or weakened cartilage. Soft stenosis is related to the reparative process after trauma, and histologically shows granulation tissue, submucosal fibrosis, and gland hyperplasia. This may be compared with congenital stenosis in which a submucosal fibrosis is noted or an anatomically small cricoid ring is apparent. Soft stenosis, if not removed or treated, may develop into hard stenosis. Treatment depends on the stage at which the stenosis is encountered.

The premature or newborn child who is intubated because of respiratory distress reaches a point where extubation is attempted. Most children, if cared for appropriately and intubated with the proper-sized tube, will be extubated without problem. Some children fail extubation because soft stenosis, in the form of tissue edema, develops in the subglottis. In the past these patients required a tracheotomy. However, if, during bronchoscopy, edema is apparent with minimal mucosal ulceration and granu-

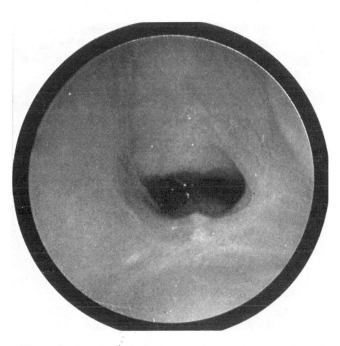

Figure 5 Acquired subglottic stenosis secondary to prolonged intubation. (Courtesy of Oxford Medical Publications.)

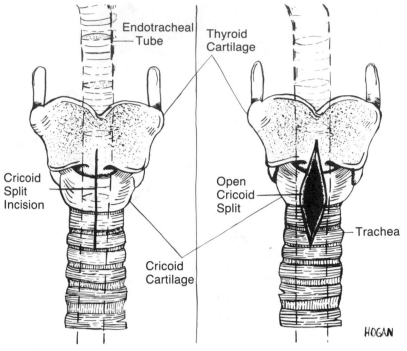

HOGAN

Figure 7 The incision line, illustrating how the cricoid decompresses after it is split.

lation, these children respond to a splitting of the cricoid cartilage, with continued intubation for 1 week and extubation (Fig. 7). The philosophy is to decompress the subglottis and trachea by releasing the cricoid and first two tracheal rings. This allows for resolution of edema and expansion by at least 1 mm of the airway. Twelve cricoid splits have been performed and 11 patients have been extubated. Patients with multiple problems requiring numerous operations after extubation probably should undergo a tracheotomy rather than a cricoid split. However, two of my 11 patients in whom the cricoid was successfully split have undergone one or two surgical procedures requiring intubation uneventfully. The importance of appropriate endotracheal tube size in the neonate is indicated by the fact that only one cricoid split has been performed in the past 2 years. Ten of 11 such procedures that were performed in the 2 years before that were related to an overzealous attending physician who was using an oversized endotracheal tube.

The child who develops subglottic tracheal stenosis requiring a tracheotomy to maintain the airway presents a difficult management problem. Dilatation is not very successful in dealing with acquired stenosis. Adjunctive injection of a depot steroid such as triamcinolone acetonide (Kenalog) into the stenosis may offer some benefit. CO_2 laser microlaryngoscopy-bronchoscopy to treat stenosis can be helpful if the stenosis is limited and not circumferential, smaller than 1 cm, and fibrous (not cartilaginous) and has not been tampered with by previous surgery. Only one area at a time is treated and multiple procedures may be necessary. Children who fail endoscopic therapies require an open procedure, after reaching at least 1 year of age.

Open laryngotracheal procedures involve conservative excision of the stenosis, with placement of an autogenous bone or cartilage graft into the open segment. Depending on the degree and extent of stenosis, additional procedures such as a posterior splitting of the cricoid cartilage for total stenosis may be beneficial. Although the use of stents is controversial, they are employed for severe stenosis. Figure 8 shows a procedure for correction of moderate subglottic stenosis utilizing rib cartilage. Figure 9 shows the correction for severe stenosis using

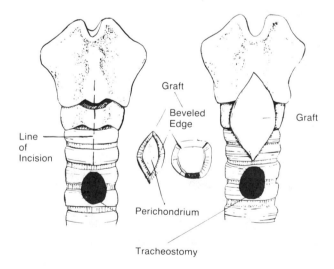

Figure 8 Insertion of sculpted rib cartilage into the tracheal lumen. The middle section shows how the graft looks on horizontal section.

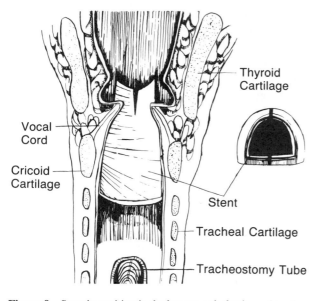

Vocal
Cord

Cricoid
Cartilage

Thyroid
Cartilage

Stent

Tracheal Cartilage

Tracheostomy Tube

Figure 9 Stent in position in the larynx, subglottis, and trachea. The stent is often contiguous with the tracheotomy tube.

a stent and a posterior cricoid splitting incision. Laryngeal stenosis is corrected in the same fashion if endoscopy is unsuccessful. Severe laryngeal stenosis almost always has a subglottic component.

The stent is left in place for 6 to 8 weeks postoperatively. Follow-up laryngoscopy is necessary to control granulation tissue and recurrent stenosis. Most airways stabilize by 6 to 12 months and decannulation can then proceed. Speech therapy is very important to help prelingual and early lingual tracheotomized children develop appropriate speech patterns. All children with tracheotomies are cared for at home after the parents have undergone rigorous training in tracheotomy care and cardiopulmonary resuscitation. Children who fail open procedures require surgical revision; some children need long-term tracheotomy.

Acknowledgment. The author would like to thank Mrs. Joan Findlay for her assistance in the preparation of this manuscript. Figures 1 to 6 are reproduced by permission of Oxford Medical Publications, London, from Benjamin B. Atlas of paediatric endoscopy, 1981.

MAPLE SYRUP URINE DISEASE

JOSEPH DANCIS, M.D.
SELMA E. SNYDERMAN, M.D.

Maple syrup urine disease is a rare autosomal recessive disease involving three essential amino acids—leucine, isoleucine, and valine—which share a common branched-chain structure. The biochemical defect interrupts the degradative pathway so that the branched-chain amino acids (BCAAs) and their keto acids (BCKAs) are elevated. The clinical onset is much more acute and violent than that of the analogous aminoacidopathy, phenylketonuria, probably because of the extreme toxicity of the branched-chain keto acids.

RATIONALE OF TREATMENT

Treatment is directed toward (1) control of intake of the BCAAs, and (2) removal of excesses of the BCAAs and BCKAs.

Control of Intake of the BCAAs

Protein foods have high concentrations of the BCAAs. Furthermore, there is no simple way of removing these from food. It is therefore necessary to use synthetic diets

prepared from amino acids. Amino acid mixtures lacking the BCAAs have been specially prepared for patients with maple syrup urine disease and are commercially available as MSUD diet powder (Mead Johnson), analog MSUD (Scientific Hospital Supplies, distributed by Ross) and MSUD, (Milupa distributed by Mead Johnson). The first two are complete in that other essential dietary constituents have been added, such as fats, carbohydrates, vitamins, and minerals. The latter formulation requires the addition of fats and carbohydrates. The BCAAs are added to both formulations in amounts that are just sufficient for maintenance and growth, avoiding the excesses that require degradation. Neither is complete in that arrest of growth follows prolonged exclusive use. There must be unknown factors that are essential for the growth of the infant that are found in milk and other natural foods. For this reason, milk is added to the diet after the infant has been stabilized on the artificial diet, generally at about 1 month of age. The amount of milk that is offered is limited to that which meets the requirement for leucine. The concentration of leucine in milk is much higher than that of isoleucine or valine. Most of the nitrogen requirement must still be met with MSUD formula.

The appropriate diet must be determined for each infant. Each BCAA must be titrated individually, avoiding excesses or deficiencies. As a rough index, the daily requirements for maintenance and growth in the newborn period are leucine 110, isoleucine 80, and valine 85 mg per kilogram. These values decrease rapidly during the first months of life. Frequent monitoring of the plasma amino acid concentrations is required for fine adjustments.

It is important to realize that elevations in plasma BCAAs may be a consequence of dietary deficiency as well as excess. Inadequate intake of an essential amino acid over a period of several days causes tissue breakdown, which releases large amounts of the BCAAs. A generalized hyperaminoacidemia commonly results.

Removal of Excesses

Measures for removing excess BCAAs include (1) a diet free of BCAAs, (2) intravenous fluids, and (3) peritoneal dialysis.

Diet Free of BCAAs. Metabolic disposal and urinary excretion of minor excesses may be enough in the relatively asymptomatic child. It is rare for the neonate to be asymptomatic.

Intravenous Fluids. The more severely decompensated infant is commonly unable to retain food, is dehydrated and acidotic, and has reduced renal flow. Symptomatic correction with intravenous fluids containing glucose and alkali may make a dietary approach possible.

Peritoneal Dialysis. The severely decompensated infant has large excesses of BCAAs and BCKAs in all body fluids. The most efficient way to remove these excesses and relieve associated symptoms is by aggressive peritoneal dialysis. Tissue BCAAs and BCKAs equilibrate rapidly across the peritoneum.

CLINICAL APPLICATION

Antepartum Diagnosis

Consistent identification of the heterozygote has not been possible. Antepartum diagnosis is therefore limited to families in which a child with maple syrup urine disease has been born. In such cases, we recommend the following:

1. Amniocentesis at 16 weeks' gestation.
2. Amnionic cells are grown in tissue culture. Analysis of amniotic fluid is not useful for diagnosis.
3. Assay of cells for BCKA decarboxylase. The assays are available at select medical centers. Diagnosis of the homozygote can be made with great accuracy.

In most instances the diagnosis can be made before 20 weeks' gestation, offering the parents the opportunity to decide whether to continue the pregnancy. Chorionic villus biopsy should make diagnosis possible during the first trimester.

Diagnosis at Birth

This is accomplished only when the condition is suspected because the family has had a previous child with maple syrup urine disease. A rapid diagnosis can be made by enzymatic assay of peripheral leukocytes.

Dietary therapy can be instituted immediately. Plasma amino acids are normal at birth, so that accumulations of BCAAs and BCKAs with associated symptoms may be avoided. The following measures are recommended:

1. Intravenous glucose in saline is begun at maintenance levels.
2. A maple syrup urine disease diet with supplementary BCAAs is introduced as soon as oral feedings are tolerated.
3. Plasma amino acids are assayed daily, and the intakes of the individual BCAAs are adjusted.

Diagnosis in the Nursery

Clinical suspicion may be raised if a maple syrup odor is detected in an infant who is doing poorly. Onset of symptoms is within the first week of life, and diagnosis is made by plasma amino acid analysis. In many states routine screening for maple syrup urine disease with a bacterial inhibition assay for plasma leucine is the rule. In theory, the diagnosis can be made by 48 to 72 hours of age. The logistics of central laboratories generally delay the diagnosis until the second week of life.

Treatment

The aggressiveness of treatment is dictated by the magnitude of elevation of the BCAAs and the severity of symptoms. Plasma leucine is regularly the highest of the three BCAAs. The acute symptoms appear to be caused primarily by the keto acid of leucine, α-ketoisocaproic acid. If the diagnosis is delayed until the second week of life, the patient is generally severely ill, with plasma leucine levels exceeding 20 mg per deciliter.

Blood volume and renal flow are restored with intravenous glucose in saline. Alkali is added for severe acidosis, and fluids are continued to maintain renal flow.

Peritoneal dialysis is instituted for the more severely ill patient. The indications are leucine levels over 25 mg per deciliter and/or the appearance of neurologic signs. The procedure should be undertaken only by someone who is experienced in the technique. Commercially available dialysate containing 1.5 percent glucose and electrolytes is instilled into the peritoneal cavity in amounts sufficient to cause abdominal distention without hampering cardiorespiratory function, generally 30 to 50 ml per kilogram. The fluid is exchanged every half hour. In 12 to 14 hours, there is obvious clinical improvement, and the plasma levels of the BCAAs and BCKAs have dropped sharply toward normal. Hemodialysis has been used in other centers.

Caloric intake is maintained with 10 percent glucose and fats, given intravenously, to avoid a negative nitrogen balance.

Oral feeding with a maple syrup urine disease diet lacking BCAAs is begun when the patient can tolerate it. The BCAAs are added as plasma levels return to normal. Supplementation is most easily accomplished with solutions of 10 g per liter water (10 mg per milliliter) of each

BCAA. The valine plasma level generally returns to normal first, so that supplementation with this amino acid is the first to be required. Supplementation with leucine may not be necessary until 7 to 10 days after the initiation of dietary therapy.

The acute response is generally very gratifying. Reversal of neurologic damage may not be possible if the diagnosis has been delayed too long. The best results are obtained in centers experienced in the care of this rare disease. Transfer to such facilities is highly desirable after the infant has been stabilized by intravenous fluids and other symptomatic measures.

MECONIUM ASPIRATION

BONNIE BOYER HUDAK, M.D.
M. DOUGLAS JONES Jr., M.D.

Meconium staining of amniotic fluid occurs frequently, in approximately 10 percent of all deliveries. Since the ability of the gastrointestinal tract to respond with effective peristalsis increases with maturity, meconium staining is encountered rarely in infants of less than 34 weeks' gestation and in as many as 40 percent of post-term infants. Current thinking is that aspiration of meconium may occur in two settings: prenatally, in an asphyxiated infant in whom asphyxia either initiates or contributes to meconium passage and then causes gasping and massive aspiration; and postnatally, when meconium in large airways is aspirated into smaller airways and alveoli in the course of resuscitation and air breathing. In the latter instance the reason for meconium passage is often unclear. It is also not clear whether the initial aspiration of meconium into larger airways is the result of birth asphyxia (in the sense of a pathologic condition), the result of mild, "physiologic" asphyxia that accompanies an apparently normal labor and delivery, or simply the result of normal fetal respiratory movements. There are few experimental data to suggest whether meconium aspiration that results in the severest disease is primarily a prenatal event, a postnatal event, or both. The assumption as to which event is the most common is important because to a large extent it determines how the efficacy of postnatal tracheal suctioning is regarded.

The presence of meconium in the lung causes respiratory distress for at least three reasons. First, it leads to large and small airway obstruction and increased resistance to air flow. Partially or completely obstructed smaller airways also cause atelectasis and hyperinflation. Second, probably due to the bile salts and proteolytic enzymes that it contains, meconium causes a chemical pneumonitis. Third, it is an airway irritant and can cause bronchoconstriction.

About 15 years ago investigators began to report a marked improvement in outcome in infants with meconium-stained amniotic fluid. Mortality was reported to be 0 to 3 percent in contrast to previous figures of 4 to 9 percent. The approach responsible for that change had two elements. The first and perhaps more important was aggressive obstetric management. The second was combined obstetric and pediatric suctioning of the airway at the time of delivery. The separate importance of airway management is difficult to assess for several reasons. First, massive prenatal aspiration of meconium undoubtedly occurs and is unlikely to be ameliorated by airway suctioning at the time of delivery. Second, infants who die following meconium aspiration frequently have a clinical diagnosis of persistent pulmonary hypertension. One study has shown that such infants often have histologic evidence of the same excessive muscularization of small pulmonary arteries that is associated with fatal persistent pulmonary hypertension in other settings. Excessive muscularization would necessarily have to be prenatal in origin. This finding requires confirmation because it suggests that only some, and perhaps very few, fatalities from meconium aspiration are attributable to aspiration and meconium per se. This of course says nothing about meconium aspiration as a cause of morbidity in infants who do not die. Third, suctioning of the trachea has never been separately evaluated in an appropriately designed clinical trial. None of these considerations justifies abandonment of tracheal suctioning, but they speak for prudence in its use. Certainly, suctioning should not be done at the expense of aspects of delivery room management of the asphyxiated infant that are of established usefulness. The implications of this approach for clinical management are mentioned below.

PRENATAL PREDICTORS IN PREGNANCIES WITH MECONIUM-STAINED AMNIOTIC FLUID

Obstetric studies have focused on identifying factors that predict meconium passage and poor fetal outcome. The combination of meconium staining and fetal heart rate abnormalities is associated with increased mortality. Specific heart rate patterns predictive of poor outcome include late decelerations and loss of beat-to-beat variability. *This information mandates continuous fetal heart rate monitoring in the presence of meconium-stained amniotic fluid.* Fetal acidosis can be present even in early labor, and monitoring of fetal scalp pH is a useful adjunct to fetal heart rate monitoring in patients with disturbing heart rate patterns.

The timing and amount of meconium passage influence prognosis. In general, the larger the amount of meconium and the earlier in labor it is passed, the poorer the fetal outcome.

OBSTETRIC MANAGEMENT

The presence of meconium mandates continuous monitoring of fetal heart rate and appropriate medical intervention (Fig. 1). A scalp pH reading is obtained in any infant with moderate to thick meconium in the amniotic fluid if (1) baseline fetal heart rate variability is poor, (2) late decelerations occur, and (3) the heart rate tracing shows evidence of poor fetal reactivity. If the scalp pH is less than 7.20, the fetus is delivered. Upon delivery, the infant's upper airway should be suctioned with a DeLee catheter prior to delivery of the thorax. Suction catheters are more efficient for the retrieval of meconium than bulb syringes. Oral or combined oronasal suctioning is more effective than nasal suctioning alone. Everyone in the delivery room should be aware, however, that *vigorous pharyngeal suctioning occasionally results in bradycardia and laryngospasm.* The significance of the 1-minute Ap-

gar score in a suctioned infant is not necessarily the same as in an infant whose oropharynx has not been manipulated.

PEDIATRIC MANAGEMENT

Delivery Room

Tracheal suctioning at the time of delivery, preferably prior to the first breath, may decrease the incidence and severity of meconium aspiration syndrome and the need for mechanical ventilation. It seems plausible that not all infants with meconium-stained amniotic fluid require laryngoscopy and direct tracheal suctioning. Generally, visualization of the glottis is a benign procedure and allows the resuscitator to determine if there is meconium at the level of the vocal cords. However, reflex bradycardia may be induced during laryngoscopy and suctioning, just as it is with suctioning by the obstetrician. Thus, laryngoscopy and suctioning may necessitate further intervention. This is a problem even when the resuscitator is skilled and experienced.

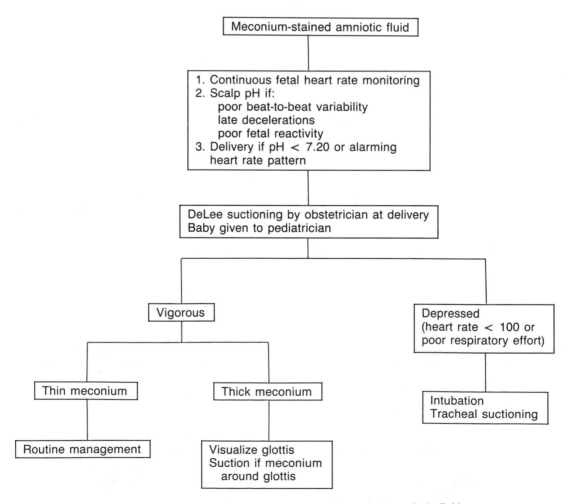

Figure 1 Scheme for managing the fetus or infant with meconium-stained amniotic fluid.

The following approach was developed in an attempt to provide appropriate intervention without subjecting the infant to unnecessary morbidity. These recommendations are based on the condition of the infant at the time he or she is handed over to the pediatrician and the consistency of meconium in amniotic fluid.

1. **Vigorous infants with thin meconium in the amniotic fluid:** No special resuscitative measures seem indicated.
2. **Vigorous infants with thick meconium in the amniotic fluid:** In these babies, we attempt to visualize the glottis and, if meconium is seen, we suction the trachea. Although these are the infants who should theoretically benefit most from tracheal suctioning, they are unfortunately the most difficult patients upon whom to perform the procedure and the ones in whom iatrogenic morbidities of induced bradycardia and traumatic intubation are most likely to occur.
3. **Depressed infants (heart rate less than 100 beats per minute or poor respiratory effort) with meconium staining:** We visualize the glottis and suction the trachea in depressed infants, regardless of the consistency of the meconium.
4. **Time limit on tracheal suctioning:** Once suctioning is complete *or* 2 minutes have elapsed from the time of delivery, whichever comes first, we stimulate and ventilate the infant. Prolonged attempts at suctioning prolong bradycardia and hypoxia. Suctioning continues in the infants with copious tracheal meconium once color has improved and the heart rate is over 120 beats per minute.

The suctioning technique commonly used is that of intubation with a 3.0-mm or 3.5-mm orotracheal tube and suctioning is through the tube by mouth with a face mask or piece of gauze to separate the resuscitator from the infant. Although this provides the largest internal diameter for suctioning, it is not safe for either the infant or the resuscitator. The risk of transmission of infectious agents is mutual. The risk to the resuscitator is obvious, but the infant is also in jeopardy. Herpes simplex virus type 1 has been transmitted to an infant at the time of airway suctioning for meconium. Face masks or gauze limit the amount of meconium ingested by the resuscitator, but these are not adequate barriers to infection.

In all infants except those with the thickest meconium, we intubate with a 3.5-mm endotracheal tube and suction the trachea with an No. 8 French suction catheter. The regulator on the suction device should be adjusted to provide "medium" or about 80 to 100 mm Hg of suction. Care should be taken to suction intermittently rather than continuously. Two potential disadvantages of this method are that it calls for suction through a catheter of relatively small internal diameter and that it exposes the airway mucosa to trauma from excessive negative pressure. Ordinarily it allows repeated suctioning without requiring multiple intubations, but infants with large amounts of thick meconium may still have to be reintubated when meconium clogs the suction catheter. Several alternative devices have recently been suggested for tracheal suctioning of meconium. One is simply an endotracheal tube attached directly to the adapter of an adult suction catheter. At present we are evaluating a similar device that allows for rapid connection of moderate level wall suction to the endotracheal tube connector but still retains the critical feature of thumb occlusion–controlled intermittent suction. Another approach is the use of a hand-powered suction unit that attaches to the endotracheal tube.

Nursery

The clinical course of infants with meconium aspiration is variable. Many are asymptomatic, and even those with symptoms demonstrate a broad spectrum of disease requiring various levels of support. Thus we feel that a highly protocolized clinical approach, especially to ventilatory management, is inappropriate.

General Measures

Since there is an association between meconium aspiration and fetal asphyxia, these infants need to be evaluated for other sequelae of asphyxia, including metabolic disturbances, polycythemia, and central nervous system, gastrointestinal, or renal dysfunction. Serum electrolytes, including calcium, and glucose levels should be monitored. Renal status often varies, and fluid and electrolyte administration must be tailored accordingly.

A conservative approach is to administer antibiotics to all infants with meconium aspiration who require intensive care. Infection may have contributed to the stress that caused the fetus to pass meconium; infectious pneumonia may coexist with meconium aspiration pneumonia, and meconium augments bacterial growth in amniotic fluid. If the infant is much improved and if tracheal and blood cultures show no growth, we discontinue antibiotics at 72 hours, even if infiltrates persist on the chest x-ray. We assume that the persistent infiltrate represents a chemical pneumonitis.

Respiratory Management

Chest physical therapy (vibration and percussion) may help to clear meconium remaining in the lung after suctioning. It should be combined with postural drainage and applied vigorously and frequently (every 30 minutes as tolerated) until the pharyngeal or tracheal aspirate is clear.

Following initial stabilization, the infant needs to be carefully monitored and evaluated for abnormalities of gas exchange. Adequate oxygenation is important. Continuous monitoring of oxygenation, either by pulse oximetry or transcutaneous PO_2, is an extremely useful adjunct to an arterial catheter. If the infant is full-term or post-term, as infants who aspirate meconium usually are, the PO_2 is maintained in the range of 80 to 100 mm Hg. The real risk of hypoxia with its deleterious effect on pulmonary vascular resistance outweighs the theoretical risk of retinal damage from brief hyperoxia, especially in an infant with incipient persistent pulmonary hypertension.

Infants with central respiratory depression or severe lung disease may require mechanical ventilation, but mechanical ventilation should be delayed as long as is practical; the risk-benefit ratio of ventilatory assistance is much higher with meconium aspiration syndrome than for more common neonatal pulmonary disorders. Since airway resistance may be high, adequate time should be allowed for expiration in order to minimize air trapping. Sedation may facilitate ventilatory assistance in a vigorous infant, and on rare occasions we paralyze the infant with pancuronium. The response to positive end expiratory pressure is individual and must be carefully evaluated. As always, but especially in meconium aspiration syndrome, it is desirable to limit inspiratory pressure in the hope of preventing air leaks. Air leaks often manifest dramatically, with an abrupt decline in oxygenation and blood pressure and worsening of skin color. Immediate needle thoracentesis followed by chest tube insertion is required. Placement of the thoracostomy tube in the midclavicular line is more likely to result in effective drainage than is the lateral approach.

Other Measures

Cardiotonic drugs (dopamine and dobutamine), pulmonary vasodilators, and extracorporeal membrane oxygenation provide additional measures for the infant with a poor response to conventional ventilatory therapy. If tolazoline is administered repeatedly or continuously, care must be taken to avoid accumulation of toxic blood levels. We administer a loading dose of 1 mg per kilogram intravenously and maintain an infusion of 0.16 mg per kilogram per hour. The infusion rate is decreased in infants with impaired renal function. Unfortunately, the benefit of vasodilators is often transitory and associated morbidity is high. Extracorporeal membrane oxygenation has been successful in reducing mortality in some centers in infants selected on the basis of a projected poor chance of survival at that same center. As has been emphasized repeatedly, projections are not necessarily transferable from one center to another.

MECONIUM ILEUS

ROBERT M. FILLER, M.D.

Meconium ileus is a form of neonatal intestinal obstruction caused by inspissated meconium in the lumen of the distal small bowel. In over 95 percent of cases, this diagnosis indicates that the child has cystic fibrosis. In the remainder, no specific cause has been found. In about 50 percent of cases, meconium ileus is complicated by association with one or more of the following: intestinal atresia, volvulus, intestinal infarction, and meconium peritonitis. The diagnosis of simple or complicated meconium ileus is made by plain abdominal x-ray films and barium enema examination of the colon. Initial emergency treatment consists of intestinal decompression with a nasogastric tube and intravenous fluid therapy, just as in any neonate with intestinal obstruction.

In cases of simple meconium ileus we believe that attempts at disimpacting the obstructing meconium by enema techniques are preferable to immediate surgical therapy, especially since these infants are so prone to develop postoperative pulmonary complications. Various enema preparations have been reported to be useful in relieving the obstruction. Gastrografin (meglumine diatrizoate with 0.1 percent polysorbate 80), a hypertonic (1,900 mOsm per liter) iodine solution combined with a wetting agent, has received the most attention in the literature since its first successful use in meconium ileus in 1969.

The success of Gastrografin in relieving intestinal obstruction is presumably due to its high osmolarity, which draws fluid into the bowel from plasma, dislodging the abnormally adherent meconium. The wetting agent may also aid in separating the meconium from the intestinal wall.

The hyperosmolarity of Gastrografin is also responsible for shock, the one major complication associated with its use. When used as an enema, the hypertonic solution can cause sufficient fluid to shift from plasma into the intestinal lumen to produce hypovolemic shock, especially in small infants. When this agent is used, the infant must therefore be adequately hydrated before it is instilled, and intravenous fluid therapy must be maintained during the enema with 5 percent dextrose in 0.2 percent normal saline at 10 ml per kilogram per hour. The child's blood pressure and pulse are carefully monitored.

Because of its potential for producing hypovolemia, we no longer use Gastrografin to treat meconium ileus. Instead, we now employ a solution of 25 percent sodium diatrizoate (Hypaque) or non-ionic contrast material with 5 percent N-acetylcysteine (Mucomyst), made by mixing equal amounts of 10 percent N-acetylcysteine and 50 percent sodium diatrizoate. The osmolarity of the final solution is about 700 mOsm per liter, and this combination appears to be just as effective as Gastrografin in breaking up the obstruction. Even though the mixture is still hypertonic with respect to plasma, fluid shifts associated with its use have apparently not been excessive, and fluid therapy during the enema is not necessary in the well-hydrated neonate.

The therapeutic enema is a procedure best performed in the radiology department. Since a treatment takes at least 15 minutes and may last an hour, it is important that the infant be protected from hypothermia by maintaining a high room temperature (80° F) or by providing direct heat with an infrared heating lamp.

We insert a No. 8 Foley catheter with a 3-ml balloon into the rectum and strap the buttocks together to minimize loss of enema fluid. Some centers do not use a Foley catheter for this procedure for fear of rectal perforation, but we have not observed this complication. The radiopaque fluid is drawn up in a 30-ml syringe and injected into the rectal catheter under radiologic control. The objective of treatment is to separate the adherent meconium from the ileal wall and have the irrigating solution enter the dilated intestine above the point of obstruction. As the colon fills and the irrigating solution reaches the obstructed area, increased resistance to injection is encountered. When the injection of small additional quantities of fluid meets significant resistance, the enema is discontinued and the bowel allowed to evacuate spontaneously. To avoid intestinal perforation, the small caliber colon and terminal ileum must not be overfilled.

The instillation procedure is repeated after each evacuation, provided the child's condition is stable. Only a fraction of the obstructing meconium can be eliminated at each attempt, so one can anticipate that at least five or 10 instillations will be necessary. Failure of the contrast material to reach the dilated intestine may mean that all of the inspissated meconium has not been dislodged or that there is an underlying intestinal atresia. Therefore, considerable judgment is needed to determine how long to persist with the intestinal irrigation. Usually about 50 to 200 ml of enema fluid is required, depending upon the amount of fluid lost around the rectal catheter and the total number of times the instillation and evacuation procedure is repeated. Intestinal obstruction is relieved by this technique in about half the cases of simple meconium ileus.

If the initial irrigations fail to relieve the obstruction and the child's condition remains stable with no evidence of peritonitis, then we continue nasogastric suction and intravenous fluid therapy before repeating the procedure in 12 to 24 hours. Failure at this time signifies that operation is necessary to relieve the obstruction.

In those infants in whom simple rectal irrigations are successful, nasogastric suction and intravenous fluid therapy are continued for 2 to 3 days to allow complete decompression of the dilated intestine. Oral feeding is started only when the child is having spontaneous bowel movements, indicating that the chronically obstructed distended small bowel is capable of effective peristaltic activity. We use Pregestimil for feedings of all infants with cystic fibrosis, since it does not require pancreatic enzymes for absorption.

Operative treatment is required for all infants with complicated meconium ileus as well as for those with simple meconium ileus in whom enema therapy has failed. Many surgical methods have been used to relieve the meconium obstruction. At present, we employ enterotomy and irrigation for simple meconium ileus. At surgery, the dilated terminal ileum is opened just proximal to the point of obstruction. A straight No. 16 French catheter is inserted into the lumen of the dilated, obstructed bowel, and the intestine is irrigated repeatedly with 15 to 30 ml aliquots of 5 percent N-acetylcysteine. Between instillations, the catheter is aspirated and drained, but if the thickened

meconium does not pass through the tube, it is manually milked out of the intestine at the enterotomy site. This irrigating and evacuating procedure is continued until the small meconium pellets obstructing the terminal ileum are dislodged, allowing irrigating fluid to enter and distend the colon. The molasses-like meconium that remains upstream is also evacuated, so that the upper intestine is completely decompressed through the enterotomy. After the obstruction has been relieved, the opening in the intestine is sutured, the bowel returned to the peritoneal cavity, and the abdominal wall closed. Our experience indicates that this procedure relieves obstruction in over 90 percent of cases. If the intraoperative irrigations fail, a stoma must be created proximal to the point of obstruction. In these cases, irrigations are continued after surgery, as described below.

Instead of performing a simple enterotomy and evacuating the meconium at the operating table, some surgeons prefer to create an intestinal stoma and delay irrigations of the intestinal tract until the postoperative period so as to avoid contaminating the wound and peritoneum. A number of different procedures have been described. As a first step, the dilated ileum, just proximal to the point of obstruction, is resected. The two cut ends of the intestine are brought out to the skin as a double-barreled ileostomy. As an alternative, one cut end is brought out to the skin and the other is anastomosed to the side of this limb, the "chimney" operation described by Bishop and Koop, and Santulli. After surgery, when the infant's condition is stable, the intestinal stoma and the rectum are irrigated daily with 5 percent N-acetylcysteine to remove the obstructing meconium. When the bowel obstruction is relieved and the patient is stable, usually 2 to 3 weeks later, the stoma is closed at a second operation. Sometimes a "chimney" will close spontaneously or it can be closed at the bedside by placing a ligature around its base.

In patients with complicated meconium ileus, the atretic, infarcted, or perforated intestine is excised at the time of surgery. It is usually unwise in these cases to attempt intraoperative irrigations and primary end-to-end anastomoses because of the likelihood of anastomotic complications. The procedure involving creation of a double-barreled ileostomy or "chimney" stoma, postoperative irrigations, and late closure of the stoma is preferable.

The postoperative management of infants who require surgery is similar, regardless of the type of corrective procedure employed. Nasogastric suction is maintained until bowel movements begin (by rectum or by ileostomy) and nasogastric tube output is minimal. Oral feeding is then started with Pregestimil. Prophylactic antibiotics (gentamicin 5 mg per kilogram per day and ampicillin 100 mg per kilogram per day) are started just prior to surgery and continued for 24 hours postoperatively in uncomplicated cases. In patients with necrotic intestine or frank peritonitis, antibiotic therapy is continued for 7 days and clindamycin (50 mg per kilogram per day) is added to the regimen.

A significant number of infants with complicated meconium ileus requiring intestinal resection develop prolonged malabsorption. Often they do not tolerate a full diet for several weeks after surgery, so that nutrition must be maintained intravenously. The likelihood of pulmonary complications must also be considered. Frequent suctioning, postural drainage, and physiotherapy should be instituted to minimize this possibility.

A sweat test to confirm the diagnosis of cystic fibrosis is performed as soon as possible. However, a satisfactory sweat test is not possible in most cases until a sufficient quantity of sweat can be collected, usually not until the infant is 3 to 4 weeks old.

MYELOMENINGOCELE

RALPH A.W. LEHMAN, M.D., F.A.C.S.

Approximately one in 500 children is born with spina bifida, evident as a midline skin defect or cyst overlying defects extending into the spinal canal through all soft tissue and posterior spinal elements. This defect may be a simple meningocele without neural involvement (5 to 27 percent) or a myelomeningocele (95 to 73 percent) with malformed nerve roots and/or spinal cord. With the latter, there is usually loss of sphincter and sexual function, as well as varying degrees of sensory and motor loss in the lower extremities. In addition, myelomeningocele often is associated with other malformations, including hydrocephalus, malformations of the brain, orthopaedic abnormalities (including foot deformity, hip dislocation, gibbus, and kyphoscoliosis), and ocular muscle imbalance, as well as urologic and cardiac anomalies. The multitude of primary and secondary medical problems, and the associated financial and social difficulties attendant upon the care of many of these children, mandate a team approach.

TREATMENT

The Spinal Defect. Initial management of these infants is almost always neurosurgical. In the hours and days following birth, the pressing problems are related to the defect in the back and the presence of hydrocephalus. Most neurosurgeons attempt to repair the back within the first 24 hours after birth in order to prevent meningitis and ventriculitis, as well as to preserve existing neurologic function. However, this reasoning is still open to debate. Leakage of spinal fluid from the back is a clear indication for rapid repair shortly after birth. Because the skin becomes colonized with bacteria by 36 hours after birth, repair should be delayed if the infant is first seen 36 hours or more after birth and neural tissues are exposed. Surgery should be put off until the exposed neural elements (which will be internalized at surgery) can be rendered relatively sterile. During this delay, wet to dry dressings of the back are applied. Antibiotics are administered if spinal fluid leakage occurs.

The greatest controversy surrounds decisions to limit early surgery to those infants judged not to have a "dismal" prognosis. If this policy is pursued, untreated infants are re-evaluated at some future date (e.g., 1 month of age), and the back is then repaired in the survivors. Selection of patients for treatment is discussed below. An alternative is early shunting for hydrocephalus with delayed closure of the back in those infants in whom healing does not occur. This has never been a popular approach.

Operative technique is aimed at preservation of all neural elements that might be intact, followed by a multi-layered closure of the soft tissue defect. Initially, the thin attenuated skin is removed. This may either occur in a ring around the margin of an exposed neural plate or, when there is complete epithelial cover, as a thin parchment covering a cyst containing spinal fluid and neural elements. The dural sac also participates in the defects and is splayed open posteriorly, extending laterally to fuse with the lateral margins of the abnormal skin. After the neural elements are freed from any attachments to skin, the dural sac is reconstructed as a tube surrounding them. For this purpose, flaps of dura are freed up laterally on each side and sutured together in the midline. If paraspinous fascia is not used for the dural reconstruction there may be sufficient tissue to reflect flaps over the dural closure as an additional layer of protection. Finally, the skin is closed. This may require extensive undermining of the skin and the creation of flaps if the defect is to be covered. *Only rarely does neurologic function improve postoperatively.* Rarely, worsening may occur.

Postoperatively the dry gauze dressing over the wound is protected by a sterile plastic drape with a single adhesive edge. The latter is stuck transversely to the skin between the incision and the anus so that it can be turned up over the dressing to protect it. A small hole is made in the upper portion of this plastic drape so as to provide ventilation for the dressing. The child is kept off his or her back until the incision is healed and the sutures are removed.

If the skin closure appears to be in jeopardy, as indicated by pallor or cyanosis, twice daily thin applications of 2 percent nitroglycerin ointment may enhance the circulation and prevent wound breakdown. Should the skin closure dehisce slightly, antibiotics should be given and wet to dry saline dressings applied every 4 hours.

Hydrocephalus. *Hydrocephalus occurs in more than 80 percent of children with myelomeningocele but is rare when only a simple meningocele is present.* Although measurements of head circumference may be helpful in detecting hydrocephalus, often *the ventricles enlarge be-*

fore the head size is much greater than normal. Consequently other means of making this diagnosis are desirable and permit earlier treatment. Although computed tomographic (CT) scanning is helpful, ultrasonography is used because it is simple to perform and permits both ready diagnosis and convenient postoperative follow-up. Ultimately CT scanning or magnetic resonance imaging is done in order to obtain greater definition of the intracranial structures and provide a baseline for the future.

If hydrocephalus is diagnosed early, a shunt can be placed immediately after repair of the back under the same anesthesia. Shunting relieves intracranial pressure. It permits the brain to expand and the ventricles to contract toward normal size. This, in turn, allows mental development to improve, perhaps even up to the limits set by any other abnormalities of brain structure that may be present.

A shunt consists of a catheter inserted into one cerebral ventricle and extending through the skull to connect with a distal catheter that runs subcutaneously to a drainage site. The drainage site chosen is usually the peritoneum, but on occasion the distal end of the system is placed into the jugular vein and right atrium or elsewhere. Incorporated within this system is a reservoir, a valve, and a pump chamber. The reservoir may be tapped under sterile conditions to permit aspiration, irrigation, injection, or measurement of ventricular pressure. The valve regulates the flow characteristics of the shunt and permits fluid to flow in only one direction, out of the ventricles. Consequently, *pumping the shunt chamber provides an indication as to its function.* If the pump does not compress easily, distal outflow probably is obstructed. Of course if this obstruction is of a low degree, such as the enclosure of the peritoneal end of the shunt in a cyst, the pump may still compress relatively easily under the pressure exerted by one's finger. If the pump chamber does not refill readily after being compressed, inflow from the proximal ventricular catheter may be obstructed. However, this may also occur if the shunt is functioning exceedingly well and causing the ventricles to become slit-like.

Since the shunt is usually fixed at its point of entry through the skull, its distal end gradually shortens relative to the body as the child grows. This procedure usually results in the child's "out-growing" the shunt, with ventriculoatrial shunts ending up high in the superior jugular vein and clotting shut and ventriculoperitoneal shunts ending up outside the abdominal cavity and thereby failing to function. As a result, regular radiologic follow-up is necessary so that shunts may be lengthened before they obstruct.

For the most part, complications are due to shunt malfunction with acute or gradual increase of intracranial pressure manifesting as lethargy, coma, irritability, seizures, failure to achieve developmental milestones, decreased school performance, nausea or vomiting. Assessment includes physical examination for abnormalities such as abnormal shunt pump, unusual increase in head circumference, full fontanelle, papilledema, abducens or upward gaze paresis, and lethargy. CT (or magnetic resonance imaging or ultrasound) scan may reveal ventricular enlargement. Doubtful cases may sometimes be resolved by tapping the shunt reservoir and determining whether there is spontaneous egress of fluid and measuring its pressure. On occasion, injection of contrast agent or radioactive tracers is helpful. Malfunctioning shunts require revision.

Infection of the shunt is always a possibility. If no other source of fever is discovered, a child with a shunt should have the reservoir tapped in order to obtain cerebrospinal fluid for culture and other studies. There is usually no nuchal rigidity. Usually, high fever (over 38.5° C) is not due to shunt infection. Shunt infections are best treated with appropriate intravenous antibiotics (cerebrospinal fluid drug levels monitored by Schlichter's test against the previously isolated organisms). After cerebrospinal fluid cultures become sterile, the entire shunt is replaced and intravenous antibiotics are continued for another 7 to 10 days.

As a rule, shunts should not be removed or prevented from functioning in order to see whether the child can manage without one. This is true even if the shunt does not seem to function any longer, as this impression may be incorrect. In general, children with even a partially functioning shunt remain dependent upon it for their well-being. Children with shunts should probably receive prophylactic antibiotics for a day before and several days after any procedures that may be associated with transient bacteremia, such as dental work.

Sphincter and Genital Problems. The large majority of patients with myelomeningocele are incontinent of urine and may require intermittent catheterization, medication, or other maneuvers in order to expedite urinary voiding and diminish the risks of urinary stasis and infection, secondary changes in the bladder, ureteral reflux, and chronic renal failure. Frequent diapering and, for males, external collecting devices are helpful. Ultimately various operations on the urethra or bladder or some form of ureteral diversion may prove necessary.

Defecation usually can be regulated with a rectal suppository or rapid small hypertonic enema given postprandially at the same time each day. Eventually, abdominal pressure or massage (or digital stimulation of the rectum) following one specific meal each day should prove sufficient. A number of dietary and medical regimens can be used to modify the consistency and decrease the bulk of the stool.

Great emphasis should be placed on the training of the parents and ultimately of the child to establish a regular program of bladder and bowel care. They should be taught the need for diligent hygiene and rapid cleansing whenever incontinence occurs. Acidification of the urine, protective ointments for the skin, and frequent changes of diapers or other protective garments should become routine. These children eventually learn to rely upon others as well as themselves to detect unseemly odors, so that cleansing and changes of clothes can be done rapidly and efficiently in order to avoid any social stigma.

Most individuals with a myelomeningocele have genital anesthesia and males only rarely have effective ejaculation. However, orgasm and erection are often possible, and patients of both sexes frequently are capable of producing children. The risk of a similar or associated malformation in the offspring is approximately 3 to 4 percent.

Orthopaedic Problems. Along with the loss of sphincter function, most patients with myelomeningocele suffer from paraparesis of some degree. It appears that knee extension as well as hip flexion are minimal requirements for ambulation. Consequently, *there is little hope that patients with loss of function up through the third lumbar spinal cord level will ever ambulate.* Even with lesions below this level, many children often prefer to use a wheelchair because of lack of motivation, spinal curvature, lower extremity deformities, or other factors. Body and leg braces or casts, surgical correction of lower extremity deformities, muscle transfers, release of contractures, crutches, and physical or play therapy are all useful adjuncts providing increased mobility. Training in walking is delayed in accord with each individual's handicaps.

Any uncorrected kyphus should be protected by a soft doughnut whenever the child is in a position to put pressure on it, and precautions should be taken to prevent decubitus ulcers. Surgical correction of kyphosis and scoliosis is delayed or avoided by using body jackets for as many years as possible. Because these children usually have anesthesia of the skin of sitting surfaces, great care must be exercised to avoid decubitus ulcers.

Other Complications. Many other problems may occur with myelodysplasia. Among these are seizures, late onset of progressive paralysis, and early apnea.

Seizures are usually of the grand mal type and respond to anticonvulsants. Shunt malfunction with increased intracranial pressure occasionally manifests with seizures, and the need for shunt revision should always be considered when a child with myelodysplasia has fits.

Progressive loss of lower or even upper extremity function and, rarely, isolated deterioration of bladder function may be due to a variety of causes, including shunt malfunction, syringomyelia, intraspinal lipoma, dermoid or teratoma, diastematomyelia, and tethered cord. These lesions often are responsive to additional surgery and should be sought with appropriate radiologic studies if progressive loss occurs.

Respiratory difficulty may occur in the infant and young child and can be of neurogenic origin. This may take the form of upper airway obstruction with stridor and may lead to sudden death. In these instances, the cause is usually paralysis of the vocal cord abductors, and immediate endotracheal intubation may be necessary. The ultimate cause appears to be increased intracranial pressure with hindbrain displacement related to the Arnold-Chiari malformation. Consequently, treatment requires ventricular drainage by tap, followed by shunt placement or revision. If vocal cord function does not return after this, tracheostomy may be necessary for an extended time.

In other cases, there may be periodic apnea, usually during sleep. This also may necessitate intubation and requires assisted ventilation. A ventricular tap should be done, and if there is increased intracranial pressure or ventricular enlargement, shunt placement or revision is necessary. It should be noted that, even though episodes of spontaneous apnea may resolve spontaneously over time,

they also can lead to death. Infants should be monitored at all times if the apnea continues to occur after treatment or has not been severe enough to require treatment.

In cases in which either form (stridor or apnea) of respiratory difficulty is present, there may be no increase of intracranial pressure, or the child may fail to respond to the establishment of a satisfactory shunt. In such instances, local compression at the level of the foramen magnum must be considered, and decompression of the occipital and high cervical regions may be warranted.

PROGNOSIS

Since it is usual to close the back defect and even to install a ventriculoperitoneal shunt within the first 24 hours of life, the infant's parents are confronted with a bewildering, unexpected, and difficult series of medical problems and decisions very early on. Often the child has been transported from another hospital for treatment, with the mother staying behind and the father shuttling back and forth between the two. With the time limitation for treatment and the frequent absence of the mother, it is difficult for the physician to convey a balanced presentation of the infant's immediate and long-range outlook or even the current therapeutic options and suggestions. It is considerably more difficult for the parents to comprehend them.

Although opinions vary and have changed in differing directions in the past, controversy still continues over the question of selective or unselective treatment. Usually the immediate management of the myelodysplastic infant hinges on the consensus of the pediatrician and neurosurgeon. The initial recommendation to operate or not that is offered to the family often is specific to the infant being considered.

A number of physicians think that children with the worst prognosis, i.e., paraplegia to or above the third lumbar spinal cord level combined with hydrocephalus of marked degree, should not be treated surgically until after 1 month of age to determine whether their defects are compatible with survival. It is my opinion that, given adequate nourishment and physical care, almost all infants will survive for this period and that early operation is more apt to result in somewhat better quality of survival. *Although the quality of survival of some of these infants may ultimately be judged unsatisfactory, it is probably better and more manageable in the future if they are treated thoroughly from the beginning.* Consequently I recommend that, with very rare exceptions, myelodysplastic infants be treated vigorously and aggressively from the first days of life. The above explanation, some of the uncertainty regarding the child's future, and information regarding known deficits are conveyed to the parents.

Early deaths are usually due to infection with meningitis or ventriculitis. Later deaths are due to shunt malfunction and, as the child ages, tend to be due to renal failure.

Periodic check-ups and care of these children involve the pediatrician, neurosurgeon, orthopaedist, urologist, physical and occupational therapist, a social worker or a nurse versed in these problems, a psychologist, and at times other specialists. Routine visits to a team specializing in these problems are an especially effective means of long-term management.

The recurrent and persistent problems of these patients create a great financial and emotional drain upon families, and it is possible that the incidence of divorce among the parents of such children is much higher than average. Parents should receive genetic counseling and be aware of the increased risk of similar and related defects (1 to 5 percent) in subsequent children.

SUGGESTED READING

Charney EB, Weller SC, Sutton LN, Bruce DA, Schut LB. Management of the newborn with myelomeningocele. Pediatrics 1985; 75:58–64.
French BN. Midline fusion defects of formation. In: Youmans JR, ed. Neurological surgery. Philadelphia: WB Saunders, 1982: 1276–1380.
McLaughlin JF, Shurtleff DB, Lamers JY, Stuntz JT, Hayden PW, Knopp RJ. Influence of prognosis on decisions regarding the care of newborns with myelodysplasia. N Eng J Med 1985; 312:1589–1594.
Shurtleff DB. Myelodysplasia: Management and treatment. Curr Probl Pediatr 1980; 10(3)1–98.

NECROTIZING ENTEROCOLITIS

EDMUND F. LA GAMMA, M.D., F.A.A.P.

PATHOGENESIS

Technologic and therapeutic advances have revolutionized medical care in virtually every area of perinatal medicine in the past 20 years. Despite this, necrotizing enterocolitis (NEC) remains an unabated complication of newborn intensive care that results in a characteristic pattern of necrosis of large segments of affected intestine. Moreover, with increased survival of extremely immature neonates (less than or equal to 1,000 g at birth), NEC has emerged as an important factor in determining overall neonatal morbidity and mortality. NEC occurs in up to 30 percent of "sick" neonates (Table 1), carries a mortality rate of up to 50 percent when associated with sepsis, and accounts for 3 to 8 percent of all admissions to neonatal intensive care units.

Unfortunately, the pathogenesis of NEC remains obscure. Nevertheless, several generalizations on etiology are accepted. For example, NEC occasionally erupts as an epidemic, is largely a problem of premature infants, and, in virtually all cases, NEC damage to the gut manifests itself almost exclusively *after* birth, despite a functionally active intestine while the fetus is in utero. Consequently, the pathogenesis of necrotizing enterocolitis appears to derive from a dynamic interaction between exposure of the immature intestine to the abnormal conditions of the non-uterine environment and various ex utero processes of gut colonization. Recent studies, although recognized as a departure from traditional teachings, have raised doubts about previous theories that impaired blood flow and the initiation of enteral feeding are necessary prerequisites for causation in this illness. It is, however, universally agreed that enteral feeding is contraindicated at any age in a patient with evidence of compromised bowel.

Empiric and experimental evidence links causation of necrotizing enterocolitis in some cases to hyperosmolar formula (or to nonmanufacturer formula additives that can increase osmolarity; such as vitamins or phenobarbital), to ischemic or hypoxic injury, to embolic complications of umbilical artery catheterization, to portal venous congestion (after umbilical vein catheterization), to the microcirculatory failure of polycythemia (or its treatment by exchange transfusion), and to severe hypothermia or dehydration.

In each of these pathogenic conditions the clinical history and circumstances existing at the time of diagnosis of necrotizing enterocolitis are protean, but they represent plausible causative mechanisms. In contrast, certain other situations exist in which no single obvious mechanism can be invoked to explain the occurrence of NEC in infants who were *never* fed, in infants who were *fed breast milk*, in growing ("stable") infants several *weeks after an asphyxial episode*, or in infants who were *never stressed* at birth.

In addition, by temporal analysis, in full-term infants the most common time of occurrence of NEC is during the first few days of life (when it is associated with cyanotic heart disease, polycythemia, or severe birth asphyxia). In contrast, in infants born weighing less than 1,500 g, NEC occurs later (most commonly within the first 2 postnatal weeks), and as already stated, is not universally associated with signs of oxygen deprivation or perfusion stress. By occurrence, since NEC is reported at as much as a fourfold higher rate in preterm patients compared with term infants, the clinical entity may, in fact, actually represent the *"final common pathway"* of several entirely unrelated pathologic processes.

Following along this line of thought, a fruitful approach to defining disease-producing mechanisms should begin by carefully selecting patient cohorts (e.g., Table 1) and then deriving unbiased new theories of pathogenesis for prospective testing. These ideas should be based on principles of development and on an expanded examination of the interaction between the gut, and developing immune system, the microbiologic environment, and the role of oral intake as part of the continuum of trophic factors acting during development. Further expansion of the use of current state-of-the-art cell and molecular biologic tools to probe these issues is warranted. Of particular note

**TABLE 1 Illness Scale; Increased Risk for Neonatal Necrotizing Enterocolitis
If >21**

Factor	Day 1	Day 2	Day 3
Birth weight $\leq$1,500 g = 1 <1,000 g = 2			
Gestational age $\leq$ 32 weeks			
Apgar score $\leq$5 at 5 minutes			
Requires O_2 > 21%			
Requires respirator			
Requires O_2 > 21% or respirator for > 2 days			
Low blood pressure for age and weight			
Intraventricular hemorrhage or seizures			
Patent ductus arteriosus			
Umbilical artery catheter			
Umbilical vein catheter			
Daily Sum		+	+

Total Risk Score =

From LaGamma EF, Ostertag SG, Birenbaum H. Failure of delayed oral feedings to prevent necrotizing enterocolitis. Am J Dis Child 1985; 139:385–389.

is the historical emphasis on studying the gut as a vehicle for providing nutrition, which has served to impair new insights. It may prove to be more productive to circumvent the issue by parenteral nutrition and then to directly attack the more fundamental biologic questions concerning organ growth, its maturation, and its unique susceptibility.

For example, what are the underlying reasons for the unique perinatal vulnerability of the immature intestine? If gut immaturity is an issue, can we exploit the long-recognized observation that maturity and differentiation can be induced through the use of hormones (e.g., glucocorticoids, thyroid hormones) or possible other neurohumoral regulatory factors (e.g., gut peptides such as gastrin, vasoactive intestinal polypeptide, or cholecystokinin)? Using a current understanding of the principles of infectious disease and immunobiology, can gut flora be manipulated to achieve a more desirable balance of bacterial flora in the sick neonate? On a more speculative note, do oxygen free radicals and tissue deficiencies of antioxidants play a role? If so, how do they act? Do other mediators of perinatal tissue damage exist of which we are unaware (e.g., tumor necrosis factor, leukotrienes)? Is NEC not a single entity but really the final common pathway of many disease states? These and other questions can only be resolved by further expansion of basic and applied research programs in developmental biology of the gut and through collaborative prospective clinical research trials.

NEONATAL NUTRITION

The optimal rate of ex utero growth is unknown. Consequently, efforts directed at providing postnatal nutrition for "normal" growth are empirically defined by rates approximating in utero accretion in the absence of complications. With this vague general guideline, it is important to recognize that because energy requirements differ, neonatal growth will never achieve the in utero accretion rate. On the other hand, in a substantial amount of literature it is argued that the provision of sufficient calories, electrolytes, water, and vitamins facilitates recovery from illness and therefore an aggressive intervention should be started on the first day of life. Due to the limitations of the functional capacity of the immature intestine (and because of other coexisting medical problems), achievement of nutritional goals usually cannot be accomplished orally. This limitation often dictates supplementation of oral nutrition via the parenteral route.

To define the proper proportion of total nutrition to be provided via the enteral or parenteral route, it is necessary to review certain clinical and developmental issues. No attempt is made to document a thoroughly comprehensive guide to nutrition; only practical concerns are covered, relevant factors identified, and comments targeted at sick, very low birth weight neonates (see Table 1).

Oral Intake

Sucking in the immature infant is characterized by short burst that are either followed by or preceded by swallows. In the mature infant a more regular pattern of sucking and then swallowing occurs. The immature pattern can be matured considerably by allowing non-nutritive sucking. Immature infants also have decreased tone of the lower esophageal sphincter, a poorly organized gag reflex (which matures by approximately 32 postconceptional weeks), and they frequently become apneic 15 to 20 minutes following feeding. Despite these limitations, early in pregnancy and at term, a normal fetus can swallow as much as 150 ml per kilogram per day of amniotic fluid, a somewhat surprising degree of mature, integrated function when compared with that of the ex utero neonate.

Therefore, after birth, in view of the well-documented delays in gastric emptying time (worsened by stresses of a difficult birth and commonly occurring respiratory insufficiency), it may be prudent to delay enteral intake on the first day of life in sick, very low birth weight neonates (see Table 1). On the other hand, at a later time, it seems reasonable to base the initiation of enteral feeding on *physiologic grounds* defined by the individual patient. For example, our criteria include:

1. Absence of retrograde flow: no nasogastric drainage or emesis.
2. Peristaltic activity: presence of bowel sounds, passing stools.
3. No signs of peritonitis: no abdominal distention, no tension, and no tenderness.
4. No signs of obstruction: absence of masses.
5. No evidence of bleeding: passing heme-negative stools.

6. Establishing respiratory, cardiovascular, and hematologic stability (predictability) during assisted ventilation (most important).

Deliberately delaying enteral feeding for several weeks (or up to a month after birth as is occasionally recommended) delays achievement of normal ontogenetic milestones acquired in utero while swallowing amniotic fluid and promotes disuse atrophy of the brush border, with concomitant down-regulation of enzymes (starvation pattern). Since it is unusual for the neonate to achieve stability (i.e., predictability) until several days after birth, it is prudent to wait until then before introducing any new, entirely elective intervention (i.e., feeding). Therefore, the strategy is to make use of the prior "stable" baseline status as a point of departure for evaluating the effects of initiating oral intake. Often a period of stability is achieved only following 4 to 7 days of intensive care therapy or longer in some cases.

A conservative approach to the introduction of oral intake is outlined in Table 2. Although a discussion of continuous nasogastric infusions (nasojejunal infusions are associated with more feeding intolerance, difficult placement requiring radiologic confirmation, and an inability to routinely change the catheter position) is presented, a suitable alternative would be to follow the same schedule using intermittent bolus volumes summed every 2 hours. Furthermore, because of delayed gastric emptying and greater success (less intolerance), it is preferable to gavage feed the preterm infant by gravity (approximately 10 cm of water pressure) in the prone or right lateral decubitus position.

In order to monitor progress or tolerance of feeding, stomach contents should be aspirated and examined for residual formula at least every 2 hours. If the aspirate is less than half the total desired intake, replace the aspirate plus the volume needed to achieve the desired total volume. If intermittent feeding is selected (every 2 hours), clamp the tube immediately after instilling formula for a half hour. Then unclamp the tube and connect it to straight drainage to measure reflux. If the reflux is more than half the volume administered (and/or it persists on several occasions), discontinue oral gavage feeding. Similarly, discontinue feedings if drainage shows bilious material, since retrograde flow through the outlet sphincter of the stomach is *never* normal (except, of course, when using nasojejunal tubes). Success of enteral feeding should be monitored as indicated in Table 3.

Discontinued feedings for observations outlined in Table 4 and place the patient on straight drainage via the nasogastric tube. Do not resume enteral feeding unless drainage is less than 4 to 5 ml of clear secretions per 8-hour period, bowel sounds have returned, the abdominal examination is benign, stools are heme-negative, and no emesis is present. Then, depending on the patient's clinical presentation, an abdominal x-ray film is warranted (see Diagnosis of NEC). The observation period should extend to a minimum of 12 to 24 hours and constitutes what we commonly refer to as a "NEC Alert."

Other prudent routine approaches to daily manage-

TABLE 2   Suggested Nasogastric Feeding Schedule for Infants Less Than 1,500 g at Birth With High Illness Score (> 21)

Days of Enteral Feeds	Concentration of Formula/Breast Milk	Rate of Constant Infusion
1	Sterile H_2O	1 ml/hr
2	2.5% Dextrose	1 ml/hr
3–4	Half Strength	1 ml/hr
5–6	Full strength	1 ml/hr
7	Full strength	2/hr

* Recommended whey-predominant formulas as of 1988: Similac Premature 24, Mead-Johnson 24, or Premie SMA 24.

† After day 7, increase volume 1 ml/hr each day as tolerated (see text), up to a total of 150–170 ml/kg/day. Discontinue intravenous fluids after 100 ml/kg/day orally.

ment include consulting with nurses before advancing either volume or strength of oral intake and always being wary of potential problems when experimenting with a new formula preparation.

The nutritional value of breast milk varies over time after birth, and it is not a complete source for intake in very low birth weight infants. However, breast milk has several distinct non-nutritive advantages that make it the superior choice over formula. In general, breast milk is felt to be better absorbed and results in fewer episodes of gastrointestinal intolerance. More important it contains iron, thyroid hormone, phagocytic cells (macrophages), and immunocompetent T and B cells (active if milk is collected in plastic, not glass, and never frozen). In combination, these components may amplify bacterial defenses by providing C3 and C4 complement, lysozyme, lactoferrin, and secretory IgA (which is not destroyed by gut enzymes). Moreover, breast milk promotes the growth of *Lactobacillus bifidus* (which may impair colonization by pathogens) even in the presence of broad-spectrum antibiotics. Breast milk may also have trophic effects important in promoting gut maturation ex utero or play a central role in modifying gut colonization, immune competence, or other effects to be defined, all requiring further investigation.

To maintain cellular competence, stored milk should be refrigerated for less than 48 hours and should be cultured on arrival. Practitioners should also be aware that virtually all drugs, environmental toxins, and most viruses are excreted in breast milk.

Parenteral Nutrition

It is necessary to institute a *dextrose* infusion shortly after birth to sustain blood glucose levels upon termination of placental blood flow in very low birth weight neonates. This is customarily started at a dose of 8 to 10 g per kilogram per day of dextrose. This can be increased 1 g per kilogram per day to maintain the blood glucose level at less than or equal to 150 mg per deciliter and trace to negative glucose in the urine.

Fluid volume is administered at 80 to 100 ml per kilogram per day on day 1 and advanced every 12 hours to sustain a urine output of 1 to 2 ml per kilogram per hour and a stable weight (less than or equal to 10 percent weight loss in the first 3 days). Electrolytes can be initiated after urination (usually by 24 hours of birth) at a ratio of 3:1:1 for sodium:potassium:calcium (initially balanced with half chloride and half acetate and phosphate). In the first 72 hours after birth, serum and urine electrolyte readings should be obtained every 12 hours to estimate salt balance and appropriateness of fluid therapy. This approach to metabolic balance proves accurate, since preterm neonates lose free water principally through evaporation (not sweating), and in the absence of substantial output of stool or gastric drainage they have no other body fluids except urine, and thus no other electrolyte losses.

Protein is provided by a mixture of crystalline amino acids (e.g., FreAmine II or Trophamine), which can be administered after 1 to 2 days of age at an initial rate of 0.5 g per kilogram per day, increasing in increments of

TABLE 3   Clinical Monitoring During Enteral Feeding

1. Check for gastric residuals at least every 2 hours; supplement residual with formula up to the desired volume.
2. Replace nasogastric tube every 12 hours (use No. 5 or No. 8 French size).
3. Measure abdominal girth every 2 hours.
4. Perform abdominal examination every 2 hours for distention/tension/tenderness/bowel sounds/masses.
5. Record frequency and consistency of stools.
6. Check stools for occult blood (Hematest) each bowel movement; exclude artifacts, anal fissures.
7. Check for reducing substances with Clinitest tablets at least once per day.

TABLE 4   When to Discontinue Feeding for "NEC Alert" Surveillance

1. Residuals $\geq 50\%$ of interval volume $\times$ 2 to 3 feedings.
2. Abdominal/distention/decreased bowel sounds/abdominal mass.
3. Occult or gross blood in the stools.
4. Frequent apnea/respiratory deterioration.
5. Hypotension (shock)/poor peripheral perfusion.
6. Persistent hypoxemia.
7. "Unstable" patient.
8. Reducing substances present in stool.*

* Consider changing formula to lactose-free product.

0.5 g per kilogram per day to a maximum of 2.5 or 3.0 g per kilogram per day. The best nutritional or "safe" protein intake is not clearly established; however, these guidelines approach in utero accretion rates without causing metabolic acidemia. Excessive protein (6 g per kilogram per day or higher) is associated with lower IQ scores and strabismus at 4 to 6 years of age. Excessive amino acids are obviously dangerous, as evidenced from brain damage associated with inborn errors of metabolism (e.g., phenylketonuria, Hartnup's disease).

The chief advantage of providing protein early in life goes beyond growth requirements. Urea derived from protein turnover also assists in establishing the countercurrent multiplier system of the renal medulla augmenting urine concentrating ability.

Intravenous fat emulsions (10 percent or 20 percent suspension: Intralipid or Liposyn) should be the last parenteral component to be instituted. Various reports link its use to impaired immune defenses, lipoid pneumonia, increased pulmonary vascular resistance, decreased platelet adhesiveness, and dissociation of unconjugated bilirubin from protein-binding sites. Although these potential complications merit consideration, intravenous fats are an important caloric source (1.1 or 2.2 kcal per milliliter, respectively) and provide essential fatty acids as linoleic acid. Fats are cleared by lipoprotein lipase more slowly in preterm and small for gestational age than in term infants. Thus, it is recommended that serum turbidity checks be performed prior to instituting the next dose. In addition, infusions must be given as close to the infusion site as possible, distal to the in-line filter, and preferably over 12 to 20 hours (emulsions are not stable when mixed with protein solutions and electrolytes). Liver function tests need to be followed at least weekly. Intravenous fat therapy is discontinued for any evidence of liver dysfunction (elevated serum glutamic-oxaloacetic transaminase or serum glutamic-pyruvic transaminase levels) or cholestatic jaundice. In general, the dose of intravenous lipid is started and maintained at 0.5 g per kilogram per day (to provide essential fatty acids) even for respirator-dependent neonates. In clinically stable (predictable) infants without liver dysfunction, advances of 0.5 g per kilogram per day are made daily until 30 to 50 percent of total calories are provided by fat.

Vitamins and trace elements are conventionally added to parenteral solutions according to standard guidelines and formulations (e.g., M.V.I.-Pediatric, Multivitamin Infusate-12, and Table 5).

General Comments on Nutrition

It is recommended that all very low birth weight neonates should be gavage fed until they regain their birth weight and achieve a weight of more than 1,500 g or if the respiratory rate is more than 60 breaths per minute (nothing by mouth if it is more than 80 breaths per minute). In most circumstances it is advisable to begin a combination of both oral (see Table 2) and intravenous (see Table 5) nutrients. Early in life, the intravenous route of nutrition predominates, with the transition to oral intake (more than 50 percent of calories plus fluids given by mouth) occurring at approximately 2 weeks of postnatal age. Once at least 80 kcal per kilogram per day (or maximal guidelines) is achieved by the intravenous route (and full-strength formula orally), as the volume of oral intake increases, the intravenous volume of infusate is decreased in equivalent amounts to maintain fluid balance. At this point there is no need to recalculate parenteral solutions; the patient is simply weaned from the intravenous route by adjusting corresponding volumes (infusion rates) and oral intake. If oral feeding is not tolerated, the intravenous solution is adequate for all nutritional requirements and the rate is simply increased while oral fluids are reduced.

Peripheral veins are adequate for dextrose solutions less than or equal to 12 percent. Higher dextrose concentrations, calcium infusions, and high potassium concen-

TABLE 5   Daily Nutritional and Vitamin Requirements for Low Birth Weight Infants*

Total Nutrients	Per 100 Cal	Per kg/day	Vitamins	Total (Vitamins) Per Day†
Calories	100	100–140	A	1,400–2,500 IU
Water	—	130–200 ml	Thiamine	0.4 mg
Protein	1.8	3–4 g (10–15%)	Riboflavin	0.5 mg
Carbohydrate	—	10–15 g (45–55%)	Pyridoxine	0.25 mg
Fat	3.3	5–7 g (30–45%)	B_{12}	1.0 μg
Sodium	0.9	2–4 mEq	C	30–50 mg
Chloride	1.6	0.5–2 mEq	D	400 IU
Potassium	2.1	0.5–2 mEq	E	5–100 IU
Calcium	50 mg	20–40 mg	Niacin	6.0 mg
Phosphorus	25 mg	20–30 mg	Panthenol	—
Magnesium	6 mg	3–6 mg	Folic acid	0.35 mg
Iron	—	6 mg/day	K	1.5 mg

* Adapted from Klaus MH, Fanaroff AA. Care of the high-risk neonate. Philadelphia: WB Saunders, 1986.
† Start vitamin supplementation between the fifth and tenth days of life.
‡ Adequate to maintain normal urine output of 1–3 ml/kg/hr.

trations (greater than or equal to 60 mEq per liter) are more likely to cause phlebitis or to slough fragile skin if they infiltrate. Therefore, it may be advisable to convert to a central venous catheter (never arterial) if prolonged parenteral nutrition is anticipated (e.g., more than 75 percent of fluids and nutrition are to be provided parenterally for more than 1 to 2 weeks). In all cases, a vascular access route should be dedicated to nutrition and not used for drug or blood product administration. Daily adjustments of electrolytes and medications can be delivered through an alternative intravenous site maintained with a heparin lock.

DIAGNOSIS OF NECROTIZING ENTEROCOLITIS

Feeding Intolerence

Early evidence of feeding intolerence is manifested by the clinical signs outlined in Table 4. It is prudent to withhold feedings for at least 12 to 24 hours after complete resolution of these findings and to convert to total parenteral nutrition during this time. Then during the period of observation, additional information is accumulated to assist in making subsequent decisions. This includes:

1. Abdominal x-ray films every 6 to 8 hours until abnormal signs resolve.
2. Serial blood counts and differential and platelet counts every 12 to 24 hours to look for falling hematocrit values or decreasing total white blood cell count, increasing bands, and dropping platelets—evidence of infection or bleeding.
3. Serial electrolyte determinations every 8 to 12 hours for signs of third spacing; urine specific gravity check after every voiding.
4. Hourly vital signs for evidence of shock.
5. Serial arterial blood gas determinations at least every 4 hours to identify developing metabolic acidosis.
6. Nasogastric tube connected to straight drainage: normal is less than 4 to 5 ml of clear secretions per 8-hour period; bile is *never* normal. Continuous suction for more than or equal to 5 ml per 8 hours.
7. Document abdominal examination and girth every hour.
8. Test all stools for heme.
9. Follow fluid balance carefully for evidence of third-spacing (edema, unexplained increase in body weight).
10. Stool culture to assist in early diagnosis of infection or for planning antibiotic therapy if it becomes necessary (outbreaks are reported with *Escherichia coli, Klebsiella, Salmonella*, clostridial species, *Staphylococcus epidermidis* and viruses).

Necrotizing Enterocolitis

It is clinically useful and a practical guideline (for house staff teaching) to define the clinical entity of NEC in only two ways:

1. The *classic clinical triad* of bile-stained emesis (or nasogastric drainage), abdominal distention or tenderness (ileus), and heme-positive or grossly bloody stools.
2. *Necrotizing enterocolitis with pneumatosis* as indicated by x-ray examination or by surgical pathology.

Approximately 10 to 20 percent of sick, very low birth weight neonates have feeding intolerance ("NEC Alert", see Table 4) requiring withholding feedings for evaluation at least once. If intolerance persists in the absence of the clinical triad or if the infant looks toxic, feedings are withheld and management proceeds according to the NEC protocol. The presence of portal venous gas and detection of new intra-abdominal masses are often early signs consistent with a diagnosis of NEC.

MEDICAL MANAGEMENT OF NECROTIZING ENTEROCOLITIS

Once the diagnosis is established, major management issues include abdominal decompression by nasogastric suction, administration of broad-spectrum antibiotics (ampicillin and gentamicin) as treatment for possible infection, circulatory support (dopamine/dobutamine and packed red blood cells, as indicated), and maintenance of hemostasis (serial platelet counts, prothrombin and partial thromboplastin times, then fresh frozen plasma and platelets as necessary). Because of extreme instability plus rapid progression of NEC, oral intake and parenteral nutrition (protein and fat) are converted to dextrose with electrolytes until the infant becomes stable again and liver function tests return to normal.

Other considerations include provision of additional *antibiotic coverage* (e.g., vancomycin) for *Staphyloccus epidermidis* organisms because of its recent emergence as a commonly recognized pathogen. On the other hand, it is not advisable to use oral aminoglycoside antibiotics prophylactically or therapeutically because of the emergence of resistant organisms, variable absorption through damaged intestinal mucosa, and poor distribution during the absence of peristaltic activity. Choices for intravenous antibiotics other than those recommended are targeted at organisms recovered from the blood or peritoneum at surgery or at those bacteria endemic to the intensive care unit service. The treatment is continued for 2 weeks even in the face of negative cultures. Because of the possibility of impaired renal function, aminoglycoside blood levels should be monitored regularly and doses adjusted accordingly.

Initially, to *support blood pressure* we recommend fresh frozen plasma (10 ml per kilogram per dose) if the hematocrit is adequate because it provides colloid volume (protein) as well as nonspecific blood components that may assist in resisting infections plus clotting factors. Serial assessment of clotting function requires excessive amounts of whole blood (typically 2.5 to 3.0 ml). Therefore an alternative to this test is to follow clotting status by placing 0.5 ml of whole blood in a plain glass tube. If the clot lyses within 2 hours at room temperature, the fibrinogen levels are below 50 mg per deciliter, and fresh frozen plasma should be administered.

Packed red blood cells (15 ml per kilogram per dose) are recommended to maintain the hematocrit above 40 ml per deciliter to ensure abundant oxygen delivery to compromised bowel, especially in respirator-dependent patients. As always, when considering administration of any blood product good judgment should be exercised to minimize risks of exposure to transfusion reactions, hepatitis virus, cytomegalovirus, and acquired immunodeficiency virus (HIV). Blood should be screened for each of the potential pathogens prior to administration.

Pharmacologic support of blood pressure can be provided by dopamine or dobutamine infusion at standard doses only after volume expansion (i.e., maintenance of central venous pressure at 5 to 10 cm of water). Rarely are exchange transfusions recommended to remove "toxins" in support of the circulation.

If *metabolic acidosis* persists, and before instituting therapy, it is important to distinguish among problems of oxygen delivery (vasodilation or hypovolemia causing low blood pressure, decreased cardiac output, or anemia), bacterial toxins (affecting cellular oxidative metabolism), and acidemia due to massive tissue necrosis or renal failure. In this context, bicarbonate infusions should be viewed as temporary support until more specific treatment (e.g., transfusion, blood pressure support) can be provided that will help reduce the production of metabolic acids (e.g., lactate).

Fluid and electrolyte disturbances are extremely common as a result of gastric suctioning, third spacing, and frequently associated renal failure following circulatory collapse. Serum, gastric, and urine electrolytes, body weight, hematocrit, urine output, urine specific gravity, and fluid administration must be regulated frequently (every 12 hours) in the first 48 hours after the diagnosis of NEC is made. For estimating colloid osmotic pressure, a convenient accurate measure of total serum solids from capillary tubes (capillary total proteins) can be obtained by tapping out serum on to a standard refractometer lens (at the time that capillary hematocrits are checked); then the total protein value is read directly.

Surgical Management

As with most issues concerning decision-making in NEC, there are divided opinions on the indications for surgery. A reasonable approach is to delay intervention if the infant is clinically stable unless evidence of free air in the abdomen indicates perforation of the viscus. At this time the surgical task of delineating boundaries of necrotic bowel in an evolving picture can be more readily achieved.

Abdominal masses or peritonitis are not absolute indications for surgery. These findings occur frequently and may resolve spontaneously without surgery. However, surgery should be considered in infants who have particularly toxic signs with evidence of necrosis (high serum potassium level in the absence of renal failure and in the absence of excessive potassium administration) or have persistence of a single dilated loop of bowel for more than 24 to 48 hours. Empiric consideration for surgery in these circumstances is important before the problem evolves into a picture of complete deterioration, including shock and renal failure, in which surgical mortality is virtually assured. Contributing equally to the dilemma is that too early entry into the abdomen may reveal no surgically treatable problem and can be a mistake in an extremely unstable patient.

Enthusiasm has waxed and waned for peritoneal lavage by paracentesis (as an aid in decision-making) for examination of peritoneal fluid for evidence of peritonitis or perforation (white blood cells, bacteria, bile, or meconium). The major short coming of this approach is the risk of bowel perforation during transcutaneous puncture in the face of ileus. Similarly, placement of peritoneal drains for perforation in unstable nonoperative extremely low birth weight patients remains a last resort, preferably to be avoided.

Surgery involves removal of necrotic tissue and creation of venting ostomies that are also sometimes useful to inspect visually in the postoperative period as an index of continued gut viability. (This is of practical value if the gut looks healthy; if not, it may have no significance). Efforts are made to preserve as much contiguous normal bowel as possible. Unfortunately, this is difficult to achieve because diseased, transmurally necrotic gut is often interspersed with unaffected areas without necrosis ("skip areas"). Recently, attempts have been made to preserve several of the healthy skip areas with the intention of performing subsequent re-anastomosis. A wider experience is necessary before recommending this approach. Finally, every effort should be made to preserve the ileocecal valve and distal ileum to facilitate surgical revisions and normal bowel habits in the future as well as to provide a surface for vitamin, iron, and bile resorption.

LONG-TERM OUTCOME

Overall recovery in the neonatal intensive care unit should be higher than 80 percent using current clinical approaches. Typical problems include malabsorption and the short gut syndrome (especially in surgically-treated patients), requiring prolonged periods of parenteral nutrition. In these circumstances, it is important to provide supplementation for trace elements, vitamin K, and vitamin B_{12}.

Fortunately, many infants can undergo reanastomosis before discharge from the neonatal intensive care unit and can therefore leave on full oral fluids. In some cases it is necessary to discharge the patient on supplemental parenteral nutrition to be administered at home. Long-term survivors have shown that as little as 10 to 15 cm of proximal bowel can hypertrophy enough after 5 years of age to permit parenteral support to be discontinued.

Surgical complications of medically managed NEC may also emerge with time and include strictures, adhesions, and bowel obstruction.

SUGGESTED READING

Brown EG, Sweet AY. Preventing necrotizing enterocolitis in neonates. JAMA 1978;; 240:2452–2454.

Clark DA, Thompson JE, Weiner LB, et al. Necrotizing enterocolitis: Intraluminal biochemistry in human neonates and a rabbit model. Pediatr Res 1985; 19:919–921.

Kanto WP Jr, Wilson R, Breart GL, et al. Perinatal events and necrotizing enterocolitis in premature infants. Am J Dis Child 1987; 141:167–169.

Klaus H, Fanaroff AA. Feeding and selected disorders of the gastrointestinal tract. In: Care of the high-risk neonate. Philadelphia: WB Saunders, 1986:pp 113–134.

Kliegman RM, Fanaroff AA. Necrotizing enterocolitis. N Engl J Med 1984; 310:1093–1101.

Kosloske AM, Pathogenesis and prevention of necrotizing enterocolitis: A hypothesis based on personal observation and a review of the literature. Pediatrics 1984; 74:1086–1092.

LaGamma EF, Ostertag SG, Birenbaum H. Failure of delayed oral feedings to prevent necrotizing enterocolitis. Am J Dis Child 1985; 139:385–389.

Lawrence G, Bates J, Gaul A. Pathogenesis of neonatal necrotising enterocolitis. Lancet 1982; 1:137–139.

Lucas A, Bloom SR, Green AA. Gastrointestinal peptides and the adaptation of extrauterine nutrition. Can J Physiol Pharmacol 1985; 527–537.

Ostertag SG, La Gamma EF, Reisen CE, Ferrentino FL. Early enteral feeding does not affect the incidence of necrotizing enterocolitis. Pediatrics 1986; 77:275–280.

NEONATAL ABSTINENCE SYNDROME

LORETTA P. FINNEGAN, M.D.

Infants born to heroin- or methadone-dependent mothers have a high incidence of neonatal abstinence syndrome. Less potent opiates or opiate-like agents also have been identified as precipitating neonatal opiate abstinence. These include propoxyphene hydrochloride, codeine, and pentazocine. A number of nonopiate central nervous system depressants have been implicated, including alcohol, barbiturates, bromide, chlordiazepoxide, diazepam, ethchlorvynol, diphenhydramine, and imipramine.

Neonatal opiate abstinence (from narcotics and barbiturates) is a generalized disorder characterized by signs and symptoms of central nervous system hyperirritability, gastrointestinal dysfunction, respiratory distress, and vague autonomic symptoms that include yawning, sneezing, mottling, and fever.

The time and onset of abstinence in infants exposed to psychoactive drugs in utero vary from shortly after birth to 2 weeks of age, but symptoms usually appear within 72 hours after birth. Many factors influence the time of onset in individual infants, including the type of drug used by the mother, the dosage, time of use before delivery, character of labor, type and amount of anesthesia or analgesia used during labor, maturity, nutritional status, and the presence of intrinsic disease in the infant. Late presentation of neonatal methadone abstinence has been observed, however, with symptoms appearing between 2 and 4 weeks of age in several infants. Fetal accumulation and delayed excretion of the drug due to tissue binding may account for such a delayed onset of symptoms.

Abstinence may be mild and transient, intermittent, delayed in onset, increasing in severity, stepwise, or biphasic, with acute withdrawal followed by improvement and then the onset of subacute withdrawal. Withdrawal seems to be more severe in infants whose mothers have taken large amounts of drugs for a long time. In general, *the closer to delivery a mother takes the drug, the greater the delay in onset of and the more severe the symptoms.*

The maturity of the infant's metabolic and excretory mechanisms plays an important role in the duration of symptoms, which can range from 6 days to 8 weeks. Although the infants are discharged from the hospital following drug therapy, symptoms of irritability may persist for 3 months or more. The infants may have hyperphagia, increased oral drive, sweating, hyperacusis, irregular sleep patterns, loose stools, and poor tolerance to being held or to abrupt change in position.

PHARMACOLOGIC MANAGEMENT

Many pharmacologic agents have been used in the treatment of neonatal abstinence, and some appear to be effective in relieving symptoms. The agents most commonly employed have been paregoric, phenobarbital, and diazepam.

Paregoric has been used for over 70 years with the rationale that narcotic abstinence symptoms are relieved most specifically by narcotic substitution. It can be orally administered, has no known adverse effects, and can provide a level of sedation that inhibits bowel motility, diminishing the loose stools frequently accompanying abstinence. Sucking has been found to be much closer to normal among paregoric-treated infants than among those treated with phenobarbital or diazepam. Disadvantages associated with paregoric are that high doses are often necessary, and the duration of therapy can often be longer with paregoric than with other drugs.

Phenobarbital has been used extensively for neonatal abstinence, since it suppresses the major symptoms through a nonspecific central nervous system depression. Phenobarbital is especially effective in controlling irritability and insomnia. Occasionally an infant paradoxically becomes more irritated after treatment, and although central nervous system symptoms are prevented by barbiturates, they do not prevent loose stools. It has been shown that some infants are not fully controlled even at doses that produce plasma levels considered to be in the toxic range.

Diazepam therapy has also been advocated in the treatment of neonatal abstinence and has been reported to be safe and effective in a short course of therapy. However, infants treated with diazepam have become severely obtunded and their sucking reflex is markedly diminished in comparison to infants treated with other drugs. Seizures have been seen more often in infants treated with diazepam than in those treated with paregoric.

Our experiences and research with neonatal abstinence show that treatment for infants exposed to only *narcotic* agents in utero is more often successful with paregoric than with either phenobarbital or diazepam. Paregoric is able to control withdrawal symptoms in over 90 percent of infants, whereas phenobarbital is successful in about 50 percent of infants, and diazepam is not at all successful in the treatment of any infant whose prenatal drug exposure is limited to narcotics. Treatment for infants exposed prenatally to multiple drugs is more often successful with phenobarbital than with paregoric or diazepam. Phenobarbital treatment is successful in about 90 percent of these infants, whereas paregoric is successful in 60 percent and diazepam in 40 percent.

Therefore, paregoric appears to be the drug of choice for the control of abstinence symptoms due exclusively to narcotic use. This supports the supposition that narcotic abstinence symptoms are most specifically relieved by narcotic substitution. Phenobarbital is most efficacious when the infant has been exposed perinatally to multiple drugs particularly when sedatives are used excessively. If multiple drugs are used but the primary drug of abuse is a narcotic, paregoric has been shown to be most useful. Diazepam appears to be the least efficacious of the three drugs.

NEONATAL ABSTINENCE SCORING SYSTEM

The scoring system is used to monitor the passively addicted neonate in a comprehensive and objective way, and it is essential for assessing the onset, progression, and diminution of symptoms of abstinence. The score is used to monitor the infant's clinical response to pharmacotherapeutic intervention necessary for the control of withdrawal symptoms as well as for detoxification (Fig. 1).

There has recently been an epidemic of cocaine use among women. One should be cautioned that the individual using cocaine frequently uses other psychoactive agents. In assessing neonatal abstinence in these cases, the clinician should be aware that abstinence may occur due to the narcotics and depressants that the mother may have used concomitantly with cocaine. When cocaine is the primary drug of abuse, most clinicians have not seen symptoms of abstinence significant enough to treat pharmacologically. Infants may react similarly to those exposed to amphetamines and show symptoms of lethargy intermittently with irritability, poor sucking patterns, and sleep disturbances. If narcotics and barbiturates have been used excessively along with the cocaine, indications for observation are the same, and the baby should be observed for 4 days. When cocaine is the primary drug, from a purely physical standpoint the infant need not stay in the nursery longer than the general requirement. Unfortunately, family disfunction, inadequate housing, and lack of infant supplies may often necessitate a longer period of observation.

The abstinence score lists 21 symptoms most commonly seen in the passively-addicted neonate. Signs are recorded as single entities or in several categories if they occur in varying degrees of severity. Each symptom and its associated

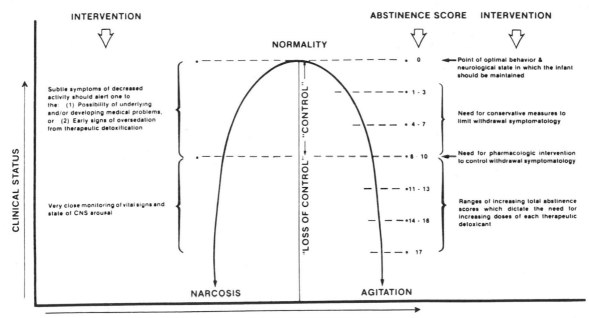

Figure 1 Management of the Neonatal Abstinence Syndrome.

degree of severity have been assigned a score. Higher scores are assigned to symptoms found in infants with more severe abstinence with consequent increased morbidity and mortality. The total abstinence score is determined by adding the score assigned to each symptom observed throughout the entire scoring interval. The scoring system is dynamic rather than static; that is, all of the signs and symptoms observed during the 4-hour intervals at which infant symptoms are monitored are point-totaled for that interval. Infants are assessed 2 hours after birth and then every 4 hours. If, at any point, the infant's score is 8 or higher, every 2-hour scoring is instituted and continued for 24 hours from the last total score of 8 or higher. If the 2-hour scores continue to be 7 or less for 24 hours, then 4-hour scoring intervals may be resumed.

If pharmacotherapy is not needed, the infant is scored for the first 5 days of life at the prescribed 4-hour intervals. If pharmacologic intervention is required, the infant is scored at 2- or 4-hour intervals, depending on whether the abstinence score is less than or greater than 8, as described above, throughout the duration of the therapy. Once therapy is discontinued, if there is no resurgence in the total score to 8 or higher after 3 days, scoring may be discontinued. If there is a resurgence of symptoms with scores consistently equaling 8 or higher, then scoring should be continued for a minimum of 4 days following discontinuation of therapy to ensure that the infant is not discharged prematurely with the consequent development of abstinence at home. **Note:** Because our studies have shown that 96 percent of children have the onset of withdrawal by the fourth day, we have decreased the length of stay from 5 to 4 days. Moreover, an additional day, although encompassing 100 percent of children is not financially feasible under DRGs.

The Neonatal Abstinence Scoring Sheet can be seen in Figure 2. Symptoms are listed on the left, with their respective scores listed to the right. Times of each evaluation are listed at the top, and the total score is listed for each evaluation. A new sheet should be started at the beginning of each day. The complete scoring system allows scoring as frequently as every 2 hours for a full 24-hour period on each sheet.

A "Comments" column has been provided so that the nursing and medical staff can record important notes regarding the infant's scoring and treatment and can make reference to relevant progress notes recorded in the infant's chart. Some important points to remember when using the score sheet are

1. The times designating the end of the scoring intervals (whether every 2 or 4 hours) have been left blank to permit the nursing staff to choose the most appropriate times for the scoring intervals in relation to effective planning and implementation of nursing care.
2. The first abstinence score should be recorded approximately 2 hours following the infant's admission to the nursery. This score reflects all infant behavior from admission to that first point in time when the scoring interval is completed (this is the first time indicated on the score sheet).
3. All infants should be scored at 4-hour intervals, except

when high scores indicate more frequent scoring.
4. All symptoms exhibited during the entire scoring interval, not just a single point in time, should be included.
5. The infant should be awakened to elicit reflexes and specified behavior. Sleeping should never be recorded for a scoring interval except under extreme circumstances when the infant has been unable to sleep for an extended period of time: more than 12 to 18 hours. If he or she is crying, the infant must be quieted before assessing muscle tone, respiratory rate, and the Moro reflex.
6. If the infant is awakened to be scored, one should not score him or her for diminished sleep after feeding.
7. Respirations are counted for one full minute.
8. The infant is scored if prolonged crying is exhibited, even though it may not be high-pitched in quality.
9. Temperatures should be taken rectally (mild pyrexia is an early sign indicating heat produced by increased muscle tone and tremors).
10. If the infant is sweating solely because of conservative nursing measures (e.g., swaddling), a point should not be given.

Before pharmacotherapy is initiated, one must rule out other common neonatal metabolic alterations that can mimic or compound abstinence (e.g., hypocalcemia, hypomagnesemia, hypoglycemia, and hypothermia). Serum glucose and calcium tests are indicated before therapy is initiated. Toxicologic examination of the urine, for a total of 25 ml collected immediately after birth, is necessary to ensure appropriate choice of pharmacotherapy. Urine collected after 24 to 36 hours of life is likely to be negative for qualitative toxicologic assessment.

Pharmacologic intervention is not indicated if consecutive total abstinence scores or the average of any three consecutive scores continues to be 7 or less. If pharmacotherapy is not indicated, the infant must be scored for a minimum of the first 4 days of life.

The total scores have been categorized into ranges of scores indicating the severity of abstinence in relation to functional disturbances in various physiologic systems. The total abstinence scores dictate the specific dose of the pharmacotherapeutic agents used to detoxify infants in two management regimens. In the score-dose titration approach, the initial dose of a specific pharmacotherapeutic agent (i.e., paregoric or phenobarbital) and all subsequent doses are determined by and titrated against the total abstinence score. In the phenobarbital loading dose approach, an initial dose of 20 mg per kilogram is administered in an attempt to achieve an expected therapeutic serum level with a single dose.

The need for pharmacologic intervention is indicated when the total abstinence score is 8 or higher for three consecutive scorings (e.g., 9–8–10) or when the average of any three consecutive scores is 8 or higher (e.g., 9–7–9). Once an infant's score is 8 or higher, the scoring interval automatically becomes 2 hours, so that the infant exhibits symptoms that are out of control for no longer than 4 to 6 hours before therapy is initiated.

If the infant's total score is 12 or higher for two con-

NEONATAL ABSTINENCE SCORING SYSTEM

SYSTEM	SIGNS AND SYMPTOMS	SCORE	AM						PM							COMMENTS
CENTRAL NERVOUS SYSTEM DISTURBANCES	Excessive High Pitched (Or other) Cry	2														Daily Weight:
	Continuous High Pitched (Or other) Cry	3														
	Sleeps < 1 Hour After Feeding	3														
	Sleeps < 2 Hours After Feeding	2														
	Sleeps < 3 Hours After Feeding	1														
	Hyperactive Moro Reflex	2														
	Markedly Hyperactive Moro Reflex	3														
	Mild Tremors Disturbed	1														
	Moderate-Severe Tremors Disturbed	2														
	Mild Tremors Undisturbed	3														
	Moderate-Severe Tremors Undisturbed	4														
	Increased Muscle Tone	2														
	Excoriation (Specific Area)	1														
	Myoclonic Jerks	3														
	Generalized Convulsions	5														
METABOLIC/VASOMOTOR/RESPIRATORY DISTURBANCES	Sweating	1														
	Fever<101 (99-100.8 F./37.2-38.2C.)	1														
	Fever>101 (38.4C. and Higher)	2														
	Frequent Yawning (> 3-4 Times/Interval)	1														
	Mottling	1														
	Nasal Stuffiness	1														
	Sneezing (> 3-4 Times/Interval)	1														
	Nasal Flaring	2														
	Respiratory Rate > 60/min	1														
	Respiratory Rate > 60/min with Retractions	2														
GASTRO-INTESTINAL DISTURBANCES	Excessive Sucking	1														
	Poor Feeding	2														
	Regurgitation	2														
	Projectile Vomiting	3														
	Loose Stools	2														
	Watery Stools	3														
	TOTAL SCORE															
	INITIALS OF SCORER															

* Finnegan, L.P. Neonatal Abstinence Syndrome: Assessment and Pharmacotherapy Neonatal Therapy: An Update, Rubaltelli, F.F., and Granati, B., (Eds.), Exerpta Medica, Amsterdam-New York-Oxford, 1986.

Figure 2 Neonatal Abstinence Score sheet.

secutive intervals or the average of any two consecutive scores is 12 or higher, therapy should be initiated at the appropriate detoxicant dosage for that score before more than 4 hours elapse.

In summary, it is important to remember that all infants who meet the scoring criteria for pharmacologic intervention should have the prescribed detoxicant regimen started no longer than 4 to 6 hours following loss of control. The more severe the abstinence, as reflected by the total score, the greater the need to initiate pharmacotherapy as soon as possible. Finally, the longer the delay in initiation of appropriate pharmacologic intervention, the greater the risk of increased infant morbidity.

PHARMACOTHERAPEUTIC REGIMENS

Score-Dose Titration Approach

Once the criteria are met to initiate pharmacotherapy (indicated by the total abstinence scores), the total scores dictate the specific detoxicant dose as prescribed in Table 1. Because "steady state" levels of paregoric are not achieved, serum concentrations are not helpful in managing the infant. Serum levels of phenobarbital should be determined using micromethod blood samples every 24 hours throughout the treatment phase and until the serum concentration reaches a homeopathic level during detoxification.

Dosage adjustments and timing of dosage changes must be carefully monitored. An increase in a detoxicant dose is necessary at any time after the initiation of therapy when there have been three consecutive total scores of 8 or higher or an average of any three consecutive total scores of 8 or higher.

When a change in dose is indicated, the time intervals for the administration of the next dose should remain the same as the prescribed dosing schedule. For example, if the total withdrawal score indicates that an increase in dose is needed, the adjusted dose should be given on schedule (i.e., 4 hours following the previous dose with paregoric and 8 hours following the previous dose with phenobarbital). These stepwise increases in dosage should be implemented every 4 to 8 hours (i.e., 4-hour increments with paregoric and 8-hour increments with phenobarbital) until the total abstinence scores consistently fall below 8.

TABLE 1 Titration Dosage Schedule According to Abstinence Score

Abstinence Score	Detoxicant	
	Paregoric	Phenobarbital
8–10	0.8 ml/kg/day: every 4 hours	6 mg/kg/day: every 8 hours
11–13	1.2 ml/kg/day: every 4 hours	8 mg/kg/day: every 8 hours
14–16	1.6 ml/kg/day: every 4 hours	10 mg/kg/day: every 8 hours
17 or above	2.0 ml/kg/day: every 4 hours; continue at 0.4 ml increments until control is achieved	12 mg/kg/day: every 8 hours

Substantial changes in the weight of the infant indicate a need to recalculate the base dose. This will necessitate weight-related dosage adjustments during any phase of pharmacologic intervention (i.e., dosage increases, maintenance doses, and dosage reductions).

Once abstinence is controlled using the prescribed dosage schedule, the following procedures should be implemented to (1) maintain control for 72 hours, and (2) initiate the detoxification process. If paregoric is the agent used, the dose administered to achieve control should be maintained for 72 hours before a dosage reduction schedule (i.e., detoxification) is initiated. Detoxification is achieved by decreasing the total daily dose by 10 percent every 24 hours. When dosage levels reach 0.5 ml per kilogram per day, paregoric may be discontinued. If an infant's abstinence scores remain low (1 to 3 range) after a minimum of 72 hours of detoxification, usually a rare event, the detoxification rate may be increased with caution to 15 to 20 percent and should never exceed 20 percent.

If phenobarbital is used, the dose administered to achieve the phenobarbital serum level necessary to control abstinence should be noted. If the infant is metabolizing and excreting phenobarbital at an expected rate, the infant should have a $1:1\pm2$ ratio between milligrams of phenobarbital administered and micrograms per milliliter of phenobarbital in the blood serum. This ratio or an increase in the blood serum provides the data necessary for detoxification from phenobarbital.

The objective in detoxifying an infant with phenobarbital is to allow the phenobarbital serum level to fall approximately 10 percent every 24 hours. This is accomplished by shifting from the score-dose titration schedule to the following dosage schedules, assuming the aforementioned $1:1\pm2$ dose to serum level ratio exists:

1. Maintenance of the same phenobarbital serum level is achieved by administering phenobarbital 4 to 6 mg per kilogram per day in three divided doses (every 8 hours).
2. A 10 percent decrease in the phenobarbital serum level is accomplished with 1 to 3 mg per kilogram per day in three divided doses (every 8 hours).

The rationale for the foregoing maintenance and/or detoxification approach is based on our current knowledge of the kinetics of phenobarbital. Continuation of the total daily dosage (in three divided doses) required to achieve control of the abstinence will result in a continuous increase in the phenobarbital serum level beyond that serum level at which control was achieved. For example, if phenobarbital, 10 mg per kilogram per day in three divided doses, was administered for 3 days to achieve control and phenobarbital serum levels of 28 μg per milliliter, we know that continuation of this same dose would most likely result in a rapid rise in the phenobarbital serum levels and overcontrol of the symptoms.

Phenobarbital Loading Dose Approach

Important definitions include:

Loading Dose. This term refers to the administration of a single priming dose of phenobarbital (i.e., 20 mg per kilogram per day) in a quantity sufficient (i.e., achieving a serum level of 18 to 22 μg per milliliter) to provide for drug distribution throughout the body compartments as well as a therapeutic level in the brain and cerebrospinal fluid.

Steady State. This is a state in which the amount of phenobarbital absorbed and distributed per dosing interval is equal to the amount eliminated (excreted and metabolized) per dosing interval, thus resulting in a constant therapeutic level, as determined by serial measurements of plasma concentration.

Maintenance Dose. Once the effective dose of phenobarbital is determined (i.e., control of abstinence with plasma concentrations between 20 and 70 μg per milliliter), the maintenance dose is the amount of phenobarbital (usually 2 to 6 mg per kilogram per day) administered every 24 hours to maintain the effective steady state level.

Dosage Increase. Once the loading dose has been administered, it is often necessary to increase the plasma concentration of phenobarbital to attain control. This may be accomplished by administering phenobarbital 10 mg per kilogram as frequently as every 12 hours until control or a plasma concentration of 70 μg per milliliter has been reached, or signs of clinical toxicity appear.

In some "atypical" infants, the amounts of phenobarbital prescribed in this protocol are insufficient to either maintain an effective steady state level or increase the serum levels at the predicted rates. See Figure 3 for the dynamics of the phenobarbital loading dose regimen.

If an infant meets the criteria for initiation of therapy, a loading dose of 20 mg per kilogram followed by micromethod blood samples is given to determine phenobarbital serum levels at 12 and 24 hours after administration of the loading dose. A loading dose of 20 mg per kilogram

should be administered *only once* and should result in the desired therapeutic serum phenobarbital level of 20 μg per milliliter ± 2 μg per milliliter (i.e., 18 to 22 μg per milliliter). Occasionally levels ranging from 15 to 25 μg per milliliter are observed following the loading dose.

If the **total withdrawal score is** <**8** (i.e., control is achieved) after the desirable therapeutic serum level (i.e., 18 to 22 μg per milliliter) is attained, the level is maintained for 72 hours. Dosing following the loading dose is considered maintenance and is initiated 24 hours following the initial dose.

The desirable therapeutic serum level is maintained by a daily dose of 4 to 6 mg per kilogram per day. Maintenance should be started with 5 mg per kilogram per day every 24 hours, and this dose is adjusted as necessary (i.e., increased to 6 mg per kilogram per day or decreased to 4 mg per kilogram per day) to maintain the desired steady state phenobarbital level of 18 to 22 μg per milliliter, determined by 24-hour serial measurements of plasma concentrations.

If the **total score continues to be** >**8** (poor control) after the loading dose and the desired therapeutic level of 18 to 22 μg per milliliter is achieved, the serum phenobarbital level should be increased by increments of 10 μg per milliliter per 12-hour period until control is achieved. This can be accomplished by administering phenobarbital at 10 mg per kilogram every 12 hours (12 hours following administering loading dose of phenobarbital) concomitant with verification of expected plasma concentrations of phenobarbital. This stepwise increase of 10 μg per milliliter should be continued every 12 hours only until (1) control is attained (i.e., the total score is <8), or (2) the serum level reaches 70 μg per milliliter *or* (3) the infant demonstrates signs of phenobarbital toxicity. If the total

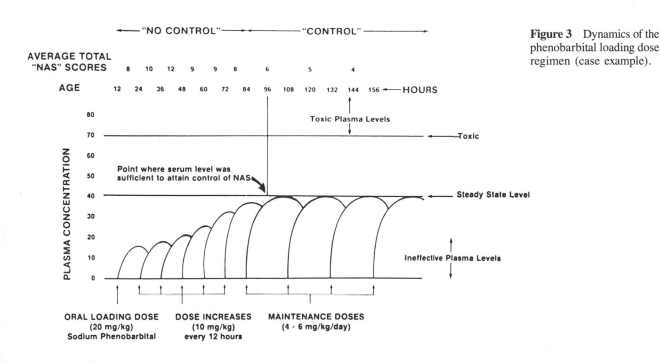

Figure 3 Dynamics of the phenobarbital loading dose regimen (case example).

serum phenobarbital level reaches 70 μg per milliliter or higher and control still has not been attained, the choice of detoxicant should be re-evaluated before attempting to exceed this level.

After 72 hours of steady state maintenance in a clinically controlled situation (verified by constant serum levels and total scores of <8), detoxification can begin by allowing the phenobarbital serum levels to decline at a rate of 10 to 20 percent per 24 hours, ideally 15 percent, by administering phenobarbital 2 mg per kilogram per day. If serum phenobarbital levels indicate that detoxification is too rapid (>20 percent in 24 hours), the maintenance dose should be increased to 3 mg per kilogram per day. If total abstinence scores escalate to 8 or higher, detoxification is stopped. The phenobarbital dose should be increased to achieve the serum level at which the infant was previously controlled. This level should be maintained, assuming the infant is controlled again, for 48 hours before detoxification is started again. If detoxification is too slow (10 percent per 24 hours), the maintenance dose should be decreased to 1 mg per kilogram per day. Once the serum level falls below 10 μg per milliliter, and the total score is <8, the phenobarbital should be discontinued.

After the phenobarbital is discontinued, the infant is observed for 72 hours for increased withdrawal symptoms. If the total score continues to be <8, the infant can be discharged. If the score escalates to 8 or higher after discontinuation of therapy, the infant is observed until control re-occurs or he or she is re-evaluated for further pharmacologic intervention.

During the initiation and maintenance of infants on paregoric or phenobarbital, observations for central nervous system depression are made. These include

1. Diminished or absent reflexes—Moro, sucking, swallowing, Galant, Perez, tonic neck, corneal, grasp (palmar or plantar)
2. Truncal (central) or circumoral cyanosis or persistent mottling not associated with cold
3. Decreased muscle tone with passive resistance to extension of extremities or decreased neck or trunk tone
4. Altered state of arousal (e.g., obtunded or comatose)
5. Diminished response to painful stimuli
6. Failure at visual following
7. Hypothermia
8. Altered respirations—irregular (periodic breathing in full-term infants), shallow (decreased air entry), decreased respiratory rate (<20 per minute), apnea
9. Cardiac alterations—irregular rate, distant heart sounds with weak peripheral pulses, heart rate of 80 to 100 beats per minute, poor peripheral perfusion (pale, grey, mottled), cardiac arrest.

Any infant who exhibits a precipitous drop in a total score of 8 points or higher should be monitored for vital signs immediately.

It is important to determine whether any underlying medical problems are developing, such as sepsis, meningitis, hypocalcemia, or hypoglycemia. Detection of underlying medical problems may be difficult because poorly controlled abstinence may mimic and/or disguise many common neonatal problems.

An infant may be increasingly depressed by a pharmacotherapeutic agent that is not drug-specific for abstinence. This situation may be reflected in the gradual development of symptoms of depression with concomitant poorly controlled abstinence and requires re-evaluation for appropriateness of pharmacologic intervention.

One must always assess the pharmacologic intervention for efficacy in a particular infant. Two common situations indicate that pharmacotherapy must be reassessed: (1) central nervous system depression, and (2) failure to achieve "control" despite aggressive pharmacotherapeutic intervention and/or near-toxic serum levels of therapeutic agents. In these situations, the following measures are indicated:

1. Evaluate the infant for metabolic derangements, sepsis, and central nervous system disturbances to detect underlying problems compounding the clinical picture. Laboratory evaluations including serum electrolyte, calcium, and glucose determinations, and blood cultures are indicated.
2. Review the maternal drug history along with both maternal and infant urine toxicology results to ensure appropriate pharmacotherapy. If the mother has abused barbiturates along with other psychoactive agents not including narcotics, phenobarbital is always the drug of choice. If the maternal drug history and toxicologic findings indicate that only opiates were administered prenatally, therapeutically administered nonopiates (even at high plasma concentrations) may be ineffective in controlling the symptoms of narcotic abstinence. A change to paregoric may be indicated. If maternal drug history and toxicologic findings indicate that narcotics are the primary drug of maternal abuse, although other addicting agents were also used, paregoric will be most efficacious.
3. If a single pharmacotherapeutic agent is ineffective in controlling abstinence symptoms, consider a combination of therapeutic agents.

In conclusion, rapid recognition, careful assessment, and appropriate treatment of neonatal abstinence will augment the satisfactory initial and long-term outcome of drug-exposed infants.

Acknowledgments: The author wishes to acknowledge the contributions of those individuals who assisted in the development of the Neonatal Abstinence Score and those who have been involved in the clinical trials in the evaluation of infants undergoing abstinence using the scoring system. These include Reuben Kron, M.D., Bonnie MacNew, B.S.N., M.S.N., the neonatal nursing staff of the Philadelphia General Hospital and the Thomas Jefferson University Hospital, the neonatology staff and the resident staff of the Philadelphia General Hospital, the Children's Hospital of Philadelphia, and the Thomas Jefferson University Hospital. The author also wishes to acknowledge the editing assistance of Dr. Sandra Tunis and Tina Wong in the preparation of the manuscript.

NEONATAL SEIZURES

DONALD YOUNKIN, M.D.

Seizures are a common neurologic problem in newborn babies. The exact incidence is unknown, but rates as high as 1.4 percent have been reported. In the intensive care nursery the incidence is much higher; up to 25 percent of the infants may have seizures. *The immature nervous system is relatively resistant to the initiation and propagation of seizures; consequently, neonatal seizures indicate a serious neurologic problem.* In animal models neonatal seizures: increase cerebral blood flow and metabolism; decrease brain pH, phosphocreatine, and ATP; inhibit DNA synthesis in the brain; and delay the achievement of normal developmental milestones. We assume that similar changes may occur in the human newborn, and believe that neonatal seizures require prompt, vigorous management.

DIAGNOSIS

The diagnosis of neonatal seizures is based on a combination of clinical observation and electroencephalographic (EEG) recording. Clinical observation can be used to divide seizures into five subtypes: subtle, tonic, focal-clonic, multifocal-clonic, and myoclonic.

Subtle seizures are the most common type and are characterized by repetitive and stereotyped oral, facial, or ocular activity. Lip smacking, tongue thrusting, eye deviation, and eye blinking are typical manifestations of subtle seizures; bicycling or pedaling movements are another manifestation. On rare occasions, cessation of motor activity and apnea can be manifestations of subtle seizure activity; however, these are usually indicative of other disorders. Since all these movements occur frequently in normal babies, it is impossible to use clinical observation alone to distinguish between normal movements and subtle seizures. Rather, *simultaneous EEG recording and observation, ideally recorded by split-screen video and EEG, is required to identify subtle seizures.*

Tonic seizures may be either focal (involving one limb) or generalized (involving the entire body). They are characterized by sudden increases in muscle tone, usually extension. Tonic seizures are described frequently as posturing or stiffening, and may be confused with decerebrate and decorticate "posturing." The latter indicates brain stem injury, not seizures. Tonic seizures are frequently related to intraventricular hemorrhage, especially in premature babies.

Focal-clonic seizures consist of repetitive jerking movements of one limb and must be carefully distinguished from "jitteriness," which is usually stimulus sensitive, abolished by changing limb position, and rhythmic.

Multifocal-clonic seizures involve clonic activity in several different body areas, frequently with irregular migration from one body part to another. *Myoclonic seizures* occur infrequently and are characterized by sudden flexion or extension of arms and legs. They may occur individually or repetitively.

Although clinical characterization of seizures is useful, only a small percentage of brain ictal activity is manifested as clinical seizures. Because of the subtle nature of most seizure activity, it is difficult to distinguish between ictal and nonictal behavior. Consequently, prolonged EEG recordings are necessary in the diagnosis and management of neonatal seizures. Serial EEGs are useful in following therapeutic response and can help in estimating the prognosis. Several different ictal EEG patterns have been described in the immature brain, including: (1) migrating sharp waves, (2) monorhythmic delta activity at 1 to 4Hz, (3) positive or negative spikes at 2 to 6Hz, (4) spike and slow wave complexes, and (5) runs of alpha activity at 6 to 10Hz with amplitudes of 25 to 30 microvolts. In addition, the interictal EEG may demonstrate abnormal background activity with excessive sharp EEG transients. Once seizure activity has been confirmed, attention should be focused on discovering the cause and instituting treatment.

ETIOLOGY

Although the etiology of neonatal seizures is extremely diverse, *most can be attributed to hypoxic-ischemic encephalopathy (about 65 percent of neonatal seizures), intracranial hemorrhage (about 15 percent), metabolic disturbances (hypoglycemia, hypocalcemia), intracranial infection, and cerebral cortical dysgenesis.*

The age at onset of seizures and the gestational age of the infant are frequently helpful in determining the cause. *Most seizures beginning within the first 12 to 24 hours in premature and full-term babies are due to hypoxic-ischemic encephalopathy from perinatal asphyxia.* Other causes of seizures during the first day are congenital infections (toxoplasmosis, cytomegalovirus, herpes, rubella), cerebral dysgenesis, stroke, and familial neonatal seizures. Pyridoxine dependency can cause in utero seizures and should be considered in any baby with early-onset seizures. In our own experience, local anesthetic intoxication (mepivacaine, lidocaine) is a rare cause of neonatal seizures, but the incidence varies, depending on patient population and management of obstetric anesthesia. Seizures caused by local anesthetics are usually tonic, occur within the first 6 hours, and are associated with apnea, bradycardia, hypotonia, and fixed, dilated pupils.

Seizures with onset between 1 and 2 days of life are frequently indicative of intracranial hemorrhage (laceration of the tentorium of the falx, cerebral contusion, intraventricular hemorrhage), metabolic abnormalities (hypoglycemia or hypocalcemia, especially in babies who are premature, small for gestational age, or infants of diabetic mothers), bacterial meningitis, or drug withdrawal.

Seizures occurring after 3 days of life are most frequently due to intracranial infection, cerebral cortical dysgenesis, or inborn errors of metabolism (urea cycle defects, amino acidemias, organic acidemia).

CLINICAL AND LABORATORY EVALUATION

A complete physical examination should be performed in all babies with suspected seizures. In addition to vital signs and cardiac and pulmonary findings, the general physical examination should include notation of: (1) estimated gestational age—seizures are much more common in full-term babies and rare in premature babies of less than 34 weeks' gestation; (2) dysmorphic features that suggest cerebral dysgenesis; (3) head circumference—microcephaly may indicate congenital infection or cerebral dysgenesis, and macrocephaly suggests hydrocephalus; (4) evidence of cranial trauma—needle puncture sites on the scalp, fractures, or extreme molding; and (5) examination of the skin for rash or stigmata of neurocutaneous diseases.

The neurologic examination should include description of seizure activity and mental status (level of consciousness). An estimate of intracranial pressure can be based on fontanelle tension and cranial suture separation. Cranial nerve examination is used to evaluate brain stem function, and should include: visualization of the fundi (choreoretinitis, developmental defect, or papilledema); observation of pupillary reactivity, spontaneous and reflex eye movements; facial movements; sucking and swallowing; and gag reflex. The quality and symmetry of motor activity, muscle tone, and posture should be noted but is not very helpful in localizing brain lesions in babies.

The laboratory evaluation of any newborn with suspected seizures should include measurement of serum glucose, calcium, magnesium, and electrolytes, as well as cerebrospinal fluid analysis (glucose, protein, cell count, differential, and culture). If clinically indicated, the following studies must be obtained: ammonia; arterial blood gas measurement; urine amino acids and organic acids; and maternal and fetal titers against toxoplasmosis, herpes, cytomegalovirus, coxsackievirus, rubella, and syphilis. Infants weighing less than 1,500 g or who are suspected of having head trauma should undergo cranial ultrasonography for intraventricular and intracerebral hemorrhage. Infants suspected of having cerebral dysgenesis should also receive a computed tomographic (CT) scan or magnetic resonance imaging (MRI).

TREATMENT

As mentioned, the neonatal nervous system is relatively resistant to seizure initiation and propagation, and the presence of neonatal seizures represents serious neurologic complications. Consequently, neonatal seizures should be treated vigorously; our current approach to therapy is outlined in Table 1.

Blood glucose levels should be checked (Dextrostix) before anticonvulsants are started, and hypoglycemia corrected with 10 percent dextrose (2 mg per kilogram intravenously).

Phenobarbital is the drug of choice for managing neonatal seizures. At the first sign, it should be administered with an initial loading dose of 20 mg per kilogram, administered slowly by the intravenous route over

TABLE 1 Treatment of Neonatal Seizures

Initial Therapy

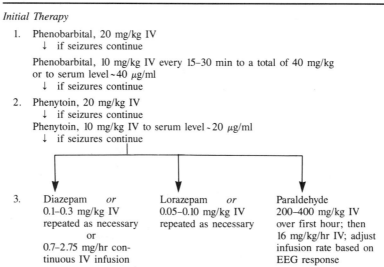

1. Phenobarbital, 20 mg/kg IV
   ↓ if seizures continue

   Phenobarbital, 10 mg/kg IV every 15–30 min to a total of 40 mg/kg or to serum level ~40 μg/ml
   ↓ if seizures continue

2. Phenytoin, 20 mg/kg IV
   ↓ if seizures continue
   Phenytoin, 10 mg/kg IV to serum level ~20 μg/ml
   ↓ if seizures continue

3.
| Diazepam *or* 0.1–0.3 mg/kg IV repeated as necessary *or* 0.7–2.75 mg/hr continuous IV infusion | Lorazepam *or* 0.05–0.10 mg/kg IV repeated as necessary | Paraldehyde 200–400 mg/kg IV over first hour; then 16 mg/kg/hr IV; adjust infusion rate based on EEG response |

Since clinical detection of seizures is frequently inaccurate, it is helpful to have continuous EEG monitoring during the initiation of therapy. The EEG is especially helpful in making decisions regarding additional diazepam or lorazepam, or in adjusting the rate of paraldehyde infusion.

Maintenance Therapy

1. Phenobarbital, 3–4 mg/kg/day IV, IM, PO starting 12 hr after loading dose
2. Phenytoin, 3–4 mg/kg/day IV starting 12 hr after loading dose
3. Primidone, 12–20 mg/kg/day

5 to 10 minutes; this usually achieves a serum level of approximately 20 μg per milliliter. If seizures persist, subsequent doses of 10 mg per kilogram should be administered intravenously every 15 to 30 minutes until the serum level is greater than 40 μg per milliliter. Maintenance therapy can be started 12 to 24 hours after the initial loading dose; the usual maintenance dose is 3 to 4 mg per kilogram per day divided every 12 hours (depending on clinical status, maintenance phenobarbital can be administered intravenously, intramuscularly, or orally). In neonates, the serum half-life is variable: e.g., the half-life of phenobarbital is approximately 100 hours after 2 weeks of therapy, but approximately 20 hours after 1 month of therapy. Consequently, phenobarbital levels should be monitored closely and the daily dose adjusted to maintain a therapeutic phenobarbital concentration.

If clinical and EEG-revealed seizures persist despite phenobarbital concentrations greater than 40 μg per milliliter, phenytoin (Dilantin) should be added. The initial loading dose of phenytoin is 20 mg per kilogram administered intravenously at a rate of 1 to 3 mg per kilogram per minute; this usually achieves a serum concentration of about 15 μg per milliliter. The electrocardiogram (ECG) should be monitored at this time, because rapid phenytoin administration may produce heart block and hypotension. If seizures persist, subsequent intravenous doses of 10 mg per kilogram can be given to achieve a serum level of approximately 20 μg per milliliter. Phenytoin is not well absorbed orally or intramuscularly, so subsequent maintenance doses must be given intravenously. The normal maintenance dose is approximately 3 to 4 mg per kilogram per day divided every 12 hours; maintenance therapy should be started 12 to 24 hours after loading with phenytoin. The serum half-life of phenytoin is also age-dependent and may fall during the immediate neonatal period from 104 hours to 4 to 5 hours; consequently, frequent blood level determinations are necessary to maintain the proper daily dosage.

Approximately 70 percent of neonatal seizures respond to phenobarbital; about 90 percent respond to a combination of phenobarbital and phenytoin. If seizures persist despite adequate levels of phenobarbital and phenytoin, other medications should be considered, including diazepam, lorazepam, paraldehyde, and primidone.

The use of diazepam (Valium) is controversial because it may increase the risk of respiratory arrest and circulatory collapse, especially when phenobarbital and phenytoin have been given. In addition, parenteral diazepam has a sodium benzoate vehicle that may uncouple the bilirubin-albumin complex, thus increasing the risk of kernicterus. Despite these concerns, we have used diazepam on several occasions without encountering these difficulties; the usual loading dose is 0.1 to 0.3 mg per kilogram intravenously. The anticonvulsant properties of diazepam are relatively short, but the sedative effect can be prolonged. Continuous infusions of diazepam are useful in treating status epilepticus in older children and adults, but we do not have experience with its continuous infusion in neonates. Successful treatment of status epilepticus in term infants has been reported with continuous intravenous infusion of diazepam at rates of 0.7 to 2.75 mg per hour for up to 11 days.

Lorazepam is another benzodiazepine that has been very effective in adults and children with status epilepticus; a single dose frequently controls seizures for several hours. A detailed investigation of the benefit of lorazepam in neonatal status epilepticus has not been published, but preliminary reports are very encouraging. The loading dose is 0.05 to 0.10 mg per kilogram, given over approximately 2 minutes. As with diazepam, lorazepam may be repeated several times if seizures persist.

Paraldehyde is also useful in treating neonatal status epilepticus, but because of difficulties with preparation and handling we use it infrequently. Paraldehyde may be administered intravenously as a 5 percent solution in D$_5$W; 200 to 400 mg per kilogram are infused over the first hour, followed by a continuous infusion of 16 mg per kilogram per hour. When we use a paraldehyde infusion, we employ continuous EEG monitoring and adjust the infusion rate to abolish EEG seizures. Paraldehyde can also be administered rectally, 2 ml mixed with 2 ml of mineral oil, but may cause rectal mucosal irritation.

Another anticonvulsant that has been effective for neonatal seizures is primidone, administered orally in a loading dose of 15 to 20 mg per kilogram with maintenance doses of 12 to 20 mg per kilogram per day. Parenteral primidone is not available. Primidone is not useful in treating status epilepticus, but may be for long-term management of neonatal seizures.

DURATION OF THERAPY

Anticonvulsant therapy must be tailored to the individual needs of the child, so it is difficult to provide definitive guidelines on the duration of therapy. *Most neonatal seizures are secondary to an acute cerebral insult and thus tend to resolve within 2 to 4 days*; therefore, most babies can be managed on a single anticonvulsant (usually phenobarbital) after the fourth day. Two to 3 days after seizures have been controlled, we discontinue phenytoin and continue phenobarbital. It is our policy to discontinue all anticonvulsants by 10 to 14 days if seizures have been easily controlled with anticonvulsants, and if the EEG, head ultrasound, CT, and clinical examination results are normal. *If there has been status epilepticus or if seizures have not been controlled with phenobarbital alone, we continue anticonvulsants for at least 3 months.* Children with cerebral dysgenesis, other parenchymal abnormalities, abnormal neurologic examination results, persistently abnormal EEG studies, inborn errors or metabolism, or familial neonatal seizures should receive maintenance phenobarbital.

PROGNOSIS

The long-term prognosis for babies with neonatal seizures is poor. With improvements in perinatal and neonatal care, the mortality rate has decreased. Most recent reports suggest a mortality rate of less than 15 percent, but these are based on seizures detected clinically. In a recent report of EEG-proved seizures, the mortality rate was 32.5 percent. The incidence of long-term neurologic sequelae in survivors varies from 30 to 50 percent. Several factors influence this, but *babies with normal clinical examination, cranial ultrasound, CT, and EEG results at 7 to 14 days usually have a good prognosis.* Estimates of the incidence of epilepsy in children with neonatal seizures vary from 15 to 20 percent; a few authors have reported rates greater than 50 percent.

SUGGESTED READING

Bergman I, Painter MJ, Hirsch RP, Crumpine PK, David R. Outcome in neonates with convulsions treated in an intensive care unit. Ann Neurol 1983; 14:642–647.

Fenichel GM. Convulsions. In: Fenichel GM, ed. Neonatal neurology. 2nd ed. New York: Churchill Livingstone, 1985:25.

Mellits DE, Holden KR, Freeman JM. Neonatal seizures. II. A multivariate analysis of factors associated with outcome. Pediatrics 1982; 70:177–185.

Mizrahi EM, Kellaway P. Characterization and classification of neonatal seizures. Neurology 1987; 37:1837–1844.

Painter MJ, Bergman I, Crumrine P. Neonatal seizures. Pediatr Clin North Am 1986; 33:91–109.

Painter MJ, Pippenger C, Wasterlain C, et al. Phenobarbital and phenytoin in neonatal seizures: Metabolism and tissue distribution. Neurology 1981; 31:1107–1112.

Rowe JC, Holmes GL, Hafford J, et al. Prognostic value of electroencephalogram in term and preterm infants following neonatal seizures. Electroencephalogr Clin Neurophysiol 1985; 60:183–196.

Scher MS, Painter MJ. Controversies concerning neonatal seizures. Pediatr Clin North Am 1989; 36:281–310.

Volpe J. Neonatal seizures. In: Volpe J, ed. Neurology of the newborn. 2nd ed. Philadelphia: WB Saunders, 1987:129.

NOSOCOMIAL INFECTIONS

JEROME O. KLEIN, M.D.

Nosocomial infections are those that are hospital-acquired; signs appear during the hospital stay or become apparent after discharge. Hospital-acquired infection is of particular concern for the neonate. The nursery is a small community of highly susceptible patients cared for by many adults, including mothers, nurses, and physicians. After arrival in the nursery, the newborn may become infected by various pathways involving either human carriers or contaminated materials and equipment. *Nursery-acquired infection is frequently epidemic, and a common source may be identified by simple epidemiologic techniques.* The purpose of this review is to discuss the problem, the need for a policy that anticipates and prevents infection, and specific issues of management when nosocomial infection occurs.

THE PROBLEM

Transmission of infection to newborn infants from human sources includes droplet spread of respiratory viruses, hand carriage of organisms (*Staphylococcus* species and *Streptococcus* species and fecal contaminants), and direct contact with infectious lesions due to herpes simplex virus, group A *Streptococcus*, and *Staphylococcus aureus*. Blood products used for replacement or exchange transfusion are potential sources of cytomegalovirus infection, hepatitis B, and human immunodeficiency virus (HIV).

Equipment has been implicated in nosocomial infection. The most common factors involved in transmission of infection in such instances have been contaminated solutions used in nebulization equipment, room humidifiers, and bathing solutions. Several gram-negative bacteria, including *Pseudomonas* species, *Serratia marcescens*, and *Flavobacterium* species, have been so troublesome that they have been termed "water bugs" because of their ability to multiply in aqueous environments.

New techniques may also pose significant problems of hospital-acquired infection for the neonate. Catheterization of the umbilical vein and artery has been associated with sepsis, umbilical cellulitis, and abscesses. Intravenous alimentation using central venous catheters has been associated with significant infection.

POLICIES FOR CONTROL OF INFECTION

Various texts and manuals (published by the American Academy of Pediatrics, the Centers for Disease Control, and others) provide guidelines for infection control in the nursery. Each nursery should have a program that incorporates standard guidelines. Selected features of importance follow.

Surveillance for Infection

A program should be in place that provides current information about occurrence of infection in infants. Since some infections may not be apparent until after discharge, the program must *include a method of identifying infection after discharge.* Various techniques can be used, including postcards, telephone calls, and records of visits to physician's offices. A sample of discharged infants of 50 percent or more is necessary for useful information.

Routine Cultures

Cultures of skin and mucous membranes of infants for detection of staphylococcal, streptococcal, or other bacterial infection on a routine basis are usually unnecessary if adequate surveillance for infection is available. Culture of specimens from equipment and personnel is not recommended either.

Antimicrobial Susceptibility Data

Frequent reports of antimicrobial susceptibility of organisms causing disease should be available to guide initial therapy for the infant with suspected sepsis. Although antibiotic susceptibility data based on strains obtained from neonates are optimal, *the pattern of antibiotic susceptibility of strains obtained from other areas of the hospital is usually adequate to monitor changes and emergence of strains with new patterns of susceptibility.* Emergence of a bacterial strain with a new or different pattern of antimicrobial susceptibility may be an important epidemiologic marker in tracing spread of organisms in the nursery.

Surveillance of Personnel

The employee health service should receive clear guidelines from the director of the nursery for exclusion of employees with selected infectious diseases. I recognize that some practices are a compromise between the ideal and the practical. The medical and nursing care of the infants cannot be jeopardized because of community-wide infections of the respiratory and gastrointestinal tracts. However, personnel with communicable diseases that pose a threat to the infants under their care must be excluded from the nursery. *Individuals with an acute respiratory infection, a nonspecific febrile illness, or open or draining lesions of the skin should be excluded from patient care responsibilities* for the duration of the period of disease communicability.

Hospital employees may acquire infections from neonates, and policies should be instituted to protect employees from known infectious hazards. Serologic screening of female hospital personnel for rubella antibodies should be done at the time of employment. Vaccination is advised for nonpregnant females who are seronegative and may come in contact with infectious children. All hospital employees, including those working in nurseries, should be skin-tested with tuberculin annually. Those whose test results are positive should have periodic chest roentgenograms. Allocation of pregnant nurses to duties involving minimal contact with infectious patients should be considered.

Employee Education

All medical and nursing personnel should participate in periodic discussions of infection control. Criteria for isolation procedures should be reviewed. The importance of simple preventive measures, such as compulsive hand-washing and appropriate use of gloves, must be emphasized. Appropriate techniques for use of new equipment and materials should be reviewed.

Blood and Secretion Precautions

Bloodborne pathogens of the neonate include HIV and hepatitis B virus. Neonates should be managed as potentially carrying infectious agents communicable by blood or blood-containing fluids. Gloves should be worn for contact with blood or secretions that may contain blood and for procedures that may lead to exposure to blood. Exposure to urine, stool, and nasal secretions does not require gloves (except if these materials contain blood). These recommendations may be modified, depending on the acceptable level of risk in the community for HIV or hepatitis B infections.

MANAGEMENT OF OUTBREAKS

The medical and nursing staff must be alert to the possibility of common source outbreaks of infection. Prevention of disease is based on the level of awareness of personnel. Infection in previously well infants who lack high-risk factors associated with sepsis must be viewed with suspicion. *Several cases of infection occurring within a brief period or in close physical proximity or caused by an unusual pathogen should also be cause for concern.* An epidemiologic survey is often sufficient to identify the source.

The hospital laboratory can assist in providing specific methods of identification of pathogens, or strains may be sent to laboratories of the community, state, or Centers for Disease Control. Similar isolates from multiple cases can be established by bacteriophage for *Staphylococcus aureus*, serotyping for *Escherichia coli* and groups A and B streptococci, and DNA fingerprinting for herpes simplex viruses.

MANAGEMENT OF INFANTS WITH HOSPITAL-ACQUIRED INFECTION

Clinical signs of nosocomial infection in the neonate may present as early as 3 to 4 days and as late as 3 to 4 months of age. Hospital-acquired infection must be considered in infants who develop local or systemic signs during this period of time.

The choice of antimicrobial agents for the treatment of suspected sepsis before the epidemic agent is identified is based on knowledge of the prevalent organisms responsible for sepsis in the nursery and the patterns of their antimicrobial susceptibility. Treatment of the infant who becomes septic after day 4 should include coverage for hospital-acquired organisms such as *S. aureus* and gram-negative enteric bacilli including *Pseudomonas* species and *Serratia*.

Staphylococcal Infections

Most strains of S. aureus that cause disease in neonates produce beta-lactamase and are thereby resistant to penicillin G, ampicillin, carbenicillin, and ticarcillin.

These organisms are sensitive to the penicillinase-resistant penicillins and cephalosporins, and these drugs must be considered when staphylococcal disease is known or suspected. Methicillin-resistant staphylococci that are cross-resistant with other penicillinase-resistant penicillins (and in most cases cephalosporins) have been encountered in nurseries in the United States. Bacterial resistance must be monitored by surveillance of strains of *S. aureus* causing infection and disease in the nursery. Bacterial resistance must also be considered as a possible cause of therapeutic failure whenever a patient with staphylococcal disease who is receiving an adequate dosage schedule of a penicillinase-resistant penicillin does not respond favorably. Most of these strains are sensitive to vancomycin, and some are sensitive to gentamicin.

Hexachlorophene bathing decreases the rate of colonization of infants with *S. aureus*. Although hexachlorophene should not be used for routine bathing because of reports of neuropathologic toxicity when large amounts are absorbed percutaneously, it is a valuable adjunct in controlling epidemic staphylococcal disease in the nursery. *A daily bath of the diaper area with a 3 percent solution of hexachlorophene should be used during epidemic periods.* Because neuropathologic changes were seen only in small premature infants, it is best to exclude premature infants from the hexachlorophene bathing program. Hexachlorophene is ineffective against gram-negative enteric bacilli, but there is no evidence that an increase in disease due to these occurs in bathed infants.

The use of systemic antimicrobial agents administered to all infants admitted to the nurseries for a limited period may be necessary to halt nursery outbreaks. A penicillinase-resistant penicillin for outbreaks of *S. aureus* and penicillin G for group A *Streptococcus* have been successful when other methods of control have failed.

Staphylococcus epidermidis may be a cause of infection from prosthetic devices such as shunts for cerebrospinal fluid. Most strains produce beta-lactamase. Many are also resistant to methicillin and other penicillinase-resistant penicillins and cephalosporins. Initial therapy for disease that may be caused by *S. epidermidis* must be considered carefully: vancomycin may be used and the initial choice re-evaluated when results of susceptibility tests are available. Removal of the device is often necessary to effect a cure.

Gram-Negative Enteric Bacilli

The choice of antibiotics for infections due to gram-negative enteric bacilli depends on the pattern of susceptibility in the hospital or nursery. These patterns vary in different hospitals or communities and from time to time within the same institution. The aminoglycosides kanamycin, tobramycin, gentamicin, netilmicin and amikacin are highly effective against most isolates of *E coli, Enterobacter, Klebsiella*, and *Proteus* species. All but kanamycin are also active against *Pseudomonas aeruginosa*. The third-generation cephalosporins (cefotaxime, ceftriaxone, and ceftazidime are now available in the United States for use in newborn infants) have excellent in vitro activity against gram-negative enteric bacilli and are the drugs of choice if meningitis is known or suspected to be due to these bacteria. Because the third-generation cephalosporins have variable activity against gram-positive cocci and are ineffective against infections due to enterococcus and *Listeria monocytogenes*, a penicillin must be added if a third-generation cephalosporin is used before results of cultures are available. Clinical studies are in progress to identify the role of these new drugs in neonatal sepsis.

Diarrheal Disease

Outbreaks of diarrhea are usually of infectious origin and due to viruses, *Salmonella, Shigella*, or toxigenic or enteropathogenic strains of *E. coli*. All infants with diarrhea should be isolated from well infants. Strict enteric precautions must be instituted and observed. *Vicious hand washing is undoubtedly the most important part of any control program.* When diarrhea occurs in a single case, the infant should be isolated from others in the nursery. When multiple cases occur, the room should be closed to further admissions and a separate nursing staff provided for the affected infants. If epidemic disease involves more than one room in the nursery, *it may be necessary to close the nursery to further admissions*. The nursery is reopened when a room is available with a separate nursing staff to receive new admissions.

During an outbreak of enteropathogenic strains of *E. coli*, oral nonabsorbable antibiotics such as neomycin or colistin may be administered to infants with diarrhea and may be of value as prophylaxis for unaffected infants.

OBSTRUCTIVE APNEA

BRADLEY T. THACH, M.D.

Clinically significant apnea in infancy is usually defined as absent ventilation for 20 seconds or longer, or absent ventilation of any duration, if associated with

bradycardia or cyanosis. Upper airway obstruction is a frequent cause, or partial cause, of such episodes. This chapter deals with several forms of "obstructive" and "mixed" apnea in infants. A generally accepted and clinically useful classification system for infantile apnea is nonexistent. Apneic episodes are often classified according to mechanism: "obstructive," "central," or "mixed" apnea. In so-called "central" apnea, respiratory effort is absent. In "obstructive" apnea, respiratory efforts are present but there is no air flow because of airway obstruction. In "mixed" apnea, during part of the apneic episode, the infant makes no respiratory attempts, and the rest of the time respiratory attempts are ineffective because of airway obstruction. Apneas are also commonly classified by triggering phenomena; e.g., gastroesophageal reflux apnea and feeding apnea. Other classifications are based on predisposing factors (e.g., sepsis-related apnea, apnea of prematurity), the age of the infant (e.g., apnea of infancy, neonatal apnea), or the state of consciousness (e.g., sleep apnea, awake apnea). These various classifications generally have limited practical applications as far as clinical management of the patient is concerned. Accordingly, the focus of the present discussion is upon three common apnea syndromes that have distinctive clinical features and require different therapeutic approaches. Although upper airway obstruction appears to be a factor in each of these three forms of apnea, successful management of these patients does not necessarily depend on precise classification of apnea mechanism, or on documenting the exact amount or duration of obstructive or mixed apnea episodes. What is important is prompt recognition of the clinical syndrome. Since errors in diagnosis are common, we emphasize this aspect.

APNEA ASSOCIATED WITH A NARROW UPPER AIRWAY

In 1934 Pierre Robin first described a syndrome of impaired ventilation in infants born with a hypoplastic mandible and in children with adenoid hypertrophy. Robin attributed the problem to "glossoptosis" — backward movement of the tongue causing pharyngeal airway obstruction. In recent years, obstructive apnea of this variety has been described in association with numerous conditions, all of which have in common an anatomic narrowing of the nasal or pharyngeal airway (Table 1). The condition of these patients closely resembles Robin's "glossoptosis" syndrome from the standpoint of pathophysiology and symptomatology.

A hallmark of the narrow upper airway syndrome is the variability of the obstruction: one minute the patient is healthy and breathing normally, the next the airway is totally obstructed. In normal individuals, pharyngeal patency is maintained by the airway-dilating force of the upper airway muscles. Thus, muscular tension opposes the airway-constricting effect of suction during inspiration. However, when the lumen of the airway is reduced in diameter by choanal stenosis, for example, resistance to air flow is increased and inspiratory suction increases downstream from the constriction. Periodically, this suction overcomes the force exerted by the airway-maintaining muscles, and the walls of the oropharynx collapse inward. Such obstructive episodes usually occur during sleep. Presumably, this is because the airway-maintaining muscles have diminished activity during sleep. Hence, glossoptosis in infants with the narrow upper airway syndrome apparently results from the inability of the tongue muscles to overcome pharyngeal suction forces. Also, in some infants with obstructive apnea the narrowing of the air-

way is minimal or absent. In these patients, it can be speculated that motor control of tongue muscles or local airway maintenance reflexes may be abnormal. Some of these infants have neuromuscular disorders resulting in muscular weakness.

Patients with this form of obstructive apnea are frequently symptomatic at birth, if the cause of the upper airway narrowing is a congenital defect, such as mandibular hypoplasia or choanal stenosis. In other patients, obstructive episodes may go unrecognized, only to be diagnosed later after they have been discharged from the newborn nursery. Still other infants may first present symptoms when an upper respiratory tract infection increases nasal resistance.

Infants with the narrow upper airway syndrome characteristically have episodes of obstructive apnea during sleep. The site of the obstruction is the oropharynx. As a rule, many spells occur during a 1- to 2-hour sleep cycle. A typical episode of obstruction in these patients lasts 2 to 20 seconds. Respiratory efforts increase in intensity during the course of the obstructive episode and are apparent as subcostal or substernal retractions. Bradycardia often is not severe, but cyanosis may occur toward the end of the episode. Pulse oximetry or transcutaneous oxygen monitors indicate that arterial desaturation always accompanies such episodes. Recovery from the episode is often associated with signs of arousal, such as a startle or postural change. Indeed, a history of very restless sleep may be an early clue to diagnosis.

Associated with episodes of complete upper airway obstruction are episodes of decreased ventilation, presumed to be caused by partial airway obstruction, termed "hypopneas." In some infants, these hypopneas may represent a midinspiratory closure of the airway, with only the early part of the inspiratory effort contributing to effective ventilation. In other patients, transient inspiratory narrowing of the upper airway may reduce inspiratory air flow and limit tidal volume on the basis of increased airway resistance.

Obstructive episodes in very young infants are typically accompanied by harsh upper airway inspiratory sounds, with a stridulous quality. After about 3 months of age, this sound is supplanted by a more typical snoring sound, which is almost universal in the older infant with this form of sleep apnea. A history of mouth breathing while awake is frequently obtained in older infants with this syndrome. In the neonatal period, the cessation of obstructive symptoms with oral breathing or crying is often the initial observation that suggests the correct diagnosis.

A number of factors can increase symptoms of airway obstruction in children with the narrow upper airway syndrome. Position often plays an important role in obstructive episodes. Micrognathic infants almost invariably have more symptoms when they are supine. Neck flexion is also associated with increased symptoms, as is upper respiratory tract infection. In infants with micrognathia, symptoms are often markedly aggravated during feedings; the causal mechanism is unknown.

In attempting to confirm the diagnosis of obstructive apnea, one should always examine patients during their sleep to assess upper airway noises and respiratory retrac-

TABLE 1 Primary Diagnoses and Sites of Airway Narrowing
in Narrow Upper Airway Sleep Apnea Syndrome

Presumed Location of Airway Narrowing	Condition
Nostrils	Fetal warfarin syndrome
Nose	Nasal septal hematoma
	Choanal atresia or stenosis
	Crouzon's disease
	Nasal septal deviation
	Nasal congestion
Nasopharynx	Adenoid hypertrophy
	Obesity
	Postpalatoplasty
Pharynx	Mandibular hypoplasia (Pierre Robin syndrome, Treacher Collins syndrome, Cornelia de Lange's syndrome and others)
	Down syndrome
	Achondroplasia
	Tonsillar hypertrophy
	Macroglossia (Beckwith-Wiedemann syndrome and others)
Degree of airway narrowing minimal, absent, or unknown	Hypotonic cerebral palsy
	Congenital myopathy

tions. Infants should be examined in a supine posture and when the neck is slightly flexed. Episodes of complete upper airway obstruction may be easily detected by observing the chest and abdominal movements while auscultating inspired air flow at the neck. Detection of prolonged obstructive episodes by this method is diagnostic of obstructive apnea, but detection of individual, isolated, obstructive breaths may be suggestive of this diagnosis. Inspiratory retractions, in particular, retractions in the neck over the carotid triangle (Tonkin's sign), are indicative of partial or complete pharyngeal collapse. Additionally, in some infants the cheeks may be sucked in during obstructive episodes, and glossoptosis may be present. Glossoptosis is recognized by posterior position and rotation of the tongue within the mouth. Rotation is evidenced by the tongue tip, which points directly upward toward the hard palate rather than forward toward the lower lip.

Examination of the upper airway should be undertaken to evaluate the patency of the nose and pharynx. The time-honored test of nasal patency made by passing a catheter through the nostrils and into the pharynx is useful to diagnose choanal atresia or marked stenosis, but does not rule out obstructive apnea due to partial airway narrowing. Cineradiography of the upper airway during sleep to document the site of obstruction may be useful in some patients. Polysomnography may further document the frequency and severity of obstruction during sleep. In this evaluation, respiratory air flow is recorded with a carbon dioxide sampling catheter at the nose and mouth, or with thermistors, flow meters, or a combination of these. Documentation of intermittent hypoxemia by pulse oxim-

etry or transcutaneous oxygen is also useful. Such techniques give a more precise documentation of the frequency and duration of obstructive episodes than can be obtained by physical examination alone. However, clinical experience suggests that, given a history indicating obstructive apnea combined with positive physical findings, including documentation of obstructive episodes by auscultation, the diagnosis of obstructive apnea can be made without the need for polysomnography.

Successful management of this variety of obstructive apnea calls for close monitoring of the patient's condition and eliminating, if possible, the anatomic source of airway narrowing. In many patients, surgical correction of the airway is possible. In cases in which surgical correction is not feasible, alternative measures to prevent pharyngeal collapse can be taken. Maintaining a prone posture and avoidance of neck flexion are important. Additionally, nasopharyngeal or nasoesophageal tubes that prevent pharyngeal closure have been used with success. Some infants can be managed with oropharyngeal airways, although most do not tolerate these for extended periods. Nasal positive pressure delivered by nasal prongs or cannulas may be effective in some infants. Such pressure provides a pneumatic splinting effect on the collapsible upper airway segment. Bypassing the upper airway entirely by nasal tracheal intubation or tracheostomy may be needed if other less invasive measures fail. The key to success is often trial and error, adjusting the therapy to the needs and tolerances of the individual patient. During this initial evaluation period, an intensive care environment with electronic monitoring of respiration, heart rate, and arterial oxygenation is crucial. Such close observation is important, since serious prolonged obstructive episodes can occur suddenly and without warning.

During the first postnatal month, infants with obstructive apnea secondary to micrognathia tend to improve their airway-maintaining ability. This appears to be due not only to growth of the jaw but also to improved regulation of the upper airway musculature. Infants with other primary anatomic defects may experience similar improvement, although this is less well documented. Effects of maturation on upper airway function are variable. Some infants with choanal stenosis, for example, have been known to remain symptom free in the neonatal period owing to reliance on oral breathing from the time of birth.

During the first few postnatal weeks or months, specific airway therapy, such as nasal positive pressure, may be discontinued as the child begins to improve airway-maintaining ability. In some special situations, we have sent infants home after parents have been trained to manage their children by using a nasopharyngeal airway. However, discharge from the hospital is usually contingent on the infant being able to maintain airway patency in the prone position or on having a tracheostomy.

Respiratory embarrassment during feedings in some infants with the narrow upper airway syndrome is well documented. In the case of choanal stenosis or atresia, its origin is clear, as the infant is totally dependent on the nasal airway during feeding. In other situations, the pathophysiology is less clear. Such feeding problems are initially managed by gavage feedings or occasionally by gastrostomy, if symptoms appear to be long term. Such feeding difficulty is usually transient and the infant can often be gradually weaned to oral feedings by 3 to 4 months of age.

It is important to recognize that infants diagnosed as having obstructive apnea of this kind may have recurrent symptoms after initial discharge from the hospital. Although their long-term course may be that of improved regulation of upper airway patency, upper respiratory infection or growth of tonsils and adenoids may exacerbate obstructive symptoms. General anesthesia and sedatives should be used only with great caution. Generalized growth retardation and developmental delay are well-known symptoms of obstructive sleep apnea in infants. Cor pulmonale, which can rapidly progress to pulmonary edema, has long been recognized as part of the syndrome. Therefore, infants should be followed closely for evidence of growth failure, cardiac symptoms, or recurrent signs of obstructive sleep apnea.

Unlike older patients with obstructive sleep apnea, young infants with micrognathia and obstructive apnea have, in recent times, had a very high mortality. Deaths have often occurred suddenly and unexpectedly when the infants appeared to be improving and had been discharged from the hospital. In these patients, evidence of aspiration of gastric contents is sometimes seen at postmortem examination; in others there are only minimal findings. Acute airway obstruction is the presumed, although unproved, cause of these deaths. It is our practice to recommend a home monitoring program for the first 9 to 12 months of life for infants diagnosed as having obstructive sleep apnea in whom definitive surgical correction cannot be performed.

INFANTILE BREATH-HOLDING RESPONSE (INFANTILE SYNCOPE)

Breath-holding spells are a common and well-known cause of apnea in the 1- to 5-year-old child. They are less frequently considered as a cause of apnea in infants under 3 months of age. Such episodes in the very young infant are often diagnosed as obstructive apnea and are confused with apnea secondary to gastroesophageal reflux or epileptic seizure. We have found breath-holding apnea to be common in young infants, including preterm infants and those who have endotracheal airways, who have had tracheostomies, or who have chronic lung disease.

The pathophysiologic basis for this form of apnea appears to be transient interruption of the respiratory activity of thoracic and airway muscles by generalized motor activity or crying. The Valsalva maneuver is a physiologic component of vigorous motor activity in young infants. Moreover, a Valsalva response usually occurs with painful, frightening, or annoying stimuli. Apneic spells, associated with "squirming" motor activity in preterm infants and breath-holding spells in older infants appear to consist of a single, prolonged Valsalva maneuver, or a series of briefer maneuvers. Thus, the normal breath-holding Valsalva response to pain or emotional stimuli, which usually results in a brief reduction in ventilation, progresses to severe asphyxia with loss of consciousness in certain infants. In a simple breath-holding spell, an infant who is crying suddenly holds his breath until cyanosis appears. In contrast, during severe breath-holding spells, this cyanotic phase is rapidly followed by a syncopal episode and often a brief seizure. The pathophysiology of respiratory and circulatory events during such spells is complex. Loss of consciousness and the seizure are the result of cerebral hypoxemia. The hypoxemia results from reduced arterial oxygen tension, reduced cerebral perfusion, or a combination of these.

In preterm infants, such spells have been termed "squirming apnea" or "disorganized breathing." In addition to the Valsalva maneuver, these infants often have obstructive inspiratory efforts, and hence most of these spells are a form of mixed apnea. During such episodes in preterm infants, bradycardia may suddenly occur. The entire sequence of events during squirming apnea is similar to the older child with breath-holding spells, a major difference being that the preterm infant's spells are rarely preceded by crying.

It is important to recognize that the primary inhibitory influence on breathing during such spells is probably not upper airway obstruction per se, but rather the prolongation of expiration inherent in the Valsalva maneuver. Consequently, endotracheal intubation or tracheostomy usually does not reduce the frequency or severity of these episodes. In fact, bypassing the upper airway with tracheostomy often makes episodes worse, possibly by lowering lung volume. On the other hand, when severe spells are encountered, tracheostomy may facilitate resuscitation of the infant.

A critical point in managing these patients is to avoid misdiagnosis. When episodes are associated with posturing or seizure, it is important to recognize that hypoxemia is the cause of the seizure, and not vice versa; otherwise, an incorrect diagnosis of epileptic seizure may be made. In order to reduce the frequency of episodes, the first approach is to identify and eliminate, if possible, noxious stimuli that may be triggering the spells. Some excessively irritable infants have responded to mild sedation or analgesia for painful procedures. In infants who are intubated, we have not infrequently noted improvement in spell frequency and severity following extubation. In preterm infants, apnea of this type often occurs in association with otherwise typical apnea of prematurity, and it is our impression that theophylline or caffeine may be useful in these patients. Since iron deficiency anemia may predispose to breath-holding spells, infants should be evaluated and treated, if necessary.

Breath-holding spells in children over 1 year of age are generally regarded as benign. However, the prognosis is uncertain for severe breath-holding spells (e.g., spells that involve loss of consciousness) in infants under 6 months of age. Accordingly, our approach is generally to consider this type of apnea to be life-threatening in the very young infant.

PROLONGED APNEA DURING FEEDINGS

Apnea associated with feedings has received widespread attention only recently. Many seemingly healthy, normal full-term infants develop mild to moderate cyanosis during their first feeding. In the great majority of patients, the symptoms rapidly resolve. Occasionally, certain infants continue to have prolonged apnea, cyanosis, and bradycardia during feedings. The mechanism of the apnea is not entirely clear; it has been reported to be central by some investigators and mixed or obstructive by others. Such apnea is believed to be unrelated to aspiration, although aspiration of very small amounts of the feeding has in no way been ruled out. In some cases, an abnormality of the swallow mechanism has been reported in which there is intranasal reflux of formula during swallowing. Not infrequently, infants with feeding-related apnea have also had prolonged apnea and bradycardia during sleep. During the typical feeding, in both term and preterm infants, there is a normal tendency toward decreased ventilation during the early phase of the feed. Therefore, infants with symptomatic apnea during feeding may represent one extreme in the range of physiologic feeding behavior. It is also speculated that feeding may trigger laryngeal chemoreflexes that cause airway obstruction and apnea. Preterm infants clearly are at increased risk for apnea during feedings and many have a history of apnea of prematurity.

Management of these patients should be influenced by the observation that this form of apnea in most cases represents a functional abnormality of the control of breathing. Symptoms are usually transient in both term and preterm infants. Recovery often occurs in several days, but complete resolution of symptoms may take several weeks. In patients in whom spells are persistent and severe, radiographic and/or endoscopic studies of the upper airway and esophagus should be performed to rule out anatomic defects. Also, one should always be alert to the possibility that some spells may involve gross aspiration during feedings.

In cases that have a functional basis, we may elect to gavage feed the infant until coordination of feeding and breathing matures. In patients with only mild symptoms, we continue feedings while monitoring oxygen saturation, heart rate, and respiration during the feed. The feeding is interrupted at the first indication of apnea. Some infants have responded to slow feedings in which the nipple is removed frequently to allow time for breathing.

In our experience, the long-term prognosis for this form of apnea is excellent. However, in the absence of prospective long-term follow-up studies of such infants, conclusive statements regarding prognosis cannot be made at the present time.

SUGGESTED READING

Abu-Osba YK, Brouillette RT, Wilson SL, Thach BT. Breathing pattern and transcutaneous oxygen tension during motor activity in preterm infants. Am Rev Respir Dis 1982; 125:382–387.

Guilleminault C, Coons S. Apnea and bradycardia during feeding in infants weighing >2000 gm. J Pediatr 1984; 104:932–935.

Marsh JL, Vannier MW. Comprehensive care for craniofacial deformities. St. Louis: CV Mosby, 1985:319.

Rosen CL, Glaze DG, Frost JD. Hypoxemia associated with feeding in the preterm infant and full term neonate. Am J Dis Child 1984; 138:623–628.

Thach BT. Sleep apnea in infancy and childhood. Med Clin North Am 1985; 69:1289–1315.

PERSISTENT PULMONARY HYPERTENSION

ROBERT M. WARD, M.D.

Persistent pulmonary hypertension of the newborn (PPHN) is the pathophysiologic condition in which pulmonary vascular resistance (PVR) is equal to or greater than systemic vascular resistance (SVR) in the newborn, causing systemic hypoxemia due to right-to-left prepulmonary vascular shunting through the ductus arteriosus or foramen ovale. PPHN usually presents within the first 18 hours after birth with marked cyanosis out of proportion to underlying lung disease, and must be distinguished from cyanotic cardiac malformations. When first described in the United States, PPHN was designated "persistent fetal circulation" (PFC). Subsequent investigators have considered PPHN to be a more accurate and inclusive term for this disorder of neonatal pulmonary perfusion.

Although severe ventilation-perfusion mismatch from pulmonary infections or hyaline membrane disease may produce profound hypoxemia and pulmonary vasoconstriction, we will discuss PPHN as a distinct clinical entity associated with right-to-left vascular shunting due to increased PVR. Some neonates develop PPHN *without* apparent associated problems, such as sepsis or meconium aspiration, and some workers in this area have suggested that the term PFC be reserved for these patients as a subset of all neonates with PPHN.

PATHOPHYSIOLOGIC CLASSIFICATION

A variety of disorders may ultimately lead to increased pulmonary vascular resistance, right-to-left prepulmonary vascular shunting, and decreased pulmonary perfusion–PPHN. A review of the physiologic factors that determine organ perfusion will help to organize the abnormalities associated with PPHN. These factors will be grouped by altered physiologic variable, possibly arbitrarily and naively, owing to our continued ignorance of the basic mediator(s) that control pulmonary vascular tone. Such a grouping around physiologic variables will demonstrate the wide range of clinical problems associated with PPHN and may suggest therapeutic approaches directed at the specific disorder.

Physiology of Organ Blood Flow and Shunting

The physiologic principles governing the circulation through an organ, such as the lung, are the same as those of the physics of electrical current flow and fluid mechanics. A brief review of these principles will illustrate the factors that contribute to increased pulmonary vascular resistance and right-to-left vascular shunting. Blood flow from the heart can be reduced to the product of two variables: heart rate and stroke volume.

$$\text{Flow (cardiac output)} = \text{HR (heart rate)} \cdot \text{SV (stroke volume)}$$
$$\text{ml/min} = \text{beats/min} \cdot \text{ml/beat}$$

Ohm's law can now be adapted to describe the pressure drop (Δ pressure) observed as flow (cardiac output) passes through a capillary bed displaying a specific resistance to flow.

Ohm's Law

$$\text{Current} = \text{Voltage drop/Resistance}$$
$$\text{Flow (cardiac output)} = \Delta \text{ Pressure/Vascular resistance}$$

For the pulmonary vasculature alone, resistance (PVR) is defined by the following equation, in which pulmonary venous pressure is often equated with pulmonary artery wedge pressure, which is easier to measure.

$$PVR = \frac{\text{Pressure}_{\text{pulmonary artery}} - \text{Pressure}_{\text{pulmonary vein}}}{\text{Cardiac output}}$$

Like electrical current being distributed between two parallel circuits, flow between two branching vessels, such as the patent ductus arteriosus (PDA) and the pulmonary artery, is distributed in proportion to the reciprocals of their resistances. This is illustrated in Figure 1, where vascular resistances (PVR and SVR) are represented by symbols for electrical resistance ($\wedge\wedge\wedge$), right ventricle output is Q or flow, and the PDA represents the connection between the two parallel circulations.

Assume that: (1) PVR is twice as high as SVR (PVR = 2SVR); (2) aortic and pulmonary pressures are equal; (3) pulmonary venous and right atrial pressures are equal, so the pressure drop (Δ Pressure) is equal in the systemic and pulmonary circulations.

$$\text{Flow (cardiac output)} = \Delta \text{ Pressure/Vascular resistance}$$
$$\text{Flow}_{\text{systemic}} = \Delta \text{ Pressure/SVR}$$
$$\text{Flow}_{\text{pulmonary}} = \Delta \text{ Pressure/PVR}$$
$$= \Delta \text{ Pressure/2SVR}$$
$$\text{Flow}_{\text{pulmonary}} = \tfrac{1}{2} \times \text{Flow}_{\text{systemic}}$$

Poiseuille's Law explains the proportionality of viscosity, vessel number, radius and length to resistance to flow of a fluid through a narrow tube, comparable to arterioles. Although blood is a rather complex fluid, containing proteins and red blood cells, the principle described by Poiseuille for ideal fluids helps to relate several factors that have an impact on vascular resistance.

$$\text{Resistance} \propto \frac{8(\text{Viscosity})(\text{Vessel length})}{\pi (\text{No. of vessels})(\text{Vessel radius})^4}$$

The most important feature of PPHN is increased pulmonary vascular resistance (PVR). As can be seen from the equations above, several factors can affect this parameter. Within the pulmonary circulation, resistance varies directly with blood viscosity and pulmonary ves-

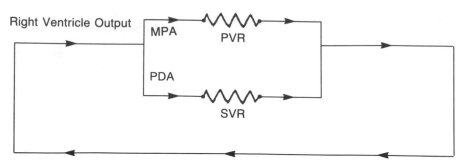

Figure 1 Fundamental division of perinatal right ventricular output into parallel circuits. MPA = main pulmonary artery; PDA = patent ductus arteriosus; PVR = pulmonary vascular resistance; SVR = systemic vascular resistance.

sel length and inversely with the number of vessels. Note especially, however, that changes in vessel radius are amplified to the fourth power in their effect upon resistance. Thus, *a 50 percent decrease in vessel radius increases the resistance 16-fold.*

Classification of Causes of PPHN

As may be anticipated, these factors translate into clinical problems that may lead to PPHN and which may be used to organize some of the disorders that lead to PPHN.

DIAGNOSIS

General

As shown in Table 1, many disorders can be associated with PPHN. Cyanosis remains the predominant presenting sign and is typically more severe than the pulmonary findings would indicate. Despite this generalization, PPHN may complicate aspiration syndromes, (especially of meconium), and neonatal sepsis/pneumonia, especially with group B streptococcus (GBS). Thus, the chest radiograph may actually be completely free of infiltrates, may lack peripheral vascular markings, may show mild interstitial infiltrates or atelectasis, or may show prominent infiltrates of GBS pneumonia or meconium aspiration.

Cardiac Evaluation

Any neonate with severe hypoxemia unresponsive to increased oxygen, especially without sufficient respiratory disease to explain the hypoxemia, should be evaluated for structural cyanotic cardiac disease. Evaluation should begin with a careful history of pregnancy and delivery followed by a thorough cardiac examination, with special attention to the apical impulse and equality of pulses. Studies should include a chest radiograph, electrocardiogram (ECG), and two-dimensional Doppler echocardiogram. The echocardiogram is most important for detection of cardiac malformations and signs of increased PVR, and for examination of cardiac function. It is often impossible to visualize all four pulmonary veins, so *partial anomalous PVR can seldom be ruled out echocardiographically.* Most other cyanotic congenital cardiac malformations may be accurately delineated by echocardiography.

Echocardiographic evidence of PPHN may be prominent or subtle. The ductus arteriosus is usually widely patent. The right ventricle and right atrium may be dilated. Tricuspid insufficiency is also consistent with increased PVR and is, in fact, a poor prognostic sign. Contraction of the right ventricle against an increased distal resistance (afterload) may prolong the systolic time interval, although it is influenced also by ventricular contractility, preload, and heart rate. If the right ventricular systolic time interval is markedly increased, it may be diagnostic of PPHN. (Since several other factors may also prolong the systolic time interval, some cardiologists feel that a single measurement of the right ventricular systolic time interval is not sufficiently accurate to establish the diagnosis of PPHN.) In contrast, some neonates with PPHN demonstrate only paradoxical bowing of the atrial septum to the left during diastole. Contrast echocardiography often shows paradoxical right-to-left atrial shunting at a time when left atrial pressure should exceed right atrial pressure and close the foramen ovale.

Electrocardiographic results may be completely normal with PPHN. In many patients with PPHN, however, the ECG shows signs of right-sided volume and force overload with evidence of right atrial hypertrophy, right ventricular hypertrophy, or ST-T wave changes of subendocardial ischemia. ECG abnormalities usually revert to normal as the infant's condition improves. Arrhythmias are infrequent.

When PPHN is suspected, it is important to seek evidence of right-to-left ductal shunting. Physical examination, oximetry, transcutaneous oxygen monitoring, or simultaneous right radial and aortic PaO_2 may be used to detect a step down in oxygenation from the right arm (usually preductal) to the lower extremities or descending aorta (postductal), which indicates right-to-left ductal shunting. If right-to-left shunting occurs at the atrial level, no such difference in oxygenation will occur. *Right-to-left ductal shunting without cardiac malformations seen by echocardiography strongly suggests PPHN.*

TABLE 1 Pathophysiologic Classification of PPHN

Physiologic Abnormality	Clinical Disorder
Increased viscosity	Polycythemia (Hct $\geq$ 65)

Decreased vessel number (decreased lung mass)	Intrathoracic mass lesions
	   Congenital diaphragmatic hernia
	   Cystic adenomatoid malformation
	   Pleural effusion

	Absence of fetal breathing
	   Werdnig-Hoffmann disease
	   Absence of phrenic nerve or diaphragm
	   Severe neurologic dysfunction

	Thoracic constriction
	   Oligohydraminos due to renal agenesis/dysplasia
	   Oligohydraminos due to chronic amniotic fluid leak
	   Asphyxiating thoracic dystrophy

	Primary pulmonary hypoplasia

Decreased vessel radius	Reactive
	   Pulmonary vasoconstriction—idiopathic PFC
	   Group B streptococcus sepsis/pneumonia

	Narrowed vessel lumen—normal/decreased flow
	   Chronic in utero hypoxemia (presumed) with
	      increased pulmonary arteriolar muscularization

	Narrowed vessel lumen—increased flow
	   Premature closure ductus arteriosus
	   Arteriovenous malformation (usually cerebral)
	   Endocardial cushion defect (shunting left ventricle
	      to right atrium)
	   Supradiaphragmatic total anomalous pulmonary
	      venous drainage

	Pulmonary venous obstruction
	   Infradiaphragmatic total anomalous pulmonary
	      venous drainage
	   Incomplete hypoplastic left heart syndrome

TREATMENT

General

Since GBS infections are sometimes subtle, cyanosis suggestive of PPHN with mild respiratory symptoms is an adequate indication for sepsis evaluation and treatment with antibiotics, if this has not been done previously.

Nursing care of infants with PPHN is a critical part of their management. Every effort must be made to minimize episodes of hypoxemia, which increase PVR and worsen the right-to-left shunt. The decision to suction the endotracheal tube for secretions must be made quite deliberately, after first considering the potential for hypoxemia and irreversible worsening of the shunt. Some infants increase their right-to-left shunt in response to external stimuli such as touching or loud noises, which should be minimized in caring for the infant.

Tissue oxygenation, not only of the lungs, but of the entire body, must be optimized in the treatment of PPHN. After treating cardiac output by improving stroke volume and heart rate, oxygen-carrying capacity and preload may be increased by transfusing to maintain a hematocrit of 45 percent.

Oxygenation

Oxygen is the mainstay of treatment for PPHN that presents with cyanosis mimicking cyanotic congenital heart disease. In the patient with PPHN and clear lung fields on chest radiograph, cyanosis is the result of right-to-left shunting, so that pulmonary venous oxygen concentrations are usually normal and increase with increased inspired oxygen concentrations. Clearly, patients with pulmonary parenchymal abnormalities from bacterial infections or aspiration syndromes require increased inspired oxygen.

Theoretically, little is gained with a right-to-left shunt lesion by increasing the pulmonary venous oxygen concentrations above 100 percent saturation, since the PaO_2 is determined from the percentage admixture of desaturated blood and the hemoglobin saturation of the admixed blood. In reality, some neonates with high pulmonary venous oxygenation (based on right radial artery oxygen concentrations) worsen with small decreases in inspired oxygen concentration.

Mechanical Ventilation

Whenever possible, we utilize the infant's spontaneous respirations as long as possible. Some infants with PPHN require mechanical ventilation because of their pulmonary parenchymal disease. Others tire from their work of breathing in response to a hypoxic drive superimposed on relatively minor pulmonary parenchymal abnormalities. In these situations, mechanical ventilation often improves pulmonary mechanics, possibly through re-expansion of areas of atelectasis, and decreases the infant's work of breathing. Although the infant's spontaneous ventilation often contributes a large portion of total minute ventilation, which is lessened by sedation, sedation is often helpful in infants who require mechanical ventilation for PPHN. Many of these infants react to direct handling or environmental stimulation by increasing the right-to-left shunt and desaturating further. We try to avoid actual paralysis, since it usually increases the requirements for mechanical ventilation, as well as edema formation.

Sedation

Treatment of mechanically ventilated infants with a hypnotic-sedative such as pentobarbital, chloral hydrate, or morphine sulfate may be helpful. No ideal hypnotic-sedative is available that preserves rapid-eye-movement sleep, does not depress myocardial contractility or respiratory drive, and can be administered parenterally and enterally. Chloral hydrate decreases respiratory drive the least, but is not available in a parenteral preparation. Pentobarbital doses must often be repeated to achieve sedation. Pentobarbital may depress myocardial contractility, and its sedation occasionally lasts for days. Morphine sulfate has the usual narcotic depressant effects upon smooth muscle action and may produce ileus and urinary retention. Morphine releases histamine and may produce hypotension and local urticaria at the site of injection. (Such urticaria with morphine is not equivalent to a hypersensitivity reaction, as long as the urticaria is localized.) Fentanyl, a very potent narcotic usually reserved for surgical anesthesia, may improve the survival of infants with congenital diaphragmatic hernia and postoperative PPHN. During induction of anesthesia, *fentanyl may induce severe muscle rigidity,* designated "stiff man syndrome," to a degree that prevents spontaneous ventilation, as well as intubation, if the patient is treated before mechanical ventilation is initiated. This can be reversed with narcotic receptor antagonists.

Mechanical Hyperventilation

Mechanical hyperventilation to marked respiratory alkalosis of pH 7.55 to 7.60 and $PaCO_2$ of 20 to 25 mm Hg often relaxes the pulmonary vasculature in neonates with PPHN and abolishes the right-to-left shunt. Early studies of this observation described the use of pulmonary vascular catheters and confirmed that pulmonary arterial pressure equaled or exceeded aortic pressure and decreased with hyperventilation. Although hyperventilation with 100 percent oxygen has been advocated as a clinical test to establish the diagnosis of PPHN, enough patients with PPHN fail to respond to this maneuver to make it unreliable as a test to rule out PPHN. On the other hand, when PaO_2 increases rapidly from 30 to 40 mm Hg to greater than 100 mm Hg within minutes after beginning hyperventilation, it usually reflects rapid changes in the degree of shunt and strongly supports the diagnosis of PPHN.

Clearly, mechanical hyperventilation with ventilator pressures and rates adequate to lower $PaCO_2$ to the teens or 20s may improve oxygenation by increasing mean airway pressure. Atelectatic alveoli may be recruited, and *the short expiratory times that accompany mechanical hyperventilation may prevent complete expiration and produce inadvertent positive end-expiratory pressure (PEEP) at an alveolar level.* The amount of hidden PEEP may induce barotrauma and may vary markedly with changes in the respirator flow and respirator rate, or with changes in the expiratory airway time constant resulting from secretions, bronchoconstriction, or bronchodilatation.

Severe alkalemia related to mechanical hyperventilation is often lethal in adults. Similar outcomes have not been seen in neonates, but it is still a relatively understudied therapy. In adults and animals, respiratory alkalosis induces a marked decrease in serum and urine phosphorus to levels that may affect ATP production. Hypokalemia may be expected because of shifts of potassium from extracellular to intracellular fluid, and may be severe enough to alter transmembrane potentials and contribute to arrhythmias and ileus. Replacement of the extracellular potassium to normal concentrations during marked alkalosis, however, produces an increase in total body potassium stores. Sudden cessation of the alkalosis from a mechanical airway problem, such as a pneumothorax or bronchial plug, may decrease the pH, shift potassium out of cells, and acutely increase serum potassium to lethal concentrations.

Many patients who are hyperventilated respond as if their capacitance vessels are widely dilated, and so require large infusions of volume expanders to maintain urinary output and a central venous pressure at 3 mm Hg or more. Urinary specific gravity is often increased during hyperventilation, suggesting prerenal underperfusion, despite volume expansion to 40 to 50 percent of predicted intravascular volume.

Initial follow-up studies of neonates who have PPHN treated with hyperventilation indicated no problems. Later studies have detected an increased occurrence of hearing loss in these infants. Additional studies are needed, but close follow-up of all survivors with severe PPHN is indicated.

Bicarbonate Therapy

The effectiveness of hyperventilation may relate more to the blood pH than to the low $PaCO_2$. Despite reports of intraventricular hemorrhage following infusions of hyperosmolar bicarbonate solutions, bicarbonate may be useful to treat PPHN in two situations. During mechanical hyperventilation to alkalotic pH values that are sustained for more than a few hours, renal excretion of base will increase to compensate for this perturbation of pH. *Infusion of bicarbonate in place of a portion of maintenance NaCl may help to maintain the alkalotic pH.* Instead of hyperventilation to achieve alkalosis, infusions of bicarbonate diluted 1:1 or 1:2 with sterile water to produce metabolic alkalosis may successfully lower the PVR and reverse the shunt of PPHN. This may relate both to the change in blood pH and to increased cardiac output from the acute volume expansion.

Cardiovascular Support

A brief review of cardiac physiology illustrates how cardiac function may be altered to improve pulmonary perfusion. Cardiac performance is determined by preload, afterload, and cardiac contractility. The volume of blood filling the atrium during diastole largely determines preload, and reflects the circulating vascular volume and state of constriction of the venous capacitance vessels. Afterload reflects the distal vascular resistance against which the ventricles are contracting. Constriction of peripheral vessels increases afterload, stiffens the ventricle wall, and increases myocardial oxygen consumption. The rate of myocardial muscle fiber movement/time and degree of fiber stretch define myocardial contractility. Muscle fibers contract more slowly and less effectively when stretched to a long fiber length, as occurs with increased vascular resistance, increased end-diastolic volume, cardiac failure, and cardiomegaly. Muscle fiber motion (Δlength/Δtime) is difficult to measure accurately without invasive procedures, but useful clinical indices of contractility can be obtained from careful examination of the pulse contour by palpation, determination of heart size on chest radiography, and echocardiographic determination of myocardial motion and ejection fraction, end-diastolic chamber size, and systolic time interval.

Whenever possible, preload should be monitored with right atrial pressures. Accurate atrial pressure measurements are difficult and require careful attention to placement of the transducer at the level of the right atrium. An absolutely optimal right atrial filling pressure is not determined for these patients, but a CVP between 3 and 10 mm Hg in patients without right heart failure has generally produced adequate atrial filling. With right heart failure and a stiff ventricle, filling pressures may need to be maintained closer to 10 mm Hg.

If cardiac contractility must be supported pharmacologically, it is theoretically better to use a drug that increases systemic vascular resistance more than pulmonary resistance. Since peripheral vasculature is dilated slightly by dobutamine and markedly by isoproterenol, *we favor the use of dopamine to support contractility while increasing systemic vascular resistance.* Studies of dopamine in the neonate are limited, but they show improvement in systolic and diastolic pressures as well as urinary output at 4 μg per kilogram per minute. To increase systemic vascular resistance, we often increase doses to 10 to 15 μg per kilogram per minute. Theoretically, high doses of dopamine in neonates may cause constriction of renal vasculature and possibly pulmonary vasculature through predominance of alpha-receptor stimulation. Despite many dogmatic statements that this effect occurs at doses of 15 to 20 μg per kilogram per minute, this range has not been studied or defined for the neonate. During treatment with dopamine to improve cardiac contractility, serum ionized calcium should be monitored and maintained in the high normal range.

Pharmacologic Pulmonary Vasodilatation

Ideal Pulmonary Vasodilator

Optimal treatment would utilize a drug that inhibits the specific mediator responsible for the pulmonary vasoconstriction of PPHN. *This mediator is still not identified, but recent studies have shown higher leukotriene concentrations in pulmonary secretions of infants with PPHN than in size-matched control infants without PPHN.* Until the final mediator of fetal-neonatal pulmonary vasoconstriction is identified and an inhibitor developed, pharmacologic treatment should use a drug that selectively dilates constricted pulmonary vessels without affecting the systemic vasculature. This drug should also increase cardiac output to further improve pulmonary perfusion. Unfortunately, no agent has been found that meets these criteria. Thus, treatment of PPHN has proceeded empirically and will continue as such until basic physiologic studies explain pulmonary vascular control and thus direct our therapeutic approach.

Various Pulmonary Vasodilators

The history of pulmonary vasodilators is a story of empirical therapies directed toward a vascular bed that actively autoregulates. Initial decreases in right-to-left shunt, reflected in improvements in aortic oxygenation, have usually been followed by loss of the response or the occurrence of side effects that prevented further treatment. Some of the vasodilators that have been tried for treatment of PPHN and then largely abandoned include acetylcholine, chlorpromazine, prostaglandin D_2, and bradykinin. Nitroprusside is still used in many institutions as a first-line pulmonary vasodilator, although the vasodilatation it provides is not specific for the pulmonary vasculature. Accumulation of cyanide and thiocyanate, especially with oliguria, limit its usefulness.

Tolazoline

Background. Tolazoline remains the most frequently used pharmacologic pulmonary vasodilator in neonates, and one of the more effective pulmonary vasodilators in adults. Like many therapies in pediatrics, tolazoline therapy for neonates developed empirically from treatment of adults with pulmonary hypertension. The history of its clinical use has some relevance for neonatologists today.

Tolazoline was developed and released in 1939 as a structural analogue of histamine and phenylethylamine, the parent structure of the catecholamines, and it possesses attributes of both. In 1944 it was reported to be as potent as histamine for stimulation of gastric acid secretion. A few years later, it was found to vasodilate ischemic extremities and to be more effective in the more ischemic areas. During the poliomyelitis epidemics, hundreds of patients were treated with tolazoline to improve skin perfusion and heal stasis ulcers. As might be predicted from the 1944 report, this was associated with gastritis and gastrointestinal hemorrhage in 79 percent of patients. When tolazoline therapy for PPHN was adopted by neonatologists in the 1970s, we had to rediscover the effects of tolazoline upon gastric acid secretion from neonates who developed gastritis, gastrointestinal ulceration, and perforation.

Adverse Effects. Side effects to tolazoline have been numerous. A recent review of tolazoline's pharmacology in the neonate presented adverse effects in 132 neonates from three clinical series treated with tolazoline infusions of 1 to 2 to 1 to 10 mg per kilogram per hour. The adverse effects are shown in Table 2.

Overall, the highest rates of adverse effect occurred in the study using the highest doses. The high prevalence of adverse effects from tolazoline therapy for neonates may relate to excessive doses without regard to its kinetics in the neonate. The infusion doses now in general use (2 to 10 mg per kilogram per hour) are six- to sixty-fold higher than doses based on documented neonatal kinetics without adjustment for oliguria (see below). The efficacy of these kinetically-derived reduced doses has not been studied in many patients, but neither has the efficacy of the higher doses that have gained popular use.

With such a high prevalence of adverse effects, why do neonatologists persist in using tolazoline for treatment of PPHN? In most reported series of tolazoline-treated neonates, PaO$_2$ improves initially in 60 to 70 percent after treatment with tolazoline bolus doses. Despite this initial favorable response, PPHN still carries an overall mortality of 40 to 70 percent.

Dosage for Neonates. The history of tolazoline dosage for neonates illustrates how therapy without the guide of pharmacokinetic and pharmacodynamic data inexorably leads to progressively higher doses. Tolazoline was first administered in pulse doses of 1 to 2 mg per kilogram, but reported doses quickly increased to 5 mg per kilogram. When patients were noted to become less responsive to later doses, tolazoline was infused continuously in doses of 1 to 2 mg per kilogram per hour. Infusion rates later reached as high as 10 mg per kilogram per hour. This naturally-progressive increase in dosage occurred before the *first* study of tolazoline kinetics in neonates was made!

A study of tolazoline kinetics in neonates showed wide variation in the agent's half-life, but the longest half-life occurred in the sickest patient. A later study confirmed this wide variation in tolazoline's half-life in neonates (1.5 to 42 hours) and found that oliguria and renal dysfunction (especially acute renal tubular necrosis) prolong tolazoline's half-life. In addition, the study provided values for tolazoline distribution volume and disposition rate constant, beta, in neonates as shown in Table 3 (mean ± SEM).

Both adverse effects and failure to sustain initial improvement with tolazoline therapy for PPHN may reflect inappropriate dosage. Earlier studies as well as our own indicate that high concentrations of tolazoline (21.8 to 56.8 mg per liter) are lethal in animals. In addition, plasma tolazoline concentrations appear to increase in neonates receiving tolazoline infusions in doses of 2 to 10 mg per kilogram per hour. We have assumed that tolazoline's effects are related to its plasma concentration. In about 65 percent of tolazoline-treated infants, aortic oxygenation is improved initially with doses of 1 to 2 mg per kilogram,

TABLE 2   Adverse Effects Associated with Tolazoline Treatment of Neonates

Clinical series	1	2	3
Patient no.	46	47	39
Tolazoline doses (mg/kg/hr)	1–2	1–2	1–10

	Percentage of Patients		
Overall Incidence	30		82
Gastrointestinal			
Distention		9	
Distention/hemorrhage	13		
Mild hemorrhage		55	8
Extensive hemorrhage	7		3
Renal			
Hematuria		23	
Oliguria		11	
Failure	4		
Hyponatremia		40	
Cardiovascular			
Hypotension	2	19	67
Hypertension	2		
Bone marrow			
Thrombocytopenia	4	45	31
Central nervous system			
Hyperactivity		6	
Seizures		30	
Pulmonary			
Hemorrhage	2	6	13

Modified from Ward RM. Pharmacology of tolazoline. Clin Perinatol 1984; 11:710.

TABLE 3   Neonatal Tolazoline Pharmacokinetic Parameters

Parameter	Mean ± SEM
Apparent volume of distribution, beta	1.61 ± 0.21 L/kg
*Disposition rate constant, beta—all patients	0.0027 ± 0.0007 min^{-1}
Disposition rate constant, beta—urine output ≥ 0.9 ml/kg/hr	0.0034 ± 0.0006 min^{-1}
Disposition rate constant, beta—urine output < 0.9 ml/kg/hr	0.0013 ± 0.0004 min^{-1}

* Beta = 0.693/elimination half-life

so we have assumed that the serum tolazoline concentrations produced after such doses are part of its effective concentration range. Using the values for beta listed in Table 3, infusion doses to maintain this concentration constant may be calculated. At the very least, these doses will avoid progressive accumulation of tolazoline to potentially toxic or even lethal concentrations.

The formulas and the kinetic constants listed in Table 3 may be used to estimate the tolazoline concentration achieved with a tolazoline bolus dose and the infusion rate to maintain that concentration constant. (The weight of the proprietary form of tolazoline, tolazoline-HCl, includes the weight of the hydrochloride salt and is only 81.6 percent parent compound, which is the form measured with tolazoline assays.)

Since every 1.0 mg per kilogram loading dose of tolazoline-HCl increases the plasma tolazoline concentration an average of 0.5 mg per liter, the plasma tolazoline concentration following a loading dose that has improved oxygenation can be estimated. The estimated concentration can then be used with the standard pharmacokinetic formulas shown in Table 4 to calculate an infusion rate that avoids steadily increasing tolazoline concentrations which may be toxic, if not lethal. Thus, a tolazoline-HCl infusion rate of 0.16 mg per kilogram per hour for every 1.0 mg per kilogram loading dose should avoid accumulation in neonates. Further dose reductions may be needed for patients with oliguria or acute renal tubular necrosis.

Tolazoline should not be administered to hypotensive neonates until the blood pressure has been restored to normal. Some clinicians feel that volume expansion should precede tolazoline administration, since systemic hypotension from its nonspecific vasodilatation will prevent an improvement in PVR and may even worsen the shunt. We favor volume expansion with 10 ml per kilogram saline or lactated Ringer's solution over 10 to 20 minutes just prior to a 1 to 2 mg per kilogram dose of tolazoline infused over 1 to 2 min. (With a half-life as long as that of tolazoline in the newborn, this agent will rapidly distribute throughout the circulation, so there is no pharmacologic reason to infuse it into the superior vena cava in order that it passes through the lungs first.) If the infant improves, we proceed to hyperventilation which is often more successful at that time. If additional bolus doses of tolazoline are required, they are usually followed by tolazoline infusions at 0.16 mg tolazoline-HCl per kilogram per hour for every 1.0 mg per kilogram tolazoline-HCl bolus dose previously administered. If oxygenation is successfully maintained for 8 to 12 hours and the inspired oxygen has been weaned to less than 0.70, the tolazoline infusion will be halved and discontinued over the next 12 hours. The infant will then be maintained on mechanical hyperventilation for 1 to 2 days before it is tapered slowly over another 1 to 2 days.

Extracorporeal Membrane Oxygenation

Extracorporeal membrane oxygenation (ECMO) therapy for neonates has advanced rapidly over the last 5 years, so that it represents a therapeutic option for the neonate with PPHN who has failed to respond to more conventional treatment. The techniques for ECMO vary widely from center to center. Infants who were clearly dying from PPHN associated with the meconium aspiration syndrome or with right heart failure have survived with ECMO therapy. Long-term morbidity, however, remains uncertain. Complications such as cerebral hemorrhage and necrosis, as well as severe sepsis and empyema, have been observed. Many investigators worry about the cerebral effects of unilateral carotid artery ligation. It is too early to endorse ECMO without reservation. More important, it is

TABLE 4   Pharmacokinetic Dosing of Tolazoline for Neonates

$$
\begin{aligned}
\text{Plasma tolazoline conc} &= \text{Dose} \times 0.816^*/\text{Volume of distribution} \\
\text{(mg tolazoline base/L)} &= \text{(mg tolazoline} - \text{HCl/kg)/(L/kg)} \\
\text{Infusion rate} &= \text{beta} \cdot \text{Vd} \cdot \text{Conc} \cdot 1/0.816^* \\
\text{(mg tolazoline-HCl/kg/hr)} &= 1/\text{min} \cdot \text{L/kg} \cdot \text{mg/L} \\
&= 0.0027/\text{min} \cdot 60 \text{ min/hr} \cdot 1.61 \text{ L/kg} \cdot 0.5 \text{ mg/L} \cdot 1/0.816 \\
&= 0.16 \text{ mg tolazoline-HCl/kg/hr}
\end{aligned}
$$

* 1.0 mg tolazoline-HCl = 0.816 mg tolazoline parent drug

clearly *too early to claim that it is unethical to continue randomized trials comparing ECMO with other treatments* until prolonged follow-up is available for comparison of morbidity rates.

SUGGESTED READING

Philips JB III, ed. Neonatal pulmonary hypertension. Clin Perinatol 1984; ll:515–776.

PHENYLKETONURIA

SELMA E. SNYDERMAN, M.D.

It is most important to confirm the diagnosis of phenylketonuria before initiating specific therapy. *A positive result in the newborn metabolic screening program is not diagnostic*; it simply indicates which infants should be further evaluated with the proper confirmatory procedures. This would also include the special procedures necessary to differentiate those forms of hyperphenylalaninemia that are caused by defects in the synthesis and maintenance of tetrahydrobiopterin, the cofactor for phenylalanine hydroxylase and for neurotransmitter synthesis. These defects require a completely different form of therapy, substitution therapy with dopamine and 5-OH-tryptophan, and tetrahydrobiopterin.

A confirmed diagnosis of phenylketonuria involves a team effort of physician, nutritionist, social worker, and a laboratory capable of performing accurate phenylalanine determinations. Therefore, therapy should not be carried out by individual physicians but by special centers where all these services are available and there is experience in treating this disorder. Treatment should be instituted as soon as the diagnosis is confirmed; there is little doubt that the best results have been obtained with very early treatment. *We make every effort to see the infant on the day the positive screening result is reported and usually have the infant on a treatment regimen by 7 to 14 days of age.*

PRINCIPLES OF TREATMENT

The aim of therapy is to limit the phenylalanine intake while still providing enough to meet the requirement of this essential amino acid. Since it is not possible to provide enough protein without greatly exceeding the phenylalanine requirement, special formulas, either low or devoid of phenylalanine, are required. The formula that has been most widely used in the United States and the one with which we initiate therapy is Lofenalac. This formula contains adequate amounts of all nutrients with the exception of phenylalanine. Our usual procedure is to give enough to provide 125 cal per kilogram per day. This is provided by 27 g of the powder, which also provides 4 g of protein and 20 mg of phenylalanine per kilogram of body weight. This formula has the disadvantage of a high protein intake; however, we have not seen the sequelae of a high renal solute load when it is fed in the recommended dilution of

20 cal per ounce. If a greater caloric intake is required, carbohydrates should be added instead of increasing the amount of formula. This phenylalanine content is approximately one-quarter the requirement for this age group, and hence the plasma phenylalanine level can be expected to fall rapidly. The time required to approach the normal range depends on the height of the level and the age of the infant when therapy is initiated. It takes somewhat longer for the level to fall in older infants whose levels have been elevated for a prolonged period.

When the phenylalanine level drops to the normal range, usually 3 to 5 days after therapy is started, supplementation with phenylalanine is necessary to provide the requirement. We have always used a carefully measured amount of whole milk for this purpose. We prefer this to evaporated milk or any other infant formula, since a relatively small amount is used daily and thus one can avoid wasting the remainder. Rarely, if an infant is sensitive to cow's milk protein, a soy or hydrolyzed casein formula can be substituted to provide the phenylalanine requirement. Initial supplementation is usually calculated to provide a total phenylalanine intake of 80 mg per kilogram per day (~20 from Lofenalac and 60 from milk). Blood is then drawn every 2 to 3 days to determine phenylalanine level and thus ascertain the adequacy of intake. Since it requires about this length of time for equilibrium to be established, there is no need to perform blood determinations more frequently. The intake is then adjusted either up or down, according to the plasma phenylalanine level. During the first weeks of treatment, changes of intake of 5 mg per kilogram per day are usually sufficient to bring about the desired changes in phenylalanine level.

We have always tried to maintain the phenylalanine level as close to the normal range as possible. There is no need to keep the level above normal to avoid phenylalanine deficiency if the laboratory determinations are accurate enough to distinguish deficient from normal levels. The recommendation of maintaining levels above the normal range was originally made as a result of insensitive laboratory methods. It is our impression and experience that *rigid control during the early months of life results in the best intellectual outcome for the infant.*

Available Formulas

There are at present three other products on the American market designed for the treatment of phenylketonuria. Phenyl-Free is also made by Mead Johnson and differs from Lofenalac in that it is completely free of phenylalanine and contains a higher percentage of nitrogen. If used as the only food in the newborn period, the provision of adequate calories would result in an excessive protein intake. This problem can be avoided by supplementing the formula with carbohydrate. It may be advantageous to initiate therapy with this formula, since it is frequently used at a later age to allow the intake of more natural foods of low protein content. Occasionally it may be difficult to make this shift because some children who accept Lofenalac willingly may find Phenyl-Free quite distasteful. Two other products that can be used for the treatment of infants are now available in the United States: PKU 1, made by the Milupa Corporation of Germany and marketed by Mead Johnson, and Maxamaid XP, produced by Scientific Hospital Supplies Inc. of Great Britain and distributed in the United States by Ross. Both contain an amino acid mixture free of phenylalanine; they also contain vitamins, minerals, and a small amount of carbohydrate. Carbohydrate and fat must be added to provide adequate calories for infants, and hence their preparation is more difficult and time-consuming. Both have the advantage, at later ages, of the low caloric content and can be used to prevent or treat obesity in these children. The contents of the dietary products are listed in Table 1.

The phenylalanine requirement, when expressed in terms of body weight, falls rapidly during the first months of life and hence frequent readjustments of intake are necessary. Average requirements of phenylalanine are listed in Table 2.

Introduction of Other Foods

Since these products (with the exceptions already noted) are complete foods, routine supplementation is not necessary. An occasional infant does require an iron supplement. Solid foods can be introduced at the usual times; we have usually started with fruits, which are virtually free of phenylalanine and require no readjustment of phenylalanine intake. Rice cereal, the lowest protein-containing cereal, is usually introduced next. When properly treated—with appropriate protein, caloric, and phenylalanine intake—these infants do very well. They should maintain their respective growth curves (e.g., height, weight, head circumference); if this does not occur, causes other than phenylketonuria should be sought.

Termination of Therapy

The length of time that dietary treatment should be continued is still under investigation and debate. Termination of treatment will result in the reappearance of high phenylalanine levels and other abnormal metabolites. However, the effect of these abnormalities on the brain at later ages is not known. It has been suggested that once brain development and myelinization are virtually complete, at approximately 6 to 8 years of age, they are no longer susceptible to untoward influences. However, clinical experience with dietary termination has suggested that this may not be so. Slow but significant reduction in I.Q., the onset of behavior problems, and the development of learning problems in patients who do not have a drop in I.Q. have all suggested that adverse effects of high levels of phenylalanine may occur at any age. Although these consequences of dietary termination have not been universally observed, they have occurred with significant frequency. Our inability, at present, to determine which patients may be adversely affected emphasizes the need for continuing biochemical control. *It has been our policy to continue therapy indefinitely if cooperation can be obtained.* However, we have allowed the plasma phenylalanine level to rise to levels higher than are usually recommended during the first years of life in order to permit a slightly less restricted diet.

HYPERPHENYLALANINEMIA

Hyperphenylalaninemias are states in which there is some detectable residual activity of phenylalanine hydroxylase. Since routine enzyme determinations cannot be performed, these states are usually differentiated from classic phenylketonuria by the level of the blood phenylalanine on a normal diet. There has been a good deal of controversy about the need for treatment of the patients whose phenylalanine levels remain under 20 mg per deciliter. It has been *our policy to treat infants with levels that remain over 10 with the same dietary therapy as that used in classic phenylketonuria.* Because the plasma level usually falls rapidly in these infants, supplementation with phenylalanine may be required as early as 24 or 48 hours after the institution of treatment. Many of these children do not require therapy indefinitely and can tolerate a normal diet at 2 to 3 years of age. This can be ascertained by the use of a phenylalanine challenge.

A significant number of infants have lesser degrees of phenylalanine elevation. It has been our policy not to alter the diet of those whose levels remain under 4 mg per deciliter. We have advocated some degree of protein restriction in those with higher phenylalanine levels, between 5 and 10 mg per deciliter. This can be accomplished by the use of standard infant formulas, limiting the protein to 2 g per kilogram per day and adding carbohydrate to maintain the caloric intake. This type of restriction is usually necessary only for the first months of life.

MATERNAL PHENYLKETONURIA

The effect of maternal phenylketonuria on the fetus may be an increasing problem. There were relatively few pregnancies in phenylketonuric women until recently because the severe degree of retardation in these untreated patients resulted in the majority spending their lives in institutions. Inasmuch as universal screening for phenylketonuria was instituted in the 1960s, a number of women were diagnosed and treated early and are now normal and approaching childbearing age.

There is *no doubt of the profound untoward effect of untreated maternal phenylketonuria on the fetus.* Data obtained from a retrospective study of all known cases of maternal phenylketonuria revealed that over 90 percent of the offspring were mentally retarded. There was also a high incidence of microcephaly, and the incidence of congenital heart disease, spontaneous abortions, and low birth

TABLE 1 Contents of Preparations Used in Treatment of Phenylketonuria in Infants (per 100 g of powder)

	Lofenalac*		Phenyl-Free*		PKU 1[†]		Maxamaid XP[‡]	
Energy	460	cal	406	cal	272	cal	350	cal
Protein equivalent	15	g	20.3	g	50.3	g	25	g
Fat	18	g	6.8	g	0		0	
Carbohydrate	59.6	g	66	g	17.6	g	60	g
L-amino acids								
Alanine	0.68	g	0		2.4	g	1.08	g
Arginine	0.55	g	0.69	g	2.0	g	2.33	g
Aspartic acid	1.4	g	5.2	g	5.7	g	1.95	g
Cystine	0.059	g	0.35	g	1.4	g	0.75	g
Glutamic acid	3.98	g	1.88	g	12.0	g	2.53	g
Glycine	0.38	g	3.35	g	1.4	g	1.86	g
Histidine	0.47	g	0.47	g	1.4	g	1.34	g
Isoleucine	0.87	g	1.10	g	3.4	g	1.79	g
Leucine	1.66	g	1.73	g	5.7	g	3.06	g
Lysine	1.65	g	1.89	g	4.0	g	2.34	g
Methionine	0.52	g	0.63	g	1.4	g	0.5	g
Phenylalanine	0.08	g	0		0		0	
Proline	1.42	g	0		5.4	g	2.16	g
Serine	0.94	g	0		3.0	g	1.33	g
Threonine	0.78	g	0.94	g	2.7	g	1.5	g
Tyrosine	0.81	g	0.94	g	3.4	g	2.7	g
Tryptophan	0.20	g	0.28	g	1.0	g	0.6	g
Valine	1.37	g	1.26	g	4.0	g	1.95	g
Glutamine	0		4.82	g	0		0.23	g
Vitamins								
A	1,151	IU	2,030	IU	933	IU	1,000	IU
Thiamine	0.36	mg	0.6	mg	2.7	mg	1.1	mg
Riboflavin	0.43	mg	1.0	mg	4.0	mg	1.2	mg
Pyridoxine	0.3	mg	0.5	mg	2.2	mg	1.0	mg
Cobalamin	1.4	μg	2.5	μg	6.7	μg	4.0	μg
Niacin	5.8	mg	8.0	mg	54	mg	12	mg
Ascorbic acid	37.0	mg	53	mg	234	mg	67	mg
D	288	IU	406	IU	1,000	IU	480	IU
E	7.0	IU	10	IU	34	IU	6.5	IU
Biotin	0.04	mg	0.03	mg	0.1	mg	0.12	mg
Choline	61	mg	86	mg	434	mg	110	mg
Folic acid	72	μg	102	μg	334	μg	150	μg
Inositol	22	mg	30	mg	500	mg	56	mg
Pantothenic acid	2.2	mg	3	mg	25	mg	3.7	mg
K1	72	μg	102	μg	167	μg	45	μg
Minerals								
Calcium	432	mg	609	mg	2,400	mg	810	mg
Chloride	324	mg	500	mg	1,647	mg	450	mg
Copper	0.4	mg	0.6	mg	6.7	mg	2.0	mg
Iodine	0.032	mg	0.04	mg	0.234	mg	0.134	mg
Iron	9.0	mg	12	mg	34	mg	12	mg
Magnesium	50.0	mg	71	mg	521	mg	200	mg
Maganese	0.7	mg	1	mg	2.4	mg	1.3	mg
Phosphorus	324	mg	457	mg	1860	mg	810	mg
Potassium	468	mg	711	mg	2,332	mg	840	mg
Sodium	216	mg	254	mg	1,067	mg	580	mg
Zinc	3	mg	4	mg	26	mg	13	mg
Molybdenum					0.107	mg	0.06	mg

* Mead-Johnson.
† Milupa, distributed by Mead Johnson Laboratories.
‡ Scientific Hospital Supplies, distributed by Ross Laboratories.

weight was also significantly increased. This study also suggested that *pregnant women who do not have classic phenylketonuria but have significant degrees of hyperphenylalaninemia may also be at risk for having similarly affected infants.* At present, the exact relationship between the degree of elevation of the maternal phenylala-nine level and the occurrence of damage to the fetus is not known. The situation is further complicated by the fact that all amino acids are concentrated on the fetal side, the fetal-maternal ratio being approximately 1.5 to 1.0 for phenylalanine.

There is as yet limited experience with the outcome

TABLE 2 Average Phenylalanine Requirements During the First Months of Life

Age (months)	Requirement (mg/kg/day)
Premature	120–150
0–2	65–90
3	42–65
4	38–62
6	30–55
8	26–45

of pregnancy in phenylketonuric women under treatment. The best present information indicates that treatment should be started before the onset of pregnancy and be carefully controlled. Treatment instituted later in the course of pregnancy has not been successful in preventing all the sequelae of maternal phenylketonuria on the fetus. The data are limited, and more information, especially from a prospective well-controlled study, is needed. However, planned pregnancy after good control of the plasma phenylalanine level would seem to be the best advice that can be given at present.

Large supplements of tyrosine have been suggested for these pregnancies, in addition to the usual treatment to control the phenylalanine level. Tyrosine is an essential amino acid for the phenylketonuric because of the site of the enzyme block, and hence tyrosine has been included in all formulas used for the treatment of phenylketonuria. However, the need for large supplements has not been justified. Plasma tyrosine levels during normal pregnancies are lower than those of nonpregnant women of the same age. Any supplementation should be adjusted to maintain the tyrosine level in the same range as that of normal pregnancy but not to attempt to raise it to nonpregnancy levels with extremely high tyrosine intakes. There is little information about the effect of high tyrosine levels on the fetus, and to impose another metabolic strain is not justified by the present state of knowledge.

The need for treatment of pregnant phenylketonuric patients is another reason to continue treatment indefinitely in girls. *The dietary products used in therapy usually continue to be well-accepted by those treated from early infancy. However, once they are discontinued, most patients find it difficult to start taking these products again at a later age.*

PHENYLKETONURIA: EXPERIENCE IN PENNSYLVANIA

CHESTON M. BERLIN Jr., M.D.
KAREN M. BLACKBIRD, R.D.

Phenylketonuria (PKU) refers to a group of biochemical diseases associated with enzymatic blocks in the conversion of phenylalanine to tyrosine. These diseases are autosomal recessive in inheritance. The enzyme system necessary for this reaction is complex; the oxidative enzyme phenylalanine hydroxylase is required, which in turn requires two cofactors, $NAD^+/NADH$ and biopterin (in a reduced form as tetrahydrobiopterin). Classic PKU consists of absence of phenylalanine hydroxylase. Patients with this condition have serum levels of phenylalanine (PA) above 20 mg per deciliter. Dietary limitation of protein (and hence PA) has been very effective therapy for the last 20 years.

Other variants involve only partial loss of enzyme activity and result in lesser levels of PA, termed hyperphenylalaninemia. The latter in itself seems to be a complex group of conditions. Patients with hyperphenylalaninemia are now described whose defect is in the biopterin system (at least three different defects being described). These patients do not respond to a low PA diet; they have significant and rapid neurologic deterioration in early infan-

cy. Provision of the cofactor biopterin has been partially successful. Biopterin deficiency may result in deficiencies of the neurotransmitters dopamine and serotonin; hence, some of these patients may need to be given the precursors L-dopa and 5-hydroxytryptophan. *Cofactor screening should be carried out as part of the initial evaluation of any patient with hyperphenylalaninemia.*

DIAGNOSIS

All 50 U.S. states now routinely screen all newborns for PKU. The screening test used is the Guthrie, a microbiologic assay method. In Pennsylvania in 1986, 27 of 160,000 newborns were diagnosed as having a "screening" serum PA level above 4 mg per deciliter (*overall incidence of 1 in 6,000*). Eighteen of these patients are receiving dietary therapy (level above 14 mg per deciliter), an incidence of 1 in 9,000. The diagnosis must be supported by a quantitative assay of PA and tyrosine, as determined by the McCaman-Robins fluorometric assay. The serum PA concentration at which diet is started varies from center to center; *we treat initial levels that rise to 14 mg per deciliter or above.*

Human milk is low in PA (14 mg per ounce versus 45 mg per ounce for cow's milk and 22 mg per ounce for commercial formula); hence, *serum levels may rise very slowly (over 10 to 14 days) in the breast-fed baby.* It is most important to perform weekly (or more frequent) McCaman-Robins testing in infants, whether breast- or bottle-fed, whose initial levels put them in the "hyper" group (4 to 14 mg per deciliter). If the level remains below 14 mg per deciliter after 2 months of age, it is unlikely that the infant will require dietary therapy. All patients placed on dietary therapy should be challenged between the ages of 9 and 12 months with a load of 180 mg per kilogram per day of PA. Egg and milk are incorporated into the formula, so that no foods are introduced that a child may not later be allowed to have. This not only will confirm the diagnosis, but may give a hint as to the patient's future protein tolerance.

TELLING THE FAMILY

Because dietary therapy is reasonably straightforward (at least in infancy and the toddler age group), *it is easy to misjudge the serious emotional impact this diagnosis has on the family.* Initial news that a child has PKU is invariably given over the telephone and even sometimes through the family physician. We try to see the patient and family as soon as possible, even scheduling a late afternoon or evening session to fit parents' job demands or travel time; it is important to include grandparents and siblings. At the first visit considerable information is given to parents, in the form of pamphlets and dietary counseling. Parents are encouraged to keep lists of questions for future visits. All members of the PKU center staff have crucial roles in managing these patients. Considerable support can be given by the secretary, social worker, dietitian, and public health nurse, as well as the physicians. Because of the need to monitor diet weekly, *the dietitian is usually the person who develops the most important rapport with the family.*

Patients on diet are tested weekly by the Guthrie method for the first 4 to 6 months of life or until levels are stable; serum PA levels should be between 2 and 6 mg per deciliter, but realistically, levels below 10 mg per deciliter are accepted. Children are seen monthly for the first 6 months; the purpose of these visits is mostly educational and supportive. From 6 months to 2 years of age they are seen every 6 months, and yearly thereafter.

DIET

The diet consumed by patients with PKU must be low in PA but should contain adequate protein for growth. We use 3.7 to 4.2 g per kilogram per day of protein until the infant is 2 months of age, then 2.5 to 3.0 g per kilogram per day from 2 to 12 months of age. Caloric needs are 120 calories per kilogram per day until 2 months of age, when 100 to 110 calories per kilogram per day are given if adequate growth is occurring; growth and serum PA levels are the guidelines for the remainder of infancy and childhood. The infant's diet is started with a calculation of 40 to 70 mg per kilogram per day of PA in the form of Lofenalac (Mead Johnson), which contains just 3.5 mg of PA per ounce and is balanced nutritionally in every other respect. Mothers can successfully continue breast feed-

ing with Lofenalac supplementation four or five times in 24 hours to provide needed calories and protein. Children being breast-fed may receive a lower daily total of protein because of lower protein content in human milk (10 g per liter versus 23 g per liter for Lofenalac). Evaporated milk is used to provide added protein and PA as determined by the above calculations. The level of PA in the diet is altered according to the weekly Guthrie levels.

If serum PA falls below 2 mg per deciliter with beginning of the diet, which it invariably does, we add 104 mg of PA (1 oz of evaporated milk) per day to the infant's total formula. If the level exceeds 10 mg per deciliter, 104 mg of PA is removed from the total daily formula. After 4 months of age smaller adjustments are made (usually one-half of the above amounts).

Solid foods are introduced at 4 to 6 months of age with emphasis on fruits, vegetables, and iron-fortified cereal. All meats, dairy products, fish, eggs, nuts, and legumes are prohibitively high in protein (and hence PA) for consumption at any age (see later under "Maternal PKU"). Total daily amounts of PA per kilogram decrease as the child gets older and growth velocity decreases. *We are always impressed by the wide variation in PA consumption from patient to patient* in the attempt to keep the serum PA within an acceptable range.

COMPLIANCE

Compliance can be a serious problem in a very small number of patients (in our experience 10 percent or less of those receiving dietary therapy). Reasons vary: (1) refusal to accept the diagnosis, (2) multiple caretakers with differing degrees of understanding of the condition and the need for dietary therapy, (3) cheating by older children, and (4) family physicians who suggest dietary additions in infancy as if the child were normal. All of these can be successfully managed with patience and persistence, except the first. *It is a great and continuing frustration to deal with a hostile, suspicious family who cannot understand either the condition or its treatment.*

LENGTH OF DIETARY TREATMENT

Most centers are now keeping patients on the diet until at least age 12 years. Formerly it was considered safe to terminate the diet at age 6 years, but several studies have shown significant slippage in IQ testing (5 to 10 points) from ages 6 to 12 years when the patient is off the diet. There is a cogent argument for *continuing dietary treatment in females until they have passed their childbearing years.* Pregnant patients with PKU must have their levels controlled before conception if there is to be any hope of having an undamaged infant. Reinstituting the diet later in life is very difficult; the formula is very unpalatable, and attempts to disguise the somewhat metallic, potato-like taste with flavoring agents are only partially successful. The financial cost of the decision to prolong treat-

TABLE 1 Distribution of IQ Values Versus Age in PKU Patients on Dietary Treatment

Score	18 mo	3 yr	5 yr	7 yr	10 yr
< 50	2%	—	1%	2%	—
51–75	9%	4%	5%	16%	15%
76–90	22%	33%	40%	37%	30%
91–110	42%	41%	35%	30%	46%
111–125	20%	20%	8%	14%	7%
> 126	5%	2%	—	—	—
Average	97	93.2	93.3	95.6	90.2

Data courtesy of Drs. J.C. Ramer and D. E. Tinker.

ment beyond age 6 years is $2,000 to $3,000 per year per patient.

PSYCHOLOGICAL TESTING

We perform the following psychological evaluations:

Age	Test
18 months	Bayley
3 years	Stanford-Binet
5 years	Stanford-Binet
7 years	WICS-R
10 years	WISC-R

Like all other published groups, we can identify a relationship between serum PA levels and IQ. In general, patients who have been well-controlled (levels below 10 mg per deciliter) test within normal limits. However, even in well-controlled patients, low average IQ results may be obtained and learning problems may occur during the school ages. *In Pennsylvania 90 percent of PKU patients receiving dietary treatment are functioning at least in the low-average range.* Distribution of IQ is shown in Table 1.

MATERNAL PKU

For 30 years it has been appreciated that women with untreated classic PKU give birth to infants with multiple problems: low birth weight, microcephaly, mental retardation, and an increased incidence of congenital heart disease. There is no question that the risk in pregnant women with uncontrolled levels above 20 mg per deciliter is virtually 100 percent. A safe level has not yet been determined; it may be 10 mg per deciliter or lower. All workers are agreed that attempts must be made to lower serum PA levels to as close to normal as possible *before* conception. A National Collaborative Study has been launched to study the effectiveness of this approach.

There are over 200 affected females of reproductive age in Pennsylvania. Management of pregnancies in these patients is very complicated, frustrating, and expensive. Cost of formula alone is about $3,000 per 9 months; it is not clear who will pay for it. Registered dietitians are becoming depressed at the idea of keeping patients continuously on diet through their child-bearing years, but are also discouraged by attempts to make women resume the diet who are no longer accustomed to the taste of the low-PA formula. *The management of maternal PKU is a major problem in the clinical care offered by PKU clinics.*

PULMONARY INTERSTITIAL EMPHYSEMA

KEITH H. MARKS, M.B., B.Ch., F.C.P., Dip. Paed., M.R.C.P., Ph.D.

Air leak outside the pulmonary air spaces occurs in approximately 30 percent of preterm infants who require assisted ventilation with high airway pressures for severe lung disease. The aberrant air is not available for respiratory gas exchange and may encroach upon the normal anatomy of the thorax to cause life-threatening ventilatory and hemodynamic compromise.

Embryologically, the bronchopulmonary buds grow into the splanchnic mesoderm, which is prolonged later-ally into the developing mediastinum and lung as the perivascular and peribronchial connective tissue sheaths. The anatomic relationships of the investing perivisceral fascia constitute a potential space and "connecting highway" between the visceral and parietal pleura, pericardium, mediastinum, peritoneal cavity, and soft tissues of the neck. The intrathoracic extra-alveolar gas may remain in the perivascular and peribronchial connective tissue sheaths (pulmonary interstitial emphysema) or it may dissect toward the mediastinum (pneumomediastinum), pleural cavity (pneumothorax), pericardium (pneumopericardium), peritoneal cavity (pneumoperitoneum), or into the fascial planes of the neck (subcutaneous emphysema). Perforation of the pharynx or esophagus should be included in the differential diagnosis when an aberrant gas collection is seen on the chest x-ray film. The amount of air leak can vary in extent from minimal (asymptomatic) to massive (bronchopleural fistula).

PRINCIPLES OF TREATMENT OF PULMONARY INTERSTITIAL EMPHYSEMA

General

Pulmonary air leak should be suspected in any infant with respiratory distress who has a sudden deterioration in clinical status. Individuals responsible for the care of the distressed neonate must anticipate and be capable of managing a medical emergency if a tension pneumothorax develops. The availability of a high-intensity transillumination light (Chun Gun Transilluminator, Model 291-A, TI Radiation Measurements Inc., P. O. Box 327, Middleton, WI 53562) can be used to make a rapid noninvasive diagnosis of air in the pleural cavity. If there is circulatory collapse and severe respiratory distress, tension pneumothorax should be suspected, diagnosed with transillumination, and treated without waiting for radiologic confirmation. Small pneumothoraces, pulmonary interstitial emphysema, and pneumomediastinum are more reliably diagnosed by chest x-ray examination, particulary in the term infant with a relatively thick chest wall. All infants with pulmonary air leak require close observation and monitoring. Untreated infants with pneumothorax should not be transported in unpressurized aircraft because the decrease in atmospheric pressure may result in catastrophic enlargement of the pneumothorax to the point of seriously compromising ventilatory and cardiac functions. Attention must be given to the essentials of supportive care of the neonate with pulmonary air leak, including prompt resuscitation, circulatory support, oxygenation, temperature control, glucose hemostasis, and fluid and electrolyte balance.

Prevention

Pneumothorax may occur spontaneously but is more common in infants with related problems in the perinatal period. Risk factors for the development of pneumothorax include

1. resuscitation for fetal distress,
2. infants with respiratory distress due to hyaline membrane disease, congenital pneumonia, meconium aspiration syndrome, diaphragmatic hernia, and pulmonary hypoplasia,
3. mechanical ventilation, and
4. rarely, ruptured esophagus.

Individuals responsible for neonatal resuscitation in the delivery room should be skilled in rapid and accurate evaluation of the newborn condition as well as proficient in airway management, laryngoscopy, endotracheal intubation, artificial ventilation, suctioning of airways, cardiac massage, biochemical resuscitation, and maintenance of thermal stability. Equipment for intubation and resuscitation of the newborn must be functioning properly. The delivery room should be equipped with endotracheal tubes that are marked with a circumferential black ring at 3 cm proximal from the tip to facilitate proper placement of the endotracheal tube well above the carina. Alternatively, a Cole's tube, which has a shoulder to prevent passage of the tube beyond the tracheal bifurcation, can be used. Inadvertent intubation of the right main stem bronchus is dangerous and must be avoided because of barotrauma to the right lung.

Every infant with significant meconium aspiration requires immediate suctioning of the nasopharynx by the obstetrician as soon as the head appears in the perineum. Immediately after delivery the cords should be visualized by laryngoscopy and the trachea suctioned directly by means of the endotracheal tube. This procedure should be repeated to ensure removal of as much material as possible. Positive pressure and stimulation to elicit a cry should be avoided in these infants until adequate laryngotracheal toilet has been performed, to prevent pushing meconium farther into the small airways.

Adequate ventilation with oxygen should be provided by positive pressure in asphyxiated infants. Approximately 10 to 25 cm of water pressure is needed to inflate the lungs of a normal newborn infant, but pressure twice as high may be necessary initially. Initial lung inflation may require 30 to 40 cm of water pressure, but less pressure is needed for succeeding breaths, which should be provided at a rate of approximately 40 to 60 times per minute. Adequacy of ventilation is judged by symmetric movement of the apices of the chest. The resuscitation bag, flowmeter, suction equipment, and connectors should be checked for proper functioning. The connection from endotracheal tube or face mask to bag is preferably separated by a T-piece, which allows interposition of an aneroid manometer to estimate inflation pressure. A wall oxygen source and a Y-connector to the infant's airway must not be used to inflate the chest, because wall oxygen has a line pressure of approximately 3,500 cm of water pressure and will rupture the lung.

In general terms, the prevention of perinatal events related to the development of air leak include the obstetric management and prevention of preterm labor and delivery; the induction of pulmonary surfactant with maternally administered steroids to reduce the incidence of hyaline membrane disease; and gentle effective resuscitation in the delivery room. The assisted ventilation strategy should *aim to reduce barotrauma by following an aggressive weaning policy.* Treatment of hyaline membrane disease by administering animal or human surfactant to the lung appears promising.

Conservative Therapy

Nonintervention, but with close observation and monitoring of the infant's clinical status, should be used only in term infants with a small pneumothorax causing mild distress. The air in the pleural space will be reabsorbed spontaneously, since the sum of the partial pressures of the gases in the pleural space (i.e., arterial pressure = 760 mm Hg at sea level) is greater than the sum of the partial pressures of gases in end-capillary blood due to the low end-capillary PO_2. The nitrogen washout technique can be used by administering 100 percent oxygen to the infant via an oxyhood. This treatment may hasten resolution of the pneumothorax by creating a large diffusion gradient for nitrogen from the air in the pleural space to the blood. This technique should only be used in term infants with mild distress. Serial x-ray studies should be performed to ensure that the pneumothorax has resolved.

Needle Aspiration

Aspirating a tension pneumothorax in an emergency can be accomplished using a 23-gauge butterfly needle with a three-way stopcock and a 30- to 50-ml syringe. The equipment should be immediately available for use. After preparing the skin with a povidone-iodine swab, the needle is inserted in the pleural space at the level of the second to third intercostal space anteriorly at the midclavicular line. As much air as possible should be withdrawn into the syringe and the stopcock turned so the air can be rapidly evacuated through the open port. The procedure is repeated until one can no longer withdraw any additional air. A thoracostomy tube should be placed when the appropriate equipment and facilities are available. The presence of pulmonary interstitial emphysema at the time of first pneumothorax is an extremity sensitive index of later contralateral pneumothorax. Failure of the lung to re-expand despite aspiration of air indicates that there is a large continuing air leak through a communication between the pleural space and the lung. In this circumstance, a closed thoracostomy tube is essential.

Closed Chest Tube Drainage

In the presence of underlying lung disease, or if a pneumothorax develops during assisted ventilation, closed thoracostomy tube drainage is almost always needed. A sterile technique is used to administer a local anesthetic (1 percent lidocaine) into the skin and subcutaneous tissues, and a 1-cm skin incision is made with a pointed blade over the third or fourth intercostal space in the anterior or midaxillary line. A No. 10 or No. 12 French thoracic catheter is mounted on the trochar to facilitate its introduction. Create an oblique passage by tunneling toward the midclavicular line under the pectoralis major, which will collapse and seal as the chest tube is removed. Be careful not to tunnel through and thereby damage the breast, which is just medial to the incision. Avoid the nipple. Holding the trochar and catheter vertically over the second intercostal space, place the thumb and index finger just behind the side hole of the catheter to act as a guard. Push the trochar and catheter into the pleural space deeply enough so that the side holes are within the pleural cavity. *Direct the catheter anteriorly if air is to be drained or posteriorly if fluid is to be drained.* Remove the trochar and attach the catheter to a one-way valve system (see below). The catheter is then secured by using the pursestring suture technique (4-0 silk) and adhesive tape or Opsite. A chest x-ray film must be obtained immediately to determine the thoracostomy tube placement and its effectiveness in allowing the lung to re-expand. No air must be introduced into the pleural cavity during aspiration or intercostal drainage. Appropriate antibiotics are given for the associated pulmonary disease process.

The Use of Chest Tube Suction

Intercostal drainage must be closed (under water) to allow air to escape from the chest yet prevent its entry into the pleural space. The basic and time-honored components of the three-bottle suction system have been ingeniously incorporated into the Pleur-evac disposable 3-bottle unit. The rate of evacuation through the Pleur-evac is proportional to the negative pressure applied to the thoracostomy tube and the radius of the tube. The air flow rate (bubble rate) through the Pleur-evac is of minor importance in affecting the rate of evacuation. The Pleur-evac is filled to 10 to 20 cm of water in the suction control chamber. With the application of negative pressure of 20 cm of water (as suggested by the manufacturer), the Pleur-evac has the capacity to evacuate more than 4 L of air per minute, depending on the size and number of the thoracostomy tubes. This evacuation rate is probably adequate under most conditions. However, in the event of a large air leak such as a bronchopleural fistula, higher evacuation rates may be necessary. Under these circumstances, assuming that the thoracostomy tubes are patent and the accumulating air is in continuity with the thoracostomy tubes and not loculated elsewhere (e.g., in the subpleural space), one could *add water to the suction control chamber to increase the negative pressure and thus the evacuation rate. If this does not produce the desired result, a larger thoracostomy tube or second tube should be placed.* The small-bore thoracostomy tubes used in small infants impose significant resistance to air flow.

A Heimlich's chest drain flutter valve has been used in neonates as an alternative one-way valve system. This equipment is recommended for use on transports or if no underwater seal is available. A potential problem with the Heimlich's valve is serous drainage from the chest tube "gluing" the rubber valve together with accumulation of air in the pleural cavity. Suction should not be applied to the open end of the Heimlich's valve because if the negative suction pressure exceeds the positive outflow pressure from the tube, the soft rubber valve will collapse and drainage will cease. The Heimlich's valve is ideally suited for chest drainage of a pneumothorax during transport.

The chest tube should be left in place until no bubbling in the air-fluid level chamber has been observed for at least 24 hours. The chest tube is then placed to underwater seal by shutting off the suction being applied to the Pleur-evac for an additional 24 hours. The thoracostomy tube should be withdrawn with Vaseline-coated gauze wrapped around the tube to plug the chest incision, thereby preventing entrance of air; prevent the baby's vigorous crying to decrease the risk of recurrent air leak. A chest x-ray study should be obtained if clinical deterioration occurs.

Physical Therapy and Postural Effects

Often this is the only modality of therapy one has to offer the infant when the air leak is limited to pulmonary interstitial emphysema. If the interstitial emphysema is unilateral, one can try selective intubation of the main stem bronchus. In many infants, this procedure results in deterioration of the overall status and has to be abandoned. If it is tolerated, the infant may gradually improve over the next 24 to 48 hours. The oxygen-breathing infant with unilateral interstitial emphysema should be positioned so that the affected lung is dependent and the good lung uppermost until improvement occurs.

Surgery

In rare instances, bullous emphysema of an affected lobe may require lobectomy. Thoracic surgery may be necessary to repair bronchopleural fistula. In general, surgery is not recommended for acquired cystic disease of the lung, which is best managed conservatively. Surgery is the treatment of choice for congenital cystic disease of the lung.

Experimental Therapy

Future therapy, which at this stage remains experimental, includes high–frequency oscillatory ventilation to provide more uniform lung inflation and less acute barotrauma, the use of extracorporeal membrane oxygenation in severe pulmonary interstitial emphysema, and surfactant replacement therapy. These therapies should be used only by centers equipped for formal evaluation of these techniques.

RENAL CYSTIC DISEASE

CHARLES L. STEWART, M.D.
LEONARD I. KLEINMAN, M.D.

Renal cystic disease is a heterogeneous group of disorders, some of which may have distinctive morphologic, radiologic, or clinical features. The pathogenesis, clinical manifestations, importance, and approach to therapy of renal cysts in the newborn are variable. Many attempts have been made to classify renal cystic disease; Table 1 is based on the classification of Bernstein and Gardner, highlighted to show those cystic conditions of importance in the neonate. This classification system attempts to incorporate radiologic, clinical, genetic, and morphologic information.

CLINICAL DIAGNOSTIC APPROACH

The increasing use of sonography to monitor fetal-maternal health and growth has resulted in an increased recognition of structural abnormalities in the fetal urinary system; the presumptive diagnosis of conditions such as polycystic disease, multicystic dysplasia, and hydronephrosis is now commonly made prenatally, with postnatal imaging used to confirm (or refute) the prenatal diagnosis. A renal or other abdominal mass in the newborn may also be suspected from findings on physical examination of the abdomen. Again, sonography is the most useful imaging tool to define masses and is the imaging procedure of first choice to define cystic disease in newborn kidneys. In addition to the findings on abdominal examination, other aspects of the neonatal physical examination may lead to the suspicion of urinary tract abnormalities. A single umbilical artery has been noted to be associated with an increased incidence of renal anomalies, as have abnormalities of the external ears, and these findings may prompt the neonatologist to order renal sonography. Infants with multiple congenital abnormalities are also at higher risk for urinary tract abnormalities, especially hydronephrosis and renal cystic disease.

The correct diagnosis and a reasonable approach to therapy of renal cystic disease can usually be made on the basis of physical examination, sonographic findings, and the evaluation of renal function and urinalysis. Other imaging modalities, such as radionuclide renal scans, voiding cystourethrograms, and occasionally excretory urograms, may be useful to define functional and anatomic abnormalities of the kidney(s) with cystic disease and to rule out the possibility that a contralateral kidney, which perhaps appears sonographically normal, may have an abnormality requiring further attention. Table 2 lists the modalities used in the diagnosis of cystic disease, and Table 3 lists the prominent features of the major cystic renal diseases found in the newborn.

CYSTIC DYSPLASIA

Dysplasia implies an abnormality in morphogenesis and differentiation that is characterized by abnormal renal parenchymal development. Although dysplasia is not a specific malformation associated with a specific developmental abnormality, it is commonly associated with fetal urinary tract obstruction. Abnormalities of the ureter, bladder, or urethra are seen in about 90 percent of cases. The dysplastic kidney is not always cystic in nature.

The multicystic, dysplastic (MCD) kidney is almost always associated with obstruction or atresia of the ureter. Although MCD is most frequently unilateral, bilater-

TABLE 1 Classification of Renal Cysts

Polycystic disease
    Autosomal recessive polycystic kidney disease
        Polycystic disease of newborns and young infants
        Polycystic disease of older children and adults
    Autosomal dominant polycystic kidney disease

Renal cysts in hereditary syndromes
    Tuberous sclerosis complex
    Orofaciodigital syndrome I
    von Hippel-Lindau disease
    Zellweger's cerebrohepatorenal syndrome and Jeune's
        asphyxiating thoracic dysplasia
    Cortical cysts and syndromes of multiple malformations
    Glomerulocystic disease of newborn (in part)

Simple cysts, solitary and multiple

Segmental and unilateral cystic disease

Acquired cystic disease

Renal medullary cysts
    Hereditary tubulointerstitial nephritis
    Medullary sponge kidney

Renal dysplasia
    Multicystic and aplastic dysplasia
    Diffuse cystic dysplasia
    Cystic dysplasia associated with lower urinary tract
        obstruction

al MCD kidneys are possible and other anatomic abnormalities of the contralateral kidney, such as ureteropelvic junction obstruction, can occur. The MCD kidney usually appears as a large cystic mass on prenatal sonography or as a unilateral abdominal mass on physical examination of the newborn. Frequently, the multiple cysts, described as resembling a bunch of grapes, can be palpated. Sonography usually shows the diagnostic features described in Table 3. The major diagnostic distinction is between MCD kidney and unilateral, severe hydronephrosis; in a MCD kidney the cysts may be arrayed to mimic a dilated renal pelvis with peripheral dilated calyces. A nuclear scan with dimercaptosuccinic acid is useful to resolve this differential diagnosis; a MCD kidney does not usually concentrate any of this material, whereas a hydronephrotic kidney does. Once the diagnosis of a MCD kidney is made, it is necessary to evaluate the function and anatomy of the contralateral kidney, which is more likely to have vesicoureteral reflux or ureteropelvic junction obstruction. An intravenous nuclear study with diethylenetriaminepenta-acetic acid, followed by diuresis with furosemide, is useful to evaluate the contralateral kidney for obstruction. In addition, a voiding cystourethrogram (VCU) should be performed; if reflux is present in a unilateral functioning kidney, then antibiotics for prophylaxis against urinary tract infection are warranted, and surgical correction of the reflux should be considered. A nuclear VCU results in less radiation dose to the infant than a contrast VCU, but the nuclear study does not image the posterior urethra and bladder well. In MCD kidneys, however, the obstruction is virtually always at the ureteral level; posterior urethral valves are not associated with MCD disease. Lower urinary tract obstruction can result in renal dysplasia and cyst formation, with the cysts present in the subcapsular area and along the columns of Bertin. Male infants with this pattern or an intermediate or indefinite pattern should have a contrast rather than a nuclear VCU to evaluate the possibility of

TABLE 2 Diagnostic Modalities in Cystic Renal Disease

Physical examination

    Size, contour, texture of renal mass
    Other physical anomalies

Prenatal sonography

    Useful in early detection of hereditary
    renal masses, hydronephrosis, MCD kidneys

Postnatal renal sonography

    Imaging examination of first choice for neonatal renal mass. Usually sufficient
    for diagnosis of cystic renal disease. Also useful for follow-up evaluation to
    assess progression of disease process.

Nuclear renal scans
    Diethylenetriaminepenta-acetic acid: useful in detecting functional renal blood
    flow and in evaluating possibility of and level of obstructive uropathy.
    Dimercaptosuccinic acid: used to determine presence of functioning renal
    cortical tissue.

Intravenous urography

    Not useful in neonates. In older infants, useful to assess quality of renal function
    and to define anatomy.

Abdominal CT scan

    May be used for assessing cystic disease whose anatomic pattern is not
    determinable by other modalities.

Voiding cystourethrogram

    Used to detect vesicoureteral reflux.

TABLE 3   Characteristics of Cystic Disease

Disease	Sonographic Features	Renal Function	Associated Findings
Multicystic dysplastic	Multiple cysts of varying size Interfaces between cysts Nonmedial location of larger cysts Absence of indentifiable renal sinus Usually no demonstrable communication between cysts	Normal if contralateral kidney normal	High incidence (25–30%) of obstructive involvement of contralateral kidney
Autosomal rescessive polycystic kidney disease	Bilateral, frequently massively enlarged kidneys Increased uniform echogenicity Occasionally small cysts in the dense, echogenic medullary area	May range from normal to significant azotemia; if azotemia, usually progressive	Hepatic disease, hepatic fibrosis, portal hypertension Frequent hypertension
Autosomal dominant polycystic kidney disease	Bilateral renal enlargement Cysts of varing size, depending on stage of lesion A normal study in patient with positive family history does not preclude the later development of renal enlargement cysts	Slowly progressive renal dysfunction	15% have aneurysms of cerebral blood vessel Antibiotic-resistant urinary tract infection Hypertension

posterior urethral valves. A single MCD kidney with a normal functioning contralateral kidney is only rarely associated with other clinical abnormalities. With time, the large cysts may involute and the mass become smaller. Rarely, hypertension has been reported to occur as a result of MCD kidneys, but only occasionally has the hypertension been "cured" with nephrectomy; this implies that the contralateral kidney, which we know is more likely to have anatomic abnormalities, is probably producing renin and may have sustained reflux nephropathy or hydronephrosis, which can cause hypertension. Some have also reported that with time there may be a higher incidence of malignant changes in MCD kidneys. However, these reports are anecdotal and far from conclusive. Nevertheless, most pediatric surgeons and urologists remove these MCD kidneys when the patient is about 1 year of age. In contrast, some centers are now opting to wait and to follow the natural history of MCD kidneys, so that further refinements in the role of surgical therapy should be forthcoming. Follow-up sonographic evaluation of the remaining functioning kidney should be done yearly or twice yearly to ensure adequate compensatory growth.

Bilateral MCD kidneys are not compatible with life; since these kidneys are not functional from relatively early in gestation, infants with bilateral involvement may display the effects of oligohydramnios, such as hypoplasia of the lungs and Potter's facies. If the infant's pulmonary function is adequate to support life, then chronic peritoneal dialysis may be instituted as renal replacement therapy. In addition, aggressive, meticulous attention to nutritional requirements and prompt therapy of intercurrent infections may allow the infant to survive to an age at which renal transplantation can be undertaken. Bilateral nephrec-

tomy is often done to decrease the amount of space filled by these large, nonfunctioning organs. This form of therapy for infants requires extreme dedication on the part of the parents as well as many hours of involvement on the part of the entire pediatric dialysis/transplant team.

AUTOSOMAL RECESSIVE (INFANTILE) POLYCYSTIC KIDNEY DISEASE

Autosomal recessive (infantile) polycystic kidney disease is a heterogeneous group of inherited disorders characterized by small, cystic dilatations of the collecting ducts of the kidneys that extend from the corticomedullary junction to the capsule, with the medullary pyramids containing dilated ducts. Also present in this disorder is bile duct hyperplasia in the portal areas of the liver.

Most infants with autosomal recessive polycystic kidney disease are recognized either by prenatal sonography, which shows enlarged fetal kidneys and perhaps increased renal echogenicity, or by the observation on physical examination of a distended abdomen and the presence of large renal masses. The liver may also be enlarged in these patients. Many infants with autosomal recessive polycystic kidney disease have a history of oligohydramnios and are born with Potter's facies. The kidneys may be so massively enlarged that intrapartum dystocia occurs. Because of the oligohydramnios, pulmonary hypoplasia may exist.

Once the renal masses are recognized, sonography is the major diagnostic tool. With sonography, renal size can be reproducibly determined and small cysts recognized as an increase in renal echogenicity (see Table 3). If the physical examination and renal imaging studies are not sufficient for diagnosis, a renal biopsy may be required. A biopsy of the liver would also demonstrate characteristic portal findings. Some of these infants have significant azotemia and should have regular evaluation of their blood urea nitrogen and creatinine levels. Other causes of bilateral renal enlargement are listed in Table 4.

Infants with autosomal recessive polycystic kidney disease may have progressive renal insufficiency, failure to thrive, hypertension, and congestive heart failure. Many infants and children have mild to moderate polyuria because of their tubular disease. The rate of decline of renal function is variable, and some children have problems related to their hepatic involvement, such as portal hypertension.

Therapy is supportive. Hypertension is common, and physicians should be aggressive in controlling blood pressure, since hypertension may quicken the decline of renal function. If the hypertension is mild, hydralazine, alone or in combination with a diuretic or a beta-adrenergic antagonist, may be sufficient. Captopril, an angiotensin-converting enzyme inhibitor, is frequently effective in controlling blood pressure. Antihypertensive agents useful in treating infants with autosomal recessive polycystic kidney disease are listed in Table 5. Nutritional support is also extremely important to minimize growth retardation, bone disease, and anemia associated with progressive renal insufficiency. In spite of renal insufficiency, these infants may continue to be polyuric, and access to fluids must be maintained, especially during intercurrent viral infec-

tions, in order to prevent dehydration. When signs of end-stage renal insufficiency ensue, these infants and children can be successfully dialyzed and receive kidney transplants.

AUTOSOMAL DOMINANT (ADULT) POLYCYSTIC KIDNEY DISEASE

Although rare in infancy, autosomal dominant (adult) polycystic kidney disease has been diagnosed in the neonate and by prenatal ultrasonography. Seventy-five percent of persons with this disease have a positive family history; the remaining 25 percent may represent spontaneous mutation. Cysts may occur in any part of the nephron, but glomerular cysts seem to be more common in infants than in older patients. This disorder is the third most common cause of renal failure in adults. The most frequent manifestation reported in infants is an abdominal mass, which may be detected by prenatal sonography or on the newborn physical examination. Cysts can occur in other organs, such as the liver, pancreas, spleen, thyroid, seminal vesicles, and ovaries. Hepatic cysts, unlike in autosomal recessive polycystic kidney disease, are not typically associated with portal hypertension. Imaging findings are noted in Table 3. Of note is that 15 to 30 percent of patients with autosomal dominant polycystic kidney disease may have berry aneurysms of the cerebral blood vessels.

The treatment of this disorder is largely supportive. Regular assessment of renal functional parameters, such as blood urea nitrogen and creatinine, is advisable to monitor disease progression. Hypertension should be aggressively managed, as described in the previous section. Urinary tract infections may be quite serious, as antibiotics frequently do not reach adequate levels in infected renal cysts. Lipid-soluble antibiotics, such as chloramphenicol or trimethoprim, may be necessary to eradicate cystic infections. Antibiotic therapy based on sensitivity for the infecting organism should be used, but if symptoms, signs, or microbiologic evidence of infection persists, the lipid-

---

TABLE 4 Causes of Bilateral Renal Enlargement

Autosomal dominant polycystic kidney disease
Autosomal recessive polycystic kidney disease
Bilateral multicystic dysplastic kidney
Bilateral hydronephrosis
Bilateral renal tumor (Wilms')
Bilateral renal venous thrombosis

TABLE 5 Oral Neonatal Antihypertensive Agents

Drug	Dose	Note
Hydralazine	1–6 mg/kg/day orally, divided in 4–6 doses	Can cause reflex tachycardia requiring beta-adrenergic antagonist
Propranolol	0.5–3.0 mg/kg/day orally, divided in 4 doses	Use with extreme caution in patients with congestive heart failure, arrhythmias, and bronchospastic disease
Captopril	0.1 mg/kg/dose, given 3–4 times/day; dose may be increased to 4 mg/kg/day	Closely monitor renal function; use cautiously in patients with single kidneys
Minoxidil	0.2 mg/kg, given once a day; increase dose up to 1 mg/kg/day if needed	Usually requires diuretic; causes hirsutism
Furosemide	1–4 mg/kg/day in 1–3 divided doses	Monitor for hypercalciuria, electrolyte abnormalities
Hydrochlorothiazide	2 mg/kg/day in 1–2 doses	Not useful in renal insufficiency or immediate newborn period

soluble antibiotics may be required. Appropriate precautions for these antibiotics in the newborn period should be used. The progression toward end-stage renal disease does not usually ensue until adulthood. Early diagnosis is very helpful in genetic counseling. If a family with autosomal dominant polycystic kidney disease has an infant with radiologically normal kidneys, this does not ensure freedom from the disease. Family members should be followed at regular intervals with sonographic studies.

OTHER HEREDITARY SYNDROMES

Renal cysts are found in several inherited conditions (see Table 1), and although they are usually multiple in number, the kidneys should not be regarded or labeled as "polycystic." Small cortical cysts are found in Zellweger's syndrome, trisomy D, and trisomy E syndromes and are usually of no particular clinical significance. Cystic disease in Ehlers-Danlos syndrome and orofaciodigital syndrome can on rare occasion lead to significant functional impairment. Morphologically distinctive renal cystic disease, leading to hypertension and azotemia, has been described in neonates as the first clinically apparent manifestation of tuberous sclerosis. These patients have benefited from surgical decompression of their cysts, resulting in resolution of their hypertension and improvement in their renal function.

OTHER CYSTIC DISEASE

The cysts found in most other hereditary disorders listed in Table 1 are not detectable in the newborn period. Similarly, acquired renal cysts are found as life progresses and are not present in the newborn. On occasion, isolated or multiple simple renal cysts are found in newborns. Renal function is almost always normal with this cystic abnormality, and only routine (yearly) sonographic follow-up is necessary.

RETINOPATHY OF PREMATURITY

DALE L. PHELPS, M.D.

As neonatologists, one of our delights is the vigorous, growing, premature infant, safely past the perilous times of ventilation, intracranial hemorrhage, patent ductus, and feeding difficulties. As discharge home comes closer, screening for retinopathy of prematurity (ROP, previously known as retrolental fibroplasia) and hearing loss is carried out, and potential neurologic or visual sequelae are discussed again with the family. Fortunately, most infants grow to be normal adults, but as many as 5 percent of those weighing less than 1 kg at birth may be virtually blind from ROP. As the number of survivors in the lower and lower birth weight categories continues to climb, the number of potentially affected infants also increases. There are few established facts about the etiology, prevention, and treatment of ROP. The resulting policies are the practical product of our current understanding or misunderstanding of ROP, and are always evolving on the basis of results of ongoing investigations.

DEVELOPMENT

Retinopathy of prematurity consists of the abnormal proliferation of small retinal vessels. These vessels normally begin to grow out from the optic disc around 16 weeks of gestation. They should grow in a steady wave of differentiation, remaining within the maturing retinal substance, and reach the far edge of the retina near term. The smaller the area of the retina that these vessels have covered at the time of birth, the more likely is it that something will go wrong with the process of vascularization and that ROP will occur.

The condition seems to be initiated when the delicate growing vessels are injured, most likely owing to oxygenation changes, asphyxia, shock, and other stresses surrounding the time of birth. We infer this because of the association between ROP and other morbid conditions when compared within weight groups of the smallest infants. The normal orderly progress of vessel growth is thus disrupted, and the vascularization of the maturing retina must be accomplished through a repair response rather than normal angiogenesis. After a delay of 4 to 6 weeks, this response becomes visible upon ophthalmic examination as early ROP. *The lower the gestational age at birth, and therefore the larger the area of retina that is not yet normally vascularized, the more likely is ROP to occur.* As many as 80 to 100 percent of infants born weighing less than 1 kg have been reported to develop ROP of some degree.

Once started, there are several directions that ROP can take. It can disappear (regress) within a few weeks, progress to more severe manifestations and then regress over a period of many weeks, or progress to severe proliferation, "plus" disease and permanent sequelae. The more complex and unstable an infant's hospital course, the more likely is severe progression to occur. This, along with laboratory observations, supports the belief that infants' condition during the healing process, and therefore their care, may affect the outcome of ROP.

SEQUELAE

Infants who have had mild ROP, but then fully vascularize the retina without visible sequelae, are often considered recovered—end of follow-up. However, *these infants must not be dismissed from ophthalmic follow-up because they have a higher than usual incidence of refractive errors and strabismus* that can lead to amblyopia. The neonatologist should emphasize to parents the need to keep ophthalmic follow-up appointments because of these problems.

When ROP regresses slowly and leaves visible residual scars in the retina, the incidence of these sequelae rises, with severe myopia leading the list. Without glasses, these infants have impaired visual learning, and if the myopia is unilateral, they will develop amblyopia as well. These sequelae in the early years occupy the attention of the families and physicians, but tend to be forgotten as the visual changes stabilize under treatment. However, as the children grow, *the diagnosis of ROP retinal scars should not be forgotten* and each of these children should learn their histories. These former premature infants must continue to undergo annual ophthalmologic follow-up. The areas of residual retinal scars are subject to later degeneration and late retinal detachments, typically in the teenage or young adult years. These changes occur far more slowly than acute ROP, and can often be effectively treated by retinal surgeons. A late partial detachment that goes undetected for some time is particularly tragic in a young adult who is already blind in the other eye.

When acute ROP progresses to retinal folds involving the macula, or large retinal detachments, the infants become visually impaired to a severe degree. Each of these children needs ongoing evaluation for the degree of vision loss, placement in programs for the visually impaired, and continuing education of the family regarding the child's potential for independent function. Sometimes significant peripheral vision is retained or perhaps only light-dark perception, but each level of residual visual function should be used to the child's fullest advantage.

Pediatricians and family, as well as ophthalmologists, need to be aware that the *infant with total retinal detachments can develop acute glaucoma.* The young infant with ROP who appears to be in pain and is suddenly rubbing the eyes should be immediately evaluated by the ophthalmologist for control of this complication, often unsuspected in an infant who cannot express this pain, and whose eyes may be small and frequently rubbed anyway. On a less acute basis, infants who retain some vision can lose even that, owing to the cataracts that sometimes develop in severe ROP. Thus, it behooves the pediatrician to ensure the ongoing ophthalmic follow-up of even those infants who seem to be blind in an end stage of ROP.

PREVENTION

Prevention of prematurity itself would clearly be the most effective method of eliminating ROP. However, for infants who are born early, it seems likely that minimizing complications of the neonatal period may substantially decrease the incidence of severe ROP, through the reduction of initial injury and whatever adverse effects subsequent complications of the hospital course may have on the healing process. The monitoring of oxygen administration has been the primary focus of pediatricians in this regard since the 1950s; however, more recent evidence suggests that we may also need to consider light, nutritional status, and perhaps other drugs or conditions of care.

Oxygen

Monitoring of oxygen administration has been accepted as critical since the demonstration that routine administration of over 50 percent oxygen for 4 weeks without regard for an infant's respiratory status increased the incidence of ROP several times. Thus, current practice requires that oxygen be given to premature infants only when they would be hypoxic without it, and that frequent, appropriate monitoring such as arterial or capillary blood gas determinations, or transcutaneous oxygen monitoring and/or pulse oximetry, shows that oxygen is still needed. *Several attempts to establish levels of arterial oxygen that are safe in respect to ROP have failed, and we increasingly recognize that oxygen is only one component of a complex series of events that are active in this disease.*

Antioxidants

The recognition that prolonged excess oxygen causes a higher incidence of ROP has led to the belief that exogenously administered antioxidants may spare the retina from this (presumably) oxidant injury–induced disorder. However, *controlled trials testing the lipid antioxidant, vitamin E, have been disappointing.* Although vitamin E seemed to have a small beneficial effect on the incidence of severe disease in some trials, it had none in others. In no trial has it convincingly reduced the overall incidence of this disease. In order to use vitamin E effectively against ROP, it would have to be given prophylactically to the more than 36,000 infants born annually weighing less than 1,500 g, although only 1,000 or 2,000 of those are destined to have ROP sequelae. Since a large majority (over 90 percent) of premature infants do not develop severe ROP, all would be exposed to the risk of prophylactic Vitamin E (a low incidence of side effects has been reported in infants given large doses of vitamin E), while only a few could possibly benefit, even if it were definitely effective. Therefore, large doses of vitamin E for prevention of ROP should not be given at this time.

Prophylactic administration of D-penicillamine, a heavy metal-binding antioxidant, has been noted to reduce the incidence of ROP in both an initial study and a confirming randomized trial in Hungary. However, these observations in a single unit require replication in other settings, and further investigation into risks and side effects, before the widespread use of this agent can be recommended.

Light Exposure

There has been a recent report of a reduction in ROP when light exposure was reduced in two nurseries. Unfortunately, the controls were sequential rather than concurrent, weakening this evidence and making it difficult to use as a basis for policy. Specific randomized testing of the effect of light in the 1940s failed to show any adverse effect of light exposure on ROP. However, it seems reasonable, and without recognizable risk, to avoid direct bright light exposure of the face in all infants. There is no strong evidence to support patching the eyes of all premature infants or to justify extreme reduction of light levels in the nursery at this time.

CLASSIFICATION

The International Classification of Retinopathy of Prematurity (ICROP) should now be used by all ophthalmologists examining premature infants. It describes the disorder in three new dimensions (amount of avascular retina, extent of the disease, and "plus" component) and facilitates communication between physicians over a particular case and comparison of different studies. A multicenter study currently in progress is using the ICROP system to collect prospective sequential ophthalmic data on thousands of extremely premature infants. The *amount of avascular retina seen on an early examination and recorded in zones 1, 2, or 3 will likely prove to be a strong predictor of the risk* in a particular infant for developing severe disease.

When ROP has developed, the *extent of the proliferation around the retina is recorded in clock hours* of disease. This measure of extent is likely to prove as important as the stage of that disease. The old staging of the amount of vasoproliferation (Stages 1 to 3) remains in the ICROP.

The concept that *some additional component of ROP exists, a "plus" component*, seems likely to prove critical to our understanding of the pathophysiology and prognosis. Progressive disease often develops a turning point when the proliferative process suddenly becomes aggressive with an apparent inflammatory component, including clouding of the vitreous, exudation along the retinal vessels, and increased flow of blood through those vessels and the iris. This has been termed "plus" disease, a more ominous form of ROP, but one that can still fully regress in many cases.

Finally, a descriptive classification of partial or total retinal detachments has also been developed that is coordinated with ICROP, as well as the traditional classification used by retinal surgeons for detachments caused by other diseases. This addition uses Stage 4 ICROP for classifying partial retinal detachments and Stage 5 for total detachments.

EXAMINATIONS

The reasons for ophthalmic screening of premature infants are to set aside concerns about potential vision loss as soon as possible if there is no ROP, to ensure appropriate follow-up if early ROP is detected and *to detect severe disease in time for treatment with cryotherapy which has proven effective in reducing vision loss.*

Who Should be Examined? In my opinion, all infants of less than 32 weeks' gestation should be examined, because of the degree of retinal vascular immaturity likely to be present at this gestational age. Premature infants over 31 weeks who have required ventilation and oxygen or who have had otherwise complicated medical courses also deserve examination to rule out ROP. *Infants over 36 weeks' gestation (i.e., 37+ weeks) are unlikely to develop ROP* and, unless they are also small for gestational age, need not be screened for ROP.

When Should Examinations be Performed? Active ROP cannot be seen until 4 to 7 weeks after birth, and it has been argued that there is little point in examining an infant before that time. However, if an infant is ready to go home, the examination should be done before discharge because many older premature infants who have done well are found to have retinal vessels that reach the far periphery or are very close to it. Since the vasculature is past the point at which ROP can develop, the parents and staff can be immediately reassured that ROP is no longer a concern. *When the retinal vasculature is complete and there has been no ROP, standard ophthalmic follow-up with the pediatrician is all that is needed.* If there is a significant amount of avascular retina, a more cautious counseling and ophthalmic follow-up is indicated. Occasional exceptions can be made to this examination-before-discharge policy if the parents can be utterly depended upon to return for follow-up.

If an infant remains in the hospital for more than 4 to 7 weeks and is not examined, ROP can develop and progress to retinal detachments without the chance for surgical intervention. *Transscleral cryotherapy (freezing) of the avascular peripheral retina in severe ROP reduces the chance of retinal detachments from about 50 percent to about 25 percent.* While this treatment certainly will not prevent all vision loss, it offers significant hope to those with severe ROP, and screening exams must be done in a timely fashion in order for cryotherapy to be tried before retinal detachments occur.

INTERVENTIONS

Before Retinal Detachment

Current research suggests the presence of an angiogenic substance released from the avascular retina that sustains and drives the vasoproliferation in ROP. *Trans-scleral cryotherapy or photocoagulation to ablate the avascular retina is aimed at destroying the source of this angiogenic substance, and therefore arresting the retinopathy.* In this procedure, the peripheral neuroretina is permanently destroyed, with the goal of maintaining attached retina in the posterior pole and retaining central vision from the macular area. Physicians in Japan and Israel and a few in North America had earlier believed this treatment to be effective, and in February 1988 United States investigators declared an early termination to a confirmatory multicenter, randomized trial of cryotherapy for a defined threshold level of ROP incorporating one eye as a control in each infant. The long-term outcome in those infants treated is still ongoing (see the chapter *Cryotherapy for Retinopathy of Prematurity*).

After Retinal Detachment

There is no proven treatment for the early retinal detachments associated with severe ROP. If a retinal detachment has occurred, a few retinal surgeons recommend that a scleral buckle be placed around the eye to push the sclera closer to the retina. This would be combined with a cryotherapy procedure to hold the retina in place with scar tissue. However, to be effective, the buckle must be done before the detachment carries the retina too far from the sclera, and it is unlikely to succeed if there is extensive fibrous tissue in the vitreous cavity, since that tissue will continue to contract and pull the retina into a tight ball behind the lens, the retrolental mass. An additional complication is that the buckle must be removed later in the first year to permit the eye to continue to grow to reach adult size.

If total detachment occurs, the visual prognosis is reduced, at best, to light perception only. Because of the hopelessness of this situation, *heroic efforts have been made in some patients to perform extensive vitrectomy procedures in which the lens and then the fibrous vitreous are laboriously removed, in an attempt to release, retain, and replace the retina. This is far from a standard procedure, and there is vigorous debate among retinal surgeons as to whether it should be attempted at all*, and if so when. Proponents for performing the procedure soon after detachment has occurred feel that they should try to replace the retina before critical ages for visual development have passed, and to prevent the extensive retinal degeneration that occurs with a prolonged retinal detachment. Proponents of waiting several months before attempting the surgery point out that early procedures are likely to be complicated by hemorrhage and recurrence of the vitreous mass of scar tissue, causing the detachment to recur.

The risks of these procedures consist of infection and loss of the eye. If this occurs, and if the eye has had any residual function, it is lost. *Without an eye, the orbit grows poorly, creating a cosmetic defect.* On the other hand, as a natural part of severe ROP and retinal detachments, the eye may also sometimes fail to grow, resulting in a similar cosmetic effect, even though the eye be retained.

RICKETS IN INFANTS

WINSTON W.K. KOO, M.B.B.S., F.R.A.C.P.
REGINALD C. TSANG, M.B.B.S.

Rickets during infancy in the Western world occurs in growing very low birth weight (VLBW) infants, in full-term infants who have received prolonged exclusive breast-feeding and little sunshine exposure, and in some infants who have required prolonged parenteral nutrition. Other less common causes of rickets in infancy include neonatal hepatic disease and inborn errors of metabolism. Only the management of the more frequent causes of rickets is discussed.

The classic clinical features of rickets are craniotabes, palpable enlargement of the costochondral junctions (the "rachitic rosary"), thickening of the wrists and ankles, and deformities of the spine, pelvis, and legs. Laxity of ligaments, hypotonia, delayed (and abnormal) dentition, and delayed motor milestones also occur in infants with rickets. Most of the clinical signs occur relatively late in the development of the disease. Craniotabes is often a nonspecific feature, particularly in VLBW infants. Serum alkaline phosphatase measurements suffer from variations in technique of measurement, the presence of alkaline phosphatase of nonbone origin, and wide ranges of normal in the growing infant, particularly the VLBW infant. The only practical definitive diagnosis of rickets is made by radiologic methods. However, radiology does not distinguish among the multiple causes of rickets; specific disorders, such as the less common inherited vitamin D–resistant hypophosphatemic rickets, need to be considered, and if one is present, appropriate specific therapy should be undertaken.

TREATMENT

Nutritional Rickets in Very Low Birth Weight Infants

The frequency of nutritional rickets in VLBW infants (birth weight less than 1,501 g) may be 30 percent or higher. The frequency of rickets may vary inversely with the birth weight and gestational age of the infants and directly with the degree of illness experienced by these infants. The time of presentation is usually between 3 and 6 months of age, presumably at the time of rapid growth after the initial acute illness and when the rate of bone mineralization lags behind general skeletal growth. Clinically there are few signs, although fractures may occur in the ribs and extremities, particularly in the distal forearms and legs. Often the condition is detected coincidentally during x-ray examination of organ systems other than bone. Biochemically, serum phosphorus concentrations may be low, but serum calcium concentrations are usually normal. Serum alkaline phosphatase concentrations are often elevated above childhood values, but as described earlier, these values are difficult to interpret. Rickets may occur in VLBW infants fed human milk, commercially available cow's milk, or soy formula. The major cause of rickets in these infants appears to be combined deficiency of calcium (Ca) and phosphorus (P).

Vitamin D Supplementation

Vitamin D is converted to 25-hydroxyvitamin D (25 OHD) in the liver. Some VLBW infants appear to have low serum 25 OHD concentrations. In general, however, VLBW infants with rickets have serum 25 OHD concentrations in the range of older normal children. These values are comparable to those in VLBW infants without rickets and are similar whether they are receiving 400 or 800 IU vitamin D_2 (ergocalciferol) daily. In addition, serum 1,25-dihydroxyvitamin D ($1,25[OH]_2D$, the most active vitamin D metabolite derived from 25 OHD) concentrations are elevated in nutritional rickets of VLBW infants as compared with concentrations in healthy children and adults. Thus it appears that defects in vitamin D metabolism are unlikely as usual causes for rickets in VLBW infants. Therefore, a daily supplement of 400 IU vitamin D_2 orally should be adequate in the prevention or treatment of rickets in VLBW infants when used with mineral supplementation protocols (to be discussed). Serum 25 OHD concentrations can be measured at 1- to 2-month intervals and the dose of vitamin D_2 adjusted if needed until complete healing of rickets occurs.

Calcium and Phosphorus Supplementation

During the last trimester of pregnancy there is a major maternal-fetal transfer of Ca and P. The VLBW infant is "deprived" of this significant Ca and P supply postnatally, and this deprivation is thought to be the major reason for the development of rickets in such infants. Although VLBW infants with rickets may have low serum phosphorus concentrations, the administration of a P supplement alone may precipitate hypocalcemia and should be used with caution. In addition, since lack of Ca and P appears to be the major reason for rickets in VLBW infants, ideal therapy appears to be combined Ca and P supplementation, providing a balanced approach to improve bone mineralization (Fig. 1).

The optimal quantity of Ca and P required in the treatment of rickets in VLBW infants is not known. The use of Ca and P supplements at a ratio of less than 2:1 (by weight) has been reported to be associated with hypocalcemia; at a Ca:P ratio of more than 2:1, and final concentration of calcium in the milk (>1600 mg per liter), intestinal obstruction has been reported. Generally, the aim has been to attempt to deliver a quantity that approximates the loss of intrauterine mineral accretion because of premature birth. In general, supplementation of elemental Ca (100 mg per kilogram per day) and elemental P (approximately 50 mg per kilogram per day) in divided doses with feeds, in addition to the standard milk feeding (maternal

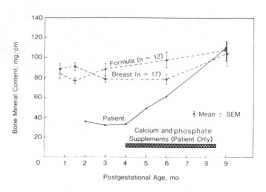

Figure 1 Bone mineral content of left radius shows response to Ca and phosphate supplementation. For comparison, bone mineral content values of 12 full-term bottle-fed infants (a standard proprietary cow's milk formula, Similac, 20 calories per ounce and 17 full-term breast-fed infants are included. (From Greer F et al. Calcium and phosphate supplements in breast milk-related rickets. Am J Dis Child 1982; 136:581, with permission.)

or commercial), may constitute adequate treatment. The Ca and P supplement should be commenced at half the desired dosage to minimize potential side effects such as diarrhea. The dose may be increased by 25 percent of the initial dose every 3 to 4 days. Alternatively, it is possible that the doses of Ca and P required for the treatment of rickets may be lower than the traditionally recommended quantities based on intrauterine mineral accretion data. In anecdotal instances, P intakes of approximately 30 mg elemental P per kilogram per day apparently may be sufficient to maintain normal serum biochemical measurements with reversal of rickets (Fig. 2). The duration of treatment with Ca and P supplement is usually about 3 months.

The type of Ca and P preparation best suited for use in a VLBW infant with active rickets depends on (1) the solubility of the Ca and P product, (2) the volume needed to deliver the required amount of Ca and P, (3) osmolality, and (4) potential for acid-base disturbance.

Generally, liquid preparations may be better absorbed than the water-insoluble powder preparations. Water-insoluble calcium phosphate powders also may sediment in the bottle or feeding tube, especially if the infant is being fed by the continuous infusion technique. The actual quantity absorbed may be less than that from the liquid preparation.

A suitable Ca preparation may be calcium glubionate (115 mg elemental Ca per 5 ml) or calcium gluceptate (90 mg elemental Ca per 5 ml). Because of its syrup base, calcium glubionate contains about 70 percent sucrose, which may be a significant carbohydrate and osmolality load for very small infants. In VLBW infants who are at risk for necrotizing enterocolitis, the use of calcium glubionate is probably undesirable. The gluceptate preparation, when added to the feeding, appears to be a suitable preparation for use as a Ca supplement.

The more soluble form of P (sodium monobasic phosphate) has a potential for causing acidosis if used in rela-

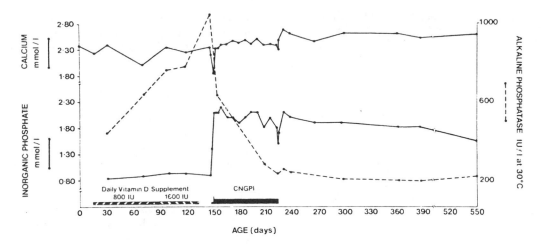

Figure 2 Serial changes in serum Ca, inorganic phosphate, and alkaline phosphatase during various treatment regimens and on follow-up. During continuous nasogastric phosphate infusion (CNGPI) of 100 mg elemental P daily, serum inorganic phosphate concentration was elevated rapidly and maintained within normal ranges without hypocalcemia, whereas serum alkaline phosphatase concentration rapidly decreased. Radiologic rickets resolved on completion of CNGPI. Conversion: serum calcium 1 mM per liter = 4 mg per deciliter; serum inorganic phosphate 1 mM per liter = 3.1 mg per deciliter. (From Koo WWK et al. Continuous nasogastric phosphorus infusion in hypophosphatemic rickets of prematurity. Am J Dis Child 1984; 138:172, with permission.)

tively high doses. Liquid preparations containing a mixture of mono- and dibasic (less soluble) phosphate may be used (sodium or potassium phosphate, 93 mg elemental P per ml). However, immediate precipitation with Ca may occur when these preparations come in direct contact with Ca salts. Precipitation may be prevented by first mixing the P with milk or administering the Ca and P separately, i.e., before and after each feeding. The mixed mono- and dibasic phosphate solution theoretically is less likely to induce acidosis than is the pure monobasic form; however, acidosis may still occur secondary to increased bone mineralization. The "liquid" Ca and P formulation, when mixed with a volume of pooled expressed breast milk equivalent to 150 ml per kilogram per day, has a measured osmolality of approximately 400 mOsm per kilogram and should not pose a problem with respect to the osmolar load on the gastrointestinal tract. The volume needed to deliver the desired quantity of Ca and P supplement should be well tolerated.

In a few patients treated with liquid Ca and P preparation, hypokalemia (serum potassium concentrations of less than 3.5 mM per liter) has been noted even in the presence of metabolic acidosis (unpublished observations). Hypokalemia might be theoretically due to the deposition of potassium along with Ca and P in bone. The low serum potassium level appears correctable with additional potassium; spontaneous correction of hypokalemia and metabolic acidosis also may occur on cessation of the Ca and P supplement. Prevention of hypokalemia may be achieved by the use of a mixture of approximately equal portions of phosphate salts of sodium and potassium.

The doses of Ca and P supplement used may be adjusted by the measurement of serum Ca and P concentrations and urinary Ca and P excretion (Table 1). Nutritional hypophosphatemic rickets typically is associated with absent or minimal urinary P excretion (fractional excretion of P less than 3 percent and markedly elevated urinary Ca excretion (more than 8 mg per kilogram per day). Adequate treatment may be reflected by normalizing serum Ca and P concentrations and rapidly decreasing serum alkaline phosphatase and serum $1,25[OH]_2D$ concentration to the normal ranges. The return of elevated serum $1,25[OH]_2D$ concentration to normal reflects the provision of adequate Ca and P intake, thereby removing the signals for increased production of this vitamin D metabolite. Upon adequate Ca and P supplementation, the urinary Ca excretion should be lowered. We also aim to maintain the urinary fractional excretion of P at 3 to 5 percent. The serum biochemical measurements, urinary Ca excretion, and fractional P excretion should be monitored once or twice weekly until the dose of Ca and P supplement is stabilized; thereafter, these measurements may be made at 1- to 2-week intervals until the rickets is healed. Recently it has been demonstrated that measurements of bone mineral content by infant-adapted photon absorptiometry are useful in evaluating the adequacy of bone mineralization. This may be done at monthly intervals. Standard radiographs of wrists and knees at 2- to 3-month intervals help to confirm the healing of rickets.

Other sources of Ca and P are available. Powder mineral fortifier containing Ca and P may be used as an additive to human milk. Infant formulas designed specifically for small preterm infants have high Ca and P content and are available in a high caloric density (81 kcal per ounce) form. These formulas should be vigorously shaken immediately prior to administration in order to maximize the amount of Ca and P suspended in the milk and thus their delivery to the infants. There are some potential drawbacks with the use of these formulas in the treatment of rickets. It is difficult to titrate the amounts of Ca and P that can be delivered to the infant without affecting the delivery of other nutrients. The safety and

TABLE 1 Monitoring During Treatment of Nutritional Rickets in Very Low Birth Weight Infants

Test	Frequency
Serum	
Ca, P, Na, K, creatinine	Once or twice a week
Urine	
Ca, P, creatinine	Once or twice a week
Acid-base status	Once a week
Serum	
25 OHD	Once a month
1,25(OH)$_2$D	Once every 1 to 3 months
X-ray films	
Wrists or knees	Once every 1 to 3 months
Other sites	Upon clinical indication

efficacy of its prolonged use in preterm infants greater than 3 kg is not known and, as with all infants receiving high Ca and P supplementation, chronic diuretic usage should be avoided, because of the potential development of nephrocalcinosis.

Frequently, VLBW infants with rickets have concomitant fractures of ribs and extremities involving particularly the humerus, distal radius and ulna, and distal tibia and fibula. These appear to be related to chest percussion and local compression areas associated with blood collection procedures. Care should be taken to avoid excessive vigor in handling any VLBW infants. These fractures may occur in the absence of radiologic rickets. Radiologic evidence of callus formation can occur even in the presence of active radiologic signs of rickets. The treatment of fractures in VLBW infants is generally similar to that for the active rickets. Splints and casts usually are not required, and many fractures are diagnosed after healing has been noted.

Spontaneous healing of rickets has been reported. In an otherwise well infant with uncomplicated rickets, close observation of the progress for several months to determine spontaneous healing might be justified.

Documented trace element deficiency such as copper deficiency causing rickets in VLBW infants is rare. Generally, no routine additional trace element supplementation is needed in the treatment of rickets in VLBW infants.

Nutritional Rickets in Infants Born at Term

Term infants with nutritional rickets may present with typical skeletal changes of rickets such as swollen wrists and/or a large head. More frequently, they present with nonspecific features such as failure to thrive, difficulty in walking, or refusal to walk. They may also be asymptomatic and the rickets diagnosed as part of family screening because of an affected sibling or during evaluation for other illness. Term infants with rickets usually have received prolonged breast-feeding exclusive of other dietary intake and have experienced little exposure to sunshine. In contrast to VLBW infants, vitamin D deficiency appears to be the major cause of this form of rickets. Successful treatment has been reported with the use of vita-

min D (ergocalciferol), 400 to 2,000 IU per day, for periods varying from 3 months to a year or more. The use of a single high dose of vitamin D, for example, 60,000 IU, does not offer an added advantage in the treatment of vitamin D–deficient rickets, and theoretically it may be complicated by hypercalcemia and the possible development of metastatic calcification. There are insufficient data concerning the use of Ca and P supplements in these infants. However, intake approximating recommended daily intake of these minerals from their diet should be ensured.

Some of the rachitic infants also may have evidence of healed fractures on x-ray films. A few also may have developed skeletal deformities on initial presentation, and orthopaedic consultation would be needed. The family members, especially the siblings, also should be screened for rickets and other nutritional deficiencies if there is a history of "food fads" in the family. The screening of family members would also be important to rule out genetic forms of hypophosphatemic rickets.

Prolonged Total Parenteral Nutrition

Infants who develop rickets during prolonged total parenteral nutrition (TPN) usually also have concomitant liver dysfunction and hypophosphatemia. The most important treatment is reduction of TPN and introduction of oral feeding as soon as possible. If the infant tolerates oral feeding, the diet and vitamin supplementation are oriented toward that of any patient with liver dysfunction. Vitamin D supplementation is useful in view of possible malabsorption of vitamin D and 25 OHD (impaired enterohepatic circulation) and liver hydroxylation problems. The dosage ranges from 1,000 to 4,000 IU per day and varies with the serum 25 OHD concentration. We recommend keeping serum 25 OHD concentrations in the 20 to 40 ng per milliliter range. Serum 25 OHD concentrations reflect the vitamin D status of the body and the intestinal absorption and hepatic hydroxylation of vitamin D. Since there may be an element of malabsorption with hepatic dysfunction, Ca and P supplementation also may be required if there is no evidence of improvement of serum Ca and P concentrations in the presence of normal serum vitamin D metabolite concentrations. The dose of Ca and P supplement used would be similar to that mentioned above, with doses adjusted according to criteria listed in Table 1.

For infants who are unable to be weaned from TPN, additional Ca and P may be added to the TPN solution. The quantity of Ca and P that can be delivered in the TPN solution is limited by their precipitation when Ca and P are present in excess quantity. We have used Ca and P in the concentration of 20 mM each in TPN solutions. Potential problems, however, include clogging of barium-impregnated catheters, presumably because of formation of insoluble barium phosphate complexes, which form a nidus for further precipitation of minerals. Metastatic calcification also is a potential problem associated with excessive Ca and P supplements. The use of lower concentrations of Ca and P—between 10 and 15 mM—may prevent these complications while maintaining normal serum Ca and P concentrations. Excessive sodium and glucose loads in the TPN solution may aggravate urinary losses of Ca and P. Therefore, the monitoring of urinary excretion of sodium, Ca, and P may help to achieve an optimal intake of Ca and P.

Trace element deficiencies occur in infants who receive TPN solutions free of these elements, and all TPN solutions should contain adequate quantities of trace elements, particularly zinc and copper.

Theoretically, vitamin D, because of its major action on gut absorption of Ca and P, may be unnecessary for infants on TPN. Furthermore, excessive vitamin D in the TPN fluid theoretically may aggravate bone losses, since the other major action of vitamin D is the mobilization of Ca and P from bone. However, some vitamin D activity may be essential in bone mineralization, and we suggest that a dose of 25 IU vitamin D_2 per kilogram per day might be reasonable for infants receiving prolonged TPN.

PREVENTION

There are inadequate data concerning the prevention of rickets in VLBW infants. These infants should continue to receive optimal general nutrition at all times and vitamin D (400 IU per day) supplementation. Ca and P sup-plementation holds promise as an additional measure in the prevention of rickets in VLBW infants. Intestinal mineral absorption may be impaired in VLBW infants fed soy formula, and therefore the prolonged use of soy formula in these infants should be avoided. Chronic diuretic therapy with increased renal calcium loss may contribute to the impairment of skeletal mineralization in preterm infants and should also be avoided.

Full-term infants fed human milk in the first 6 months of life and presumably exposed to adequate sunshine may have sufficient serum concentrations of vitamin D metabolite and bone mineral content similar to those who receive supplemental vitamin D. Without adequate sunshine exposure, vitamin D deficiency may occur in exclusively breast-fed infants during late infancy. Daily supplementation of 400 IU of vitamin D during the first year serves as an adequate prevention for vitamin D deficiency as reflected by normal serum 25 OHD concentrations in both the full-term and the VLBW infant.

The prevention of rickets in infants on TPN currently involves the introduction of oral feeding as soon as possible, since there is insufficient information with regard to manipulating the vitamin D, Ca, and P content of the infusate.

SEPSIS

LUIS M. PRUDENT, M.D.
NESTOR E. VAIN, M.D.

The incidence of neonatal sepsis (defined as a positive blood culture in a sick infant less than 28 days of age) ranges from 1/1,000 live births in the full-term infant to as high as 160/1,000 in very low birth weight (VLBW) babies and is influenced greatly by a number of risk factors. Perinatal complications, such as maternal infection, prolonged rupture of membranes, and premature delivery increase the incidence of the so-called "early onset" infections (beginning in the first 3 to 4 days of life). The organisms responsible are usually a reflection of the maternal flora. *Infants who become septic after the fourth day of life usually have a hospital-acquired infection.* Hence, the nursery environment and local epidemiology play an important role in determining the type and incidence of such nosocomial infections.

Mortality rates vary between 10 and 50 percent and are highest in VLBW infants and in fulminant, early onset sepsis, such as that associated with group B *Streptococcus*. Since the initial clinical signs of infection are commonly subtle and nonspecific, a high index of suspicion, a thorough investigation, and prompt initiation of appropriate treatment are essential to improve the outcome.

ANTIMICROBIAL TREATMENT

The choice of antimicrobial agents must be based on knowledge of the pathogens most frequently responsible for sepsis, as well as the patterns of their antibiotic sensitivity. However, the rapid progression of sepsis in the newborn and its high mortality demand that treatment be started as soon as the diagnosis is suspected, after appropriate cultures have been obtained. Of necessity, this policy requires the treatment of many infants who will not, subsequently, be proved to have bacterial sepsis. Although an abnormal leukocyte count and differential may suggest bacterial infection, isolation of a pathogen from the blood is the only specific method of diagnosis. *Since meningitis accompanies sepsis in up to one-third of cases, examination and culture of the spinal fluid should always be performed.* Cultures from other sites such as urine, other body fluids (pleural, peritoneal, joint), or tissue may be of great diagnostic help in specific clinical situations. Examination of buffy-coat smears for bacteria or detection of antigen by counterimmunoelectrophoresis or other rapid diagnostic tests may suggest a diagnosis of bacteremia. Early and frequent visual inspection of blood culture bottles, a Gram's stain, and a subculture from the bottle to solid culture media between 6 and 12 hours after collection can accelerate the characterization of the pathogen. Reliable interpretation of results and effective communication between the clinician and the laboratory are important to the rapid selection of the most appropriate therapeutic regimen.

Early Onset Infection

For initial therapy of early onset sepsis we use ampicillin and gentamicin, because this combination offers coverage for the most frequently found pathogens (*Escherichia coli,* other gram-negative enteric bacilli, and groups B and D *Streptococcus*) as well as for less common agents (*Listeria monocytogenes, Haemophilus influenzae,* and *Streptococcus pneumoniae*). Ampicillin is administered intravenously 50 mg per kilogram per day in two doses for infants under 1 week or 100 to 150 mg per kilogram per day in three doses for infants 1 to 4 weeks of age (Table 1). Gentamicin sulfate is given intravenously or intramuscularly twice daily in a dosage of 5 mg per kilogram per day in infants under 1 week or 7.5 mg per kilogram per day divided into three doses for infants 1 to 4 weeks of age (Table 1). Monitoring of serum concentrations of aminoglycosides may become necessary to the clinical management of VLBW infants or those with renal failure, for whom the dosage interval may have to be lengthened (every 18 to 24 hours or longer). Ototoxicity and nephrotoxicity have rarely been associated with the prolonged use of aminoglycosides in the neonatal period, but evaluation of renal status and auditory function, particularly among low birth weight babies, is recommended.

An alternative approach for infants born to mothers with premature rupture of membranes and prolonged antibiotic therapy is the combination of cefotaxime or ceftriaxone and ampicillin. This regimen offers coverage for resistant strains of gram-negative bacteria as well as the other common etiologic agents or early onset infections. *Once a pathogen is isolated and its antimicrobial sensitivity determined, therapy is altered, if necessary, taking into account the clinical condition of the infant.* As a general rule a single bactericidal antimicrobial is preferred unless synergistic effects are expected through a combination of drugs (i.e., penicillin or ampicillin and gentamicin against enterococci or tolerant strains of group B *Streptococcus*).

If initial culture results are negative and the infant is asymptomatic, we stop therapy after 3 to 5 days and *observe the patient closely. If the infant has clinical or laboratory evidence of bacterial infection (such as leukopenia) but culture results are negative, we continue antibiotics for 7 to 10 days.* Infants whose culture results are positive receive 10 days of therapy in the absence of meningitis. When multiple systems are involved or clinical response is slow, treatment is continued for a minimum of 2 weeks.

Late Onset Infection

Late onset septicemia in high-risk infants is frequently a hospital-acquired infection. Exposure to invasive lifesaving procedures, intravenous fluids, humidifiers, respiratory equipment, and personnel contributes to nosocomial bacterial infection rates as high as 10 to 20 percent. These infections reflect prior colonization of the infants and contamination by fomites with predominantly gram-negative bacteria and staphylococci. Previous broad-spectrum antibiotic therapy may predispose to the development of resistant organisms. Management should include removal of indwelling catheters (arterial, venous, or vesical), appropriate cultures, discon-

tinuation of current antibiotics, and initiation of alternative antimicrobials. We restart antibiotic treatment in this particular situation with a cephalosporin (cefotaxime, ceftriaxone, or ceftazidime) and amikacin. This combination is used because of the excellent activity of these cephalosporins against enteric bacilli, particularly *Klebsiella* spp., and the frequent resistance of these organisms to gentamicin (15 to 40 percent). In addition, synergistic activity of these agents has been shown for some species of *Klebsiella.*

Ceftriaxone has a substantially longer half-life than other cephalosporins, is very active against gram-negative bacilli, *H. influenzae,* group B *Streptococcus,* and *S. pneumoniae,* and has excellent diffusion into spinal fluid. This drug is an excellent therapeutic choice for the treatment of serious infections (sepsis and meningitis).

Ceftazidime (a derivative of cephalosporin C) has also been recommended for the empiric treatment of hospitally acquired infections, especially if *Pseudomonas aeruginosa* is suspected as the etiologic agent. Since a synergistic effect between ceftazidime and the aminoglycosides against *Pseudomonas aeruginosa* has been observed in vitro, this combination is the therapeutic choice in these cases.

Imipenem (*N*-formimidoil thienamycin) is a new betalactam drug with a broad-spectrum activity against grampositive and gram-negative organisms as well as anaerobic agents. Although this drug appears to be potentially useful for the empiric treatment of nosocomial infections, it has not yet been sufficiently evaluated in neonates.

We use vancomycin if staphylococcal infections are prevalent in the unit or are suspected on clinical grounds. This drug is particularly effective for the treatment of infections caused by *Staphylococcus aureus* resistant to methicillin and multiply resistant *Staph. epidermidis,* an increasingly common pathogen in North America. Blood cultures are repeated 24 to 48 hours after initiation of treatment. If they remain positive, the choice of the antibiotics should be reevaluated, since drug resistance is the most common cause of persistent bacteremia. A thorough search for an unidentified focus of infection should also be undertaken. If lateonset sepsis is documented, treatment should continue for a minimum of 10 days to 2 weeks.

Anaerobic infections, although uncommon, are being recognized with increased frequency, particularly in infants with necrotizing enterocolitis, if suspected, an active drug against these organisms should be used. Many antibacterial agents demonstrate activity against anaerobic organisms (chloramphenicol, metronidazole, clindamycin, and cefoxitin), but no controlled clinical trials have yet been conducted to prove their efficacy in severe neonatal infections. Chloramphenicol and metronidazole have been used extensively in clinical practice. Chloramphenicol, although effective, is a bacteriostatic rather than bactericidal agent and has a dose-dependent toxicity. Determinations of serum concentrations are mandatory to allow for dose adjustments (see Table 1). Metronidazole is remarkably effective, possibly through its bactericidal action and good tissue diffusion (including cerebrospinal fluid). Its toxicity appears to be low.

Neonates with serious underlying illness who are on broad-spectrum antibiotic therapy, receiving a parenteral nutrition, or with indwelling catheters in place are at risk for systemic *Candida albicans* infections. After removal of

TABLE 1 Antimicrobial Agents in Neonatal Sepsis*

Drug	Dose (per kg)	Age (days)	Weight	Interval	Preferred Route	Comments
Penicillin G	25,000 U	0–7 7–28 7–28 with meningitis		q12h q8h q6h	IV	Double to triple dose for meningitis.
Ampicillin	25–50 mg	0–7 7–28 7–28 with meningitis		q12h q8h q6h	IV	Double dose for meningitis.
Carbenicillin	100 mg	0–7 7–28 7–28		q12h q6h q8	IV	Should not be mixed with gentamicin.
Ticarcillin	75 mg	0–7 7–28 7–28	<2,000 g	q12h for <2,000 g q8h for >2,000 g q6–8h		
Mezlocillin	75 mg	0–7 7–28		q12h q8h		
Methicillin	25 mg	0–14 15–28 0–14 15–28	<2,000 g <2,000 g >2,000 g >2,000 g	q12h q8h q8h q6h	IV infusion 15–30 min	Unstable in acid solutions. Renal function to be monitored because of nephrotoxicity.
Cefotaxime	25 mg	0–7 7–28 0–7 7–28	<2,000 g <2,000 g >2,000 g >2,000 g	q12h q8h q8h q6h		
Cefuroxime	25 mg			q8h	IV	Double to triple dose for meningitis.
Ceftriaxone	50 mg			q12h	IV	Longest half life of all cephalosporins (2–7 times).
Kanamycin†	<2,000 g: 7.5 mg >2,000 g: 10 mg/kg	0–7 7–28	>2,000 g	q12h q8h	IM IV slow infusion over 30 min	Peak levels 15–25 μg/ml
Gentamicin†	2.5 mg	0–7 7–28		q12h q8h	IM IV slow infusion over 30 min	Blood levels to be monitored. (Peak levels 4–8 μg/ml through levels should be <2 μg/ml)
Amikacin†	7.5 mg	0–7 7–28		q12h q8h	IM, IV slow infusion over 30 min	Peak levels 15–30 μg/ml.
Chloramphenicol	25 mg	7–28 0–14 15–28 15–28 15–28 with meningitis	<2,000 g >2,000 g <2,000 g <2,000 g	q12h q24h q12h q24h q12h	IV	Blood levels to be monitored. Peak 2–25 μg/ml.
Vancomycin	15 mg	0–7 7–28		q12h q8h	IV	Nephrotoxic, especially when given in combination with aminoglycosides.
Metronidazole	15 mg loading 7.5 mg maintenance	0–7 7–28		q12h q12h	IV	Maintenance dose is started after 24 hr in term and 48 hr in preterm infants following the loading dose.
TMX Sulfa	5 mg 3 mg TPM 10 mg SMC (loading) 1 mg TMP 3 mg SMC (maintenance)			q12h		For pathogens resistant to other antibiotics. Good CSF levels.
Amphotericin B	See text					
5 Fluorocytosine	25 mg			q6h	PO	

* Based on McCracken et al, Klein et al, and other pharmacodynamic studies.

† Blood levels should be monitored in babies with renal failure and in very low birthweight infants ($\leq$ 1,500 g). Peak serum levels of antimicrobial agents are determined within 1 hour following administration of a dose. Through levels should be obtained prior to the next dose.

catheters and discontinuation of antibiotics, blood, urine, and cerebrospinal fluid cultures should be repeated. If persistent candidemia, candiduria, and/or meningitis confirms systemic infection, specific therapy should be initiated with amphotericin B. The recommended dosage for total treatment is 25 to 30 mg per kilogram. The initial dose of 0.25 mg per kilogram per day is increased every other day to a maximum of 1 mg per kilogram per day. The drug is given intravenously, diluted in 5 percent glucose (a precipitate will form in saline), usually over a 6-hour period. Both the bottle and the tubing should be protected from light. Nephrotoxicity, the most important side effect of the drug, appears to correlate with the total dose administered. Convulsions and cardiac arrhythmias during infusion have been observed when administration is too rapid or the concentration of the drug exceeds 0.1 mg per milliliter of diluent. Hypokalemia and anemia also occur. In vitro synergism between amphotericin B and 5-fluorocytosine suggests that the combination of the two agents may have a beneficial effect. 5-Fluorocytosine (flucytosine), at a dose of 100 mg per kilogram per day, is used orally in four divided doses. Bone marrow depression and hepatocellular damage may occur with this drug.

Infections observed in normal full-term infants after discharge from the hospital and with no history of perinatal complications are usually acquired from a household contact. Epidemiologic data are important to select the appropriate treatment. Urinary tract infection should always be ruled out in these infants. Group B *Streptococcus, L. monocytogenes*, and *S. pneumoniae* are frequent causes of late onset neonatal sepsis after the second week of life in infants without urinary tract infections. Since an increased incidence of infections due to *H. influenzae* has been reported lately in infants after hospital discharge, a third-generation cephalosporin should be included in the management of these infants. At present we use ceftriaxone as a single drug in household-acquired infections because of its excellent coverage and its simplicity of administration.

Dosage recommendations of the various antibiotics are summarized in Table 1.

Supportive Care

Careful attention must be given to supportive care of these ill neonates: control of thermal environment, fluid balance, and glucose metabolism is essential. Since septic infants may develop respiratory failure or become apneic, mechanical ventilation may be necessary to maintain normal blood gas values and decrease the work of breathing. Hypoxia, acidosis, hypovolemia, and the vascular effects of endotoxins may lead to septic shock. Hypotension is commonly absent initially because peripheral vasoconstriction temporarily sustains blood pressure. Tachycardia, abnormal capillary refill, decreased urine output, and metabolic acidosis should alert the clinician to cardiovascular collapse. Whole blood, plasma, salt-poor albumin, dextran, and normal saline may be needed to expand circulating blood volume in septic shock. Because of their beneficial effect on cardiac function, adrenergic agonists such as dopamine and dobutamine are being used with increasing frequency. Continuous monitoring of vital signs, arterial blood pressure, central venous pressure, blood gases, and hourly urine output provide the information necessary to adjust the amount and type of fluids and drugs to be administered. Noninvasive methods recently developed for cardiac output (such as pulsed Doppler ultrasound) may allow a more rational approach to the management of septic shock and should permit ongoing evaluation of various therapeutic interventions. The treatment of metabolic acidosis is the treatment of the cause (usually hypoxemia and hypovolemia). If acidosis persists in spite of adequate oxygenation, 0.5 M solution of sodium bicarbonate may be administered slowly in a dose of 2 to 3 mEq per kilogram. Dopamine and bicarbonate should not be mixed in the same solution and dopamine is preferably given through a central line to avoid the complications of tissue extravasation and ischemia.

Disseminated intravascular coagulation, with its attendant thrombocytopenia, may accompany severe septicemia. The treatment of disseminated intravascular coagulation is the treatment of the underlying cause (sepsis).

Anemia frequently accompanies bacterial infections, and the hematocrit should be maintained above 40 ml per deciliter to provide adequate oxygen-carrying capacity. Frequent determinations of body weight, serum electrolytes, osmolality, urine output, and specific gravity are necessary for appropriate management of fluid balance.

Adjunctive Therapy

In spite of the wide array of antimicrobial agents available and the correct application of intensive care techniques, the mortality rate from bacterial infections is high, particularly in the fulminant early onset type and in premature infants. The reason for this frustrating outcome is most likely related to compromise of the newborn's host defenses, and various therapies directed at improving these specific deficits have been proposed. Decreased levels of immunoglobulins and complement, as well as poor chemotactic and opsonic activity of the neonatal serum, have led to the use of fresh frozen plasma. Although in vitro studies show that plasma infusions correct some of these deficits, their efficacy in modifying the course of sepsis has not been proved. Whole blood transfusions have also been used for immunologic purposes. In group B *Streptococcus* sepsis, *large transfusions of fresh blood improve survival only when the presence of the specific opsonic antibody is demonstrated in the donor's blood.*

Several metabolic abnormalities, including decreased chemotaxis, phagocytosis, and bactericidal activity of leukocytes, have been documented in stressed neonates. Furthermore, in fulminant bacterial infections, leukopenia and exhaustion of bone marrow polymorphonuclear leukocytes are common. Some studies have suggested that polymorphonuclear leukocyte transfusions improve the survival rate in this group of patients. Other authors have been unable to show advantages with this therapy. Pulmonary complications have been described, and there are several potential risks, such as transmission of viral diseases and "graft versus host" reaction. Furthermore, appropriate methods for polymorphonuclears (leukapheresis) are not regularly available in many hospitals. Christensen has demonstrated that a double-volume exchange transfusion with very fresh whole blood provides a number of leukocytes similar to one unit of polymorphonuclear leukocytes prepared by leukapheresis.

The course of septicemic newborn infants who develop sclerema is almost invariably fatal. Therapeutic trials with fresh whole blood exchange transfusions have been conducted in this situation. The rationale behind this therapy has been its potential effect for removing bacteria and toxins, improvement of oxygen transport, and enhancement of the immunologic response. Results, though preliminary and uncontrolled, show promise. *We perform exchange transfusions only in infants with sclerema who are rapidly deteriorating, in spite of adequate antibiotic treatment and full supportive care.* This technique and polymorphonuclear leukocyte transfusion await further controlled evaluation, and precise recommendations concerning their use cannot be made at present.

Based on the low levels of immunoglobulins found in low birth weight infants and some evidence from experimental studies in animal models, intravenous immunoglobulins appear to be a promising alternative for the prevention of bacterial infections. Some recent preliminary clinical reports have suggested that intravenous immunoglobulins may be efficacious in the prevention of late onset sepsis among low birth weight infants. Double-blind, randomized, placebo-controlled trials are only now being conducted to prove the efficacy and safety of intravenous immunoglobulins, so we are not using them at the present time, either for prevention or for treatment of neonatal sepsis, and we cannot recommend their use until well-designed studies are completed.

SPINAL CORD INJURY

HARRY J. BELL, M.D.

Most authors agree that with improved obstetric technique, the incidence of neonatal spinal cord injury has decreased. However, postmortem studies of newborns who died within the first weeks of life have shown that approximately 10 percent have evidence of significant mechanical trauma to the cervical spinal cord and/or brain stem. This percentage has remained relatively constant over the past 18 years.

The most comprehensive clinical and pathologic study of spinal cord injury in the newborn was done in 1969 by Towbin. In this work, three outcome groups are described. First are the newborns with an upper cervical or brain stem lesion presenting as stillborn or with rapidly ensuing death in the first days or weeks of life. Second are the newborns with significant respiratory compromise who survive into the early months or years of childhood, eventually succumbing to recurrent pneumonias and respiratory arrest. Third are the neonates who survive long term. It is the third patient group that requires lifelong management of the multiple medical, developmental, and functional problems resulting from injury.

Speculation exists regarding a fourth group of neonates. In this group, injury to the spinal cord may be incomplete and unsuspected. Long-term neurologic sequelae manifested by motor dysfunction may be attributed to the birth asphyxia that often complicates difficult deliveries in which risk of spinal cord injury is highest.

The prognostic category into which a newborn falls is determined by a combination of factors. Most important are (1) the anatomic level of the spinal cord lesion, (2) the presence or absence of damage to vital brain stem centers, and (3) the presence of other medical complications such as birth asphyxia. The impact of more recent advances in the medical management of neonates with acute and chronic respiratory insufficiency on long-term prognosis remains to be seen. As more spinal cord–injured infants survive the acute phase of their course, it will fall upon the pediatric rehabilitation team to maximize functional outcome and provide for long-term needs.

PATHOMECHANICS

In autopsy studies, Towbin demonstrated that ligamentous laxity in the newborn vertebral column makes the relatively inelastic spinal cord vulnerable to forces generated during the delivery process. It was found that vertebral bodies and supporting ligamentous structures may stretch up to 2 inches longitudinally, whereas the spinal cord reaches the limits of elasticity at one-half inch. Excessive longitudinal stretch, torsional forces, and flexion-extension forces can result in disruption of the dura, the vascular supply, and neuronal structures. In addition, poorly developed cervical musculature and horizontal orientation of the facet joints in the immature spine allow significant subluxation and the possibility of spinal cord compromise through forces of compression.

Risk of injury to the newborn spinal cord is maximal when it is subjected to the forces generated during vaginal delivery of a breech presentation. However, risk is likewise significant in other malpresentations. Recent attention has been focused on fetal transverse lie with neck hyperextension and spinal cord injury after delivery by cesarean section. Forces generated during a middle to high forceps delivery may also be significant. Postmortem studies often show evidence of epidural hematoma, infarction, and laceration. More detailed descriptions of pathology and pathomechanics are available elsewhere.

INITIAL PRESENTATION AND DIAGNOSTIC EVALUATION

Clinically, in the case of a difficult breech delivery and an infant with profound hypotonia, absent deep tendon reflexes, paradoxical breathing, and an obvious sensory level, little doubt exists regarding the presence of a spinal cord injury. However, the circumstances of delivery and initial physical findings may not always be clear.

A high index of suspicion may not be present after a difficult forceps extraction with superimposed birth asphyxia. The asphyxiated neonate with a spinal cord lesion may display a triple flexion withdrawal to a noxious stimulus in the lower extremities. Determination of a sensory level may be exceedingly difficult. The exact nature of the neurologic lesion may therefore be in question. The clinician may turn to further diagnostic testing to localize the problem more accurately.

Documentation of a spinal cord injury in the newborn can be difficult using standard diagnostic procedures. The characteristic ligamentous laxity makes actual fracture-dislocation unlikely. Several studies exist demonstrating normal standard x-ray studies in documented cord lesions. Fracture-dislocation is seen in less than 1 percent of cases. The additional diagnostic yield from conventional myelography is reportedly small. Current experience with computed tomographic scanning and magnetic resonance imaging is limited but these should prove to be useful adjuncts. Somatosensory evoked potentials have been of value diagnostically when x-ray examinations, metrizamide computed tomographic scans, and electromyogram results were inconclusive. In the case of severe cortical damage due to birth asphyxia, differentiation may be difficult.

MANAGEMENT

Clinical presentation, long-term survival, and functional outcome are most directly related to the level of the cord lesion. For the purpose of this discussion, management has been divided into three phases: acute, subacute, and long term (Table 1). Management in all phases is complex and best handled in a tertiary care setting where a multidisciplinary team approach is available. Questions regarding infant transport and the need for spinal precautions may arise. In those cases in which the spine is unstable, adequate immobilization of the head and trunk is necessary. However, this population is small, and a determination regarding stability is best made by an orthopedist or neurosurgeon. If any doubts exist, it is best to immobilize the patient.

Acute management in the newborn with high cervical or brain stem involvement will likely be complicated by paralysis of respiratory musculature and the presence of autonomic dysfunction. Establishment of an airway and of adequate ventilation should proceed, minimizing the risk of further injury to the spinal cord. Manifestations of autonomic dysfunction may include blood pressure instability due to alterations in vascular tone. The use of volume expanders and pressor agents may be needed. If vital brain stem centers are damaged, the prognosis is poor. The likelihood of long-term ventilator dependency is high in this population.

Also of immediate concern in the acute phase is management of the urinary tract. A neurogenic bladder invariably results from cord injury, and adequate bladder drainage must be ensured. Most urologists feel that the use of abdominal pressure, or the Credé method, risks reflux of urine into the ureters and should be avoided in both acute and long-term settings. The use of an indwelling catheter is recommended, particularly when fluid therapy and accurate input and output are critical.

Acute management should also include proper positioning to help maintain skin integrity and joint range of motion.

Management issues in the subacute phase are an extension of the problems faced by neonates who survive the newborn period. With stabilization of autonomic function, pulmonary management remains a prime consideration. Long-term ventilator dependency with all its complications is almost assured in the newborn with a complete high cervical lesion. The infant with a midcervical lesion and respiratory insufficiency requiring initial ventilation may successfully be weaned as spinal cord dysfunction secondary to edema and inflammation resolves. However, as Towbin describes, this group may be susceptible to frequent pneumonias and respiratory arrest secondary to underlying respiratory insufficiency. Strong consideration should be given to obtaining sleep studies, training parents in cardiopulmonary resuscitation, and using home apnea monitors. Respiratory status may be less of a concern in lower cervical lesions, although lack of movement indicates that good pulmonary toilet and frequent position changes are needed.

Neurogenic bladder management continues to be an issue in the subacute phase. Depending on the nature of the spinal cord lesion, a newborn may display evidence of either upper or lower motor neuron bladder dysfunction. This is most effectively evaluated utilizing a cystometrogram with sphincter electromyogram. Monitoring bladder residual volumes is also useful. In the presence of bladder/sphincter dyssynergia, use of a smooth muscle relaxant and early institution of an intermittent catheterization program may be necessary. However, in the case of a bladder that spontaneously empties adequately with no evidence of dyssynergia or recurrent infection, management using diapers alone may decrease the introduction of bacteria into the bladder. A baseline voiding cystogram and renal ultrasonogram may also be indicated. Early urologic consultation and regular follow-up as part of the multidisciplinary approach are recommended.

Appropriate positioning and handling techniques both on the part of professional personnel and of parents become increasingly important in the subacute phase. As a result of sensory loss and paralysis, excessive pressure may lead to skin breakdown. Paucity of movement and the development of spasticity, although usually occurring later, may lead to joint contractures. A program of passive range of motion exercises and splinting of joints in a neutral position may be helpful in preventing future deformity. Multisensory stimulation and handling by parents and professional staff as medical stability allows should be encouraged.

TABLE 1 Management of the Neonate with Spinal Cord Injury

Acute Phase	Subacute/Long Term
Pulmonary: respiratory depression or paralysis common	*Pulmonary:* possible ventilator dependency, frequent pneumonias, need for aggressive pulmonary toilet
Autonomic dysfunction: temperature and vasomotor instability common	*Urinary tract*: cystometrogram/electromyogram evaluation, monitor residuals, clean intermittent catheterization, frequent urinary tract infections, urologic follow-up, yearly renal function evaluations
Urinary tract: neurogenic bladder intermittent or indwelling catheter	*Orthopedic concerns*: related to growth and spasticity, scoliosis, extremity deformities.
Orthopedic/Neurosurgical: assessment of spine stability needed	*Rehabilitation concerns:* mobility, self-care, communications, cognitive/developmental, psychosocial/family.

With advances in acute and subacute management of neonates with pulmonary insufficiency, it is likely that a higher percentage of severely spinal cord–injured neonates will survive long term. Problems encountered both acutely and subacutely may persist as long-term problems. The level of the cord lesion and its effect on pulmonary function are probably the single most important long-term considerations. Ventilator dependency remains a long-term management problem limiting both survival and functional outcome. Aggressive pulmonary toilet remains a good management strategy in the nonventilator–dependent population. The role of nighttime ventilation in patients with marginal pulmonary status remains to be seen, as the use of accessory muscles of respiration may allow weaning from ventilation during the day.

Although little long-term follow-up data exist, management of neurogenic bowel and bladder in these patients probably parallels the experience in the spina bifida population. Clean intermittent catheterization has been shown to be an effective long-term management technique. In the patient with a severely spastic, small capacity bladder, medication of surgical procedures may be needed. Close urologic follow-up is needed, with regular assessment of bladder and renal status. Neurogenic bowel management is usually accomplished through a combination of dietary manipulation and regular use of suppositories. Stool softeners, stimulants, and enemas may be used in combination if needed.

With long-term survival of the spinal cord–injured neonate, growth-related problems that are primarily orthopedic in nature arise. In the spinal cord that has sustained significant and diffuse vascular compromise, large infarcted areas may result in flaccidity, with subsequent deformities secondary to unopposed gravitational forces. In the case of a transection producing an upper motor neuron picture, deformities mediated by muscle imbalance and spasticity may predominate. The most critical and widely studied growth-related problem is that of scoliosis. Early detection and close follow-up by an orthopedist with experience in scoliosis management are recommended. Appropriate seating, positioning, and bracing may be of value in the early management of scoliosis. However, in a patient with already compromised respiratory status, restrictive molded body jackets may not be tolerated. In long-term follow-up studies, most patients have required early surgical intervention.

Later changes in neurologic status, years after injury, are known to occur. This is usually manifested by increasing weakness or loss of function. Traumatic syringomyelia or other spinal cord abnormalities may be responsible. Follow-up by a neurosurgeon on a regular basis is necessary and should be a part of the multidisciplinary approach to management.

REHABILITATION MANAGEMENT

Acute and subacute phase management appropriately revolves around medical concerns. Many of these concerns remain as long-term management issues. However, with increasing percentages of patients surviving into childhood, issues concerning developmental and functional outcome are brought into focus. The term "functional outcome" in this sense refers to the development of skills in the areas of mobility, self-care, communication, cognition, and psychosocial interaction. Identification of functional deficits, development of intervention strategies, and implementation of treatment programs to facilitate acquisition of age-appropriate skills to the maximum extent possible are tasks best managed by an interdisciplinary pediatric rehabilitation team. Because the ongoing medical concerns are complex, medical leadership by a pediatric physiatrist or other pediatric rehabilitation specialist is necessary. Other team members include those from physical therapy, occupational therapy, speech therapy, psychology, social work, and child life and rehabilitation nursing. Although the anatomic level of the cord lesion is an important prognostic indicator, functional outcome is the result of a complex interaction between cognitive capabilities, the family support system, and the sophistication of the medical and rehabilitative systems.

SUGGESTED READING

Bell HJ, Dykstra DD. Somatosensory evoked potentials as an adjunct to diagnosis of neonatal spinal cord injury. J Pediatr 1985; 106:298.

Bucher HU, Bolthauser E, Friderich J, Isler W. Birth injury to the spinal cord. Helv Paediatr Acta 1979; 34:517.

Koch BM, Eng GM. Neonatal spinal cord injury. Arch Phys Med Rehabil 1979; 60:378.

Towbin A. Latent spinal cord and brainstem injury in newborn infants. Dev Med Child Neurol 1969; 11:54.

TETANY

ROGER E. SHELDON, M.D.
PANKAJA S. VENKATARAMAN, M.B.B.S.

The diagnosis of tetany, a condition characterized by neuromuscular irritability leading to carpopedal spasm, cramps, Chvostek's sign, laryngeal stridor, and tonic seizures, is seldom made in neonates. However, many infants have tremulousness and irritability that do not progress to the full-blown tetanic syndrome. Many more infants have few if any symptoms, and these children are detected to be hypocalcemic only by "routine" chemical testing. It is currently unclear whether all these infants should be treated with calcium supplements, and if so, at what levels of serum calcium concentration.

Infants at risk of developing hypocalcemia include preterm infants, asphyxiated infants, and infants of diabetic or hyperparathyroid mothers. Treatment with sodium bicarbonate, hyperventilation, or large volumes of citrated blood may also predispose to hypocalcemia. Tetany, or a similar complex of physical findings, can be seen in hypocalcemia, hypomagnesemia, and hypoglycemia. We are limiting this discussion to calcium and magnesium metabolism.

NORMAL CALCIUM DYNAMICS

The divalent cations have a unique role in stabilizing the neuromuscular junction and cell membrane—too little can lead to excitation, and too much may depress activity and alertness, as well as nerve conduction. These minerals are also involved in the maintenance of skeletal composition and integrity. Calcium plays a major role in cellular signal transduction, and is involved in hormone release and function. Additionally, calcium contributes to skeletal muscle contraction via interaction with the troponin complex, and to smooth muscle contraction via calcium-calmodulin activation of myosin light-chain kinase.

Normal serum calcium concentrations in adults range from 9 to 11 mg per deciliter. Neonates have usually been regarded as hypocalcemic when total serum calcium falls below 8 mg per deciliter (2 mmol) in term infants or 7 mg per deciliter (1.75 mmol) in preterm infants. About 40 to 45 percent of the total serum calcium is protein bound, and 5 to 10 percent is complexed with anions such as citrate, sulfate, bicarbonate, phosphate, and lactate. About 45 to 50 percent of the total serum calcium is in the ionized form (Ca^{++}); this is the physiologically important fraction of calcium in the blood. The *calculation* of blood ionized calcium concentration from various formulas or nomograms does not accurately predict blood ionized calcium concentration. Hence, measurement of blood ionized calcium level, by using electrodes sensitive to Ca^{++}, is desirable, and makes it possible to follow the ionized fraction itself and to correlate it with the physiologic situation. In the past, ionized calcium levels less than 3.5 mg per deciliter (0.875 mmol) were usually interpreted as indicating hypocalcemia. However, more recent data, using newer calcium ion electrodes, provide norms for blood ionized calcium in the range of 4.8 to 5.2 mg per deciliter (1.2 to 1.3 mmol).

EARLY NEONATAL HYPOCALCEMIA

Early neonatal hypocalcemia occurs during the first 3 days after birth and is related to the abrupt cessation of calcium supply from the mother via the placenta. Elevation of serum calcitonin concentration, transient relative hypoparathyroidism, and target organ unresponsiveness to parathyroid hormone have all been implicated in the etiology of early neonatal hypocalcemia.

The postnatal fall in serum calcium concentration occurs in normal infants, but is greater after asphyxia, after preterm birth, and in infants of diabetic mothers. Treatment with calcium supplements has typically been given to infants with serum calcium concentrations less than 7.0 mg per deciliter (1.75 mmol). Most neonatologists use this approach to raise calcium levels, to avoid further falls in Ca^{++} concentration, and to prevent cardiovascular instability, tremors, irritability, and seizures. There is little controlled evidence that this policy is effective or necessary.

LATE NEONATAL HYPOCALCEMIA

The late form of neonatal hypocalcemia results from ingestion of cow milk or even cow milk–based formulas with lower calcium-to-phosphorus ratios than human milk. It has been suggested that this leads to the ingestion of relatively large amounts of phosphorus, with a resulting calcium-phosphorus imbalance and hypocalcemia. Calcium supplementation corrects this situation.

HYPOMAGNESEMIA

Hypomagnesemia has been implicated in the etiology of early neonatal hypocalcemia. Infants at risk of hypomagnesemia include growth-retarded infants, infants of alcoholic or diabetic mothers, and those exposed to chronic diuretic use or multiple exchange transfusions. Magnesium is primarily an intracellular cation, so that serum magnesium levels may not accurately indicate total body magnesium status. Relative hypoparathyroidism related to chronic magnesium deficiency is one possible explanation for the hypocalcemia noted in these infants. Magnesium levels less than 1.5 mg per deciliter (0.625 mmol) are low in most laboratories. Magnesium supplementation typically repairs both the hypomagnesemia and the hypocalcemia.

CARDIAC ISSUES

Abnormal cardiac rhythm and function during hypocalcemia has been a concern of many neonatologists. Although the QoTc interval (the elapsed time from the electrocardiographic Q wave to the onset of the T wave, corrected for heart rate) may be prolonged in hypocalcemia, the relationship is not consistent. We studied eight normokalemic, normonatremic preterm infants with birth weights less than 1,500 g. A decline in serum calcium to 6.0 mg per deciliter (1.5 mmol) was not associated with documentable alteration in echocardiographic cardiac function. In these very low birth weight infants, who were also hypoproteinemic and hypoalbuminemic, the decline in serum total calcium was associated with relative defense of blood ionized calcium concentration (mean of 3.8 mg per deciliter.) We caution against extrapolating these findings to other groups of infants and other clinical situations. In an earlier study of larger preterm infants, left ventricular systolic time intervals, heart rate, and blood pressures increased after calcium infusions. Ionized calcium concentrations were not reported in that study.

THERAPY

When the decision is made to supplement the child's calcium intake, details are important. Oral supplementation is possible, but attention must be given to the compound and its mode of administration. Gastric irritation, ileus, and mucosal injury, possibly leading to necrotizing enterocolitis, may be minimized by using 10 percent calcium gluconate (the intravenous preparation) orally and by diluting it or giving it with a feeding. Calcium chloride should be avoided, since it can injure the gastric mucosa and cause metabolic acidosis. Calcium glubionate syrup (Neo-Calglucon) may cause loose stools.

Parenteral supplementation requires similar care. The intravenous cannula must be working perfectly, since the extravasation of calcium-containing fluid can produce tissue necrosis and ulceration. Hence, the site of the infusion should be watched carefully and the infusion discontinued if extravasation is suspected. Unfortunately, subtle extravasation may not always be detectable. With this in mind, intravenous locations over the hands, forehead, and scalp should be avoided as much as possible.

Cardiac rate should be monitored throughout the infusion of concentrated calcium solutions with a stethoscope or electronic monitor while the calcium is being "pushed" intravenously. Slowing of heart rate is reversed by slowing the infusion.

Discontinuation of calcium treatment also requires close attention. After serum calcium levels return to normal, and preferably after oral feeding has begun, parenteral calcium should be *tapered*. First the dose should be halved, and the serum calcium measured after 24 hours. If the level is normal, the dose may be reduced to one-fourth of the original dose; otherwise, the half-dose should be continued for another day. Twenty-four hours later, a normal calcium level would allow discontinuation of the supplement. Such stepwise tapering of the calcium therapy enables the infant's own homeostatic mechanisms to function and maintain normocalcemia.

In a recent study of very low birth weight infants, parenteral 1,25-dihydroxy vitamin D_3 (calcitriol) at doses up to 3 μg per kilogram per day failed to ameliorate early neonatal hypocalcemia. Higher doses may be effective, but at these doses the risk of calcitriol toxicity may outweigh any possible benefits. Hence, calcitriol currently is not advocated for the treatment of early neonatal hypocalcemia.

Our Approach

Our approach to the treatment of hypocalcemia still includes supplementation with calcium on a regular schedule in infants in whom hypocalcemia is confirmed biochemically.

After the ionized calcium level has been initially restored to normal by a "push" infusion of 10 percent calcium gluconate (usually 100 mg per kilogram or 9 mg of elemental calcium per kilogram), regular infusions are begun using 400 mg per kilogram per day of calcium gluconate initially, increasing to 600 mg if needed. This solution is incompatible with sodium bicarbonate and certain phosphorus mixtures (calcium carbonate or phosphate can precipitate). Prolonged calcium therapy may lower serum phosphate concentration, so it should be monitored regularly. It is important to realize that calcium infusions can stop seizures even when they are of nonhypocalcemic origin.

We do not use arterial catheters for calcium infusions at any time. Transhepatic umbilical venous catheters, i.e., those located in the inferior vena cava, are acceptable, but only when peripheral intravenous infusion is impossible. Infusion into the hepatic portal system carries the risk of tissue damage and necrosis; infusion too near the heart (S-A node) risks bradycardia and other arrhythmias. If umbilical venous catheters are used for calcium infusion, they should be carefully labeled, and calcium-containing fluids should not be flushed rapidly through them. All containers of calcium-containing solutions should be clearly labeled to avoid inadvertent admixture of bicarbonate or other solutions that may precipitate with calcium.

PERSISTENT HYPOCALCEMIA

If calcium supplementation fails to restore serum calcium levels to normal, hypomagnesemia should be suspected. Magnesium sulfate can be given in a dose of 0.1 to 0.2 ml of 50 percent solution intramuscularly every 12 hours to repair the hypomagnesemia; this usually restores the calcium level as well.

Serum magnesium levels should be monitored every 12 hours. If hypocalcemia persists in spite of these treatments, other diagnoses should be considered. These include maternal hyperparathyroidism, maternal vitamin D deficiency, and hypoparathyroidism in the child, which can be either idiopathic or associated with thymic and branchial arch abnormalities (DiGeorge's syndrome).

SUGGESTED READING

Mirro R, Brown DR. Parenteral calcium shortens the left ventricular systolic time intervals of hypocalcemic neonates. Pediatr Res 1984; 18:71–73.

Tsang RC, Steichen JJ, Chan GM. Neonatal hypocalcemia: Mechanisms of occurrence and management. Crit Care Med 1977; 5:56–61.

Venkataraman PS, Tsang RC, Greer FR, et al. Late infantile tetany and secondary hyperparathyroidism in infants fed humanized cow milk formula. Am J Dis Child 1985; 139:664–668.

Venkataraman PS, Tsang RC, Steichen JJ, et al. Early neonatal hypocalcemia in very low birth weight infants: High incidence and refractoriness to supraphysiologic doses of 1,25 dihydroxy-vitamin D3. Am J Dis Child 1986;140:1004–1008.

Venkataraman PS, Wilson DA, Sheldon RE, et al. Effect of hypocalcemia on cardiac function in very low birth weight infants—studies in blood iCa, echocardiography, and cardiac effects of intravenous Ca therapy. Pediatrics 1985; 76:543–550.

THERMAL AND CALORIC BALANCE

KEITH H. MARKS, M.B., B.Ch., F.C.P., Dip.Paed., M.R.C.P., Ph.D.

PREGNANCY

The temperature of the human fetus at term, as measured in utero or immediately following delivery, is normally about 0.5 °C higher than the maternal temperature. Effective heat-dissipating mechanisms via placental heat exchange are required to maintain the fetomaternal temperature gradient. A pregnant woman who develops a high fever increases her skin blood flow and ventilation at the expense of blood flow to the uterus and placenta. This reduces the heat removal efficiency of the placenta and results in a high fever in the fetus. It is now known that fetuses exposed to hyperthermia early in pregnancy are usually lost, and that a later insult (4 to 14 weeks' gestation) may have a teratogenic effect on the developing fetus, including central nervous system and facial defects. An increased frequency of spontaneous abortions, stillbirths, and prematurity has been noted after maternal illnesses that provoke high fevers. It appears that under ordinary circumstances, hot summer temperatures, bathing, and sauna bathing (which is usually limited to less than 10 minutes) or uncomplicated upper respiratory viral infections are not necessarily dangerous unless unusually pronounced or prolonged maternal hyperthermia occurs. Aggravating factors include employment in a laundry or foundry, long-distance running, or repeated exposure to heat, as in undulating or biphasic fevers, which have been shown experimentally to have particularly severe effects. The most important steps in the treatment of pyrexia are those measures that uncover and remove the underlying disease or functional disturbance. Because of few side effects, acetaminophen (Tylenol) has been used as an effective analgesic/antipyretic agent during pregnancy (600 mg by mouth).

Adverse maternal or fetal effects from acetaminophen use in pregnancy have not been reported, but formal clinical or epidemiologic studies of its use have yet to be conducted.

THE DELIVERY ROOM

It is common practice to maintain the ambient thermal environment of the delivery room for the comfort of the mother and medical personnel. Under usual delivery room conditions, newborn infants lose heat rapidly because of large radiant, convective, and evaporative heat losses from their warm, wet skin. The infant's skin temperature may fall precipitously by 0.3 °C per minute, whereas rectal temperature falls more slowly. Asphyxia, anesthesia, maternal sedation, infection, and birth injury may all have adverse effects on thermal stability of the newborn. Because of the limited ability of infants to generate an adequate thermogenic response to a cool environment over the first 12 hours of life, heat losses should be minimized during this period, even in healthy term babies. Measures taken to reduce heat loss after birth include the following:

1. Dry the baby completely with clean, dry, prewarmed towels. The head and face, which constitute a large surface area, are particularly important.
2. Use a radiant heater above the baby and a warming mat-

tress to add extra warmth and to promote a heat-gaining environment.

3. Swaddle the baby with a dry, warm blanket. An aluminum wrap or bubble plastic bag to insulate the skin from the dry room air also reduces heat loss but cannot provide a heat-gaining environment in already cold infants.

4. A radiant heat source or prewarmed blanket over the mother and baby are effective means of preventing cooling in babies kept with their mothers in the delivery room. When these methods are used, the infant may be partially dressed or nude while lying next to the mother on the delivery table.

5. Infants should not be bathed or washed until thermal stability is assured, and circumcision should never be performed in the delivery room.

THERMAL ENVIRONMENT AFTER BIRTH

Normal term infants in bassinets should be dressed and blanketed. Table 1 shows the air temperature of the room necessary to provide adequate warmth for babies nursed clothed and well wrapped in a bassinet in a draft-free room of moderate humidity (35 to 60 percent).

It is normally safe to assume that any environment that seems reasonably warm to an adult will be equally appropriate for a comparably clothed infant over 3 months old.

Incubators

The air temperature of the incubator should be adjusted manually to provide an air temperature within the thermoneutral zone (Table 2). Recent studies indicate that the neutral temperature, especially during the first week of life, depends more on gestational age at birth than on birth weight. In Figure 1, the environmental temperatures shown will maintain stable core and skin temperatures that are within normal limits. Note that these incubator air temperatures were determined in the laboratory under optimal conditions and serve only as a general guide for locating the neutral temperature inside the incubator. The incubator air temperature should be recorded simultaneously with the infant's axillary or skin temperature (measured with a skin hermistor) so that changes in the infant's temperature can be interpreted appropriately. Normal axillary and rectal temperatures range from 36.5 to 37.5 °C. The axil-

lary temperature is taken by placing a clinical thermometer deep in the axilla while the arm is held gently but firmly against the chest for 3 minutes. Rectal temperatures generally should not be taken. Plexiglass hoods, bubble blankets, clothes, or double-wall incubators may be used to reduce heat loss from naked infants inside incubators and are particularly useful for infants weighing less than or equal to 1,500 g.

Infants in incubators who are receiving phototherapy should have their skin temperatures maintained at 36.0 to 36.5 °C by using a servocontrolled incubator. When servocontrol is used, the skin probe must be dry, taped securely to the exposed surface of the infant, and protected from the heat by an aluminum patch. Servocontrolled incubators can cause overheating if the skin sensor becomes loose; they may obscure the signs of early septicemia and, theoretically at least, subject an infant with a raised thermoregulatory set point to appreciable cold stress.

Available evidence suggests that a moderate relative humidity of about 50 percent probably provides suitable conditions for the newborn baby.

Radiant Warmers

Radiant infant warmers are frequently used because they facilitate contact with the infant, particularly critically ill infants who require cardiorespiratory support and monitoring, intensive care after surgery, and various procedures. A significant increase in insensible water loss and a small increase in metabolic rate occur in infants under radiant warmers. The changes vary according to the infant's weight and condition, and no predetermined increase in fluid intake is recommended. Fluid requirements should be regulated according to clinical and biochemical criteria. Infection has not been found to be a significant problem for infants nursed under these conditions.

When used for more than a few minutes, these warmers should only be used in the servocontrol mode with the abdominal skin temperature maintained at 36.0 to 36.5 °C. The thermistor must be covered with an aluminum patch (to prevent the radiant heat source from directly heating the thermistor itself) and securely taped to the anterior abdominal wall. Other potential dangers associated with the use of open radiant heaters include hyperthermia, burns, unstable temperature control, difficulties using other equipment (x-ray, phototherapy), and overheating of personnel working with the infant.

TABLE 1 Required Air Temperature for Term Infants

Birth Weight (kg)	Room Temperature		
	29.5°C (85°F)	26.5°C (80°F)	24°C (75°F)
1.0	for 2 weeks	after 2 weeks	after 1 month
1.5	for 2 days	after 2 days	after 2 weeks
2.0	—	for 1 week	after 1 week
3.0	—	for 1 day	after 1 day

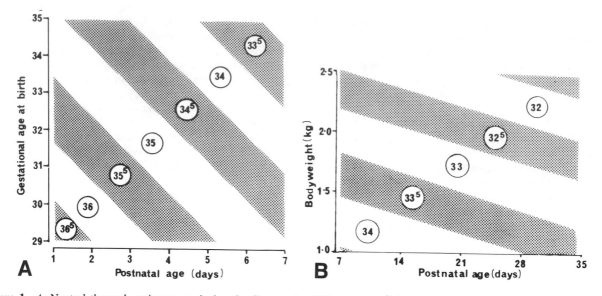

Figure 1 *A*, Neutral thermal environment during the first week of life, calculated from the measurements. *B*, Neutral thermal environment (°C) from day 7 to 35. For this figure, the neutral temperature was defined as the ambient temperature at which the core temperature of the infant at rest was between 36.7 and 37.3 °C. Dew point of the air was 18 °C, flow 10 L per minute. Body weight is current weight. Values for body weight greater than 2.0 kg are calculated by extrapolation. (From Sauer PJJ, Dane HJ, Visser HKA. New standards for neutral thermal environment of healthy very low birthweight infants in week one of life. Arch Dis Child 1984; 59:18–22.)

Hyperthermia

Hyperthermia can be produced by infection and dehydration as well as by excessively high environmental temperatures in improperly regulated incubators and radiant warmers (sometimes the result of improper placement or fixation of servocontrol probes). Radiant heat from phototherapy lights and sunlight overheats the infant without initially warming the air in the surrounding environment. Measurement of the skin temperature of the anterior mid-lower leg simultaneously with the core temperature helps to differentiate pyrexia due to disease from that due to environmental overheating. A core-leg temperature difference of more than 1.7 °C in a term infant suggests a disease-related fever. Hyperthermia produces an increase in metabolic demands with increased oxygen requirements and sweating in the full-term and older premature infant.

The treatment of hyperthermia consists of cooling the infant as rapidly as possible. When the skin temperature is between 37.5 °C and 39 °C, undressing and exposing the infant to room temperature is usually all that is necessary. If the skin temperature is above 39 °C, the patient should be undressed and sponged with tepid water at approximately 35 °C until skin temperature is less than 38 °C.

Hypothermia

Hypothermia exists when the core temperature is below 36.5 °C or the skin temperature is below 36 °C. Severe hypothermia produces neonatal cold injury. These infants appear red and edematous and may have sclerema. Lethargy, hypoglycemia, acidosis, azotemia, and pulmonary hemorrhage also occur. Chronic but mild cold stress in the newborn infant is associated with a decreased growth rate and an increased metabolic rate, oxygen requirement, and mortality rate. Hypothermic infants must be warmed, but whether this should be done slowly or rapidly is still controversial. Therefore during warming in a heat-gaining environment hypothermic infants should be monitored for hypoxia, acidosis, hypoglycemia, shock, and clotting disorders.

Temperature Control in Special Circumstances

Infants with cyanotic congenital heart disease generally have a diminished metabolic response to cold stress, whereas those with acyanotic congenital heart disease, especially those in congestive heart failure, are frequently diaphoretic, have a high metabolic rate, and can easily become hyperthermic. Infants born to mothers who have received high doses of diazepam have a blunted response to thermal stress, and hypothermia is common. Swings in body temperature (thermolability) are more common than stable pyrexia in infants with sepsis.

Special attention should be given to adequately warming and humidifying all inspired gas. When gas is delivered via an oxyhood, the temperature in the oxyhood should be similar to that in the neutral thermal environ-

TABLE 2   Neutral Thermal Environmental Temperatures*

Age and Weight	Starting Temperature (°C)	Range of Temperature (°C)	Age and Weight	Starting Temperature (°C)	Range of Temperature (°C)
0–6 Hours			72–96 Hours		
Under 1,200 g	35.0	34.0–35.4	Under 1,200 g	34.0	34.0–35.0
1,200–1,500 g	34.1	33.9 34.4	1,200–1,500 g	33.5	33.0–34.0
1,501–2,500 g	33.4	32.8–33.8	1,501–2,500 g	32.2	31.1–33.2
Over 2,500 g	23.9	32.0–33.8	Over 2,500 g	31.3	29.8–32.8
(and >36 weeks)			(and >36 weeks)		
6–12 Hours			4–12 Days		
Under 1,200 g	35.0	34.0–35.4	Under 1,500 g	33.5	33.0–34.0
1,200–1,500 g	34.0	33.5–34.4	1,501–2,500 g	32.1	31.0–33.2
1,501–2,500 g	33.1	32.2–33.8	Over 2,500 g		
Over 2,500 g	32.8	31.4–33.8	(and >36 weeks)		
(and >36 weeks)			4–5 days	31.0	39.5–32.6
12–24 Hours			5–6 days	30.9	29.4–32.3
Under 1,200 g	34.0	34.0–35.4	6–8 days	30.6	29.0–32.2
1,200–1,500 g	33.8	33.3–34.3	8–10 days	30.3	29.0–31.8
1,501–2,500 g	32.8	31.8–33.8	10–12 days	30.1	29.0–31.4
Over 2,500 g	32.4	31.0–33.7	12–14 Days		
(and >36 wccks)			Under 1,500 g	33.5	32.6–34.0
24–36 Hours			1,501–2,500 g	32.1	31.0–33.2
Under 1,200 g	34.0	34.0–35.0	Over 2,500 g		
1,200–1,500 g	33.6	33.1–34.2	(and >36 weeks)		
1,501–2,500 g	32.6	31.6–33.6	2–3 weeks		
Over 2,500 g	32.1	30.7–33.5	Under 1,500 g	33.1	32.2–34.0
(and >36 weeks)			1,501–2,500 g	31.7	30.5–33.0
36–48 Hours			3–4 weeks		
Under 1,200 g	34.0	34.0–35.0	Under 1,500 g	32.6	31.6–33.6
1,200–1,500 g	33.5	33.0–34.1	1,501–2,500 g	31.4	30.0–32.7
1,501–2,500 g	32.5	31.4–33.5	4–5 weeks		
Over 2,500 g	31.9	30.5–33.3	Under 1,500 g	32.0	31.2–33.0
(and >36 weeks)			1,501–2,500 g	30.9	29.5–32.2
48–72 Hours			5–6 weeks		
Under 1,200 g	34.0	34.0–35.0	Under 1,500 g	31.4	30.6–32.3
1,200–1,500 g	33.5	33.0–34.0	1,501–2,500 g	30.4	29.0–31.8
1,501–2,500 g	32.3	31.2–33.4			
Over 2,500 g					
(and >36 weeks)	31.7	30.1–33.2			

* Generally speaking, the smaller the infant in each weight group, the higher the temperature required. Within each time range, the younger the infant, the higher the temperature required. For this table, scopes had the walls of the incubator 1 to 2 degrees warmer than ambient air temperatures.

ment. Gases delivered directly via endotracheal tubes should be warmed to about 36°C.

Temperature Control for Special Procedures

In-house transport to and from the operating room or the radiology department may be done using a transport incubator or a regular incubator with the infant lying on a heated mattress and covered by a thermal blanket. A similar system (or a circulating warm water mattress) can be used to keep the infant's temperature stable during surgical procedures, computed tomographic scans, radiologic procedures, and cardiac catheterization.

Temperature Control During Transport

The transport incubator air temperature should be set to maintain a thermoneutral environment (see Table 2). In cold environments it is helpful to use a double-walled incubator or to cover the infant with a thermal blanket. Transport incubators with radiant warming hoods are also effective.

THROMBOCYTOPENIA

BARBARA A. MILLER, M.D.

Mean platelet counts of healthy full-term and premature infants are within the normal adult range (150,000 to 450,000 per cubic millimeter). *Platelet counts below 100,000 per cubic millimeter are abnormal and should be investigated.* A small number of normal infants have platelet counts in the range of 100,000 to 150,000 per cubic millimeter. Since a decline in the platelet count can be an early sign of systemic illness, platelet counts in this range should be repeated with additional evaluation based on the infant's clinical condition. Causes of thrombocytopenia include (1) increased platelet destruction from immune (autoimmune or isoimmune) or nonimmune disorders, (2) decreased platelet production (megakaryocyte hypoplasia, congenital leukemia), or (3) a combination of both. It is important to identify the cause of thrombocytopenia in order to select appropriate therapy.

THROMBOCYTOPENIA SECONDARY TO INCREASED DESTRUCTION

Neonatal Immune Thrombocytopenia

Immune thrombocytopenia in the newborn is secondary to maternal antiplatelet antibodies that cross the placenta. These antibodies are of two types: (1) in autoimmune thrombocytopenia, autoantibodies produced by the mother's immune system recognize common platelet antigens present on maternal, fetal, and most random donor platelets; (2) in isoimmune thrombocytopenia, the mother produces antibodies to paternal antigens present on neonatal platelets but absent on maternal platelets. Autoimmune neonatal thrombocytopenia can also be associated with drug-induced thrombocytopenia and with systemic lupus erythematosus in the mother. Immune thrombocytopenia in the infant can last from hours to several months, depending on clearance of IgG antibodies, which have a half-life of 21 days. Infants are usually well and have a normal physical examination except for skin and mucosal bleeding.

Immune Thrombocytopenia Secondary to Maternal Autoimmune Thrombocytopenia

Mothers with autoimmune disease at risk of having an infant with thrombocytopenia are usually identified before the delivery. However, neonatal thrombocytopenia can be the first manifestation of autoimmune thrombocytopenia in the mother; conversely, neonatal thrombocytopenia can occur years after successful treatment of the mother for childhood idiopathic thrombocytopenic purpura (ITP). *The most important management issue in the mother with active disease or a history of autoimmune thrombocytopenia is the method of delivery,* since the greatest risk to the thrombocytopenic infant is intracranial hemorrhage from the stress of vaginal delivery. The maternal platelet count is a poor indicator of the fetal platelet count. The level of unbound maternal antiplatelet antibodies has been shown to correlate with fetal-neonatal thrombocytopenia, as has maternal platelet-bound IgG in some studies. None of these measurements is a reliable indicator of the fetal platelet count. *The most accurate test to identify the infant at risk for thrombocytopenia is measurement of the platelet count on fetal scalp blood.* If the fetal scalp platelet count is greater than 50,000 per cubic millimeter, vaginal delivery can proceed safely. If the platelet count is less than 50,000 per cubic millimeter or a reliable fetal scalp platelet count cannot be obtained, cesarean section should be performed. A short course of corticosteroids (20 to 40 mg per day of prednisone given to the mother 10 to 14 days before delivery) has been shown to raise the fetal platelet count of infants of some women with immune thrombocytopenia. Treatment failures occur and measurement of fetal scalp platelet counts is still necessary. A concern is that such treatment may displace maternal platelet-associated IgG, thereby increasing circulating antiplatelet antibody and worsening neonatal thrombocytopenia. Further experience is necessary before firm recommendations for steroid use can be made.

The second issue of management is bleeding in the thrombocytopenic infant. Frequently the infant's platelet count continues to fall for several days after delivery, possibly because of the increasing function of the reticuloendothelial system. Neonatal platelet counts should be checked twice daily for the first several days, and then less frequently after an upward trend is noted. Treatment is reserved for infants with platelet counts of less than 20,000 or evidence of bleeding. Use of steroids (1 to 2 mg per kilogram per day of prednisone or an equivalent agent for 1 to 3 weeks) is controversial. *We recommend steroids primarily for infants showing clinical evidence of bleeding,* although some hematologists use thrombocytopenia alone as an indication for treatment. Administration of high-dose intravenous gamma globulin (0.4 g per kilogram per day for 5 days) has been markedly effective in treatment of childhood ITP, resulting in a higher, faster rise in the platelet count with less complications than steroids. Several reports of successful treatment of neonatal immune thrombocytopenia have been published. More experience in the newborn is needed, but *treatment with gamma globulin should be seriously considered for infants with platelet counts less than 20,000 or bleeding secondary to immune thrombocytopenia.* The value of transfusion of random donor and maternal platelets in autoimmune thrombocytopenia is limited, because these platelets are destroyed by maternal antiplatelet antibodies. However, in the bleeding infant, even though platelet survival is shortened, transfusion of 1 to 2 units of random donor platelets may help transiently with hemostasis, and should be given. In infants with persistent bleeding, exchange transfusion with fresh (not maternal) blood may be considered, since by removing circulating antibody and providing platelets, bleeding may be controlled. The effect lasts a maximum of several days, since IgG has a diffuse intravascular and extravascular distribution (half-life of 21 days), and the subsequent course of disease is unaffected. *Irradiation of blood used for exchange transfusion or intrauterine transfusion is recommended* because graft-versus-host (GVH) disease has been reported in this setting.

Isoimmune Neonatal Thrombocytopenia

Isoimmune neonatal thrombocytopenia occurs when the infant's platelets carry a platelet-specific antigen inherited from the father but absent in the mother. The mother is immunized to the paternal antigens on the infant's platelets, and antibody subsequently crosses the placenta to destroy fetal platelets. The antigen responsible for more than half of the cases is PL^{A1}; other rarer antigens include PL^{E2}, Duzo, and Bak. Although 50 percent of cases occur in the first pregnancy, infants from 75 percent of subsequent pregnancies are affected. *The diagnosis should be suspected in well infants with thrombocytopenia whose mothers have normal platelet counts.*

The two major issues are (1) management of delivery of the mother in whom a previous pregnancy resulted in isoimmune thrombocytopenia and (2) management of thrombocytopenia in the infant. The approach to delivery of a mother with a previously affected infant is similar to that in autoimmune thrombocytopenia. Because management of future pregnancies is altered, an attempt should be made to diagnose isoimmune thrombocytopenia definitively in the first affected infant by performing maternal and paternal platelet antigen typing, and testing the maternal serum for antibodies to paternal and maternal platelets. A fetal scalp platelet count should be taken in mothers with previously affected infants. If the platelet count is less than 50,000, a cesarean section should be performed; if greater than 50,000, vaginal delivery can proceed.

Indications for treatment of infants in whom the diagnosis is suspected are a matter of controversy. The greatest risk to the infant is intracranial hemorrhage secondary to birth trauma. Indications for platelet transfusions are not universally agreed on; *we recommend a platelet transfusion if the infant's platelet count is less than 30,000 or if bleeding occurs. These should be maternal platelets,* since they do not carry the paternal-fetal antigen recognized by circulating antibody. Since the most common antigen that causes neonatal thrombocytopenia, PL^{A1}, is present in 97 percent of the population, most random donor platelet transfusions carry the antigen and have a short survival time. Random donor platelets should be used only to control bleeding until maternal platelets are available. Maternal platelets should be washed to remove antibody present in maternal plasma and resuspended in AB-negative plasma. If facilities for washing platelets are not available, a unit of maternal blood can be transferred to a center at which the platelet transfusion can be prepared. Maternal platelets have a normal platelet survival time (7 to 10 days) in the infant, and measurement

of a normal platelet survival time helps confirm the diagnosis. One unit of platelets transfused into a 3-kg infant should result in a rise of the platelet count to 50,000 to 75,000 per cubic millimeter. In the absence of increased platelet destruction, transfused platelets will decline by 10 percent a day, reaching pretransfusion levels in 1 week. To establish the platelet survival time, platelet counts should be measured at 1 hour, 12 hours, and 24 hours after transfusion, subsequent measurements being based on the rapidity of disappearance from the blood. Repeat platelet transfusions are rarely necessary unless the platelet count falls again to less than 20,000, or bleeding persists. In pregnancies with previously affected infants, a unit of blood should be drawn from the mother before delivery, the red cells reinfused to the mother, and the platelets prepared for administration to the infant if necessary. Since GVH disease has been described in an infant given maternal platelets, platelets should be irradiated before administration, if possible. Treatment with corticosteroids or exchange transfusion is frequently unsuccessful. We use corticosteroids only in an infant with severe bleeding in whom maternal platelets are not available and random donor platelets are being given. Several reports have demonstrated the efficacy of high-dose intravenous gamma globulin (0.4 g per kilogram per day for 5 days) to treat neonatal isoimmune thrombocytopenia. Its use should be considered in infants with persistent thrombocytopenia (platelet counts less than 20,000) or bleeding. Splenectomy for this self-limited disorder, as in neonatal thrombocytopenia secondary to maternal autoimmune disease, is contraindicated.

Thrombocytopenia Secondary to Increased Platelet Destruction from Nonimmune Causes

Disseminated intravascular coagulation (DIC) is the second most frequent cause of neonatal thrombocytopenia after immune causes, and may be secondary to birth asphyxia, hyaline membrane disease, infection, hypothermia, necrotizing enterocolitis, severe hemolysis, and vascular lesions including hemangiomas. Infections also cause thrombocytopenia in the absence of diagnosable DIC by other mechanisms, including direct damage to platelet or endothelial surfaces, binding of IgG to the platelet surface with subsequent clearance by the immune system, and decreased production. Responsible infections include bacterial infections, TORCH infections (toxoplasmosis, rubella, cytomegalovirus, herpes simplex) and congenital syphilis. Exchange transfusions can result in thrombocytopenia, owing to the dilutional effect of few viable platelets in stored blood; this effect can be minimized by using blood less than 12 hours old.

The clinical picture frequently suggests the etiology of platelet destruction from nonimmune causes, and therapy is aimed at correction of the underlying process. Platelet transfusions are given in the infant with bleeding or a platelet count of less than 20,000. While one unit of platelets should increase the platelet count to at least 50,000, platelet survival is shortened and repeat transfusions are frequently necessary to control bleeding. Corticosteroids or other therapies usually are not indicated.

THROMBOCYTOPENIA DUE TO DECREASED PRODUCTION

Decreased platelet production secondary to megakaryocyte hypoplasia may be associated with the TAR syndrome (thrombocytopenia with absent radii), trisomy 13, trisomy 18, microcephaly, constitutional aplastic anemia (Fanconi's anemia, which rarely presents at birth), or amegakaryocytic thrombocytopenia. Mothers of infants with the TAR syndrome should be advised of a 25 percent chance of recurrence in subsequent pregnancies, since inheritance is autosomal recessive. If a child with the TAR syndrome survives, gradual improvement in the platelet count occurs toward the end of the first year of life. The Wiskott-Aldrich syndrome, characterized by immunodeficiency, thrombocytopenia, and eczema, can also present in the newborn. In this syndrome, thrombocytopenia is due to decreased platelet production, as well as intrinsically abnormal platelets with a short life span. Because of the underlying immune deficiency, only irradiated blood product support should be offered.

In this group of disorders we recommend supportive treatment for bleeding, including platelet transfusion and red blood cells. These patients have persistently low platelet counts and are chronically at risk for bleeding. Prophylactic platelet transfusions for platelet counts less than 20,000 may result in sensitization to platelet antigens, with subsequent failure of response to platelet transfusions when needed for clinical bleeding. Therefore, we administer platelets *only* for bleeding. The exception is immediately after vaginal delivery, when a platelet transfusion should be given for platelet counts less than 30,000. Transfused platelet survival is normal; 1 unit should increase the platelet count by 50,000 to 75,000, with a return to baseline in 7 to 10 days, unless platelets are actively consumed. Mean platelet age in thrombocytopenia due to decreased production is older than in thrombocytopenia due to increased destruction, in which platelets are younger and larger and have better function at equivalent platelet counts. This should be taken into account when making a decision on platelet transfusions. Steroids have no role in the treatment of this group of disorders.

TOTAL ANOMALOUS PULMONARY VENOUS CONNECTION

WELTON M. GERSONY, M.D.

Total anomalous pulmonary venous connection (TAPVC) is a relatively uncommon congenital cardiac anomaly that can occur in the context of a number of anatomic and physiologic variations. Embryologically, the defect appears to be the result of the *failure of incorporation of the common pulmonary vein into the left atrium*. Venous drainage of the lungs thus depends on the persistence of some anatomic components of the fetal venous system. The dominant pathway that remains patent determines the course of pulmonary venous return to the right atrium. *As with most severe congenital heart abnormalities, circulation during fetal life is not affected with TAPVC*. Regardless of the location of the anomalous pulmonary venous connections, the minimal pulmonary blood flow prior to birth simply joins the blood which has been oxygenated via the placental circulation as it enters the right atrium and right ventricle and reaches the systemic circulation via the ductus arteriosus. After birth, however, the hemodynamic derangements are usually severe.

Pulmonary venous blood flow reaches the right side of the heart by one of a number of pathways. *Anomalous pulmonary veins are classified as supracardiac (50 percent), cardiac (25 percent), infracardiac (20 percent), and mixed (5 percent)*. The supracardiac return may be to the left superior vena cava, reaching the right atrium via a vertical vein, innominate vein, and right superior vena cava, or directly into the right superior vena cava. The cardiac connections primarily drain into the coronary sinus, but direct communication to the right atrium may occur in rare cases. Infracardiac connections reach the heart via the portal vein and inferior vena cava. Mixed connections are less common.

The most important factor in determining the severity of circulatory dysfunction in the neonatal period is the degree of pulmonary venous obstruction. Significant stenosis at any site from the common pulmonary vein to the right atrium results in pulmonary venous and capillary hypertension, and if obstruction is severe, pulmonary edema and pulmonary artery hypertension ensue. *Virtually all the infants with infracardiac connections and approximately one-half of the patients with supracardiac pulmonary venous return have significant obstruction and are in severe distress early in the neonatal period.* The majority of infants have only mild to moderate pulmonary venous obstruction, and right ventricular and pulmonary blood flow and pressures are increased. Rarely, an older infant or child with no pulmonary venous obstruction has increased pulmonary blood flow and normal pulmonary artery pressure. Thus, there are three basic physiologic types of patients with total anomalous pulmonary venous return (Table 1).

TYPE I: SEVERE PULMONARY VENOUS OBSTRUCTION, PULMONARY HYPERTENSION, LOW PULMONARY BLOOD FLOW

Babies with severe pulmonary venous obstruction, most of whom have infracardiac connections present within the first few days of life, rarely survive untreated for more than a week or two. At the time of diagnosis, these infants are critically ill with pulmonary edema and associated severe clinical manifestations. Survival depends on early recognition of respiratory distress and cyanosis by the primary physician and immediate transfer to a medical center where there are facilities to manage neonates with congenital heart disease. *Differentiation from pulmonary disease may be difficult.* In most instances cardiac catheterization is carried out to make the diagnosis and determine the site of the abnormal connections. In some cases, echocardiographic study alone, without hemodynamic or angiographic studies, has been sufficient to plan surgical management. Medical management generally is not helpful in improving the clinical status of these babies. Oxygen should be administered and diuretic therapy utilizing individual doses of furosemide (1 to 3 mg per kilogram intravenously) is appropriate for babies with frank pulmonary edema. Early ventilation and intravenous catecholamines may be required. However, in the presence of mechanical obstruction, *little improvement can be expected until relief of obstructed pulmonary venous return is provided surgically.*

With supracardiac and infracardiac connections, *the aim of surgical management is to reincorporate the common pulmonary vein into the left atrium.* Since this chamber may be small, correction is carried out with a wide parallel incision between the posterior aspect of the atria and the anterior wall of the common pulmonary vein. The atrial septum is then reconstituted to the right of the anastomosis to enlarge the functional left atrium. The anomalous connection is simply ligated and divided. This procedure is done on an urgent basis after the diagnosis is made, usually within the first week of life. In the presence of severe obstruction to pulmonary venous return, there are no alternative nonsurgical approaches that can achieve success.

TYPE II: MILD PULMONARY VENOUS OBSTRUCTION, PULMONARY ARTERY HYPERTENSION, AND HIGH PULMONARY BLOOD FLOW

Babies of this physiologic type usually have supracardiac or cardiac connections. Although pulmonary venous obstruction is mild, *pulmonary artery hypertension is severe, and there is markedly increased pulmonary blood flow.* These patients usually develop signs of congestive heart failure within the first 3 or 4 weeks of life. As with other infants with congestive heart failure attributable to large left-to-right shunts, improvement may be noted with medical management. However, chronic congestive heart failure and failure to thrive lead to debilitation and early death. *Without an operation, the great majority of infants succumb* with cardiac cachexia, heart failure, and pulmonary disease.

Initial medical management may be more helpful for

TABLE 1 Basic Physiologic Types of TAPC

Type	Features
Type I	Severe pulmonary venous obstruction Pulmonary artery hypertension Decreased pulmonary blood flow
Type II	Mild to moderate pulmonary venous obstruction Pulmonary artery hypertension Increased pulmonary blood flow
Type III	Absence of pulmonary venous obstruction Absence of pulmonary artery hypertension Increased pulmonary blood flow

this group of babies than for those with severe pulmonary venous obstruction. After initial treatment with diuretics and perhaps digoxin, a reparative operation, as already described, is carried out. The common pulmonary vein is anastomosed to an enlarged functional left atrium. When anomalous pulmonary venous connections are to the coronary sinus, the roof of the coronary sinus is excised widely into the left atrium, and the atrial septum is reconstituted to the right of the coronary sinus.

Some centers have advocated enlargement of the foramen ovale by balloon septostomy to allow greater flow from the right atrium to the left side of the heart and a reduction in pulmonary blood flow. A medical regimen is instituted and surgery delayed until after the first year of life. This approach may be helpful in some cases, but the great majority of infants do not have obstruction of the foramen ovale, so that enlargement of this communication does not result in significant improvement. In general, *it is most advantageous to carry out surgery within the first month or two of life* to avoid the severe symptoms and complications that inevitably occur if operation is not performed.

TYPE III: ABSENCE OF PULMONARY VENOUS OBSTRUCTION, NORMAL PULMONARY ARTERIAL PRESSURE, INCREASED PULMONARY FLOW

In the absence of pulmonary venous obstruction, *the hemodynamic pattern is essentially that of a patient with a large atrial septal defect and no pulmonary hypertension.* The pulmonary blood flow is so large that blood reaching the left side of the heart via the foramen ovale has a relatively high oxygen saturation, and cyanosis is not apparent. Congestive heart failure and growth retardation do not occur, so that this cardiac defect may remain unrecognized for many months or even years. Repair is carried out electively at low risk by the surgical techniques previously described.

A number of factors that might result in long-term complications after surgical correction of total anomalous pulmonary venous return have been suggested: (1) the development of chronic pulmonary vascular obstruction because of long-standing pulmonary hypertension, which is not reversed by surgical correction, (2) hypoplasia of the left atrium and ventricle, as judged at preoperative studies, and (3) technical factors related to the surgical procedure (e.g., a narrow anastomosis between the common pulmonary vein and the left atrium) leading to persistent pulmonary venous obstruction. Postoperative hemodynamic studies have indicated that these concerns are rarely translated into late complications among infants who have had successful surgery.

It has been shown that *pulmonary artery hypertension present in infants prior to surgery is completely reversible after anatomic correction of the anomalous pulmonary venous drainage.* Rarely, significant pulmonary arteriolar constriction may persist after what appears to be an unobstructed surgical anastomosis between the common pulmonary vein and left atrium. This has proved to be reversible with time, usually within a few weeks after surgery. In some cases of acute severe pulmonary arteriolar vasoconstriction in the immediate postoperative period, the use of intravenous vasodilator therapy may be advantageous (tolazoline 1 mg per kilogram as a single dose, repeated as indicated).

When the left atrium is suitably enlarged at the time of surgery, this chamber, as well as the left ventricle, grows normally. Late hemodynamic studies have shown the left side of the heart to be normal.

Occasionally, the surgical anastomosis between the common pulmonary vein and left atrium is inadequate. Such patients require postoperative echocardiographic, angiographic, and hemodynamic study to make this diagnosis and to delineate the precise anatomy at the site of the surgical anastomosis. If obstruction is significant, reoperation must be carried out. Rarely is hypoplasia of the pulmonary veins so severe that relief of pulmonary venous obstruction is not possible at the initial surgical procedure. No cases have been reported in which a well-documented unobstructed anastomosis has narrowed with time.

Significant late rhythm disorders are not often seen after repair of TAPVC. Some patients have nonsinus atrial rhythms, and there are occasional infants who show manifestations of "sick sinus syndrome." However, in contrast to babies with transposition of the great arteries who have had early Mustard operations, this has been an unusual disturbance in patients after repair of anomalous pulmonary venous return.

Rarely is late medical management or surgical reintervention necessary among infants with TAPVC in whom an initial excellent surgical result has been accomplished. It has become clear that *TAPVC has the most favorable long-term prognosis of all the critical congenital heart lesions that require urgent surgery in the neonatal period.*

TOTAL ANOMALOUS PULMONARY VENOUS CONNECTION: SURGICAL ASPECTS

RICHARD A. JONAS, M.D.
ALDO R. CASTANEDA, M.D., Ph.D.

Total anomalous pulmonary venous connection (TAPVC) consists of both an anatomic and a physiologic spectrum of anomalies. Management of TAPVC varies from a low-risk, relatively elective, technically simple procedure, such as for TAPVC to the coronary sinus, to the most urgent of neonatal cardiac surgical emergencies, carrying a high risk of death, as obstructed infradiaphragmatic TAPVC. The heterogeneous nature of this anomaly can be easily explained by its embryologic origin. Failure of the primitive common pulmonary vein to merge with the splanchnic plexus of veins surrounding the developing lung buds results in a *persistent splanchnic venous connection to almost any point in the central cardinal or umbilical-vitelline venous systems.*

CLINICAL PRESENTATION AND INDICATIONS FOR SURGERY

As long as there is unobstructed return of pulmonary venous blood to the right atrium, the neonate is likely to show few clinical signs other than cyanosis due to mixing of pulmonary and systemic venous return at atrial level. As pulmonary resistance falls during infancy, there is a progressive increase in left-to-right shunt, with resulting tachypnea and failure to thrive. Since *surgical results for unobstructed TAPVC appear to be uninfluenced by age,* we believe that surgery should be performed at a convenient time in infancy before there is a chance for developmental delay, pulmonary vascular disease, or permanent myocardial decompensation.

By contrast, the neonate with obstructed pulmonary venous return may be extremely sick from the moment of birth. The child will be severely hypoxic with an arterial PO_2 of less than 20 mm, and a metabolic acidosis may ensue. Chest x-ray film will reveal bilateral pulmonary edema. Two-dimensional echocardiography can usually provide accurate diagnosis. It is undoubtedly advantageous to avoid cardiac catheterization and angiography in these severely compromised children. *This is almost the only congenital heart anomaly that cannot be palliated in the neonate by the use of prostaglandin E_1.* There is only one reasonable course, namely, rapid accurate diagnosis, preferably by two-dimensional echocardiography alone, followed by immediate surgery.

ANESTHESIA FOR OBSTRUCTED TAPVC

The hypoxic, acidotic neonate with obstructed TAPVC requires meticulous anesthetic management. Pulmonary resistance should be minimized by hyperventilation with 100 percent oxygen. Anesthesia is induced with high dose fentanyl, which will decrease pulmonary vasoreactivity. If an inotropic agent is required, isoproterenol is preferred so long as the patient does not become unduly tachycardic. In view of the mildly hypoplastic nature of the left heart, however, a rapid heart rate of up to 200 beats per minute may in fact be necessary to maintain adequate cardiac output. Metabolic acidosis should be aggressively treated with bicarbonate or tromethamine (THAM). There may be a large calcium requirement and blood glucose may be labile. Occasionally, there is associated sepsis and renal failure. *Digoxin probably is not useful and lowers the threshold for ventricular fibrillation.*

EMERGENCY SURGICAL MANAGEMENT OF OBSTRUCTED INFRACARDIAC TAPVC

Adequate venous access and an arterial monitoring line, preferably in an umbilical artery, are essential. A pulse oximeter also provides extremely useful information. It is best to avoid surface cooling, because these desperately ill children may fibrillate at a relatively high core temperature (greater than 30°C), particularly if large doses of digoxin have been given. The chest is opened by a median sternotomy, and at least one lobe of the thymus, usually the left, is excised. A patch of anterior pericardium is harvested. This can be treated with 0.6 percent glutaraldehyde for 30 minutes, which considerably improves ease of handling. It is essential that there be minimal disturbance of the myocardium after the pericardium is opened. Even the slightest retraction of the ventricular myocardium can result in ventricular fibrillation.

After systemic heparinization, bypass is commenced with an arterial cannula in the ascending aorta and venous return via a single cannula inserted into the right atrial appendage. Immediately after bypass is begun, the ductus arteriosus is dissected free and ligated. This should be done in all cases irrespective of whether ductal patency has been demonstrated. During body cooling, the heart should be gently retracted out of the chest to allow dissection of the anomalous descending vertical vein. Retraction should not be excessive; otherwise it will cause kinking of the coronary arteries and interfere with myocardial perfusion. *A heavy ligature is tied around the vertical vein at the point where it pierces the diaphragm. The vertical vein is divided and filleted proximally to the level of the superior pulmonary veins* (Fig. 1). The heart is now replaced in the pericardium. By the time the rectal temperature is less than 20°C, the esophageal temperature will be 13 or 14°C and tympanic temperature will be approximately 18°C. The ascending aorta is clamped, and cardioplegic solution is infused into the root of the aorta. Bypass is ceased and blood is drained from the child. The venous cannula is removed.

A *transverse incision is made from the right atrial appendage and carried posteriorly through the foramen ovale into the left atrium.* Because the right pulmonary veins do not anchor the left atrium, excellent exposure of the previously dissected vertical vein is now obtained. The incision in the posterior wall of the left atrium is carried inferiorly parallel to the vertical vein (see Fig. 1). It may

also be extended superiorly into the base of the left atrial appendage. The common pulmonary vein to left atrium anastomosis is performed using continuous 6–0 absorbable polydioxanone suture. Excellent exposure is obtained by the approach described and there is no possibility of kinking or malalignment, as may be the case with the alternative technique of performing the anastomosis with the heart everted from the chest. The foramen ovale and the more posterior part of the right atriotomy can be closed with a pericardial patch. Direct suture closure of the foramen ovale has a tendency to narrow the anastomosis and should be avoided. Before the atrial septal defect is closed, the left heart should be filled with saline, and air can be vented through the cardioplegia site in the ascending aorta. After closure of the right atriotomy, the right heart is filled with saline, the venous cannula is reinserted, and bypass is recommenced. The aortic cross clamp is released with the cardioplegia site bleeding freely. During rewarming, a pulmonary artery monitoring line is inserted through a horizontal mattress suture in the infundibulum of the right ventricle. Insertion of a left atrial monitoring line through a pulmonary vein should be avoided because of the small size of the pulmonary veins. It is, however, possible to insert a left atrial line through the left atrial appendage.

WEANING FROM CARDIOPULMONARY BYPASS

Once rewarming to a rectal temperature of at least 35°C is completed, the patient can be weaned from cardiopulmonary bypass. Although this should be uneventful in any patient after elective surgery, it can be a critical phase in the management of one who is acutely ill and previously obstructed. Such *patients tend to have markedly labile pulmonary vascular resistance.* Their response to cardiopulmonary bypass is frequently a substantial, though brief, temporary increase in pulmonary resistance. It is therefore useful to monitor pulmonary artery pressure in addition to aortic pressure and left atrial pressure at the time of weaning from bypass. It is not uncommon for pulmonary pressure to be close to systemic levels for the first 10 to 15 minutes after weaning from bypass. During this time, ventilatory management is critical. Once again, the patient should be maintained on 100 percent oxygen, and PCO_2 should be lowered to at least 30 mm. Isoproterenol is frequently useful as an inotropic agent in further lowering pulmonary resistance. Because of the mildly hypoplastic nature of the left ventricle and left atrium, it may be necessary to maintain relatively high left atrial pressures, perhaps as high as 15 to 20 mm Hg. In the presence of a widely open anastomosis, pulmonary pressure should fall to less than two-thirds to one-half systemic within 15 to 30 minutes of weaning from bypass. If pulmonary pressure remains elevated, a high suspicion of an obstructed anastomosis should be entertained. Intraoperative two-dimensional echocardiography can give excellent visualization of this area.

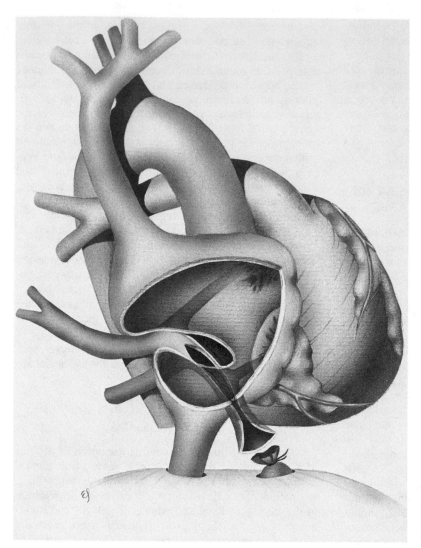

Figure 1 Operative exposure obtained with infradiaphragmatic TAPVC using an approach from the right.

ELECTIVE SURGICAL MANAGEMENT OF NONOBSTRUCTED SUPRACARDIAC TAPVC

The general operative approach to nonobstructed supracardiac TAPVC is similar to that for infracardiac TAPVC. Deep hypothermic circulatory arrest in the infant provides optimal exposure, and therefore the most consistently wide-open anastomosis. The horizontal pulmonary venous confluence is dissected free during the cooling period. In this case, after cessation of cardiopulmonary bypass and removal of the venous cannula, *the right atrial transverse incision is carried across the atrial septum at the level of the foramen ovale into the left atrium. It is then continued transversely, extending into the base of the left atrial appendage. A longitudinal incision, parallel to the posterior wall of the left atrial incision, is made in the horizontal pulmonary venous confluence* (Fig. 2). A direct anastomosis is fashioned between the left atrial and pulmonary venous confluence using continuous 6–0 polydioxanone suture. The anastomosis is begun at the most leftward point, using a continuous technique and working toward the right. Once again, it

is best to *close the foramen ovale with a patch of autologous pericardium.* This avoids any narrowing of the anastomosis and also helps to supplement the size of the small left atrium (Fig. 3). Pulmonary hypertension is rare after such elective cases in which pulmonary artery pressure has usually been only mildly elevated before surgery.

ELECTIVE SURGICAL MANAGEMENT OF TAPVC TO THE CORONARY SINUS

It was previously thought that obstruction of TAPVC to the coronary sinus was extremely rare, but a recent review at this hospital revealed a surprisingly high incidence of 22 percent of such cases. Two-dimensional echocardiography should therefore carefully assess the point of junction between the pulmonary veins and the coronary sinus, which was the most common point of obstruction in our series. If there is any doubt about this area, cardiac catheterization should be performed. In the absence of obstruction, a simple unroofing procedure of the coronary sinus will suffice. The *tissue between the fora-*

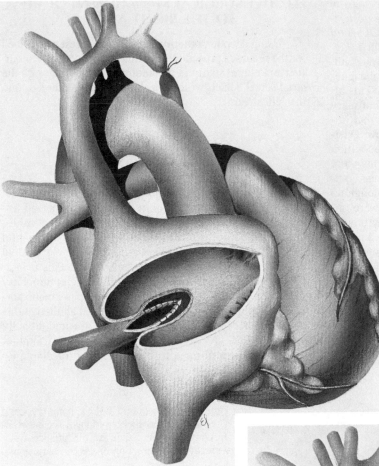

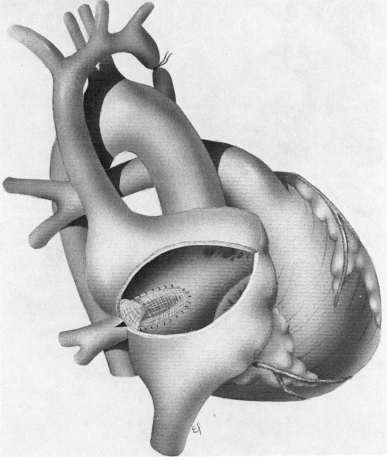

Figure 2 Excellent exposure of the horizontal pulmonary venous confluence is obtained by a single atrial incision extended through the foramen ovale into the left atrium for supracardiac TAPVC.

Figure 3 Autologous pericardium is used to close the foramen ovale, supplement the anastomosis, and enlarge the left atrium in supracardiac TAPVC.

men ovale and coronary sinus is incised, and the incision in the roof of the coronary sinus is carried to the posterior wall of the heart (Fig. 4). The resulting atrial septal defect is closed with an autologous pericardial patch (Fig. 5). In an attempt to decrease the incidence of bradyarrhythmias following this procedure, Van Praagh and colleagues in 1972 suggested the "fenestration" procedure. This allows for preservation of the tissue between the coronary sinus and foramen ovale, where it was thought that important internodal conduction pathways may have existed. The experience at this hospital with this operation between 1972 and 1980 revealed that in 10 patients there was no decrease in the incidence of bradyarrhythmias compared with the more traditional procedures. Although no cases of restriction at the point of fenestration were observed at this hospital, this has been reported by others.

If two-dimensional echocardiography reveals a potential site of obstruction at the junction of the coronary sinus with the horizontal confluence, an operation similar to that for supracardiac TAPVC should be performed. The horizontal confluence should be filleted, and a parallel incision should be made in the posterior wall of the left atrium, extending into the left atrial appendage. A direct anastomosis can be fashioned using continuous absorbable polydioxanone suture.

ELECTIVE SURGICAL MANAGEMENT OF TAPVC TO THE RIGHT ATRIUM

Using deep hypothermic circulatory arrest as outlined for the previous procedures, an autologous pericardial baffle can be used to direct the anomalous veins through the atrial septal defect, which may be surgically enlarged, into the left atrium.

FAILURE TO WEAN FROM CARDIOPULMONARY BYPASS

If the right ventricle appears to be incapable of generating the high pressures required in the early period following weaning from bypass, it may be useful to consider the application of extracorporeal membrane oxygenation (ECMO) for a period of several days to allow a gradual decrease in pulmonary vascular resistance. This principle has been successfully applied for the high pulmonary resistance encountered in neonates with diaphragmatic hernias. Although this procedure has not been applied at this hospital for obstructed TAPVC, there are undoubtedly some children who would benefit from ECMO. Cannulation could be performed as recommended for diaphrag-

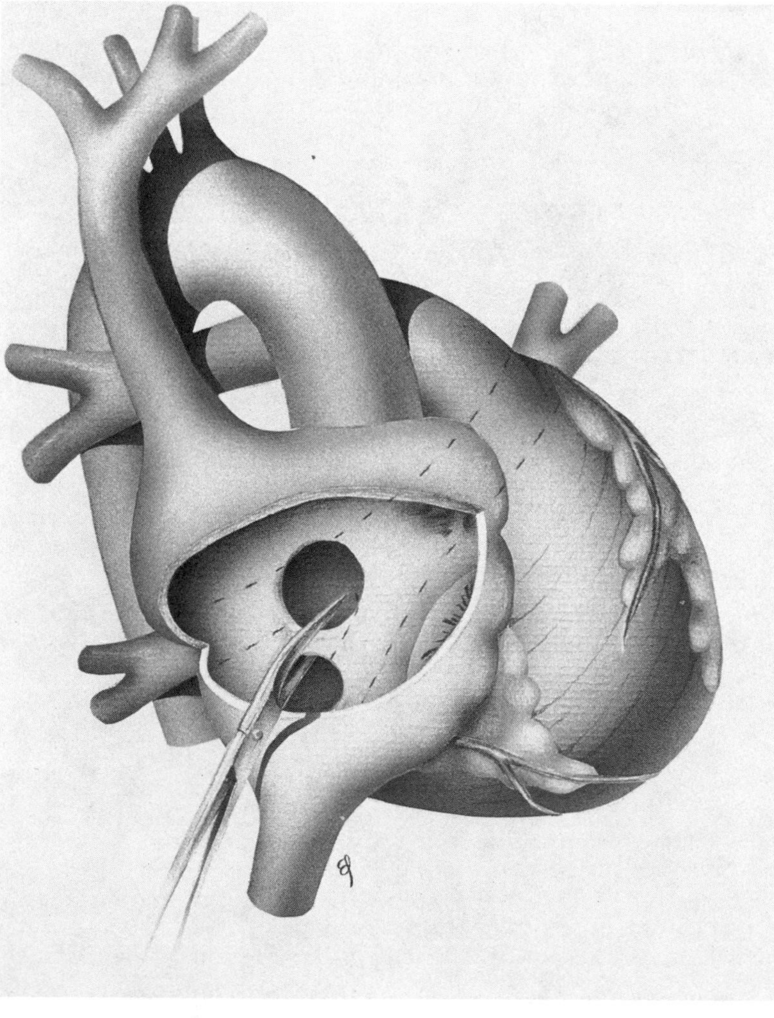

Figure 4 Unobstructed TAPVC to the coronary sinus is treated by incision of the tissue between the coronary sinus ostium and the foramen ovale with complete unroofing of the coronary sinus.

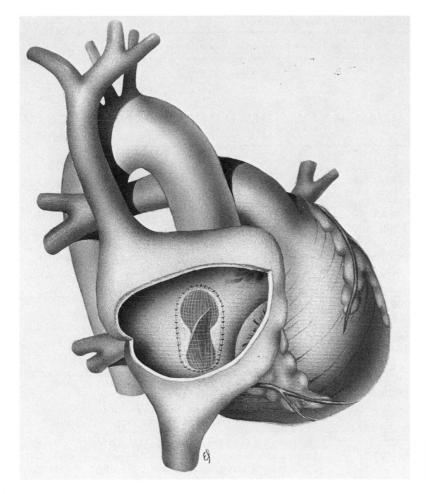

Figure 5 Autologous pericardium is used to close the resultant atrial septal defect in TAPVC to the coronary sinus.

matic hernia, with arterial cannulation of the carotid artery and venous return via a multifenestrated tube inserted into the right atrium through the internal jugular vein.

INTENSIVE CARE MANAGEMENT

The heavily muscularized pulmonary arterioles of the child with obstructed TAPVC remain particularly labile for up to several days after corrective surgery. During this period, pulmonary resistance should be minimized by appropriate ventilatory management. The stress response of pulmonary vasoconstriction should be minimized by maintaining a constant state of anesthesia, using a fentanyl infusion supplemented with hourly boluses of pancuronium, 0.1 mg per kilogram. Arterial PCO_2 should be maintained at approximately 30 mm, and the inspired oxygen concentration should be titrated so as to *achieve a pulmonary pressure, as measured by the indwelling pulmonary artery line, of less than two-thirds systemic.* A low-dose isoproterenol infusion of up to 0.1 μg per kilogram per minute may also be continued for 24 to 48 hours for its pulmonary vasodilatory effects. After 24 to 48 hours of hemodynamic stability, the level of anesthesia may be lightened, with careful observation for pulmonary hypertensive crises. These are particularly likely to occur in

response to the stress of endotracheal tube suctioning, which should be performed carefully after hyperventilation. Assuming that the child remains hemodynamically stable, ventilatory weaning can be commenced. When an intermittent mandatory ventilation (IMV) rate of four breaths per minute can be tolerated, the child will usually withstand extubation.

Throughout intensive care management, it is essential that caloric intake be maintained at at least 125 percent of basal requirements. Electrolyte status, including ionized calcium levels, should be carefully monitored and maintained.

LONG-TERM FOLLOW-UP

Despite an initial satisfactory course, a small percentage of children develop pulmonary venous obstruction after surgery for TAPVC, often within 3 to 6 months after surgery. Most commonly this takes the form of an obliterative intimal fibrous hyperplasia affecting the pulmonary veins close to their junction with the original common pulmonary vein, and therefore somewhat remote from the actual line of anastomosis with the original true left atrium. This entity is particularly difficult to deal with surgically and is also unresponsive to balloon dilatation. Attempts

TABLE 1 Distribution of TAPVC

Connection	No. of Cases	Early Deaths	Late Deaths
Supracardiac	28	2	0
Infracardiac	16	3	1
Coronary sinus	17	0	2
Right atrium	3	0	0
Mixed	3	1	1
Total	67	6	4

at pericardial patch plasty have generally been unsuccessful. Patching techniques using flaps of atrial tissue may be more successful in relatively mild cases.

Anastomotic obstruction due to inadequate growth of suture lines can occur in spite of the use of absorbable sutures or interrupted suture technique. This form of obstruction can usually be readily managed by repeat surgery. Generally, there is dilation of a secondary chamber behind the anastomosis. Simple incisions connecting the two chambers followed by endocardial approximation generally suffice to deal with this problem.

Echocardiography has proved to be an important noninvasive adjunct for detection of such pulmonary venous problems and should be aggressively employed when clinically indicated.

RESULTS OF SURGICAL MANAGEMENT

Over the 10-year period between 1977 and 1986, 67 children with TAPVC underwent repair at Boston Children's Hospital. This total excludes children with complex multiple anomalies including TAPVC, usually as part of the heterotaxy syndrome. Table 1 illustrates the distribution of the various anatomic forms of TAPVC. It can be seen that the most common form was supracardiac TAPVC, which made up 42 percent of the entire group. There was no early mortality among the 20 patients with

TAPVC to the coronary sinus or right atrium, although there were two late deaths due to obstruction in the coronary sinus group. There was a 7 percent mortality rate among patients with supracardiac TAPVC. The highest mortality was seen with infracardiac TAPVC, in which three of 16 patients died early.

SUGGESTED READING

Gold JP, Jonas RA. Lang P, et al. Transthoracic intracardiac monitoring lines in pediatric surgical patients: A ten year experience. Ann Thorac Surg 1986; 42:185–191.

Hickey PR, Hansen DD, Wessel DL, et al. Blunting of stress responses in the pulmonary circulation of infants by fentanyl. Anesth Analg 1985; 64:1137–1142.

Jonas RA, Smolinsky A, Mayer JE, Castaneda AR. Obstructed pulmonary venous drainage with total anomalous pulmonary venous connection to the coronary sinus. Am J Cardiol 1987; 59:431–435.

Norwood WI, Hougen TJ, Castaneda AR. Total anomalous pulmonary venous connection: surgical considerations. In: Engle MA, ed. Pediatric cardiovascular diseases. Philadelphia: FA Davis, 1981: 353.

Pacifico AD, Mandke NV, McGrath LB, et al. Repair of congenital pulmonary venous stenosis with living autologous atrial tissue. J Thorac Cardiovasc Surg 1985; 89:604–609.

Van Praagh R, Harken AH, Delisle G, et al. Total anomalous pulmonary venous drainage to the coronary sinus. J Thorac Cardiovasc Surg 1972; 64:132–135.

Whight CM, Barratt-Boyes BG, Calder AL, et al. Total anomalous pulmonary venous connection. J Thorac Cardiovasc Surg 1978; 75:52–63.

TRACHEOESOPHAGEAL FISTULA

EUGENE D. McGAHREN, M.D.
BRADLEY M. RODGERS, M.D.

Esophageal atresia with tracheoesophageal fistula (TEF) was first recognized in 1697 by Thomas Gibson. It was a uniformly fatal congenital defect for nearly 2 ½ centuries until 1939, when Ladd and Levin, working independently, performed successful staged repairs of this

anomaly. Haight performed the first successful primary repair in 1941. Since then, operative technique and overall management principles have been refined to the point at which, barring other associated anomalies, most infants with tracheoesophageal defects can be expected to proceed with relatively normal lives after repair.

The incidence of TEF is approximately 1 in 3,500 live births. Fifty percent of these infants have an associated anomaly. The most common of these anomalies are cardiovascular (60 percent) and gastrointestinal, particularly imperforate anus (30 percent). Approximately 10 percent of infants with TEF have anomalies comprising the VATER association; this generally is not regarded as a true syndrome, but consists of *v*ertebral, *a*nal, *t*racheo*e*sophageal, *r*enal, and *r*adial bony abnormalities.

Knowledge of the anatomic varieties of TEF is important for planning initial therapy and operative correction. The five categories of TEF, traditionally classified A to E, are listed below in order of frequency:

1. Type C: Esophageal atresia with distal TEF (80 percent).
2. Type A: Esophageal atresia without TEF (8 percent).
3. Type D: Esophageal atresia with fistulas to both pouches (7 percent).
4. Type E: H-type TEF without esophageal atresia (4 percent).
5. Type B: Esophageal atresia with proximal TEF (1 percent).

Infants with TEF are placed in one of the following Waterston categories at the time of diagnosis in order more accurately to assess prognosis and plan management:

1. Category A: Infants over 5½ lb (2,500 g) birth weight and otherwise well.
2. Category B: Infants between 4 and 5½ lb (2,000 to 2,500 g) birth weight and otherwise well, or infants over 5½ lb birth weight with severe anomalies or severe pneumonia.
3. Category C: Infants under 4 lb (2,000 g) birth weight, or birth weight between 4 and 5½ lb with severe anomalies or severe pneumonia.

SIGNS AND SYMPTOMS

The presenting signs and symptoms of an infant with TEF vary according to the specific anatomic form of the lesion. However, with few exceptions, the signs and symptoms present soon after birth. It is noteworthy that polyhydramnios during pregnancy may occur if the fetus has an atretic distal pouch without tracheal communication, as seen in Types A and B. Infants with esophageal atresia, with or without a tracheal fistula, present with excessive drooling of saliva. Feeding results in regurgitation, coughing, and choking. In the absence of a distal TEF the abdomen is scaphoid, since no air can enter the gastrointestinal (GI) tract. When present, a fistula to the distal esophageal pouch allows air to enter the GI tract and gastric contents to reflux into the trachea. Thus, the infant may experience respiratory distress secondary to chemical pneumonitis and abdominal distention, which compromises the motion of the diaphragm. The presence of a fistula to the proximal esophageal pouch, with direct aspiration of feeds, compounds these symptoms, causing more severe pulmonary complications.

Patients with the Type E anomaly, often referred to as an H-type fistula, sometimes present later in life. They may experience "gassiness" as air enters the GI tract through the fistula and is then cleared by burping. However, coughing, choking, and recurrent respiratory infections, resulting from the entrance of swallowed foods and saliva into the trachea, are the classic symptoms of this defect and are often what brings the child to medical attention. Liquids tend to cause greater problems than solids in this regard. A patchy, dependent pneumonitis is often present, or will most likely develop if the condition is left untreated. These findings may mimic those of more common disorders, such as gastroesophageal reflux, esophageal stenosis, vascular ring, or esophageal dysfunction.

DIAGNOSIS

The diagnosis of TEF can be established by attempting to pass a small feeding tube into the stomach. Resistance is met in the presence of atresia. Occasionally, if the catheter is not stiff enough, it may coil in the pouch and appear to have passed into the stomach. In addition, the catheter may sometimes be mistakenly placed into the trachea, whereby it may pass through an existing fistula into the stomach. This should be readily apparent by a change in the tone of the infant's cry, or symptoms of coughing.

If TEF is suspected, radiographs including the infant's entire body should be obtained. One should particularly note the side of the aortic arch, since a right-sided arch will complicate the right thoracotomy usually used for repair. One should also look for the presence of air in the abdomen, which indicates the presence of a distal TEF. The pattern of abdominal gas may indicate associated intestinal obstructions. Finally, the presence of any bony or vertebral anomalies may indicate the presence of the VATER association.

The atretic proximal esophageal pouch should always be outlined radiographically by passing 1 or 2 ml of barium or metrizamide through a catheter placed in the pouch. A soft No. 8 French red rubber catheter with a single end hole is preferred, as one may then control the exact level of injection. The infant is placed in the lateral position and the contrast medium is injected under fluoroscopy until the distal portion of the pouch is distended. If contrast material enters the trachea through a fistula at this stage, the procedure is terminated and the residual contrast material is aspirated from the pouch. If no fistula is demonstrated, the infant is placed in the Trendelenburg position at 10 to 20 degrees, and contrast material is allowed to flow to the level of the arytenoids. This is necessary because many upper pouch fistulas follow an oblique, cephalad course. If no fistula is seen, the remaining contrast material is then removed.

Ultrasonography is also useful to rule out the cardiac or renal abnormalities that often accompany TEF. Thorough cardiac evaluation should precede any attempt at repair; however, full renal evaluation may be delayed until after repair.

Infants with H-type fistula may present a diagnostic dilemma, because the fistula is often small enough to be easily missed on a barium swallow. It is helpful to perform videoesophagography in infants in whom this anomaly is suspected, by placing a catheter in the prone infant's stomach and injecting contrast material while withdrawing the catheter. If the diagnosis is still suspected despite a normal esophagogram, bronchoscopy or esophagoscopy should identify the fistula.

TREATMENT

Treatment of TEF varies with the particular lesion, and in some cases with the Waterston classification into which the infant falls. However, although repair may have been delayed in the past for some of the infants in the lower Waterston classifications, today's improved anesthetic and critical care techniques allow early primary repair in most infants.

Proper preoperative preparation is essential to a successful outcome for these infants. Body temperature must be maintained. A suction catheter (No. 10 French) is placed in the proximal esophageal pouch in order to minimize aspiration, and the infant is maintained in an upright position to reduce reflux through a distal fistula. Intravenous fluids are begun immediately, using D_{10} ¼ normal saline at 75 percent of normal calculated maintenance dosage, in the assumption that cardiac anomalies or a patent ductus may be present. Broad-spectrum antibiotic coverage is initiated in the anticipation of surgical correction, using ampicillin (200 mg per kilogram per day) and gentamicin (6 mg per kilogram per day). Arrangements are then made to transfer the infant to an intensive care nursery with appropriate surgical specialists. A central venous catheter is placed immediately if a delayed repair is anticipated, or in the operating room if repair is to be undertaken immediately.

Appropriate radiologic studies are performed preoperatively to assess the possibility of associated anomalies that might influence management. The decision to institute delayed repair of the TEF is usually necessitated by the presence of complex congenital cardiac anomalies or severe pulmonary compromise from aspiration. Except in extreme cases, the size of the infant is not used as an indication for delay.

Most infants with TEF (Types B, C, and D) are repaired through a right posterior thoracotomy via the fourth intercostal space. However, if preoperative radiographs indicate the presence of a right aortic arch, repair should be accomplished through a left posterior thoracotomy. The skin incision should not extend beyond the midaxillary line, in order to avoid compromising future breast development. On dividing the intercostal muscles, the pleura is gently dissected away from the chest wall, so that the repair may be accomplished in retropleural fashion. This technique prevents infection of the entire pleural space if an anastomotic leak should occur postoperatively. The azygos vein is identified, ligated with fine silk ligatures and divided, thus exposing the posterior mediastinum. In Type C TEF, control of the distal fistula is accomplished first, in order to prevent further aspiration and to allow more effective use of positive-pressure ventilation. Care is taken during the dissection in this region to avoid injuring the vagus nerves and their many branches to the esophagus. The distal fistula is then transected, leaving a 3-mm cuff on the tracheal wall, and this defect is closed with interrupted sutures of 5–0 Vicryl. The distal portion of the esophagus is exposed with minimal dissection, since its blood supply is segmental, from posterior mediastinal vessels. Exploration of the superior mediastinum is then performed to expose the proximal esophageal pouch. This exposure may be facilitated by asking the anesthesiologist to push on the suction catheter in the proximal pouch while the surgeon palpates the mediastinum. The blood supply to the proximal esophageal pouch is abundant and arises in the neck from the thyrocervical trunk, thus allowing more freedom in this dissection. In dividing the proximal pouch from the posterior membranous trachea, one must search carefully for a proximal fistula. With sharp dissection, the proximal pouch is dissected to the level of the crycopharyngeus sphincter. Circular myotomies (Livaditis) of the proximal pouch may be helpful in relieving tension on the anastomosis. We prefer a single-layer anastomosis between the proximal and distal pouch, using interrupted 5–0 Vicryl sutures, tying the knots within the lumen. An end-to-side anastomosis with simple ligation of the fistula may occasionally be used in these infants. While the incidence of recurrent fistula is slightly higher than with the end-to-end technique, it does allow construction of a wider anastomosis, and also leaves the anastomosis secured in place by the intact fistula. If this technique is chosen, the mucosa of the fistula should be abraded with a fine rasp before ligation of this structure. After completion of the esophageal anastomosis, a small Silastic drain is left in the retropleural space and the thoracotomy is closed in standard fashion. A gastrostomy is routinely placed in infants in Waterston Class C, but otherwise is used only if the anastomosis is under tension or a prolonged recovery is anticipated.

Infants with esophageal atresia without associated fistula (Type A) usually require a delayed repair. The distal pouch is always short and rarely extends far into the thorax. Both ends of the esophagus appear to elongate with time, however, and primary repair usually can be accomplished. A gastrostomy tube is placed upon recognition of the anomaly, and a sump catheter (No. 10 French) is maintained in the proximal pouch. We prefer to utilize high-volume gastrostomy feedings, spaced as widely apart as the infant's serum glucose will allow. The associated gastroesophageal reflux then serves to elongate the distal esophageal pouch. The proximal pouch is stretched daily in the intensive care nursery with small rubber dilators. On a weekly basis dilatation is performed under fluoroscopy from above and below to monitor the gap between the esophageal segments. Once it appears that the two segments will easily meet in the posterior mediastinum, usually at 4 to 6 weeks of age, repair is accomplished in the retropleural fashion with a single-layer anastomosis. Often, a Livaditis myotomy is used to relieve tension on the anastomosis. Rarely, in situations with an extremely long gap, a colon interposition is required to establish esophageal continuity. Such an operation is usually delayed until the infant is 6 months to 1 year of age, and an early proximal esophagostomy is performed to allow the patient to be discharged home.

In patients with Type E TEF (H-fistula), the fistula usually occurs at or above the level of the second thoracic vertebra and may be approached through a low cervical incision on the right side. Identification of the fistula is accomplished preoperatively by passing a small catheter into the fistula through the bronchoscope and retrieving it through the esophagus. Rarely, multiple fistulas may be encountered. Care must be taken in the dissection of the fistula to protect the recurrent laryngeal nerve, which may pass either in front of or behind the fistula. Following division of the fistula and closure of the esophageal and tracheal defects with interrupted 5–0 Vicryl, it is useful to interpose a flap of strap muscle between the esophagus and trachea to minimize the possibility of recurrent fistula.

If the infant is in the Waterston classification B or C, with severe associated anomalies or pulmonary insufficiency, a staged or delayed repair may be elected. In the presence of a distal fistula (Types C and D), if the delay is anticipated to be less than 7 to 14 days, a simple gastrostomy may be sufficient to prevent aspiration of gastric contents. With longer delays, however, division of either the distal fistula or the stomach may be necessary to prevent aspiration until definitive surgery is appropriate.

The infant with poor pulmonary compliance (e.g., the respiratory distress syndrome) and a distal esophageal fistula presents special problems in management. Adequate ventilation may be impossible to achieve, since air preferentially enters the low-resistance GI tract through the distal fistula. In these infants, immediate bronchoscopy should be performed and a Fogerty balloon catheter placed in the fistula as a means of temporary occlusion. Early thoracotomy, either for primary repair or for operative division of the distal fistula, may be necessary to achieve survival of these infants.

POSTOPERATIVE MANAGEMENT

Most infants with TEF may be weaned immediately from mechanical ventilation. Once these patients are extubated, all the personnel involved in their management must understand the hazards associated with the reintubation of an infant with an esophageal anastomosis and tracheal closure. This reintubation should be performed by the most skilled individual available, should it become necessary. Many of these infants will be noted to have lobar collapse immediately after surgery, from operative compression of the lung. Respiratory support should be maintained with humidified oxygen and vigorous chest physical therapy. Suctioning of excessive pharyngeal secretions is allowed only with a carefully measured suction catheter, to avoid passage into the esophagus. A small sump tube is left in the proximal pouch, with the tip above the level of the esophageal anastomosis. This tube is removed and not replaced if it becomes obstructed or dislodged. Antibiotics are continued for 7 days postoperatively and intravenous hyperalimentation initiated on the first postoperative day. *We prefer not to feed these infants by gastrostomy tube immediately after surgery because of the high incidence of gastroesophageal reflux.* Seven days postoperatively a barium radiograph is obtained to ensure the integrity of the anastomosis, and at this time oral feedings may be initiated.

COMPLICATIONS

Significant postoperative complications occur in about 15 percent of infants with TEF. Anastomotic leaks occur in about 10 percent of repairs. These appear to be somewhat more frequent with single-layer repairs, as opposed to the double-layer repairs performed in the past. However, they are rarely serious and the vast majority are managed expectantly with an additional week of intravenous hyperalimentation. Transthoracic drainage is rarely necessary. Strictures at the anastomotic site also occur in about 10 percent of repairs, being more common in double-layer repairs. Strictures are also more common in infants who have suffered anastomotic leakage. Dilatation is usually successful in relieving the stricture and is currently performed using a balloon catheter under fluoroscopic control, with the infant sedated. Most infants with refractory esophageal strictures are found to have significant gastroesophageal reflux, and antireflux procedures (Nissen fundoplication) should be performed.

Gastroesophageal reflux and poor esophageal motility are characteristically seen in patients with TEF. Thus, precautions must be taken to minimize reflux, including upright feeding, elevation of the head of the bassinet, and pharmacologic manipulation (cimetidine and Reglan). Antireflux operative procedures are nevertheless often required in these infants to avoid recurrent aspiration pneumonia, refractory strictures, or failure to thrive.

Tracheomalacia is present in nearly all patients with TEF, who frequently are noted to have expiratory stridor and a "barking" cough. The resultant inefficiency of respiratory mechanics contributes to the increased frequency of pulmonary infections noted in these children. Obstruction of the soft airway by an anomalous innominate artery may be considerably more common in these infants than previously appreciated. Bronchoscopy should be performed in infants with symptoms of severe obstructive airway or persistent stridor to identify this anomaly. Innominate artery suspension may be necessary in symptomatic infants. Recurrent respiratory infections may afflict infants who have undergone repair of TEF. These infections sometimes result from aspiration secondary to gastroesophageal reflux, poor esophageal motility, or recurrent or missed TEFs. If recurrent infections occur, a thorough re-evaluation of the infant should be undertaken with appropriate radiographic and bronchoscopic studies. Recurrent TEFs occur in 4 to 8 percent of repairs. However, we believe that *many reported "recurrent" fistulas actually represent a proximal fistula missed at the first examination.* A second operation is required to repair such a fistula, performed transthoracically because of adhesions present from the initial repair.

Some infants who have undergone repair of TEF may experience chest wall deformities or scoliosis as they grow. These are thought to be secondary to growth disturbances from an early thoracotomy. The physicians caring for these children later in life should watch for these deformities, as early detection and intervention are important in their correction.

TRANSIENT DIABETES

JAMES J. McGILL, M.B.B.S., F.R.A.C.P.
DON M. ROBERTON, M.D., F.R.A.C.P.

Transient neonatal diabetes mellitus (TNDM), was first reported fully by Ramsey in 1926. Since then, over 50 cases have been reported in the medical literature. This condition has many synonyms, including congenital diabetes, congenital neonatal pseudodiabetes mellitus, congenital temporary diabetes mellitus, transient hyperglycemia of infancy, idiopathic neonatal hyperglycemia, the syndrome of transient diabetes, and transient neonatal diabetes.

TNDM is a disorder of carbohydrate metabolism characterized by transient hyperglycemia and glycosuria, presenting in the neonatal period. Ketonuria and metabolic acidosis usually are absent or mild. Although the condition is probably uncommon, its *true incidence remains unknown, partly because symptomatic patients may be unrecognized, but more importantly because it may be asymptomatic.*

CLINICAL SPECTRUM

Most patients with TNDM have been infants who were small for gestational age (SGA). Pregnancy and delivery are usually normal. Most such babies are born between 38 and 42 weeks of gestation, although TNDM has been recorded in a few premature infants. Frequently the placenta is small and calcified and there may be evidence of infarction.

The most common clinical presentation is poor weight gain or weight loss within the first few weeks of life. The infants have marked loss of subcutaneous tissues, giving the appearance of loose skin and signs of varying degrees of dehydration due to glycosuric diuresis. Polyuria is present but may not be recognized. Gastrointestinal symptoms are not a major feature of TNDM, although there may be vomiting. Affected infants are alert and remain hungry until the degree of dehydration becomes severe enough to alter the conscious state.

There may be fever and the clinical presentation may resemble severe infection with shock. The *diagnosis frequently has been made by chance from the finding of an elevated glucose concentration in urine or in cerebrospinal fluid (CSF)* collected during investigation for suspected sepsis. Skin or systemic infection may be apparent at the time of presentation, and it is not clear whether these are secondary to the underlying metabolic disturbance or have precipitated the clinical presentation. A few infants have had hypoglycemia in the first few days of life and have later developed TNDM.

Blood glucose concentrations are elevated, usually to greater than 15 mmol per liter; levels up to 140 mmol per liter having been recorded. Acidosis and ketosis are usually absent or mild. *Endogenous insulin concentrations have been shown to be inappropriate for the degree of hyper-glycemia.* Electrolyte disturbances are noted occasionally, particularly when vomiting is present.

It is not clear whether the biochemical disturbance causes some infants to be small for gestational age or whether infants who are SGA from some other cause are less resistant to the biochemical disturbance of TNDM, and are therefore more likely to become symptomatic.

A minority of published cases have been noted in babies with a birth weight appropriate for gestational age. These infants present with either poor weight gain, infection, or dehydration. We recently reported two infants in whom TNDM was asymptomatic.

DIFFERENTIAL DIAGNOSIS

Type 1 diabetes mellitus is rare in the first few months of life, and it should be possible to differentiate it from TNDM by the consistently low levels of insulin in response to glucose loads in the former condition. Ketosis and acidosis are not always marked in neonatal Type 1 diabetes mellitus, and in exceptional cases time may be the only reliable method of differentiating between these two disorders.

The iatrogenic hyperglycemia and glycosuria associated with parenteral glucose administration and hyperalimentation is easily distinguished by the rapid fall in blood glucose concentrations when the exogenous supply of glucose is interrupted.

Infants with TNDM who have severe dehydration and fever at presentation create the most difficult diagnostic dilemma. The differential diagnosis includes sepsis; inborn errors of protein, fat, and carbohydrate metabolism; the salt-losing form of congenital adrenal hyperplasia; acute gastrointestinal disorders; and disorders of renal tubular function. Clinicians should include estimations of blood and urinary glucose in their assessment of the sick neonate. Galactosemia or hereditary fructose intolerance may cause some initial confusion if reducing substances are detected in urine; however, a dipstick test specific for glucose and a blood glucose estimation will readily differentiate TNDM from these other disorders of carbohydrate metabolism.

ETIOLOGY

The etiology of TNDM is unknown. The opportunity exists for clinicians to contribute to the knowledge of the cause of this disorder and they should give some thought to this early in the course of the illness.

Numerous theories have been proposed regarding the cause of this condition. The one receiving the most support currently is that the biochemical disturbance is the result of delayed functional maturity of the beta cells of the islets of Langerhans. Plasma insulin concentrations do not respond appropriately to fluctuations in blood glucose. The mechanism of the delayed maturation is unknown but several theories exist. There is no evidence of insulin insensitivity, as affected neonates respond normally to exogenous insulin.

A flat maternal glucose tolerance curve has been

described but has not been a consistent finding in subsequent patients with TNDM. Ferguson and Milner postulated that the small, calcified, and infarcted placentas of these neonates led to a deficiency of fetal steroids; however, some placentas have been normal and plasma and urinary corticosteroids are normal. Pagliari and colleagues found that insulin secretion was stimulated by caffeine but not by glucose or tolbutamide. They postulated a defect in the adenyl cyclase–cyclic adenosine monophosphate system. The variable response of insulin in normal infants to these agents made interpretation of their findings difficult.

Insulin antibodies were suspected to be the cause of this disorder, but we and other investigators have failed to detect such antibodies. We found no evidence of autoantibodies in the serum of either our patients or their mother, and infants of mothers with insulin-dependent diabetes mellitus and insulin antibodies do not get TNDM.

GENETICS

Three families with more than one affected member have been reported. Ferguson and Milner reported three affected male siblings, and we described two male siblings with TNDM born to nonconsanguineous parents. Coffey and Killelea described three half-siblings all with the same father but with different mothers. The existence of this family, and the knowledge that TNDM may be asymptomatic and may pass unrecognized, strongly suggests autosomal dominant inheritance. In the former two families, either autosomal recessive or autosomal dominant inheritance may have been present, with the disorder unrecognized in one of the parents.

Parents of affected infants and perhaps parental siblings should be counseled that in some families TNDM is inherited, and that they therefore have a small but definite chance of recurrence in any future pregnancy. Because TNDM has such a good prognosis, the chance of recurrence is unlikely to alter these parents' reproductive decisions. However, any future child of the couple or either parent and a new partner should be monitored closely during the first month of life. There is no clear relationship between TNDM and diabetes mellitus Types 1 and 2. Although a family history positive for diabetes mellitus has been documented in many case reports, this has usually been in second-degree or more distant relatives, and no distinction has been made between Types 1 and 2 diabetes mellitus. It is interesting to note that the second of the siblings reported by Coffey and Killelea with a family history of Type 2 diabetes mellitus developed Type 1 diabetes mellitus at 15 years of age. We found no relationship between TNDM and HLA type, and in particular no relationship between TNDM and those HLA types known to be associated with Type 1 diabetes mellitus.

MANAGEMENT

The management of TNDM is dependent upon the clinical presentation. Treatment protocols range from intravenous fluids and insulin therapy for SGA infants presenting with severe dehydration, to careful monitoring only for appropriate-for-gestational age infants detected by routine urinalysis. Therapy is directed particularly toward control of fluid disturbances resulting from hyperosmolality. Associated infection should be treated appropriately.

Fluid Therapy

Intravenous fluids should be given to all infants who are 5 percent or more dehydrated at presentation. There is a tendency to overestimate the degree of dehydration because of the marked loss of subcutaneous tissue, particularly when the infant was SGA at birth.

We recommend using 0.075 mol per liter of sodium chloride (one-half normal saline) initially at a rate calculated to correct the dehydration slowly over 36 to 48 hours because of the risks of too rapid a correction of hyperosmolar dehydration, e.g., intracerebral hemorrhage. If the infant is in shock, 10 to 20 ml per kilogram of body weight of either 0.15 mol per liter NaCl or plasma protein solution should be infused over 1 hour before commencing the previously described fluid regimen.

If insulin is being given, the parenteral fluid should be changed to 5 percent dextrose/0.075 mol per liter NaCl once the blood glucose concentration has fallen below 15 mmol per liter, to minimize the risk of hypoglycemia. Serum potassium concentrations will fall as potassium moves into the cells with glucose following insulin administration, so potassium supplementation is usually necessary. Once the infant has been rehydrated it should be possible to change to oral feeds without difficulty.

Infants with lesser degrees of dehydration, particularly if their birth weight was appropriate for gestational age, may be able to be rehydrated orally with the aid of insulin to decrease ongoing losses from the glycosuric diuresis.

Insulin

The decision to use insulin depends on the degree of hyperglycemia and the clinical state of the infant. Insulin therapy should be considered for all infants except those with mild or no clinical signs at presentation. Blood glucose concentrations are very responsive to exogenous insulin.

Insulin should be started at the low dose of 1 to 2 units per kilogram per day of regular insulin in divided doses every 4 to 6 hours. If the infant is being fed orally, the insulin should be given before feeds. Blood glucose concentrations should be measured every 1 to 2 hours during the first day of insulin treatment, and at least before insulin injections in the following days. There is a considerable risk of hypoglycemia, which may cause irreversible neurologic impairment. If it is judged that larger doses of insulin are required, this should be achieved by successive small increments in dosage. Some infants have required doses of insulin in excess of 5 units per kilogram per day. Because of the potential danger of severe hypoglycemia, it is not appropriate to use higher doses of longer-acting insulin preparations.

Once the infant has been stabilized, a decision must

be made whether to continue insulin therapy. The aim of insulin treatment should be to achieve adequate growth. It is inappropriate to aim for normalization of blood sugar concentrations because of the risk of hypoglycemia. Adequate growth may be achieved with blood glucose concentrations averaging between 10 and 15 mmol per liter.

Many infants need only a short course of insulin therapy. Once an adequate growth rate has been achieved, the total daily dose of insulin should be decreased slowly by lowering the magnitude and frequency of individual doses. If symptoms recur, no further attempts at reducing the insulin dose should be made for about 2 weeks.

Some infants do not require insulin treatment: usually those with birth weights appropriate for gestational age who have been detected on routine urinalysis, or who have presented with minimal degrees of dehydration or with mild infections. Such infants should be monitored closely to ensure that they continue to grow adequately, and parents should be educated regarding the importance of seeking early medical assessment in the event of intercurrent infections.

The duration of insulin treatment has varied from a few days up to 18 months; most infants have required several weeks of such therapy. Following the cessation of insulin treatment, infants should be monitored at home two or three times weekly by urinalysis or a home blood glucose meter until the biochemical abnormalities resolve.

Subsequent Management

Infants in whom TNDM has resolved should continue to have growth monitored and, since the ultimate outcome is not yet known, should undergo occasional monitoring of glucose homeostasis throughout childhood and adult life. The occurrence of familial cases suggests a need for monitoring of affected females during pregnancy and of the offspring of affected individuals.

PROGNOSIS

The prognosis for TNDM generally is good. Neurologic sequelae have been reported in a small percentage of patients. With early recognition, controlled correction of the dehydration, and the use of low doses of insulin, combined with frequent monitoring of blood glucose concentrations to avoid hypoglycemia, the frequency of neurologic sequelae should be reduced greatly.

Only one patient, that of Coffey and Killelea, has been reported to have developed insulin-dependent diabetes later in life. Several individuals have been described as leading normal adult lives.

SUGGESTED READING

Coffey JD Jr, Killelea DE. Transient neonatal diabetes mellitus in half sisters. A sequel. Am J Dis Child 1982; 136:626–627.

Ferguson AW, Milner RDG. Transient neonatal diabetes mellitus in sibs. Arch Dis Child 1970; 45:80–83.

Gentz JCH, Cornblath M. Transient diabetes in the newborn. Adv Pediatr 1969; 16:345–363.

McGill JJ, Roberton DM. A new type of transient diabetes mellitus in infancy? Arch Dis Child 1986; 61:334–336.

Pagliara AS, Karl IE, Kipnis DB. Transient neonatal diabetes: Delayed maturation of the pancreatic beta cell. J Pediatr 1973; 82:97–101.

TRANSPOSITION OF THE GREAT ARTERIES

WELTON M. GERSONY, M.D.

Over the past 30 years, the prognosis for newborn infants with transposition of the great arteries has undergone a remarkable turnabout. In the pretreatment era, transposition of the great arteries was the major cause of death among infants with cyanotic heart disease, and few babies survived the first few months of life. At present, *80 to 90 percent of patients are long-term survivors.*

Prior to birth, oxygenation of the fetus is normal because of the presence of fetal channels and the placental circulation. However, soon after birth in babies with transposition of the great arteries and an intact ventricular septum, the minimal mixing of the systemic and pulmonary venous blood at the atrial level via the patent foramen ovale is insufficient, and severe hypoxemia ensues within the first few days or weeks of life. When a ventricular septal defect is present, sufficient mixing of oxygenated and venous blood occurs so that many babies are relatively well-saturated with oxygen in the neonatal period. These infants may not have recognizable symptoms until several weeks of age or later. Indeed, with a large ventricular septal defect, signs and symptoms of congestive heart failure may be the first manifestations, and only minimal cyanosis is observed. The following *discussion stresses the management of babies with transposition of the great arteries and intact ventricular septum,* since this is not only the most common type of transposition complex but is almost invariably diagnosed in the first few days of life before discharge from the nursery.

EARLY MANAGEMENT

A severely cyanotic newborn infant with transposition of the great arteries is a medical emergency. Immediate transfer to a medical center with a cardiac program is mandatory at the time the diagnosis is suspected. If echocardiographic diagnosis is not absolute, appropriate angiographic study should be carried out initially to confirm the diagnosis.

There are now *two basic approaches to surgical management* of transposition of the great arteries. In most major centers today, an *"arterial switch"* operation is performed. The aorta and pulmonary arteries are transected above the valves and reversed. The ductus arteriosus is ligated. The coronary arteries are then transplanted into the base of the new aorta. This operation is carried out within the first 2 weeks of life. Some surgeons continue to prefer *early palliation by Rashkind balloon septostomy, followed by the Mustard or Senning atrial switch procedure* at approximately 6 months of age.

All neonates in whom the plan of management includes an atrial switch procedure require atrial septostomy, and this should be performed as soon as possible after diagnosis. The balloon catheter is advanced to the left atrium via percutaneous catheterization of the femoral vein or through the umbilical vein, by way of the inferior vena cava, right atrium, and patent foramen ovale. The balloon is inflated to 4 cc, and with a quick firm motion, the septum primum is torn by the balloon as it is pulled back to the right atrium. Several pull-throughs are accomplished in succession, and decreased resistance is noted. Following the procedure, arterial blood gas is sampled, and a significant rise in PaO_2 level to 35 to 50 torr suggests that an adequate communication has been established that will result in improved mixing of the systemic and pulmonary venous return. In addition, lack of a pressure gradient across the atrial septum from the left atrium to the right atrium after the septostomy suggests that a sufficiently large atrial communication has been established. Prior to the procedure, the mean left atrial pressure is most often significantly higher than the right atrial mean pressure.

Patients with transposition of the great arteries with an associated significant ventricular septal defect should also undergo balloon septostomy. Some of these patients do not mix well at the ventricular level despite the ventricular communication, and others may benefit from decompression of the left atrium to alleviate the early pulmonary symptoms of left-sided heart failure.

Surgical methods (Blalock-Hanlon, Baffes, Sterling-Edwards operations) for increasing atrial mixing have been available for many years, but the balloon septostomy technique has replaced these procedures at virtually all institutions. In capable hands, the risk of the balloon procedure is low. However, complications have been described, including (1) fracture of the balloon with embolization of the foreign material into the systemic or pulmonary circulation, (2) wedging of the balloon in the inferior vena cava, and (3) inability to deflate the balloon for technical reasons. In the latter circumstances the balloon can be pierced with a wire that is projected from a second catheter lodged against the external balloon surface. In addition, the incidence of seizures and potential residual brain injury in this group of markedly hypoxemic patients is significant, although it is not clear whether the catheterization and septostomy procedures are causative factors.

Some infants are so severely cyanotic and acidotic that there is not sufficient time to assemble the cardiac catheterization laboratory staff to make preparations for the catheterization study. In this situation, *prostaglandin E_1 (0.05 to 0.10 µg per kilogram per minute) can be infused in order to maintain ductal patency* or reopen a ductus arteriosus that is in the process of closing. Adding an additional mixing site in this manner improves arterial oxygenation. Acidosis should be corrected simultaneously by infusion of sodium bicarbonate. In some instances prostaglandin administration should be prolonged even after balloon septostomy until the PaO_2 becomes stable at an acceptable level. However, infusion of prostaglandin E_1 is rarely necessary for more than a few days, and if the patient appears to be prostaglandin-dependent, plans for surgical management should be initiated.

Most patients who are to be managed by the arterial switch procedure receive prostaglandin therapy, but balloon atrial septostomy is not always done. If the patient is admitted with acceptable arterial oxygen saturation utilizing prostaglandin therapy and surgery is to be done virtually immediately, the balloon septostomy can be avoided. However, a septostomy is performed in babies who are severely hypoxemic and in whom the switch operation cannot be done at once.

FOLLOW-UP MANAGEMENT

Atrial Switch

In most instances, the baby with transposition of the great arteries improves noticeably after balloon septostomy. The infant appears to be less cyanotic and begins to eat well. However, relatively severe cyanosis may still be noted with crying. Higher arterial blood oxygen levels will reflect the infant's improved status, but fluctuations can be expected. Blood pH should consistently remain within normal limits, regardless of the PaO_2; the metabolic acidosis noted prior to septostomy should no longer be present. In some cases, PaO_2 begins to fall within hours after what appears to be a successful septostomy. Urgent invasive management, either by reballooning or by surgical alternatives, is not necessarily warranted simply on the basis of a low PaO_2, even in the range of 20 to 30 torr, assuming the baby continues to feed and gain weight, and blood pH remains normal. However, on rare occasions there may be little improvement in the baby's condition despite what appears to be a successful septostomy, and intervention is obviously required during the first few weeks or months of life. Echocardiographic studies may indicate that an inadequate atrial communication has been established. *Even when a large communication is established, pulmonary and systemic venous blood may tend to follow their original channels to their respective ventricles without adequate mixing at the atrial level.* Under these circumstances, a second balloon procedure is rarely helpful, especially if the infant is past the first month of life. Some institutions would temporize with the Blalock-Hanlon procedure or open atrial septostomy to allow mixing and carry out an open heart atrial corrective operation later (Mustard's or Senning's procedure). However, experienced surgeons can successfully perform the Mustard or Senning operation during infancy and thus avoid committing the patient to two major operations within the first year of life.

Infants with transposition of the great arteries and an intact ventricular septum or a very small ventricular septal defect can be discharged within a few days, without medications, after successful septostomy. Digoxin, diuretics, or antiarrhythmic agents are rarely required. However, close follow-up of these patients is necessary. Anemia is a serious problem that can lead to major central nervous system complications secondary to cerebral ischemia. Therefore the hemoglobin should be monitored carefully. *Hemoglobins of 11 to 13 g per deciliter represent significant anemia in patients with cyanotic heart disease.* On the other hand, severe polycythemia is rarely a clinical problem in this age group. Failure to thrive due to chronic hypoxemia, extremely severe cyanosis, or early central nervous symptoms is an urgent indication for further management. However, the majority of patients remain stable, and elective surgery can be done on a scheduled basis.

The Mustard or Senning operation for infants with transposition of the great arteries and intact ventricular septum can be performed at any age after initial balloon septostomy, whether a few days of life after a failed septostomy procedure or months later on an elective basis. These procedures reverse blood flow patterns at the atrial level, allowing systemic venous blood to reach the lungs via the left atrium and ventricle and pulmonary venous blood to cross over to the right atrium, right ventricle, and aorta. Each of these operations has its advocates, depending on the experience at a particular medical center. Elective surgery is usually done when the baby is 4 to 9 months of age. This time period is chosen because an older infant is somewhat larger and clinically stable and thus a better surgical candidate than a desperately ill cyanotic infant. Concern regarding *development of pulmonary vascular obstruction disease precludes delay* beyond this age range. Accelerated arteriolar vascular changes of the irreversible intimal type have been documented by the age of 1 year in babies with transposition of the great arteries with an intact ventricular septum, although this complication is even more likely when a large ventricular septal defect also is present.

The Mustard and Senning operations result in an early survival rate of over 90 percent. Complications include obstruction of the systemic or pulmonary veins, tricuspid valve incompetence, right ventricular dysfunction, and "sick sinus syndrome," occasionally associated with severe bradycardia or "brady-tachy" syndromes. The great majority of patients live a normal life for many decades. The average life expectancy for the survivor of the Mustard and Senning operations with good early right ventricular function and no other abnormalities is unknown, beyond the 30 years since the operations were first introduced.

Arterial Switch

The arterial switch operation (Jatene procedure) has become more widespread recently as an increasing number of pediatric cardiovascular surgeons are now capable of performing it. The indications and timing for a switch procedure vary somewhat among medical centers throughout the world. Most surgeons choose to operate in the first days of life while left ventricular pressure still remains high, due to the usual elevated pulmonary vascular resistance of fetal life. Over the past 5 years the mortality rate for this operation at experienced centers has decreased to a level where it has become the operation of choice. A successfully repaired infant will have a normal anatomic left ventricle, and the anatomic and electrophysiologic abnormalities that can be associated with the atrial switch procedures do not occur. Since long-term follow-up is not yet available for the great majority of infants who have undergone corrective switch operations, concerns remain regarding the integrity of the reimplanted coronary arteries, late aortic valve insufficiency, and supravalvular pulmonary stenosis. However, a number of patients have reached the end of the first decade of life, and late problems in these areas are infrequent. Late reoperation or balloon dilation for supravalvular pulmonary stenosis, which appears to be the most common late manifestation, can be carried out at extremely low risk.

For the great majority of infants with transposition of the great arteries and an intact ventricular septum, the left ventricular pressure remains elevated for the first weeks of life and a switch operation can be carried out. Once pulmonary resistance falls and the left ventricular pressure decreases to the levels of a pulmonary ventricle (less than 35 mm Hg), the resumption of systemic pressure after a switch procedure may be too large a burden for the left ventricle during the postoperative period. If an arterial switch procedure is contemplated after the first month of life, some surgeons carry out pulmonary artery banding in order to raise left ventricular pressure to the degree that hypertrophy is stimulated. In this way *the left ventricle is "prepared," by an artificial increase in afterload, for its role as a systemic ventricle.* A few months later the arterial switch procedure is carried out, and the pulmonary artery banding is removed. In a few such babies, a Blalock-Taussig shunt is done with the pulmonary artery banding to prevent an unacceptably low arterial oxygen saturation during the waiting period. This is also taken down at the time of the switch operation.

TRANSPOSITION OF THE GREAT ARTERIES WITH VENTRICULAR SEPTAL DEFECT

The treatment of transposition of the great arteries with a large ventricular septal defect has consisted of balloon septostomy and medical management of congestive heart failure in the early weeks or months of life. Further management is indicated by 6 months of age to prevent the onset of pulmonary vascular obstructive disease. Pulmonary artery banding has been utilized with mixed success in controlling pulmonary blood flow and congestive heart failure, as well as preventing the high pulmonary artery pressure that accelerates pulmonary vascular damage. Later, the banding must be removed and a Mustard or Senning operation with a ventricular septal defect closure is carried out. Some patients can be managed medically after banding long enough to undergo a Rastelli intraventricular repair. This procedure consists of an intraventricular baffle directing pulmonary venous blood entering the left ventricle from the left atrium to the aorta. A right ventricular–pulmonary artery conduit provides pulmonary blood flow consisting of systemic venous blood. Unfortunately there is significant overall mortality and morbidity regardless of which management plan is initiated. There are dangers in the first few months of life during medical management, and multiple complex surgical procedures also carry significant risk. Long-term survival for this group of patients has been barely 50 percent.

The switch operation is a reasonable option for patients with transposition of the great arteries and ventricular septal defect. These babies can be operated on at a few months of age without pulmonary artery banding, since the left ventricular pressure has been elevated because of the ventricular septal defect. Sufficient hypertrophy is present so that the left ventricle can assume the afterload responsibilities of the systemic ventricle without "preparation" by pulmonary artery banding. Indeed, the Jatene switch procedure was originally reserved for this combination of lesions. Mortality rates for this operation are becoming lower, and preliminary follow-up information is encouraging regarding prospects for long-term survival with good cardiac function.

TRANSPOSITION OF THE GREAT ARTERIES WITH VENTRICULAR SEPTAL DEFECT AND SIGNIFICANT PULMONARY STENOSIS

Neonates may have transposition of the great arteries with ventricular septal defect and significant pulmonary outflow obstruction. Although such patients benefit from increased mixing by means of atrial septostomy, they may also require a systemic to pulmonary artery shunt to augment pulmonary blood flow. If these procedures are successful in providing adequate systemic oxygenation, and the pulmonary pressure is documented to be within normal range, the patient can then be followed clinically for a number of years until further intracardiac surgery is planned. The Rastelli operation is the treatment of choice for late management of these patients. However, a second shunt procedure may be required as an interim measure, since the Rastelli operation is best delayed until the patient is in the 5- to 8-year age range.

VATER ASSOCIATION

JAY M. MILSTEIN, M.D.
ARTHUR W. GRIX, M.D.

The VATER association is a nonrandom association of anomalies in which similar abnormalities in embryogenesis (specifically, a common type of mesodermal defect occurring prior to 35 days of embryonic development) are implicated. The defects depicted by the usual acronym "VATER" include *vertebral defects, vascular abnormalities (such as ventricular septal defect and single umbilical artery) anal atresia, tracheoesophageal fistula with esophageal and (rarely) tracheal atresia, and radial and renal dysplasia.* Although many infants with this association fail to thrive as a result of some of their abnormalities, they generally have normal neurologic function. In addition, the risk of recurrence in affected families is low. Consequently, aggressive evaluation and treatment are indicated.

DIAGNOSTIC EVALUATION

Differential Diagnosis

Diagnostic tests are performed both to confirm the diagnosis for counseling purposes and to establish the scope of the abnormalities in order to formulate a treatment plan. This is particularly important because many of the features of the VATER association may occasionally be present in other syndromes. With the assistance of a geneticist, infants with more serious conditions such as

trisomy 18, trisomy 9, deletion 13Q, and deletion 6Q may be identified. Since these conditions have unfavorable prognoses, aggressive intervention may not be indicated. *Although bone marrow karyotyping may identify the trisomic states, it is not reliable for identifying small deletions.* Most cytogenetic laboratories can give the clinician a diagnosis in 4 to 5 days, however.

Patients with the VATER association manifest phenotypic similarities to those with other conditions, and differentiation is particularly important because of differences in heritability. *The more common heritable conditions include the CHARGE association (choanal atresia, renal and retinal, growth and ear abnormalities), the Holt-Oram syndrome (cardiac-limb syndrome), OAVD (oculo-auriculo-vertebral dysplasia), and the Klippel-Feil anomalad, each of which is occasionally an autosomal dominant disorder.* These conditions may be distinguishable on the basis of their sites of spinal involvement or other more unique choanal, auricular, or ocular abnormalities. Another condition, the *TAR syndrome (thrombocytopenia-absent radius syndrome), which is an autosomal recessive* disorder, also has some phenotypic similarities to the VATER association and warrants differentiation. The recurrence risk in the above conditions clearly justifies establishing an accurate diagnosis for counseling purposes. Similarly, it is important to identify the malformed infant of a diabetic mother with or without the caudal regression syndrome, since subsequent pregnancies can be substantially improved with careful management.

Other diagnostic considerations may be relevant, depending on which features of the VATER association are present in a given patient. For example, craniofacial involvement with ear abnormalities, choanal atresia, cleft lip or palate, and eye abnormalities have been reported in the VATER association. These findings should arouse concern that the diagnosis is other than the VATER association. Similarly, the presence of an imperforate anus without tracheoesophageal abnormalities should lead to careful evaluation of other family members for less severe involvement occurring on a genetic basis. *It is critical that minimal diagnostic criteria, usually including three features, be identified before a definitive diagnosis of the VATER association is assigned.* Because of the overlap with other conditions, further evaluation (including consultation with several subspecialists, particularly a dysmorphologist) is highly recommended.

History

In order to establish the scope of the abnormalities and a treatment plan, the diagnostic evaluation of any infant with single or multiple birth defects begins with a detailed family pedigree and pregnancy history. In terms of family history, because of the variable expression of some dominant disorders, mildly affected family members may not have been previously identified, resulting in the mislabeling of affected infants as spontaneous mutations and leading to errors in future genetic counseling. Second, in a family with a history of increased fetal wastage along with the live birth of infants with malformations seen in the VATER association, the clinician should consider a genetic condition occurring because of a chromosomal translocation or autosomal or X-linked single-gene abnormality. Third, if other family members are free of any portion of the association, a similarly affected sibling may suggest autosomal recessive inheritance.

A careful pregnancy history is essential. For example, *maternal glucose intolerance remains an important contributor to birth defects, many of which overlap those seen in the VATER association.* Second, the pregnancy history may alert the physician to specific features in the association. Polyhydramnios along with a postnatal history of excessive salivation or respiratory distress may be a clue not only to gastrointestinal atresia or upper tracheoesophageal abnormalities, but also to poor fetal swallowing secondary to a central or peripheral neuromuscular lesion. On the other hand, oligohydramnios may indicate renal dysplasia or an obstructive uropathy.

Physical Examination

Awareness of the association alerts the physician to look selectively for those physical features that encompass the association. Vertebral defects may be undetectable at birth and suspected only because of skin lesions such as cystic masses, hemangiomas, dimples, sinus tracts, hypertrichosis, or hyperpigmentation that overlie the spinal column, or may be discovered as incidental findings on the initial chest radiographs obtained for the evaluation of potential cardiac or pulmonary disease. Severe congenital scoliosis may appear as a recognizable deformity of the spine or trunk, and severe congenital kyphosis may appear as a severe angular deformity of the spine. *When craniofacial abnormalities are present, cervical vertebral abnormalities are more likely. On the other hand, when there is an imperforate anus, sacral abnormalities are more likely.*

Vascular abnormalities, including a ventricular septal defect and single umbilical artery, may be indicated by the findings of a typical murmur and increased precordial activity (although the appearance is usually delayed in the full-term infant) and a two-vessel umbilical cord demonstrable in the delivery room.

The anal abnormalities may take the form of an imperforate anus with stool presenting through ectopic rectal openings or fistulas. In the female, rectoperineal, rectovestibular, or rectovaginal fistulas are possible. In the male, rectoperineal, rectoureteral, or rectovesicular fistulas are possible. Abnormal genitalia have been reported in both sexes, leading to difficulties in sex assignment, as well as concerns regarding inborn errors of steroid metabolism.

Tracheoesophageal abnormalities may be implicated by the findings of excessive salivation, respiratory distress, and the inability to pass a nasogastric tube into the stomach. The H-type tracheoesophageal fistula may require sophisticated radiologic evaluation, but those that produce abdominal distention with bagging provide ready grounds for suspicion.

Radial abnormalities may range from complete absence of the radius and thumb to hypoplasia of the proximal radius with or without a hypoplastic thumb. Radial hypoplasia may be unilateral or bilateral and may be as subtle as thenar muscle mass hypoplasia, noted only by side-by-side comparison of the two hands. The radial defects may present as a shortened forearm with bowing of the ulna, convex and posterior to the ulnar side. Movement in the elbow is limited. The thumb may be absent or hypoplastic, with the hand deviating radially.

Renal abnormalities, of which dysplasia and obstructive uropathy are the most common, usually do not show distinct physical findings.

Laboratory Studies

Laboratory studies utilized to establish the scope of the defects and treatment plan include chromosome analysis, imaging studies consisting of plain abdominal radiographs, anteroposterior and lateral radiographs of the spine, radiographs of the forearms and hands, anterior and lateral radiographs of the chest, ultrasonographic imaging of the kidneys and bladder, possibly a voiding cystourethrogram, urinalysis, urine culture, complete blood count, and determination of blood urea nitrogen, serum creatinine, sodium potassium, chloride, total carbon dioxide, calcium, phosphorus, alkaline phosphatase, and creatinine clearance. Further cardiac evaluation, including echocardiography, is done when dictated by the physical findings.

TREATMENT

The vertebral abnormalities may have variable natural histories, depending on the types of abnormalities present. Early orthopedic consultation, along with two radiographic views of the spine is critical. Undetected congenital scoliosis may result in significant deformities affecting visceral and neurologic function as well as appearance. *Unilateral unsegmented bar deformities have the worst prognosis, and require prompt localized spinal fusion to avoid progressive deformity and loss of longitudinal growth.* Multiple unilateral hemivertebrae also have a poor prognosis and may require fusion. Mixed anomalies require documentation and close observation. Congenital kyphosis, which may present subtly or as a severe angular deformity, may be a result of failure of formation of the anterior portion of a vertebral body at single or multiple levels. This defect is always progressive and may result in severe deformity and decreased neurologic function, including possible paraplegia. Therefore, surgery is essential if progressive kyphosis is present as a result of a lack of segmentation or a posterior hemivertebra or failure of vertebral formation.

The vascular abnormalities, particularly ventricular septal defect, usually do not pose problems in the immediate neonatal period. Progressive left-to-right shunting with early congestive heart failure or later irreversible pulmonary hypertension are possible, necessitating ongoing evaluation by a pediatric cardiologist. Other cardiac defects may require immediate evaluation and treatment.

Tracheoesophageal lesions require early evaluation by pediatric surgeons. The most common anomaly is esophageal atresia with a distal tracheoesophageal fistula. The choice of primary repair, short-term delay followed by primary repair, or long-term delay with staged repair is usually determined on the basis of risk categories for such infants (see the chapter on esophageal atresia and tracheoesophageal fistula). Tracheal agenesis, an extremely rare and potentially lethal variant with bronchoesophageal fistula, may require immediate esophageal intubation or a distal tracheostomy.

Anal atresia with intestinal obstruction is more likely in male infants, whereas female infants generally have a low defect with adequate ectopic rectal openings or fistulas. In infants of either sex, but particularly in males, anatomic definition and identification of an ectopic rectal opening are pursued early. Subsequent repair is determined by these findings. Pediatric surgical involvement is essential at the onset.

The management of radial abnormalities, particularly pollicization of the index finger, is controversial and complex but dependent on elbow function. For instance, because of associated neurovascular changes, some hands function as ulnar hands; thus, pollicization of the index finger may provide no functional advantage. In order to centralize the hand in relation to the distal ulna, initial therapy may need to include passive stretching exercises and serial splinting or casting. Surgical centralization is often required in unilateral cases. Obviously, therapy should be directed by an experienced pediatric hand surgeon.

Renal dysplasia and obstructive uropathy are the most common renal abnormalities in the VATER association. Biochemical studies are routinely performed but are usually of little value initially. However, a creatinine clearance test performed later may prove helpful, and a urinalysis and urine culture should also be undertaken. Of the imaging techniques, ultrasonographic evaluation of the kidneys and bladder is an ideal initial study. Whether further imaging studies, a voiding cystourethrogram, nucleide studies, or nephrology consultation are indicated will be dictated by the findings from the initial evaluation.

WET LUNG SYNDROMES

EDMUND A. EGAN, M.D.

The fetal lung is filled with a fluid that is secreted by the lung itself at a rate of 250 ml per day in late pregnancy. Before labor, the volume of fetal lung fluid approximates the postnatal functional residual capacity, 30 ml per kilogram body weight. Normal labor initiates the reabsorption of this alveolar fluid, but about half is still present at delivery and must be absorbed after birth. Usually it takes 2 to 6 hours for the lung to absorb all the liquid from the air space and to clear it from the interstitium. For the first hour after birth, both liquid and gas are in the alveoli. In the lung interstitium, lakes of absorbed fetal lung liquid lie in areas abutting the pulmonary arteries and veins until total clearance is achieved at about 6 hours.

WET LUNG, TRANSIENT TACHYPNEA, OR TYPE I IDIOPATHIC RESPIRATORY DISTRESS SYNDROME

These three terms have been used to describe newborn infants who have some or all the clinical signs of respiratory distress: tachypnea, retractions, nasal flaring, grunting, and cyanosis in room air. The features that distinguish wet lung from respiratory distress syndrome are presented in Table 1. Typically, the symptoms are mild and the patients are mature premature infants, 34 weeks or older, or term infants born after elective cesarean section without labor. Chest x-ray film reveals normal aeration or hyperinflated lungs with streaky infiltrates, frequently with prominent fissures. *Unless cyanosis is present or unless the symptoms persist more than 4 hours after birth, we do not make a diagnosis of wet lung syndrome.* During the first 4 hours of life, mild or intermittent symptoms are acceptable normal variants of the transition to lung gas exchange.

The most important treatment for wet lung syndrome is adequate inspired oxygen to maintain normal oxygenation. Arterial, transcutaneous, or pulse oximetry monitoring is necessary. Since bacterial pneumonia cannot be excluded as a primary cause or secondary complication, a penicillin and an aminoglycoside are given after blood cultures are obtained. Treatment of the excess lung water itself is neither easy nor necessary. In some infants there is a progression of symptoms. *We make a diagnosis of respiratory distress syndrome if there is progressive hypercapnia or hypoxemia despite 50 percent oxygen or more.* Since idiopathic respiratory distress syndrome cannot always be differentiated from the wet lung syndromes initially, wet lung syndrome is a provisional diagnosis in the first hours of life. *Wet lung syndrome does not progress.* Supplemental oxygen may be necessary for 1 to 3 days, but resolution without complications or residuals is expected.

AMNIOTIC FLUID ASPIRATION

Postmortem pathologic findings of amniotic fluid debris in the alveoli, including lanugo hairs and sloughed epithelial cells, led to the conclusion that massive aspiration of amniotic fluid could produce a lethal, drowning syndrome. Actually, the gasping of a fetus who is hypoxic can result in mixing a small amount of amniotic fluid with lung liquid in the upper airway. After birth, this debris is transported to the alveoli upon lung aeration. Lung elastic properties make aspiration of a significant volume of amniotic fluid into an already fluid-filled lung nearly impossible. This syndrome is really the same as wet lung syndrome, and the lethal cases, which provided the pathologic evidence of amniotic fluid aspiration, probably died from the effects of prenatal hypoxia or persistent pulmonary hypertension, not excess lung fluid.

LUNG EDEMA IN NEONATAL DISEASES

Alveolar Edema

When hemodynamic pressures in the lung force fluid from the vascular system in excess of the maximum flow rate of the lung lymph, and the interstitial space can contain no more liquid, then a fluid similar to lung lymph floods the alveoli through epithelial ruptures. In addition, in any severe lung injury syndrome, tissue injury allows a lung lymph-like fluid to passively enter alveoli without hemodynamic abnormalities. In either situation, *a high protein fluid fills part of the alveolar volume.*

The most dramatic neonatal syndrome of alveolar edema is pulmonary hemorrhage, actually a hemorrhagic pulmonary edema, in which a large volume of high protein fluid with a hematocrit of 2 to 5 volume per deciliter gushes from the trachea. Treatment must focus on re-establishing cardiopulmonary integrity. Parenteral fluids, plasma, and saline are used to re-establish vascular volume and inotropic amines are used to normalize cardiac output.

Adequate ventilation depends on use of enough end-expiratory pressure to aerate liquid-containing alveoli. Care must be exercised, and end-expiratory pressure more than 8 cm H_2O is usually not needed. Higher end-expiratory pressures can tamponade lung blood flow. Ventilation is not effective unless the edematous lung is aerated.

Clearance of alveolar edema fluid from the air space, whether its origin is hemodynamic or secondary to lung injury, is a long process. Cardiopulmonary equilibrium can halt its progression, but reabsorption cannot be accelerated by attempting to diminish vascular volume or lung vascular pressures. The emphasis must be on careful monitoring of cardiac function and ensuring adequate ventilation. The processes that clear edema fluid from the alveolar space probably involve cellular mechanisms and not just passive hydrostatic and osmotic forces.

Interstitial Pulmonary Edema

When lung vascular pressures rise or lung disease alters the lung interstitial space, increasing its capacity to hold liquid, edema fluid accumulates in the perivascular and periairway interstitium of the lung. This fluid increases lung mass, and, if enough accumulates, it alters the normal transmural pressure gradients of small airways and venules enough to affect both ventilation and blood

TABLE 1 Features That Distinguish Wet Lung Syndrome From Respiratory Distress Syndrome

	Wet Lung Syndromes	*Idiopathic Respiratory Distress Syndrome*
Highest risk	Pre-term infants (34–37 weeks) Cesarean section without labor	Premature infants (34 weeks)
X-ray findings	Normal to increased inflation, linear infiltrates	Low lung volume Granular lung fields Air bronchograms
Respiratory function	Hypoxemia relieved by O^2	Respiratory failure Hypoxemia insensitive to inspired oxygen
Course	Nonprogressive	Increasing respiratory failure
Treatment	Added oxygen	Positive airway pressure Assisted ventilation Oxygen

TABLE 2 Pulmonary Edema in Neonatal Disease

Alveolar Edema	Alveolar and Interstitial Edema	Interstitial Edema
Pulmonary hemorrhage "Shock" lung	Hyaline membrane disease Patent ductus arteriosus with respiratory decompensation	Wet lung syndrome Bronchopulmonary dysplasia
Congenital heart disease: obstructed anomalous pulmonary venous return	Congenital heart disease: left-sided heart obstructive lesions	Congenital heart disease: other left-to-right shunts

flow. Decreased compliance, airtrapping, and ventilation-perfusion mismatching are consequences of this interstitial liquid accumulation. In neonatal patients, interstitial pulmonary edema is a significant pathophysiologic factor in several primary lung diseases and in congenital heart disease (Table 2).

When the primary cause of interstitial edema is high pulmonary blood flow through a patent ductus arteriosus, intracardiac left-to-right shunt, or congenital heart disease without separation of pulmonary or systemic arterial supply, lung interstitial edema can be diminished only by limiting lung blood flow. Recourse to systemic therapies will work only if cardiac output is diminished, since lung blood flow is a constant fraction of cardiac output.

In bronchopulmonary dysplasia or other syndromes in which lung interstitial edema results from intrinsic pathology of the lung, efforts should be made to ensure that vascular volume is not increased. Total fluid intake should be adjusted so that urine flow is 1 to 2 ml per kilogram per hour and urine specific gravity is between 1,010 and 1,020. Caloric density of feeding or intravenous nutrition should be adjusted to provide necessary calories on this restricted water regimen. The object is to maintain vascular volume and vascular venous pressure at a low nor-

mal level to keep lung interstitial fluid volumes as low as possible. For some infants even fluid restriction is not adequate to maintain necessary respiratory function, and chronic diuretic therapy is required. Furosemide (Lasix) 1 to 2 mg per kilogram once or twice daily is most effective, but *long-term therapy carries substantial risk of renal calcifications.* Chlorothiazides and spironolactones are sometimes functional substitutes. In some infants with chronic lung disease, intermittent diuretic therapy or diuresis for acute respiratory symptoms often results in substantial improvement.

The *effectiveness of diuretic therapy appears to relate to the way vascular volume is restored following diuresis.* Water is recruited to replace vascular volume from the interstitial water of organs. The organs with the highest blood flow per kilogram contribute most of the replacement volume. Since the lung has the highest blood flow per kilogram of any organ, it preferentially has more interstitial water drawn back into the vascular space after diuresis. Eventually, when intake replaces the water lost from diuresis, there is a re-establishment of the prediuresis water distribution among the organs. *No lasting diminution of lung water can be accomplished by diuretics unless they are administered chronically.*

ARTERIAL SWITCH OPERATION: CORRECTION OF SIMPLE TRANSPOSITION OF THE GREAT ARTERIES

JOHN L. MYERS, M.D.

The diagnosis of transposition of the great arteries in neonates is often made on clinical evaluation, and the anatomic condition is confirmed by echocardiography. Simple transposition of the great arteries is the term used to describe patients who have no other associated cardiac defects, such as ventricular septal defect or anatomic left ventricular outflow tract obstruction. Cardiac catheterization is not routinely performed in these infants unless other anomalies are suspected that require further investigation. A prostaglandin E_1 infusion is started to maintain ductal patency, and acidemia is corrected if present. Oxygen is not routinely administered, since oxygen is a stimulant for ductal closure. An arterial Po_2 of 20 to 30 mm Hg is acceptable, as long as there is good peripheral perfusion and provided that metabolic acidosis does not persist. Infrequently these babies require muscle relaxants, endotracheal intubation, and mechanical ventilation. In infants with simple transposition the left ventricle atrophies and loses muscle mass after 3 to 4 weeks and will no longer be able to support the systemic circulation if an arterial switch operation is performed so late. By performing the arterial switch operation earlier in the newborn period, one can take advantage of the elevated pulmonary vascular resistance present in the newborn, which maintains left ventricular pressures near systemic level. Therefore, the arterial switch operation using cardiopulmonary bypass with deep hypothermia and circulatory arrest is performed in the next 12 to 48 hours. Newborns with transposition who evidence persistent poor mixing, hypoxia, acidosis, and hypoperfusion are taken to the cardiac catheterization laboratory to undergo a Rashkind balloon atrial septostomy. Once perfusion and metabolic derangements are corrected, surgery is undertaken.

In the operating room a right internal jugular vein catheter and a urinary catheter are inserted. An umbilical artery catheter is routinely inserted in the newborn intensive care unit at the time of admission. General endotracheal anesthesia with fentanyl and pancuronium bromide (Pavulon) is administered. Surface cooling is begun using a cooling blanket at 13 °C and crushed ice in double plastic bags placed around the head. A median sternotomy incision is made and the heart exposed (Fig. 1). Heparin (3 mg per kilogram) is injected directly into the right atrium. A straight No. 8 Fr. arterial cannula is inserted into the ascending aorta just proximal to the origin of the innominate artery and secured with a pursestring suture and tourniquet. A single No. 20 Fr. cannula is inserted into the right atrial appendage for venous drainage (Fig. 1a). Methylprednisolone (30 mg per kilogram) and phentolamine (0.5 mg per kilogram) are added to the cardiopulmonary bypass prime. Cardiopulmonary bypass is instituted at a calculated flow of 1.0 liter per minute per square meter of body surface area, and the pump oxygenator arterial blood temperature is lowered to 12 °C, using a heat exchanger in the bypass circuit. Core cooling is continued for 20 to 30 minutes until the rectal temperature is 20 °C and the nasopharyngeal temperature, 15° to 16 °C. Thiopental (9 mg per kilogram) is given 5 minutes before circulatory arrest is effected. During core cooling the ductus arteriosus is exposed, doubly ligated, and divided (Fig. 1b). The main and branch pulmonary arteries are mobilized completely, extending out beyond the pericardial reflections into each hilum of the lungs. An 18-gauge angiocatheter for cardioplegia administration is placed in the midportion of the ascending aorta (Fig. 2) about 1 to 1.5 cm above the valve annulus. Cardiopulmonary bypass is then discontinued and circulatory arrest established. The aorta is cross-clamped distal to the aortic cannula and the cannula is removed. The baby is exsanguinated into the pump oxygenator through the venous cannula, which is then removed (Fig. 3).

Cardioplegia solution (St. Thomas solution, 4 °C) is infused through the 18-gauge angiocatheter in the ascending aorta. A volume equal to 15 mg per kilogram is infused at 50 mm Hg pressure. Cold saline slush is placed around the heart.

The ascending aorta is transected 1 to 1.5 cm above the aortic valve annulus (Fig. 4). The pulmonary artery is transected proximal to its bifurcation, leaving about 1 cm of distal main pulmonary artery. The semilunar valves and coronary ostia are carefully inspected. An incision is started above the left coronary ostium, and a large button of the aorta is included with the ostium (Fig. 5). A stab incision is then made above the right coronary ostium and extended circumferentially to include a large button of aorta around this ostium (Fig. 6). The proximal

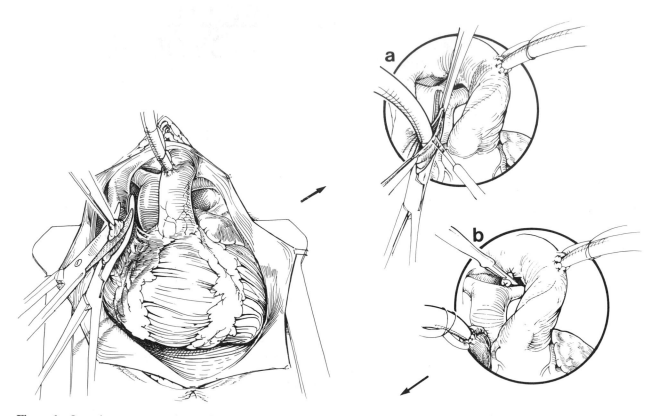

Figure 1 Operative exposure and cannulation technique for arterial switch operation: venous cannulation (*a*); ligation and division of the patent ductus arteriosus (*b*).

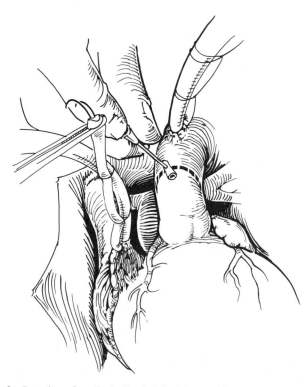

Figure 2 Insertion of cardioplegia administration needle at the level of planned aortic transection (*dotted line*).

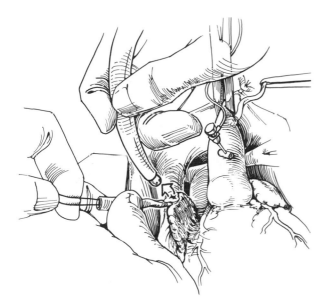

Figure 3 Deep hypothermia and circulatory arrest; administration of cardioplegia.

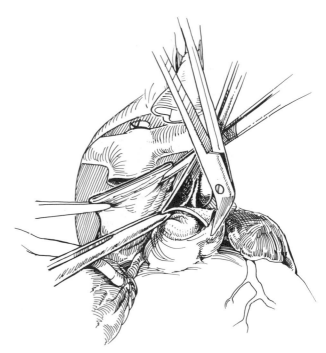

Figure 5 Excision of the left coronary ostial button.

coronary arteries are dissected free just enough to allow rotation of the ostial button to reach its recipient site on the proximal pulmonary artery without any tension, torsion, or kinking of the coronary artery.

A circular aortotomy is made in the proximal pulmonary artery (the great vessel arising from the left ventricle) with a 4.8-mm diameter punch (Fig. 7). The coronary ostial button is anastomosed with a 6–0 monofilament absorbable suture (PDS) in a continuous fashion (Fig. 8). The same procedure is carried out for the right coronary

artery anastomosis. The distal ascending aorta is then passed beneath the pulmonary artery bifurcation (Lecompté maneuver) (Fig. 9). The proximal artery arising from the left ventricle is then anastomosed to the distal ascending aorta with a continuous suture of 6–0 PDS.

The left heart is filled with cold heparinized saline solution through the patent foramen ovale while the aortic cannulation site is held open to allow egress of any air in the left heart chambers. The venous cannula is reinserted into the right atrial appendage after the right atrium is filled with cold saline solution. The aortic cannula is reinserted

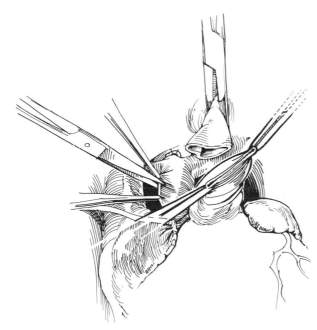

Figure 4 Transection of the great arteries.

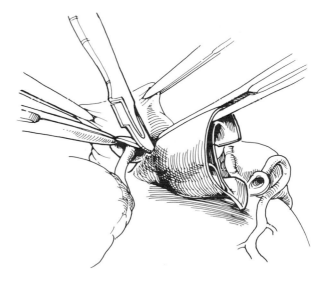

Figure 6 Excision of the right coronary ostial button.

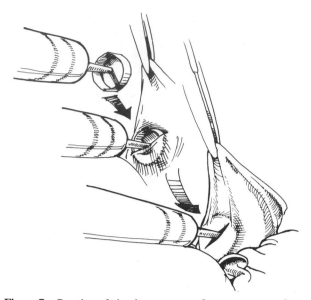

Figure 7 Creation of circular aortotomy for a coronary ostium-to-aorta anastomosis.

and cardiopulmonary bypass reinstituted. Full rewarming is begun. Phentolamine (0.25 mg per kilogram) is given to promote vasodilatation and hasten rewarming. The cooling blanket is turned to 38 °C.

Autologous pericardium is used to patch the circular defect where the right coronary artery was excised (Fig. 10a). A large piece of pericardium is likewise used to patch the donor site of the left coronary artery, and this also enlarges the diameter of the new main pulmonary artery (Fig. 10b). The distal pulmonary artery is anastomosed to the proximal aorta with a running suture of 6–0 PDS (Fig.

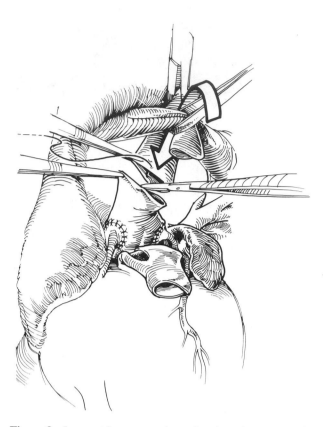

Figure 9 Lecompté maneuver (*arrow*) and aortic anastomosis.

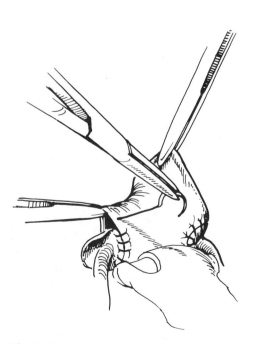

Figure 8 The right coronary artery ostium-to-aorta anastomosis.

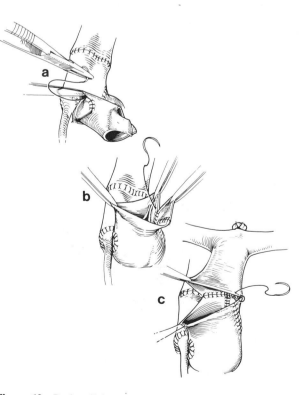

Figure 10 Pericardial patch closure of the right (a) and left (b) coronary artery donor site and pulmonary artery anastomosis (c).

10c). A monitoring catheter is inserted into the left atrium between the right superior and inferior pulmonary veins. The completed repair is shown in Figure 11.

The anatomy and the course of blood flow through the cardiac chambers before and after arterial switch operation for anatomic correction of transposition of the great arteries is shown in Figure 12.

When rewarming is completed (rectal temperature 32° to 34°C), the patient is separated from cardiopulmonary bypass and the cannulas are removed. Protamine sulfate is given to reverse the effects of heparin. Very fresh blood, obtained several hours previously, is infused as needed. When hemostasis is complete, a No. 16 Fr. mediastinal tube is inserted through the lower right anterior chest wall and positioned in the anterior superior mediastinum. The sternum is approximated with stainless steel wires. Skin closure is completed. Sterile drapes are removed and warming lights are positioned over the patient to complete rewarming. The baby is placed in a neonatal intensive care bed and transferred to the cardiac intensive care unit. Mechanical ventilatory support is usually continued for 48 to 72 hours. Standard care for newborns and infants undergoing cardiac surgery is provided. Newborns typically are extubated on the second or third postoperative day and feedings are begun. They are usually discharged 10 to 14 days after surgery.

DISCUSSION

In the past, transposition of the great arteries with intact ventricular septum was fatal in 90 percent of infants during the first year of life. The balloon atrial septostomy

pioneered by Rashkind palliated the condition of many of these infants to allow successful atrial redirection by the Senning or Mustard operation.

Reports documenting the late development of venous baffle obstruction, right atrioventricular valve regurgitation, right ventricular failure, and dysrhythmias have prompted new interest and increased application of the

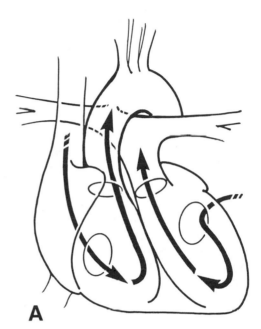

A

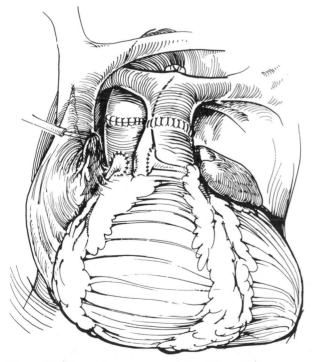

Figure 11 Complete repair: arterial switch operation.

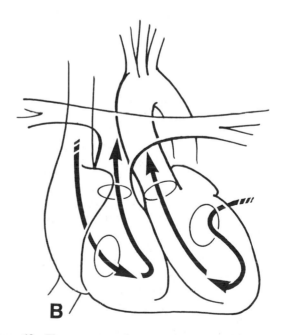

B

Figure 12 The anatomy and course of blood flow through the heart before (a) and after (b) the arterial switch operation.

TABLE 1 Arterial Switch Operation for Transposition of the Great Arteries

	TGA with IVS Intact Ventricular Neonates	TGA + VSD—Infants + Children
The Pennsylvania State University Hershey, PA	7 (0)	4 (25)
Leiden, The Netherlands J Thorac Cardiovasc Surg 1986; 92:361	23 (4)	33 (18)
Children's Hospital Boston, MA Ann Thorac Surg 1984; 38:438	14 (7)	

Numbers in parentheses indicate % mortality. TGA = transposition of the great arteries; IVS = intact ventricular septum; VSD = ventricular septal defect

arterial switch operation in many infants. These late complications are peculiar to the atrial redirection operations and are unlikely to occur after the arterial switch operation. However, the long-term fate of the aortic valve (anatomic pulmonary valve), left ventricular function, and coronary ostial anastomoses in the arterial switch operation is currently unknown. Short-term follow-up in several series supports the superiority of the arterial switch operation for transposition of the great arteries (Table 1).

SUGGESTED READING

Castaneda AR, Norwood WI, Jonas RA, et al. Transposition of the great arteries and intact ventricular septum: Anatomical repair in the neonate. Ann Thoracic Surg 1984; 38:438–443.

Martin RP, Radley-Smith R, Yacoub MH. Arrhythmias before and after anatomic correction of transposition of the great arteries. J Am Coll Cardiol 1987; 10:200–204.

Quaegebur JM, Rohmer J, Ottenkamp J, et al. The arterial switch operation. An eight-year experience. J Thorac Cardiovasc Surg 1986; 92:361–384.

BALLOON ATRIAL SEPTOSTOMY

EHUD KRONGRAD, M.D.

Patients with transposition of the great arteries manifest various degrees of clinical cyanosis immediately after birth. All are hypoxemic to a certain degree, and some patients are markedly cyanotic with rapid development of metabolic acidosis associated with clinical deterioration that may lead to death. Without treatment, less than 10 percent of infants with transposition of the great arteries are expected to survive beyond 6 months of age. Therefore prompt diagnostic and therapeutic measures are indicated when hypoxemia and clinical suspicion of transposition are present. In recent years, with improved neonatal care and the availability of monitoring techniques, the diagnosis of transposition of the great arteries is often suspected and made immediately after birth and certainly during the perinatal hospitalization period and prior to the infant's discharge home.

The main hemodynamic characteristic of transposition of the great arteries is that both the pulmonary and systemic circulations function in parallel rather than in series, as in the normal heart. This allows mixed venous blood to enter the systemic circulation and pulmonary venous blood to enter the pulmonary arterial circulation. Survival is therefore dependent on mixing the above circulations. Traditionally, this is achieved by performing a balloon atrial septostomy (the Rashkind procedure).

Since its introduction in 1966, balloon atrial septostomy remains the method of choice for creating an adequate intra-atrial communication in newborns with transposition of the great arteries. In the past, this has always been carried out as part of a diagnostic cardiac catheterization, in a cardiovascular laboratory using fluoroscopy for guiding the balloon catheter during the procedure.

A cardiac catheterization in the newborn carries with it considerable risks. These hazards should be reduced by (1) limiting the use of sedation, particularly in a very sick infant, in order to reduce the risk of cardiopulmonary depression, (2) providing a warm environment to maintain adequate body temperature by using external thermoregulating devices, (3) reducing possible cardiac and vascular trauma by minimizing intracardiac catheter manipulation, (4) reducing the risk associated with angiocardiographic studies in small hypoxemic infants to a necessary minimum, (5) controlling blood loss by taking only small blood samples and reducing the number of samples to a minimum, and (6) carefully monitoring and correcting any evidence of metabolic acidosis that may develop during the procedure when a newborn is diagnosed as having transposition of the great arteries.

Until a balloon atrial septostomy can be carried out, the infant should be maintained in a warm environment and his or her acid-base and oxygen saturation levels monitored carefully. A transcutaneous oxygen monitor is very helpful for continuous monitoring of O_2 saturation. At this time the infant may benefit from O_2 administration and occasionally from judicial use of prostaglandin E_1 infusion. For simple transposition (without associated defects), preparation for a balloon atrial septostomy should be made as soon as the diagnosis is verified.

After the infant has been transferred to the cardiac catheterization laboratory, the groin or, less frequently, the umbilicus is prepped and draped to form a sterile field. The procedure is performed without sedation in newborns to approximately 1 month of age. Occasionally some newborns may benefit from administration of morphine sulfate (0.1 mg per kilogram). Local anesthesia at the site of the needle puncture is usually sufficient to keep the child comfortable. At present, the balloon atrial septostomy is virtually always carried out by the percutaneous technique, either by the femoral venous approach or the umbilical approach, with the catheter traversing the ductus venosus to enter the right side of the heart.

Catheter manipulation and placement of the catheter tip in the left atrium are very often easier from the femoral venous approach. In this approach, a number 18-gauge or a 16-gauge Teflon catheter is inserted into the femoral vein, which is located just medial to the femoral artery pulse, at a level just about at the inguinal crease. For monitoring purposes, the femoral artery is often cannulated by placing a number 18-gauge Teflon catheter connected to a pressure gauge, which allows for constant pressure monitoring and withdrawal of blood samples throughout the procedure. After the needle has entered the femoral vein (this is verified by free flow of rather dark blood via the plastic sheath surrounding the needle), a number 0.32 or 0.38 flexible soft-tipped wire is advanced via the plastic envelope into the inferior vena cava and advanced into the right atrium. After the wire has been placed in the right atrium, the Teflon catheter is withdrawn and a number 6 or 7 French dilator and sheath with a side arm are advanced over the wire and placed in the femoral vein. The wire and the dilator are then withdrawn, and a number 6 catheter for hemodynamic and angiographic studies or a balloon catheter can then be advanced either for hemodynamic studies if desirable or for the immediate creation of an atrial septal defect using the balloon catheter. The balloon catheter is advanced via a No. 7 sheath.

Prior to advancing the balloon catheter via the sheath, the balloon is emptied of all the air present. This is done by inflating the balloon with 1 to 2 ml either of saline or of saline mixed with some contrast solution, repeatedly emptying and filling up the catheter and the balloon several times. This allows one to withdraw all the trapped air inside the catheter's lumen and to fill the lumen with fluid. The procedure is repeated several times until no air can be visualized inside the balloon. Only then is the balloon advanced via the sheath while simultaneously applying some negative pressure with a syringe attached to the catheter. This is done to reduce the balloon volume and to allow smooth transfer of the balloon catheter via the sheath.

The creation of the intra-atrial defect using a balloon catheter is carried out first by advancing the catheter under fluoroscopic guidance using both the anteroposterior and lateral x-ray views into the left atrium (Fig. 1). Occasionally, in order to facilitate the advance of the catheter into the left atrium, the stylet, which comes with the balloon catheter, can be formed to have a 45-degree curve at the distal end. This creates a curve at the tip of the catheter, allowing its easy advance from the right to the left atrium. The same stylet can also be used to puncture a balloon on the rare occasions in which it cannot be deflated. The location of the catheter in the left atrium is verified by advancing the tip toward the left side border of the cardiac silhouette or preferably even into a pulmonary vein. When possible, left atrial blood samples should be taken to determine the left atrial saturation, arterial blood gas, and intra-atrial pressures, which usually are substantially higher than right atrial pressures.

After the location of the balloon catheter is verified as being in the left atrium, it is best to start and inflate the balloon with the catheter tip just at the mouth of a pulmonary vein. Inflation of the balloon at this site usually causes a sliding motion of the catheter into the left atrium. As the inflation proceeds, the balloon should be observed to move freely within the left atrium. Occasionally, the balloon may advance into the left ventricle via the mitral valve. This should be recognized immediately, the balloon deflated, and the catheter withdrawn back into the left atrium. When a tendency for the balloon to advance into the left ventricle is recognized, the inflation can be done while the catheter is snugly secured at the interatrial septum so it is not permitted to advance downstream into the left ventricle. Less frequently, the catheter may be caught in the left atrial appendage. Inflation of the balloon at this site usually causes distortion of its shape.

In general, any distortion of the initial round shape of the balloon should indicate to the operator an unusual and basically unacceptable catheter location. If the catheter is advanced too far into a pulmonary vein and the balloon is inflated, this can be recognized by both the location of the catheter and the distortion of the balloon shape creating an elongated form within the pulmonary vein. This usually does not occur, since the balloon tends to slip back into the left atrium. Occasionally, the balloon may be inadvertently inflated in the right atrium, and from there it may tend to advance easily via the tricuspid valve into the right ventricle and bounce anterially and cephalad with each cardiac systole. This is an important position to recognize, and it is imperative that the balloon immediately be deflated and withdrawn carefully (in the deflated position) back across the tricuspid valve. Rarely, the balloon may be inflated in the coronary sinus in a posterior-inferior

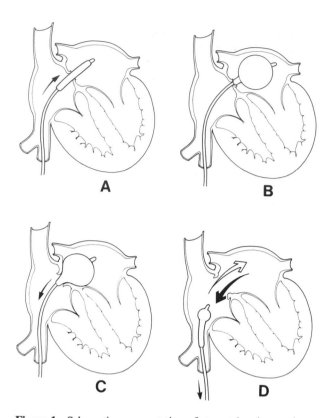

Figure 1 Schematic representation of steps taken in creating a balloon atrial septostomy. *A*, The catheter is passed from the inferior vena cava via the right atrium into the left atrium. *B*, The balloon is inflated in the left atrium. *C*, The balloon is "pulled" through the interatrial septum. *D*, The balloon is deflated, leaving a large atrial septal defect that enhances intra-atrial mixing.

aspect of the cardiac silhouette. In complex cardiac malformations with a juxtaposed right atrial appendage, the catheter may be inadvertently placed into a right atrial appendage, which is behind the great arteries and just adjacent to the left atrial appendage. Juxtaposition of the right atrial appendage to the left atrial appendage is extremely rare and usually occurs in patients with transposition of the great arteries and additional complex malformations.

After the balloon is placed in the desired site just across the interatrial septum, it is further inflated to its maximal volume of about 4 cc using a mixture of saline and contrast material. When the balloon is inflated to its maximal capacity, it should be continuously observed under fluoroscopy to assure its precise location. Both the clinical condition of the infant and the electrocardiogram are constantly monitored. Frequently, when the balloon is inflated to its maximal capacity, infants tend to develop episodes of bradycardia. Therefore inflation and withdrawal of the balloon at this phase of the procedure are done in rapid succession.

The balloon septostomy itself is done by grasping the catheter firmly and with a forceful, brisk motion of a short distance withdrawing the inflated balloon across the intra-atrial septum, from the left atrium into the orifice of the

inferior vena cava. This motion is completed by immediately advancing the inflated balloon from the mouth of the inferior vena cava into the right atrium. Thus, the entire motion of the septostomy is V-shaped: first the inflated balloon is withdrawn across the intra-atrial septum toward the inferior vena cava, and then the balloon catheter is advanced from the inferior vena cava into the right atrium. The balloon is then emptied by applying negative pressure to the syringe attached to the proximal end of the balloon catheter. The inflated balloon catheter should not be allowed to rest in the inferior vena cava, since cases in which an inflated balloon could not be dislodged from the inferior vena cava have been known to occur. This rare complication requires dextrous manipulation of the catheter and attempts to reduce the balloon volume so the catheter can be pushed back from the inferior vena cava into the right atrium. Failing that, on extremely rare occasions there has been a need to advance a second rigid guide-wire or the stylet that comes with the catheter through the other femoral vein or through the sheath alongside the balloon catheter to puncture the balloon with its rigid tip. This releases the saline-contrast mixture into the bloodstream and reduces the balloon volume so it can immediately be withdrawn from the circulation.

The withdrawal of the balloon catheter across the atrial septum is then repeated several times with the maximal tolerated volume, usually with 4 ml of a saline–contrast material mixture. Perhaps the most important withdrawal is the first "pull," which creates the initial tear. This "pull" is often felt by the operator as a typical sensation indicating a successful tear in the delicate membrane covering the foramen ovale. This tear is then enlarged with similar repetitive pulls. The likelihood of creating a tear in the membrane covering the foramen ovale is less likely with graduated soft pulls. If it does occur, either the catheter cannot be withdrawn from the left to the right atrium or the foramen ovale is just dilated, and although some beneficial short-term effects are usually seen, the long-term results of the balloon septostomy are usually unsatisfactory.

After completion of the balloon septostomy, we find it useful to verify the immediate beneficial effects of the procedure by comparing left atrial and right atrial saturations and pressures obtained afterward with values obtained prior to the balloon atrial septostomy. With a successful balloon atrial septostomy, the systemic saturation may rise 20 to 40 percent and the left atrial pressure, which is usually higher then the right atrial pressure, decreases and frequently is identical to the right atrial pressure.

Some operators tend to measure the results of the balloon septostomy by gradually inflating a balloon and withdrawing it through the newly created atrial septal defect. The volume of the inflated balloon should approximate the size of the created atrial defect. We find this maneuver unnecessary in most patients, since the size of the atrial septal defect can easily be seen on a two-dimensional echocardiogram (Fig. 2).

In the past, successful creation of an atrial septal defect was verified by performing an angiocardiographic injection into the left atrium and recording it in a left anterior oblique position with cephalad angulation. This, again,

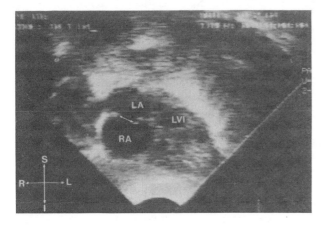

Figure 2 Two-dimensional echocardiographic view showing the size of the newly created atrial septal defect following a balloon septostomy.

has been largely abandoned in favor of verifying the size of the defect by a two-dimensional echocardiogram upon completion of the study.

The introduction of two-dimensional echocardiography as an aid in diagnostic evaluation of the newborn with transposition of the great arteries and also in catheter manipulation allows the creation of balloon atrial septostomy outside the cardiac catheterization laboratory. The echocardiographic diagnosis of transposition of the great arteries can be made with ease, and certainly without cardiac catheterization, thus eliminating the need for an elaborate diagnostic work-up and a procedure associated with considerable risk to the infant.

In recent years, the classic Rashkind procedure, carried out in a cardiac catheterization laboratory with fluoroscopic guidance, is gradually being replaced by creating an atrial septostomy with the use of two-dimensional echocardiography and manipulating the catheter without the use of fluoroscopy. This echocardiography-assisted procedure is often carried out in neonatal intensive care units but should always be carried out in medical centers with back-up cardiac catheterization laboratories and vascular and cardiac surgical services (Fig. 3).

In the infant who is beyond 4 weeks of age, the creation of an atrial septal defect using the balloon technique is often ineffective. In these infants, the same results may be obtained by creating an atrial septal defect using a blade septostomy catheter. The blade septostomy technique is very similar to the balloon atrial septostomy technique in that the blade septostomy catheter is advanced via the previously inserted sheath into the left atrium. When the septostomy catheter is placed in location, the blade, which is 1 cm long, razor thin, and enclosed at the tip of the septostomy catheter is dislodged by manipulating a wire at the proximal site of the septostomy catheter. When the blade protrudes out of the catheter tip it creates a triangle, the base of which is the catheter, and the two arms include the blade itself and an anchoring wire that anchors the blade to the catheter. After the blade has been dislodged and the proper position verified, it is withdrawn across the interatrial septum, this time gently by pulling it slowly across. After an initial incision with the blade has been made, this tear is enlarged by the previously described balloon atrial septostomy technique and by repeatedly pulling an inflated balloon from the left to the right atrium. Occasionally, in an older child without an atrial communication the blade septostomy catheter can be advanced only after creating an interatrial septal defect (Brockenbrough's technique). This can be created by advancing a needle contained within a dilator and a long sheath especially developed for this purpose (Mullin's system). After the needle, dilator, and sheath cross the interatrial septum, the dilator and the needle are withdrawn, whereas the tip of the sheath remains in the left atrium. The blade septostomy catheter can then be advanced through this sheath into the left atrium. Extreme care should be exercised with the use of long sheaths because of the large volume of air contained within the sheath. This should be emptied by applying negative pressure and being mindful at all times of its potential hazards.

Although in most medical centers the balloon atrial septostomy remains the treatment of choice for initial management of patients with transposition of the great

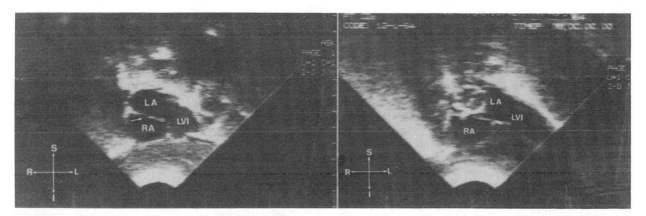

Figure 3 Two-dimensional echocardiographic views showing a nearly intact interatrial septum (*arrow*) on the left and on the right an echocardiographic presentation of an inflated balloon catheter inside the left atrium.

arteries, some centers have recently begun to perform complete surgical repair during the neonatal period. The surgical approach is an anatomic correction of the defect by which the aorta and the pulmonary artery are transected and switched to create left ventricular-aortic continuity as well as right ventricular to pulmonary artery continuity. When this procedure is performed in the neonatal period, an atrial septostomy may not be required. This innovative and new approach is performed today only in a few selected centers. The majority of centers caring for infants with transposition of the great arteries continue to perform the balloon atrial septostomy as the initial life-saving procedure in the management of such infants.

SUGGESTED READING

Rashkind WJ, Miller WW. Creation of an atrial septal defect without thoracotomy. Palliative approach to complete transpositions of the great arteries. JAMA 1966; 196:991–992.

Steeg CN, Bierman FZ, Hordof A, et al. "Bedside" balloon septostomy in infants with transposition of the great arteries. New concepts using two-dimensional echocardiographic techniques. J Pediatr 1985; 107:944–946.

BILIRUBINOMETRY

ROBERT E. SCHUMACHER, M.D.

Jaundice is one of the most frequently encountered physical findings in newborns, but is of little long-term consequence for most infants in whom it is present. However, for a minority of patients the jaundice serves to signify the presence of significant underlying hyperbilirubinemia and the potential adverse sequelae associated with it. Because of the devastating outcome (e.g., kernicterus) associated with certain cases of hyperbilirubinemia, a great deal of effort is spent attempting to identify those infants at risk. Various screening tests have been devised and used in attempts to separate the population of infants that has significant hyperbilirubinemia from the population that does not. Tests used have ranged in sophistication from simple visual inspection of the infant to routine blood sampling in all infants. Transcutaneous bilirubinometry, in theory, should serve as an excellent means for screening and identifying infants who may have significant hyperbilirubinemia.

In broadest terms, there are three methods for performing transcutaneous bilirubinometry, which vary in degrees of sophistication. First and simplest is visual inspection, with the presence of jaundice serving as the "action point" or "cut point" used to order further tests, most commonly serum bilirubin determination. It is clear, however, that many variables can and do affect visual estimates of jaundice. These include intensity and spectral characteristics of environmental light, skin color, the presence or absence of plethora or anemia, and the clinical experience of the observer. A refinement of this technique (a simple visual estimate) includes using the phenomenon of the cephalocaudal progress of jaundice to redefine action or cut points. Using such a scheme, jaundice to the level of a body landmark, such as the nipples or umbilicus, rather than the simple absence or presence of jaundice, serves to define a cut point. Such an approach has yielded credible results, with rough estimates of sensitivity, specificity, and positive and negative predictive values (see below) being 100, 25, 50, and 100 percent respectively.

A second method or technique for performing transcutaneous bilirubinometry is to combine visual estimates of jaundice against a reference device. We recently evaluated the utility of such a device (an Ingram Icterometer) as a screening tool for hyperbilirubinemia. This commercially available device consists of a strip of clear plastic on which are painted yellow stripes of graded hue. By pressing the plastic against the baby's skin, the color of the skin can be compared with the yellow stripes and a jaundice score assigned. Using this device, hyperbilirubinemia (serum bilirubin greater than 12.9 mg per deciliter) was classified with a sensitivity of 82 percent and a specificity of 74 percent. Predictive values of positive and negative tests were 38 percent and 94 percent, respectively. The efficacy of the icterometer has been documented in white, Oriental, and black newborns. Drawbacks to this technique include all the variables mentioned above that affect visual estimates of jaundice. Accordingly, although such devices are useful aids to clinical acumen, it is recommended that they be used under controlled lighting and that the characteristics of the infant, such as race and gestational age, be taken into account when normative values for each yellow stripe or hue are generated. *Separate data bases for each race and gestational age are recommended.* Most important, *it is critical that each individual user generate his or her own normative data*, as the precision of the device is in part secondary to the individual user's ability to distinguish between shades of color.

A third method for transcutaneous bilirubinometry is the use of spectral reflectance in which skin color is quantified by measuring that color as a function of reflected light wavelength. The Minolta/Air-Shields Jaundice Meter is such a device that is commercially available. It is a hand-held rechargeable unit that, when pressed against the infant's skin emits a flash of light from a xenon tube. The light emitted penetrates and reflects from the skin. The reflected light returns to the instrument, where photo cells convert the light to electrical signals and produce a digital display of the transcutaneous bilirubin index in arbitrary units. The efficacy of this device has been documented by many different investigators. As with other methods mentioned, several factors affect the values obtained while using this instrument, including gestational age, chronologic age, and race. The site at which the measurement is taken is also important, as different skin sites have different characteristics that affect meter readings. In babies with rapidly rising serum bilirubin values (e.g., with hemolysis), transcutaneous values tend to lag behind serum values and, as such, the meter should not be used when jaundice appears on the first day of life. Similarly, when phototherapy is used, changes in transcutaneous measurements may precede serum value changes, although the use of an opaque skin patch may alleviate this difference. The meter is not reliable in the immediate postexchange transfusion period. Care must be taken to keep the probe at a 90-degree angle to the reading site, and it is recommended that several readings be taken on each infant to improve accuracy. Because of the potential variation in the response of different jaundice meters, regression lines and 95 percent confidence limits should be generated for each instrument used, using serum bilirubin values as the independent variable and the transcutaneous index values

as the dependent variable. Instructions for generating such lines are provided with the instrument.

Although the jaundice meter is marketed as a screening device and should be used as such, it is also useful in following jaundiced infants. An infant whose jaundice meter index value does not change is not likely to show a significant change in serum bilirubin values.

The three transcutaneous techniques described for screening for hyperbilirubinemia (direct visual, icterometer-assisted visual, and electronic spectral reflectance) have not been the subject of many comparison studies. Thus, it is difficult to say with assurance that the jaundice meter is better than the naked eye when screening for hyperbilirubinemia. We compared the icterometer and the Minolta/Air-Shields Jaundice Meter as screening tests for hyperbilirubinemia and concluded that, for the *individual* clinician, the icterometer performed as well as the more complex and expensive jaundice meter. However, the electronic jaundice meter offers the distinct advantage of having no interobserver variability, and as such should prove more useful in large nurseries where multiple caretakers are present for each infant.

TABLE 1 Predictive Value Model for a Screening Device for Hyperbilirubinemia

	Patients with Positive Test Result	Patients with Negative Test Result	Totals
Patients with significant hyperbilirubinemia	TP	FN	TP + FN
Patients with hyperbilirubinemia	FP	TN	FP + TN
Totals	TP + FP	FN + TN	TP + FP + TN + FN

TP = True positives: number of patients with hyperbilirubinemia correctly classified by the test

FP = False positives: number of patients without hyperbilirubinemia misclassified by the test

TN = True negatives: number of patients without hyperbilirubinemia correctly classified

FN = False negatives: number of patients with hyperbilirubinemia misclassified

Sensitivity: If a patient has disease, how likely is there to be a positive test?:

$$\frac{TP}{TP + FN}$$

Specificity: If a patient does not have disease, how likely is there to be a negative test?:

$$\frac{TN}{FP + TN}$$

Positive predictive value: If a patient has a positive test, how likely is there to be disease?:

$$\frac{TP}{TP + FP}$$

Negative predictive value: If a patient has a negative test, how likely is there to be no disease?:

$$\frac{TN}{TN + FN}$$

Regardless of the transcutaneous method, any test used to screen for hyperbilirubinemia should possess certain qualities. Factors such as risk and relative cost are important. None of the methods used for transcutaneous bilirubinometry pose significant risk to infants. The Ingram Icterometer costs approximately $10, while the Minolta/Air-Shields Jaundice Meter retails for about $2,000. It is important that each institution using a screening device quantify performance at every cut point value chosen in terms of sensitivity, specificity, and predictive values. These terms are defined in Table 1. At any cut point, the net value of the screening procedure is given by the formula

$$V_s = (V_{tp} \times T_p) + (V_{fp} \times F_p) + (V_{tn} \times T_n) + (V_{fn} \times F_n),$$

where V_s equals the health value of the device to society, V_{tp} equals the health value of one true-positive finding, V_{fp} the health value of one false-positive finding, and so on. Cut points should be chosen in response to the consequences of different test results. If the adverse value of a false-negative test result increases relative to the value of a false-positive result, the cut point chosen should be such that sensitivity is high (less stringent). Similarly, if the adverse value of a false-negative test result decreases relative to the adverse value of a false-positive result, a cut point with greater stringency should be favored. If the device chosen is used to screen all newborns, the prevalence of hyperbilirubinemia will be less than if the device is used only in visibly jaundiced infants. If the former is the case (low prevalence), the cut point chosen should strive to minimize false-positive results. If the latter is the case (higher prevalence), the cut point could shift a little to reduce the number of false-negative results.

Given the technology available today, transcutaneous bilirubinometry is recommended as a useful screening device to identify significant neonatal jaundice. At present, we choose to screen only infants who are visibly jaundiced and, defining hyperbilirubinemia as a serum bilirubin level greater than 12.9 mg per deciliter, set our cut point at that index that yields approximately 20 false-positive results for every false-negative result. However, decisions about who should be screened and what constitutes the best cut point are best left to individual health care providers.

CONTINUOUS DISTENDING PRESSURE

MARK MONTGOMERY, M.D., FRCPC
VICTOR CHERNICK, M.D., FRCPC

Continuous distending pressure (CDP) can be defined as the theapeutic application of an increased transpulmonary pressure that is designed to increase the functional residual capacity (FRC) of a poorly compliant lung or to prevent early airway closure during expiration. The transpulmonary pressure is the pressure difference between the airway and the pleural space. Thus, an increase in transpulmonary pressure may be generated either by increasing the pressure within the airways (as with continuous positive airway pressure, CPAP) or by decreasing the pleural pressure (as with the application of subatmospheric pressure to the chest wall, continuous negative pressure, CNP). CDP improves arterial oxygen tension (PaO$_2$) in patients of all ages who have a diffuse lung parenchymal abnormality characterized by a low compliance and reduced FRC. We will discuss the use of CDP in spontaneously breathing neonates.

CDP has been used extensively in the management of hyaline membrane disease. Harrison and colleagues reported that neonates with this disease would lose the ability to grunt after intubation, with a subsequent decrease in PaO$_2$. They speculated that this phenomenon was due to the loss of previously maintained positive end-expiratory airway pressure (spontaneous PEEP), which was necessary to prevent alveolar collapse and maintain an adequate FRC. Gregory and colleagues found that application of CPAP resulted in an increase in PaO$_2$ in neonates with hyaline membrane disease, and allowed a reduction in the concentration of inspired oxygen. The improved PaO$_2$ with a lower concentration of inspired oxygen improved the outcome and reduced the long-term morbidity from this disease.

The appropriate level of CDP decreases the work of breathing, and improves the matching of regional ventilation and perfusion and arterial oxygenation, without compromising cardiac performance. The primary alteration in lung mechanics that occurs with CDP in neonates with hyaline membrane disease is that of an increased FRC, due to enhanced alveolar stability and prevention of atelectasis. The work of breathing is reduced, since there is no need for re-expansion of collapsed areas of lungs. Gas exchange is improved because of improved matching of regional ventilation and perfusion. Previously underventilated areas once again contribute to gas exchange, thus decreasing right-to-left shunting in the lung. CDP may also improve arterial oxygenation in the presence of pulmonary edema. The mechanism for this improvement does not result from a decrease in lung water per se, but rather from a greater alveolar surface area for oxygen diffusion and a thinner layer of lung liquid in the alveolus acting as a barrier to oxygen diffusion. The incidence of air leaks (pneumothorax, pneumomediastinum) is reduced with CDP as compared with mechanical ventilation, but still requires vigilance and prompt treatment if lung rupture occurs.

Excessive levels of CPAP may decrease cardiac output. CPAP increases the mean airway pressure, which may be transmitted to the pulmonary interstitium and vasculature and then to the pleural space. The increased pleural pressure (i.e., less negative) decreases systemic venous return, thus reducing right ventricular stroke volume. Also, right ventricular afterload may be increased when excessive levels of CPAP compress the pulmonary vessels, thereby increasing the pulmonary vascular resistance. The increased force of right ventricular contraction required to overcome the pulmonary vascular resistance may cause the interventricular septum to bulge into the left ventricle. Also, pulmonary venous return may be decreased by the elevated pulmonary vascular resistance, which may decrease blood flow through the lungs. Hence, left ventricular stroke volume may be compromised, owing to decreased pulmonary venous return into a left ventricle reduced in size because of bulging of the interventricular septum. Thus, CPAP should be used with caution in order to avoid a reduced cardiac output and oxygen supply to the tissue.

DEVICES FOR APPLYING CPAP

Continuous distending pressure may be provided by either CPAP or subatmospheric pressure applied to the chest wall (continuous negative pressure, or CNP). There are several systems that may be used to deliver CPAP.

Endotracheal Tube

An endotracheal or nasotracheal tube provides a reliable means of direct delivery of a known level of CPAP to the lungs. In addition, with an endotracheal tube in place mechanical ventilation can be initiated easily if necessary. The disadvantages relate primarily to the tube itself, which must be properly positioned in the trachea; this may be determined by the equality of breath sounds over both hemithoraces, but is best documented by chest radiography. An endotracheal tube is a foreign body in the trachea, and will impair ciliary activity and induce mucus secretion. Frequent suctioning of the endotracheal tube is required to maintain tube patency and prevent bacterial colonization and suprainfection of secretions. Suctioning per se may cause damage to airway epithelium. The endotracheal tube must be securely taped to prevent movement of the tube and subsequent subglottic or nasal scarring. Because of these problems, most neonatologists prefer other methods of administering CPAP, particularly nasal prongs, unless the infant is being weaned from a ventilator.

Nasal Prongs

There are short and long nasal prongs. The theoretical advantage of long nasal prongs that extend into the nasopharynx is maintenance of patency, since obstructing nasal secretions are bypassed. However, the long nasal prongs may kink, thereby obstructing the delivery of CPAP. Short nasal prongs are an attractive means to deliver CPAP, since neonates are preferential nose breathers. Unfortunately, with either type of prongs the level of CPAP can fluctuate, since it is reduced to atmospheric pressure whenever the infant's mouth is open or when the nasal prongs are dislodged. Leakage or blow-off through the mouth restricts the use of CPAP to levels below 10 to 12 cm H_2O. Gastrointestinal distention is common, and all infants undergoing nasal CPAP should receive intermittent gastric suctioning.

Face Mask

The use of a face mask to deliver CPAP to neonates is fraught with hazard. The application of the mask must be sufficiently secure to prevent leaks when movement occurs. The rim of the mask may produce pressure necrosis of the facial nerve or skin, and pressure on the occiput may impair venous return from the head and contribute to intracranial hemorrhage. The face mask increases anatomic dead space, which in turn increases the $PaCO_2$ unless the flow of gas through the system is sufficient to wash out the CO_2. Finally, the face mask makes the detection of vomiting and oropharyngeal suctioning difficult and thus increases the likelihood of aspiration. At present there is no role for the face mask in delivery of CPAP to neonates.

Head Chamber

A head chamber has been developed to deliver CPAP to neonates. There are variations on this method, such as a face chamber, head hood, or head bag, but although they obviate the need for an endotracheal tube, there are several disadvantages. There is reduced access to the infant's head for venipuncture, suctioning, or endotracheal intubation. An orogastric tube should be inserted to prevent gastric distention. The flows within a head hood can produce a noise level of 90 decibels, which may be harmful to the developing ear. The iris neck seal in the head hood, if too loose, prevents adequate levels of CPAP and oxygen; if it is too tight, it reduces venous drainage from the head, possibly predisposing the infant to intracranial hemorrhage.

METHODS OF INCREASING AIRWAY PRESSURE

Gregory first described a system that uses a flow of warmed humidified air-oxygen mixture from a gas blender, reservoir bag, pressure gauge, and safety blow-off valve; this is still widely used. A simpler system using a Carden valve has gained some popularity because it is lightweight, easy to use, and adaptable to any device producing CPAP. The valve is inserted into the gas supply line, and any level of CPAP is generated by changing the resistance to expiratory flow, altering the resistance through a series of holes drilled in the expiratory port. Another method that is simple but noisier, because of continous bubbling, is to submerge the expiratory tube in water. The distance from the top of the water column to the tip of the expiratory tube is the level of CPAP achieved.

CONTINUOUS NEGATIVE PRESSURE

The application of continuous negative pressure (CNP) has been used to supply CDP, especially in larger infants. It does not require endotracheal intubation but does have significant disadvantages. There is restricted access to the patient's body, although access to the head is satisfactory. The development of subatmospheric pressure in the body compartment demands that the compartment be leak free. Thus, CNP is lost when the iris seal ports are opened to gain access to the neonate, and CDP must be provided by CPAP. As well as reducing the level of CNP, leaks in the body compartment draw in room air that cools the infant and subsequently increases oxygen consumption. The iris seal separating the head from the body compartment must not be too loose, to prevent a decrease in oxygen or cooling of the face, or too tight, which would decrease venous return from the head. Because of these difficulties, most centers have abandoned the use of CNP in favor of CPAP, usually by the nasal prong method.

CLINICAL APPLICATIONS

There are several clinical applications for CDP in neonates. It has been used most frequently in the management of newborns with hyaline membrane disease. These infants have poorly compliant lungs, and CDP increases the FRC. CDP may decrease the work of breathing, improve PaO_2, and decrease FRC in infants with bronchiolitis. In bronchiolitis, CPAP splints the small airways open during expiration, allowing for a more complete expiration; this decreases FRC and, since the lung is less distended, improves compliance. CPAP is also effective in splinting open the airways in neonates with tracheomalacia or bronchomalacia. The aspiration of meconium leads to areas of atelectasis and overinflation because of inspissated meconium, as well as bronchial wall inflammation and edema. CPAP has been used in the management of meconium aspiration, and acts to splint airways open in much the same way as in an infant with bronchiolitis. CPAP has been employed for both central and obstructive apnea during sleep in adults, and for apnea of prematurity in neonates, and has been efficacious in some individuals. The mechanism of reducing central apnea with CPAP is unknown but may be related to stimulation of pharyngeal mechanoreceptors, vagal afferents, or the reduction in the costophrenic inhibitory activity seen in newborn infants. The concern with CPAP in this population who usually have normal lungs is that the increased airway pressure will be transmitted to the lung interstitium, compressing pulmonary vessels, decreasing blood flow through the lungs, and decreasing cardiac output. However, infants with apnea of prematurity usually respond to low levels of CPAP, say 2 to 5, cm H_2O.

COMMENTS ON USE OF CDP

The early use of CDP in the course of hyaline membrane disease reduces the duration of respiratory distress, the mortality rate, and long-term morbidity. A candidate for CDP as initial therapy in hyaline membrane disease should be spontaneously breathing, have a birth weight over 1,250 g, be free of respiratory acidosis (pH greater than 7.30), and require an FIO_2 greater than 0.5 to maintain PaO_2 above 50 mm Hg. A rising $PaCO_2$ and consequent respiratory acidosis, often present in neonates under 1,250 g in birth weight who have hyaline membrane disease, may be aggravated by CDP and requires mechanical ventilation for correction. Oxygen plays a major contributory role in the development of bronchopulmonary dysplasia. The use of CDP when the FIO_2 is greater than 0.5 allows a reduction in FIO_2 and consequent reduction in the incidence of bronchopulmonary dysplasia. Principles of care for any ill neonate apply to those receiving CDP therapy. A neutral thermal environment should be maintained to minimize oxygen and calorie consumption. Fluid balance must be meticulously followed to prevent fluid overload, since there is a tendency to retain fluid with CDP. Sufficient calories should be provided to prevent tissue catabolism, and should take into account the increased requirements due to the increased work of breathing. Oxygen delivery to the tissues depends on cardiac output and arterial oxygen content. Since cardiac output may be compromised, frequent assessment of blood pressure and capillary refill is vital. Indwelling lines to determine central venous or arterial pressure may be required to assess cardiac performance. Arterial oxygen content depends on the amount of hemoglobin and the degree of saturation of the hemoglobin with oxygen. The hemoglobin level should be maintained above 100 g per liter while the neonate is receiving CDP to optimize arterial oxygen content. Pulse oximetry provides a reliable means of monitoring oxygen saturation (SaO_2), which should be maintained between 85 and 95 percent. The transcutaneous monitoring of PO_2 is an alternative to monitoring SaO_2, and when coupled with transcutaneous PCO_2 monitoring displays changes in the respiratory status of the newborn infant. Serial arterial blood gas determinations are essential to validate the results of the transcutaneous monitors.

The following guidelines are helpful regarding the use of CDP; however, their use must be tailored to each patient and the practice and experience of each neonatal unit. FIO_2 and the level of CDP should be adjusted to maintain PaO_2 between 50 and 80 mm Hg. A reasonable initial level of CDP is 5 cm H_2O. CDP can be increased in 2-cm H_2O increments to a maximum of 10 to 15 cm H_2O, and FIO_2 can be changed by 5 percent decrements to maintain the PaO_2 between 50 and 80 mm Hg. Failure of CDP occurs when respiratory acidosis develops or the PaO_2 persists below 50 mm Hg, despite an FIO_2 above 0.60 and a CDP level of 15 cm H_2O. Mechanical ventilation must be initiated in these patients, or if there are frequent severe apneic episodes.

Weaning from CDP entails a gradual reduction in both the pressure and FIO_2. Continuous monitoring of oxygen saturation (maintained between 85 and 95 percent) or transcutaneous PO_2 (maintained between 50 and 80 mm Hg) is useful during the reduction in CDP. Generally, the FIO_2 should be reduced to less than 0.40 in 0.02 to 0.05 decrements as tolerated every 1 to 2 hours. Once an FIO_2 of 0.40 is reached, the CDP can be reduced in 2-cm H_2O decrements every 1 to 2 hours.

When weaning a neonate from endotracheal CPAP, it must be remembered that an endotracheal tube prevents the development of spontaneous PEEP. Therefore, CPAP should not be discontinued in an intubated neonate. Instead, the CPAP should be reduced to 2 cm H_2O, the neonate extubated, and CPAP supplied by nasal prongs at 3 to 5 cm H_2O. Weaning from the nasal prongs then proceeds by 1 to 2 cm H_2O decrements every 1 to 2 hours. An FIO_2 increase of 0.10 is often required to prevent a fall in PaO_2 when CPAP is discontinued. CPAP is also used when weaning patients from mechanical ventilators. The ventilator rate is weaned to zero with an optimal CDP. When the patient's condition allows, he or she is then weaned from CDP as described above.

OPTIMAL CDP

The optimal level of CDP may be defined as that pressure which is associated with a marked increase in PaO_2 without changing $PaCO_2$ or interfering with cardiac output. The optimal pressure of CDP is variable. Clinically *there is a marked reduction in indrawing or grunting when the optimal level of CPAP is achieved.* An accurate means of assessing optimal CPAP is to use an esophageal pressure probe. Optimal CDP is then determined to be the point at which airway pressure is transmitted to the esophageal pressure probe. When optimal CDP is exceeded, PaO_2 at a fixed FIO_2 does not increase but $PaCO_2$ rises.

OUTCOME

Since the institution of CDP during spontaneous ventilation and the application of PEEP during mechanical ventilation, there has been a striking reduction in the mortality rate of infants with hyaline membrane disease. Whereas at one time 80 percent of such infants would die, the overall mortality rate now is less than 20 percent and is noted largely in infants weighing less than 1,000 g at birth. In addition, CDP during spontaneous ventilation has not increased the risk of lung rupture, but has reduced the incidence of bronchopulmonary dysplasia. Early institution of CDP has decreased the duration and mortality rates of disease in patients with hyaline membrane disease. However, CDP should be used with appropriate caution to avoid pressures that are too high.

SUGGESTED READING

Berg TJ, Pagtakhan RD, Reed MH, et al. Bronchopulmonary dysplasia and lung rupture in hyaline membrane disease: influence of continuous distending pressure. Pediatrics 1975; 55:51.

Carden R, Levin K, Fisk G, Vidyasagar D. A new method of applying continuous positive pressure breathing in infants. Pediatrics 1974; 53:757.

Gregory GA, Kitterman JA, Phibbs RH, et al. Treatment of idiopathic respiratory distress syndrome with continuous positive airway pressure. N Engl J Med 1971; 284:1333.

Harrison VC, Heese DV, Klein M. The significance of grunting in hyaline membrane disease. Pediatrics 1968; 41:549.

CRYOTHERAPY FOR RETINOPATHY OF PREMATURITY

EARL A. PALMER, M.D.

Retinopathy of prematurity (ROP) is a leading cause of blindness among prematurely born infants. It is characterized by an abnormal proliferative neovascularization at the leading ends of developing vessels in the premature retina, and may lead to blindness after detachment of the retina as early as 2 to 3 months from birth. ROP is a discouraging disease for ophthalmologists, because an eye that appears normal in an infant 1 month of age may have a completely detached retina within a few months. Since the survival rate for extremely premature infants has been on the increase, there has been a corresponding increase in the number of cases of ROP.

In 1972, early reports suggested that photocoagulation or cryotherapy might ameliorate the course of ROP. Cryotherapy was thought to have favorable effects in many infants if applied during the acute phases of ROP, before retinal detachment occurs.* However, other investigators found little or no effect from the treatment. Because of these conflicting results and conclusions, along with the surgical risk

in such tiny patients, cryotherapy was not accepted as standard treatment for ROP in the United States during the early 1980s.

Most of the early reports of cryotherapy suffered from lack of a uniform classification system for ROP. There now exists an International Classification, which divides the retina into 12 clock-hour sectors and 3 anteroposterior zones for location purposes. This classification contains five progressive stages of severity, with the final two stages describing retinal detachment, from partial to complete.

As a further impediment to our interpretation of the efficacy of cryotherapy, insufficient data were initially available on the natural course of the disease to permit accurate prediction of outcome. The retinopathy may progress to an alarming stage of severity and then spontaneously subside, leaving the eye with good vision. It has been estimated that 80 percent of infants with severe (Stage 3) ROP experience this favorable natural resolution. For such an unpredictable disorder, *any* therapy may appear effective in many cases.

An objective assessment of cryotherapy can only be achieved by (1) selecting eyes in which the severity of ROP

---

* Alternative terminology has appeared. The terms "cryopexy" or "cryoretinopexy" are inappropriate here, since "pexy" refers to fixation. The meaning of this suffix would be appropriate in referring to the treatment of retinal detachment that has already occurred. "Cryocautery" is another term that is unclear, because it connotes heat as well as cold.

is similar, and then (2) following the clinical course of eyes that have been randomly assigned to receive cryotherapy, as well as those randomly assigned *not* to receive it. Small-scale attempts at randomized trials prior to 1985 were essentially inconclusive, although one series in Philadelphia showed a statistically significant benefit. Although important, that study was flawed, because the assignment of the eye to receive cryotherapy was made arbitrarily by the surgeon, rather than by any randomization scheme, and outcome was thus potentially biased.

Even though a patient may be described as having "symmetric" disease, experienced examiners have observed that there are frequently subtle differences between the two eyes. We do not yet know how to interpret these differences with regard to how the eye may respond to therapy. This is another reason that randomization is imperative in evaluating surgery for ROP.

To resolve these uncertainties about the value of cryotherapy, a randomized multicenter trial was organized in the U.S. in 1985. This trial of cryotherapy for retinopathy of prematurity (CRYO-ROP) was begun in January, 1986, under the sponsorship of the National Eye Institute, and is continuing into the 1990s (Table 1). The study was launched with the prospective examination of the ocular fundi of premature infants weighing less than 1,251 g at birth. The eyes were observed until the retinopathy (if any) reached a specified threshold degree of severity, and then one eye was randomly selected to receive cryotherapy. If only one eye was severely affected, that infant was considered an "asymmetric" case, and the one eye with threshold severity of ROP was randomized into either the control or cryotherapy group. (If the fellow eye went on to develop severe ROP, it was eligible to receive cryotherapy whenever the first eye was randomized to control. *In no case did both eyes receive cryotherapy under the study protocol.*) The multicenter trial was also designed to study the natural course of ROP, so that outcome predictions could be refined for clinical use and for future studies.

In CRYO-ROP, each eye was observed as it developed progressive acute ROP until it reached a specified degree of severity that had been estimated to lead to a 50 percent risk of severe visual impairment. This threshold point was defined in the study protocol as Stage 3 ROP in Zone 1 or 2, for a total of eight clock-hour sectors, or involving a minimum of five confluent sectors (by the International Classification), along with the presence of "plus disease." Once threshold severity was reached, it was considered ethically sound to randomize for a treatment that had promise of benefit, but was not yet *proven* beneficial. Had cryotherapy been applied at a lower threshold of severity than Stage 3, it was likely (spuriously) to *appear* effective, in the judgment of the planning committee. Accordingly, the sample

TABLE 1 Participating Centers in the CRYO-ROP Study

State and City	Contact Physicians
Alabama: Birmingham	Frederick Elsas, M.D.
California: Sacramento	Alan Roth, M.D.
Florida: Miami	John Flynn, M.D.
Illinois: Chicago	Marilyn Miller, M.D.
Indiana: Indianapolis	Forrest Ellis, M.D.
Kentucky: Louisville	Charles Barr, M.D.
Louisiana: New Orleans	Robert Gordon, M.D.
Maryland: Baltimore	Michael Repka, M.D.
Michigan: Detroit	Jack Baker, M.D.
	Michael Tress, M.D.
Minnesota: Minneapolis	C. Gail Summers, M.D.
New York: Rochester	Dale Phelps, M.D.
Buffalo	James Reynolds, M.D.
Syracuse	Paul Torrisi, M.D.
North Carolina: Durham	Edward Buckley, M.D.
	Susie Wong, M.D.
Ohio: Cincinnati	Miles Burke, M.D.
Columbus	Gary Rogers, M.D.
	Don Bremer, M.D.
Oregon: Portland	Earl Palmer, M.D.
Pennsylvania: Philadelphia	Graham Quinn, M.D.
	David Schaffer, M.D.
Pittsburgh	Albert Biglan, M.D.
South Carolina: Charleston	Richard Saunders, M.D.
	Linda Christmann, M.D.
Tennessee: Nashville	Stephen Feman, M.D.
Texas: Dallas	Rand Spencer, M.D.
San Antonio	Wichard van Heuven, M.D.
Utah: Salt Lake City	Jane Kivlin, M.D.
District of Columbia: Washington	David Plotsky, M.D.
	William Gilbert, M.D.

In the Outcome Study of Cryotherapy and Retinopathy of Prematurity, the 23 Centers listed here will continue to follow the patients enrolled in the cryotherapy trial.

size required to demonstrate a statistically significant benefit would need to be much larger than if randomization were done at the more serious level of retinopathy finally selected by CRYO-ROP. More importantly, earlier treatment would have subjected more infants to needless intervention.

In CRYO-ROP, the outcome after cryotherapy or control management was formally assessed 3 months after randomization, and then again 9 months later, via masked reading of fundus photographs, as well as clinical fundus examination. Of course, all infants with severe retinopathy were observed more frequently, if indicated, for any perceived complications. For example, infants who suffer retinal detachment from ROP may develop pain from glaucoma and corneal opacity. These complications can sometimes be ameliorated by medical and surgical management, although additional research is required concerning these problems and their management.

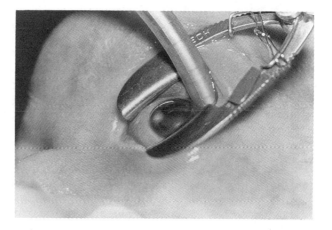

Figure 1 A cryoprobe is shown applied to a premature infant's eye.

STUDY RESULTS

The results of the CRYO-ROP were evaluated through a masked photographic comparison of the incidence of certain objectively visible adverse findings, such as macular fold, retinal detachment, or retrolental mass. Preliminary *study findings showed such a positive response to cryotherapy that the study's data and safety monitoring committee recommended early termination* of enrollment. Within weeks of stopping enrollment, the study results were disseminated across the nation via a "medical alert" notice mailed out by the National Eye Institute to neonatologists and ophthalmologists who treat premature infants. The preliminary results were published 3 months after enrollment ceased.

Three-month outcome findings on 172 of the 291 randomized infants showed that *cryotherapy significantly reduced the frequency·of adverse outcome, from 43 percent to 21.8 percent.* Full outcome data for both 3 and 12 months after randomization are not published at this writing.

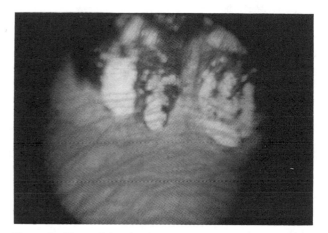

Figure 2 The peripheral retina shows pigment clumping ("scarring") a few weeks after cryotherapy.

WHAT IS CRYOTHERAPY?

Cryotherapy (cold treatment) is essentially a destructive procedure. For the eye, it is ordinarily applied through the sclera by placing a cryoprobe onto the surface of the sclera (Fig. 1), then activating the probe to produce a small "ice ball" on the choroid and retina, which form the inner lining of the sclera. The freezing of these delicate intraocular tissues produces necrosis, while the sclera itself is resistant to damage from cryotherapy. Cryotherapy is commonly used by ophthalmologists to destroy pathologic lesions in the choroid and retina, and to create tissue adherence that inhibits retinal detachment. In ROP, *the theory is that by destroying the portion of the peripheral retina that has not yet received its destined blood supply* (Fig. 2), *the production of some presumed vasoproliferative factor will be reduced,* causing a subsidence of the neovascularization that may lead to detachment of the retina.

In ROP, numerous spots of cryotherapy are briefly applied in contiguous fashion while the retina is directly visual-

ized under local or general anesthesia. Shortly after each application of cryotherapy, the retina blanches permitting the clinician to observe where previous freezes have been applied. The peripheral avascular retina takes on a spotted appearance by fundus examination, and later undergoes patchy atrophy (see Fig. 2).

HOW SHOULD INFANTS WITH ROP BE MANAGED?

First, premature infants at risk for ROP should have an eye examination by an ophthalmologist at some point between 4 and 6 weeks of life. *The earlier recommendation that initial screening examination be done between 7 and 9 weeks must be abandoned, since treatment must now be considered during the active phase of the disease.* Any ROP detected should be carefully monitored, at least every two weeks, until it regresses or becomes more severe. If the infant's ROP reaches a "prethreshold" state of ROP (Zone 1, any stage; or Zone 2, Stage 3), then examination is recommended at maximum intervals of one week, as the disease is highly unpredictable at this point.

Once a patient is diagnosed with bilateral ROP at the threshold level of severity, it is suggested that a confirming examination be performed by a second ophthalmologist whenever any doubt exists as to staging. If confirmed, cryotherapy should be immediately considered.

I am not yet firmly recommending treatment of both eyes in all cases of threshold disease because the data on long-term effects of cryotherapy are not yet available and caution is warranted. If cryotherapy were completely innocuous, its widespread prophylactic application to every threshold (perhaps even prethreshold) eye might be reasonable. On the contrary, cryotherapy requires additional expense, causes damage to developing tissue (with unknown long-term consequences), and is stressful to the infant. Therefore, even though cryotherapy is effective, it should be applied only to the eyes of infants at risk for visual damage. Until long-term analyses are complete, the ophthalmologist must individually judge the appropriateness of cryotherapy for a particular eye in a particular patient.

In following severe ROP, with or without cryotherapy, the ophthalmologist needs to monitor for retinal detachment and other sequelae of ROP, including refractive error, glaucoma, amblyopia, nystagmus, and strabismus. *Parents should be urged to maintain regular contact with the ophthalmologist, since many sequelae of regressed ROP are treatable.*

SUGGESTED READING

Cryotherapy for Retinopathy of Prematurity Cooperative Group. Multicenter trial of cryotherapy for retinopathy of prematurity: preliminary results. Pediatrics 1988; 81(5):697–706.
Patz A, Palmer EA. Retinopathy of prematurity. In: Ryan S, ed. Retina, Volume II Medical Retina. St. Louis: CV Mosby, 1989.

ECHOCARDIOGRAPHIC EVALUATION OF CONGENITAL HEART DISEASE IN THE FETUS AND NEWBORN

RICHARD A. MEYER, M.D.

The single most important technologic advance in the diagnosis of cardiac disease of the newborn in the past two decades has been echocardiography. The advent of two-dimensional echocardiography, Doppler, and (most recently) color flow has enhanced our ability to diagnose cardiac disease accurately, painlessly, and with little risk to the fetus and newborn. In addition, this technology has permitted the cardiologist to distinguish signs and symptoms of respiratory disease, sepsis, metabolic derangement, and abnormalities of hemoglobin from those of congenital or acquired cardiac disease in a controlled environment at the bedside. Most recently, color flow mapping has been added to the armamentarium of the clinician. It will be impossible in the space allotted to provide an in-depth discussion of the technology and its application, so I shall provide only a brief overview of the state of the art. For a more in-depth discussion, the reader is referred to several monographs on the subject.

SAFETY

Since diagnostic ultrasonography is accurate and free of pain, it has tremendous appeal to the perinatologist as a noninvasive diagnostic tool in premature and full-term infants, as well as in the fetus. The dictum "do no harm" assumes clear significance today as this technology becomes more widespread. To date, no adverse effects resulting from the application of diagnostic ultrasonography in any patient have been reported. However, with the increased application of pulsed Doppler, color flow, and other technologies that utilize greater intensities of ultrasound energy, concerns about the safety of ultrasonography, particularly in the fetus, have been heightened. As responsible clinicians and research investigators, we must take into account the potential, albeit small, adverse effects of diagnostic ultrasonography. Current research into the bioeffects of ultrasonography has failed to document or confirm adverse biologic effects in humans. Nevertheless, efforts to study and monitor these bioeffects in the fetuses and in premature infants must continue.

TECHNIQUES AND VIEWS

The standard views obtained for imaging include the long-axis plane (Fig. 1*A*) of the left ventricle; the short-axis plane (Fig. 1*B*) of the left ventricle; the short-axis plane of the great arteries (Fig. 1*C*); the apical four-chambered plane (Fig. 1*D*); the subcostal four-chambered plane (Fig. 1*E*); and the suprasternal notch plane of the great vessels (Fig. 1*F*). Originally, the equipment always placed the apex of the sector at the top of the video screen (Fig. 1*A–C*). The apex corresponds to the transducer face that rests on the skin. However, for the apical and subcostal views, it is easier to understand the images if they are inverted, since they more closely relate to the underlying anatomy as we view the patient from the front. Most equipment today permits one to invert the images if desired (Fig. 1*D, E*).

Doppler and color flow permit detection of the flow of blood cells. By convention, flow signals that come toward the transducer are red (see Fig. 9) and above the horizontal baseline. Signals that go away from the transducer are blue or below the baseline.

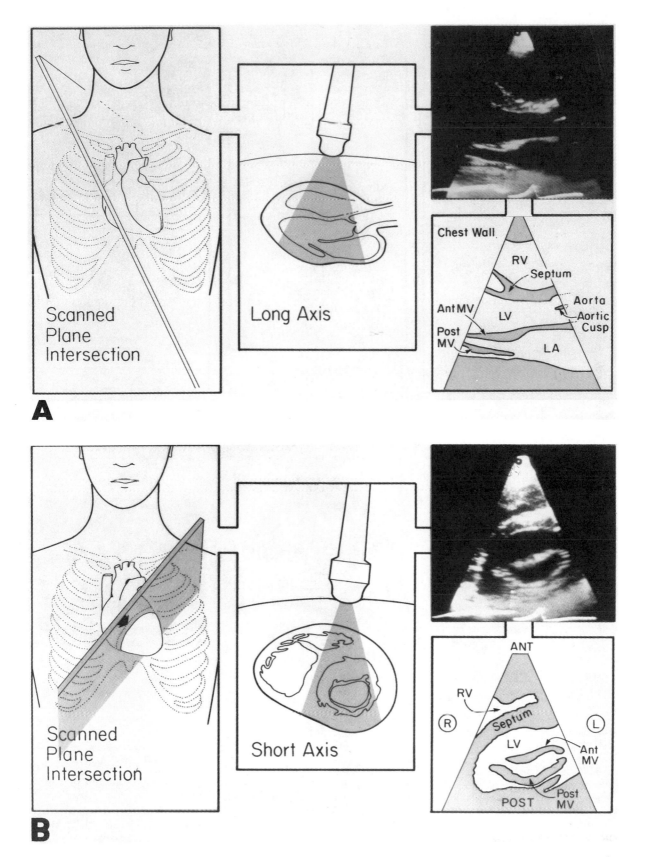

Figure 1 *A* and *B*, Typical examination planes used for two-dimensional imaging. These planes will serve as a reference for the following examples of diseases. AO, aorta; innom A, innominate artery; LA, left atrium; LCA, left carotid artery; LPA, left pulmonary artery; LPV, left pulmonary vein; LSA, left subclavian artery; LV, left ventricle; MPA, main pulmonary artery; MV, mitral valve; RA, right atrium; RPA, right pulmonary artery.

Figure continues on following page

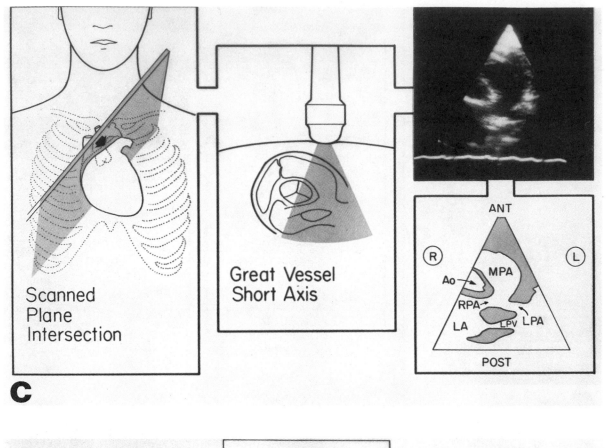

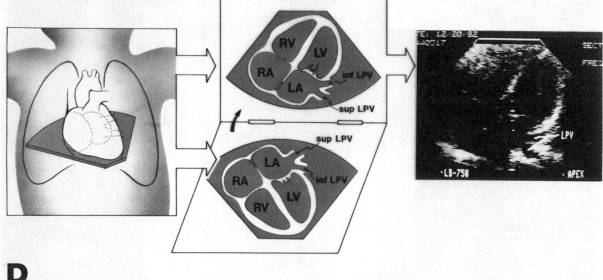

Figure 1 *C* to *F*, Typical examination planes used for two-dimensional imaging. These planes will serve as a reference for the following examples of diseases. AO, aorta; innom A, innominate artery; LA, left atrium; LCA, left carotid artery; LPA, left pulmonary artery; LPV, left pulmonary vein; LSA, left subclavian artery; LV, left ventricle; MPA, main pulmonary artery; MV, mitral valve; RA, right atrium; RPA, right pulmonary artery. (Reproduced with permission from Meyer RA. Echocardiography. In: Adams FH, Emmanoulides GC, Riemenschneider TA, eds. Moss' heart disease in infants, children and adolescents. 4th ed. Baltimore: Williams & Wilkins, 1989.)

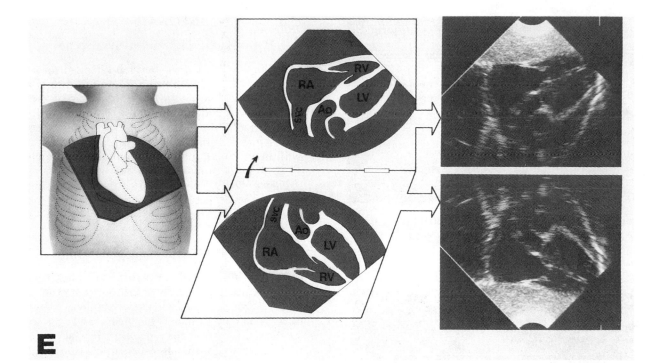

E

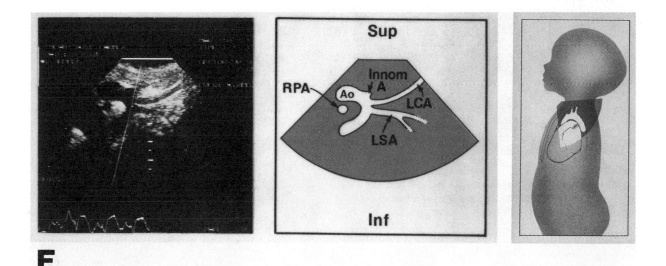

F

FETUS

Fetal echocardiography has become routine in many institutions. Awareness of complex congenital heart defects and rhythm disturbances in utero usually permits judicious medical and surgical management of these problems. For example, a supraventricular tachycardia in a fetus (Fig. 2) who is developing hydrops may be converted to sinus rhythm by administering antiarrhythmic drugs to the mother. On the other hand, bradycardia in an infant may be due to complete heart block, resulting from systemic lupus erythematosus in the mother. The correct diagnosis in this case can be made by echocardiography, which properly allows the baby do remain in utero, to grow and develop normally until term. For the most part, severe cardiac defects such as tricuspid atresia (Fig. 3) are easily recognized in the fetus. In these cases, early detection allows appropriate planning for intrapartum or postpartum

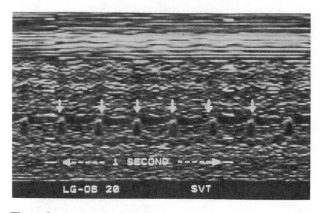

Figure 2 A supraventricular tachycardia (240 bpm) in a 31-week fetus. The arrows point to the mitral valve echo.

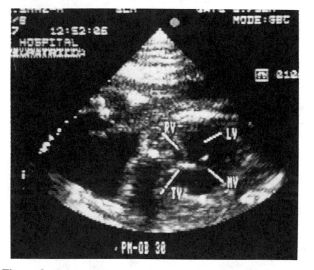

Figure 3 Tricuspid valve (TV) atresia in a 30-week fetus. In this apical plane the right ventricle (RV) is small and the TV appears as an immobile plate, whereas the mitral valve (MV) moves freely and is thin. LV = left ventricle.

management. Small ventricular septal defects or transposition of the great vessels may be more difficult to diagnose accurately in utero, even after several examinations.

It is important to understand that fetal echocardiography is not simple, but requires an experienced sonographer to perform and interpret the study. Since these examinations are usually obtained because of a history of congenital heart disease or death in a previous pregnancy or a high-risk pregnancy, the family is greatly concerned and emotionally volatile. Therefore, only our most experienced individuals perform these examinations and speak to the family; it should be emphasized that this diagnostic procedure is associated with the highest rate of litigation. Hence, we perform fetal echocardiography only when specific medical indications exist and in close collaboration with an obstetrician well versed in ultrasonography.

NEONATE

Hypoplastic Left Heart Syndrome

Newborns who suddenly develop symptoms of poor peripheral perfusion and cyanosis after a few days of life most likely have some variant of aortic and/or mitral atresia. These entities are accurately diagnosed by echocardiography that demonstrates an ascending aorta less than 5 mm in diameter and/or absence of a mitral valve (Fig. 4). In our hands, *cardiac catheterization and angiography have not been required to establish this diagnosis since the mid-1970's*. This is not to say that this is a simple diagnosis to make, but it can be made confidently, once sufficient expertise and competence has been gained.

Cyanotic Lesions

Cyanosis in the newborn period most often results from transposition of the great arteries, tricuspid atresia, pulmonary atresia, or total anomalous pulmonary venous connection. In transposition of the great vessels, the aorta is visualized arising from the right ventricle while the pulmonary artery arises from the left ventricle (Fig. 5A). In

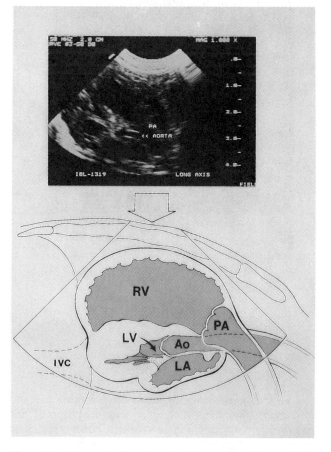

Figure 4 A long-axis view of aortic (Ao) atresia and hypoplastic left ventricle (LV) in a newborn. IVC = inferior vena cava; LA = left atrium; PA = pulmonary artery; RV = right ventricle.

addition, the aorta now resides slightly anterior and to the right of the pulmonary artery (Fig. 5B). This diagnosis is likewise made with confidence by echocardiography and, under ordinary circumstances, cardiac catheterization is performed, not to make a diagnosis but, rather, to perform a palliative balloon septostomy. When the infant is critically ill and unstable, we have performed septostomy under echo guidance in the nursery incubator. Once the baby has been stabilized, a complete cardiac catheterization can be undertaken electively. Conal truncal abnormalities (Fig. 6), such as tetralogy of Fallot, truncus arteriosus, and pulmonary atresia, likewise can be recognized and diagnosed with certainty by echocardiography.

Persistent Pulmonary Hypertension of the Newborn

The syndrome of persistent pulmonary hypertension of the newborn must be distinguished from congenital

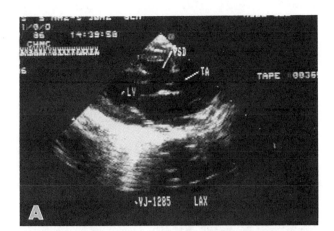

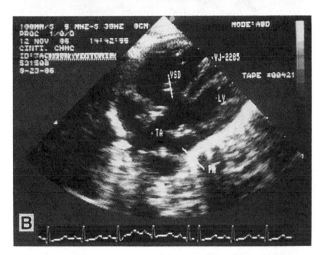

Figure 6 Echogram of a 6-week-old infant with truncus arteriosus. *A,* Long-axis view showing the single truncal vessel (TA) overriding the septum. The ventricular septal defect (VSD) was easily seen. *B,* The pulmonary artery (PA) can be visualized arising from the TA in this subcostal view. The VSD is also well seen. LV = left ventricle.

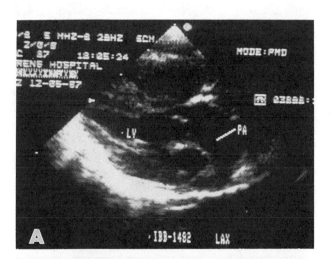

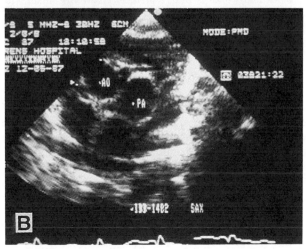

Figure 5 Echogram of a newborn with D-transposition of the great vessels (D-TGV). *A,* Long-axis view of the pulmonary artery (PA) arising from the left ventricle (LV). *B,* Short axis view of the aorta (Ao) slightly anterior and to the right of the PA, characteristic of D-TGV.

cardiac defects when evaluating a cyanotic newborn. For the most part, *echocardiography has eliminated the need for cardiac catheterization in these critically ill neonates.* The advent of extracorporeal membrane oxygenation to treat this disease, however, has placed *an increased burden on the cardiologist to exclude total anomalous pulmonary venous drainage before placing these infants on bypass therapy.* The diagnosis of this disease by two-dimensional echocardiography has been facilitated by the application of Doppler to verify the presence or absence of pulmonary venous drainage into the left atrium. The recent addition of color flow mapping has increased the accuracy of confirming the presence of normal pulmonary venous drainage.

M-mode echocardiography (Fig. 7) continues to be a reliable means of sequentially assessing the state of the pulmonary vascular bed. The ratio of the pre-ejection period to the ejection time of the pulmonary artery

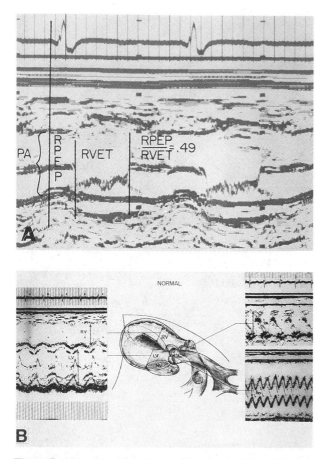

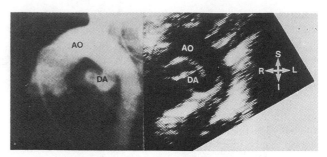

Figure 8 This composite demonstrates a patent ductus arteriosus (DA) arising from the aorta (Ao) on an aortogram and companion echogram of the long axis plane of the aorta taken from the suprasternal notch. (From Smallhorn JF, Huhta JC, Anderson RH, et al. Suprasternal cross-sectional echocardiography in the assessment of patent ductus arteriosus. Br Heart J 1982; 48:321–330. By permission of the British Medical Association.)

Figure 7 Echogram of newborn with pulmonary hypertension. *A*, The expected elevated right-sided systolic time intervals ratio of the pulmonary artery (PA). The normal ratio should not exceed 0.35 RPEP = right pre-ejection period; RVET = right ventricular ejection time. *B*, Sagittal view of the heart with corresponding M-mode echograms of great vessels and chambers for reference. Ao = aorta; LA = left atrium; LV = left ventricle; MV = mitral valve; RV = right ventricle.

decreases over time as pulmonary vascular resistance decreases. Otherwise, the right-sided systolic time intervals ratio remains elevated, if the resistance is increased. The normal newborn has elevated ratios (greater than 0.35) in the first 36 to 48 hours, but by 72 hours the ratio returns to normal (less than 0.30 to 0.35).

Patent Ductus Arteriosus

The patent ductus arteriosus has assumed a major role in neonatal cardiology. The ability to close or open the ductus arteriosus has changed the management of premature infants and of those with ductal-dependent cardiac lesions such as pulmonary valve atresia. Thus, characterization of the ductus arteriosus has assumed even greater significance. It is *now possible to visualize the patent ductus arteriosus (Fig. 8) and to confirm any shunting through it by Doppler* when the characteristic continuous flow is detected in the pulmonary artery (Fig. 9). Color flow has facilitated recognition of the ductus and of the characteris-

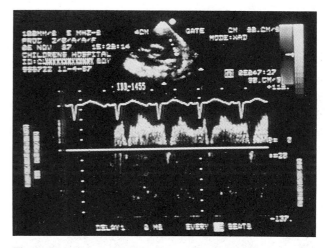

Figure 9 This color flow Doppler echogram (reproduced here in black and white) is from a premature newborn infant with a patent ductus arteriosus (PDA) and was obtained in the short-axis view of the great vessels. The sample volume on the two-dimensional image is positioned in the ductal flow, and continuous flow toward the transducer (above the horizontal line) is detected.

tics of its flow patterns. In addition, we still use M-mode echocardiography along with two-dimensional imaging to quantify the hemodynamic effects and left ventricular function.

Obstructive Lesions

Systolic ejection murmurs in a newborn usually signal some form of left ventricular or right ventricular outflow obstruction. Often the precise location of the obstruction is difficult to determine by examination at the bedside. Two-dimensional echocardiography with Doppler has done much to clarify the nature of these lesions (Fig. 10*A*). If it is unclear by two-dimensional imaging whether the aortic valve or the pulmonic valve is affected, Doppler

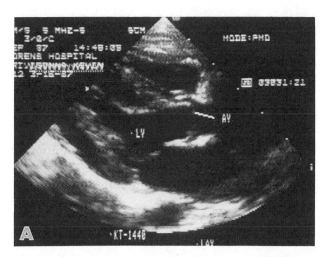

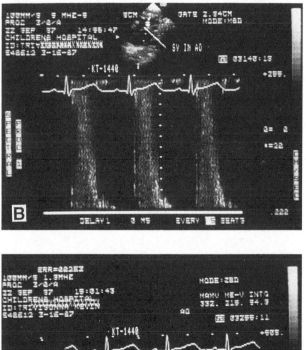

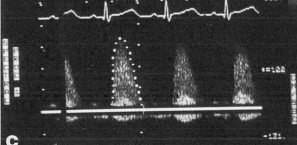

evaluation usually points to the valve producing turbulence in the artery (Fig. 10B). Also, it is possible with Doppler to quantitate the severity of obstruction by applying the modified Bernouilli equation ($P = 4V^2$, where $P =$ mm Hg and $V =$ velocity in cm per second) to the derived Doppler velocity (Fig. 10C), in order to arrive at an assessment of the severity of the gradient. In this patient the peak instantaneous gradient was 44 mm Hg and the mean gradient was 18 mm Hg.

Intracardiac Shunts

Large atrial septal and ventricular septal defects (see Fig. 6) are usually visible with two-dimensional echocardiography. On occasion, a very small ventricular defect may be difficult to image, but by using color flow mapping (Fig. 11A) it is possible to locate the defect more easily

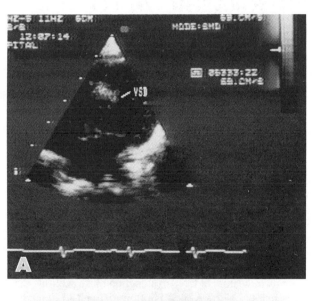

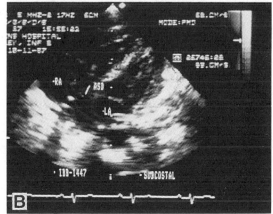

Figure 10 These echograms are from a 6-month-old infant with aortic stenosis. *A*, A long-axis view of the left ventricle (LV) shows doming of the thin aortic valve (AV) cusps characteristic of valvar disease. *B*, A pulsed Doppler study showing the sample volume (SV) in the aorta (Ao) on the two-dimensional image and simultaneous turbulent Doppler signal consistent with obstruction going toward the transducer (above the horizontal line). *C*, A continuous wave Doppler signal from the same patient. Tracing the envelope of the Doppler signal provides calculated peak and mean velocities of 332 and 215 cm per second (see text).

Figure 11 Echograms of color flow imaging (reproduced here in black and white) in two newborns. *A*, A tiny midseptal ventricular septal defect (VSD) was located only by using color flow. *B*, A secundum atrial septal defect (ASD) shows dominant left-to-right shunting and approximate size of the defect. LA = left atrium; RA = right atrium.

and accurately and then visualize it. In addition, the flow direction, the character, and some estimate of size can be determined by color flow techniques (Fig. 11*B*).

SUGGESTED READING

Berman W Jr. Pulsed Doppler ultrasound in clinical pediatrics. Mt Kisco, NY: Futura Publishing, 1983.

DeMaria AN. Color Doppler flow imaging 1987: Principles and practice. Echocardiography 1987; 4:465–467.

Goldberg SJ, Allen HD, Sahn DJ. Pediatric and adolescent echocardiography. A handbook. 2nd ed. Chicago: Year Book, 1980.

Kimball TR, Weiss RG, Meyer RA, et al. Color flow mapping to document normal pulmonary venous return in neonates with persistent pulmonary hypertension being considered for extracorporeal membrane oxygenation. Pediatr 1989; 114:433–437.

Meyer RA. Echocardiography. In: Adams FH, Emmanoulides GC, Riemenschneider TA, eds. Moss' heart disease in infants, children and adolescents. 4th ed. Baltimore: Williams & Wilkins, 1989:56.

O'Brien WD Jr. Biological effects of ultrasound: Rationale for the measurement of selected ultrasonic output quantities. Echocardiography 1986; 3:165–179.

Powis RL, Powis WJ. A thinker's guide to ultrasonic imaging. Baltimore: Urban & Schwarzenberg, 1984.

Smallhorn JF, Huhta JC, Anderson RH, et al. Suprasternal cross-sectional echocardiography in the assessment of patent ductus arteriosus. Br Heart J 1982; 48:321–330.

ELECTROENCEPHALOGRAPHIC/ POLYGRAPHIC/VIDEO MONITORING

ELI M. MIZRAHI, M.D.

CLINICAL PROBLEM

The incidence of seizures is greater in the first month of life than at any other time in childhood, and seizures are often the first clinical sign of central nervous system (CNS) dysfunction in the newborn. Failure to recognize seizures as such may delay neurologic evaluation and essential treatment, whereas an incorrect designation of a clinical event as a seizure may lead to unnecessary diagnostic procedures and anticonvulsant therapy.

Both the high incidence of seizures and their importance as indicators of CNS dysfunction make accurate diagnosis critical. However, it is often difficult to determine whether a neonate has had, or is having, a clinical seizure. Because many neonatal seizures are poorly organized, random, or subtle clinical events, the clinician's threshold of suspicion concerning repetitive and stereotypic behaviors of newborn infants is high. Thus, diagnosis is a significant clinical challenge.

Similar clinical problems in older infants, children, and adults have been resolved with the development and application of time-synchronized electroencephalographic (EEG)/video monitoring techniques, which provide the basis for the detection, characterization, classification, and quantification of various types of seizures. EEG/video monitoring has been useful in the clinical investigation and management of disorders such as infantile spasms, absence seizures, complex partial seizures, pseudoseizures, and nonepileptic disorders such as disturbance of sleep.

In the past, it was necessary to transport patients to a specially equipped laboratory for monitoring, which meant that sick neonates could not be studied routinely. However, *the recent development of portable monitoring instrumentation has allowed newborns suspected of having seizures to be monitored in neonatal intensive care units (NICUs) without disrupting their critical care.* Although cribside monitoring of the newborn is relatively uncommon, it will increase in frequency as the instrumentation and expertise in its use become more available. This report is based on EEG/polygraphic/video monitoring of more than 600 neonates at Texas Children's Hospital, Houston, Texas.

Basis of Monitoring

The purpose of monitoring is to record the suspected abnormal clinical event and the EEG simultaneously, so that the character of the clinical event can be analyzed objectively, any changes in the EEG can be characterized, and the relationship between the clinical and electrical events can be determined. The presence of EEG seizure activity concurrent with the clinical event suggests that the behavior is epileptic in origin, whereas its absence would suggest that other pathophysiologic mechanisms are operant. In order for monitoring to provide clinically useful information on which to base a diagnosis, a suspected seizure must be recorded. Thus, to capture the clinical events, some monitoring sessions may need to be prolonged.

Clinical Character of Neonatal Seizures

The most common reason for requesting a monitoring study is to determine whether a particular paroxysmal clinical event is a seizure. *Clinical seizures in the neonate are unique in character compared with those in older infants and children.* Some seizures are primarily *clonic*—rhythmic, repetitive contractions of muscles. *Tonic* seizures, either focal or generalized, are characterized by sustained posture of limbs, trunk, head, or eyes. *Myoclonic* seizures are either focal or generalized single jerks or slowly repetitive jerking movements of circumscribed muscle groups or of the trunk. A group of behaviors have been

Supported by grant NS11535 and by Teacher-Investigator Development Award NS00810 from the National Institute of Neurological and Communicative Disorders and Stroke, National Institutes of Health.

referred to as "subtle" seizures or "*motor automatisms*;" these include oral-buccal-lingual movements, ocular movements, and progression movements of the arms or legs. *An important feature of neonatal seizures is the activation of the autonomic nervous system during, or as the sole manifestation of, the clinical event.* Autonomic nervous system manifestations include elevation in arterial blood pressure, changes in heart rate, pupillary dilatation or constriction, salivation or drooling, pallor or flushing, and possibly changes in respiration.

Because of the wide range of physiologic changes that may occur during clinical seizures, a number of parameters are recorded simultaneously with the EEG and video. These are polygraphic tracings that appear as additional channels of recorded data on the EEG. Routinely, they include recordings of respiratory movement and air flow, heart rate, muscle movement, and eye movements. In special circumstances, recordings are made of arterial blood pressure and of end-tidal Pco_2 and Po_2 by pulse oximetry. Thus, monitoring in the neonate is most accurately designated as time-synchronized EEG/polygraphic/video monitoring.

INSTRUMENTATION

The monitoring instrument in use in our laboratory is shown in Figure 1. Its components are mounted onto a standard 16-channel electroencephalograph.

Electroencephalograph. Twelve channels of the EEG are routinely recorded from electrodes placed on the frontal, temporal, and occipital regions of the scalp. A single sequence of EEG derivations (a montage) is used throughout the recording.

Polygraphic Recording. Several parameters are recorded to characterize specific changes in the clinical state of the infant. Respirations are recorded on two additional channels of the EEG. Thoracic and/or abdominal respiratory movements are recorded either by use of strain gauges around each region or by impedance measurement across the chest. Air flow is measured by a sensing device (thermistor) placed at one nostril. End-tidal Pco_2 and pulse oximetry may also be recorded and displayed as tracings on the EEG. The electrocardiogram (ECG) is recorded from electrodes placed on the chest and is displayed on one channel of the EEG. The electromyogram (EMG)

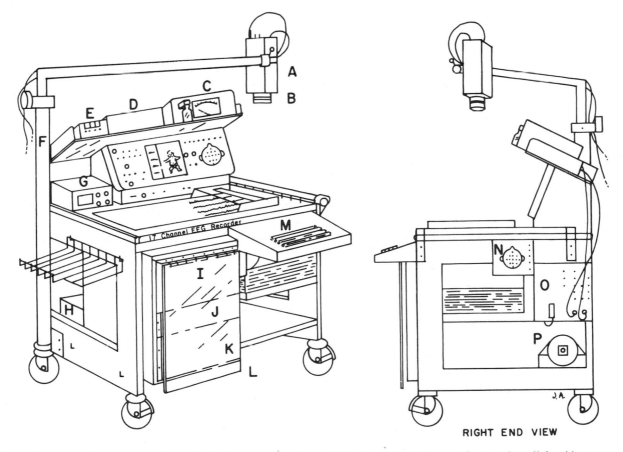

Figure 1 Schematic drawing of the cribside, time-synchronized, EEG/polygraphic/video monitor. *A*, Low-light video camera; *B*, automatic aperture lens; *C*, Pco_2 monitor; *D*, storage area for monitoring accessories; *E*, videocassette recorder; *F*, adjustable camera boom; *G*, Po_2 monitor; *H*, isolation transformer; *I*, area for blood pressure monitoring instrumentation; *J*, time clock and video titler; *K*, waveform reformatter; *L*, Plexiglas protective equipment cover; *M*, keyboard assembly for titler; *N*, EEG headboard; *O*, EEG interface panel (standard Nihon Kohden); *P*, calibration gas cylinder and regulator for Pco_2 monitor. (Reprinted, with permission, from Kellaway P, Frost JD Jr. Monitoring at the Baylor College of Medicine, Houston. In: Gotman J, Ives JR, Gloor P, eds. Long-term monitoring in epilepsy (EEG Suppl. No. 37). Amsterdam: Elsevier, 1985:403.

may be recorded from electrodes placed over specific muscle groups and displayed on one EEG channel. Eye movements (electro-oculogram) are recorded from electrodes placed medial and lateral to one eye and displayed on another channel of the EEG. Systemic blood pressure (BP) may be recorded from an umbilical artery transducer; a BP tracing is displayed on one EEG channel. Not all polygraphic parameters are recorded in each infant; specific parameters are selected, depending on the clinical situation.

Video Recording. A low-light, black-and-white video camera is mounted onto a camera boom, which can be placed above the infant. Videotaping is performed without special lights, under ambient conditions of the NICU. Color cameras are not used because they require continuous adjustment and additional lighting. A portable, four-head, one-half-inch VHS videocassette recorder is used. The television monitor is mounted in the EEG console.

Time Synchronization. The EEG and the polygraphic parameters must be time-locked to the videotaped image of the infant. This is accomplished by a time clock that simultaneously displays the time digitally (to 1 sec) on the video image and in analog code on the EEG.

Video Display. The infant is displayed on one-half of the television monitoring screen, and several of the EEG or polygraphic channels are displayed on the other half. This is accomplished by a screen-splitting device and a waveform reformatter. In addition, patient identification information and the EEG channel designations are displayed by a video titler and a keyboard mounted on the monitor console.

Instrument Maintenance. When establishing a monitoring service, the need to maintain the instrumentation is often overlooked. However, when the basis of the monitoring service is the capability to record fleeting clinical events on an emergency basis, the monitoring instruments must always be in working order. Thus, mechanical engineers with expertise in EEG and video instrumentation are as important as the instruments themselves. They perform routine maintenance and are on call around the clock.

MONITORING PROTOCOL

Availability. To be an effective clinical tool, monitoring must be available on a 24-hour, 7-day-a-week, emergency basis. At Texas Children's Hospital, a monitoring instrument is stored in the NICU and can be brought easily and quickly to cribside (a back-up unit is located in the Clinical Neurophysiology Laboratory). A group of specially trained technologists are continuously on call. A clinical neurophysiologist is also on call and at cribside for interpretation of each study as it is being performed.

Timing of Monitoring. The best time to monitor an infant is when the suspected clinical events are occurring—ideally, before anticonvulsant therapy has been started. Thus, a rapid response by the monitoring team is required.

History Taking. It is important to determine the features of the clinical events that prompted the request for the monitoring study so that they can be looked for during the study. This may require discussions with referring physicians, house officers, nurses, or others who may have witnessed the suspicious clinical event.

Infant Observation. An important aspect of monitoring is the direct observation of the infant by the technologist and the clinical neurophysiologist. A written log is maintained during monitoring, with notations made of the time and type of clinical care given and blood assays obtained. Because some abnormal, nonepileptic behaviors may be evoked by tactile stimulation or suppressed by restraint, the technologist or clinical neurophysiologist must be ready to perform these maneuvers.

Monitoring During Critical Care. Because many of the neonates who require monitoring may be critically ill, it is important that the monitoring not disrupt the clinical management. For this reason, the instrument and monitoring protocols have been designed to allow complete access to the infant.

DATA ANALYSIS

The monitoring studies are interpreted both at cribside, to provide immediate clinical information, and later, to characterize EEG, polygraphic, and video findings more precisely. When clinical events have been recorded, they are viewed in real time, in slow motion (to evaluate components of the movements), and at high speed (to determine less apparent patterns of repetition of behavior).

The EEG is evaluated for the presence and character of seizure activity and its relationship to clinical events, for background activity, for developmental characteristics, and for waveforms that may be abnormal but not epileptogenic.

CLINICAL RELEVANCE OF MONITORING

Seizure Detection. The finding of EEG seizure activity that has a close and consistent relationship to paroxysmal clinical signs is the clearest indication that a seizure of epileptic origin is occurring. Although this may seem obvious, there are circumstances in which seizure activity may be noted in the EEG without accompanying EEG seizure activity (see below). Thus, the finding of EEG seizure activity, alone, does not imply that any observed abnormal movements of the patient represent an epileptic seizure. *It is the correlation of the electrical seizure with the clinical event that is crucial for diagnosis.*

Seizure Characterization and Classification. Monitoring can be helpful in characterizing and classifying neonatal seizures. Clinical events can be described precisely and even shown (on videotape) to those caring for the infant. Thus, seizure frequency and the emergence of new types of clinical seizures can be determined. The classification of seizures also has clinical relevance, since certain seizure types appear to be associated with certain etiologic factors, prognoses, and pathophysiologic mechanisms of initiation and elaboration (see below).

Seizure Quantification. Determination of the effectiveness of therapy is important in the management of neonatal seizures. For example, in an untreated newborn, the clinical seizures may be closely associated with EEG seizure activity. However, in response to anticonvulsants, the clinical seizures may be "decoupled" from the electrical seizures; i.e., the clinical seizures are suppressed, but the electrical seizures persist. If the end point of anticonvulsant therapy is the elimination of the clinical seizures, clinical observation is adequate to quantify a response. However, if the end point is the elimination of the epileptic activity in the brain, further EEG monitoring is required (see below).

CURRENT CONCEPTS OF NEONATAL SEIZURES AND CRIBSIDE MONITORING

Although EEG/polygraphic/video monitoring is not yet widely available for the routine management of neonatal seizures, its application to the investigation of this disorder has provided new data concerning seizures and neonates with CNS dysfunction. By means of EEG/polygraphic/video monitoring techniques, neonatal seizures have been characterized and an electroclinical classification system has been devised. Two major categories of clinical seizures and one category of electrical seizures were identified (Table 1).

Clinical Seizures with a Consistent Electrocortical Signature

Clinical events that consistently occur in association with EEG seizure activity constitute approximately one-third of the clinical seizures of the newborn. They include *focal clonic* seizures (unifocal, alternating, migrating, or hemiconvulsive); *focal tonic* seizures (tonic eye deviation, tonic posturing of one limb, or asymmetric posturing of the trunk); and some *myoclonic* seizures (focal or generalized).

The movements of focal clonic seizures are rhythmic and regular, and cannot be suppressed with light restraint. Focal clonic seizures are most often seen in infants who are awake and alert, have normal background EEG activity, and have etiologic factors characterized as focal structural or irritative lesions. The short-term outcome for these infants is relatively good.

Seizures with a consistent electrocortical signature are most clearly epileptic in origin. Anticonvulsants are indicated; however, because of the "decoupling" effect of the anticonvulsants, the appropriate end point of therapy (elimination of clinical seizures versus elimination of electrical seizures) has not been established.

Clinical Seizures with No Electrical Signature

These seizures include generalized, *symmetric tonic* seizures, almost all "subtle" seizures (currently referred to as *motor automatisms*), and some generalized and focal myoclonic seizures. This group represents approximately two-thirds of the clinical seizures of the newborn.

TABLE 1 Electroclinical Classification of Neonatal Seizures*

I.   Clinical seizures with a consistent electrocortical signature
   A. Focal clonic
     1. Unifocal
     2. Multifocal
       a. Alternating
       b. Migrating
     3. Hemiconvulsive
     4. Axial
   B. Myoclonic
     1. Generalized
     2. Focal
   C. Focal tonic
     1. Asymmetric truncal
     2. Eye deviation
II. Clinical seizures with no electrocortical signature
   A. Motor automatisms
     1. Oral-buccal-lingual movements
     2. Ocular movements
     3. Progression movements
       a. Pedaling
       b. Stepping
       c. Rotary arm movements
     4. Complex purposeless movements
   B. Generalized tonic
     1. Extensor
     2. Flexor
     3. Mixed extensor/flexor
   C. Myoclonic
     1. Generalized
     2. Focal
III. Electrical seizures without clinical seizures

* Infantile spasms and episodic apnea (associated with EEG seizure activity) may also occur as neonatal seizures, but they are rare and currently do not warrant major classifications.

Some neonates with tonic posturing or motor automatisms have characteristic responses to stimulation and restraint. Tactile stimulation may evoke clinical seizures, and light restraint or repositioning of the limbs, trunk, or head may suppress the clinical event. Tonic posturing and motor automatisms occur most often in infants who are lethargic or obtunded, have depressed and undifferentiated background EEG activity, and have etiologic factors consistent with diffuse neuropathology (most frequently, hypoxic-ischemic encephalopathy). The short-term outcome for infants with these types of seizures is relatively poor, with high incidences of both neurologic abnormality at the time of hospital discharge and mortality.

The clinical features of infants with tonic posturing and motor automatisms, the characteristic response of these behaviors to tactile stimulation and restraint, the character of the background EEG activity, and the absence of EEG seizure activity suggest that these clinical events are not generated or elaborated by an epileptic pathophysiologic mechanism. The findings are more consistent with primitive, reflex behaviors, referred to as "brainstem release phenomena." This supposition, that tonic posturing and motor automatisms are nonepileptic in origin, indicates that anticonvulsant therapy may not be required.

Electrical Seizures Without Clinical Seizures

Electroencephalographic seizure activity in the absence of clinical seizures may occur in infants who are pharmacologically paralyzed for respiratory care, in infants already treated with anticonvulsants, and in untreated infants who have severe encephalopathies. In the last instance, infants are obtunded or lethargic and have depressed and undifferentiated background EEG activity. Electrical seizure activity, unaccompanied by clinical signs, in an infant not yet treated with anticonvulsants is indicative of a poor prognosis.

A particularly difficult clinical dilemma is posed by EEG seizure activity without associated clinical signs. Electrical seizure activity can be remarkably resistant to anticonvulsant therapy. With increasing dosages, the infant's state of alertness and background EEG activity may become depressed, yet the electrical seizure activity may persist. In some instances the depressant effects of the anticonvulsants may be so great as to render the infant obtunded and the EEG virtually isoelectric except for the electrical seizure activity. The desire to avoid undue depression of the neonatal CNS is tempered by the recognition that some animal studies have suggested that electrical seizure activity in the immature brain may be detrimental. Specific criteria for therapy under these circumstances have not yet been established.

WHAT IS A NEONATAL SEIZURE?

Throughout this discussion, neonatal seizures have been described in both clinical and electrical terms. Clinical seizures have been described as occurring both in close association with EEG seizure activity (epileptic in origin) and without accompanying EEG seizure activity (presumably nonepileptic in origin). Are both types of clinical events seizures, and should they continue to be referred to as such in clinical practice? In the classic use of the term "seizure," all the clinical events described here are seizures; they are paroxysmal, abnormal clinical behaviors. However, neonatal seizures are not a homogeneous group. Certain seizure types may have specific underlying pathophysiologic mechanisms that may ultimately indicate specific therapies. Thus, although all the clinical events discussed here are "seizures," not all are necessarily *epileptic* seizures.

It should be emphasized, however, that regardless of the type of clinical seizure or the pathophysiologic mechanism responsible for its elaboration, all the clinical seizures described indicate the presence of significant CNS dysfunction. In this regard, the findings of monitoring studies do not change a fundamental concept concerning seizures of the newborn: that *each newly diagnosed neonatal seizure represents a neurologic emergency.*

SUGGESTED READING

Gotman J, Ives JR, Gloor P, eds. Long-term monitoring in epilepsy (EEG Suppl. No. 37). Amsterdam: Elsevier Science Publishers BV, 1985.

Kellaway P, Frost JD Jr. Monitoring at the Baylor College of Medicine, Houston. In: Gotman J, Ives JR, Gloor P, eds. Long-term monitoring in epilepsy (EEG Suppl. No. 37). Amsterdam: Elsevier Science Publishers BV, 1985:403.

Kellaway P, Hrachovy RA. Status epilepticus in newborns: a perspective on neonatal seizures. Adv Neurol 1983; 34:93.

Kellaway P, Mizrahi EM. Neonatal seizures. In: Lüders H, Lesser RP, eds. Epilepsy: electroclinical syndromes. New York: Springer-Verlag, 1987:13.

Meldrum BS. Metabolic factors during prolonged seizures and their relationship to nerve cell death. Adv Neurol 1983; 34:261.

Mizrahi EM, Kellaway P. Characterization and classification of neonatal seizures. Neurology 1987; 37:1837.

Volpe JJ. Neurology of the newborn. Philadelphia: WB Saunders, 1986:129.

Wasterlain CG. Inhibition of cerebral protein synthesis by epileptic seizures without motor manifestations. Neurology 1974; 24:175.

EXCHANGE TRANSFUSION

PHILIP J. LIPSITZ, M.D.

Exchange transfusion (ET) was first popularized in 1951 by Diamond, who inserted a plastic catheter in the umbilical vein of a newborn with hemolytic disease and hyperbilirubinemia. The technique was universally accepted and the procedure soon became part of the armamentarium of neonatal medicine. *Over the last decade, the number of ETs performed has significantly decreased because of the rare occurrence of Rh-hemolytic disease of the newborn and the prophylactic and therapeutic use of phototherapy* in newborn nurseries and neonatal intensive care units. In our large tertiary neonatal unit over the past few years, the use of ET has been limited to two to three per 1,000 of all admissions.

INDICATIONS

At present, there are only two major indications for ET in the newborn: (1) replacement of blood components without major perturbation of hemodynamic parameters, and (2) removal of excess circulating bilirubin.

ET has occasionally been performed in the newborn with severe sepsis as part of the medical management. It has also been used for removal of other circulating toxins, but more recently hemodialysis and continuous arteriovenous hemofiltration have been used in the newborn and are probably more effective than ET.

This review does not comment on the absolute indications for ET, as each perinatal center has established definitive criteria for its use.

PREPARATION OF THE NEWBORN FOR ET

Current obstetric practice identifies in utero the newborn who is severely affected by hemolytic disease. It would be prudent for such a patient to be delivered in a perinatal center.

The newborn with hemolytic disease who is severely compromised in utero and would require an ET is rapidly stabilized after delivery with correction of asphyxia, hypoxia, and acidosis. The newborn who has gradually developed a potential toxic level of bilirubin necessitating ET is usually clinically stable and may have had several feedings before the procedure needs to be performed. If an ET is anticipated, feeding should be held for 4 hours. However, if this is not possible, the gastric contents should be aspirated before the ET is performed to prevent vomiting and aspiration. The nasogastric tube is left in place. The preference in this center is to start an intravenous infusion of 10 percent dextrose in water and electrolyte solution at the onset of the procedure.

An ET in a sick, low birth weight newborn may present an additional risk. Careful attention to the respiratory and hemodynamic status is necessary during the ET. The use of a transcutaneous Po_2 electrode or oxygen saturation monitor is of great benefit in this circumstance. In some of these patients, it may often be necessary to buffer the donor blood with bicarbonate 1.0 mEq per 100 ml of blood if acidosis is present, as determined by arterial blood gases obtained prior to and during the procedure. The use of 0.3 molar tris- (hydroxymethyl) aminomethane (THAM) has also been advocated for correction of the mixed metabolic and respiratory acidosis of donor blood.

The newborn is placed on a radiant warmer, and monitor electrodes are applied for continuous heart and respiratory rate recording. The skin temperature also needs constant monitoring. Blood pressure may be recorded from an umbilical artery catheter already in place or a cuff applied to a limb for oscillometric measurement. The unit is cycled to give readings every 2 to 3 minutes. Equipment for resuscitation is readily available. A nurse is in attendance to record the vital signs and the volumes of blood exchanged.

TYPE OF BLOOD USED FOR EXCHANGE TRANSFUSION

Heparinized blood is the most ideal donor blood to use, but it is not readily available. Heparinized blood has no effect on serum calcium, magnesium, or blood glucose levels, and clots do not form in the catheter. There is a transient rise in nonesterified fatty acids after transfusion of the heparin.

Acid citrate dextrose anticoagulated blood, when infused into the circulation of a vigorous term newborn, is readily buffered, the excess CO_2 eliminated by the lungs, and the citrate metabolized. In the compromised preterm newborn, however, adequate compensation may not occur.

Citrate phosphate dextrose anticoagulated blood is generally used in most centers. However, even after 1 to 2 days, potassium levels are greatly increased in stored blood. These may be lowered by washing the red blood cells before reconstitution. Most blood banks now have available fresh red blood cell concentrates that require reconstitution with fresh frozen plasma.

The donor red blood cells should be compatible with both maternal and newborn antibodies and are reconstituted with AB, Rh-positive donor fresh frozen plasma. The desired hematocrit of the reconstituted blood should be indicated. This can be readily achieved by the blood bank technologist by means of a relatively simple calculation using the volume (weight) of the red blood cells, the hematocrit of the red blood cells, and the volume (weight) of the fresh frozen plasma. The volume of blood requested is usually twice the approximate blood volume of the newborn patient. Estimates of blood volume average 85 ml per kilogram in term infants and 100 ml per kilogram in preterm infants.

TECHNICAL CONSIDERATIONS

As originally described, ET was performed in a sterile operating room. The procedure is now performed in the neonatal intensive care unit but requires the same sterile techniques as used in an operating room.

A commercially available kit is used. The umbilical cord area is washed with a povidone-iodine solution. The periumbilical area is covered with sterile drapes. The umbilical cord is cut with a blade, and the umbilical vein is identified as the large and least muscular-walled vessel. Blood clots noted should be removed, and the No. 8 French catheter in the term newborn or No. 5 French catheter in the perterm infant is gently inserted into the umbilical vein. Rarely a supraumbilical cutdown on the vein or a cutdown on a peripheral vein may be necessary.

If an umbilical artery catheter is already in position, it may be used for the procedure if the umbilical vein cannot be identified.

CATHETER PLACEMENT AND MEASUREMENT OF VENOUS PRESSURE

The catheter is pushed to a depth that allows for easy blood return, usually 6 cm (first marking). There is no technical difficulty in performing the ET at this position. If difficulty is encountered, gently rotate the catheter, as the vessel wall may adhere to the side hole during withdrawal. If the catheter is pushed in farther, it may enter the portal sinus within the liver. In 50 to 70 percent of newborns, the catheter may pass through the ductus venosus into the inferior vena cava, and at 10 to 12 cm in the full-term infant it will reach the right atrium. Portal venous pressure is usually plus or minus 10 cm H_2O and central venous pressure is plus or minus 2.0 cm H_2O. Changes in pressure with respiration may be useful in determining the site of the catheter tip. The pressure rises on inspiration and falls on expiration. An x-ray film is not necessary to confirm the position of the catheter tip if the venous pressure is measured. *Most newborns requiring ET are not hypervolemic, and careful consideration should be given to removing and infusing equal volumes.*

PROCEDURE

Donor blood is warmed to 37°C (98.6°F) before infusion. The tubing from the donor blood is connected to a coil of plastic tubing (commercially available) and put in a 37°C waterbath. Frequent checks of the waterbath temperature are desired to assure warm blood for the severely compromised infant. The plastic bag of donor blood frequently should be gently mixed to prevent sedimentation of red cells.

The "push-pull" method is most commonly used. Various other techniques have been described using pumps that simultaneously withdraw and infuse the blood. A two-way exchange using the umbilical artery for withdrawal and the vein for infusion may be used in the very unstable newborn to eliminate the swings in blood volume and pressure that occur with the push-pull method.

The umbilical vein catheter is removed at the end of the procedure unless it has been ascertained to be in the inferior vena cava and needs to be used as a central line for the infusion of hypertonic solutions. If a repeat ET is indicated, the same technique is used. Prophylactic antibiotic therapy is not indicated.

The first aliquot of blood is labeled "pre-exchange blood" and is used for the determination of bilirubin, a complete blood count, and electrolyte content. Some of the blood should be saved for other tests that may be indicated. An equal volume of donor blood is then given and the procedure continues with exchange of equal aliquots. *It is generally recommended not to exceed the removal of more than 10 percent of the infant's circulating blood volume at one time.* Most commonly 10 to 20 ml aliquots are used. Monitoring of the heart rate and blood pressure should alert one to significant hemodynamic changes.

The ET is a flushing out of the intravascular space. Initially the removal of blood is mainly the infant's blood, but later in the procedure most of the donor's blood is also removed. It is, therefore, suggested that using large aliquots of blood out and in would be more efficient in removing more bilirubin and exchanging more of the infant's blood. This may lead to the removal of a dangerously large volume of blood and stress the cardiovascular adaptive mechanisms, and it is not more effective than the use of the recommended aliquots. It has been estimated that the efficiency of removal of the newborn's blood volume is approximately 85 percent using the procedure as described.

The rate of ET has been studied. *The most satisfactory rate producing the least hemodynamic changes is 5 ml per kilogram per 2 to 3 minutes.* The total procedure is usually performed in 60 to 90 minutes, during which time the vital signs of the infant are carefully monitored and recorded. Any significant change warrants stopping the ET and a thorough physical examination of the newborn.

ASSOCIATED DERANGEMENTS DURING EXCHANGE TRANSFUSION

In the very compromised newborn, significant morbidity such as apnea, bradycardia, cardiac arrest, cardiac arrhythmias, and vasospasm with thrombosis may be noted. Resuscitation equipment should therefore always be immediately available. The incidence of morbidity during ET has varied from 5 to 10 percent.

The procedure is safe in most instances, but due to the infrequent need for ET in the late 1980s and therefore less experience with the technique on the part of the physician, it is possible that the mortality and morbidity rates may increase. It is appropriate to inform parents of the risks.

The citrate in the donor blood may produce significant changes in the divalent cations, calcium, and magnesium. It has been recommended that calcium gluconate be administered during the ET to counteract citrate binding, but this does not significantly affect serum ionized calcium. During the ET many newborns manifest episodes of crying or irritability and even jitteriness, but these cannot be correlated with low ionized calcium levels. Like others, *we do not administer calcium gluconate during the* ET and have not noticed any adverse effects in the newborn. Changes in serum magnesium do not result in clinical symptoms and do not require correction unless there has been a previously recognized hypomagnesemia.

POSTEXCHANGE MANAGEMENT

Thirty minutes after the ET, a blood sample is obtained for bilirubin level, complete blood count, platelet count, electrolytes, and calcium concentration. Perturbations in serum electrolytes have been noted after exchange. This may be avoided by careful processing and selection of the donor blood.

Necrotizing enterocolitis has occurred in the newborn following ET. *The policy in our center is to keep the baby on nothing by mouth for 12 hours after ET.* The peripheral intravenous solution of 10 percent dextrose in water and electrolytes is maintained in order to administer the fluid requirements related to age and weight. When started the feeding is usually 15 to 30 ml and it is increased as tolerated; the intravenous line is discontinued at an appropriate time.

In the newborn with hemolytic disease a screening of the blood glucose is obtained every 30 minutes after exchange for a 2- to 3-hour period, since hypoglycemia has been frequently noted. If hypoglycemia is demonstrated, the intravenous infusion rate is increased to administer 6 to 8 mg per kilogram per minute of glucose. The blood glucose level is checked frequently and when the infant is euglycemic, the intravenous rate is gradually decreased.

Bilirubin levels are determined every 4 to 6 hours after exchange. ET removes 75 to 80 percent of the albumin-bound bilirubin, but extravascular bilirubin equilibrates within 30 minutes and produces a rebound of serum bilirubin to 60 percent of the pre-exchange level. Administration of albumin before or during ET has been recommended to enhance the removal of bilirubin, but conflicting results of its efficacy have been reported. It should be used with caution in the severely compromised newborn, as it may produce acute pulmonary edema and hemorrhage.

A moderate transient thrombocytopenia commonly occurs following exchange and, because in most blood banks platelets have been removed from the donor blood, platelet transfusion may be required when the newborn platelet count is less than 20,000 per cubic millimeter, or other bleeding manifestations are noted.

Donor blood should be carefully screened for sickle trait or disease because of reports of massive intravascular sickling after ET with the inadvertent use of such donor blood.

LATE COMPLICATIONS

The generally accepted definition of mortality related to an ET is death within 6 hours of the procedure. In the National Institute of Child Health and Human Development collaborative phototherapy study, the mortality was 0.53 percent and 0.3 percent per procedure.

Graft versus host disease may occur in the newborn following ET if intrauterine transfusions have been given. In the immunologically compromised newborn a similar clinical syndrome may occur following a postnatal ET.

Donor red blood cells for ET should be irradiated before administration in any of these newborns.

There have been previous reports of viral infections following ET, this may be avoided by careful screening of donor blood, as performed in most blood banks now.

SUGGESTED READING

Aranda JV, Sweet AY. Alterations in blood pressure during exchange transfusion. Arch Dis Child 1977; 52:545–548.

Diamond LK, Allen FH, Thomas WO. Erythroblastosis fetalis. VII. Treatment with exchange transfusion. N Eng J Med 1951; 244:39–49.

Farquhar JW, Smith H. Clinical and biochemical changes during exchange transfusion. Arch Dis Child 1958; 33:142–159.

Phibbs RH. Advances in the theory and practice of exchange transfusions. Calif Medicine 1966; 105:442–453.

Sotelo-Avila C, Brouillette RT, Gould SD. The hematocrit of reconstituted blood for exchange transfusion in newborn infants. J Pediatr 1982; 100:971–974.

Sproul A, Smith L. Bilirubin equilibration during exchange transfusion in hemolytic disease of the newborn. J Pediatr 1964; 65:12–18.

GRANULOCYTE TRANSFUSION

FRANCESCO LAURENTI, M.D.

NEONATAL SEPSIS

The failure of antibiotics and supportive therapy to eradicate neonatal death from sepsis encourages investigation in the area of host defense mechanisms. Antibodies and complement, as well as neutrophils, are the factors most implicated in defense against extracellular bacteria. They cooperate subsequently in elimination of germs through opsonization (first line of defense) and phagocytosis (second line of defense). In neonates both these mechanisms are impaired, which suggests that an adequate reconstitution could be effective in the treatment of neonatal sepsis.

The first report on the use of granulocyte transfusion (GT) dates back to 1978 and concerns a 1.4-kg infant with *Klebsiella* sepsis. The surprising, successful response to a single transfusion unit prompted us to initiate more extensive trials and to standardize the best management.

In this article some basic concepts about the treatment of neonatal sepsis with GT are briefly reviewed, as well as the clinical results and a critical evaluation of the problems emerging after a 10-year experience.

Rationale

The most intuitive indication for GT in neonatal sepsis is the detection of *neutropenia and/or bone marrow depletion* in severe infections. This condition is quite unusual in Italy, probably because of the infrequent occurrence of group B *Streptococcus* sepsis. Therefore, we focused our attention on another apparently less obvious, but far more common, indication: the recently recognized *multifactorial impairment of neonatal neutrophils.* In neo-

nates several neutrophil activities show a basic impairment of function, especially chemotaxis and killing of selected microbial species. More recent findings emphasize that this basic defect can further decay in the course of sepsis or other disorders: it may be that the bacterial and/or toxin overload, together with hypoxia, hypoperfusion, and acidosis, induce a primary perturbation of neutrophil membranes followed by deactivation or autoxidation.

Also, in our experimental and clinical experience, infants with severe infections or other stressful conditions (more so in the case of preterms) showed a relevant fall of neutrophil activities, and could be compared with neutropenic patients, even when their circulating granulocytes were above the normal range.

Clinical Studies

In subsequent communications we have reported the results of different clinical trials. In this article we illustrate the final data obtained by the overall number of proved cases of sepsis, collected over about 10 years, and treated with GT. In addition, we hint at a pilot study concerning the treatment of neonatal meningitis with GT.

We should specify that our studies must be considered as controlled but not prospectively planned, at least according to the usual definition. In fact, our design treated with GT all the eligible infants, and considered as controls the infants who could not be treated for reasons independent of our wishes, such as the unavailability of appropriate granulocyte donors. This plan was chosen by considering the basic difficulty in obtaining concentrates for all the patients, and a certain number of infants thus escaped.

However, in the final evaluation we ended up with an equal number of treated and untreated babies (Table 1): 92 patients met more properly the usually accepted criteria for sepsis, whereas the remaining 16 presented with septic shock.

TABLE 1 Comprehensive Clinical Material in 108 Neonates: Positive Blood Culture

	GT	No GT
Total number	54	54
Sepsis	48	44
Septic shock	6	10

The treated and untreated groups were quite comparable in risk factors: birth weight and gestational age distribution (Table 2) and the severity injury score (Table 3).

Management

Table 4 shows how the concentrates were prepared: in the first period granulocytes were collected by leukofiltration and subsequently by centrifugation. Although this second method of collection is more reliable, we never had the impression that the granulocytes so prepared were more effective or safe.

The treatment protocol is shown in Table 5.

Tables 6 and 7 illustrate the usually accepted diagnostic criteria for sepsis and septic shock.

Analysis of Results

By considering the total number of patients, the case fatality rate was significantly lower in treated than in untreated patients (43.7 percent versus 68.1 percent; $p < 0.02$).

Selecting the results on the basis of the different risk factors, more detailed data emerged.

Case Fatality Rate According to Birth Weight (Table 8). A more significant difference was found in the group with birth weight ranging from 1 to 2.5 kg; under 1-kg mortality was quite high in both series. Therefore, the most favorable results occurred in non-neutropenic preterm infants, in whom a functional decay of neutrophil chemotaxis and killing is easily established, as demonstrated in most of them.

On the other hand, the very low birth weight (VLBW) infants (<1 kg) continue to be habitual victims of the bacterial septicemias. In these cases the critical factor is not only the profound impairment of the defense mechanisms, but also the extreme dysfunction of reactivity and homeostasis, which determines the easy occurrence of severe complications, such as intraventricular hemorrhage (IVH), ischemic-necrotic areas, disseminated intravascular coagulation (DIC), necrotizing enterocolitis (NEC), and systemic hypoperfusion.

Case Fatality Rate According to Bacterial Etiology (Table 9). *A significantly lower case fatality rate was demonstrated in treated infants with sepsis due to Klebsiella.* The number of patients with sepsis due to *Pseudomonas* or *Staphylococcus* species was limited, but no trend toward a possible difference in mortality was apparent. Cases with other etiologies were too scattered to allow any suggestion; unfortunately, no data emerged about group B *Streptococcus* and *Escherichia coli*, since these bacteria were hardly represented in our material.

TABLE 2 Birth Weight (BW) and Gestational Age (GA) Distribution in Neonates With and Without GT

	No. of Patients	BW (g)	GA (wks)
500–1,000 g			
GT	11	939 ± 63	27.5 ± 2
No GT	8	827 ± 108	27.0 ± 2
1,001–2,500 g			
GT	32	1,697 ± 427	31.7 ± 3
No GT	27	1,795 ± 483	32.0 ± 3
> 2,500 g			
GT	5	3,142 ± 257	39.0 ± 1
No GT	9	3,095 ± 428	38.2 ± 2

TABLE 3 Severity Injury Score in Neonates With and Without GT*

	GT (%)	No GT (%)
Respiratory distress syndrome	36	49
Intraventricular hemorrhage	19	10
Asphyxia	21	23
$FiO_2 > 0.70$	19	23
Mechanical ventilation	56	64

* Difference in incidence is never significant.

TABLE 4 Preparation of Granulocyte Concentrates

Isogroup donors monitored for: Syphilis, BHV, CMV,
EBV, HIV

Collection ⌈ Leukofiltration (lymphocytes 2–5%)
⌊ Centrifugation* (lymphocytes 10–20%)

* Irradiation = 1,500–2,000 rad.
CMV = cytomegalovirus; EBV = Epstein-Barr virus; BHV = hepatitis B virus; HIV = human immunodeficiency virus.

TABLE 5 GT Protocol

Standard transfusion unit: 20 ml/kg ($0.5-1 \times 10^9$ cells)
Rate: 1 unit every 12 or 24 hrs
Treatment period: usually 5–7 days or more if required

TABLE 6 Eligible Infants: Early Diagnostic Requirements

At least three of the following criteria for inclusion in the GT protocol:*

Maternal fever, prolonged rupture of membranes
Otherwise unexplained depression, gray color, abdominal distention, sclerema, vomiting, apneic spells
Neutropenia ($< 1,500/\mu l$); I/T ratio > 0.20; vacuolizations and toxic granulations

* Final inclusion only when blood culture was positive. I/T = immature/total granulocytes.

TABLE 7 Septic Shock: Diagnostic Requirements

Signs of systemic hypoperfusion
Gray color, respiratory failure, oliguria, central nervous system depression (otherwise unexplained)
Intractable hypotension
Sudden onset and deterioration

As far as *Klebsiella* is concerned, this strain circulated in our intensive care unit (ICU), was resistant to all the in vitro tested antibiotics, and caused a sequence of cross-infections showing an insidious but slow progression; worsening occurred only in the ultimate phase. The excellent results observed in *Klebsiella* sepsis probably had several causes: the slow clinical progression, the prevalent destruction of the organisms by means of the transfused phagocytes, and the low capacity of this strain to release endotoxin, as suggested by the unusual or late occurrence of endotoxemic shock.

The bacterial species represents a very critical point in the management of infections, as its invasiveness, initial germ load, antibiotic sensitivity, and specific resistance to host defense mechanisms deeply affect the efficacy of the treatment. Toxin generation is another relevant point because, when endotoxemia occurs, appropriate measures against this condition are a priority, and granulocyte supply may be only a second line of defense.

Case Fatality Rate According to Associated Severe Disorders (Table 10).   The concurrent presence of severe disorders, such as hyaline membrane disease (HMD), massive IVH, and birth asphyxia, modifies the effects of GT, partly suppressing its benefit. In fact, a markedly better outcome was noted in treated than in untreated infants when the above conditions were absent, whereas differences were small and statistically insignificant when they were present.

Case Fatality Rate in Patients with Septic Shock. All the six treated infants as well as the 10 untreated infants who presented with the typical picture of septic shock had a lethal outcome. However, the treated infants had the chance to receive only one granulocyte unit in preagonic conditions. It is difficult to speculate whether the death could be avoided with a quicker availability of the concentrates. Septic shock, indeed, still represents an enormous unsolved problem, being the chief obstacle to the lowering of the neonatal mortality. In such instances the

TABLE 8 Case Fatality Rate According to Birth Weight

	GT	No GT
500–1,000 g	9/11 (82%)	8/8 (100%)
1,001–2,500 g	11/32 (34%)	17/27 (63%)*
2,500 g	1/5 (20%)	5/9 (55%)
All patients	21/48 (43%)	30/44 (68%)†

* $p < 0.003$.
† $p < 0.002$.

TABLE 9 Case Fatality Rate According to Bacterial Etiology

	GT	No GT
Klebsiella	9/26 (34%)	14/18 (78%)
Pseudomonas	6/7 (85%)	6/6 (100%)
Staphylococcus	3/8 (37%)	4/10 (40%)
Other organisms	3/7 (43%)	5/10 (50%)

* Group A *Str.*: 3; group B *Str.*: 1; group D *Str.*: 3; *Str. viridans*: 1; *Proteus*: 2; *Enterobacter*: 2; *E. coli*: 5

TABLE 10 Case Fatality Rate According to Associated Severe Disorders (HMD, IVH, Asphyxia)

	GT	No GT
Isolated sepsis	5/17 (22%)*	11/15 (73%)
Sepsis plus associated disorders	16/31 (52%)	19/29 (66%)

* p < 0.02. HMD = hyaline membrane disease; IVH = intraventricular hemorrhage.

sudden onset and the overwhelming outcome hinder the timely onset of antibacterial treatment, and the explosive development of an uncontrolled inflammatory reaction wastes the metabolic circuits and causes irreversible systemic mitochondrial damage.

NEONATAL BACTERIAL MENINGITIS

From 1979 to 1983 a pilot study was performed in 23 patients consecutively admitted to the ICUs of two hospitals in Rome. In the whole series there were only 2 deaths, with a case fatality rate of 8.6 percent. The 21 patients who survived were followed up to the age of 3 years at least. Mild handicap was found in three patients and moderate to severe handicap in the remaining six.

The promising observation of this pilot study does not allow definite conclusions, but offers scope for further investigations.

The utility and limits of GT can be summarized by: (1) in general, a significant improvement of the case fatality rate; (2) an excellent result in the slow-progressing septicemias of premature infants weighing from 1 to 2.5 kg, and in sepsis due to *Klebsiella* species; and (3) an unsatisfactory effect in septic shock, in VLBW infants, and in sepsis associated with other severe conditions.

However, the present results can be applied only in well-defined circumstances, and different effects can be expected in diverse conditions. In view of the enormous range of aspects related to the treatment of neonatal infections, a definitive judgment is not yet possible. In contrast with animal experimentations, in which several conditions can be kept constant, in human trials a tremendous number of intriguing variables can affect mortality and must be carefully taken into account.

Therefore, isolated studies are presently inadequate to solve all the aspects of the problem, considering the few cases observed in each single ICU, the difficulty in rapid identification of organisms, and the numerous variables confusing the trial results.

A definitive answer to all the clinical questions can be obtained only by a well-designed and carefully conducted randomized multicentric trial.

SIDE EFFECTS

In more than 1,000 GT procedures performed in 10 years, clinically evident untoward effects never occurred:

neither early transfusional reactions (chills, fever, rash) nor late adverse effects, such as graft-versus-host disease (GVHD) and alloimmunization.

In order to better substantiate the risk of side effects, a study was carried out in 33 infants who had received several GT procedures in the first 3 weeks of life. In all the patients no clinical and laboratory sign of immunization, immunologic dysfunction, or GVHD was detected, as compared with the control group.

As neonatal tissues are elective targets for oxygen toxicity, GT can increase the risk of lytic-oxidative damage, since phagocytes release lysosomal proteases and oxidizing free radicals. This occurs particularly when granulocyte aggregation is established. In fact, neutrophils can aggregate intravascularly under the effect of various mediators (C5a, thromboxane, leukotrienes, bacterial toxins) profusely generated in the course of sepsis by the host inflammatory reaction. Although we never observed shock lung or other early manifestations of leukoaggregation, a study was performed in 14 patients in order to detect direct or indirect signs of leukoaggregation. Neither alteration of clinical state nor changes in peripheral white blood cell count, chest radiograph, $Ptco_2$ (transcutaneous Pco_2), heart rate, and mean arterial pressure occurred in all the patients monitored continuously during and after the GT. Also, in those infants in whom plasma granulocyte aggregating activity was detected, no clinical alteration appeared, suggesting that the packed white blood cells became in some way hyporeactive to the aggregating challenge. Indeed, a number of factors can impair aggregation, such as premedication of the donors with corticosteroids, the procedure used for collection, or the addition of substances that improve the granulocyte storage but inhibit function (e.g., calcium chelating agents).

Therefore, the risk of leukoembolization seems to be reasonably low, and probably is only present when a high concentration of plasma aggregating factors in the recipient is associated with a perfect responsiveness of the supplied cells.

In the area of neonatal GT, there are several unanswered questions that deserve further investigation: the silent risk of long-term lytic-oxidative tissue injury, the intimate routes by which transfused granulocytes operate in vivo, and finally the possible impairment of the macrophage system when overloaded by the granulocyte debris.

SUGGESTED READING

Laurenti F. WBC transfusion in the treatment of neonatal sepsis: 8 year experience. In: Three hot topics in neonatology. Special Ross Conference, Washington, DC, Dec. 15–18, 1985.

Laurenti F, Ferro R, Isacchi G, et al. Granulocyte transfusion in very small newborn infants with sepsis. In: Stern L, ed. Intensive care in the newborn. Vol 3. New York: Masson 1979:175.

Laurenti F, Ferro R, Isacchi G, et al. Polymorphonuclear leukocyte transfusion for the treatment of sepsis in the newborn infant. J Pediatr 1981; 98:118–123.

Laurenti F, La Greca G, Ferro R, Bucci G. Transfusion of polymorphonuclear neutrophils in a premature infant with *Klebsiella* sepsis. Lancet 1978; 2:111–112.

Stegagno M, Pascone R, Colarizi P, et al. Immunologic follow-up of infants treated with granulocyte transfusion for neonatal sepsis. Pediatrics 1985; 76:508–511.

HIGH-FREQUENCY VENTILATION

IVAN D. FRANTZ III, M.D.

High-frequency ventilation (HFV) has aroused much interest as a means of therapy for infants as well as older patients with respiratory failure. A number of techniques have been lumped together under the title HFV. Although these techniques have in common their use of higher than physiologic respiratory rates, they differ greatly in their means of application, tidal volume delivered, and perhaps mechanism of gas exchange. In this chapter I define the various techniques that have been referred to as HFV, describing the equipment involved and, where known, the physiologic interaction with the subject's respiratory system. In addition, I will try to indicate where these techniques may have application to infant respiratory disease.

There are four principal techniques that have the word "high" included in their names: high-frequency positive pressure ventilation (HFPPV), high-frequency jet ventilation (HFJV), high-frequency flow interruption (HFFI), and high-frequency oscillation (HFO) (Table 1). Most of what has been described can be fitted into one of these categories with some degree of overlap. HFFI and HFO differ most markedly from conventional techniques.

HIGH-FREQUENCY POSITIVE PRESSURE VENTILATION

HFPPV is the oldest of the techniques, having been described and used in Sweden for more than 10 years. The frequencies used have been 60 to 120 min^{-1}, hardly high by neonatal standards. The technique involves insufflation of air into the endotracheal tube by means of a catheter inserted into the tube or by direct connection of the endotracheal tube to a ventilator circuit with low compressible volume. *The tidal volumes used, although probably smaller than with conventional ventilation, are larger than the dead space* of the subject, and gas exchange probably occurs by bulk flow and convection, as with conventional ventilation.

Several advantages have been attributed to HFPPV, but the chief one is that it allows both the anesthetist and the surgeon access to the airway simultaneously. For instance, the insufflation catheter may be attached to a bronchoscope so that adequate ventilation can be continued during bronchoscopy. Other benefits, such as decreased interference with cardiovascular function, seem less clear and less well substantiated.

HFPPV per se has not been extensively evaluated in infants. Manual ventilation with an anesthesia bag or ventilation with a conventional ventilator at faster than usual rates has been used with some success to treat infants with respiratory distress syndrome (RDS), pulmonary interstitial emphysema, and persistent fetal circulation but does not represent a radical departure from conventional therapy. There is no reason why HFPPV should not be a useful adjunct to bronchoscopy in infants, as it has been in older subjects.

HIGH-FREQUENCY JET VENTILATION

HFJV represents an outgrowth of HFPPV. The rates used clinically have been somewhat higher, up to 250 to 300 min^{-1}, but substantially higher rates (to 1,000 min^{-1}) have been used in laboratory studies. In this technique, gas is injected through a small-bore cannula into the airway at a high flow rate. The injector may be located anywhere from the endotracheal tube adapter to close to the tip of the endotracheal tube. *The tidal volume produced by the jet itself may be relatively small, but because gas entrainment occurs (due to the high flow of gas through a venturi), the tidal volume delivered to the subject is increased.* In the frequency range used clinically tidal volumes are greater than dead space, and as with HFPPV, gas exchange is by convection.

HFJV has had the widest clinical use of any of the new techniques, although most of that has been in adults. As with HFPPV, jet ventilation has been useful in the operating room, particularly during bronchoscopy. The major disease in which it has been said to have efficacy is bronchopleural fistula, although convincing trials have not been published. Much of the use of HFJV in infants has been limited to uncontrolled experiences in which clear benefits have not been demonstrated, although large numbers of infants have been treated. Early use of jet ventilation was complicated by difficulty in achieving adequate humidification and by tracheal damage. These problems appear to be resolved, and at least one device has now been approved by the Food and Drug Administration for clinical use. A tendency for functional residual capacity to increase in some situations remains a concern. This

TABLE 1 Comparison of Techniques for High-Frequency Ventilation

Technique	Frequency (min^{-1})	Tidal Volume*	Gas Exchange Mechanism
HFPPV	60–120	$V_T > V_D$[†]	Convection
HFJV	100–300[‡]	$V_T > V_D$	Convection
HFFI	120–3,000	$V_T < V_D$	Convection plus augmented diffusion
HFO	120–3,000	$V_T < V_D$	Convection plus augmented diffusion

* V_T = tidal volume.
† V_D = dead space volume.
‡ Higher frequencies may be possible and desirable.

appears to be related to the duration of the expiratory phase, but the limits on duration of expiration at various tidal volumes have not yet been established. Pneumothoraces and significant cardiovascular compromise may occur.

Jet ventilation is the easiest of the new techniques to carry out, both because of simplicity of equipment and because of ease of achieving adequate gas exchange. Adequate settings can be found for almost any patient through trial and error.

HFJV may not reach its ultimate value until its use at frequencies higher than those currently popular has been explored. *At sufficiently high frequencies and low tidal volumes, jet ventilation may have the same potential for reducing pulmonary barotrauma as HFO.*

HIGH-FREQUENCY FLOW INTERRUPTION

This technique is an offshoot of HFO, developed to take advantage of simplicity of design of flow interrupters over oscillators. With this technique, a ball or poppet valve interrupts a bias flow of gas. The nature of the oscillations produced by a flow interrupter differs from those of a piston-type oscillator in that there is no to-and-fro movement of gas, but the physiologic effects and mechanisms of gas exchange are probably similar. HFFI has not been submitted to a controlled clinical trial; however, substantial experience in infants with air leaks and in whom there has been failure of conventional ventilation is being gathered.

HIGH-FREQUENCY OSCILLATION

HFO represents the biggest departure from conventional techniques of ventilation in terms of frequency, tidal volume, and mechanisms of gas exchange. Frequencies used have been up to 3,000 min^{-1}, but 600 to 900 min^{-1} has been the range most used in clinical studies. More exceptional than frequency, however, is the fact that *tidal volumes used are less than the dead space* of the subject. Such tidal volumes obviously imply that the mechanism of gas exchange must be different from that with conventional ventilation.

In HFO, oscillations of a bias gas flow are created. The devices used have relied on piston pumps, diaphragms, or loud-speakers to create the oscillations. HFO has been studied in a large multicenter controlled trial in premature infants with a need for mechanical ventilation. This trial did not demonstrate a beneficial effect on risk of mortal-

ity or occurrence of bronchopulmonary dysplasia. Reasons for this lack of beneficial effect include the fact that most infants received a period of conventional ventilation prior to being placed on HFO, many infants were crossed over from one technique to the other, some centers had no previous experience with HFO, and the technique may not have been optimally applied. Based on this study, HFO cannot be recommended as the treatment of choice for all infants needing ventilation, but it still may play a role in those infants with air leaks.

GAS EXCHANGE DURING HIGH-FREQUENCY VENTILATION

Although frequently presented as mysterious, gas exchange during HFV probably depends on the same basic mechanisms as during conventional ventilation: convection plus diffusion, with the balance between them being different. Since tidal volumes with HFPPV and jet ventilation are greater than dead space, there is no need to invoke other than conventional mechanisms for gas exchange, that is, convection in the proximal airways with diffusion in the alveoli. When tidal volumes are less than dead space, as with HFO, diffusion must take on a larger role. Convection still moves gas in and out of the largest airways and may even ventilate some alveoli. In addition, there is probably convective mixing between terminal units due to asynchronous filling. This phenomenon, known as *pendelluft*, may result in peripheral lung units exchanging gas several times with one another for each time they exchange with the trachea. Finally, however, there is probably an augmentation of diffusion caused by turbulent mixing at high flow rates. This results in gas transport by diffusion over a much longer portion of the airways than during conventional ventilation. The proportions of total gas exchange during HFO through bulk flow in the trachea, mixing between units, and augmented diffusion have not been established.

APPLICATION TO INFANTS

There is not at present an established indication for HFV in infants (Table 2). Its potential advantage is in situations in which pulmonary trauma due to pressure may occur or has occurred. Chronic lung disease has been described after prolonged conventional ventilation of infants for a variety of primary conditions, indicating that HFV may be beneficial in all of them. Severe pulmonary interstitial emphysema has responded well to HFV in

TABLE 2   Indications for HFV

Technique	Established	Probable	Potential
HFPPV	Bronchoscopy		Virtually any infant lung disease
HFJV	Bronchoscopy	Bronchopleural fistula	Virtually any infant lung disease
HFFI		Pulmonary interstitial emphysema	Virtually any infant lung disease
		Bronchopleural fistula	
HFO		Pulmonary interstitial emphysema	Virtually any infant lung disease
		Bronchopleural fistula	

uncontrolled studies and is a leading candidate for a disease that may be a specific indication for HFV.

Specification of ventilator settings is not yet possible because of limited experience. The variables to be manipulated include bias flow, frequency, amplitude of oscillations, waveform of oscillations, and mean airway pressure.

In choosing the mean airway pressure at which to ventilate, it is important to consider that *the pressure amplitude with HFO or HFFI is too low to overcome atelectasis. The lungs must therefore be inflated prior to starting HFO or HFFI and then brought down to a lung volume (mean airway pressure) that maintains alveolar patency.* If alveoli are allowed to collapse as suggested by falling PaO_2, the inflation must be repeated, and a higher mean pressure chosen. Amplitude of oscillation affects both oxygenation and carbon dioxide elimination; thus increasing amplitude through either increasing stroke volume or flow through an interrupter valve will improve both oxygenation and carbon dioxide elimination. Swings in alveolar pressure diminish with increasing frequency, and swings in tracheal pressure are at a minimum at the resonant frequency for any given flow rate. This presents a dilemma in the choice of the appropriate frequency for ventilation. To minimize tracheal barotrauma, one would ventilate at the resonant

frequency (approximately 1,000 min^{-1} in infants with RDS), but to minimize alveolar barotrauma, one would choose the highest frequency at which adequate gas exchange can be obtained.

HFV cannot be recommended as the treatment of choice for any infant lung disease at this time. Studies of oscillation mechanics of the infant respiratory system and gas exchange during HFV may soon indicate optimal methods of application. Pulmonary interstitial emphysema appears to be the most likely condition in which benefit will be seen.

SUGGESTED READING

Boynton BR, Hammond MD, Fredberg JJ, Buckley BG, Villanueva D, Frantz ID. Gas exchange in healthy rabbits during high frequency oscillatory ventilation. J Appl Physiol 1989; 66:1343–1351.
Carlo WA, Chatburn RL, Martin RJ. Randomized trial of high-frequency jet ventilation versus conventional ventilation in respiratory distress syndrome. J Pediatr 1987; 110:275–282.
Frantz ID, Werthammer JW, Stark AR. High frequency ventilation in premature infants with lung disease: adequate gas exchange at low tracheal pressure. Pediatrics 1983; 71:483–488.
The HIFI Study Group. High frequency oscillatory ventilation compared with conventional mechanical ventilation in the treatment of respiratory failure in preterm infants. N Engl J Med 1989; 320:88–93.

MECHANICAL VENTILATION

JEN-TIEN WUNG, M.D.

Early continuous positive airway pressure treatment of infants with respiratory distress may avoid the subsequent need for mechanical ventilation. However, mechanical ventilation is still a common therapy in neonatal intensive care units worldwide. Approaches to management and the incidence of related complications, such as lung rupture and bronchopulmonary dysplasia, vary considerably from institution to institution. Because of the possibility that the incidence of complications is related to the technique employed, the approach to artificial ventilation of the newborn infant merits special attention.

Protocols emphasizing modest but adequate ventilator settings should logically result in lower risk for complications. Ventilator functioning in the intermittent mandatory ventilation (IMV) mode allows spontaneous breathing and gradations of ventilatory support according to the degree of respiratory failure. Hence, the ventilator cycling frequency is less with IMV than in the control mode, and barotrauma and cardiovascular compromise are minimized and weaning is facilitated.

TYPE OF VENTILATOR

Most infant ventilators currently in use are time-cycled, pressure-limited, continuous flow devices, such as the BabyBird, Bourns BP200, Bear Cub, Healthdyne 105,

or Sechrist IV-100B infant ventilator. Their design features are similar in many respects. For successful treatment of respiratory failure, it is important that the involved personnel be familiar with the function of each parameter of the ventilator (FIO_2, flow rate, peak inspiratory pressure, positive end expiratory pressure [PEEP], IMV rate, and inspiration time.) The Healthdyne 105 ventilator is used in our neonatal intensive care unit. In clinical practice, *this ventilator can be regarded simply as a continuous gas flow T-tube circuit* (Fig. 1). The proximal end connects

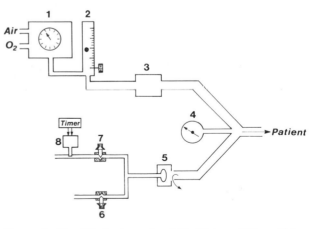

Figure 1 Simplified schematic of Healthdyne 105 ventilator. 1, oxygen blender, 2, flowmeter, 3, heated humidifier, 4, manometer, 5, exhalation valve, 6, PEEP/continuous positive airway pressure control, 7, inspiration pressure control, 8, solenoid valve with electronic timer.

to the oxygen blender and flowmeter, which permits the desired concentration of oxygen to flow continuously through the circuit. An exhalation valve with a time-cycling device is placed at the distal end. Controlled breaths are delivered by intermittently pressurizing the exhalation valve. this is accomplished by a solenoid-operated pilot valve and the inspiratory pressure control. *Between mechanically delivered breaths the infant can breathe spontaneously* through the circuit. The levels of peak inspiratory pressure and PEEP are set by varying the pressure in the exhalation valve using inspiratory pressure control and PEEP control, respectively. The rate and inspiration time are set by an electronic timer using the setting of rate control and inspiration time control.

Indications for mechanical ventilation (Table 1) are marked retractions, frequent apnea while on continuous positive airway pressure, a PaO_2 of less than 50 mm Hg with an FIO_2 of 80 to 100 percent, a $PaCO_2$ greater than 65 mm Hg, or an intractable metabolic acidosis with a base deficit greater than 10 mEg per liter, despite bicarbonate therapy. Other situations in which cardiovascular function is severely compromised or there is a neuromuscular disorder are also indications for ventilator support.

AIRWAY CARE

Nasotracheal intubation provides better fixation of the tube and permits better oral hygiene to be carried out. Supplemental oxygen should be administered during intubation either by using an oxyscope or by taping a tube on top of the laryngoscope blade. The endotracheal tube is guided into the trachea using alligator forceps. Satisfactory positioning of the tube is verified by listening to the air exchange with a stethoscope over the tip of the tube and auscultating both axillae. The placement is then further confirmed by a chest roentgenogram taken with the infant's head in the neutral position. The end of the tube should be about 1 to 2 cm above the carina, depending on the size of the infant.

Maintenance of adequate humidity is essential to prevent tube occlusion from thick secretions. The Bennett cascade humidifier gives a relative humidity of 100 percent at the water temperature inside the cascade. The water temperature is kept between 90 and 100°F.

The endotracheal tube is suctioned every 2 to 3 hours and more frequently if there are a lot of secretions. The suction catheter is advanced only 3 to 5 cm beyond the end of the endotracheal tube, depending upon the size of

the infant, in order to prevent perforation of the lung by the catheter. Each main stem bronchus is suctioned by turning the head to the opposite side.

INITIAL SETTINGS OF VENTILATOR

For the initial settings (Table 2), we have arbitrarily selected a flow rate of 5 to 7 L per minute. The *minimum flow rate needs to be at least 2.5 times the patient's minute ventilation (about 200 ml per kilogram).*

The fraction of inspired oxygen depends on the clinical condition of the infant or the previous level being administered. It should be quickly adjusted to *maintain the arterial oxygen tension between 50 and 70 mm Hg.*

The rate of IMV depends on the patient's ability to breathe spontaneously. It is usually started at between 20 to 30 breaths per minute and then adjusted to avoid excessive respiratory effort by the patient as well as to *maintain an arterial carbon dioxide tension in the range of 50 to 60 mm Hg.* This higher level of carbon dioxide is accepted because it allows a lower level of minute ventilation and thus reduces the risk of barotrauma. The patient soon adapts to this and breathes spontaneously between the respirator cycles.

An inspiratory time in the range of 0.6 sec has been chosen. It is used for IMV rates of up to 40 breaths per minute.

The peak inspiratory pressure applied depends on the compliance of the lung. The *pressure is adjusted so that adequate but not excessive chest excursion is visible.* It is usually in the range of 20 to 30 cm H_2O. If the inspiratory pressure is too low, the patient will develop intrapulmonary shunts and will become more hypoxic. If, on the other hand, the inspiratory pressure is too high, it will cause barotrauma, impede venous return, and decrease the cardic output. If the infant remains hypoxic in the face of good chest excursion, it is of great importance to exclude other causes of hypoxia, such as cyanotic heart disease or persistent fetal circulation (PFC), and not just continue to increase the peak pressure.

The PEEP is initially set at 5 cm H_2O.

ADJUSTMENT OF RESPIRATOR SETTINGS

Improvement in the patient's clinical condition is indicated by decreasing tachypnea and retractions and improving blood gas values. The *IMV rate is lowered by*

TABLE 1 Indications for Mechanical Ventilation

Marked retractions on continuous positive airway pressure
Frequent apnea on continuous positive airway pressure
PaO_2 < 50 mm Hg with FIO_2 80–100%
$PaCO_2$ > 65 mm Hg
Base deficit > 10 mEq per liter after treatment with sodium
   bicarbonate
Cardiovascular collapse
Neuromuscular disorder

TABLE 2 Initial Settings of Ventilators

1. Flow rate 5–7 liters per minute
2. FIO_2 to keep PaO_2 at 50–70 mm Hg
3. IMV rate
   Usually 20–30/min
   Avoid excessive labored breathing
   Maintain $PaCO_2$ at 50–60 mm Hg
4. Inspiration time 0.6 sec
5. Inspiration pressure
   Adequate chest excursion
   Usually 20–30 cm H_2O
6. PEEP 5 cm H_2O

2 to 5 breaths per minute as the $PaCO_2$ falls into the range of 50 mm Hg or lower and there are no excessively labored spontaneous breaths. The *inspiratory pressure is lowered by 2 to 5 cm H_2O for excessive chest excursion, and the inspired oxygen is lowered by about 1/10 of the inspired oxygen concentration if the arterial oxygen tension is greater than 60 mm Hg.* PEEP, inspiratory time, and flow rate remain the same.

Increasing severity of illness is evidenced by worsening hypoxia, a $PaCO_2$ rising above 60 mm Hg, or excessively labored breathing. For worsening hypoxia, the FiO_2 is raised and/or peak pressure is gradually increased if chest excursions are not adequate. For a rising $PaCO_2$ or excessively labored breathing, the IMV rate is gradually increased up to a limit of 40 breaths per minute. For severe retractions observed during spontaneous breathing, PEEP may be increased in increments of 2 cm H_2O to a limit of 10 cm H_2O, but this is rarely necessary. Inspiration time is not changed and is kept in the region of 0.6 sec.

MANAGEMENT OF THE MOST SEVERELY ILL INFANT

In the most severely ill infants, an arterial oxygen tension of between 50 and 70 mm Hg cannot be maintained even when the infant is ventilated with 100 percent oxygen and/or the $PaCO_2$ rises above 70 mm Hg, despite an inspiratory pressure greater than 35 cm H_2O and an IMV rate of 40 breaths per minute. For these infants, the following ventilator settings are tried: the ventilator rate is increased to 100 and the inspiratory time is reduced to 0.3 sec. The inspiratory pressure should be lowered by 5 to 10 cm H_2O from the earlier setting and the flow rate increased to 10 to 20 L per minute. If the patient's condition improves as indicated by the blood gases or a more stable oxygen tension monitored on the transcutaneous PO_2 ($TcPO_2$) recording, these settings are maintained.

If, on the other hand, there is no improvement and hypoxia remains a problem, we return to the former settings and try increasing the inspiration time to from 0.8 to 1 sec. This is very rarely necessary, probably in less than one in 100 infants ventilated.

Rarely the $PaCO_2$ remains high (> 70 mm Hg) despite a high respirator rate. This is probably due to a high physiologic dead space. Attempting to lower the $PaCO_2$ by increasing the ventilator settings is not beneficial and only serves to inflict lung damage. *If hypoxia is not a problem, the high $PaCO_2$ can be tolerated.* As the patient's condition improves, the $PaCO_2$ will gradually fall.

WEANING

An attempt to wean the infant from mechanical ventilation is begun as soon as it is started. The concentration of inspired oxygen is lowered in decrements of 2 to 10 percent to maintain an arterial tension of between 50 and 70 mm Hg. The IMV rate is lowered in decrements of 2 to 5 breaths per minute, keeping the $PaCO_2$ between 50 and 60 mm Hg.

Inspiratory pressure is lowered to prevent excessive

chest excursion and avoid barotrauma as the patient's clinical status improves.

If the patient is being ventilated at a rate of 100 breaths per minute, the peak inspiration pressure is gradually lowered to 20 cm H_2O, at which point the management is changed back to the conventional settings with an IMV rate of 40 breaths per minute. Thereafter, the infant is weaned as described above.

It is important to wean aggressively and not to leave the infant on the same settings as improvement takes place. The settings should be reviewed and modified constantly, depending on the infant's clinical status.

EXTUBATION

Extubation is undertaken when the rate of IMV is down to 6 breaths per minute. At this stage, the patient usually requires an FiO_2 of less than 40 percent with a PaO_2 between 50 and 70 mm Hg and a $PaCO_2$ between 50 and 60 mm Hg, and the general condition is stable. It is not unusual after extubation to see the $PaCO_2$ fall to a lower level than was present with an IMV of 6 breaths per minute. This is probably because of the decreased airway resistance to spontaneous breathing after the tube is removed. Extubation is performed under direct laryngoscopy with supplemental oxygen provided as previously described. *When the tube has been removed the larynx is painted with racepinephrine (Vaponefrin) to decrease postextubation edema.* Nasal continuous positive airway pressure at 5 cm H_2O pressure is then applied, and the concentration of inspired oxygen is increased by 5 percent.

For the very low birth weight infant, continuous positive airway pressure through the endotracheal tube is tried for 15 minutes prior to extubation, with the inspired oxygen concentration increased by 5 percent. This is to check whether the infant may develop apnea. If the infant breathes satisfactorily, he or she is then extubated. If apnea and bradycardia occur with endotracheal tube continuous positive airway pressure, then an intravenous bolus of aminophylline is administered in a dose of 3 mg per kilogram. A further trial of 15 minutes of continuous positive airway pressure is undertaken before extubation. However, aminophylline is rarely needed during the weaning process.

MISCELLANEOUS

The position of the head is occasionally important, particularly in low birth weight infants. The degree of chest excursion may be affected by different head positions because of the bevel of the endotracheal tube resting against the wall of the trachea, causing obstruction

During mechanical ventilation, continuous recording of the transcutaneous oxygen tension or saturation is essential, since the infant's response to a change in the ventilator setting can be observed immediately. The physician then knows whether the change is in the right direction. This is particularly important for the very unstable infant or for determining the cause of deteriorating blood gas values.

We do not administer muscle relaxants to paralyze the

infant, because with spontaneous breathing there is a better match between ventilation and perfusion of the lungs. For the paralyzed patient who is lying in the supine position, the anterior portion of the lungs is ventilated more whereas the posterior-dependent portion is perfused more. Furthermore, ventilation can be achieved at a lower rate in the nonparalyzed patient, thus minimizing barotrauma to the lung. Finally, the clinical status of the infant can be assessed by his or her activity. If the patient appears to be fighting the respirator, this may indicate that something is wrong. The endotracheal tube may be blocked by secretions and need suctioning or it may be misplaced. This may also indicate that the respirator settings are incorrect or that the respirator is malfunctioning. Another possible reason for the patient's restlessness and hypoxia is a pneumothorax. Whatever the cause, it should be carefully sought rather than just paralyzing the patient. Once a cause is determined and corrected, the patient may become quiet and breathe synchronously with the mechanical ventilator. If there is no obvious cause, *the patient may merely need tender loving care or a pacifier.*

MORPHINE INFUSION

GIDEON KOREN, M.D., A.B.M.T.
MONICA BOLOGA, M.D.

Because of obvious ethical and practical considerations, drugs are almost always introduced first in adult medicine, then in pediatrics, and only much later in the neonatal period. Morphine is no exception. Despite being one of the most ancient drugs in clinical medicine, only during the last decade have we witnessed an initial attempt to introduce it to perinatal medicine. The use of morphine for analgesia in the newborn period is controversial, as is the concept of pain in this age group. We will present our own experience with this opioid in the context of indications, relevance, and side effects.

THE PHARMACOLOGY OF MORPHINE

Morphine acts specifically on the μ opioid receptor in the central nervous system (CNS) to produce analgesia, respiratory depression, mood alterations, and mental changes. *Unlike many other classes of drugs affecting the CNS, it produces analgesia without loss of consciousness. Moreover, other sensory functions, such as vision, hearing, touch, and vibration, are not impaired.* The effect on respiration stems from a direct effect on brain stem respiratory centers. Both respiratory rate and minute volume are depressed, and even *doses that are not capable of producing analgesia can cause deleterious respiratory effects.* Typically, and most important for the perinatal period, morphine is capable of producing important pupillary miosis. When asphyxia is produced, however, mydriasis may occur and may confuse the clinical picture. Other important pharmacologic effects of this opioid include nausea and vomiting from a direct stimulation of the medullary chemoreceptor trigger zone. In the gastrointestinal tract, morphine has been largely used for relief of diarrhea by decreasing motility. It is capable of increasing biliary tract pressure as well as causing release of histamine, thus inducing sweating, pruritus, and urticaria.

Of specific interest for the neonatologist and pediatrician, morphine in high doses has been shown in several species to produce seizures due to excitation of specific groups of neurons, especially pyramidal cells. It has been suggested that narcotic-induced seizures may not involve the same receptors that are responsible for opioid-induced analgesia.

Physical Dependence and Withdrawal

When morphine is administered chronically, the well-described physical dependence and subsequent withdrawal syndrome generally occur. In the perinatal context, opioid dependence and withdrawal are the outcome of maternal exposure in late pregnancy. In the therapeutic situation discussed below, it is crucial to try to prevent these untoward effects by careful monitoring of pain and limited exposure to the drug.

DOES THE NEWBORN INFANT SUFFER FROM PAIN?

This question, which may sound strange to some clinicians, has been the focus of a heated debate in recent years. On the one hand, there is a school of thought supported by both pediatricians and surgeons claiming that painful procedures such as circumcision, endotracheal intubation, and even explorative surgery are not perceived as painful by the newborn infant. On the other hand, a steadily increasing number of researchers have shown by monitoring crying intervals, changes in heart rate, body movement, and other parameters that even "simple" procedures such as heel lance cause the neonate to perceive pain. Although the evidence is far from unequivocal, it appears that *the more careful the observation, the more convincing the evidence is that infants suffer from pain.*

The obvious missing link in the study of pain in infancy is self-reporting, leaving the clinician with indirect evidence. The question is much more complicated in the case of the critically ill infant, who is often intubated and subjected to neuromuscular blockade, thus losing most of the reactions that are likely to occur during pain.

MORPHINE PHARMACOKINETICS

Morphine, like other opioids, is readily absorbed from the gastrointestinal tract, nasal mucosa, and by inhalation. Because of a significant "first-pass effect," a large proportion of the orally administered drug is metabolized in the liver before reaching the systemic circulation. The use of oral morphine has been studied in adults and children but not in the newborn infant. After reaching the systemic circulation, about 30 percent of the drug is bound to plasma proteins in adults; however, no data are available with respect to newborn infants. *Because it is the free fraction of the drug that is distributed to various tissue compartments, including the brain, a higher fraction of unbound protein in the newborn infant may cause a more intense effect.* Because protein binding of some other drugs has been shown to decrease in infancy, it will be important to measure this parameter in this age group.

Morphine is detoxified in the liver by conjugation to glucuronide. Most of the metabolite is excreted by the kidney, whereas in adults 7 to 10 percent is eliminated through the biliary system. Some degree of enterohepatic circulation of morphine occurs due to β-glucuronidase activity in the gut, introducing more drug into the circulation.

DISPOSITION OF MORPHINE IN NEWBORN INFANTS

Two recent studies contain the first evidence that newborn infants eliminate the opioid differently from older infants, children, or adults. Both studies were conducted in neonates recovering from surgery.

In a group of 12 neonates of gestational ages from 35 to 41 weeks, postnatal ages of 1 to 49 days (mean 9.5 days), and weight 2.2 to 4.2 kg, we found the mean half-life (Tl/2) of the drug to be 13.9 $\pm$ 6.4 hours (range 5.2 to 28 hours) when calculated from all concentration time points after cessation of morphine infusion. However, "terminal" Tl/2 calculated from the two terminal points only was significantly longer (24.8 $\pm$ 4.6; range 11 to 30 hours) and may be explained by enterohepatic circulation of the drug (Fig. 1). These values of Tl/2 are significantly longer than those obtained in older children and adults (2 hours). Lynn and coworkers studied the disposition of morphine in 10 infants born after 36 to 41 weeks' gestation between 1 day and 10 weeks of age. The newborn group (0 to 7 days of age) differed significantly from the group of older infants in elimination Tl/2 (6.8 versus 3.9 hours). These differences could be attributed to a *slower clearance rate in younger infants* (6.3 versus 23.8 ml per minute per kilogram mean value). These two independent studies indicate that a maturation process of morphine metabolism takes place during early infancy. A similar trend is found in neonates with many other drugs and is *consistent with immaturity of hepatic conjugation of morphine in the newborn.*

Our study documented improvement in morphine clearance over time in some children, which may represent gradual improvement in the general status of the neonate

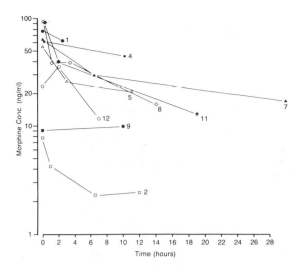

Figure 1 Concentration time curves of morphine after cessation of morphine infusion in neonates. (Reprinted from J Pediatr 1985; 107:963–967, with permission of CV Mosby Co.)

after surgery and specifically in cardiac output and hepatic blood flow (Fig. 2).

The fact that newborn infants eliminate the drug much more slowly than older children or adults because of lower clearance rates indicates that proportionally higher serum concentrations of the opioid are present in neonates receiving the same dose.

Indeed, Lynn and associates found that after 24 hours of infusion of 20 μg per kilogram per hour of morphine in older children, mean (plus or minus standard deviation) levels were 17 $\pm$ 9 ng per milliliter. In our patients receiving the same infusion rate for at least 24 hours, levels were 52 $\pm$ 31 ng per milliliter. These differences may have

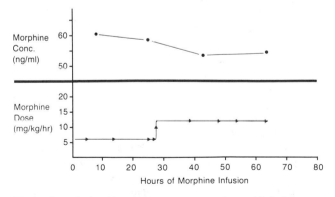

Figure 2 Relationship of plasma concentration and infusion rate of morphine in neonates. *A,* In the neonate receiving an unchanged rate of infusion, plasma concentrations tended to decrease, suggesting an improvement in clearance rate. *B,* In this neonate, concentrations remained unchanged despite a twofold increase in infusion rate of morphine, suggesting improvement in clearance rate of the drug. (Reprinted from J Pediatr 1985; 107:963–967, with permission from CV Mosby Co.)

important clinical implications, because sensitivity to morphine is believed to be enhanced in newborn infants and newborn rats. This issue is further discussed under adverse effects of morphine.

THE RATIONALE OF MORPHINE INFUSION

Historically, morphine was administered to adults intravenously as a bolus, with the dose repeated every 1 to 2 hours if necessary. With increasing knowledge of pharmacokinetic and pharmacodynamic characteristics of the drug, it became apparent that a bolus is capable of producing high initial peak concentrations, often in the toxic range, followed by rapid decrease of levels, according to the half-life, into the subtherapeutic range. Thus patients are likely to be exposed for a good part of the dosing interval to either potentially toxic levels or to subtherapeutic levels associated with inappropriate pain control.

During the last decade, the advantages of continuous morphine infusion have been appreciated by most authorities. If carefully designed, this modality permits stable levels within the therapeutic window, thus avoiding both dangerous peaks and subtherapeutic troughs. *When a drug is infused at a certain rate, it takes about five "half-lives" to achieve a steady state level.* The level (Css) achieved by a certain infusion rate (dose) depends solely on the clearance rate (Cl) of the drug, according to the equation:

$$Css = \frac{Dose\ (\mu g/kg/hr)}{Cl\ (ml/kg/hr)}$$

Consequently, in an infant with a morphine half-life of 10 hours, it would take 50 hours to achieve a steady state level. A simple way to overcome the prolonged time needed for achievement of a steady state is to administer a loading dose as a bolus at the initiation of therapy. This dose will fill in the distribution volume of morphine and substantially shorten the time needed to achieve a steady state.

In our studies, a bolus of 50 to 100 μg per kilogram was given to some infants, followed by an infusion at a rate of 6.2 to 32 μg per kilogram per hour. Lynn and Slattery administered morphine infusion at rates between 20 and 100 μg per kilogram per hour. As described below, adverse effects occurred in two infants who received a loading dose plus the highest infusion rates (32 and 40 μg per kilogram per hour, respectively) and who had high serum concentrations of morphine (61 and 90 ng per milliliter). As a result, *we currently feel that in this age group the infusion rate should not exceed 20 μg per kilogram per hour and that a loading dose should be avoided.*

ADVERSE EFFECTS OF MORPHINE INFUSION

Apart from occasional mild hypotension and respiratory depression in acute overdose, morphine has been safely used for many years. CNS hyperexcitability has been reported in animals and humans and extremely high doses of morphine and its surrogates produce seizures in animals.

Previously, seizures have been reported with morphine in one child. In addition, fentanyl, a relatively new narcotic analgesic, has been shown to cause convulsions.

In our series, none of the neonates exhibited CO_2 retention, respiratory depression, or hypotension associated with morphine therapy. For those receiving mechanical ventilation, lack of respiratory depression was determined during periods of disconnection from the respirator. Even with serum concentrations as high as 100 ng per milliliter, the infants responded to tactile stimulation. After tracheal extubation, all patients showed good sucking, coughing, gag reflex, and response to painful stimuli. However, two infants had generalized seizures and bradycardia associated with the morphine administration.

Case 1

Baby RB was born to a 19-year-old married prima gravida at 41 weeks' gestation after an uncomplicated pregnancy and uneventful delivery. The infant weighed 3.95 kg and had Apgar scores of 8 at both 1 and 5 minutes of age. An imperforate anus and omphalocele were diagnosed, but no other congenital abnormalities were noted. In fact, no other physical or neurologic problems were detected prior to surgery. He was premedicated with atropine, muscle relaxation was achieved with succinylcholine, and anesthesia was maintained with N_2O/O_2. At operation at 1 day of age, a duplicated terminal ileum and appendix were resected, and a loop colostomy and omphalocele closure were performed. The operation was uneventful. On his return to the neonatal intensive care unit, 0.4 mg (0.1 mg per kilogram) of morphine was administered intravenously and an infusion of 40 μg per kilogram per hour of morphine was commenced for analgesia. Six and a half hours after commencing the narcotic infusion, a generalized seizure occurred. This was followed by two additional seizure episodes 40 minutes later. The child was given phenobarbital 20 mg per kilogram intravenously, and the morphine infusion was stopped. Serum calcium, electrolytes, blood glucose, bilirubin, and hemoglobin levels were all normal. Blood gases showed a pH of 7.35, a PaO_2 of 67 mm Hg, and a $PaCO_2$ of 38 mm Hg, bicarbonate and base excess 18 mEq per liter and 6. Cerebral ultrasonography, an electroencephalogram, and CSF and chromosome examinations were subsequently normal. Serum concentration of morphine at the time of the seizures was 90 ng per milliliter. Five hours and 20 minutes later a further brief generalized seizure occurred and an additional 10 mg per kilogram of phenobarbital was given intravenously. No further seizures occurred and no further phenobarbital was given. At follow-up examination at 7 months of age, the infant has had no further seizures and was normal.

Case 2

Baby BQ born to a 25-year-old gravida 2 para 1 at 35 weeks' gestation by cesarian section after a pregnancy complicated by polyhydramnios and a documented fetal duodenal atresia. The infant weighed 2,400 g and had

Apgar scores of 6 and 8 at 1 and 5 minutes, respectively. Apart from the clinical features of Down's syndrome, including duodenal atresia, no other congenital abnormalities were noted.

Under general anesthesia with isoflurane and N_2O and muscle relaxation with d-tubocurarine, a duodenojejunostomy was performed at 2 days of age and the infant returned to the neonatal intensive care unit. For analgesia 0.1 mg per kilogram of morphine was administered intravenously, and an infusion of 20 μg per kilogram per minute was commenced. However, the apparent morphine dose given to the neonate averaged 32 μg per kilogram per hour for the next 3 hours. Three hours and 35 minutes later a generalized grand mal seizure occurred, lasting for 5 minutes, then recurred twice over the next 20 minutes, and continued sporadically over the next 5 and one-half hours. The seizures were treated with both phenytoin 18 mg per kilogram and phenobarbital 20 mg per kilogram but stopped only after paraldehyde was administered. Blood glucose, electrolytes, calcium, bilirubin and hemoglobin levels were all normal. Blood gases showed a pH of 7.36, a PaO_2 of 50 mm Hg, a $PaCO_2$ of 39 mm Hg, bicarbonate 21 mEq per liter, and base excess, 3.0. Because of the possible association between morphine and the seizures, the drug was discontinued a few minutes after the commencement of seizure activity.

The following morning the electrocardiogram was diffusely abnormal with some paroxysmal bursts, but 5 days later it was normal. CSF examination and cerebral ultrasonography were normal. Morphine serum concentration at the time of the convulsions was 61 ng per milliliter. Anticonvulsants were discontinued after 2 days, and no further seizures occurred. At 6 months of age the infant was doing well with no further seizures and had mild hypotonia and developmental delay usually seen with Down's syndrome.

The appearance of seizures in the absence of respiratory depression in our patients may be explained by the suggestion that narcotic-induced convulsions may not involve the same receptors that are responsible for opioid-induced analgesia.

In newborn rats it was suggested that incomplete blood-brain barrier results in greater penetration of morphine in brain target cells. It is possible that increased blood concentrations due to lower clearance rates coupled with higher cerebrospinal fluid penetration and/or higher CNS sensitivity result in a higher risk of convulsions in newborns.

SUGGESTED READING

Duggan AW, North RA. Electrophysiology of opioids. Pharmacol Rev 1983; 35:219–282.

Jaffe JH, Martin WR. Opioid analgesics and antagonists. In: Gilman AG, Goodman LS, Rall TW, Murach F, eds. The pharmacological basis of therapeutics. 7th ed. New York: Macmillan Publishing Co, 1985.

Koren G, Butt W, et al. Postoperative morphine infusion in newborn infants: Assessment of disposition characteristics and safety. J Pediatr 1985; 107:963–967.

Kupferberg HJ, Way EL. Pharmacologic basis for the increased sensitivity of the newborn rat to morphine. J Pharmacol Exp Ther 1963; 141:105–112.

Lynn AM, Slattery JT. Morphine pharmacokinetics in early infancy. Anesthesiology 1987; 66:136–139.

Owens ME. Pain in infancy: Conceptual and methodological issues. Pain 1984; 20:213–230.

NEAR INFRARED SPECTROPHOTOMETRY

JANE E. BRAZY, M.D.

In 1977, Frans Jöbsis first introduced a technique for noninvasive monitoring of cerebral oxygenation using near infrared light. Although originally applied as a technique for monitoring older patients during anesthesia, it is particularly well-suited for monitoring small neonates. In contrast to adults, in whom only a small wedge of cortex can be monitored, the small thin-boned head of the preterm neonate allows temple-to-temple transmission of light, thus providing information about a significant area of the anterior cerebral cortex.

Although *near infrared spectrophotometry (NIRS) is currently available only for research*, it has several advantages over other monitors commonly used for the assessment of oxygen sufficiency. Unlike most other oxygen monitors, it provides direct information about the organ of greatest concern, the brain. Within this tissue it provides information on both *oxygen delivery* and *oxygen utilization*. At the same time it provides information on changes in *blood volume*, allowing one to appreciate alterations in the flow of blood to and from the brain. Thus, the near infrared (NIR) technique provides a unique opportunity to observe normal physiologic and pathologic processes as they influence cerebral cellular respiration on a moment-to-moment basis.

BACKGROUND

The transmission of light through biologic material is determined by a combination of light reflectance, scattering, and absorption. Specular reflectance is predominantly influenced by the angle of the light meeting a surface. Diffuse reflectance and scattering are functions of certain properties of inhomogeneous materials such as particle size and shape, differences of index of refraction between water and particulate matter (e.g., cell membranes and mitochondria), and wavelength. Scattering decreases with increasing wavelength, making NIR light (wavelength 700 to 1,300 nm) more favorable for transmission through biologic material than light of shorter wavelengths, such as the visible range (400 to 700 nm). Absorption is determined by the molecular properties of the material in the path of the light and is wavelength-specific.

Monitoring with NIRS takes advantage of many of these principles. Specifically, NIR light penetrates skin and bone, accessing cerebral tissue for study. Within tissue very few biologic compounds absorb NIR light, but among those that do are hemoglobin and cytochrome c oxidase, better known as cytochrome aa_3; in fact, *hemoglobin and cytochrome aa_3 are the only detectable compounds absorbing NIR light that react to changes in oxygenation.* Thus, by separating the light absorbance of cytochrome aa_3 from that of hemoglobin, it is feasible to monitor cerebral oxygenation not only in the intravascular space but also within the neurons.

Within the NIR range, hemoglobin has differential light absorbance in its oxygenated and deoxygenated state, designated HbO_2 and Hb, respectively (Fig. 1A). At wavelengths below 815 nm, deoxyhemoglobin has greater light absorbance, whereas above 815 nm, oxyhemoglobin predominates. The point of equal light absorbance, approximately 815 nm, is known as the isobestic point for hemoglobin. Hence, the contribution of oxy- and deoxyhemoglobin can be determined by selecting two or more specific wavelengths within this range.

Also within the NIR range cytochrome aa_3 changes its light absorbance from the oxidized to the reduced state (Fig. 1B). When this enzyme is oxidized, an absorbance band is present in the 780 to 900 nm range with the maximal absorption at 820 to 840 nm (Fig. 2); this band disappears with reduction. Cytochrome aa_3 is the terminal member of the mitochondrial electron transport chain, which accounts for over 90 percent of cellular oxygen utilization in aerobic metabolism. This enzyme, therefore, is an *indicator of mitochondrial oxygen sufficiency within the brain tissue* as its absorption characteristics change in relation to oxygen delivery and mitochondrial function. To determine if cytochrome aa_3 is a sensitive indicator of cerebral hypoxia in animals, Sylvia and coworkers compared changes in the cytochrome aa_3 redox state, determined by light spectrophotometry, with amounts of phosphocreatine during graded hypoxia. Both cytochrome aa_3 and phosphocreatine had similar patterns of response as oxygenation decreased. However, the reduction of cytochrome aa_3 began sooner, demonstrating that *cytochrome aa_3 is both an early and a sensitive indicator of cerebral hypoxia.*

INSTRUMENTATION

Our NIRS monitor is the NIROSSCOPE (near infrared oxygen sufficiency scope, Duke University, Department of Physiology). It uses three or four diode lasers as sources of different wavelengths of NIR light. The lasers are pulsed sequentially at 1 kHz for 200 nsec each. The light from the lasers is captured in glass fiberoptic strands that form a fiber bundle carrying the light to one temple of the head (see Fig. 2). The light traverses the head, where

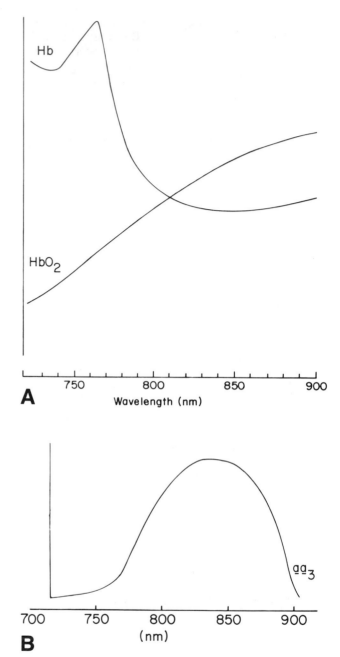

Figure 1 Absorption spectra of oxyhemoglobin and deoxyhemoglobin (*A*) and cytochrome aa_3 (*B*). The ordinates of A and B have no designated units because the optical path length of the light is indeterminate due to scattering of photons. In animal studies using NIRS, that path length may vary from six to 13 times the actual linear distance; therefore, the number of absorbing units or concentration of absorbers in the path length of the signal cannot be determined.

a second fiberoptic bundle, attached to the opposite temple, collects the transmitted light photons and conducts them back to a photomultiplier. The signals are next demodulated, amplified, expressed as a ratio of a reference signal, and converted into logarithmic form. These *raw signals are then converted into information regard-*

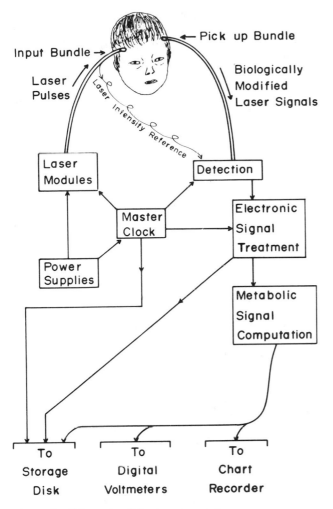

Figure 2 Schematic of the instrumentation.

INTERPRETATION OF SIGNALS

The *NIROSSCOPE does not provide data in terms familiar to the clinician, such as PaO$_2$ or percent saturation; it provides information as relative changes and directional trends.* Likewise, it does not measure cerebral blood flow in ml per 100 g tissue per minute; rather, *alterations in hemodynamics are detected as changes in cerebral blood volume.* The blood volume signal is the sum of the two hemoglobin signals, oxyhemoglobin and deoxyhemoglobin. One can use the relative distribution of these components of the blood volume signal to determine the nature of the change in blood volume. Thus, with increased blood flow to the brain, oxyhemoglobin contributes significantly to the increase in blood volume, whereas with obstruction to cerebral venous return, deoxyhemoglobin contributes solely or predominantly to the increase in blood volume.

Table 1 summarizes the factors that commonly lead to specific signal changes. In each case more than one factor may be responsible for a specific directional change. For oxyhemoglobin (tHbO$_2$), either an increase in the oxygen saturation of the blood or an increase in blood flow to the monitored portion of the brain, without a change in oxygen saturation, causes an increase in tHbO$_2$. The opposite conditions—decreased oxygen saturation and reduced blood flow to the monitored tissue—cause a decrease in the tHbO$_2$ signal.

Like tHbO$_2$, deoxyhemoglobin responds to changes in oxygen saturation and to changes in cerebral hemodynamics. It increases with the inflow of desaturated blood and with obstruction to outflow of venous blood. Changes in deoxyhemoglobin mirror those of tHbO$_2$ when there is no change in blood volume; thus, with mild decreased oxygen desaturation a rise in deoxyhemoglobin occurs simultaneous with the fall in tHbO$_2$. Because deoxyhemoglobin normally reflects changes in predominantly venous blood, it is a sensitive indicator of

ing the relative contributions of oxyhemoglobin, deoxy-hemoglobin, and cytochrome aa$_3$ using mathematical algorithms developed by Jöbsis. The signals are updated every 200 msec and displayed on a multichannel chart recorder with additional channels for electrocardiogram, blood pressure, respiration, and transcutaneous oxygen signals adapted from bedside monitors. The hemoglobin signals are from the arterial-venous mix of the blood in the regional cerebral circulation. To emphasize that they arise from the blood in the *tissue* they are designated tHb and tHbO$_2$.

Because light scattering within the head prevents definition of the exact optical path and thereby the concentration of light absorbers, the resulting information is given in relative (variation in density) rather than absolute (optical density) units. One variation in density unit (v/d) represents an order of magnitude change in each signal. Although v/d units cannot provide information in terms of absolute concentrations, they do provide a linear correlation with concentration changes. Thus a 2 v/d change in blood volume signifies an increase in cerebral blood twice as large as a 1 v/d unit change.

TABLE 1 Factors Causing Signal Changes

Increased deoxyhemoglobin

  Decrease in oxygen saturation
  Obstruction to cerebral venous return
  Increase in flow of desaturated blood
  Increase in concentration of deoxyhemoglobin

Increased tHbO$_2$

  Increase in oxygen saturation
  Increased cerebral blood flow
  Increased concentration of oxyhemoglobin

Increased blood volume

  Increase in cerebral blood flow
  Obstruction to cerebral venous return
  Increase in concentration of hemoglobin

Increased cytochrome aa$_3$ oxidation

  Increase in oxygen delivery to cells
  Increased metabolic activity of cell with oxygen sufficiency
  Decrease in supply of electrons to respiratory chain

conditions altering cerebral venous return, increasing with obstructed venous return and decreasing with accelerated venous return.

The blood volume signal represents the sum of the deoxyhemoglobin and $tHbO_2$ signals. Reciprocal changes in deoxyhemoglobin and $tHbO_2$ unaccompanied by alterations in cerebral blood flow do not cause a change in blood volume signal because a decrease in one hemoglobin signal is balanced by an increase in the other. However, any disproportionate change between the deoxyhemoglobin and $tHbO_2$ signals does cause a change in the blood volume signal, as does a simultaneous change in deoxyhemoglobin and $tHbO_2$ in the same direction. Thus, the blood volume increases whenever cerebral blood flow increases, as normally occurs with hypoxia and hypercarbia.

Blood volume also increases with any impedance to cerebral venous return. Preterm neonates have frequent changes in deoxyhemoglobin that appear to reflect alterations in cerebral venous return. These occur with gagging, crying, and movement-associated hypertensive peaks. Similarly, changes in body position affect the rate of venous return. Thus, cerebral blood volume increases if the infant is moved to the head-down position and decreases with the infant in the head-up position.

Because the blood volume is determined from hemoglobin in the NIRS technique, any marked change in hemoglobin concentration will be interpreted as a change in the blood volume signal. For example, a rapid infusion of packed red blood cells will cause an increase in the blood volume signal even if there is no change in the true blood volume of the transilluminated field. Likewise, significant hemodilution will cause a decrease in the blood volume signal.

The cytochrome signal reflects mitochondrial respiration; changes in cytochrome oxidation represent changes at the cellular level. The steady state balance of cytochrome aa_3 is the net result of the electron inflow rate along the respiratory cytochrome chain and the outflow of electrons to oxygen. Inflow is usually a stable process since there is adequate provision of electrons from substrates such as glucose. Outflow is more labile, responding to changes in available oxygen. *Cytochrome aa_3 is reduced when the supply of oxygen to the cells in the monitored field is decreased.* Hence, cytochrome aa_3 becomes more reduced with a decrease in oxygen saturation and/or a decrease in blood flow to the cells delivering the signal. In sick preterm neonates, we have seen an occasional shift to cytochrome reduction with little or no change in $tHbO_2$. In this case, we presume that shunting or abnormal flow patterns within the monitored tissue prevent the oxygenated blood from reaching the cells that are delivering the signal.

Glucose is the usual substrate that ultimately supplies electrons to the respiratory chain and contributes to the steady state flow of electrons. In animals with hypoglycemia, cytochrome aa_3 shows a slow and gradual oxidation. With the administration of glucose, it rapidly shifts to a more reduced state.

A change in cytochrome oxidation might also occur if the metabolic demands of the cells suddenly increase, as occurs with seizure activity. In induced seizures in animals using visible light spectrophotometry, cytochrome aa_3 oxidation increases as long as oxygen is sufficient, but as supplies are exhausted, reduction ensues. This effect, however, has not yet been demonstrated with the NIRS technique. If a similar response occurs, it is apparently much diminished in size.

Animal studies by Mela and colleagues demonstrate that the concentration of mitochondrial cytochrome oxidase increases with fetal age, and a second phase of respiratory chain activity begins immediately after birth. Data are needed to define the expected degree of cytochrome activity in the human neonate at different gestational and chronologic ages and to determine which patterns of response are indicative of impending cell injury or at what point metabolic recovery is impossible. *Until more is known about cytochrome activity in young animals, changes in the cytochrome aa_3 redox state must be interpreted with great caution.*

USEFULNESS OF NIRS IN NEONATOLOGY

Preliminary observations using NIRS demonstrate that this technique is a sensitive indicator of oxygenation that responds rapidly to changes in delivered oxygen. Of equal or greater importance, NIRS identifies circumstances of altered cerebral hemodynamics. The real value of NIRS, however, lies in its ability to provide this combination of information in "real time" so that it can be correlated with other monitored or observed parameters in the infant. Together these provide a better understanding of the problems of the neonate. Through serial monitoring of 25 neonates in the Intensive Care Nursery, we have found NIRS helpful in answering the following questions.

Are trends in cerebral oxygenation being adequately reflected in blood gases or by other oxygen monitors? Oxygenation assessed by NIRS correlates significantly with that assessed by transcutaneous oxygen monitors in stable infants without significant pulmonary disease. NIRS information may differ from that of other forms of oxygen monitoring in conditions causing differential perfusion to organs because sites monitored by other techniques (skin and peripheral pulse) are usually distant from the cerebral circulation. We have found poor correlation between NIRS and other forms of oxygen monitoring in infants with right-to-left ductal shunts and in infants with poor peripheral perfusion.

Are periods of apnea and/or bradycardia significant for cerebral oxygenation? The cerebral response to apnea varies among infants and in the same infant over time. Some infants have periods of apnea of 20 sec or longer with little or no change in $tHbO_2$ or cytochrome aa_3 oxidation, whereas others show a decline in $tHbO_2$ and a shift to cytochrome reduction in less than 10 sec. In general, infants with significant pulmonary disease tolerate episodes of apnea poorly, whereas infants with more pulmonary reserve take longer to desaturate hemoglobin. Regardless of lung disease, most infants tolerate sequential apneas poorly, with a more rapid fall in $tHbO_2$ and cytochrome aa_3 and a slower recovery to baseline with each successive pause in breathing.

Bradycardia usually affects cytochrome aa₃ immediately because it alters cardiac output as well as oxygen saturation. Even mild bradycardia may cause significant cytochrome reduction in some infants. For example, in one infant with a large ductus arteriosus, a drop in heart rate to the 110 to 120 beats per minute range from 160 caused marked cytochrome reduction before any change in tHbO₂ was apparent. This response probably reflects failure of forward cerebral flow during the diastolic phase of the cardiac cycle due to syphoning of blood by the ductus. Thus, any extension of the time spent in diastole leads to failure to deliver oxygen to the cells, even though the blood is adequately oxygenated. This decrease in cellular oxygenation would not have been detected by standard methods of oxygen monitoring and is, therefore, "silent." We have observed other episodes of silent cytochrome reduction (a shift to cytochrome reduction unaccompanied by a decrease in tHbO₂) without obvious clinical correlates. We speculate that these represent periods of shunting or redistribution of blood flow within the brain.

What is the pattern of metabolic response to decreased oxygen delivery? A decrease in tHbO₂ is usually accompanied by cytochrome aa₃ reduction; cytochrome aa₃ reoxidizes with the return of hemoglobin oxygenation. During the period of cytochrome aa₃ reduction blood volume increases, suggesting a matching of blood flow to metabolic demands (Fig. 3). Blood volume returns to base-

line with return of cytochrome aa₃ oxidation. Animal experiments and studies of healthy adults suggest that this is the expected pattern of response. However, NIRS monitoring of sick neonates reveals circumstances when this does not occur. With long hypoxic episodes (several minutes) or sequential hypoxic episodes, recovery of cytochrome aa₃ oxidation may lag behind the return of tHbO₂ by seconds or minutes. Although the significance of delayed cytochrome recovery is unknown at this time, it might represent cellular dysfunction.

Are therapeutic maneuvers to improve oxygenation successful? As with other oxygen monitors, the nurse or physician can observe the oxygenation response to an intervention while the intervention is taking place. Unlike other methods, however, one can also observe metabolic recovery. Since recovery of oxygenation and return of cytochrome oxidation to baseline may not be simultaneous, the therapeutic intervention can continue until both parameters have recovered fully. When a delay in cytochrome recovery occurs, nursing procedures can be organized to allow longer periods for recovery before the next activity takes place, and special efforts can be made to avoid hypoxic stresses to the infant.

Is brain blood volume relatively constant or are marked changes occurring with activity or manipulation? Probably the most valuable aspect of NIRS monitoring of neonates is its ability to detect changes in blood volume simultaneous with changes in cellular oxygenation, giving a dynamic display of how alterations in blood flow patterns and oxygen utilization affect each other. NIR monitoring of sick neonates reveals that *marked and sudden changes in cerebral blood volume occur frequently in neonates.* Some of these changes relate to blood pressure. Hypertensive peaks, first described by Lou in 1979, are sudden elevations in blood pressure, often 30 to 200 percent, which occur with coughs, gags, seizures, abdominal palpation, bladder Credé, blocked ventilator breaths, and most major movements. NIR monitoring of sick preterm neonates demonstrates that these hypertensive peaks are associated with abrupt elevations in brain blood volume (Fig. 4). Deoxyhemoglobin is the major contributor to this increase. This suggests that during these activities increased intrathoracic pressure causes relative obstruction of cerebral venous return. In addition to the increase in the blood volume signal, cytochrome aa₃ frequently shifts to a more reduced state, indicating a transient imbalance between oxygen delivery and cellular oxygen utilization. The apparent inability of the preterm infant to protect the brain from these surges in blood volume and the failure to regulate cerebral oxygenation during these episodes may be important factors in the susceptibility of preterm neonates to intraventricular hemorrhage and cerebral ischemia.

Crying is another activity accompanied by significant fluctuations in blood volume. It is a complex state associated with marked swings in intrathoracic pressure, from significantly negative during inspiration to highly positive during the period of strain. The period of strain is also accompanied by an increase in intracranial pressure and a decrease in pulse pressure. The blood volume and oxy-

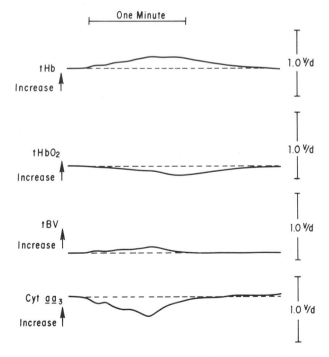

Figure 3 Period of spontaneous hypoxia in preterm infant. With the episode, there is a shift to more deoxyhemoglobin (tHb) and less oxyhemoglobin (tHbO₂). Cytochrome aa₃ becomes more reduced simultaneous with the fall in tHbO₂. During the period of cytochrome aa₃ reduction, blood volume (tBV) rises. Cytochrome aa₃ and blood volume return to their baseline as tHbO₂ increases.

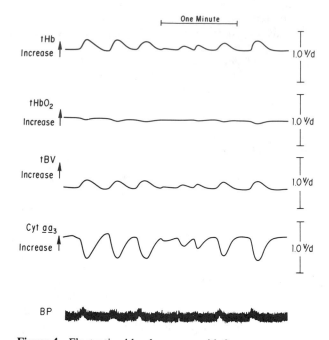

Figure 4 Fluctuating blood pressure with frequent movement-associated hypertensive peaks. Each peak is followed in 1 to 2 sec by an abrupt rise in blood volume of tissue (tBV) within the optical field and simultaneous reduction in cytochrome aa_3 (cyt aa_3). The change in tBV is predominantly from deoxyhemoglobin (tHb).

genation responses seen with NIRS parallel these changes. With the initial deep inspiration of the cry, cerebral blood volume decreases but quickly returns to baseline. During the remainder of the cry, blood volume remains elevated but fluctuates with respiration, peaking during prolonged exhalations. The $tHbO_2$ and cytochrome aa_3 responses appear to reflect the chronologic age of the infant and the presence or absence of pulmonary disease. Healthy infants over 3 days of age usually demonstrate an increase in $tHbO_2$ and greater cytochrome aa_3 oxidation during crying, whereas infants with pulmonary disease usually show a decrease in $tHbO_2$ and cytochrome aa_3 reduction. Healthy infants less than 3 days of age have a more variable response and may show no change in cytochrome oxidation.

NIRS can detect other situations of increased cerebral blood volume and altered cerebral venous return. For ex-

ample, one can identify when excessive end-expiratory pressure is obstructing venous return by a sudden decrease in cerebral blood volume and a rise in cytochrome aa_3 when the pressure is removed. Likewise, the position of the infant alters venous return and hence blood volume; the head-down position increases the blood volume signal, whereas the head-up position decreases it. With increased awareness of the circumstances associated with obstruction to venous return and elevations in cerebral blood volume, activities causing them can be minimized.

NIRS shows great promise as an oxygen monitor because of its ability to detect other states of cellular oxygen inadequacy in addition to conditions of decreased oxygen saturation. Even more important, NIRS gives us the information necessary to understand how changes in cerebral hemodynamics, both incoming blood flow and cerebral venous return, affect cellular metabolism. However, before NIRS is used for routine clinical monitoring, further information is needed on the normal state of cytochrome aa_3 oxidation in the neonate. Only then can the clinician interpret abnormal responses accurately. *Once NIRS is in clinical use, neonatologists will need to learn to identify patterns of response, much as obstetricians have learned to do for fetal heart monitoring.*

SUGGESTED READING

Brazy JE, Lewis DV. Changes in cerebral blood volume and cytochrome aa_3 during hypertensive peaks in preterm infants. J Pediatr 1986; 108:983–987.

Brazy JE, Lewis DV, Mitnick MH, Jöbsis-Vander Vliet FF. Noninvasive monitoring of cerebral oxygenation in preterm infants. Preliminary observations. Pediatrics 1985; 75:217–225.

Delpy DT, Cope MC, Cady EB, et al. Cerebral monitoring in newborn infants by magnetic resonance and near infrared spectroscopy. Scan J Clin Lab Invest 1987; 47(Suppl 188):9–17.

Jöbsis FF. Noninvasive, infrared monitoring of cerebral and myocardial oxygen sufficiency and circulatory parameters. Science 1977; 198:1264–1267.

Jöbsis FF. Noninvasive near infrared monitoring of cellular oxygen sufficiency in vivo. Adv Exp Med Biol 1986; 191:833–841.

Jöbsis-Vander Vliet FF, Fox E, Sugioka K. Monitoring of cerebral oxygenation and cytochrome aa_3 redox state. In: Tremper KK, ed. Advances in oxygen monitoring; International anesthesiology clinics. Boston: Little, Brown, 1986.

Mela L, Goodwin CW, Miller LD. Correlation of mitochondrial cytochrome concentrations and activity to oxygen availability in the newborn. Biochem Biophys Res Commun 1975; 64:384–390.

Sylvia AL, Piantadosi CA, Jöbsis FF. Energy metabolism and in vivo cytochrome c oxidase redox relationships in hypoxic rat brain. Neurol Res 1985; 7:81–88.

NEONATAL EXTRACORPOREAL MEMBRANE OXYGENATION

BILLIE LOU SHORT, M.D.

Extracorporeal membrane oxygenation (ECMO) has been successfully used to treat respiratory failure in over 1,000 newborn infants since the first survivor was documented in 1975. The key component of ECMO therapy is to supply extracorporeal cardiopulmonary support, allowing "lung rest" so that diseased lungs heal without the iatrogenic effects of high oxygen and ventilator therapy. The cardiopulmonary bypass concept was developed in the early 1950s. Devices used at that time were bubble or disc oxygenators with a direct oxygen-blood interface, resulting in marked hemolysis after a few hours of bypass, precluding their use for long-term problems. With the development of the first membrane oxygenator by Clowes and colleagues in 1956, prolonged cardiopulmonary bypass became feasible.

The design of the membrane lung and the technical aspects of the procedure were worked out during the 1960s and 1970s. It was during this period that a nine-hospital collaborative study was organized by the National Heart, Lung and Blood Institute to study ECMO therapy in adults with acute pulmonary insufficiency. Unfortunately, the survival rate was not improved (9.5 percent in patients receiving ECMO and 8.3 percent in the controls). The study noted several problems, including the continuation of intensive ventilator support on bypass. A recent study in the adult population in which pulmonary management was dramatically changed from the collaborative study design to keep the lungs "at rest" showed a survival rate of 48.8 percent. Although this study was not controlled, it does indicate that further studies in the adult population should be considered, with emphasis on pulmonary management and early treatment.

In the late 1960s the technique was used in the premature infant with hyaline membrane disease, the concept being that ECMO would act as the "artificial placenta."

Unfortunately, the systemic heparinization required for the procedure caused all the infants to die from intracranial hemorrhage. It was not until Bartlett and colleagues pioneered the treatment for term or near-term infants in respiratory failure that ECMO entered its successful phase. This early work has been confirmed by Bartlett's further work and that of others, present-day survival rates being more than 80 percent in infants with a predicted mortality of over 80 percent (Table 1). It must be noted that infants treated in centers today meet criteria developed from *historical controls* predicting 80 to 100 percent mortality. Two randomized controlled studies published to date include Bartlett and colleagues at the University of Michigan and the *randomized trial* conducted at The Children's Hospital, Boston. Both show an improved survival with ECMO (data presented at the 5th Annual ECMO Symposium, February 1989). Because of the moribund nature of this population, many centers have chosen to use historical controls to develop their criteria. To evaluate the effect of ECMO on morbidity, the University of Michigan is currently conducting a randomized controlled trial comparing conventional therapy with ECMO in a population whose predicted survival rate is 50 percent. When complete, these studies may help answer many of the questions concerning the lack of a controlled randomized study.

PATIENT POPULATION AND CRITERIA

Currently, the appropriate ECMO target patient population is the term or near-term infant (35 to 40 weeks of gestation) who fails maximal ventilatory and medical support and who, by institutional criteria, has only a 20 percent or less chance of survival. The infant must be free from congenital heart disease (CHD). Since systemic heparinization is required, infants with any major bleeding disorder, including a significant intracranial hemorrhage, must be excluded. The lung disease must be potentially reversible within a 10- to 14-day period. Severe chronic lung disease cannot be reversed within the time limits of present-day ECMO therapy, and therefore these infants should be excluded.

Most infants who are candidates for ECMO have, as

TABLE 1 ECMO Central Registry Summary, November 1987

Diagnosis	% of Total Population	% Survival
Meconium aspiration syndrome	43.0	89.9
Respiratory distress syndrome	14.0	75.7
Congenital diaphragmatic hernia	15.0	62.0
Sepsis	8.0	73.8
Persistent pulmonary hypertension	14.0	85.1
Cardiac	1.4	50.0
Other	2.6	80.8
Total patients	1,134	80.7

Courtesy of Robert H. Bartlett, M.D., University of Michigan.

an underlying process, persistent pulmonary hypertension (PPHN), which results in right-to-left shunting through the foramen ovale, the ductus arteriosus, or both. This condition occurs in diseases such as meconium aspiration syndrome, sepsis, severe hyaline membrane disease, idiopathic PPHN, and congenital diaphragmatic hernia (see Table 1). Maximal medical therapy varies from institution to institution, but it usually includes attempts at alkalinization, by either ventilatory or metabolic means (sodium bicarbonate drips), and therapy with vasodilating drugs such as tolazoline. High-frequency ventilation may be appropriate before ECMO therapy is considered. When all methods of conventional therapy have been exhausted, appropriate candidates for ECMO are those whose predicted survival rate is less than 20 percent. *We have found the alveolararterial oxygen difference, P(A-a)O$_2$ (related to time) to be the most accurate in predicting mortality in our institution.* The criteria used at Children's Hospital National Medical Center (CHNMC) are listed in Table 2. Others have found the Oxygen Index (Fig. 1) with time or Po$_2$ less than 50 mm Hg over time to be equally predictive. Infants must meet the criteria in force at the ECMO institution, because such criteria reflect that specific institution's methods of conventional therapy. Criteria should be applied only after maximal therapy and should be linked to time.

EQUIPMENT

There is no standard "ECMO machine." The system must be designed from cardiopulmonary bypass equipment. *The membrane lung used today is a silicone membrane* (Sci-Med, 0.8 m² silicone, Sci-Med Life Systems

---

TABLE 2   ECMO Entry Criteria

Patient must meet all of the following criteria:

1. Weight greater than 2 kg
2. No more than 7 days of assisted ventilation
3. Reversible lung disease
4. No major intracranial hemorrhage or severe, uncorrected coagulopathy
5. Failure of maximal medical management (100% oxygen, hyperventilation/alkalosis, tolazoline trial)
6. PLUS one of the following:
   AaDO$_2^*\geq$ 610 for 8 hr (80% mortality)
   PIP $\geq$ 38 plus AaDO$_2$ $\leq$ 605 for 4 hr (84% mortality)

---

* P(A − a)O$_2$ measured when F$_1$O$_2$ = 1.00. AaDO$_2$ = Barometric pressure (mm Hg) − 47 mm Hg − Po$_2$ − Pco$_2$.

$$OI = \left[\frac{Mean\ airway\ pressure \times F_1O_2}{PaO_2} \right] \times 100$$

$\geq$ 40, 80% Mortality (× 3 ABG)
20–25, 50% Mortality

Figure 1   Formula for Oxygen Index (OI).

Inc., Minneapolis, MN). Essential components include a tubing pack individually designed for each system; a 50-ml venous reservoir bag (Sci-Med Life Systems, Inc.); a system that monitors venous return and sounds an alarm if there is a significant drop; a 4- to 6-inch roller head occlusion pump; a membrane lung; oxygen and CO$_2$ flow meters; an oxygen blender; and a heat exchanger with a heating unit.

PROCEDURES

The currently accepted ECMO procedure is venoarterial (VA) bypass (Fig. 2). Veno-veno and single-catheter techniques hold promise, but are still in the experimental stages of development and are not discussed here.

The first step in the ECMO procedure is the preparation of the bypass circuit. It is assembled and primed with an albumin-blood mixture adjusted to the appropriate pH. While this is being done the infant is anesthetized with fentanyl (10 to 15 micrograms per kilogram) and paralyzed with pancuronium. Catheters are placed in the right internal jugular vein and right common carotid artery, with the venous catheter advanced so that it rests in the right atrium, and the arterial catheter advanced to the entrance of the aortic arch. Catheter placement is confirmed by radiography or ultrasonography. The most common catheter sizes are Nos. 8 to 10 Fr. in the artery and Nos. 12 to 14 Fr. in the vein. After completion of these two procedures, the catheters are connected to the bypass circuit, care being taken that no air is introduced during this step. The infant is slowly placed on bypass by increasing the bypass flows over a 20-minute period to the point where 60 to 70 percent of the cardiac output (CO) is going through the circuit. *Ventilator settings are reduced as bypass is achieved* to final settings of F$_1$O$_2$, 0.21; ventilator rate, 10 to 15 bpm; pressure limit, 15 cm H$_2$O; and positive endexpiratory pressure (PEEP), 5 cm H$_2$O. *The infant is allowed to awaken and breathe spontaneously.* All vasoactive drugs can be discontinued. *The infant must be anticoagulated,* and usually requires a loading dose of 100 to 150 units of heparin per kilogram during the cannulation procedure, with a heparin drip of 20 to 70 units per kilogram per hour. Activated clotting times (ACT) are measured every 30 to 60 minutes, with the ACT kept at two to three times baseline levels (240 to 280 sec). All fluids and hyperalimentation solutions are placed into the ECMO circuit, so that the infant requires only an arterial line to monitor blood gases and blood pressure.

Oxygenation is achieved by the ECMO circuit's taking over more of the infant's cardiac output, thus replacing the deoxygenated blood with oxygenated blood. The system also supplies cardiac support for infants who may have marginal cardiac function secondary to ischemia.

Since CO$_2$ is more diffusible than O$_2$, and the CO$_2$ gradient between blood and ventilating gas is small, CO$_2$ is efficiently removed and must usually be added to the system to maintain a Pco$_2$ of 40 mm Hg.

WEANING FROM ECMO

For the first 1 to 2 days, *60 to 80 percent of the cardiac output (CO) must flow through the circuit in order to keep*

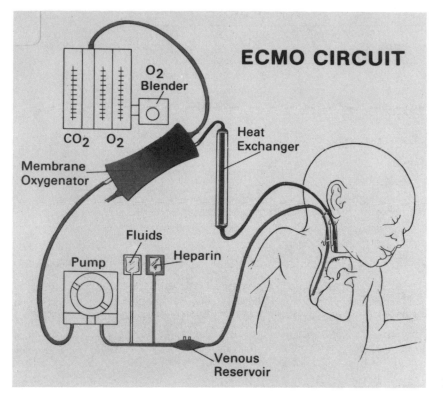

ECMO CIRCUIT

O₂ Blender

Heat Exchanger

Membrane Oxygenator

CO₂ O₂

Fluids

Heparin

Pump

Venous Reservoir

Figure 2   Venoarterial ECMO circuit.

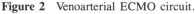

the patient's Po₂ *between 75 and 80 mm Hg.* As the lungs improve, the Po₂ increases and the ECMO flow can be decreased gradually. *Once the infant reaches bypass flows equal to only 10 percent of the CO, we speak of the infant-ECMO circuit as "idling."* This idling period continues for 8 to 12 hours to ensure that the patient is ready to be weaned from the circuit. The decannulation procedure requires that the infant be paralyzed and anesthetized. Usually a short or intermediate neuromuscular blocker is used so that the infant will awaken, allowing for faster extubation. The ventilator usually has to be increased at this time to FiO₂ of 30 to 40 mm Hg, respiratory rates of 40 to 50 bpm, and pressure limits of 15 to 20 cm H₂O. The average time to extubation at CHNMC is 24 hours, with supplemental oxygen required for 5 to 6 days.

COMPLICATIONS

Most complications of ECMO therapy are related to the use of heparin and its systemic effects. Congenital diaphragmatic hernia repairs can be extensive, and these infants, if placed on ECMO early (within 12 hours after surgery), can have significant bleeding that necessitates early removal from ECMO support. The most common cause of death in the patient on ECMO is severe intracranial hemorrhage. In our population, as with others, *the incidence of severe intracranial hemorrhage is approximately 10 percent,* with an overall incidence of 20 to 25 percent (if grades I and II are considered). The pre-ECMO asphyxia and systemic heparinization places these infants at risk for such complications; hence, heparin therapy must be monitored closely.

Inability to wean from the ECMO circuit can have a number of causes: (1) *undiagnosed cardiac disease (especially, total anomalous pulmonary venous connection,* TAPVC); (2) significant patent ductus arteriosus; (3) hypoplastic lungs; or (4) mechanical factors, such as loss of pump head occlusion. The most common cause is TAPVC.

FOLLOW-UP AND OUTCOME

The severity of the pre-ECMO illness mandates extensive follow-up. Although ligation of the carotid artery has not so far appeared to be associated with early morbidity, there are currently *unresolved long-term concerns about the cerebral circulation* as these children approach adulthood. Infants should undergo routine post-ECMO neurodevelopmental and medical evaluations.

Our follow-up studies to date are extremely encouraging. In our first 200 patients treated we have an 86 percent survival rate (Table 3). Our 1-year follow-up to date includes 103 infants. Neurological examination results are normal in 75 percent, with developmental studies normal in 63 percent, using the Bayley exam. Of the 20 percent who are delayed, one infant is profoundly delayed (Mental Developmental Index and Psychomotor Developmental Index less than 50). The remaining infants are considered suspect and are being followed closely to rule out learning difficulties at school age. Neither neuroimaging nor neurologic findings indicate short-term concerns about carotid ligation. The long-term complications have not been determined.

TABLE 3 ECMO Patients at CHNMC

Diagnosis	% of Total Population	% Survival
Meconium aspiration syndrome	49.4	93.5
Respiratory distress syndrome	13.4	85.0
Congenital diaphragmatic hernia	6.7	70.0
Sepsis	16.0	87.5
Persistent pulmonary hypertension	9.4	78.5
Cardiac	5.4	40.0
Other	1.3	50.0
Total		86.0

SUGGESTED READING

Bartlett RH, Gazzaniga AB, Huxtable RH, et al. Extracorporeal membrane oxygenation (ECMO) in newborn respiratory failure — technical considerations. Trans Am Soc Artif Organs 1979; 25:173-175.

Bartlett RH, Roloff DW, Cornell RG, et al. Extracorporeal circulatory support in neonatal respiratory failure: A prospective randomized study. Pediatrics 1985; 76:479-487.

Clowes GHA Jr, Hopkins AL, Neville WE. An artificial lung dependent upon diffusion of oxygen and carbon dioxide through plastic membranes. J Thorac Surg 1956; 32:630-637.

Gattinoni L, Presenti A, Mascheroni D, et al. Low-frequency positive-pressure ventilation with extracorporeal CO_2 removal in severe acute respiratory failure. JAMA 1986; 256:881-886.

Pratt PC, Vollmer RT, Shelburne JD, et al. Pulmonary morphology in a multihospital collaborative extracorporeal membrane oxygenation project. Am J Pathol 1979; 95:191-208.

OPHTHALMOSCOPY IN THE NEWBORN

EARL A. PALMER, M.D.

Ophthalmoscopy permits examination of the interior of the eye. There are three levels of use for this examination. The most basic use is *screening* for eye anomalies, infections, or disease. In pediatric practice, this may be reduced to simply looking for the "red reflex" in an infant and is ordinarily done without pharmacologically dilating the pupils. This light reflection is most easily seen with the help of an instrument that places the examiner's line of sight nearly coaxial with the illumination. An ordinary direct ophthalmoscope set on 0 diopters can be used for this purpose, or even an otoscope can be used (the older design using a light bulb is better for this than the newer conical fiberoptic light source). One can perform this examination at any distance from the patient, from a few centimeters to a meter. In a well baby clinic, a distance of about 1 foot is satisfactory. In a Caucasian infant, the reflex (reflection) is red-orange and sometimes slightly yellowish. In the rare event of an albino baby, the red reflex is unusually bright and often even transilluminates the underpigmented iris. In an infant with one or both parents with darker pigmentation, including Hispanics, the reflex often is not red but more gray-purple and is much less bright. When the pupils are small, it may be difficult to see the fundus reflection from the eye of an infant of darker pigmentation. Sometimes the infant's skin does not appear heavily pigmented, yet the uveal tissues of the eye will be. To resolve uncertainty in such a case, the examiner should use drops to pharmacologically dilate the pupils.

DILATING THE PUPILS OF AN INFANT

The risk of producing angle-closure glaucoma by dilating the pupils is *not* significant during childhood. Angle-closure glaucoma occurs in infants only when there is externally evident eye disease present, unlike the situation in older adults, when certain subtle anatomic predispositions can escape detection until angle-closure glaucoma is precipitated. Thus, if the infant's external eyes appear normal on critical examination with a penlight or direct ophthalmoscope, one may confidently proceed to dilate the pupils, and it is recommended that one drop each of *both* an adrenergic agent (2.5 percent phenylephrine) and an anticholinergic agent (½ percent cyclopentolate or 1 percent tropicamide) be used topically in each eye for this purpose in newborns. When the iris is darkly pigmented, the anticholinergic drop may be repeated once if necessary. Use tropicamide drops when the examination can be completed within an hour of their instillation and cyclopentolate when it may take longer. Cyclomydril is a combination of cyclopentolate 0.2 percent and phenylephrine 1 percent and is useful as a single agent for infants. It may be given twice, 1 to 5 minutes apart. After each instillation of eyedrops, the excess is immediately blotted off the closed lids before the blinking mechanism pumps excess drops into the nasopharynx via the nasolacrimal duct. This regimen for eyedrops is considered safe and effective for low birth weight infants as well as for full-term infants. However, it is not necessary for routine physical examination purposes in newborn infants; *that is, the pupils should be dilated whenever it is considered indicated, but it is not mandatory to do so if the external examination and red reflex are normal and there is no clinical reason to suspect intraocular abnormalities.* The examiner should remember to observe the relative size, shape, and reactivity of the pupils prior to dilating them and be aware that they may remain somewhat dilated up to 6 hours by tropicamide and occasionally up to 2 days by cyclopentolate. The duration of action is shorter in infants than in older children.

The second level of ophthalmoscopy, beyond simply looking for the red reflex, is the *inspection of intraocular structures*, particularly the retina and optic nerve.

INSTRUMENTATION

At least three instruments are commonly used for ophthalmoscopy in infants: the *direct ophthalmoscope*, familiar to all physicians; the *monocular indirect ophthalmoscope*, an L-shaped instrument resembling an automatic pistol; and the *binocular indirect ophthalmoscope*, generally used by ophthalmologists and becoming a familiar sight to pediatricians in most institutions. The binocular indirect ophthalmoscope requires the use of a convex lens held near the patient's eye while the examiner is positioned almost at arm's length from it. Of these three instruments, probably the most practical and potentially useful for the neonatologist is the monocular indirect ophthalmoscope (American Optical Co.). This instrument permits visibility through a smaller pupil than either of the other two and provides a wider angle view than the ordinary direct ophthalmoscope, but it does not require extensive practice and experience, as does the binocular indirect ophthalmoscope. The monocular indirect ophthalmoscope is available as a cordless instrument using rechargeable batteries. This is advantageous in the nursery but has a slight disadvantage in that the expensive instrument can be easily carried away from where it may be needed later. Another disadvantage of the monocular indirect ophthalmoscope is that the optical system within the instrument must remain properly aligned in order to permit its use through a small pupil, and when inexperienced examiners treat the instrument roughly, the optics become misaligned.

Retinoscopy

This technique needs to be briefly explained in order to clear up any confusion with "ophthalmoscopy." By use of a retinoscope, an ophthalmologist or optometrist determines the refractive state of an eye. This is an objective examination relying on the fact that lateral motion of a convex lens makes an object seen through it appear to shift in the opposite direction. Conversely, the image seen through a laterally moving concave lens exhibits "with" motion, moving in the same direction *with* the lens. The retinoscopist directs a streak of light that is coaxial with the examiner's line of sight through the instrument, through the patient's pupil, and by turning the instrument slightly from side to side, "sweeps" the pupil. Depending on the patient's refractive error, the fundus reflection appears to move with or against the direction of motion of the incident light. By interposing appropriate refracting lenses, this motion can be neutralized. The power of these neutralizing lenses is arithmetically adjusted for the examiner's working distance from the eye, and the result indicates the refractive error of the patient's eye. Newborn eyes have an average refractive error of +2.00. Low birth weight infants have less hyperopia than this. Infants with regressed retinopathy of prematurity frequently are myopic (nearsighted), which requires *minus lenses* whenever glasses are used.

TECHNIQUE

Newborn infants who resist having their eyes examined make it exceedingly difficult for the examiner to retract the eyelids open manually, and the upper lid often everts. To overcome this squeezing of the eyelids by the patient, a small lid speculum is useful. The Sauer lid speculum (Storz or Weck) is proportioned suitably for small infants. With some practice, this instrument can be inserted under the upper and lower eyelid margin and will then retain itself and hold the lids open. The infant's hands are restrained by an assistant. Although it seems cruel, a topical anesthetic is not necessary and could cause the corneal epithelium to become irregular and thereby hinder the examination. If sympathy inhibits the examiner from using a speculum, it should be kept in mind that the degree of pain experienced by the infant is probably not significantly worse than that from a venipuncture and almost certainly not as severe as the pain from a circumcision. The lid speculum ordinarily should not be placed in an eye that is inflamed with purulent exudate, since a small corneal abrasion can predispose to corneal ulcer. The speculum should be sterile, and the necessary number of speculums should be obtained to permit this. In small premature infants, the spring pressure of the speculum can be excessive and unnecessarily traumatic. This problem can be circumvented by obtaining some steel suture material and twisting a small piece around the two arms of the speculum in a loop, to hold the speculum at whatever position of maximum expansion is desired. This suture material is easily cut with bandage scissors, and the short ends of this suture loop should be bent in such a way that there is no risk of injury to the eye or lids. The stainless steel restraining loop may be left in place for numerous examinations before it needs to be replaced. Other speculum designs (e.g., Cook's or Saunders') have a thumbscrew to maintain a fixed opening, which avoids the spring problem.

Either the ordinary direct ophthalmoscope or the monocular indirect ophthalmoscope should be brought close to the patient's eye during the fundus examination.

A common technical error is to try to perform the examination several inches away from the patient's face. This would be comparable to peering through a knothole in a fence from several feet away. The closer the instrument approaches the cornea, the easier it is to see through the pupil. Since the average refractive error for a newborn infant is +2.00, the numbers on the direct ophthalmoscope should read black 2, unless the examiner also has a refractive error, in which case this needs to be modified accordingly. If the examiner wears corrective lenses during the ophthalmoscopy, no additional correction need be made on the instrument. If no clear view of the fundus can be obtained, the focusing knob must then be changed until fundus vessels can be seen. *With the direct ophthalmoscope, it is difficult to see much more than the disk, unless the pupils have been dilated.* With practice, these instruments permit a reasonably good view of the disk without dilation, as long as the ambient light is dim (it should be remembered that ceiling lights shine into the supine baby's eyes). The patient's pupil constricts to the greatest degree when the examiner's light falls on the macula and to the least degree when light falls on the disk.

The highest level of ocular fundus examination requires the use of the binocular indirect ophthalmoscope. As currently designed, this instrument consists of three parts: (1) a headband supporting a light source, adjustable mirror, and optics for the examiner's eyes; these allow the bright examining light to align closely with the examiner's binocular visual axis; (2) a power transformer for the light, with an interconnecting cord; and (3) a hand-held convex lens in the power range of 20 to 30 diopters. With this system, the trained examiner with normal binocular vision can see a stereoscopic wide-angle view of the disk and macula simultaneously. The image is seen at the level of the hand-held condensing lens and fills the lens. Optically, an inverted, real aerial image of the subject's fundus is formed between the convex lens and the examiner. This instrument is difficult to master because the image is inverted; consequently, lateral movement of the condensing lens causes the image to move in the opposite direction. It takes a typical ophthalmology resident about a year to become reasonably proficient with this instrument, and 2 to 3 years to become truly comfortable with it. This practice pays off, however, both by permitting a far more detailed view of the peripheral retina (the site of most retinopathy of prematurity) and by permitting a view of the fundus in a *moving* eye, as in an infant, child, or uncooperative adult. In such difficult circumstances, the examiner uses the same mental process that is familiar to the physician who is experienced in examining the tympanic membrane or pharynx of a child: quick glimpses give a series of mental "photographs." For detailed evaluation, numerous short exposures are made and a composite is mentally constructed. The talent for accomplishing this seems to vary among humans, as does artistic talent.

The binocular indirect ophthalmoscope has become an indispensible tool to the ophthalmologist. I have personally observed malignant melanomas in adults and retinoblastomas in infants that were virtually undetectable on direct ophthalmoscopy and yet easily studied with the binocular indirect ophthalmoscope.

An ophthalmologist consulting in the nursery faces one of his or her most difficult challenges: a fundus examination in an uncooperative patient with a *small pupil*. Even when the newborn infant's pupil is well dilated, it is not very large (about 6 mm) by adult standards. Furthermore, most *ophthalmologists lacking a strong clinical pediatric background will be understandably intimidated by the apparent fragility of many newborns.* Thus, nursery examinations have become a field of "special interest" for ophthalmologists.

There are not yet enough pediatric ophthalmologists to do all nursery consultations. In many communities, a general ophthalmologist or a retina consultant has made these examinations a personal area of special interest and expertise. The neonatologist and hospital administration may need to nurture such a relationship for the benefit of the patients.

ORGAN IMAGING

DANIELLE K.B. BOAL, M.D.

As a result of expanding technology, the field of radiology, and in particular organ imaging, has undergone dramatic growth and change. Each imaging modality possesses certain properties that make it useful in diagnosis, but no single modality has prevailed to the exclusion of others. Unique to neonatal-perinatal medicine are the disease processes themselves, as well as the constraints that direct and limit the diagnostic evaluation. Imaging must be carefully tailored to yield the desired information with the least amount of disturbance to the critically ill infant. An increasing awareness of the importance of a stable environment for the infant has led to increased use of portable studies (particularly ultrasonography) and, to a lesser extent, nuclear medicine (isotopic) examinations. Three-dimensional cross-sectional images along with dynamic and functional information can now be obtained without moving the infant from the isolette.

RADIOLOGY

The x-ray study continues to be the most frequently ordered imaging study of the infant. Valuable information (endotracheal tube position, arterial line position, free air) that directly affects patient care can be obtained with a minimum of patient handling. While the radiation dose is minimal with a single portable *chest x-ray film*, one must be wary of overuse of radiology. Although the recent introduction of rare earth screens for conventional radiologic examination has significantly decreased exposure without sacrificing image detail, there is still no justification for a "routine daily chest film" in the sick neonate. Likewise, one should confine the x-ray study to the area of interest; there is no need to combine a chest and abdomen on one film. Careful positioning and technique by the x-ray technician are necessary to reduce the number of repeat examinations. The films should be exposed by the most experienced technician available with the assistance of the nurse who is caring for the infant. In most instances, a single film of the chest in the supine position to include the subglottic airway will yield the desired information. *Routine lateral chest x-ray examinations add no further diagnostic information and should be reserved for those instances of specific benefit* (e.g., position of thoracotomy tube, location of chest mass or infiltrate), although a single initial lateral x-ray film of the chest is often valuable and advocated by many radiologists. *Lateral decubitus and cross-table lateral films* (both horizontal beam technique) are useful in identifying suspected free air in the chest or abdomen. Magnification radiography has been utilized to provide better lung parenchymal detail and improved visualization of the airway.

The chest x-ray study frequently contributes to the specific diagnosis of both cardiac and pulmonary disease, but what is not often emphasized is *the role of the radiologic examination in monitoring the response to treatment and its complications*. These parameters include changes in parenchymal lung pattern suggesting superimposed infection, interstitial air and free air, progressive parenchymal damage from barotrauma and oxygen, and patent ductus arteriosus. A change in cardiac size frequently precedes the oscultatory findings of a patent ductus arteriosus. However, because of the variability of positioning, the angle of the x-ray beam, the phase of respiration and the size of the thymus, *a measured cardiothoracic ratio is not as reliable as the interpretation of cardiac size by an experienced radiologist*.

Conventional film radiography is highly effective in imaging those parts of the body with innate high contrast but remains limited in discriminating soft tissue structures such as abdominal organs. In the neonate, *skeletal surveys* remain useful in the investigation of dwarfism and suspected bone dysplasia. In suspected osteomyelitis, the skeletal survey is useful, as is nuclear medicine bone scanning. In the neonate, osteomyelitis is often multifocal despite minimal signs and symptoms, so that a wide search is necessary. On the other hand, metabolic bone disease, such as rickets or the sequelae of intrauterine infections, is uniformly spread so that a narrow survey (e.g., wrist or knee) is sufficient. It is important to remember that the first signs of metabolic disease (osteopenia and rib fractures) are often noted on the frequently obtained chest x-ray study.

Films of the skull have largely been replaced by computed tomography (CT) and cranial sonography. In instances of suspected skull fracture, congenital malformation, or craniosynostosis, selected regular skull films are useful.

Abdominal radiology is much more limited in value because of the lack of contrast between organs. To determine arterial and venous catheter placement, a single film of the abdomen suffices; subsequent films are not indicated unless the catheter position is changed. Systematic interpretation of the adominal film, (i.e., evaluation of bones, soft tissues, and bowel gas pattern; search for a mass or abnormal calcifications) will yield important information and direct the choice of further diagnostic studies. In the neonate with suspected necrotizing enterocolitis, radiologic study yields valuable information that may modify treatment. Pneumatosis intestinalis, portal venous air, and pneumoperitoneum may be seen on the film of the abdomen in the supine position. In monitoring the infant with necrotizing enterocolitis, some prefer additional cross-table lateral films of the abdomen for early recognition of free air. More subtle radiologic abnormalities often precede the symptoms of necrotizing enterocolitis.

Contrast studies in the neonate are infrequent and are tailored to the specific problem. At our institution, nonionic excretory urography has been replaced by ultrasonography and the isotopes of nuclear medicine. If excretory urography is needed, a nonionic water-soluble contrast agent (which minimizes physiologic stress) should be used. Voiding cystourethrography should be performed in instances of documented urinary tract infection and suspected obstruction or reflux. Barium studies are usually diagnostic in the infant with bowel obstruction. A barium enema should be the initial study, followed immediately by an air or barium study of the upper gastrointestinal tract when appropriate (if there is high obstruction). The barium esophagram is useful in the evaluation of suspected gastroesophageal reflux, swallowing disorder, and tracheoesophageal fistula (via tube study).

Barium sulfate is the contrast agent of choice for studies of the gastrointestinal tract. Meglumine diatrizoate (Gastrografin) should not be used except in the treatment of meconium ileus. If a water-soluble contrast agent is indicated (as in suspected perforation), isotonic sodium diatrizoate (Hypaque) or meglumine diatrizoate (Renografin) via nasogastric tube is adequate. More recently, low osmolar nonionic media have proved to be highly successful gastrointestinal contrast agents. Nonionic contrast has the unique advantage of not being absorbed from the gastrointestinal tract, but is readily absorbed from the peritoneum and excreted via the kidneys. Thus, perforation may be diagnosed by demonstrating contrast in the renal collecting system following a gastrointestinal contrast study.

ULTRASONOGRAPHY

Ultrasound imaging utilizes acoustic waves; there is no ionizing radiation. An image is created from recorded echoes at various tissue interfaces. Most important, there appears to be no significant biologic effect. Accordingly, ultrasonography is assuming an increasing role in perinatal-neonatal medicine, and the widespread use of ultrasound in obstetrics has greatly facilitated the diagnosis and management of fetal disorders of growth and development. Many developmental abnormalities are now diagnosed early in gestation and in some instances early delivery and intervention are initiated and guided by ultrasonography. *Those features uniquely suited to radiologic study, e.g., the high contrast of bone and air, are, conversely, deterrents to ultrasound imaging.*

The many advantages of ultrasonography are uniquely suited to imaging of the neonate. These include (l) lack of ionizing radiation, (2) no sedation or preparation, (3) excellent image quality due to small body structures and a paucity of body fat, and (4) flexibility in imaging variable anatomic planes. Most important is the portability of real-time sonography, which helps maintain a stable environment for the neonate while providing anatomic, dynamic, and (in some instances) functional information.

Real-time ultrasound is the modality commonly employed in imaging of the fetus and neonate. *Real-time scanning is analogous to fluoroscopy;* it provides a continuous image, resulting in dynamic, anatomic information. Bowel peristalsis, vascular pulsations, movement of solid within liquid structures, and joint motion are among those functions that may be easily analyzed. Most real-time units used in neonatology today employ a sector scan, which results in a pie-shaped wedge of displayed image. In the neonate, the most useful frequency range is provided by a 5 to 10 MHz transducer.

Cranial sonography has all but replaced computed tomography as the "gold standard" of neonatal intracranial imaging, and the anterior fontanelle is the natural "window" on the brain. Serial cranial sonography is now the routine surveillance procedure for the smaller premature infant (less than 32 weeks gestational age, less than 1500 g). We still have much to learn about the significance of intracranial hemorrhage as it relates to the developmental outcome of the infant; ultrasound clearly establishes the site and extent of hemorrhage and is valuable in monitoring ventricular size, extension of hemorrhage, and development of porencephaly. Responses to serial lumbar punctures and shunting procedures are readily monitored with ultrasound. In many institutions, ultrasound guidance is now routine in the operative placement of ventricular shunts. Developmental anomalies of the ventricular system, including defects in diverticulation, arteriovenous malformation, and hydrocephaly, are easily defined by cranial sonography. Although diagnosis of subarachnoid and subdural hemorrhage can be made with ultrasound, these hemorrhages are frequently easier to detect by computed tomography or magnetic resonance imaging (MRI). This also holds true for posterior fossa hemorrhage and cerebral asphyxia. For both of these processes, there is now a growing body of literature concerning sonographic findings, so that *ultrasound may soon replace computed tomography* in these areas as well. Recent reports describe sonographic evaluation of the dysraphic spine, including accurate determination of the level of the conus and delineation of associated spinal anomalies such as lipoma, cyst, or solid tumor.

The combination of *abdominal ultrasound* and nuclear medicine imaging now has a higher diagnostic yield than does contrast urography. The most frequently examined site after the cranium is the abdomen. Most often an abnormality is detected on a prenatal ultrasound scan. Fifty percent of all fetal abnormalities discovered by maternal ultrasound examination involve the urinary tract. Most masses appearing in the neonatal period relate to the genitourinary tract, and the two most common masses are hydronephrosis and multicystic dysplastic kidney (MCDK). The most common obstructive hydronephrosis is ureteropelvic junction obstruction, which has a characteristic sonographic appearance (a

massively dilated central pelvis with peripherally arranged smaller dilated calices). An attempt to identify the ureter and examination of the bladder and bladder neck should be routine. In this way other possibilities, such as vesicoureteral reflux, ectopic ureterocele, ureterovesical obstruction, and posterior urethral valves, will not be overlooked. As many as 30 percent of patients have an abnormality of the contralateral kidney when ureteropelvic junction obstruction or MCDK is present. Therefore, examination of the contralateral kidney must be part of the initial sonographic evaluation. Renal dysplasia (multicystic dysplastic kidney) may take several different forms, ranging from the more common irregularly sized and arranged collection of cysts without an identifiable central pelvis to a more solid and bizarre structure.

Other flank masses presenting in the neonatal period include renal vein thrombosis and adrenal hemorrhage as well as the less common fetal renal hamartoma and infantile polycystic kidney disease. Each has fairly characteristic findings. In renal vein thrombosis, the kidney is enlarged and echogenic (increased echoes) with distorted internal architecture. Adrenal hemorrhage is typically sonolucent initially, with increasing and variable echogenicity as it involutes. At our institution, renal sonography is the initial screening study for detecting associated renal anomalies (e.g., an infant with the VATER complex). Not infrequently one must determine whether kidneys are present in a newborn with anuria or suspected Potter's syndrome. Real-time sonography is extremely valuable in this respect; however, one must be aware that when there is renal agenesis, the adrenals may enlarge and flatten into the renal fossa, thus mimicking renal tissue. In this instance, nuclear medicine may or may not be helpful, since severely impaired renal function cannot be distinguished from agenesis. When an arterial line is present, a hand injection of contrast material with a single film of the abdomen will often clarify the situation by delineating the vascular anatomy.

For other abdominal masses in the neonate, ultrasound is accurate in determining the organ of origin, and frequently the specific diagnosis, when the sonographic characteristics and clinical information are considered jointly. Neonatal neuroblastoma may be difficult to distinguish from adrenal hemorrhage, based only upon sonographic appearance. Relevant clinical information along with associated sonographic findings (such as hepatomegaly) is valuable in distinguishing neonatal neuroblastoma from adrenal hemorrhage. Serial sonography will show regression and changing echogenicity in cases of adrenal hemorrhage. In female infants with cystic abdominal masses, the genital tract should be considered, in addition to gastrointestinal duplication, cystic hygroma, and other less common entities. Hydrocolpos may be distinguished from ovarian cyst by the caudal extension of the vaginal mass below the symphysis pubis. Benign angiomatous tumors of the liver often result in dilatation of the upper abdominal aorta and a large celiac trunk as a result of significant increased blood flow and arterio-venous shunting; this is not present in hepatoblastoma.

Ultrasonography is useful in the evaluation of perinatal ascites, frequently identifying the etiology. Anomalies of the genitourinary and gastrointestinal tracts account for 60 to

65 percent of the cases in most series of nonimmune ascites. Gastrointestinal atresia has been identified in utero and in the newborn by ultrasound.

Newer applications of ultrasonography are playing an increasing role in newborn medicine. As an example, it is possible with ultrasound to identify the position of intravascular catheters and complications such as thrombi. Catheters can be identified in the aorta, inferior vena cava, and right atrium. Real-time imaging of the chest is used to identify pleural and pericardial effusions and to provide guidance during thoracentesis, and it is extremely useful in confirming suspected diaphragmatic paralysis and eventration. Real-time sonographic imaging of the hips is highly effective in diagnosing congenital hip dislocation and subluxation as well as in monitoring response to treatment. Although nonspecific as to diagnosis, ultrasound may be used to characterize superficial soft tissue masses as either cystic or solid and to determine their extent.

NUCLEAR MEDICINE

Nuclear medicine is a more limited but valuable adjunct in the diagnosis and treatment of neonatal problems. The *gamma camera* is the imaging instrument of choice. If available, a portable gamma camera may be used in studying the critically ill neonate. Special attachments such as pinhole and converging collimators allow image magnification. *A radioisotope (usually technetium-99m), attached to various molecules that target a specific organ, emits gamma rays that are collected and displayed.* Nuclear medicine plays a vital role in providing dynamic and functional organ information. With computer capabilities, more sophisticated analyses of data are possible, such as blood flow studies, assessment and fractionation of organ function (renal studies), and nuclear cardiology to evaluate anatomic and hemodynamic parameters.

In the neonate, nuclear medicine imaging is most commonly utilized in the evaluation of hepatobiliary and renal disorders. Because of normally low tubular and glomerular filtration rates, *the intravenous urogram may be unreliable in the first 2 weeks of life.* Quantification of functional impairment with renal scintigraphy is possible in the newborn with urinary tract pathology. A technetium-labeled glomerular filtrate, DTPA (technetium-99m-Sn-diethylenetriamine pentacetic acid), is recommended. By obtaining digital and visual images every 2 seconds after intravenous bolus injection, a blood flow study permits analysis of relative perfusion along with functional information. It may be necessary to obtain delayed images (24 hours) to establish the level of function. Technetium-99m-DMSA (dimercaptosuccinic acid) attaches to renal cortical tubules, providing high quality images of the renal cortex, and it is useful for assessing renal cortical mass, often providing information when both intravenous urography and technetium-DTPA studies are unsuccessful. The more common indications for renal scintigraphy in the neonatal period include hydronephrosis, renal vein thrombosis, dysplasia, abdominal mass, and agenesis. A word of caution in the evaluation of suspected renal agenesis: nuclear medicine scanning cannot definitely differentiate severe functional impairment from agenesis. A combination of nuclear medicine and ultrasound is recommended for kidney evaluation in neonates.

Differentiating neonatal hepatitis from biliary atresia in the newborn with jaundice remains a difficult problem. Radioisotope scanning of the biliary tree is the only method of imaging that provides crucial information concerning hepato-biliary physiology. Technetium-99m diethyl-IDA and technetium-99m diisopropyl-IDA are the more commonly employed radiopharmaceuticals. Phenobarbital given orally for several days prior to the study increases the accuracy of the test. Hepatocyte function (clearance of the isotope from the blood) and hepatobiliary transit time (removal of the isotope to the extrahepatobiliary tree and ultimately to the intestine) are the criteria measured. Biliary atresia is diagnosed when there is no intestinal activity through 24 hours of imaging in the setting of adequate hepatocyte clearance. Ultrasonography supplies additional anatomic information, including evaluation of biliary tract dilatation, size of the gallbladder (a gallbladder longer than 1.5 cm is rarely present in biliary atresia), presence of choledochal cyst, and parenchymal detail.

Other indications for nuclear medicine scan of the liver in the neonate include evaluation of the infant with suspected asplenia or polysplenia. A combination of technetium-99m sulfur colloid, which images the liver and spleen, and a hepatobiliary scan, liver only, is often diagnostic as to the presence, position, and configuration of splenic tissue.

Radionuclide bone scanning may be useful in the neonate with suspected osteomyelitis. It is not a replacement for radiology; the two studies are complementary. There are many reported cases of false-negative scans in the neonate with osteomyelitis. However, neonatal osteomyelitis may be multifocal, and bone scintigraphy is often valuable in identifying additional unsuspected sites of bone involvement. The most commonly employed isotope is technetium-99m diphosphonate, with blood pool and delayed images providing valuable information.

Radionuclide angiocardiography with echocardiography has increasing application in the neonate with suspected cardiac disease, providing noninvasive means of evaluation. Radionuclide angiocardiography may be used to determine the actual amount of shunt as well as define the sequence of atrial and ventricular filling and emptying, which can often delineate the site of the shunt. Flow studies employ a technetium-labeled agent, most frequently ^{99m}Tc DTPA or pertechnetate. Myocardial imaging using thallium-201 defines the distribution of myocardial blood flow. Scintigraphy is valuable in suspected shunt lesions either right-to-left or left-to-right, in evaluation of patients with pulmonary hypertension, pulmonary stenosis, and right ventricular hypertrophy, and in the differentiation of anomalous origin of the left coronary artery from congestive myocardiopathy.

Uncommonly employed studies in the newborn include ventilation-perfusion lung scans and gastrointestinal studies to exclude Meckel's diverticulum. The evaluation of gastroesophageal reflux in the neonate includes a barium swallow, which may not always demonstrate reflux. If gastroesophageal reflux is strongly suspected, scintigraphy with technetium-99m sulfur colloid may demonstrate the reflux and, rarely, document aspiration, with the isotope appearing in the lungs on delayed scans. When available, the pH probe has proved to be the most sensitive indicator of gastroesophageal reflux. Finally, in the infant with hypothyroidism, a technetium-99m pertechnetate scan is extremely valuable for detection and localization of functioning thyroid tissue.

MAGNETIC RESONANCE IMAGING

The exact role of magnetic resonance imaging (MRI) in pediatrics is still being defined. At the present time, the greatest value of MRI in infancy and childhood is in the evaluation of the central nervous system. High resolution multiplanar imaging capabilities, superb differentiation between grey and white matter, and lack of ionizing radiation make MRI a valuable imaging tool. Widespread use of *this modality is limited by lengthy imaging time, the need for sedation, the difficulty in monitoring the infant during the study, and the expense.* Magnetic field strengths between 0.15 and 2.0 tesla are used for imaging, and the development of surface coils has improved MRI capabilities for infants. MRI is superior to CT in defining central nervous system ano-

malies, delays and disorders of myelination, disordered neuronal migration, and acquired diseases of the central nervous system, such as hemorrhage or tumor; however, MRI is not able to detect calcifications. MRI has proved its usefulness in the evaluation of spinal dysraphism. With the advent of cardiac and respiratory gating, contrast agents, and faster scanners, MRI will undoubtedly have a greater and more diverse role in imaging the infant.

SUGGESTED READING

Babcock DS. Neonatal and pediatric ultrasonography. Clinics in Diagnostic Ultrasound 24. New York: Churchill Livingstone, 1989.
Cohen M. Pediatric magnetic resonance imaging. Philadelphia: WB Saunders, 1986.
Merten DF, Grossman H. Diagnostic imaging in pediatrics: the state of the art. Pediatr Ann May 1986, 15(5):355–358.
Sumner TE, et al. Neonatal abdominal real-time sonography. Radiography 1981; 1(3):29–40.
Teele RL. Seminars in ultrasound, CT and MR. Pediatric 1984 Vol. 5, No. 1.
Treves ST. Pediatric nuclear medicine. New York: Springer-Verlag, 1985.

PARENTERAL NUTRITION

NANCY F. SHEARD, Sc.D., R.D.
W. ALLAN WALKER, M.D.

INDICATIONS FOR USE

Since the late 1960s, parenteral nutrition (PN) has been used successfully in pediatrics as a means for providing adequate nutrition to infants who are unable to attain complete enteral feedings. Newborns most likely to require some form of parenteral support are those who undergo major surgery of the gastrointestinal tract, such as repair of omphalocele, gastroschisis, intestinal atresia, tracheoesophageal fistula, and necrotizing enterocolitis. Occasionally, children born with major cardiac anomalies or pulmonary defects may be unable to feed for several weeks a complication secondary to a complicated postoperative course or labile medical condition, thereby necessitating PN.

In general, *PN is indicated in a full-term infant who has been unable to take adequate calories and nutrients via the enteral route for more than 5 to 7 days.* When indicated, a combination of enteral and parenteral nutrition can be used to ensure adequate nutrient intake during this period of rapid growth.

NUTRIENT REQUIREMENTS

Precise requirements for nutrients that are delivered intravenously are not known. Although the efficiency of digestion and absorption is not a factor to be considered,

nutrients administered via peripheral or central routes bypass the physiologic processing initially performed by the small intestine and liver. Calorie and protein requirements, however, appear to be relatively unchanged by the route of administration. Most commonly, we provide the Recommended Dietary Allowances for these nutrients, using changes in weight to modify caloric goals. Protein intakes are adjusted in accordance with kidney and liver function. Blood urea nitrogen or ammonia levels are used to assess tolerance to a given protein intake. Guidelines for electrolytes, minerals, and trace nutrients administered parenterally are shown in Table 1.

SOLUTIONS

Parenteral nutrition solutions are composed of dextrose, amino acids, electrolytes, minerals, and vitamins (Table 2). Intravenous (IV) lipid is also provided as a source both of calories and of essential fatty acids.

TABLE 1 Daily Intravenous Nutrient Requirements

Calories	105–115	kcal/kg
Protein	2–3	g/kg
Sodium	2–4	mEq/kg
Potassium	2–3	mEq/kg
Chloride	2–3	mEq/kg
Magnesium	0.25–0.5	mEq/kg
Calcium	1–2.5	mEq/kg
Phosphorus	1–2	mmol/kg
Zinc	100–300	µg/kg
Copper	20	µg/kg
Chromium	0.14–0.2	µg/kg
Manganese	2–10	µg/kg

TABLE 2 Standard Parenteral Nutrition Solutions*

	PN-10	PN-20	PN-25	PN-30
Amino acids	20 g	20 g	40 g	30 g
Dextrose	100 g	200 g	250 g	300 g
Potassium	20 mEq	20 mEq	20 mEq	20 mEq
Sodium	30 mEq	30 mEq	30 mEq	30 mEq
Calcium	15 mEq	15 mEq	15 mEq	15 mEq
Magnesium	10 mEq	10 mEq	10 mEq	10 mEq
Phosphorus	10 mmol	10 mmol	10 mmol	10 mmol
Chloride	30 mEq	30 mEq	30 mEq	30 mEq
Acetate	35 mEq	35 mEq	65 mEq	50 mEq
Zinc	1.0 mg	1.0 mg	1.0 mg	1.0 mg
Copper	0.2 mg	0.2 mg	0.2 mg	0.2 mg
Chromium	2 μg	2 μg	2 μg	2 μg
Manganese	60 μg	60 μg	60 μg	60 μg
Vitamins†	Yes	Yes	Yes	Yes
Calories	410	750	990	1,120

* All quantities given are per 1,000 ml.
† A daily dose of Pediatric MVI is added to one bottle daily for each patient.

Dextrose concentrations vary with the route of delivery and the specific caloric requirements of the child. The level of amino acids in the solution depends on the age and clinical condition of the patient. Our standard PN solutions are shown in Table 2.

Commercial amino acid solutions vary in their content of essential (EAA) and nonessential (NEAA) amino acids. The *optimal ratio of EAA to NEAA in pediatric patients is 60:40.* Newer pediatric formulations include the amino acids cystine and taurine, which may be essential for premature and newborn infants. Nonessential amino acids such as glutamate and aspartate, which are found in significant quantities in breast milk, are also included in the newer solutions.

The concentration of electrolytes and minerals contained in our standard solutions is calculated to meet the intravenous maintenance requirements of these nutrients when PN solution is provided at maintenance fluid rates. Sodium and potassium concentrations can be adjusted to meet individual needs. Significant electrolyte losses secondary to diarrhea or vomiting, chest tube drainage, or renal dysfunction are most appropriately replaced with a second intravenous solution that more closely matches the composition of the fluid being lost. Cations can be provided as either the chloride or acetate salt, as the medical condition indicates. Amino acid solutions currently in use generally contain acetate salts of the amino acids, thereby providing a significant amount of this anion in the basic PN mixture.

Maximal calcium and phosphorus concentrations are dependent on the calcium/phosphorus product. Their solubility varies with both the pH of the amino acid solution and the final protein concentration. The more acidic the amino acid solution, the greater is the amount of calcium and phosphorus that can be dissolved.

Specific parenteral trace element solutions have been designed for use in pediatric patients. Our current practice is to provide zinc, copper, manganese, and chromium in the amounts outlined in Table 2. Increased requirements for any of these trace minerals are calculated and added to the PN solution. The trace elements selenium, iron, and iodine are not provided to patients who receive parenteral nutrition for less than 1 month.

A pediatric multivitamin mixture is added to the first bottle of PN solution the infant receives each day. As a result, most infants receive the estimated daily intravenous requirement of all the vitamins, including vitamin K, vitamin B_{12}, folic acid, biotin, and pantothenic acid.

Approximately 20 to 30 percent of the estimated caloric requirement is provided daily as lipid; both 10 and 20 percent lipid emulsions are used. Owing to its cost, 20 percent lipid is reserved for patients who are fluid restricted. Lipid emulsions can be soy based, safflower based, or a combination of these two oils. Soy-based formulas contain slightly less linoleic acid but more linolenic acid.

ADMINISTRATION

Once it is evident that an infant is unlikely to receive adequate nutrition for more than 5 days, the use of PN is indicated. If this is expected to be of short duration (less than 1 week) and if peripheral access is available, PN with less concentrated formulas can be initiated. In our institution, *the maximal concentrations used peripherally are 10 percent dextrose and 2 percent amino acids.* The caloric density of peripheral solutions is low, usually necessitating the use of intravenous fat at maximal doses. In neonates, we use either 10 or 20 percent lipid emulsions to provide 3 to 4 g of fat per kilogram per day. A maximum of 50 percent of calories is provided as lipid. If the medical condition allows, PN solutions are provided at a rate equal to 1 ½ times the maintenance fluid rate. Generally, adequate calories can be provided if these fluid volumes are tolerated.

If parenteral nutrition is expected to be long term, placement of a central venous catheter is indicated. This is most frequently done in the operating room by a skilled pediatric surgeon. A Silastic catheter is placed via a cutdown into the external jugular vein, and the tip threaded into the superior vena cava. The exterior end of the catheter is tunneled under the skin exiting from the chest. This helps to prevent dislodgement of the line.

Placement of a central venous line (CVL) permits the use of more hyperosmolar solutions, which are also more calorically dense. The use of more concentrated formulas permits the delivery of adequate nutrients when these solutions are run at maintenance fluid rates. Intravenous lipid is also provided through the line, using a Y or T connector beyond the filter. In general, lipid supplies 20 to 30 percent of the estimated caloric requirements in infants receiving central PN.

INITIATION OF PARENTERAL NUTRITION

A 10 percent dextrose solution can generally be initiated at maintenance fluid rates without complication. After 8 to 12 hours, the rate of D_{10} infusion is increased to 1½ times maintenance. If a central line is in place, advancement to a 20 percent dextrose solution (to be run at maintenance) is recommended for the second day. Further increases in glucose delivery can then be managed by altering either the rate of infusion or the actual dextrose concentration. Changes are generally made every 24 hours.

Intravenous fat emulsions are commonly initiated on the second day of PN. Lipid is begun at a rate of 0.5 g per kilogram per day and infused over 24 hours. The rate is doubled every 12 to 24 hours until the maximal fat infusion rate is reached (3 to 4 g per kilogram per day).

MONITORING

Daily weights are necessary for patients receiving parenteral nutrition in order to ascertain fluid balance. Glucose tolerance is monitored by checking each urine voiding until the patient is receiving a constant level of dextrose. At this point, urine voidings are checked on each shift. If glycosuria is 2^+ or greater, a blood sugar test is taken and glucose infusion rate decreased by 10 to 20 percent, as indicated.

Routine laboratory tests are run before the initiations of PN and weekly thereafter (Table 3). More frequent monitoring of serum electrolytes, glucose, and triglycerides is performed as indicated by the clinical status of the patient. Other parameters of protein nutrition (e.g., prealbumin, transferrin) are examined and biochemical assessment of trace mineral status made as indicated by the clinical condition.

WEANING FROM PARENTERAL NUTRITION

Generally, PN support is provided until the infant is consuming 75 percent of estimated needs enterally. In older children, 50 percent of the caloric goal is used. Enteral feeds are frequently begun using half-strength formula at a constant infusion rate. After the formula is advanced to full strength, the rate is gradually increased to approximately one-half the maintenance fluid rate. This usually allows the PN to infuse at maintenance rates, thereby providing adequate nutrition. Enteral feedings are then gradually increased in rate or caloric density, as indicated by the clinical condition. Concurrently, the PN infusion rate is decreased. Although this transition can be a lengthy process, this method preserves the caloric intake of infants who are likely to develop feeding intolerance. In infants who tolerate enteral feedings early on, the PN solution is weaned over several days, generally by decreasing the PN rate as oral intake increases.

COMPLICATIONS

Mechanical complications associated with central venous catheters most frequently are due to *improper placement.* For this reason, the placement of the line is checked radiographically before it is used. Other common catheter-related problems include *line occlusion* and *catheter breakage.* These can be prevented if the proper techniques are used when handling the line.

A broken catheter is easily repaired with the correct line repair kit. Catheter breaks can be prevented by alternating the clamping sites and by using appropriate, not excessive, force when clamping the line.

Initially, we attempt to clear a blocked catheter with heparin (2.5 ml of 100 U per milliliter). If this procedure fails, urokinase (5,000 U per milliliter) is instilled into the catheter (an amount equal to the volume of the line, approximately 0.5 to 1.0 ml). This procedure can be repeated 2 or 3 times as needed. The *likelihood of clotting the CVL is increased when the catheter is used for multiple purposes* (e.g., administration or drawing of blood, or drug therapies). Infection can be a frequent and sometimes life-threatening complication in infants receiving PN. The most common pathogens associated with central venous catheters are *Staphylococcus aureus* and *S. epidermidis.* An infection that is limited to the entry site can be treated with topical or intravenous antibiotics, or both. A systemic infection that appears to be related to the central line is initially treated with systemic broad-spectrum antibiotics. Once the drug sensitivity of the organism is known, specific antibody coverage is begun through the catheter. Treatment is continued for 14 to 21 days. If the clinical condition of the patient worsens, or if fever persists for more than 24 to 48 hours despite drug therapy, the catheter is generally removed. The risk of CVL infections can be minimized by using appropriate techniques when manipulating the line and by preserving lines for a single

TABLE 3   TPN Monitoring

Glucose	Phosphorus
Sodium	TCO_2
Potassium	Albumin
Chloride	Total protein
Blood urea nitrogen	Bilirubin
Creatinine	Serum glutamate pyruvate transaminase
Calcium	Alkaline phosphatase
Magnesium	Triglycerides

use (e.g., total parenteral nutrition administration, blood drawing, or drug administration).

Metabolic complications associated with PN, such as glucose or lipid intolerance, electrolyte or fluid imbalances, and vitamin or mineral deficiencies, can be prevented by the appropriate administration of PN solutions and by careful monitoring of findings and serum biochemistries. *The long-term complications most commonly seen in infants, such as cholestasis and bone disease, are difficult to prevent because their cause is unknown at present.* Provision of adequate but not excessive amounts of all nutrients is the most rational approach to prevention of these disease entities. Beginning enteral feedings, even in very small amounts, may be of help in the management of PN–related liver disease.

PERINATAL MAGNETIC RESONANCE IMAGING

WILLIAM C. HANIGAN, M.D., Ph.D.
ROBERT M. WRIGHT, M.D.
STEVEN M. WRIGHT, Ph.D.

Although magnetic resonance imaging (MRI) has gained wide acceptance for use in the older pediatric and adult age groups, its diagnostic role in the perinatal period has not been clearly outlined. Equipment costs and unique logistical requirements have restricted its general use, and individualized scanning techniques make radiologic comparisons difficult. Despite these limitations, MRI can be used effectively in younger children. This chapter describes the applications of MRI for radiologic diagnosis in the fetus and infant (at our institution).

SCANNING FACILITY

The scanning facility is located on the ground floor in a separate, isolated section of the hospital. Since the neonatal intensive care unit is located on the fifth floor and the pediatric intensive care unit on the fourth floor, seriously ill children are at a considerable distance from the scanning facility. Although this has not prevented its use for these children, it has required that inpatients be accompanied by their nurse or resident physician, depending on the clinical situation. The facility has capabilities for cardiac monitoring and oxygen administration that are used as needed. Recently, an MRI-compatible ventilator with general anesthesia and respiratory monitoring capability has been added to the facility.

SEDATION

For prenatal imaging, pregnant patients are sedated with 10 to 15 mg of intramuscular morphine or diazepam. Fetal motion artifact has not been a problem when sedation has been used. Expedited review by the institutional review board on a case by case basis is required for all prenatal scans.

Children are sedated with oral chloral hydrate at a dose of 30 mg per pound. The medication is given approximately 1 hour prior to scanning. As outpatients, neonates are scanned in the late morning or early afternoon, so that they may be discharged later in the day. The children are allowed to eat as usual, rather then delay feeding for that day. In over 150 scans in the prenatal and neonatal age groups, there have been no complications with this regimen. Approximately 5 percent of the scans are hampered by motion artifact and have to be repeated.

Infants requiring mechanical ventilation remain a significant logistical limitation to MRI. Premature infants are not scanned, as we believe that significant physical disruption of the infant's environment outweighs the potential benefit from the added information of MRI. In the rare instance in which complete anatomic clarification for diagnostic or prognostic decisions has to be made, computed tomographic (CT) scanning has been performed. When the premature newborn is not undergoing assisted mechanical ventilation, the MRI scan is performed following sonography.

SCANNING TECHNIQUE

All scans have been performed using a Siemens Magnetom (Siemens Corporation, Iselin, NJ) at 0.35 or 0.5 tesla. The imaging protocol for all studies consists of two rapid positioning sequences, followed by one or more standard spin-echo sequences. The initial two sequences are multiplane scout scans that require images in all three orientations for accurate positioning information. By using the FLASH technique and proper selection of imaging parameters, both T1- and T2-weighted positioning scans at the midline of all principal imaging orientations are obtained in approximately 1 minute with a 128×256 matrix. The T1-weighted sequence uses a repetition time (TR) of 90 msec, an echo time (TE) of 13 msec, and a radiofrequency (RF) tip angle of approximately 75 degrees. The T2-weighted sequence uses a TR of 220 msec, a TE of 35 msec, and an RF tip angle of 25 degrees.

Following the positioning sequences, multiecho, multislice imaging is performed in all studies. Congenital anomalies of the central nervous system, hydrocephalus, and intracranial hemorrhage are demonstrated with relative T1-weighted sequences, e.g., repetition times of 0.9 sec and echo times of 35 and 70 msec. Disorders of myelinization and neoplasms require T2-weighted sequences with repetition times of 1.9 to 3.0 sec and echoes of 35 and 140 msec. In the study of vascular lesions in the chest, relative T1-weighted sequences usually suffice. In the abdomen, both T1- and T2-weighted sequences are used. For the examination of the kidneys, a heavily T1-weighted single-echo sequence is used with a repetition time of 0.3 to 0.7 sec and a 15 msec echo.

Chloral hydrate sedation usually allows enough time for two to three T1-weighted sequences or two T2-weighted sequences. *Total scanning time has been reduced to an average of 30 to 45 minutes.*

When practical, image quality can often be improved by the use of specialized radiofrequency surface coils. Since it is not always practical to place a close-fitting surface coil around the patient's head or other regions, the manufacturer's standard head coil may be substituted. Spine, body, and extremity imaging may be performed in the head coil if the patient is small enough to fit inside. The configuration of the coil is almost ideal, allowing the infant to be loosely packed on both sides, thereby minimizing motion with full access and visibility from both ends. For larger infants, standard surface coils can be used. A 12×4 inch single-turn coil, used as a back coil on adults, and a 6×6 inch two-turn coil are needed for imaging of the abdomen, hips, and legs.

Since the surface coils can decrease the intensity variation across an area of interest, several identical coils can be connected in parallel and one placed above and one below the patient. The use of parallel coils can significantly improve the signal-to-noise ratio in the center of the abdomen or hip joints, which are often at the edge of a usable region of a single surface coil.

SCANNING OF THE INFANT IN UTERO

Without question, ultrasonography remains the procedure of choice for imaging the infant in utero. At the request of the sonographer, MRI may be performed for anatomic clarification when the organ pathology does not involve the central nervous system. For lesions involving the central nervous system, however, a specific diagnosis should be given; ventriculomegaly will not suffice. If the ultrasonographer cannot be more specific, MRI is performed (Fig. 1). A precise diagnosis can usually be made, although the accurate delineation of the level or extent of spina bifida, for example, remains an imaging problem. In addition, we have not been successful with accurate diagnosis prior to 30 weeks of gestation. Given these caveats, we have found that precision in the anatomic diagnosis enables the perinatologist, neonatologist, neurosurgeon, and parents to deal more effectively with a child with a central nervous system anomaly.

SCANNING OF THE CENTRAL NERVOUS SYSTEM IN THE NEONATE

Our indications for magnetic resonance (MR) scanning in the neonatal period are listed in Table 1. We have found that for congenital abnormalities and intracranial hypertension, including hydrocephalus, intracranial hemorrhage (Fig. 2), and seizure disorders, the MR scan is the neuroradiologic procedure of choice. The indications for its use in the evaluation of seizure disorders are similar to those for any specific neuroradiologic examination, e.g., focal or complicated seizures in the neonatal period. For all practical purposes, *MRI has replaced myelography* in the neonate for evaluation of such entities as lipomyelomeningoceles or tethered cords, as well as preliminary staging for central nervous system tumors. The scan may also be used as follow-up for the effectiveness of shunting for hydrocephalus or the extent of tumor removal.

MRI has been useful for the evaluation of the sequelae of neonatal trauma and hypoxia-ischemia, including cerebral atrophy, delayed myelination, or porencephaly. However, its role in the evaluation of acute brain injury

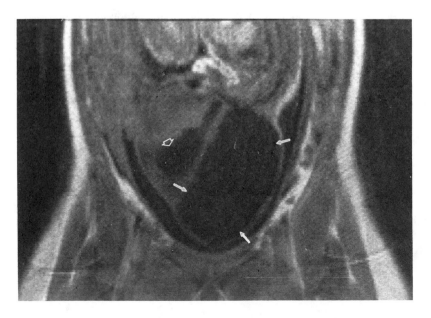

Figure 1 MR scan in a fetus at a gestational age of 34 weeks. The fetus is facing to the right. A posterior fossa cyst (white arrows) with an enlarged lateral ventricle (hollow arrow) outlines the Dandy-Walker malformation. (Reprinted from Pediatr Neurosci 1985–86; 12:154.)

TABLE 1 Clinical Indications for MRI of the Central Nervous System in the Neonate

Definite:

Hydrocephalus
Intracranial hemorrhage
Developmental abnormalities
Seizure disorders

Probable:

Birth injury and sequelae
Postasphyxial syndrome
Neurocutaneous disorders

Unknown:

Degenerative disease
Infectious disease

degenerative or infectious conditions of the central nervous system and therefore cannot evaluate the scan's usefulness. From previous reports we anticipate that the scan will demonstrate increased diagnostic capabilities in the evaluation of central nervous system infections, including herpes simplex encephalitis.

SCANNING OF OTHER ORGAN SEGMENTS

Although the MRI has been used predominantly for imaging diseases involving the central nervous system, it has also demonstrated excellent potential for visualizing pathology in other organ systems. Abdominal motion is a problem even with adequate sedation, but MRI has provided diagnostic information, at least equivalent to that of computed tomographic scanning, for the abdominal and retroperitoneal viscera. Because of its multiplane capability, it is excellent for demonstrating anomalies of the genitourinary system and rectum (Fig. 3). In addition, MRI

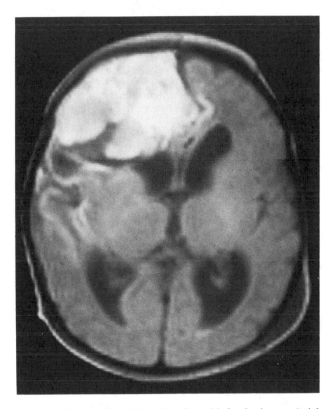

Figure 2 Twelve-day-old female infant with focal seizures. Axial MRI at the level of the foramen of Monro demonstrated a large right frontal lobe hemorrhage without mass effect. A 6-month follow-up showed resolution of the hematoma without evidence of a vascular anomaly. The child is meeting developmental milestones.

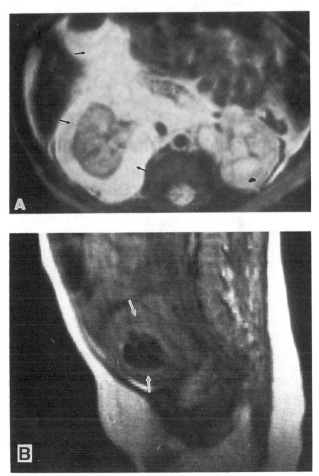

Figure 3 Two-month-old infant with a 9-day history of intermittent vomiting and abdominal distention. *A*, Coronal MRI (viewed from below) at the level of the first lumbar vertebra demonstrated massive urine ascites (black arrows) that appears to arise from the right kidney. The left kidney was hydronephrotic (black arrowhead). *B*, Sagittal MRI demonstrated a thickened bladder wall consistent with chronic urinary obstruction or a neurogenic bladder (white arrows).

(e.g., cerebral infarction or edema) has not been clearly defined. Recent evidence suggests that sonography may be more specific in premature infants, whereas MRI may be superior in the full-term newborn. Finally, our experience indicates that MRI is superior to computed tomographic scanning for the evaluation of neurocutaneous disorders.

We have very little experience scanning newborns with

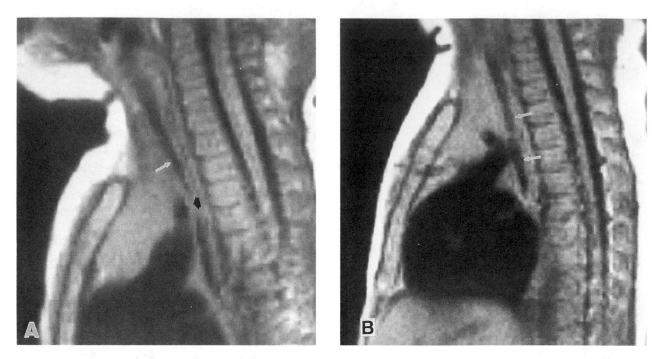

Figure 4 A 4-month-old infant with inspiratory stridor since birth. *A*, Sagittal MRI demonstrated compression of the trachea (white arrow) by the innominate artery (black arrowhead). *B*, Postoperative sagittal MRI showed the innominate artery suspended anterior to a patent trachea (white arrows).

is capable of accurately depicting vascular anomalies in the chest (Fig. 4) and can provide a good image of intercardiac anatomy with appropriate "gating" (i.e., triggered by an electrocardiogram) techniques.

DISADVANTAGES

The disadvantages of MRI include relatively high patient cost, logistics, and biological risks associated with the use of radiofrequency energy. The cost of the scan is approximately twice that of an enhanced computed tomogram. Certainly, routine MRI should be avoided, but over a period of time more specific indications, greater physician experience, and volume-driven declining costs should improve its cost-effectiveness. Logistics, such as longer scanning time and patient transport, can be solved on an individual basis. However, *the inability to use ferromagnetic materials in the vicinity of the scanner (e.g., mechanical ventilation or equipment for general anesthesia) remains a significant problem.* Finally, the biological risks of using radiofrequency energy in magnetic fields of up to 1.5 tesla in the perinatal period are unknown; although there is not a high risk-benefit ratio in the neonate, the risk of in utero imaging is sufficiently unknown to limit

its application only to the fetus with sonographically confirmed abnormalities, following appropriate informed parental consent.

FUTURE APPLICATIONS

Active research continues to refine the applications of MRI in young children. Newer scanning techniques (such as gating, pseudogating, and flow rephasing) have been designed to reduce motion artifact for cardiac and abdominal imaging, as well as for cerebrospinal fluid flow. The developmental patterns of myelinization in the normal central nervous system have been described with the goal of establishing a reference base for comparison with pathologic changes during the perinatal period. MR spectroscopy has been used to determine changes in brain metabolism following seizures or asphyxia in the newborn. Finally, the use of other ions (for example sodium) as a substitute for proton imaging suggests that the MR scan may offer extended possibilities for imaging both organ structure and function.

Acknowledgement. The authors gratefully acknowledge the secretarial assistance of Mrs. J. Gass and Mrs. Janet Arbuckle.

PHOTOTHERAPY

JERALD D. KING, M.D.
AUGUST L. JUNG, M.D.

TABLE 1 Jaundice Meter Criteria for Obtaining a Serum Bilirubin Reading

Age	Meter reading
<24 hr	12 or higher
24–48 hr	16 or higher
>48 hr	20 or higher

The conflicting evidence surrounding the level of serum bilirubin leading to kernicterus or more subtle forms of neurologic damage has left the physician without orderly, scientific guidelines for the management of hyperbilirubinemia. Hence, each clinician is left to interpret the expanding literature and to determine his or her own individual approach, or, alternatively, to choose from a number of published guidelines. In addition, a practical need exists to make the medical guidelines cost-effective.

The recent trial of phototherapy conducted by the National Institutes of Child Health and Human Development (NICHD) did not solve the basic dilemma of the relationship between the serum bilirubin level and developmental outcome, but it did draw some useful conclusions regarding phototherapy. *Phototherapy was found to be effective in controlling hyperbilirubinemia* and reducing (but not eliminating) the need for exchange transfusion in infants weighing less than 2,000 g even with hemolysis present. Larger infants were similarly benefited except in the case of hemolysis. The authors speculated that if phototherapy had been used earlier, as in infants with birth weights less than 2,000 g, it would have been proved even more effective. They *reconfirmed the short-term safety of phototherapy* when contrasted with the incidence of serious clinical problems associated with exchange transfusion, especially when sicker infants were compared.

Although other studies could be cited, these NICHD conclusions summarize our approach to phototherapy: If kernicterus or some subtle neuronal injury does occur at serum bilirubin levels less than 20 mg per deciliter, it is most likely to occur in sick, small, or immature infants. These infants are also most at risk for complications from an exchange transfusion. Until more is known, *we institute phototherapy to control the serum bilirubin level and reduce the need for exchange transfusions early in sick infants, whereas in healthy, term infants we do not begin phototherapy until it appears that the rising serum bilirubin concentration may reach 20 mg per deciliter.*

HYPERBILIRUBINEMIA IN HEALTHY, TERM INFANTS

Diagnosis

All mother and infant blood types and Rh and the infant's Coombs' test and hematocrit reading are routinely performed on day 1. We obtain a *transcutaneous bilirubin index (Minolta Airshields Jaundice Meter) once daily* as part of routine nursing care. If the jaundice meter readings meet our criteria (Table 1), the nurse obtains a serum bilirubin level. If the serum bilirubin is at or above our threshold for phototherapy for age and weight (Fig. 1), the nurse notifies the physician.

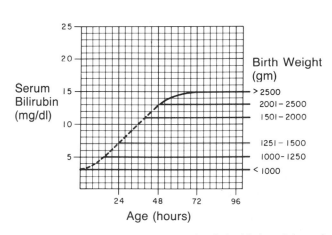

Figure 1 Suggested phototherapy levels by birth weight and age.

If the infant appears well and has one or more obvious risk factors for hyperbilirubinemia (Table 2), no further laboratory tests are done. Otherwise, additional diagnostic tests are undertaken and the etiology is algorithmically determined (Fig. 2), if possible. The additional tests include a total and direct serum bilirubin reading, a complete blood count and differential, a blood smear, platelet and reticulocyte counts, and testing for urine-reducing substances. A careful family history is also important.

Instituting Therapy

We generally start formula-fed infants on phototherapy when the total serum bilirubin level exceeds 15 mg per deciliter. However, when ABO or Rh sensitization exists with evidence of hemolysis, the physician may initiate

TABLE 2 Common Risk Factors for Neonatal Jaundice

Prematurity
Low birth weight
Maternal diabetes
Birth asphyxia
Cephalohematoma or bruising
Blood type incompatibility
Polycythemia
Sepsis
Breast-feeding

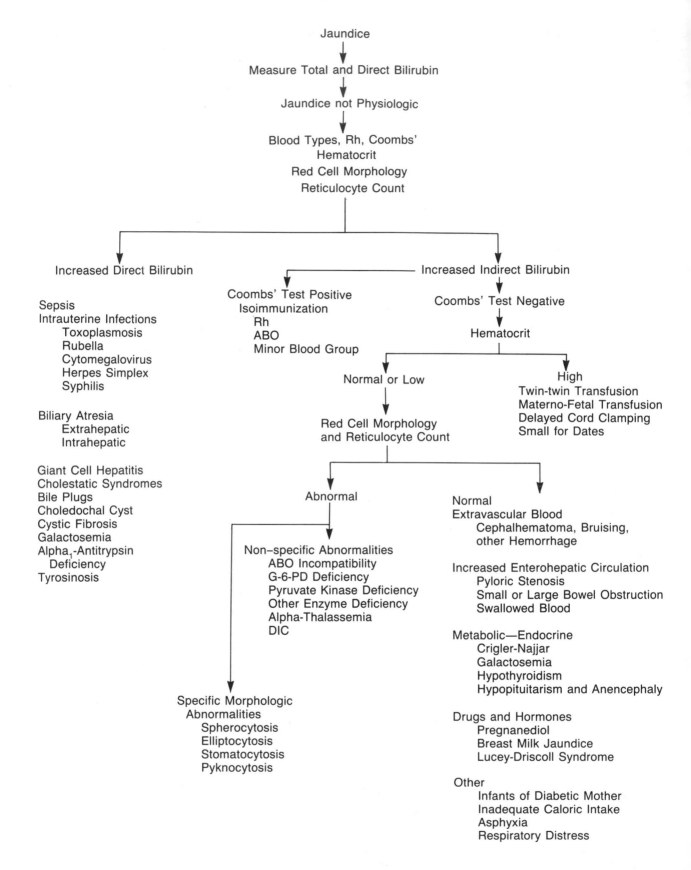

Figure 2 Diagnostic algorithm for hyperbilirubinemia. (From Maisels MJ. Neonatal jaundice. In: Avery GB, Neonatology, pathophysiology, and management of the newborn. 3rd ed. Philadelphia: JB Lippincott, 1987:559.

phototherapy when the serum bilirubin value first reaches phototherapy level for age (see Fig. 1).

Breast-fed infants (with presumed breast milk jaundice) whose bilirubin level exceeds 15 mg per deciliter are managed by interrupting breast-feeding for 24 to 48 hours. If the mother does not accept this, then phototherapy is started as in formula-fed infants.

Our protocol for phototherapy incudes clothing the infants in a diaper and placing them on a bubble mattress, applying eye patches securely, recording the infants' temperature frequently, positioning the phototherapy lights, and turning them on. Phototherapy is interrupted for laboratory work, diaper changes, feedings, and parent visits. If initial phototherapy fails to slow the rise of the serum bilirubin or the level is approaching 20 mg per deciliter, the infant's diapers are removed and a second phototherapy light is added.

We use both fluorescent and nonfluorescent lights. The fluorescent lights are generally used if the infant is in an open crib. Each "bank" has four special blue lamps placed in the center of the unit and two daylight lamps on either side. The bank of lights is positioned about 16 inches above the infant and if needed, a lower bank can be positioned 6 to 12 inches below the infant. The nonfluorescent "spotlight" we use is marketed by KDC-Healthdyne. It is positioned about 30 inches from the infant. Measurement of irradiance (μW/cm^2) or spectral irradiance (μW cm^2/nm) of the lights is done with a photometer. A review of the subject by Hammerman is useful for interpreting the readout of the photometer. The minimum acceptable spectral irradiance is approximately 4 μW per square centimeter per nanometer in the blue spectrum. The response increases until a saturation point is reached at about 10 to 12 μW per square centimeter per nanometer. Levels of both the upper and lower bank of lights (measured at the infant) should be kept in this range. We measure the spectral irradiance at intervals to ensure optimal dosing and arrive at a timely maintenance schedule.

Phototherapy is usually administered in the special care areas of the nursery. It may be performed in the mother's room if the infant's only problem is hyperbilirubinemia and the mother meets our criteria for rooming in (Table 3). The mother receives instructions (Table 4) from the nursing staff, who also continue to monitor the infant's temperature, activity, intake and output, and position of the eye patches at regular intervals. Home phototherapy is an extension of this policy, but the infant must meet additional criteria (Table 5). Home phototherapy is a particularly useful alternative when mothers desire an early discharge (within 24 hours of delivery). We have found these alternative methods for administering phototherapy to be safe when used with these restrictions.

Discontinuing Phototherapy

We monitor the serum bilirubin level at least every 12 to 24 hours while the infant is under phototherapy and continue treatment until the serum bilirubin level has been reduced to less than 12 mg per deciliter and the threat of an exchange transfusion has passed. Generally, 48 hours

TABLE 3 Maternal Criteria for In-Room Phototherapy

The mother must:
1. Be motivated and capable of understanding the additional care of the newborn.
2. Be alert and able to take action in emergencies such as choking.
3. Be willing to keep the infant in her room 24 hours a day.
4. Complete the instructional checklist and give consent.

TABLE 4 Instructional Checklist for In-Room Phototherapy

The nurse must:
1. Explain and demonstrate the placement of eye patches and state that they must be in place when the infant is under the lights.
2. Explain the clothing to be worn (diaper under lights, dress and wrap when away from the lights).
3. Explain the importance of taking the infant's temperature regularly.
4. Explain the importance of adequate fluid intake.
5. Explain the charting flowsheet (intake, output, eyes covered).
6. Explain how to position the lights at a proper distance.
7. Explain the need to keep the infant under phototherapy except during feeding and diaper changes.

TABLE 5 Guidelines for Home Phototherapy

We limit the use of home phototherapy to infants with the following characteristics:
1. Term infants, older than 48 hours, otherwise healthy
2. Those with a serum bilirubin level higher than 14 mg per deciliter but less than 18 mg per deciliter
3. Those in whom bilirubin is rising but less than 1 mg over 3 to 4 hours
4. Those with no elevation in direct-reacting bilirubin
5. Those with normal complete blood counts and differentials prior to discharge (leaving other diagnostic tests to be done as an outpatient, if needed)

Adapted from Committee on Fetus and Newborn Statement on Home Phototherapy in Pediatrics 1985; 76:136.

or more is needed. Infants with hemolysis may require extended time under phototherapy.

Exchange Transfusion

If phototherapy fails to prevent the rise of the serum bilirubin level to 20 mg per deciliter, or in the case of hemolysis, where the rate of increase will probably carry the bilirubin to an exchange level, we perform an exchange transfusion.

Follow-Up

Hospitalized infants are usually discharged soon after phototherapy is discontinued. No significant "rebound" in the serum bilirubin is seen in infants over 2,000 g, so the need to resume phototherapy is very remote. However, parents should be taught to expect the (bleached) skin color to appear yellow again when the infant is taken off phototherapy. Instructions should also include consulting the physician if the jaundice is marked or persists longer than 1 week. Some physicians ask parents to bring the infant back for a "bili check" in 12 to 24 hours.

The ever-increasing popularity of early discharge after delivery presents a new challenge: managing an infant's hyperbilirubinemia as an outpatient. Parents need to be instructed on how to recognize jaundice and when to consult their physician. If the infant becomes jaundiced at home, he or she should be brought in to see the physician and have a bilirubin check (and any other indicated laboratory tests). If the infant is already jaundiced and has a rising bilirubin level at time of discharge, a bilirubin check in 12 to 24 hours will direct management from there. One good reason for routine visits to the physician's office at 24 to 48 hours following early discharge is to monitor hyperbilirubinemia. Practice may vary, but the physician must maintain contact until the potential problem is resolved.

HYPERBILIRUBINEMIA IN SICK, PREMATURE, OR LOW BIRTH WEIGHT INFANTS

Diagnosis

The process of identification and evaluation of hyperbilirubinemia is identical to that already described for healthy, term infants. However, *we do not routinely use the transcutaneous jaundice meter in premature or low birth weight infants because of wide variation in normal ranges* at different gestational ages and birth weights.

Institution of Phototherapy

Our nomograms for starting phototherapy by birth weight and age are presented in Figure 1. Although these may suffer the shortcomings of any general guidelines, they impose some consistency in approach while satisfying our goal for early phototherapy in these infants. Prophylactic phototherapy from birth is used for very low birth weight infants who have one or more of the risk factors listed in Table 2.

Discontinuing Phototherapy

Our goal is to keep the serum bilirubin a safe distance from an exchange transfusion level until the hyperbilirubinemia is controlled. *We monitor the serum bilirubin level at least every 12 to 24 hours while the infant is under phototherapy* and continue treatment until it has been reduced to below the point on the nomogram at which phototherapy was started. Phototherapy is restarted if levels increase again above this baseline.

Exchange Transfusion

The above guidelines usually obviate the need for exchange transfusion, except in some cases of severe hemolytic disease, overwhelming sepsis, or in very low birth weight infants with significant soft tissue or internal hemorrhage or both.

ADJUNCTS TO PHOTOTHERAPY

Decreased fluid and caloric intake and delayed passage of meconium both work to increase serum bilirubin levels. Decreased fluid intake may decrease renal clearance of water-soluble bilirubin fractions and photo-oxidation products. Decreased caloric intake may decrease hepatic clearance and increase intestinal absorption of bilirubin. Delayed passage of meconium and decreased intestinal transit time also increase the intestinal absorption of bilirubin. We encourage early and frequent feedings, and supplement breast-fed infants with dextrose and water. Those infants with hyperbilirubinemia who have not spontaneously passed meconium or who are already under phototherapy and do not regularly pass meconium stools receive a suppository.

SIDE EFFECTS OF PHOTOTHERAPY

Phototherapy has many biologic effects. The acute effects are thought to be insignificant, although studies support certain precautions such as eye patches and careful monitoring of temperature and fluid status. Associated effects such as a transient rash, lethargy, abdominal distention, and loose stools may be observed in some treated infants. The bronze discoloration of the skin that occurs if phototherapy is continued despite an elevated conjugated bilirubin level is considered to be benign at present, although more long-term studies are needed.

PNEUMOGRAMS

CARL E. HUNT, M.D.

The pneumogram is a two-channel recording of respiratory pattern and heart rate. In most instances respiratory pattern has been obtained from thoracic impedance recordings. Regardless of whether abdominal (diaphragm) or thoracic movement is being recorded, the respiratory channel of the pneumogram is simply an indicator of respiratory pattern. The amplitude of the respiratory signal cannot be assumed to be representative of tidal volume and this respiratory signal is insensitive to interruptions in air flow (obstructive apnea). Pneumograms are overnight recordings that always include nocturnal sleep and variable portions of daytime nap intervals. Although pneumograms may be continuous 24-hour recordings, only quiet baseline intervals are generally analyzed, thus focusing primarily on sleep-related cardiorespiratory events. Due to the simplicity of these recordings, pneumograms can be performed at home as well as in the hospital. Pneumograms can be directly recorded on hard copy for immediate hand scoring or on a standard tape cassette for later scoring by hand or by computer analysis. *There are no universally applicable normative data.* Because of the many variations in methods for performing and analyzing pneumograms, normal values must be derived for each center.

PERFORMANCE AND ANALYSIS STANDARDS

Performance

One of the major difficulties in defining the clinical usefulness and validity of pneumograms has been the lack of uniform performance standards. It has been suggested that hyperthermic room temperature might facilitate identification of respiratory pattern abnormalities, but there are no available data on which to recommend an optimal room temperature or, if it matters, to standardize the room temperature at which pneumograms are performed. There are anecdotal unpublished reports that home pneumograms might be more likely to demonstrate respiratory pattern abnormalities than pneumograms performed in the hospital. In the only systematic evaluation to date, however, Keens and coworkers did not observe any difference in the number of abnormal pneumograms recorded in the hospital versus at home. Daytime nap recordings, generally performed in a sleep laboratory setting, may yield significantly fewer respiratory pattern abnormalities than nocturnal recordings.

The method utilized for apnea detection may result in differing degrees of sensitivity. Most respiratory pattern recordings are based on thoracic impedance, but an abdominal pressure capsule has also been used. No studies are available comparing the performance of thoracic impedance and abdominal pressure capsule methods of apnea detection either with each other or with a known standard.

Although no attempt was made to compare their performances, MacFadyen and Simpson did study the performance of capacitance pads and abdominal pressure capsules and found that both methods of apnea detection had problems with both false-positive and false-negative alarms.

There is no uniform recommendation for the age at which pneumograms should be performed for prospective evaluation of potential risk of sudden infant death syndrome (SIDS). Although the peak incidence for SIDS is 2 to 4 months of age, most pneumograms in at-risk infants have been performed in neonates. In infants who subsequently die of SIDS, would pneumograms performed during the vulnerable period be more abnormal than when performed at 0 to 4 weeks of age? Does respiratory pattern mature during infancy in normal infants, but fail to show maturational improvement or even deteriorate in infants who eventually succumb to SIDS? Although the number of available recordings is too few for any definitive conclusions, subsequent recordings at age 6 weeks in the Southall study did identify three of seven SIDS victims. Limited normative data are available for asymptomatic full-term infants, but most of the data were obtained in the neonatal period; *longitudinal pneumogram data throughout infancy are very limited in normal infants and virtually nonexistent in SIDS victims* who have died after 6 weeks of age.

Analysis

Considerable variations also exist in regard to methods for scoring and analysis. Since there are no standard definitions in general use for respiratory pattern and no standardization of printing or scoring methods, each center has evolved its own definitions and scoring methods. Although there is internal consistency if the same definitions and analyses are utilized for clinical assessment as for derivation of the normal standards, one cannot assume that normative standards from different centers are interchangeable. Computer scoring of pneumograms is now generally available, but each center must verify that the computer results are comparable to hand-scored results and that appropriate normative data are available for comparison.

A major variable in pneumogram analysis is whether awake events are included and how sleep intervals, if analyzed separately or exclusively, are identified. Harper and colleagues reported 80 percent accuracy in differentiating wakefulness, active sleep, and quiet sleep based on heart rate and respiration recordings compared with polysomnogram recordings. However, there is no uniform pneumogram definition of quiet baseline time and, thus, no established correlation between total sleep time and quiet baseline time. In the British studies, no attempt was made to separate sleep and awake intervals, and the denominator thus included both sleep and awake periods. It is not known whether inclusion of awake time affects the results observed in normal or abnormal infants or what the most appropriate method is for quantitating or indirectly estimating total sleep time.

There is no uniform definition for periodic breathing. Although some studies have defined periodic breathing as three respiratory pauses of at least 3 sec in duration interrupted by respiration lasting 20 sec or less, other definitions have including cyclic variations in respiratory amplitude and a longer minimum pause duration. Does the definition of periodic breathing utilized affect the ability to discriminate between normal and abnormal infants? Although cyclic or periodic variations in tidal volume would be the most physiologically relevant definition of periodic breathing, no studies have been done to determine the extent to which cyclic variations in amplitude, as detected by pneumograms, do in fact correspond to changes in measured tidal volume.

There is also considerable variability in the definition of brief apnea and the manner in which brief apnea is quantitated. Although some studies have identified all respiratory pauses 2 sec or longer in duration, others have only identified respiratory pauses greater than 3.6, 6.0, or 10 sec. The definitions utilized for onset and end of each respiratory pause have not been standardized and often are not even reported. Some investigators mark the onset of each respiratory pause at peak inspiration, whereas others mark the onset at end expiration. Although most investigators use the beginning of the next inspiration to identify the end of the respiratory pause, in some instances apnea duration is defined as the interval between successive inspiratory peaks. It is intuitively obvious that apnea duration will be different depending on the method for identifying onset and end of each apnea, but what has not been obvious is the magnitude of these differences and the resulting significant differences in calculated values for apnea density and periodic breathing. Although each of these methods is clinically acceptable, it is essential that the normal values used for comparison be based on the same scoring method.

There is also considerable variation in the measurements utilized by individual investigators for decision making. Longest apnea is routinely utilized, as is periodic breathing. Periodic breathing, however, may be reported as episodes per 100 min, longest episode, or as a fraction of total sleep time or quiet baseline. There is even greater variability in quantitating brief apneas. Some investigators calculate an apnea density (A/D percent), the total duration of all pauses above a specified minimum duration as a percentage of total sleep time, of quiet baseline, or of recording time; the minimum duration of the respiratory pauses to be included in the calculation of A/D percent has varied from 2.0 to 10.0 sec.

Some investigators also report irregular breathing, disorganized breathing, and/or shallow breathing. These tend, however, to be only semiquantitative or qualitative assessments, without precise normative standards, and are generally without a specific physiologic correlate. Disorganized breathing, for example, is sometimes reported on the presumption that it is a manifestation of obstructive apnea. In fact, however, there are no studies to establish either the definition, normal limits, or physiologic significance of disorganized breathing. Shallow breathing is sometimes included in pneumogram reports, the presumption being

that shallow breathing, however defined in a qualitative or semiquantitative way, is indicative of insufficient tidal volume and therefore abnormal. Because of limitations inherent in thoracic impedance, however, *impedance changes cannot be assumed to be equivalent to tidal volume changes*, and no comparisons of polysomnograms and pneumograms have been performed to assess the extent to which decreases in inspiratory impedance amplitude are quantitatively related to decreases in measured tidal volume.

The second pneumogram channel is utilized to provide a continuous recording of heart rate. In addition to reporting any age-related episodes of bradycardia, some investigators have also included an analysis of tachycardia (tachycardia index). In the British prospective study, higher levels of sinus tachycardia were reported in future SIDS victims compared with control infants. However, studies have not yet been performed to determine whether the higher tachycardia index is simply related to the inclusion of more awake time in the analysis or to increased active compared with quiet sleep, or whether tachycardia is a marker of sleep-related hypoventilation or hypoxemia, or both.

CLINICAL USEFULNESS

The potential clinical usefulness of pneumograms needs to be considered separately for symptomatic and asymptomatic infants.

Symptomatic Infants

Respiratory pattern abnormalities have been reported in patients with apnea of infancy. In these infants who present with an apparent life-threatening sleep event and in whom a detailed medical evaluation fails to identify a cause, however, the clinical controversy has been whether performing a pneumogram provides any useful or necessary clinical information. *The pneumogram should not be utilized to diagnose "apnea of infancy;" this is a clinical diagnosis, established by the history and by the exclusion of other causes.* Similarly, the decision to treat or intervene in some manner should also be based on the clinical history, not on the presence or absence of a cardiorespiratory pattern abnormality. It should be noncontroversial that infants presenting with an apparent life-threatening event for which no other etiology has been identified should receive medical intervention. *If the physician has already decided that the intervention to be utilized is a home monitor, then performance of a pneumogram will not yield any information that will alter the treatment plan,* even though it may enhance one's overall understanding of the pathophysiology. Following hospital discharge, the home monitor can safely be discontinued after 3 months without any apnea or bradycardia events, so that pneumograms may be no more essential at the time of discontinuing than at the time of initiating home monitoring. In point of fact, however, most infants on home monitors do have some alarms, and it is often difficult to determine whether an apnea/bradycardia alarm is indicative of a physiologically significant event. In such infants, the pneumogram may be helpful in determining whether a cardiorespiratory pattern abnormality is indeed present.

Asymptomatic Infants

Pneumogram recordings have been performed in many infants considered to be at increased epidemiologic risk for SIDS. These asymptomatic risk groups have included siblings of previous SIDS victims, low birth weight survivors, and infants with intrauterine drug exposure. As currently performed and analyzed, however, *pneumograms have failed to demonstrate sufficient sensitivity and specificity to be useful for population-wide prospective screening of asymptomatic infants.* In addition, even though some studies have demonstrated significant group differences in cardiorespiratory pattern between asymptomatic at-risk and normal infants, appropriately designed prospective studies have not yet been performed to determine whether intervention based on the pneumogram results contributes to a reduced incidence of SIDS.

METHYLXANTHINES

Theophylline and caffeine have both been successfully used to improve or normalize respiratory pattern in apnea of prematurity. Both drugs have also been used successfully to improve abnormalities in respiratory pattern, as identified by pneumograms in patients with apnea of infancy and in asymptomatic infants at increased epidemiologic risk for SIDS. As already discussed, pneumograms are not essential to clinical management if the physician has already decided that a home monitor is to be prescribed; if treatment with a methylxanthine is being considered, however, pneumogram recordings have been very helpful. When the initial pneumogram is normal in patients with apnea of infancy, theophylline has often not been helpful in eliminating the clinical symptoms. In subjects with an abnormal initial pneumogram, however, theophylline improves the respiratory pattern in virtually all instances. Based on normal upper limits of 0.9 percent for apnea density (A/D percent), 2.9 episodes of periodic breathing per 100 min and longest apnea of 20 sec, the repeat pneumogram was normal in 94 percent of 198 infants so evaluated (Fig. 1). A/D percent failed to normalize in 8.3 percent of infants with an initial value of greater than or equal to 0.9 percent, periodic breathing failed to normalize in 3.0 percent of infants with an initial value of greater than or equal to 2.9 episodes per 100 min, and longest apnea failed to normalize in 21 percent of infants with an initial value of greater than or equal to 15 sec. In patients with apnea of infancy treated with theophylline, recurrent symptoms have been unusual and have been seen only in infants in whom the pneumogram failed to normalize completely. In asymptomatic infants whose only indication for theophylline treatment was an abnormal pneumogram, normalization of the pneumogram with theophylline has correlated with failure to develop any apparent life-threatening events.

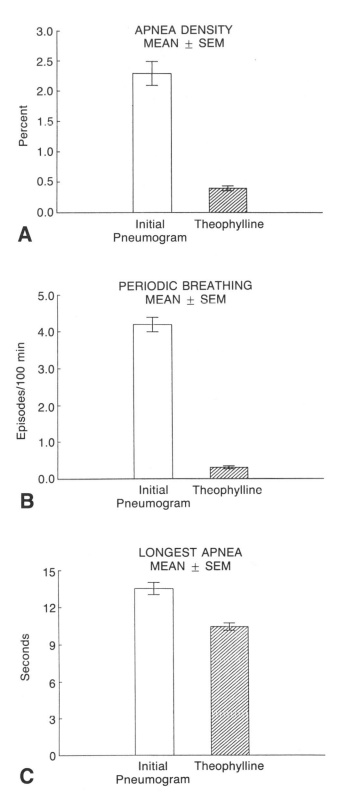

Figure 1 Effects of theophylline on respiratory pattern in 198 infants at a mean (± standard error of the mean) peak theophylline blood level of 10.2 ± 0.2 μg per milliliter. For each comparison, the decrease with theophylline is statistically significant ($p = < .005$). *A*, Apnea density (A/D percent). Upper limit of normal, 0.9 percent. *B*, Periodic breathing. Upper limit of normal, 2.9 episodes per 100 min of total sleep time. *C*, Longest apnea. Upper limit of normal, 15 sec.

DISCUSSION

An assessment of cardiorespiratory pattern is often clinically indicated as part of the evaluation of an apparent life-threatening event. Such assessments may also be helpful in developing a management strategy for symptomatic infants but are not necessary unless methylxanthine treatment is being contemplated. In asymptomatic infants, however, regardless of the epidemiologic risk group, prospective assessments of cardiorespiratory pattern compared with control infants have not yielded any differences that are of sufficient sensitivity and specificity to permit identification of future SIDS victims.

There are two general methods by which assessments of cardiorespiratory pattern can be performed—polysomnograms and pneumograms. Polysomnograms, generally performed during a daytime nap, typically include 12 channels and are carried out in a hospital setting. The advantages over pneumograms include sleep staging, quantitation of respiratory volumes, and documentation of obstructive apnea. Compared with pneumograms, however, especially home recordings, polysomnograms are more likely to alter natural sleep patterns, are more costly, and generally focus on daytime rather than nocturnal sleep.

Previous studies have shown that cardiorespiratory pattern abnormalities may be more evident during nocturnal than during daytime sleep. Since pneumograms do not require technician surveillance and thus are very practical for unsupervised overnight assessments, these two-channel recordings may provide a very useful assessment of cardiorespiratory pattern even though the scope of physiologic information that can be obtained is less than with a polysomnogram.

All published studies of home pneumograms have been based on a standard two-channel recording of heart rate and respiratory pattern. Some investigators are now evaluating the technical feasibility and potential physiologic advantages of including a channel for nasal airflow in order to also measure end-tidal Pco_2 or at least to also assess obstructive events. It is unclear, however, whether addition of an airflow channel is practical for overnight recordings without technician supervision, especially at home, and whether the additional physiologic information substantially enhances the usefulness of pneumograms either for prospective screening or for clinical management. The other refinement of the pneumogram is related to addition of an oxygen saturation channel, referred to as an *oxypneumogram*. Although oxypneumograms are now becoming practical for home as well as inpatient recordings and obviously permit a substantially greater assessment of the physiologic significance of cardiorespiratory pattern abnormalities, no data currently exist as to whether the oxypneumogram will be superior to the pneumogram in prospectively identifying potential SIDS victims or in guiding clinical management of apnea-related symptoms. Such studies are essential, however, and are currently in progress at several centers.

SUGGESTED READING

Harper RM, Leake B, Hoppenbrouwers T, et al. Polygraphic studies of normal infants and infants at risk for the sudden infant death syndrome: heart rate and variability as a function of state. Pediatr Res 1978; 12:778–785.

Hunt CE, Brouillette RT. Sudden infant death syndrome: 1987 perspective. J Pediatr 1987; 110:669–678.

Keens TG, Davidson-Ward SL, Gates EP, et al. A comparison of pneumogram recording in infants in the hospital and at home. Pediatr Pulmonol 1986; 2:373–377.

Oren J, Kelly DH, Shannon DC. Pneumogram recordings in infants resuscitated for apnea of infancy. Pediatrics 1989; 83(3):364.

Southall D, Richards JM, de Swiet M, et al. Identification of infants destined to die unexpectedly during infancy: evaluation of predictive importance of prolonged apnea and disorders of cardiac rhythm or conduction. Br Med J 1983; 286:1091.

PULSE OXIMETRY

DESMOND J. BOHN, M.B., B.Ch., F.F.A.R.C.S., M.R.C.P.(UK), FRCPC

Over the past decade significant advances have been made in the management of the critically ill infant, particularly in the treatment of the low birth weight premature infant with respiratory disease. The requirement for increased inspired oxygen concentrations in these sick newborns and the sensitivity of the premature infant to high arterial Po_2 levels have resulted in a continuing search for an accurate method of continuously monitoring arterial oxygen levels in these patients. *Direct intra-arterial Po_2 measurements from indwelling umbilical catheters or peripheral arterial lines are done on too random a basis to be able to detect either hypoxic or hyperoxic levels,* and there is also a substantial morbidity associated with their use. Consequently, there has been a continuing search to provide a form of oxygen monitoring that will accurately and rapidly reflect the PaO_2, which can be used on a continuous basis over a prolonged period. Although intravascular catheters that incorporate a Po_2 electrode at the tip are now available, their reliability in terms of long duration placement is doubtful. Their use is also associated with morbidity problems similar to those seen with regular intra-arterial lines.

The development of the transcutaneous Po_2 electrode ($PtcO_2$) in the 1970s represented a substantial advance in the monitoring of oxygenation in the newborn infant. It fulfilled some of the criteria for the ideal arterial oxygen monitor, these being (1) that it be noninvasive, (2) that it have a rapid response time, (3) that it be accurate over the range of Po_2 values seen in newborn infants (4) that the monitoring device be easy to calibrate with minimal drift after application, and (5) that there be a low morbidity associated with its use.

The PtcO2 is less than ideal, for it fails to meet some of these criteria. Although it is reasonably accurate over the Po_2 range of 30 to 100 mm Hg, there is a tendency to underread true PaO_2 values, especially in older infants with chronic lung diseases such as bronchopulmonary dysplasia. It also does not track a change in arterial oxygenation rapidly enough to detect acute hypoxic events in the neonate. There is also a lag in the response time of several minutes after a change in PaO_2. Although calibration and application are reasonably straightforward, the actual Clark's electrode at the tip of the $PtcO_2$ probe is not a robust structure and is expensive to replace when broken. Finally, although the device is noninvasive, there is still a substantial morbidity associated with its use due to trauma to the skin underlying the electrode, since the probe has to be heated to 43 to 44° C. This necessitates the position of the probe being changed every 4 hours to prevent skin burns.

PRINCIPLES OF PULSE OXIMETRY

In 1982 the noninvasive measurement of arterial saturation in the neonate on a beat-to-beat basis became available with the development of the pulse oximeter ($StcO_2$). Although oximetry, which measures arterial oxygen saturation transcutaneously, is a technique that has been used in medicine for over 20 years, it suffered many of the drawbacks associated with other transcutaneous monitors in that the response time was slow, many of the units required heating of the skin to generate accurate readings, and the oximeter probe itself was too large and cumbersome for use in newborns. Pulse oximetry, on the other hand, utilizes a single small probe that is placed over an extremity and does not require heating or calibration. It therefore overcomes most of the deficiencies associated with regular oximeters and $PtcO_2$ probes as well as providing saturation measurements with a rapid response time.

The system *combines the principles of spectrophotometry, oximetry, and plethysmography and utilizes the differing absorption bands for light of oxygenated and reduced hemoglobin.* The finger probe contains two electrodes, one of which has two light-emitting diodes and the other a single sensor. The diodes emit infrared and red light that have differing wavelengths. The absorption of the infrared wavelength changes little between oxygenated and reduced hemoglobin, whereas the absorption of red light changes markedly with hemoglobin saturation. Part of the emitted light is absorbed by tissue and nonpulsatile blood, whereas the remaining unabsorbed light is detected by the photodetector diode. This acts as a reference signal. *When pulsatile flow is present, the light received by the photodiode alters with both flow and the amount of oxygenated or reduced hemoglobin.* The measurement of the amount of oxygenated hemoglobin is then translated into a digital signal that is displayed as percent saturation, along with the pulse rate. The heart rate and saturation readings are averaged by the microprocessor from sampling intervals of 5 to 7 seconds in the standard operating mode, although this interval can be shortened or extended in most oximeter units.

The pulse oximeter only recognizes two types of hemoglobin, oxygenated and reduced, and takes no account of either carboxy- or fetal hemoglobin. Laboratory co-oximeters (e.g., IL 282), on the other hand, measure carboxyhemoglobin but cannot distinguish between this and fetal hemoglobin because of the particular wavelengths used by these machines.

CLINICAL OPERATION OF THE PULSE OXIMETER

Since *pulse oximeters depend for their operation on pulsatile blood flow,* the sensor must be applied to an extremity, whether it is the finger, the toe, or the bridge of the nose (Fig. 1). Care must be taken to ensure that the sensor is placed directly opposite the light-emitting diodes in order for the machine to function accurately. *Since the photo cell is light-sensitive, it must be shielded from strong external light sources,* such as strong sunlight, phototherapy lights, and radiant heaters, all of which are known to produce spurious results. This is best achieved by wrapping the electrode with adhesive tape. After the power is switched on, the unit will "search for" an adequate pulsation, the amplitude of which is displayed by a linear array of light emitting diodes (LED) lights or graphically by a pulse plethysmograph. In instances in which extremity pulses become impalpable because of severe hypotension or the electrode is improperly applied, the machine continues to search for an adequate pulse and does not display a heart rate. *The pulse rate displayed by the oximeter should not differ by more than 5 beats per*

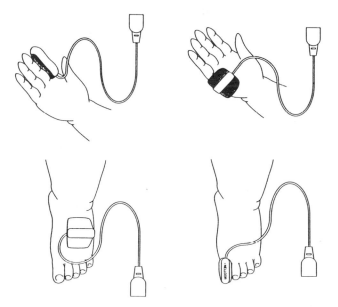

Figure 1 Methods and sites of application of pulse oximeter probes in the neonate. For accurate readings *the light-emitting diodes and the photodetector cell must be placed directly opposite each other.*

minute from the electrocardiogram recorded heart rate in order for the saturation reading to be relied on. Some idea of the dependability of the saturation reading can also be extrapolated from the amplitude of the pulse displayed on the LED lights or pulse waveform. Pulse oximeters are also rendered inaccurate by movement artifact, which may be a particular problem in the active neonate or small infant. One solution to this problem is to increase the sampling interval, which can be extended to 10 to 15 seconds in the Nelcor unit, which increases the pulse discrimination. Since the oximeter may detect and count movement as an arterial pulse, some degree of movement artifact can be eliminated by increasing the number of pulsations the machine reads before actually measuring the saturation.

PULSE OXIMETRY IN MONITORING OXYGENATION IN THE NEWBORN

Several studies have now established the efficacy of pulse oximetry in accurately monitoring oxygen saturation in the term and preterm infant with respiratory disease. Due to the shape of the oxygen dissociation curve, below a PaO_2 of 60 mm Hg a small change in PaO_2 translates to a large change in percent saturation of oxygen. Therefore oximetry measurements accurately and rapidly reflect changes in oxygenation in that important range in which the infant is at risk from hypoxia. Several studies have now shown that oximeter saturations agree with in vitro SaO_2 values, measured by co-oximetry, between the ranges of oxygenation encountered in most clinical situations (75 to 95 percent) (Fig. 2). It is therefore very accurate in rapidly detecting hypoxia and is very useful when making changes in FIO_2 or positive end-expiratory pressure levels while the infant is on mechanical ventilation. Most oximeters are portable and have an internal battery with a 1-hour life, which allows them to be used both during resuscitation in the delivery suite and for neonatal transport.

In comparative studies there is a *closer correlation between $StcO_2$ and SaO_2 than between $PtcO_2$ and PaO_2* in both newborn infants and older children. If one takes into account the more rapid response time of the pulse oximeter, this technique has distinct advantages over the $PtcO_2$ to the extent that *transcutaneous Po_2 technology is now largely obsolete.*

At the other end of the scale, the use of oximetry to prevent hyperoxia in the premature infant requires considerably more fine tuning. When oxygen saturations increase to over 90 percent, which lies along the flat part of the oxygen dissociation curve, a large increase in PaO_2 translates into only a small increase in saturation. Therefore, in the range between a PaO_2 of 60 and 100 mm Hg, there is little change in saturation. Obviously, this lack of discrimination in PaO_2 measurements is less than ideal in a situation in which small increases in PaO_2 can lead to an increased risk of retrolental fibroplasia. However, the rapid response time still makes a very useful monitoring device even in this situation where the FIO_2 can be reduced until the 90 percent saturation point is reached and the PaO_2 is then checked by an arterial sample. Many neonatal units now favor the approach of continuing to *run*

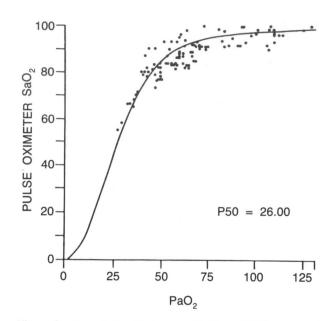

Figure 2 The relationship between $StcO_2$ and PaO_2 measured in a large series of critically ill pediatric patients on mechanical ventilation. The regression line is the classic oxygen dissociation curve, and there is an accurate correlation with PaO_2 levels of less than 30 mm Hg. (From Fanconi S, et al. Pulse oximetry in pediatric intensive care. J Pediatr 1985; 107:362. Reproduced with permission.)

oxygen saturations at no higher than 90 percent by pulse oximeter in these high-risk infants.

PULSE OXIMETRY IN NEWBORN CHRONIC LUNG DISEASE

The noninvasive monitoring of oxygenation in infants with chronic lung disease, such as bronchopulmonary dysplasia, in order to determine oxygen requirements, has proved difficult with the use of $PtcO_2$ measurements. Several studies have highlighted the problem that with increasing maturity and increasing skin and subcutaneous tissue thickness, there is a tendency toward under-reading the $PtcO_2$ measurements when compared with the actual PaO_2. It is obviously important that some reliable means be available for measuring in vivo oxygenation in infants in order that appropriate oxygen therapy can be determined. A recent study comparing $PtcO_2$ and $StcO_2$ measurements with PaO_2 and SaO_2 measured by co-oximeter in infants with bronchopulmonary dysplasia found that $StcO_2$ more accurately reflected the true in vivo oxygenation. The $PtcO_2$ measurements consistently underestimated the actual PaO_2 in this study, resulting in unnecessarily high levels of oxygen being administered.

PULSE OXIMETRY AND NEONATAL APNEA

Pulse oximetry is capable of rapidly detecting desaturations that occur with apnea in the premature and newborn infant. The rapid response time of the instrument and the fact that oxygen saturation measured and displayed at

5- to 7-second intervals means that even brief desaturations can be detected. There is the added advantage that the instrument registers the pulse rate so that the combination of bradycardia and desaturation can be accurately recorded either on the strip recorder or as part of a formal sleep study with continuous electroencephalogram and Respitrace recording (Fig. 3). The pulse oximeter has proved to be the ideal instrument for detailing apnea either secondary to prematurity or due to airways obstruction. Its rapid response time makes it superior to PtcO$_2$ for this indication.

PULSE OXIMETRY AND FETAL HEMOGLOBIN

The accurate measurement of arterial oxygen saturations by direct means is complicated in the small infant by the fact that there is a significant proportion of fetal hemoglobin (HbF). Spectrophotometric methods for measurement of hemoglobin, on which co-oximetry is based, recognize four types of hemoglobin: saturated, desaturated, carboxyhemoglobin (HbCO), and methemoglobin (MetHb). In the case of the standard co-oximeter (IL 282), the result is displayed as HbO$_2$ percent, HbCO percent, and MetHb percent, but takes no account of HbF. This discrepancy may become a problem in the newborn infant, who may have a large proportion of HbF, and there has been some doubt expressed as to whether either the co-oximeter or the pulse oximeter, which also takes no account of HbF, would accurately reflect true saturation.

Several studies have addressed this problem by comparing directly measured saturations on an IL 282 co-oximeter, on which the measurement is corrected for HbF, with StcO$_2$ measurements. In the study by Jennis, a large number of infants with measured HbF levels of 5 to 100 percent were evaluated. When HbF levels were between 50 and 100 percent, there was 2.8 to 3.6 percent inaccuracy in StcO$_2$ readings, the tendency for the error being on the side of under-reading of the StcO$_2$ values when compared with measured saturations. *Although there is a slight inaccuracy in StcO$_2$ measurements in the presence of high HbF levels, the degree of error is quite acceptable* for clinical practice.

PULSE OXIMETRY AND LOW CARDIAC OUTPUT STATES

Since pulse oximetry operates on the principle of pulsatile blood flow, the accurate measurement of StcO$_2$ depends on there being adequate peripheral perfusion for the oximeter to detect a peripheral pulse. Although this has been generally recognized as one of the limitations of pulse oximetry, in neonates it has been shown to track saturation and pulse rate accurately with mean systemic pressures as low as 20 mm Hg. It has been our experience that in situations of extremely low cardiac output seen in older children with congenital heart disease in whom the mean pressure may be higher but there is very poor peripheral perfusion with intense vasoconstriction, the

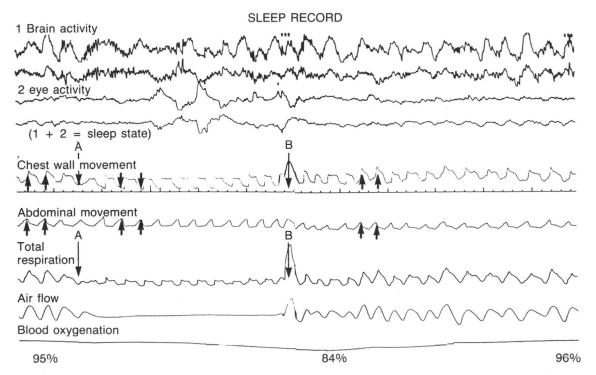

Figure 3 An example of the use of pulse oximetry for diagnosing apnea during a sleep study. In this example apnea is due to respiratory obstruction, as can be seen from the paradoxical chest/abdominal wall movement represented by the arrows. Note the rapid fall in saturation recorded by the oximeter in the lower panel, which promptly returns to normal with the resumption of normal respiration.

oximeter does not register either a saturation or a heart rate. Indeed, this is a built-in safety mechanism that ensures against a spurious saturation reading, as the $StcO_2$ *cannot be relied on unless the heart rate agrees with the monitored electrocardiogram signal within 5 beats per minute.* In contrast, the $PtcO_2$ still continues to register what is a completely erroneous number even in profound low cardiac output states.

SUGGESTED READING

Deckardt R, Steward DJ. Noninvasive arterial hemoglobin oxygen saturation versus transcutaneous oxygen tension monitoring in the preterm infant. Crit Car Med 1984; 12:935–939.

Durand M, Ramanathan R. Pulse oximetry for continuous oxygen monitoring in sick newborn infants. J Pediatr 1986; 109:1052–1056.

Fanconi S, Doherty P, Edmonds JF, et al. Pulse oximetry in pediatric intensive care: comparison with measured saturations and transcutaneous oxygen tension. J Pediatr 1985; 107:362–366.

Jennis MS, Peabody JL. Pulse oximetry: an alternative for the assessment of oxygenation in newborn infants. Pediatrics 1987; 79:524–528.

Mok J, Pintar M, Benson L, et al. Evaluation of noninvasive measurements of oxygenation in stable infants. Crit Care Med 1986; 14:960–963.

Ramanathan R, Durand M, Larrazabal C. Pulse oximetry in very low birth weight infants with acute and chronic lung disease. Pediatrics 1987; 79:612–617.

Ryan CA, Barrington KJ, Vaughan D, Finer NN. Directly measured arterial oxygen saturation in the newborn infant. J Pediatr 1986; 109:526–529.

RESUSCITATION

WILLIAM E. TRUOG III, M.D.

PATHOPHYSIOLOGY OF NEONATAL ASPHYXIA

Birth is associated with an increase in metabolic activity and oxygen consumption, a response normally modulated by the immediate postnatal increase in triiodothyronine (T_3). The risk of hypothermia with its adverse effects, including the development of a coagulopathy, is increased with asphyxia. Cold stress alone depresses arterial oxygen tension in term infants, possibly because of persistent right-to-left shunting. Cold stress may diminish oxygen availability at a time of increased oxygen need for counteracting hypoxemia.

Arterial Pco_2 rises 7 to 10 torr with each minute of apnea. Arterial Po_2 falls as oxygen consumption continues without any replacement for oxygen in the tissues. Anaerobic metabolism soon adds lactate to the acid load. The combination of respiratory and metabolic acidosis produces both constriction of the pulmonary vascular bed and eventually systemic hypotension, bradycardia, and reduced cardiac output. Without prompt intervention, the now cold-stressed and depressed fetus has difficulty reversing this situation. Chemical stimuli (e.g., elevated Pco_2) may induce gasping, but such breathing efforts are ineffectual because of persistently liquid-filled lungs.

Extremely premature infants need particular attention in the delivery room. Shiny pink skin color may not reflect satisfactory arterial oxygen tension. The premature infant's very compliant chest wall produces respiratory efforts that may be ineffectual for establishing gas-filled lungs and air flow.

ASSESSMENT OF NEONATAL WELL-BEING

The cornerstone for management of the newborn in the delivery room is serial physical examination directed toward assessing heart rate, respiratory rate and effort, *and, to a lesser extent, skin color.* Decisions for intervention can be based on these findings without waiting for any arbitrary period of time following delivery. Table 1 outlines these steps. Because *the initial approach to the depressed neonate almost always consists of establishing an airway and providing assisted ventilation*, knowing the exact cause of neonatal depression becomes more important only after the first 1 to 2 minutes of resuscitation.

The traditional approach to the assessment of perinatal transition has been to use the Apgar score. The limitations of this score are that (1) it was meant to be calculated at 1 and 5 minutes, yet resuscitative efforts should begin before 1 minute in the case of a severely depressed baby; (2) it was not designed with premature infants in mind and, hence, the evaluation of tone and even color and reflex irritability become problematic with the smaller infant; (3) it does not predict the long-term outcome from perinatal asphyxia with great accuracy; and (4) immediate attention should be focused on heart rate and breathing effort, not on the more subjective components of the scoring system, such as reflex irritability.

APPROACH TO THE ASPHYXIATED INFANT

Drying and Initial Stabilization

The infant should be dried and moved away from any convective currents. Drying also serves to help stimulate breathing. Then the infant's mouth and nares may be gently suctioned with a bulb syringe to remove any fluid. Suctioning of the mouth should occur first because stimulation of the nares may induce a sudden inspiratory gasp and cause aspiration of any remaining fluid in the mouth and lungs. Excessive suctioning produces trauma, with mucosal swelling and the potential for partial occlusion of the airways. It also diverts attention from the ongoing tasks of evaluating air entry into the lungs and monitoring heart rate.

Adequate respiratory effort is confirmed by the presence of air entry sounds on auscultation of the chest, an increase in the anterior to posterior diameter of the chest with inspiratory efforts, audible crying, absence of cyanosis of the lips and mucous membranes in the mouth, absence of marked intercostal retractions after the first

TABLE 1 Steps in Initial Evaluation of a Depressed Infant

Birth: Immediate Evaluation
Heart rate (count for 20 sec and multiply by 3)
Assess color
Assess respiratory effect
If heart rate is:

< 50 beats/min	50–100 beats/min	≥ 100 beats/min
Absent respirations	Some respiratory effects	
Color: cyanotic	Color: cyanotic	
then	*then*	*then*
Initiate immediate resuscitation. Dry the infant, suction the upper airway, and immediately apply bag and mask assisted ventilation. If there is no prompt response, reclear the infant's airway and perform orotracheal intubation.	Dry the infant and suction the airway, followed by close observation with supplemental oxygen to the face. If there is no improvement, begin bag and mask ventilation by 1 min or before if heart rate becomes progressively slower. Provide tactile stimulation.	Dry the infant. If the infant is cyanotic, use free-flowing oxygen to the face. If no obvious respirations occur, stimulate the infant by rubbing his or her back or pinching the extremities for 20 to 30 sec. If heart rate starts to fall to less than 100 beats/min, institute bag and mask resuscitation.

several minutes of life, and a pulse rate consistently maintained above 120 beats per minute. Any infant who does not demonstrate these findings on his or her own within the first minute after birth demands more evaluation and possible intervention.

Heart rate should be measured by chest auscultation or palpation of umbilical cord pulsations. A rate of more than 100 beats per minute (determined by counting the pulse for a period of 20 sec and multiplying by 3) usually indicates the absence of severe asphyxia. Ongoing serial observations without further intervention are indicated. An infant with a heart rate of more than 100 beats per minute who is still cyanotic may benefit from breathing-enriched supplemental oxygen flowing over the nose and face (see Table 1).

A pulse rate below or initially less than 100 beats per minute and, especially, less than 60 beats per minute signals the need for initiation of assisted ventilation, even if the infant is making occasional inspiratory efforts. Persistent bradycardia for the first 1 to 2 minutes following delivery is an indication to institute assisted ventilation.

Assisted Ventilation

Assisted ventilation may be delivered by one of two means: (1) a 0.5 L rubber bag attached to a molded rubber or circular plastic mask with rubber edges fitted over the baby's mouth and nares, or (2) a rubber bag connected to an endotracheal tube. The choice between bag and mask and bag and tube ventilation is based on consideration of degree of depression, cause of respiratory distress, size of the infant, and likelihood of need for prolonged resuscitation. Extremely depressed or premature babies will more likely need prolonged assisted ventilation, which can be more easily accomplished by bag and tube ventilation. The possibility of a malformation such as congenital diaphragmatic hernia should also prompt the resuscitator to perform intubation and bag and tube ven-

tilation. Many authorities, however, believe that bag and mask ventilation is sufficient for the majority of mildly to moderately asphyxiated infants. Meconium-stained and severely depressed infants benefit from intubation and suctioning of readily removable meconium from the upper airways and trachea.

Initial inspiratory positive pressure may need to exceed 20 cm H_2O and occasionally reach 50 cm H_2O to overcome surface adhesive forces in the airways. Initial assisted inspirations can be delivered slowly, with inspiration sustained for 0.5 to 1.0 sec.

Failure to mask ventilate effectively may be caused by improper face mask size precluding a tight seal on the face, airway blockage by the tongue's falling against the posterior pharyngeal wall, macroglossia (as in infants with hypothyroidism, Down syndrome, or Beckwith-Wiedemann syndrome), congenital airway anomalies, such as cleft palate or bilateral choanal atresia, or the presence of micrognathia.

Proper positioning of the infant's head is crucial for either successful bag and mask ventilation or for placement of the endotracheal tube (Fig. 1). When the infant is correctly positioned, the neck is neither flexed nor extended. Because the occiput of a full-term infant is large, the neck may become flexed when the infant is supine. Placing a small towel under the shoulders, not the neck, helps to overcome this problem. This is not, however, a problem in the smallest premature infants. The infant's chin should be extended, making him or her appear to be sniffing the air with his or her nose. Some physicians insert an oral airway during bag and mask ventilation, but its usefulness will be subverted if it becomes pressed against the posterior oropharynx. A feeding tube placed in the stomach with the proximal end open to the atmosphere helps prevent distention of the stomach, which is likely to occur with bag and mask ventilation.

Infants requiring prolonged resuscitation are best managed by placement of an endotracheal tube. If inade-

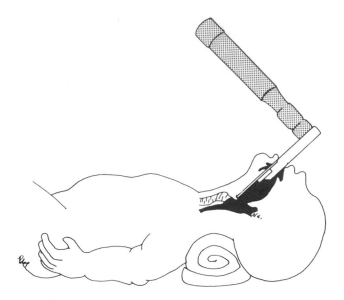

Figure 1 Proper positioning of an infant for ventilation by means of oral tracheal intubation and bag and tube ventilation. A diaper roll is placed under the shoulders to allow adequate neck extension, overcoming the natural neck flexion that occurs with supine positioning because of the term infant's large occiput. (From Truog WE. Neonatal resuscitation. In: Carlo W, Chatbum R, Lough M, eds. Neonatal respiratory care. 2nd ed. Chicago: Year Book Medical Publishers, 1988, with permission.)

should establish or restore nearly normal blood gas tensions and the concomitant onset of spontaneous respirations with normal heart rate, blood pressure, and perfusion.

For those infants in whom assisted ventilation for 1 to 2 minutes fails to restore a heart rate of at least 80 to 100 beats per minute, two additional measures are necessary: external cardiac massage and administration of bicarbonate and epinephrine.

Establishing Vascular Access

Placement of a catheter into the umbilical vein is the quickest means of obtaining vascular access. The umbilical vein can be quickly cannulated by cutting the umbilicus approximately 1 cm above the abdominal wall through Wharton's jelly. Grasping the edge of the umbilicus, the resuscitator can easily determine which is the flaccid umbilical vein and insert a catheter directly into it (Fig. 2). If the catheter can be advanced approximately 10 cm into the vein of a full-term infant or approximately 6 to 7 cm in the smallest premature infant, and if blood return occurs readily be gentle aspiration, then one can assume that the catheter has passed through the ductus venosus and inferior vena cava into the right atrium. If blood cannot be easily aspirated, then the catheter should be withdrawn until the tip is only a distance of 2 to 3 cm into the vessel. With the catheter in either position, bicarbonate and/or epinephrine can be administered (Fig. 2).

Alternative routes of administration include starting an intravenous infusion in a superficial scalp or hand vein or inserting an umbilical arterial catheter. These procedures are usually more time-consuming and technically difficult than umbilical venous catheterization.

If there is delay in establishing vascular access and the infant is continuously bradycardic, epinephrine (0.1 ml per kilogram of 1:10,000 solution increased to a volume of approximately 0.5 to 1 ml with normal saline) can be *administered via the endotracheal tube.* There is absorption into the circulation, although if the infant is profoundly acidotic, epinephrine may not have as much effect as if the pH had been corrected by adequate ventilation first followed by bicarbonate infusion.

An appropriate empirical dose of bicarbonate in a severely asphyxiated infant is 2 mEq per kilogram administered as 0.5 mEq per milliliter at a rate of infusion of approximately 1 to 2 ml per minute. Epinephrine and

quate ventilation or bradycardia persists after 1 to 2 minutes of bag and mask ventilation, oral tracheal intubation should be undertaken.

The successful intubation is performed with smooth and unhurried movements. The head should be repositioned as described above. Following resuctioning of secretions from the oropharynx, the resuscitator passes a straight infant laryngoscope blade (size 0 for the smallest babies, size 1 for full-term babies) between the base of the tongue and the anterior surface to the epiglottis, elevating the epiglottis with the tip of the blade and thereby visualizing the glottis and vocal cords. An orotracheal tube may then be passed with the tip advanced 1 cm beyond the glottis. Appropriate tube size is shown in Table 2.

Table 1 provides guidelines for the approach to the infant following the establishment of assisted ventilation. For most asphyxiated babies, establishing an airway and providing assisted ventilation for periods of 2 to 3 minutes

TABLE 2 Guidelines for Selection of Endotracheal Tube and Suction Catheters

Weight (g)	Endotracheal Tube Size (mm Outer Diameter)	Size of Suction Catheter
<1,000	2.5	5 F
1,000–1,500	2.5 or 3.0	5 F or 6 F
1,501–2,500	3.0	6 F
2,501–3,000	3.0 or 3.5	6 F or 8 F
>3,000	3.5	8 F

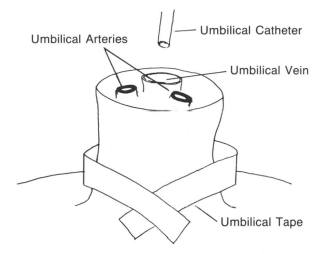

Figure 2 The cut surface of the umbilical cord (after constriction with umbilical tape to prevent blood loss) demonstrates two small muscular umbilical arteries and a single umbilical vein. (From Truog WE. Neonatal resuscitation. In: Carlo W, Chatbum R, Lough M, eds. Neonatal respiratory care. 2nd ed. Chicago: Year Book Medical Publishers, 1988, with permission.)

bicarbonate cannot be administered simultaneously by the same route, since alkalotic solutions inactivate the epinephrine. The choices then become interruption of the bicarbonate infusion, flushing of the catheter with normal saline, and then administration of the epinephrine, or administration of the epinephrine into the endotracheal tube during the bicarbonate infusion. A second dose of both may be repeated after 5 to 10 minutes, depending on the response to ongoing ventilation and massage and assessment of blood gas tensions and pH.

External Cardiac Massage

Bradycardia and cyanosis should prompt initiation of external cardiac massage by 3 minutes of age either concomitant with or immediately after the administration of the medication described above. Two techniques exist for external cardiac massage. The first involves placing the resuscitator's two thumbs over the middle third of the sternum with the fingers encircling the torso of the infant and supporting the back. The thumbs should be positioned on the sternum just below a line drawn between the nipples. The lower portion of the sternum should not be compressed because of the potential damage to the liver or spleen (Fig. 3). The second technique applies if the infant is larger or if the resuscitator's hands are too small to encircle the chest completely. Compression of the sternum is accomplished with the second and middle fingers just below the nipple line. The other hand may be needed to support the infant's back if the infant is not placed on a firm surface. The sternum is compressed approximately 1 to 2 cm at a rate of 120 times per minute. Compression should be at approximately a 1:1 ratio between compression and relaxation time. Compression should always be accompanied by positive pressure ven-

tilation, continuing at a rate of approximately 40 breaths per minute. The stimulus for forward blood flow in these circumstances may be the elevation in pleural pressure rather than forceful expulsion of the blood from the cardiac ventricles, although firm evidence for this in neonates is not available. If adequate ventilation is not being achieved during external massage, then massage should stop briefly to allow 2 to 3 inhaled breaths and then quickly resume. Once per minute spontaneous pulse rate should be determined by both listening for heart sounds and palpating a peripheral pulse.

Other Medications

Infants have rapid depletion of glucose stores, and a depressed infant has difficulty mobilizing potentially available glucose through glycogenolysis or gluconeogenesis. If ongoing resuscitation is needed beyond the first 5 to 10 minutes, a bedside reagent stick should be used to check a drop of blood for glucose concentration. An infusion of glucose (1 to 2 ml per kilogram of a 10 percent solution) may be needed, as resuscitation is unlikely to be successful in a profoundly hypoglycemic infant. Although controversy surrounds the appropriate role of glucose infusions in ameliorating hypoxic-ischemic encephalopathy, studies in neonatal animals suggest that hypoglycemia is detrimental during such stress.

The opiate antagonist naloxone (Narcan neonatal, 0.01 mg per kilogram) may be a useful adjunct to resuscitation if respiratory depression without other signs of asphyxia is present and if there is a history of maternal administration of medications likely to induce apnea (e.g., morphine or its synthetic congeners).

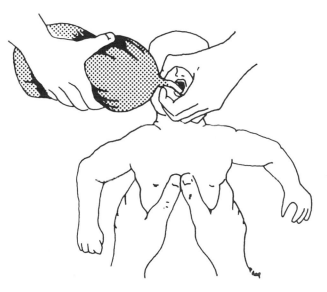

Figure 3 External cardiac compression during assisted ventilation of a neonate. This degree of resuscitation requires two trained individuals. (From Truog WE. Neonatal resuscitation. In: Carlo W, Chatbum R, Lough M, eds. Neonatal respiratory care. 2nd ed. Chicago: Year Book Medical Publishers, 1988, with permission.)

There appears to be little role for infusion of calcium salts in delivery room resuscitation. Total serum calcium levels in the newborn are actually elevated above maternal levels. It is highly unlikely that ionized calcium is low in neonates because acidosis leads to an increase in ionized calcium concentration.

Atropine, a vagolytic agent, has an unclear role in delivery room resuscitation. An empirical trial (0.01 to 0.02 mg per kilogram per dose) may be useful in persistent bradycardia, but a far more likely reason than increased vagal tone for bradycardia is depression that is unresponsive to epinephrine.

Table 3 provides a summary of potentially useful drugs in delivery room resuscitation.

Special Situations Requiring Additional Intervention

The possibility of hypovolemia contributing to asphyxia should be considered in cases of suspected placental abruption, ruptured umbilical or placental vessels, or (rarely) ruptured liver or spleen during the delivery. Pallor (difficult to appreciate with coexistent cyanosis), distant precordial heart sounds, poor peripheral capillary filling, diminished peripheral pulses, and hypotension are signs suggestive of decreased blood volume. An initially normal hematocrit does not exclude hypovolemia. Treatment consists of an infusion of fresh whole blood, either cross-matched to the mother and baby or type O, Rh negative if available, or 0.9 percent saline, or lactated Ringers solution at a dose of at least 10 ml per kilogram initially. Blood obtained from the placenta drawn into a sterile syringe containing heparin at 1 to 2 U per milliliter could be used as a last resort. Hypotension in asphyxiated infants does not necessarily mean hypovolemia, and automatic intravascular volume expansion should be discouraged in depressed neonates. Fluid overload may induce pulmonary and soft tissue edema, compounding problems with pulmonary function later on. Right atrial pressure, measured through a central venous catheter, may be helpful in interpreting intravascular volume status because of previous losses or pre-existing edema (e.g., in hydrops fetalis). Umbilical venous catheters placed in the right atrium measure central venous pressure. These catheters are most easily placed during the first 12 hours after birth.

Hydrops fetalis may require abdominal paracentesis through the lateral flank to remove ascitic fluid and allow better lung expansion. Thoracentesis for possible pleural fluid should probably be withheld until after a chest x-ray film has been obtained and examined. If the hydrops is associated with anemia, an isovolemic partial exchange transfusion with packed red cells designed to raise the hematocrit to at least 30–35 percent may be necessary shortly after birth in order to provide adequate oxygen tissue delivery.

Meconium expelled from the fetal intestinal tract in utero becomes diluted with amniotic fluid and may, occasionally be aspirated in utero or with the first breath. Aspiration produces postnatal hypoxemia and hypercarbia because of obstruction in both large and small airways. Ultimately, an inflammatory response ensues. Rapid suctioning of the oropharynx at delivery and direct laryngoscopy with suctioning of any meconium easily removable from the larynx appear to minimize the occurrence and severity of the aspiration. In this situation the physician must balance the need to remove meconium with the need to correct concomitant cyanosis and bradycardia.

Evaluation of Treatment During the Period Immediately Following Resuscitation

Immediate or severe respiratory distress in a term neonate indicates airway anomalies. These anomalies include tracheoesophageal fistula and congenital diaphragmatic hernia. In the case of esophageal atresia with or without tracheoesophageal fistula, there may be frothing of oral secretions in the mouth and immediate choking with any feeding attempt. Management of a tracheoesophageal fistula consists of placing a catheter in the proximal esophageal

TABLE 3   Potentially Useful Drugs in Resuscitation of the Neonate

Drug	Indication	Route and Dosage
Epinephrine	Prolonged bradycardia	0.1 ml/kg of 1:10,000 solution IV or via endotracheal tube
Sodium bicarbonate	Metabolic acidosis	2 mEq/kg IV as 1 mEq/2 ml fluid given at 1–2 ml/min
Dextrose	Low blood glucose	2 ml/kg of 10% dextrose in water IV = 200 mg/kg
Naloxone	Respiratory depression secondary to maternal narcotic administration	0.01 mg/kg IV or IM
Plasma-like substance (normal saline or plasma-like solution; 5% albumin in normal saline)	Low intravascular volume	10–15 ml/kg

pouch and maintaining it on continuous suction. The infant is placed in an upright and prone position. Management of congenital diaphragmatic hernia includes basic resuscitation, intubation for severe distress, evacuation of stomach contents, and confirmation of the diagnosis by radiologic studies. Early paralysis (pancuronium 0.1 mg per kilogram) may help control extreme respiratory embarrassment and minimize the risk of pneumothorax prior to surgery.

Imperforate anus, cleft lip or palate, and meningomyelocele are examples of anomalies that, while not immediately life-threatening, should be detectable immediately after birth.

COMMON ERRORS IN RESUSCITATION

Hyperextension of the neck while trying to provide a patent airway can result in occlusion of the airway and difficulty with intubation. This can be avoided by using the shoulder roll and pulling the infant's chin forward. Should effective bag and mask ventilation continue for more than 1 to 2 minutes, a common error is to fail to vent the stomach by inserting an orogastric tube with suction applied manually with a large syringe. Failure to do this can result in a restriction of lung expansion, gastric rupture, or reflux of gastric contents leading to aspiration. Unnecessary overventilation can occur with assisted ventilation. Ventilatory rates greater than 80 breaths per minute may result in pneumothorax through institution of "inadvertent positive end expiratory pressure" and/or the development of hyperventilation respiratory alkalosis, which may prolong the infant's apneic phase.

WHEN TO START OR STOP RESUSCITATION

Articles describing techniques for neonatal resuscitation routinely focus on the "hows" and "whys" but often avoid discussion about when to start or stop resuscitation.

The 1980s are a time of transition in the development of medical and societal agreement about providing intensive support for even the smallest and sickest infants. Against this background of lack of consensus, immediate decisions about whom to resuscitate must be made. *The delivery room is a poor place to make judgments about starting or stopping treatment.* At present, babies of birth weights of less than 600 g only rarely survive to discharge, whereas babies of birth weights of 750 to 800 g are much more frequent survivors, with a reasonable likelihood of normal long-term neurologic and intellectual development. It is difficult to distinguish 100 to 150 g weight differences in the delivery room. Additionally, extremely immature babies are born with a variable level of depression and a variable ability to respond to resuscitative efforts. One approach is to offer initial resuscitative efforts to liveborn infants, to continue the evaluation based on the infant's response to resuscitative efforts, and to expand the data base to include weight, gestational age, and condition of the mother at the time of delivery. No simple rules can be written to govern behavior in this situation.

The second difficult situation is determining the duration of attempts to revive an extremely depressed baby. *If a spontaneous heart rate is present and persists, resuscitative efforts should continue for at least 20 minutes.* In the absence of any spontaneous cardiac activity, no matter how slow, or any other sign of life following 2 to 3 doses of epinephrine and 10 to 15 minutes of effective resuscitation, further resuscitative efforts are unlikely to result in an infant who can be discharged alive.

Artful inactivity, so useful in medicine and, especially, in pediatrics, has little place in the delivery room when one is confronted with a depressed baby. A rapidly implemented logical approach to resuscitation may produce potentially lifelong benefits.

SURFACTANT REPLACEMENT THERAPY

DONALD L. SHAPIRO, M.D.

An article on surfactant replacement therapy in this book on neonatal therapy represents a landmark in the history of neonatology. It has been almost 30 years since a deficiency of surfactant was found to be the cause of the respiratory distress syndrome of premature infants, and since surfactant replacement was envisioned as a therapy for the disorder. This article describes the current and future picture regarding surfactant replacement therapy. However, for a complete understanding, we must know where we have been, and how the necessary information was accumulated that has led to the surfactant replacement therapy of today.

BRIEF REVIEW OF LUNG DEVELOPMENT AND THE SURFACTANT SYSTEM

The lungs begin to form early in embryologic life as outpouchings of the thoracic endoderm into the surrounding mesodermal tissue. Successive branching of this tissue to form the respiratory airways is the major morphogenic event in the lung during the first half of fetal development in the human. Once the respiratory airways have been formed by this process, the terminal functional units, the alveoli, begin to be formed between 20 and 24 weeks in the human. The alveoli are the air exchange units of the lung, and it is here that the surfactant story takes place. The alveoli are formed by structural cells known as type I alveolar epithelial cells, or type I pneumocytes. Interspersed with these type I cells are type II pneumocytes, specialized cells that produce the pulmonary surfactant.

Surfactant begins to be made by type II pneumocytes between 24 and 28 weeks of gestation in the human. An extensive amount of research has shown that this developmental process, like many others, is regulated by circulating and local hormones. These include steroids and thyroid hormone, fibroblast pneumocyte factor, and probably other factors whose effects are as yet incompletely appreciated.

When type II pneumocytes have completely developed, they have the capability of selectively taking up metabolic precursors for surfactant, synthesizing the lipid and protein components of surfactant, and packaging selected components into the storage and secretory organelle of the type II pneumocyte known as the lamellar body. When appropriate signals are received by the type II pneumocyte in response to physiologic needs, the lamellar body empties its contents into the alveolus, providing a new supply of surfactant components. Beta-adrenergic and purinergic stimuli are known to stimulate this secretory process, but there still is not a complete understanding of the physiologic, cellular, and molecular events in surfactant synthesis and secretion. Because of this, there remains some caution about surfactant replacement therapy; it cannot be predicted how various exogenous surfactants with different components will interact with the endogenous pulmonary surfactant system.

Surfactant in the alveolus is made up of a number of lipids, primarily dipalmitoylphosphatidylcholine (DPPC), and a number of surfactant-specific proteins. Phosphatidylglycerol also appears to be an important component. Although DPPC is responsible for the surface tension–lowering ability of surfactant, the surfactant lipoprotein complex must accomplish a number of other functions, all in addition to lowering surface tension. First, the film of surfactant must be able to spread easily at the air-water interface; phosphatidylglycerol and certain proteins appear to be important for this function. Second, the surfactant film must also be able to withstand compression and expansion on a breath-to-breath basis. Third, the surfactant complex must play a role in its own metabolic feedback loop, so that the cell knows when to make and secrete more surfactant. One or more of the surfactant proteins is thought to play a role in this feedback system.

The story of the type II pneumocyte and the surfactant production system is continuing to evolve in research laboratories. Progress has been very rapid within the last few years, allowing an appreciation of the complexity of this system. A relatively complete picture of the system must be obtained before surfactant replacement therapy can be optimized, because it must be known how exogenous surfactants interact with the endogenous pulmonary surfactant system. Even without this complete understanding, however, progress with surfactant replacement therapy has been steady, and there is a growing sense of security about the therapy, based on clinical experience.

EVOLUTION OF SURFACTANT REPLACEMENT THERAPY

The start of surfactant replacement therapy was the observation of Avery and Mead that infants dying of the respiratory distress syndrome (RDS) lacked pulmonary surface-active material. Because of this, alveoli were unstable and collapsed, the work of breathing increased to unsustainable levels, ventilatory failure occurred, and infants died in the absence of some intervention.

Although positive-pressure ventilation with all of its variations was then, and is now, a mainstay of supportive therapy for infants with RDS, it was envisioned almost from the beginning that surfactant might be put down into the lungs of infants with RDS and the disorder directly treated. The first such attempt was by Robillard and colleagues, who treated 10 infants with pure DPPC. They reasoned that the multicomponent surfactant mixture obtained by washing out lungs had many contaminating substances (it was known to contain albumin, clearly a serum component) and that the only active factor in the complex was DPPC. Their results were equivocal at best, but shortly afterward a research team from the Cardiovascular Research Institute in San Francisco undertook a much larger clinical trial, again using DPPC. It quickly became apparent that this substance *alone* had no significant therapeutic effect on infants with RDS.

It was not immediately known whether the failure of this clinical trial was because the hypothesis that surfactant deficiency was responsible for RDS was incorrect (an alternative explanation was suggested in which pulmonary ischemia was the major problem), or whether other components were needed for surfactant to have its full activity. The latter proved to be the case. Enhorning and Robertson used a whole surfactant complex obtained from rabbits to treat prematurely born rabbits. Pulmonary mechanics were dramatically improved. Similar studies were performed by Adams and colleagues on premature sheep. After these studies, a number of research groups became actively interested in animal experimentation using surfactants.

Although the work of Enhorning and Adams clearly showed the efficacy of surfactant, a major obstacle existed. Whole surfactant, obtained by lavage, contained approximately 10 percent protein, including albumin and other proteins. It was not known initially whether these proteins were functionally important; what *was* important was the reluctance of clinicians to administer such a large amount of foreign animal protein to human infants. Thus, a number of strategies were employed to produce surfactants that had minimal to no potentially antigenic protein. One approach, taken by Robert Notter and myself in the United States and Possmeyer, Metcalfe, and Enhorning in Canada, was to obtain whole animal surfactant by lavage and then to extract the surfactant into organic solvents, obtaining only the most lipid-like fractions of surfactant. When this was done, an extract that contained only 1 percent protein was obtained. A similar approach was taken by Fujiwara in Japan, who obtained his initial surfactant mixture by mincing and homogenizing lungs and then performing the organic solvent extraction. He had to fortify his mixture with DPPC and other components because they had become diluted in this process, but eventually his mixture was compositionally and functionally similar to the other surfactant extracts.

Two other approaches were used. Merritt, Hallman, and colleagues decided to try to avoid the problem of antigenicity by using human material. They obtained human surfactant from amniotic fluid, and have used this in a number of successful clinical trials. These have been of importance from a research standpoint, but there seems little possibility that human material can be obtained from amniotic fluid in sufficient quantity to treat all the infants who require it. A different approach to the protein problem was taken by a number of other investigators, most notably John Clements, who reasoned that the protein components of surfactant might be substituted for by nonprotein additives that could perform the same function. He has developed a synthetic mixture (Exosurf) which at least partially corrects deficiency in animal studies and is currently undergoing clinical trials.

Many people believe that the ultimate solution will be a human-type surfactant that can be made in large quantities by biotechnology. Some pharmaceutical firms are actively studying the cloning of surfactant proteins and their recombination with lipids to make clinically utilizable surfactants. The final steps in devising the perfect surfactant must await basic information about surfactant synthesis and secretion in the type II pneumocyte, so that exogenous surfactants can be designed that will integrate into the native physiologic surfactant system without adverse effects.

CURRENT CLINICAL USE OF SURFACTANT

Six major clinical trials of surfactant replacement therapy have been reported in the literature and additional information has been presented at research meetings. These trials have used all the surfactants discussed above. All have demonstrated that surfactant replacement can reverse the pulmonary insufficiency of RDS. This effect is most demonstrable when the surfactant is administered to infants in active respiratory distress; *improvement in oxygenation and compliance can be seen within minutes of surfactant administration.*

Surfactant administration has also been shown to be efficacious when given at birth before the onset of respiratory symptoms. One disadvantage of this clinical strategy is that it cannot be determined at birth who will have RDS, and many infants are given surfactant who probably do not require it. At our current stage of understanding, when the toxicity of surfactants is still a concern, there is reluctance to administer surfactant to those who might not need it.

Because of the concern about toxicity, all the early trials were designed so that infants received only one dose of surfactant, either at birth or after some respiratory symptoms had developed. After experience with these studies had alleviated some of the anxiety, the possibility of additional doses was considered. This was important, because our initial studies at the University of Rochester suggested that one dose of surfactant given at birth may not be enough for some infants. Since the surfactant deficiency of RDS is known to persist for 2 to 3 days, and the half-life of surfactant in the alveolus is usually measured in hours, it seemed reasonable that additional surfactant might be required. In a recent study we demonstrated that *significantly better results could be obtained if multiple doses of surfactant were given to infants when they required it as determined by clinical criteria.* The most striking difference in this study using multiple doses, compared with the previous one-dose study, was an improvement in survival from 71 to 94 percent in a high-risk group of infants between 24 and 29 weeks of gestation. A benefit

from multiple doses was also found in a study by Merritt and colleagues.

Some major clinical trials are currently in progress, and much more information should be available in the next 2 years about the most appropriate clinical strategies. Will it be necessary to give surfactant at birth, or can one wait until respiratory symptoms appear? Our data indicate that respiratory distress can be adequately treated by surfactant after symptoms have appeared, but RDS has a number of associated problems (bronchopulmonary dysplasia, patent ductus arteriosus, intraventricular hemorrhage), and information about the respiratory distress and its associated problems is necessary before we can provide a final answer to the question of whether surfactant administered at birth, before the onset of respiratory distress, has a significant benefit.

How many doses of surfactant are needed, and how large should the dose be? Our studies suggest that in the highest-risk group of patients, between 24 and 29 weeks of gestation, at least half the babies will benefit significantly from additional doses. *Currently used doses are approximately 100 mg per kilogram, which is five or six times more than theoretically required to cover the alveolar surface.* We do not know whether the dose of surfactant can be reduced without diminishing its effectiveness.

Is there a better way to administer the surfactant? When given at the time of birth, the surfactant easily mixes with the normal fetal lung liquid and recedes with it into the alveoli, producing almost perfect distribution. When surfactant is given after birth, however, it has to be instilled as a saline suspension. This is usually performed in aliquots, changing the position of the infant each time. Infants seem to tolerate this, but the procedure can probably be improved. One recently suggested approach is to instill the surfactant with some form of high-frequency ventilation. We are also experimenting with aerosolization of surfactants. It seems highly likely that better methods of delivery will be developed.

Although current clinical trials will surely develop more appropriate strategies, dosages, and methods of administration within the next few years, the critical issue still remains the problem of potential biologic interactions of exogenous surfactant. This is a concern both for synthetic surfactants with unphysiologic additives and for bovine-derived lung surfactant extracts. At present these concerns are largely theoretical; it is quite remarkable that in all the clinical trials to date, no serious toxicity has been found acutely. Long-term follow-up studies are currently in progress and should provide more information.

THE FUTURE

What is the future for surfactant replacement therapy? It is anticipated that within the next few years an almost complete understanding of the cellular and molecular aspects of the surfactant system will be developed. This will provide necessary information about surfactant synthesis, secretion, and recycling and their critical regulatory elements. At the same time, it should be possible to produce all the surfactant protein components in large quantity by gene cloning technology. Methods will be developed whereby these proteins can be variously recombined with lipids to make surfactants. These different surfactants will be studied in tissue culture and animal experiments to determine their effects on the pulmonary surfactant system. Finally, *when animal studies have shown that an exogenous surfactant performs its function without adverse effects on the endogenous pulmonary surfactant system and without eliciting an abnormal immunologic response, we will have the ultimate surfactant for replacement therapy.* With such a nontoxic, relatively inexpensive surfactant, many of the issues involving timing, multiplicity, and size of dose will be less relevant. It is likely then that surfactant will be given liberally in the delivery room when there is a possibility of the respiratory distress syndrome, and that when RDS occurs doses will be given frequently enough to maintain pulmonary function at near-physiologic levels. This will allow for the survival of virtually all premature infants beyond 25 weeks of gestation with a much reduced morbidity rate. I'm sure all readers will agree that this era cannot come soon enough.

SUGGESTED READING

Adams FH, Towers B, Osher AB, et al. Effect of tracheal instillation of natural surfactant in premature lambs. I. Clinical and autopsy findings. Pediatr Res 1978; 12:841.

Avery ME, Mead J. Surface properties in relation to atelectasis and hyaline membrane disease. Am J Dis Child 1959; 97:517–523.

Chu J, Clements JA, Cotton EK, et al. Neonatal pulmonary ischemia: Clinical and physiologic studies. Pediatrics 1967; 40:709–782.

Enhorning G, Robertson B. Lung expansion in the premature rabbit fetus after tracheal deposition of surfactant. Pediatrics 1972; 50:58–66.

Enhorning G, Shennan A, Possmayer F, et al. Prevention of neonatal respiratory distress syndrome by tracheal instillation of surfactant: A randomized clinical trial. Pediatrics 1985; 76:145–153.

Gitlin JD, Soll RF, Parad RB, et al. Randomized controlled trial of exogenous surfactant for the treatment of hyaline membrane disease. Pediatrics 1987; 79:31–37.

Hallman M, Merrit TA, Jarvenpaa A-L, et al. Exogenous human surfactant for treatment of severe respiratory distress syndrome: A randomized prospective clinical trial. J Pediatr 1985; 106:963–969.

Kendig JW, Notter RH, Shapiro DL. Improved survival in very premature infants treated with multiple doses of calf lung surfactant extract. Pediatrics 1987; 21:365A.

Kwong MS, Egan EA, Notter RH, Shapiro DL. Double-blind clinical trial of calf lung surfactant extract for the prevention of hyaline membrane disease in extremely premature infants. Pediatrics 1985; 76:585–592.

Merritt TA, Hallman M, Bloom BT, et al. Prophylactic treatment of very premature infants with human surfactant. N Engl J Med 1986; 315:785–790.

Robillard E, Alarie Y, Dagenais-Perusse P, et al. Microaerosol administration of synthetic dipalmitoyl lecithin in the respiratory distress syndrome: A preliminary report. Can Med Assoc J 1964; 90:55–57.

Shapiro DL, Notter RH, Morin FC, et al. Double-blind, randomized trial of calf lung surfactant extract administered at birth to very premature infants for prevention of respiratory distress syndrome. Pediatrics 1985; 76:593–599.

TISSUE pH MONITORING

RAMA BHAT, M.D.

Perinatal monitoring has undergone extensive changes during the past 10 to 15 years. These changes are the result of introduction of several new devices for continuous monitoring of hemodynamic and acid-base status. Today it is well established that intermittent monitoring of high-risk mothers in the intrapartum period and of critically ill neonates in the neonatal intensive care unit is inadequate. The trend at present is to develop monitors that can be used noninvasively. Several of the currently used monitors—namely transcutaneous Po_2 and Pco_2 and saturation devices—have been well accepted by neonatologists. Tissue pH monitoring, on the other hand, has been extensively studied in both animals and humans during the past 20 years and is still undergoing modification. The principles of tissue pH monitoring, types of electrodes, application techniques, and clinical experience and complications are reviewed in this chapter.

PHYSIOLOGIC BASIS OF TISSUE pH MONITORING

Transcutaneous monitoring of oxygen and carbon dioxide is based on the principle that both oxygen and carbon dioxide diffuse through the skin. Both these parameters can be measured noninvasively with currently available heated sensors. The *pH cannot be monitored noninvasively because the hydrogen ion (H^+) is not diffusible across the skin.* Thus the electrodes for monitoring pH have to be applied directly to the muscle surface or subcutaneous tissue. When they are applied in this fashion, the pH sensors measure the pH of the interstitial fluid. Interstitial fluid pH represents local tissue perfusion and metabolism. This fluid, which has adequate buffering capacity, is in constant contact with the underlying tissue, and is in dynamic equilibrium with the plasma. Therefore, the pH of this fluid is in balance with blood pH as long as perfusion to the tissue is adequately maintained. In cases of metabolic acidosis due to poor perfusion (e.g., hypotension, hypovolemia, and decreased cardiac output), tissue pH may show earlier and more severe acidosis than does the blood gas tension. Decreased cardiac output and subsequent decreased oxygen delivery to the tissues result in anaerobic metabolism and accumulation of lactic acid. As perfusion improves during improved circulation, tissue pH may improve faster than venous pH because of lactic acid washout form the peripheral tissues. Administration of buffers without improvement in cardiac output may show rapid changes in arterial pH with a much delayed improvement in tissue pH. Conversely, in cases of respiratory acidosis, tissue pH may immediately follow changes in arterial pH.

PRINCIPLES OF TISSUE pH MONITORING

In 1906 Cremer first reported that a glass bulb placed in an aqueous fluid-filled medium developed an electrical potential proportional to the acidity of the surrounding medium. This charge was not affected by dissolved oxygen or oxidizing or reducing agents. Subsequently this was attributed to the presence of H^+ ions. The voltage that developed was linearly and inversely proportional to the pH. However, it could not be directly measured from the surface of the glass without a reference electrode. The charge on the glass electrode changes slightly with temperature (0.03 pH units with temperature variation from 25 °C in vitro to 37 °C in body fluids) at normal pH. Hence, a temperature correction may need to be incorporated into the pH monitor. The pH electrode is connected by a specially shielded cable to the pH monitor, which has capabilities for a continuous printout.

Several types of electrodes have been developed and tested during the past two decades. These include the standard glass electrode, polyvinyl chloride polymer electrodes, needle electrodes, and paladium oxide electrodes. Experimental and clinical studies have shown that glass and polymer electrodes are sensitive and stable in biological fluids for prolonged periods. Early versions of glass electrodes were large and were intended for monitoring muscle surface pH. These electrodes needed a large skin incision (2 cm length) for placement, frequent calibration, and needed to be moved frequently. These limitations lead to their replacement by newer and smaller electrodes.

ELECTRODE DESCRIPTION AND CALIBRATION

Figure 1 represents the three different electrodes that have been introduced in recent years. Part A shows the glass electrode marketed by KONTRON (Basel, Switzer-land), originally designed by Stamm and colleagues for fetal scalp tissue pH monitoring during labor. The electrode consists of a short glass probe and a concentric reference electrode inside a common housing approximately 2.5 cm long. The pH-sensitive glass tip, about 1 mm in length, is incorporated into a hydrophilic glass shaft containing silver/silverchloride (Ag/AgCl) electrode and pH buffer solution. The glass shaft is surrounded by 4-molar potassium chloride and AgCl solution and an Ag/AgCl reference electrode. This electrode requires chemical sterilization, conditioning with potassium chloride, and calibration with standard buffers (pH 7.40 and 6.8) before application to subcutaneous tissue. This electrode is applied perpendicular to the skin's surface through a 3-mm incision. A small spiral button stabilizes the electrode to the skin. The voltage generated by the H^+ in tissue fluid on the glass membrane electrode is proportional to the pH of that tissue. Response time of the electrode under normal operating conditions is 30 sec to 1 min for +0.001 pH unit changes, and electrode drift is about 0.03 U after 6 hours of use at 37 °C. This is secondary to a decrease in potassium chloride concentration of the reference solution, due to its outflow to tissue fluid.

Polymer membrane sensors for continuous intravascular pH monitoring were first introduced by Le Blanc and coworkers in 1976. Since then, they have been modified for tissue pH monitoring. As seen in Figure 1B, the sensor consists of a silver wire, the tip of which is impregnated with chloride. Capped by a gel electrolyte, the entire tip is encapsulated in a polymer. The polymer has an H^+ selective carrier incorporated into it. The sensor also contains a reference electrode made of Ag/AgCl. The sensor is connected to an amplifier with a digital readout. The electrode is a disposable wire electrode that comes in a sterile package. It needs to be calibrated with known buffers of 6.80 and 7.40 pH, respectively, before applica-

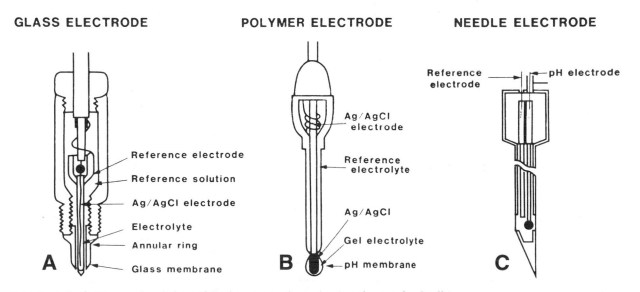

Figure 1 *A, B, C,* Cross-sectional views of the three newer electrodes (see the text for details).

tion. The electrode is easily inserted into the subcutaneous tissue (no incision is required). Although the wire electrode is about 5.5 cm long, only the 6 mm H^+-sensitive tip actually comes into contact with tissue fluid. The ease of application and disposability make this sensor appropriate for use even in preterm infants.

The newer needle electrode (Fig. 1C) described by Leuthen in 1984 consists of a glass electrode enclosed in a hypodermic needle (length 8 cm; outer diameter [OD] 0.7 mm). The beveled tip of the needle is sealed and helps in penetration of skin and tissue. The pH-sensitive tip is a spherical glass bulb with a reference electrode. This is what comes in contact with the tissue fluid through a side hole in the needle. The internal electrodes are connected via glass tubes and Ag/AgCl chloride electrodes to external cables. The electrode has been tested in animals and found to correlate well with the arterial pH (r = 0.82, p < 0.001) as well as the regular glass tissue pH electrode. The in vivo response time was 3.7 ± 2.5 min (M±SD). Studies using this electrode in humans have not yet been reported.

CLINICAL EXPERIENCE

The first clinical study using large muscle surface glass electrodes was reported in 33 adult patients undergoing reconstructive abdominal or cardiac surgery and eight healthy volunteers. The healthy volunteers were subjected to hypovolemia by withdrawing 750 ml of blood while tissue pH changes were continuously monitored for a period of 2 hours. The withdrawn blood was then reinfused; monitoring during this recovery period was continued for the next 2 hours. In these healthy adults muscle surface pH closely correlated with arterial pH. During hypovolemia, a significant decrease in muscle pH (mean change of muscle pH was −0.24 U) was seen in six out of eight volunteers. Changes in mean blood pressure were seen in only three patients. Arterial pH failed to show any significant changes. During recovery, muscle surface pH returned to normal within 30 minutes of retransfusion.

In a second group of patients undergoing vascular reconstructive surgery, a reduced flow to peripheral tissues resulted in muscle acidosis, whereas restoration of flow resulted in return of muscle pH to the normal range. These and subsequent reports in adults and children have confirmed the usefulness of tissue pH monitoring. Tissue pH monitoring has also been performed in the perinatal period.

Intrapartum Tissue pH Monitoring

Saling first reported the usefulness of fetal blood pH measurements in the evaluation of the fetus during labor in 1966. Since then several investigators have confirmed this observation, and it has become routine to monitor the fetal scalp pH in the evaluation of the fetus during labor. However, these measurements are intermittent and each require a new incision, which increases the risk of complications. Ten years later a miniaturized glass pH electrode was introduced by Stamm and his coworkers for the

continuous monitoring of tissue pH. With some modifications this electrode (KONTRON, then Hoffman-LaRoche, Basel, Switzerland) was extensively evaluated between 1975 and 1980 both in the United States and in Europe. These clinical studies in the intrapartum period have confirmed that tissue pH and blood pH are highly correlated. Correlation coefficients of r = 0.62 to 0.94 have been reported between tissue pH and scalp pH. Tissue pH was found to be lower than arterial pH by 0.026 to 0.06 pH units. This is attributable to (1) stasis and scalp edema, (2) local accumulation of lactic acid, and (3) tissue injury at the incision site. During initial trials a high failure rate (10 to 20 percent) was reported. However, in the ensuing year this decreased to less than 10 percent. Additional problems were encountered by several investigators during the evaluation period. These included scalp necrosis, local hematomas, local and generalized infections (even generalized herpes in one case), breakage of glass electrode in the tissue, and breakage before and during application. Further complications, such as deposition of blood and protein over the sensitive glass tip, can interfere with tissue pH readings. As a result of these problems, the manufacturers have withdrawn this electrode from the American market. These electrodes are still available in Europe for fetal scalp pH monitoring.

Experience in the Newborn

Continuous tissue pH monitoring was first carried out in neonates and infants in 1970. Filler and Das reported their experience using a large glass electrode (7 cm in length and 0.7 cm in diameter) in neonates and infants undergoing surgery. The electrode was found to be sensitive, reliable, and useful, although it required frequent calibration and reapplication. A large skin incision and creation of a subfascial tunnel were necessary for its application to the muscle surface. Subsequent studies have confirmed the usefulness of tissue pH monitoring in neonates, children, and adults. However, in view of its invasive nature, tissue pH monitoring did not gain widespread enthusiasm and use. Interest was subsequently revived when a new miniaturized glass electrode (see Fig. 1A) was introduced (KONTRON). We have used this electrode in critically ill neonates and found it to be a reliable indicator of peripheral perfusion. In infants with good peripheral perfusion, tissue pH correlated well with the arterial pH (r = 0.89, n = 203, y = 0.44 +0.94x, p = <0.00005). In conditions associated with poor peripheral perfusion the tissue pH was found to be significantly lower than the arterial pH. This finding was subsequently confirmed in our laboratory in puppies subjected to hemorrhage. During the period of hypovolemia, with decreased cardiac output changes in tissue pH were more pronounced than those in arterial pH. Following reinfusion tissue pH did recover, but much more slowly than arterial pH.

Although the glass electrode gives reproducible results, it has several disadvantages. Because of its construction, the electrode must be applied perpendicularly to the surface of the skin, and it needs a spiral ring to stabilize it. This is a nondisposable glass electrode requiring involved preparation prior to reuse. Even if this electrode were small enough for use in neonates, its invasive nature and the difficulty of preparation and application to preterm neonates make it unpopular among neonatologists.

Recently, a new disposable polymer electrode (see Fig. 1C) has become available (Biochem International Inc., Milwaukee). The electrode can be applied to the subcutaneous tissue through a 20-gauge Jelco catheter. When it is applied, the pH-sensitive tip comes in contact with the tissue fluid. The electrode shows a stable pH reading within 15 minutes after application. Over a 2-year period we have measured tissue pH in 40 critically ill neonates using this disposable sensor. The electrode was placed in the subcutaneous tissue of the anterior or anterolateral aspect of the thigh. The tissue pH correlated well with the arterial pH (n = 476; r = 0.84; y = 0.46 + .93x; p = < 0.00005). The sensor responded well during both respiratory and metabolic acidosis and alkalosis. During severe metabolic acidosis (arterial pH < 7.10), as seen in cases of septic shock, the tissue pH was generally lower than the arterial pH (arterial pH 6.89 ± 0.15 versus tissue pH 6.78 ± 0.23, mean + SD, p = not significant). The sensor is unheated and can be left at the same site for long periods of time (up to 117 hours in our studies) without complications. Figure 2 demonstrates the tissue pH and blood gas changes from a critically ill neonate with septic shock. The failure rate was 17.5 percent, and this was attributed to (1) kinking of the pH-sensitive tip, and (2) adherence of clots over the sensor tip. The sensors are not expensive and are disposable; therefore preparation time is negligible. Despite these advantages, the polymer electrode still needs some modifications, namely, shortening the length, improving the stability in vitro and in vivo, and a better calibration system. *At present the manufacturers have withdrawn this product from the market because the cost to benefit ratio is high.*

The needle electrode described by Leuthen has not been tested in humans in the United States. Preliminary experimental work has shown good results. Further experience with this sensor is necessary before widespread use can be advocated.

FUTURE

Clinical studies in critically ill neonates and animals subjected to different experimental conditions have all established the usefulness of continuous tissue pH monitoring. However, we still do not have an ideal or a suitable commercially available sensor for use in small, critically ill neonates. An ideal tissue pH sensor for use in neonates or during the intrapartum period should be easy to calibrate and apply, stable for prolonged periods in tissue fluid, and have a short response time. Sensors available at present do not meet all these criteria.

Transcutaneous oxygen and carbon dioxide monitoring alone do not supply the complete acid-base status of critically ill patients. Besides, these are heated electrodes that require frequent site changes. They are also affected by postnatal age. A combination of tissue pH and transcutaneous $O_2 - CO_2$ monitoring would be beneficial to the

continuous assessment of sick preterm neonates at the bedside. Technologic advances in the coming years will probably help us to achieve this goal.

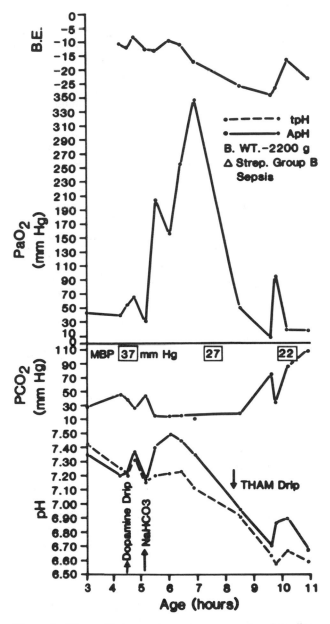

Figure 2 Tissue pH, transcutaneous oxygen and carbon dioxide, and blood gas data from a preterm neonate with β-hemolytic group B streptococcal sepsis. Mean blood pressures and treatment regimens are marked at various time points. Tissue pH was monitored using the polymer electrode applied subcutaneously in the left thigh. Tissue pH progressively decreased despite treatment with buffers and inotropic agents and was lower than arterial pH. (Birth weight = 2.2 kg, gestational age = 35 weeks.) Duration of monitoring was 7 hours (from 3 to 10 hours of age). NaHCO₃, sodium bicarbonate; THAM, trishydroxyaminomethane; tpH, tissue pH; Aph, arterial pH. (From Chaudhry U, Bhat R. Tissue pH monitoring by a disposable sensor in critically ill neonates. Am J Dis Child 1985; 139:1049, with permission.)

TRANSCEPHALIC IMPEDANCE

PATRICIA H. ELLISON, M.D.

One of the main challenges in the neonatal intensive care unit is that of measuring brain function and brain injury. The measures must capture both the *severity* and *duration* of the insult, particularly for preterm neonates who frequently sustain a series of brain insults. In the beginning weeks, the methods must disturb the neonate as little as possible, since many are critically ill. Bedside use is preferable to technologies that require transport. The measure must have the capacity for repetitive use without harming the neonatal brain. The method must be easy to use, preferably inexpensive, and applicable throughout different types of neonatal units. Otherwise, its use will be chiefly a research tool confined to small numbers of units and often to small sample sizes. To that end, we have explored the measure of transcephalic impedance (TCZ) in a series of studies in the neonatal intensive care unit.

Impedance is a measure of the energy required for the transmission of electrical current through a medium, in this instance the brain and the skull. The amount of resistance has been found to increase with age, both in the period of prematurity (24 to 40 weeks' gestation) and in the postnatal period (1 to 12 months). The amount of resistance has also been found to increase with intraventricular hemorrhage and severe asphyxia. The amount of resistance is less with hydrocephalus and in some premature neonates, particularly in those with either a severe or a repetitive series of conditions that might be considered to affect the neonatal brain.

TCZ is easily determined in neonates, although it can also be measured with more complicated instrumentation. In the latter form, it is a complex and sophisticated research tool, possibly an indicator of cerebral blood flow. The method we have used is much simpler. A small meter is utilized that contains a pair of 9-volt batteries. In our early work, the meter was constructed by the hospital biotechnician. In our later work, the meter was obtained from the Codman Company, or more recently constructed by Donald Dallman, who participated in some of the earlier studies. The more recent instruments represent a considerable improvement over the earlier models and should increase the reliability of the measures.

Needle electrodes were utilized to overcome the problem of high skin resistance in the neonate. One pair of electrodes was placed 2.5 cm just inside the anterior hairline; the second pair was placed at the inion also 2.5 cm apart. The anterior set of electrodes was directed with the tips of the needles toward the eyebrows. For the posterior set, the tips of the needles were directed downward toward the posterior neck. Each reading took less than 5 sec. We have differed in placement of electrodes from Reigel and coworkers, who used a scalp measurement. We reasoned that it would be better to make assessments on the basis of underlying brain structures using identifiable scalp landmarks rather than on scalp measures that had different relationships with different head sizes with head growth. We also differ from Reigel and associates in the use of needle rather than disk electrodes. We initially tried disk electrodes that required the abrasion of the skin to overcome skin resistance. The procedure of skin abrasion was not well tolerated by small preterm neonates with fragile skin. Skin abrasion probably precludes multiple measures because of changes in the skin. The needle electrodes are easily applied, much like a scalp intravenous line, as long as the point of the needles is maintained in good condition.

What then can we measure or, more appropriately, what should we measure? Surely, TCZ is not the best measure of intraventricular or other forms of intracranial hemorrhage. Both cerebral ultrasonography and computed tomography are much more sophisticated and appropriate technologies for such diagnoses. Similarly, TCZ may give early indication of the process of hydrocephalus, particularly as the amount of cerebrospinal fluid increases in the adjacent brain tissue. Currently we would not use it as an indicator of the size of the ventricles or as an indicator of the need for shunting procedures but would use modern brain-imaging methods. However, TCZ is helpful as an indicator of the need for an ultrasound study after shunt insertion.

We conclude from our work that *the most interesting use of TCZ is the measurement of certain processes of brain maturation in the preterm neonate,* as determined by serial weekly measurements. The nature of delays in maturation is at present open to speculation. Perhaps they involve (1) less than adequate nutrition for optimal or even adequate brain growth, (2) a slow rate of maturation of brain processes known to occur in the preterm—multiplication of glial cells and their products, and (3) changes in neurotransmitter production. Concurrent measures with TCZ and magnetic resonance imaging may yield some further clues, particularly in the development of white matter.

In our initial report, we noted lower readings of TCZ in six preterm neonates. We have more closely examined this issue in two further studies, the first a study of 22 preterm neonates in which three measures were utilized weekly (TCZ, occipital-frontal head circumference, and calories per kilogram per day). The second was a study of 51 preterm neonates in which several measures of brain function were utilized (TCZ, electroencephalogram, cerebral ultrasound, visual evoked response, occipital-frontal head circumference, and the Brazelton neonatal neurologic examination). In both studies, follow-up evaluations were made in infancy with Bayley's mental and motor scores and a neurologic evaluation.

Eight infants in the second study had no overall increase of TCZ in the first 5 weeks of life. Bayley's mental scores in infancy indicated that two had normal function and six had impaired function—four in the range of 50 to 75 developmental quotient and two with scores less than 40. The product-moment correlation between increase in TCZ and Bayley's mental scores was highly significant ($p < .001$). In the third study, four infants had an average change in TCZ less than 0.5 ohm per week at 5 weeks. One infant had a Bayley's mental score over 100, one infant had a score between 50 and 75, and two infants had scores less than 25. The correlation between the mean change per week and Bayley's mental scores was $r = .43$, significant at the level of $p < .01$. In this same study, at 8 weeks of age, only two infants had an average change of TCZ per week of less than 0.5 ohm. One infant had a score on the Bayley's mental test of 50 to 75, and one had a score of less than 25. However, one infant with a score of less than 25 now had a mean change per week of 0.85 ohm. The correlation between mean change per week in TCZ and Bayley's mental scores was .65, significant at a level of $p < .003$.

Another way to examine this issue is to compare mean differences in different categories of mental scores at particular gestational ages. Here we cite data from the 36th week of gestation because many preterm neonates are discharged around this time. The results for these outcomes are shown in Table 1. Comparison with analysis of variance indicates that the three categories in each outcome condition are significantly different except for Bayley's motor scores of 70 to 85 and over 85. However, the use of measures for separation of a particular infant may be less accurate because there is overlap among categories within a single standard deviation.

Yet another way to analyze these data is to compare means for serial measurements. Data are shown for the eighth weekly measurement for each of the three outcomes, again divided into three levels of normality/abnormality. In each of these analyses (Table 1 and Table 2) it is impossible to distinguish a middle level of abnormality on Bayley's motor score. Many premature infants score lower on Bayley's motor score than on Bayley's mental score. Their motor scores also depart significantly from the mean expected for age. The disturbance to the brain that results in mildly delayed motor function may not be as severe as the disturbance that results in mildly delayed mental function or transient neuromotor abnormalities. Thus, TCZ indicates "abnormal" motor function well but not mild delays in motor function. We consider that there is little difference between analyzing TCZ scores based on the actual age of gestation versus analyzing TCZ scores based on the number of the serial measurement in this data set.

TABLE 1 Mean TCZ and Standard Deviation at 36 Weeks' Gestation for Categories of Bayley's Mental, Motor, and Neurologic Scores in Infancy*

| | Bayley Mental | | Bayley Motor | |
	TCZ $\bar{x}$	SD	TCZ $\bar{x}$	SD
Score				
<70	24.7	±4.0	25.3	±5.0
70–85	29.8	±5.6	31.9	±2.0
>85	31.0	±3.4	31.2	±3.8
	Neurologic			
	TCZ $\bar{x}$	SD		
Abnormal	24.8	±5.1		
Transient	29.4	±2.3		
Normal	31.9	±3.8		

* All infants with birth weights less than 1,500 g, with weekly measurements.

TABLE 2 Mean TCZ and Standard Deviations at the Eighth Weekly Measurement for Categories of Bayley's Mental and Motor Scores and Neurologic Scores*

| | Bayley Mental | | Bayley Motor | |
	TCZ $\bar{x}$	SD	TCZ $\bar{x}$	SD
Score				
<70	23.0	±3.6	23.8	±4.9
70–85	28.0	±6.4	31.8	±3.1
>85	30.5	±3.0	29.5	±3.7
	Neurologic			
	TCZ $\bar{x}$	SD		
Abnormal	24.6	±6.0		
Transient	27.1	±2.8		
Normal	32.6	±1.9		

* All infants with birth weights less than 1,500 g, with weekly measurements.

This could be for any of several reasons: the composition of the data set, error in gestational age, or small sample size.

STUDIES THAT COMBINE TCZ AND OTHER VARIABLES

My experience with measurement of brain variables, such as cerebral blood flow or intracranial pressure has suggested that each method has a generous error term when measuring any individual infant. Even if technicians are trained so that the reliability of test-retest or inter-rater reliability is good, even sufficient for good scientific work, the concern that one is only approximating what one would choose to measure is not satisfied.

Second, any single method generally explained only a modest part of the outcome, i.e., accounted for only a limited part of the variance. When data are put into mathematical equations, one begins to realize the limitations of any single method of measurement.

Theoretically, *the combination of several methods of measurement would increase the percent variance accounted for and decrease the error term. We have been slow to use this approach in clinical research, although we often use it in clinical medicine.* As clinicians we often use a variety of measures to make a diagnosis: the history, the physical examination, laboratory tests, analyzing blood or urine, x-ray films, and in recent years, a variety of neuroimaging and neurophysiologic measures. Mentally we combine these tests in some way, weighting some more than others, probably varying these findings with our years of experience and diagnostic acumen. Yet in research, the majority of studies use only one measurement method or they compare one method with another (e.g., the identification of intracranial hemorrhage by computed tomography or by ultrasonography). Those qualities we seek to measure in the neonatal brain can often be categorized under one of two headings: physiologic processes (so that we may understand how something happened) and function (so that we may know that something happened). Our ability to approximate either of these qualities should increase with the use of combinations of methods of measurement.

In our first study with TCZ, which used multiple variate analysis, we examined the relationships among TCZ, calories per kilogram per week, and increase in occipital frontal head circumference per week in neonates as they related to three outcome variables: Bayley's mental score, Bayley's motor score, and neurologic condition. At this stage we were still asking the question: Which of the three predictors is most powerful? Multiple regression analyses were used. The main portion of the percent variance accounted for was clearly attributable to TCZ. The study was limited by the small sample size. In general, one assumes a risk in using multivariate analyses with small samples because the results may not replicate in a second sample measurement.

In our second study with several neonatal measures, TCZ was combined with measurements of electroencepha-

TABLE 3 Variables for Assessment of Brain Function in the Preterm Neonate: Scoring and Correlations with Mental, Motor, and Neurologic Outcome

Variables	Scoring	Mental	Correlations (r Value) Motor	Neurologic
VER slope of N_1 weeks 31–38	$< -40 = 1$ -40 to $23.5 = 2$ $\geq 23.5 = 3$	.24	.44$_b$	.34$_a$
VER slope of N_2 weeks 31–38	$< -61 = 1$ -61 to $35.5 = 2$ $\geq 35.5 = 3$	.29	.30	.33$_a$
Brazelton's Interactive (rescored)	$< 1.9 = 1$ $\geq 1.9 = 3$	.65$_c$	.69$_c$	.66$_c$
Brazelton's State Control	$2, 3 = 1$ $1 = 3$	.35$_a$	.41$_a$	.43$_b$
Brazelton's Motor (rescored)	Abnormal $= 1$ Mildly abnormal $= 2$ Normal $= 3$	.61$_c$	.58$_c$	.71$_c$
IVH grade	$4,5 = 1$ $2,3 = 2$ None $= 3$	.49$_c$	.53$_c$	.60$_c$
Ventricular dilatation	Moderate to marked dilatation $= 1$ Normal, mild dilatation $= 3$	.11	.10	.36$_a$
Serial EEG category	Severely abnormal $= 0.6$ Markedly abnormal $= 1.4$ Mildly abnormal $= 2.2$ Normal $= 3$	.70$_c$	.65$_c$	.76$_c$
Clinical seizures	None $= 1$ Observed $= 3$	.31$_a$	.35$_a$	.45$_b$
Birth weight	< 800 g $= 1$ 800 to $1,000 = 2$ $> 1,000 = 3$	.53$_c$	.46$_b$	.55$_c$
Weeks in NICU	$> 12 = 1$ 8.5 to $12 = 2$ $< 8.5 = 3$	.61$_c$	.60$_c$	.73$_c$
Initial percentile OFC	$< 25 = 1$ $> 25 = 3$	.11	.28$_a$	.33$_a$
Proportion of time OFC $<$ first percentile First 8 weeks	Mental: $\geq 0.6 = 1$ $< 0.6 = 3$ Motor: $[> 0.35 = 1]$ Neurologic: $[\leq 0.35 = 3]$	.59$_c$	.55$_c$	.63$_c$
Proportion of time OFC 10–25th percentile first 8 weeks	$< 0.35 = 1$ $\geq 0.35 = 3$	.37$_b$	.26	.33$_b$
Proportion of time OFC > 25th percentile first 8 weeks	$< 0.1 = 1$ $\geq 0.1 = 3$	.24	.32	.39$_b$
Mean percentile OFC weeks 2–8	$\leq 10 = 1$ $> 10 = 3$	.40$_b$	.44$_b$	.54$_c$
TCZ increment weeks 1–7	$< 0.5 = 1$ 0.5 to $1 = 2$ $> 1 = 3$	.35$_a$	.41$_b$	.53$_c$
TCZ—slope weeks 3–8	$\leq 1.35 = 1$ $> 1.35 = 3$	.28$_a$	.36$_b$	.41$_b$

Key: $a = p < .05$; $b = p < .01$; $c = p < .001$; VER = Visual evoked response; IVH = Intraventricular hemorrhage; NICU = Neonatal intensive care unit; OFC = Occipital frontal circumference.
From Ellison P, Horn JL, Heimler R. Prediction models in brain function in the preterm neonate. In: Oh W, Friis-Hansen B, Stern L, eds. Physiologic foundations of perinatal care. New York: Elsevier, 1987.

lography, cerebral ultrasonography, occipital frontal head circumference, visual evoked response, and Brazelton's neonatal neurologic examination. Again, each infant was assessed at age 1 year or older (corrected gestational age) with Bayley's mental score, Bayley's motor score, and a neurologic examination. Each method of assessment was examined extensively in relationship to each outcome. Similar analyses were made for those described earlier for TCZ. We tried to determine the best predictive period for each technology and the best measurement aspect of each method. Those methods of measurement that were the best predictors were then combined in several ways, seeking the best possible prediction for each outcome. In these analyses, the selected predictors were given equal weights when added for a total score. This was a deliberate choice based on the knowledge that the sample size was small; that any multivariate analyses would yield weights that might not replicate (see Ellison and co-workers), and that replicability in scores was more likely if the prediction or measurement variables were given equal weights (each was given 1, 2, or 3 points—see Table 3—for three gradations of normality/abnormality). TCZ was incorporated in the scores for prediction of mental function and neurologic condition (Tables 4 and 5). TCZ was not incorporated in the score for prediction of motor function. The reasons for this can be seen in Tables 1 and 2. In Tables 4 and 5, the outcome scores are listed for each level of neonatal score. In general, infants who had normal outcome scores had higher neonatal scores; children who had low neonatal scores had poor outcome scores. Cutoff points could be selected below which infants were abnormal, e.g., a mental score of 10 or less included only infants with abnormal mental function. One infant with

TABLE 4 Bayley's Mental Scores and Neonatal Score Levels*

Neonatal Scores	Bayley's Mental Scores	Neonatal Scores	Bayley's Mental Scores
15	130	13	128
	124		117
	119		103
	113		101
	112		95
	109		84
	104	12	93
	99		93
	97		84
	95		57 (FN)[†]
	91	11	98
	89		80
	89	10	67
	83		26
	78	9	69
14	128		67
	119	7	23
	98	5	21
	92		
	75		

* Based on electroencephalogram, ultrasonography, Brazelton's Interactive rescored, OFC < first percentile, and TCZ. Correlation between neonatal scores and Bayley's mental scores ($r = .75$, $p < .001$).

† FN = False negative.

From Ellison P, Horn JL, Heimler R. Prediction models in brain function in the preterm neonate. In: Oh W, Friis-Hansen B, Stern L, eds. Physiologic foundations of perinatal care. New York, Elsevier, 1987.

TABLE 5 Neurologic Condition Scores and Neonatal Scores*

Neonatal Scores	Neurologic Condition Scores	Neonatal Scores	Neurologic Condition Scores
15	1	13	1
	1		1
	1		1
	1		2
	1		3
	1	11	1
	1		1
	1		2
	1		2
	1		3
	1	10	2
	1		2
	2		2
	2	9	4
14	1	8	4
	1		4
	1		2 (FP)[†]
	1	7	4
	1	5	4

* Based on electroencephalogram, ultrasound, Brazelton's motor rescored, OFC < first percentile, and TCZ. Correlation between neonatal scores and neurologic condition scores ($r = -.82$, p < .001).

† FP = False positive.

From Ellison P, Horn JL, Heimler R. Prediction models in brain function in the preterm neonate. In: Oh W, Friis-Hansen B, Stern L, eds. Physiologic foundations of perinatal care. New York, Elsevier, 1987.

a neonatal score of 12 had an abnormal score on mental functions (which we would consider a false-negative score). The correlation between the neonatal score and Bayley's mental score was $r = .75$ ($p < .001$). Similar relationships were noted between the neonatal score and the neurologic condition. The correlation between the neonatal score and the neurologic score was $r = -.82$ (p < .001). A cutoff point of 9 or less indicated abnormal neurologic condition (spasticity or moderate to severe hypotonia) with the exception of one infant with transient neuromotor abnormalities (which we consider a false-positive score).

This type of work is expensive and time-consuming. It required a remarkable amount of cooperation among neonatologists, nurses, research technicians, and parents. As with all other work, it needs replication. We consider that it may never be replicated. However, other investigators may choose to replicate the methodology and use several measures of brain function or physiologic processes in their studies. Prematures can best be measured with several indicators; serial measurements generally yield more information. Each indicator has its own optimal time of measurement. The best combination of measures should be formed on the basis of their relationship to outcome in infancy (10 months of age or older), not on the basis of any variable in the neonatal unit. It is simply not possible to make sufficiently reliable assessments in the neonatal unit for use as outcome variables of brain function. Combinations of measures tested in this way could *then* be used to measure brain function in the neonatal unit.

We still consider that we have only approximated brain function or physiologic processes. We are gaining in understanding of how we can measure these entities, but a large amount of research remains to be done. In many neonatal units several conditions may hamper this type of work. The sample sizes of neonates with birth weights in selected categories may be small. The premature neonate may spend only a short time in the unit before transfer to a level II unit, making serial studies very difficult. In some units, the neonates may come from great distances or from segments of the population such that there is serious attrition in follow-up to even 10 months of age, which this investigator would consider minimal for answering these complicated questions. Then the investigator may as well seek another area of investigation.

We conclude on the basis of the work thus far that TCZ is a measure that should be incorporated in further studies of measurement of brain function for prematures. TCZ should be used serially, preferably weekly. There is excellent indication that it is measuring some quality about the neonatal brain that is related to later function. As with most measures of neonatal brain physiology and function, TCZ is best used in combination with other variables.

Acknowledgment. Special thanks to Dr. Richard Andrews, Division of Pediatric Neurology, University of Nebraska College of Medicine, for his helpful comments and critique of the manuscript.

SUGGESTED READING

Ellison P, Evers J. Transcephalic impedance in the neonate: An indicator of intracranial hemorrhage, asphyxia and delayed maturation. J Pediatr 1981; 98:968–971.

Ellison P, Heimler R, Franklin S. The relationships of transcephalic impedance, head growth and nutritional intake to outcome in preterm infants. Acta Paediatr Scand 1984; 73:820–827.

Ellison P, Horn JL, Franklin S, Jones MG. The results of checking a scoring system for neonatal seizures. Neuropediatrics 1986; 17:152–157.

Ellison P, Horn JL, Heimler R, et al. Prediction models for brain function in the preterm neonate, with and without use of ultrasound. In: Grauel EL, Syllm-Rapaport I, Wauer RR, eds. Research in Perinatal Medicine. Leipzig: VEB Georg Thieme, 1986.

Ellison P, Horn JL, Heimler R, et al. Prediction models for brain function in the preterm neonate. In: Oh W, Friis-Hansen B, Stern L, eds. Physiologic Foundations of Perinatal Care. New York: Elsevier Science, 1987.

Horn JL. Equations representing combinations of components in scoring psychological variables. Acta Psychol 1963; 21:184–217.

O'Halloran J, Sandman C, Eisenart R, et al. A new noninvasive measurement of regional cerebral blood flow in the neonate. Ann Neurol 1986; 20:411A.

Reigel DH, Dallman DE, Scarff TB, Woodford J. Transcephalic impedance measurement during infancy. Dev Med Child Neurol 1977; 19:295.

Siddiqui SF, Brown DR, Dallman DE, et al. Detection of neonatal-intraventricular hemorrhage using transcephalic impedance. Dev Med Child Neurol 1980; 22:440.

Weindling AM, Murdoch N, Rolfe P. Effect of electrode size on the contribution of intracranial and extracranial blood flow to the cerebral electrical impedance plethysmogram. Med Biol Eng Comput 1982; 20:545–549.

UMBILICAL ARTERY CATHETERIZATION

BOYD W. GOETZMAN, M.D., Ph.D.

Catheterization of an umbilical artery has become a routine procedure in the care of sick newborn infants. Each year an estimated 1 to 2 percent of all newborns in the United States, about 30 to 40 percent of those admitted to newborn intensive care units, undergo this procedure. It is an easily learned procedure that requires only simple pieces of equipment and a modicum of technical skill. The usual indications for catheterizing an umbilical artery are the need for frequent sampling of arterial blood to monitor oxygen and carbon dioxide tensions and acid-base status, and the need for arterial blood pressure monitoring. Less common indications include the need for vascular access for exchange transfusion or angiography. *Umbilical catheters are not placed for the primary purpose of fluid and nutrient administration*, except perhaps in immature infants of 26 weeks' gestation or less. However, once in place, they may be used for these purposes and the administration of some medications. The use of umbilical catheters for these purposes is attended by a variety of complications, and the risk-to-benefit ratio for each patient must be considered before undertaking this procedure. *The development of noninvasive techniques for monitoring blood gas tensions, oxygen saturation, and blood pressure has reduced the need to use the umbilical artery.* These alternatives should be considered in each patient before a catheter is inserted, as well as after failure to accomplish catheterization. They are especially important when there are relative contraindications to the use of umbilical vessels, such as when anterior abdominal wall defects are present. While catheters can remain functional for long periods, the usual policy is to remove them as soon as they are no longer needed for the major purpose. The decision to remove a functioning catheter is more difficult in a very small premature infant in whom its secure vascular access leads to decreased handling of the infant, avoidance of painful stimuli, improved skin care, and uninterrupted provision of fluid and nutrients. Thus, in some infants weighing under 800 g the catheter may be maintained for as long as 4 to 6 weeks. When major thrombotic complications have occurred, removal of the catheter is indicated. Of course, nonfunctioning catheters are removed and replaced as necessary.

TECHNIQUE

Sterile technique using gown and gloves, povidone-iodine skin and cord preparation, and proper draping is recommended for catheter insertion in all but the most emergent of situations. The size, or diameter, of the catheter is selected on the basis of the infant's weight. The 5.0 French size is used only in infants weighing more than 1500 g while the smaller 3.5 French outside diameter size can be used in infants of any weight, if desired. The catheters are radiopaque and marked in 1-cm increments, which aids in determining how far they have been inserted. The depth of insertion is estimated so that the tip of the catheter will come to lie in the aorta at the level of the third to fourth lumbar vertebral bodies. This distance is approximately 7 to 8 cm, 9 to 10 cm, or 11 to 13 cm for infants weighing less than 1,000 g, 1,000 to 2,000 g, and more than 2,000 g, respectively. Another useful yardstick is to measure the umbilicus-to-inguinal ligament distance and to double that value. Alternatively, published graphs are available that use other body measurements such as umbilicus-to-shoulder distance. *For infants weighing less than 750 g, we advance the catheter an additional 4 to 5 cm so that its tip lies in the thoracic aorta at about the level of the eighth thoracic vertebra.* Some practitioners prefer this position for larger infants as well. The literature does not clearly favor the use of one position or the other for reducing major sequelae or prolonging catheter life. However, *in general, we prefer to keep the tip below the aortic branches supplying major organs.* In the case of the smallest infants, it is our clinical impression that catheter patency is maintained longer in the high position. In any event, radiographic or ultrasonographic confirmation of the location of the tip is necessary at the end of the procedure. Proper adjustment can then be made, but only by withdrawing the catheter to a lower position.

Identification of the thin-walled, patulous umbilical vein and the two thicker-walled, constricted arteries is quite easy once the umbilical cord has been severed with a scalpel blade at about 0.5 to 0.75 cm from the skin insertion of the cord. A length of umbilical tape looped around the base of the cord and loosely knotted can be used for hemostasis, if necessary. One of the arteries is selected, and its lumen gently is probed and dilated with the blade(s) of an iris forceps. When sufficiently dilated, the tip of the umbilical catheter, which has been attached to a three-way stopcock and filled with saline solution containing 1 unit of heparin per milliliter, is inserted and advanced to the predetermined depth. Inability to advance the catheter beyond 1 to 2 cm is usually due to failure to enter the lumen of the vessel. Failure to advance beyond 4 to 6 cm is usually due to perforation of the arterial wall just under the abdominal skin where it turns sharply toward the pelvis. Catheterization is made easier by having an assistant elevate the cord in a cephalad direction to minimize the angulation of the artery. The other artery can be used if catheterization of the first fails. If the second vessel is also perforated, one artery can be further dilated with a catheter in place through the perforation. A second catheter, 3.5 French diameter, can then usually be advanced beside the first catheter and past the perforation. When the second catheter has been advanced sufficiently into the aorta, it can be held in place while the first catheter is removed. Successful catheterization of one or the other of the umbilical arteries can be anticipated in about 90 percent of the infants selected to undergo this procedure. A sub-

umbilical cutdown technique, in which the cord structures are identified just under the skin of the abdomen and an artery is entered through a small incision in its lateral wall, can increase the overall success rate to about 95 percent. However, in some infants the alternative of catheterizing a peripheral artery, such as the radial artery, will be necessary.

The catheter is held in position by placing a purse-string suture of 3-0 or 4-0 silk, using an atraumatic needle, in the cord substance around the entire periphery of the cord. An additional knot is placed by tying a knot in the ends of the suture about 1 cm above the knot in the pursestring and then tying directly around the catheter to anchor it. Subsequently, a tape bridge is usually added for security. Until the location of the tip is confirmed radiographically, infusions are limited to glucose and electrolyte solutions containing one unit of heparin per ml. We use 0.5 unit per milliliter for infants under 1,000 g whose fluid requirements are higher because of their high insensible fluid loss. Of course, blood sampling and blood pressure monitoring may be begun immediately. It is best to avoid infusion of vasoactive substances, glucose concentrations greater than 12.5 percent, and blood through the umbilical catheter whenever possible. The presence of an umbilical catheter is not a contraindication to enteral feeding, and a causal relationship with necrotizing enterocolitis has not been established. When a catheter is to be removed, it is best to withdraw it until 3 to 4 cm remain in the vessel, and then wait 10 to 15 minutes before withdrawing the remainder. Only occasionally is a suture required for hemostasis.

COMPLICATIONS

Complications of umbilical artery catheters continue to occur and can be serious or minor. They can be generally classified as thromboembolic, mechanical/vasospastic, infectious, or miscellaneous. Serious *thrombosis* involving a major artery can lead to loss of part or all of a lower limb, kidney, or intestine. The entire aorta can thrombose, causing serious systemic hypertension. Until recently, this was considered a lethal complication if untreated. Surgical removal and the use of thrombolytic therapy with urokinase have been reported to be successful in some patients. In addition, spontaneous resolution has been seen. Ultrasound imaging has made the diagnosis and monitoring of this complication easier and is recommended for suspect cases. Infarction of the anterior spinal cord with immediate and permanent paraplegia has been reported. Skin and gluteal muscle necrosis is not as serious and, as in spinal cord necrosis, it is difficult to determine whether vasotoxic substances were injected directly into these areas through catheters whose tips inadvertently came to lie near, or within, their supply vessels. Interestingly, *if thrombotic complications are going to occur, they usually do so during the first few days* that the catheter is in place. Also, the serious complications occur more often in the premature infants below 1,000 g and the large, severely asphyxiated term or post-term infants. Curiously, the common minor complication that was most obvious, embolism of vessels in the foot digits leading to blue toes and even gangrene of the tips of the toes, has nearly disappeared from many nurseries. The explanation remains enigmatic. *Vasospastic complications*, such as transient blanching of extremities or toes, usually resolve spontaneously or with blood volume expansion, and usually do not necessitate catheter removal. Tolazoline infusion via the catheter, 250 mg per kilogram per hour, has also been used successfully to treat vasospasm of the leg vessels. *Perforation* of an iliac artery, or even the left ventricle, with major occult blood loss has led to death in a few infants. Of course, blood loss due to disconnected lines and open stopcocks can occur and can be serious enough to require transfusion. *Septicemia* can occur and is more often associated with administration of parenteral nutrition via the umbilical catheter. Mycotic aneurysms of the aorta have been noted, and septic emboli have led to joint space infections in both knees and hips. Chemical hazards due to plasticizer toxicity and electrical hazards are primarily theoretical or rare. However, significant hypoglycemia can occur when an infusion of glucose is abruptly discontinued. In addition, hyperglycemia can be overdiagnosed when the feet are used for collecting blood samples by the heelstick technique during infusion of 10 percent glucose solutions.

Minor complications may arise in nearly half of the premature infants undergoing umbilical artery catheterization, and serious complications in 4 to 5 percent of all infants with this procedure. The use of catheters made of thromboresistant materials such as polyurethane or Silastic has not yet seemed to reduce thrombotic complications effectively enough to displace the more commonly used polyvinyl chloride catheters. Theoretically, the smaller surface area provided by the 3.5 French catheter should be attended by less pericatheter thrombosis than the larger exposed surface of the 5.0 French catheter, but this has not been established experimentally. Heparinization of infusates does increase the duration of catheter patency, but does not seem to reduce thrombotic complications. Currently decreased trauma during catheter insertion, attention to maintenance of blood volume and blood pressure, use of the newer microvolumetric infusion pumps, avoidance of vasotoxic drug and blood infusions, and meticulous catheter care are probably all important in reducing the complication rate associated with the use of umbilical catheters.

Alternatives to umbilical artery catheterization with fewer associated risks are available, and should be considered for each infant requiring blood pressure and blood gas monitoring. However, no single complete alternative is available. Thus, some combination of Doppler or oscillometric blood pressure monitoring devices, oximeters, transcutaneous gas tension monitors, peripheral arterial cannulation, and peripheral venous access is needed. In addition to decreased risks, several of these techniques have the added advantage of providing for continuous monitoring of important variables. Often these techniques are not available in smaller community hospitals where many critically ill infants are stabilized before transport to a tertiary center. During transport, use of these techniques also may not be practical. Thus, broader use of umbilical artery catheters can be expected in these settings. However, even in the larger centers, the secure vascular access and ease of nursing care offered by the use of umbilical catheters continue to make them useful and practical in spite of their known complications and sequelae.

WEANING FROM THE RESPIRATOR

RICHARD J. MARTIN, M.B., F.R.A.C.P.
WALDEMAR A. CARLO, M.D.

The widespread acceptance of assisted ventilation in neonatal intensive care has resulted in the use of criteria for initiating mechanical ventilation that vary widely among institutions and even within one center. Unfortunately, it is usually easier to begin than to wean or discontinue assisted ventilation, and barotrauma is a well-recognized complication of its excessive use. Thus, the need for weaning should be constantly on the minds of the medical staff caring for ventilated infants.

FACTORS INFLUENCING THE LIKELIHOOD OF SUCCESSFUL WEANING

General Condition of the Infant

Three major components of the infant's medical status are of primary concern: degree of immaturity, severity of respiratory disease, and neurologic status. Poor nutritional status and severe immaturity in the very low birth weight infant interact to aggravate ventilator dependence. The net result appears to be inability to sustain effective contraction of the respiratory muscles, especially the diaphragm, and, to a lesser extent, the intercostal, abdominal, and upper airway muscles. Respiratory drive has been indirectly measured in spontaneously breathing infants by quantifying the ventilatory response to respiratory stimuli such as increased inspired CO_2 concentrations. However, an impaired ventilatory response to respiratory stimuli can result from either immaturity of the respiratory center or from mechanical failure of the respiratory muscles. Thus *the frequent failure of weaning in very low birth weight infants has a multifactorial etiology and cannot be readily related to a single component of the respiratory system* (Table 1). Decreased lung compliance and increased airway resistance frequently occur in infants who are difficult to extubate. Infants born very prematurely or those who have undergone asphyxia may have a decreased ventilatory drive and thus fail attempts at extubation. A patent ductus arteriosus may manifest with congestive heart failure and inability to wean from the ventilator. Finally, septic infants, especially those with meningitis or pneumonia, may require prolonged ventilatory therapy.

It is important to optimize nutritional status by early and even aggressive use of enteral or intravenous alimentation. Mechanical ventilation and the presence of indwelling arterial lines are not contraindications to nasogastric feeding in very low birth weight infants. Our practice is to start small-volume feedings very early but then increase cautiously so as not to overload the immature gastrointestinal tract. Overenthusiastic use of intravenous alimentation may cause fluid overload and predispose to congestive cardiac failure, especially in association with a patent ductus arteriosus. This should be vigorously controlled prior to weaning.

Ventilator weaning is often unsuccessful in preterm infants with grade III or IV intraventricular hemorrhage or in term infants with hypoxic ischemic encephalopathy. Excessive ventilator dependency may be an early indication of subsequent neurologic compromise in these patients. Nonetheless, frequent attempts at weaning must be pursued. Concurrent anticonvulsant therapy should not affect weaning adversely, provided that blood levels remain within recommended therapeutic ranges.

Specific Ventilator Settings

Pulmonary function is not typically measured, but the infant's ventilatory settings and oxygen requirement should be indications of his or her lung function and likelihood of successful weaning. Intermittent mandatory ventilation permits both assisted and spontaneous ventilation to occur concurrently, allowing a gradual transition from the former to the latter. *Termination of ventilatory support should be attempted when the ventilation provided by the ventilator is relatively minimal compared to the infant's spontaneous ventilation.* In infants with resolving respiratory distress this can usually proceed when the following

ventilator settings have been achieved: peak inspiratory pressure less than or equal to 18 cm H_2O, frequency less than or equal to 10 breaths per minute, and inspired oxygen concentration less than or equal to 40 percent.

When a low intermittent mandatory ventilation of around 10 breaths per minute is well tolerated, *a short trial of endotracheal continuous positive airway pressure (CPAP) at 2 to 4 cm H_2O is attempted prior to extubation.* A 5 to 10 percent increase in inspired oxygen concentration may be of benefit at this time. Prolonged (greater than 30- to 60-minute) periods of endotracheal CPAP are usually unsuccessful in very immature infants with resolving lung disease. This is due to the additional work of breathing associated with the increased airway resistance and dead space of the endotracheal tube. *Nasal CPAP may be beneficial for a period of hours to days following extubation.* Steroids are of no proven benefit during extubation; however racemic epinephrine aerosols may relieve stridor caused by laryngeal edema.

Use of Computer-Assisted Ventilator Management During Weaning

Because blood gases reflect efficacy of gas exchange, we have attempted to develop an organized strategy for weaning infants from assisted ventilation based on results of blood gas analysis. A flow chart that considers blood gas results and ventilator settings has been adapted to a microcomputer to create an artificial intelligence program that facilitates weaning from assisted ventilation. The program is used by residents, nurses, and respiratory therapists as a consultation tool. We observe that resolution of blood gas derangement occurs more frequently when ventilatory management is in agreement with the computer program than when an alternate decision is followed. This beneficial effect is due to the successful weaning of assisted ventilation in infants with hyperoxemia or hypocapnia (Fig. 1). Furthermore, unnecessary increases in

TABLE 1 Major Causes of Weaning Failure

Respiratory	Nonrespiratory
Impaired respiratory drive	Nutritional compromise
Respiratory muscle failure	Neurologic problems
Abnormal pulmonary mechanics	Intercurrent infection (sepsis)
Localized atelectasis	Congestive heart failure

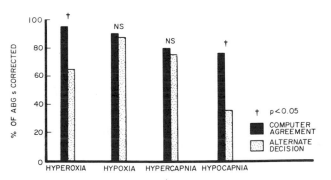

Figure 1 Percentage of abnormal arterial blood gases (ABGs) corrected by ventilator changes suggested by the computer program versus those that followed alternate decisions. Ventilator changes in agreement with the computer program are more effective in improving blood gas readings during episodes of hyperoxemia or hypocapnia.

ventilatory support occur less often when ventilatory changes are guided by the computer program.

One of the major limitations of this computer program for weaning is that it is based exclusively on blood gas results and does not take into consideration other important clinical findings, such as respiratory effort and degree of immaturity. These clinical data certainly need to be considered and, while they are more difficult to quantify, they add an essential component to the art of weaning.

Pharmacologic Agents

The methylxanthines (theophylline, caffeine) are widely used to improve the chances for successful extubation of sick infants. *Successful extubation appears to be associated with increased minute ventilation and respiratory frequency and decreased PaCO$_2$.* The beneficial effect is probably secondary to enhanced respiratory drive or respiratory muscle effectiveness. Doxapram has been used as an alternate respiratory stimulant to aminophylline but appears to offer no clear-cut advantage during weaning and may cause hypertension or other as yet unproven complications.

Whatever regimen is used for weaning, it may fail. If further weaning is impossible, assisted ventilation should continue at the lowest ventilator pressures and inspired oxygen concentration at which cardiorespiratory function is optimal and growth can be sustained. It is hoped that this can be achieved at values for both PaO$_2$ and PaCO$_2$

of around 50 cm Hg, although cor pulmonale can develop in some infants at a PaO$_2$ of less than 55 to 60 mm Hg. Reintubation can be traumatic, so several days or more should elapse before re-extubation is attempted, especially in very low birth weight infants. Meanwhile, a treatable cause for failure of extubation (such as segmental atelectasis) should be sought in an attempt to prevent its recurrence. Noninvasive blood gas monitoring, including transcutaneous PCO$_2$ and transcutaneous PO$_2$ pulse oximetry, is extremely useful, since indwelling arterial lines are frequently removed long before extubation. However, transcutaneous PO$_2$ typically underestimates PaO$_2$ in infants whose postnatal age is beyond 2 months, and pulse oximetry is of limited usefulness in identifying hyperoxemia.

Should all very low birth weight infants remain intubated and be allowed to grow until they reach a minimum weight (e.g., 1,000 g)? Current data offer no answer, although it is our practice to proceed with cautious weaning *regardless* of the infant's degree of immaturity, since *chronic lung disease is too high a price to pay for needlessly prolonged assisted ventilation.*

SUGGESTED READING

Carlo WA, Martin RJ. Principles of neonatal assisted ventilation. Pediatr Clin North Am 1986; 33:221–237.

Carlo WA, Pacifico L, Chatburn RL, Fanaroff AA. Efficacy of computer-assisted management of respiratory failure in neonates. Pediatrics 1986; 78:139–143.

INDEX